The Essential Guide to Prescription Drugs

THE ESSENTIAL GUIDE TO PRESCRIPTION DRUGS

1992 EDITION

James W. Long, M.D.

HarperPerennial

A Division of HarperCollins*Publishers*

THE ESSENTIAL GUIDE TO PRESCRIPTION DRUGS 1992. Copyright © 1977, 1980, 1982, 1985, 1987, 1988, 1989, 1990, 1991 by James W. Long. All rights reserved. Printed in the United States of America. No part of this book may be used or reproduced in any manner whatsoever without written permission except in the case of brief quotations embodied in critical articles and reviews. For information address HarperCollins Publishers, Inc., 10 East 53rd Street, New York, N.Y. 10022.

Designed by C. Linda Dingler

Library of Congress Catalog Card Number 87-657561
ISSN 0894-7058
ISBN 0-06-271534-8   91 92 93 94 95 HC 10 9 8 7 6 5 4 3 2 1
ISBN 0-06-273090-8 (pbk.) 91 92 93 94 95 HC 10 9 8 7 6 5 4 3 2 1

Contents

SECTION SIX:
Tables of Drug Information

Author's Note
for the 1992 Edition

As with each previous edition of the Guide, the information prepared for 1992 has been enlarged in scope and enhanced in pertinence for the audience it serves. Such changes are in keeping with the ever growing public interest in all aspects of health and medical care. The new additions are consistent with the basic premise of this book: to provide information on medicinal drugs of major importance that will enable the patient to (1) use appropriate drugs with maximal safety and effectiveness, and (2) communicate with medical personnel in a spirit of mutual understanding and cooperation.

Because of its increasing frequency and its complexity of management, lupus erythematosus is the subject of a new Disorder Profile added to Section Two. This chronic disorder of major importance requires substantial effort by the patient to gain the knowledge and understanding necessary to achieve satisfactory management of drug therapy. The principal drugs currently used to treat lupus have been added to the Drug Profiles in Section Three.

Additional new Drug Profiles include newly released medications for the treatment of allergic disorders, bronchial asthma, glaucoma and a wide spectrum of serious infections. Also added are four new medications representing the more recently developed and more effective classes of drugs used to manage hypertension (high blood pressure).

The increasing desire and ability of the consumer to actively participate in the conduct of medical care have prompted the addition of a new category of information to each Drug Profile in Section Three:

Possible Effects (of this drug) on Laboratory Tests. The remarkable advances in medical knowledge generally, and in drug therapy particularly, make it incumbent upon both physician and patient to be knowledgeable, responsible and communicative. Examples of critical physician–patient interaction in the management of drug therapy (involving laboratory tests) are numerous: the treatment of cholesterol disorders, depression, diabetes, epilepsy, gout, hypertension, lupus, psoriasis, rheumatoid arthritis, schizophrenia; the use of anticoagulants; the monitoring of drugs with a significant potential for damage to blood cell production, liver and kidney function; urine testing by the patient (for sugar, pregnancy, etc.). Of growing concern to more than 10 million people in targeted occupations is the issue of urine screening tests for drug abuse: which medicinal drugs (legally prescribed and used) may cause a positive result in a screening test initiated in the workplace? Twenty-three such drugs are among the Drug Profiles in Section Two. The information included in this new category is primarily patient-oriented. It is limited to tests of practical significance for those who wish to assume a role in the management of drugs prescribed for them.

As noted in each previous edition, no claim is made that all known actions, side-effects, adverse effects, precautions, interactions, etc., for a drug are included in the information provided in the six sections that comprise this book. While diligent care was taken to ensure the accuracy of the information provided during the preparation of this revision, the continued accuracy and currentness are ever subject to change relative to the dissemination of new information derived from drug research, development, and general usage.

1

HOW TO USE THIS BOOK

2

GUIDELINES FOR SAFE AND EFFECTIVE DRUG USE

1

How to Use This Book

Your physician has advised you to take a drug (or drugs), or you have been directed to administer a drug (or drugs) to someone under your care. The kind and amount of information you have been given about how to use these drugs, and what to expect from them, will vary tremendously. In many instances it will not be practical or possible for the physician to provide you with *all* the information that could be considered appropriate and useful, or it will be difficult for you to remember it. From time to time you will find it desirable—even necessary—to seek clarification and guidance about some aspect of drug action or drug use. The aim of this book is to give you the kind of information you may need to supplement the direction and guidance you receive from your physician.

The book consists of six sections. The first section will give you the orientation and insight necessary to appreciate the complexities of modern drug therapy and help you to make the best use of the information contained in Sections Two through Six.

Section Two presents useful information regarding the role of drugs in treating 26 common chronic disorders that require long-term drug therapy. A synopsis of each disorder is followed by information categories that cover drug selection, the goals of drug treatment and an overview of drug management during the period of therapy. A list of the disorders reviewed is found in the introduction to the section.

Section Three is a compilation of Drug Profiles covering 225 prescription drugs used widely in the United States and Canada. The selection of each drug is based upon three considerations: the extent of its use; the urgency of the conditions for which it is prescribed; the volume and complexity of the information essential to its proper utilization. The Drug Profiles are arranged alphabetically by generic name. (Some generic names have spellings similar to other generic names; be careful not to confuse one with another.)

The Profile of each drug is presented in a uniform sequence of information categories. (When you become familiar with the format, you will be able to quickly find specific items of information on any drug, without having to read the entire Profile.) Each Drug Profile contains 45 (or more) separate categories of information. The principal categories include the following.

Year Introduced

This tells you how long the drug has been in general use. The older the drug, the more likely its full spectrum of actions is known and the less likely its continued use will produce new surprises. The date given represents the year the drug was introduced for human use anywhere in the world.

Drug Class

This identifies the principal therapeutic class(es) to which the drug belongs. When appropriate, the chemical and/or pharmacological class designations are also given. You will find it helpful to recognize the class of the drug you are taking because many actions, reactions and interactions with other drugs are often shared by drugs of the same class. Throughout this book (and in most literature on drug information) you will find reference to drugs by their class designation. (Section Four provides alphabetically arranged listings of the classes of drugs referred to in this guide.)

Prescription Required

This indicates whether a drug is a prescription or a nonprescription (over-the-counter) purchase. Because there are significant differences in prescription requirements between the United States and Canada, the designation for each country is given when appropriate.

Controlled Drug

Drugs subject to regulation under the Controlled Substances Act of 1970 (those with potential for abuse) are so designated by the particular schedule that governs their dispensing in the United States. A corresponding schedule is also given for Canada when applicable. A description of the Schedules of Controlled Drugs is found inside the back cover of this guide.

Available for Purchase by Generic Name

Increasing interest in the availability of prescription drugs for purchase by their generic names has been prompted by two issues of major significance. The first is concerned with the cost of prescription drugs. The comparison shopper realizes that in general the cost of prescription medication is significantly less when a generic equivalent of a brand name product is purchased. The second issue relates to what is termed "bioavailability and bioequivalence"—the comparative composition, quality and effectiveness of the generic versus the brand name drug product. Further discussion of bioavailability and bioequivalence of drug products will be found in the Glossary, Section Five.

Brand Names

These are provided to confirm that you are consulting the correct Drug Profile. They may also help you to recognize a brand name that identifies this drug as one that produced in you an unfavorable reaction on previous use. Brand names are listed for the United States and for Canada (♦). A combination drug (a drug product with more than one active ingredient) is identified by [CD] following the brand name.

In a few instances a particular brand name in current use in both the United States and Canada will represent entirely different generic drugs (in a single drug product), or a significantly different mixture of generic ingredients (in a combination drug product). The generic composition of such brand name products is identified by country in the index. Travelers between the two countries who obtain their medications by brand name in either country are advised to ascertain that they are being provided the intended generic drug(s) in every instance.

Benefits versus Risks

A deliberate attempt is made here to crystallize the "pros" and "cons" for each drug. The format adopted for this category utilizes capital letters to give weight (emphasis) to the drug's principal benefits and risks, and lower case letters are used for benefits and risks of lesser significance. A glance reveals the comparative "weights" of the two columns and provides an initial and tentative impression as to whether a drug's benefits exceed its risks, or vice versa, or whether its benefits and risks seem to be roughly equivalent.

This presentation is not intended to be the principal basis for decision on whether or not to use the drug. Its purpose is to enjoin the reader to be more circumspect and discriminating in his or her use of drugs. The failure to give adequate attention to the individualization of drug selection and dosage is perhaps the greatest weakness seen in the current management of drug therapy.

Principal Uses

A drug may be available as a single drug product or in combination with other drugs. In this section of the Profile under the designation As a Single Drug Product, you will find the primary use(s) of the drug when used alone. Under the designation As a Combination Drug Product [CD], you will find the primary use(s) when combined with other active drugs within the same tablet, capsule, etc. The uses stated are those determined by consensus within the medical community and substantiated by current scientific study. Combination drugs have been developed because some conditions that warrant drug therapy have more than one cause, are characterized by a variety of symptoms, or may be treated in more than one way. Where appropriate, in this guide, the logic for combining certain drugs to enhance their therapeutic value is explained. When you find the designation for Combination Drugs [CD] in the Brand Name list at the beginning of the Drug Profile, read under the Principal Uses section to learn more about the drug's use in combination products.

How This Drug Works

This simplified explanation is limited to consideration of how the drug acts to produce its principal (intended) therapeutic effect(s). If a specific method of action has not been established, the currently held theory is given.

Available Dosage Forms and Strengths

This represents a composite of available manufacturers' dosage forms (tablets, capsules, elixirs, etc.) and strengths, without company identification. Included are those dosage forms appropriate for use by outpatients and in extended care facilities and nursing homes. Dosage forms limited to hospital use are not included. Refer to Dosage Forms and Strengths in the Glossary for an explanation of those few abbreviations used to designate the strengths of each dosage form.

Usual Adult Dosage Range

The dosage information given represents a carefully derived consensus by appropriate authorities and is the currently recommended standard. It is provided as a guide that indicates the amount of the drug that is reasonably expected to be both effective and safe when properly used for its intended purpose. Under certain circumstances, your physician may elect to modify this "standard" dosage scheme. Adhere strictly to his or her prescribed dosages and schedules.

Dosing Instructions

Specific guidance is given here regarding the timing of oral medication with regard to food intake. In addition, there are occasions when an individual finds it difficult or impossible to swallow a tablet or a capsule, and the drug to be taken is not available in a liquid dosage form. On those occasions when the patient's condition urgently requires the medication, one may wish to crush the tablet or open the capsule and mix the contents with a palatable food or beverage for administration. Many of today's drugs are available in a bewildering array of solid dosage forms, some of which should *not* be altered to accommodate administration. This information category identifies those dosage forms of each drug that may be and those that should not be altered for administration. In addition, your pharmacist can provide appropriate guidance if you should need it.

Usual Duration of Use

Many factors influence the period of time required for any drug to exert beneficial effects. Among them are the nature and severity of the symptoms being treated, the formulation and strength of the drug, the presence or absence of food in the stomach, the ability of the patient to respond and the concurrent use of other drugs. The information in this category is helpful in preventing premature termination of medication in treatment situations where improvement may seem to you to be unreasonably delayed. Where appropriate, limitations in the duration of use are given.

This Drug Should Not Be Taken If

This category consists of the *absolute* contraindications to the use of the drug (see Contraindications in Glossary). It is most important that you alert your physician or dentist if any information in this category applies to you.

Inform Your Physician Before Taking This Drug If

This category lists the *relative* contraindications to the use of the drug. Here again, it is important that you communicate all relevant information to your physician or dentist.

Possible Side-Effects

This category describes the natural, expected and usually unavoidable actions of the drug—the normal and anticipated consequences of taking it. It is important that you maintain a realistic perspective that balances properly the occurrence of side-effects and the goals of treatment. Consult your physician for guidance whenever side-effects are troublesome or distressing, so that appropriate adjustments of your treatment program can be made.

Possible Adverse Effects

This category includes those unusual, unexpected and infrequent drug effects that are commonly referred to as adverse drug reactions. For the sake of evaluation, adverse effects are classified as mild or serious in nature. It is always wise to inform your physician as soon as you have reason to suspect you may be experiencing an adverse drug effect. Serious adverse reactions usually announce their development initially in the form of mild, unthreatening symptoms. It is important that you remain alert to significant changes in your well-being when you are taking a drug that is known to be capable of producing a serious adverse effect. It is also possible to experience an adverse reaction that has not yet been reported. Do not discount the possibility of an adverse effect just because it is not listed in this category. Following standard practice, some adverse reactions (and interactions) of certain drugs are listed, as a precaution, because these reactions are associated with the use of a particular class of drugs. Although the literature may not document such reactions in connection with the use of an individual drug within that class, the possibility of their occurrence must be considered.

A word of caution is appropriate here. You have consulted your physician for medical evaluation and management. He or she has advised you to take a drug (or administer it to someone else). It is important that you recognize and understand that *in the vast majority of instances a properly selected drug has a comparatively small chance of producing serious harm.* Most of the drugs included in this book produce serious adverse effects rarely. Knowledge that a drug is capable of causing a serious adverse reaction should not deter you from using it when it has been properly selected and its use will be carefully supervised.

Possible Effects on Sexual Function

The growing interest and concern of the medical community and the general public regarding the potential effects of many drugs on sexual function justify this designated category for the provision of relevant information. This aspect of drug performance has not received the professional scrutiny or public disclosure commensurate with its importance. Currently available information (often inadequate and vague) from all reliable sources is presented for consideration. In the interest of compliance and effective management, both physician and patient are well advised to discuss frankly the full significance of any potential effect that proposed drug therapy could have on all aspects of sexual expression.

Adverse Effects That May Appear Similar to Natural Diseases or Disorders

The failure to recognize that a given symptom or disorder is actually drug induced occurs with surprising frequency. Quite often this inadvertent error is compounded by the administration of yet another drug to relieve the "symptoms" (unrecognized manifestations) of a drug being taken on a regular basis. For milder symptoms (*e.g.*, the nasal congestion and diarrhea caused by reserpine), the oversight may not be too serious. But in the case of parkinsonlike effects of some drugs, the mistake can be devastating. This category can alert you to this common flaw in the management of drug therapy.

Natural Diseases or Disorders That May Be Activated by This Drug

Similar to the situation described in the previous category, many drugs in common use are capable of "activating" latent disorders that may not be recognized as drug induced. The development of a new and seemingly unrelated disorder during the course of any treatment program should arouse suspicion that it may be drug related.

Possible Effects on Laboratory Tests

Most of the drugs in current use have multiple and significant effects on body chemistry and organ system functions. Some of these effects are intended and beneficial (therapeutic); others are unintended, unavoidable and potentially harmful. Many of these effects can be detected and evaluated by a variety of specific laboratory tests. The timely use of appropriate tests enables the physician to monitor the performance of a drug and the course of the condition being treated. The tests included in this category are limited to those of practical importance for effective physician–patient communication and cooperation in managing the use of certain drugs. Knowledge of selected test results can greatly enhance the patient's understanding and skill in the proper use of medications. (See the Author's Note at the beginning of this edition.)

Caution

This category provides information on certain aspects of drug action and/or drug use that require special emphasis. Occasionally these warnings may relate to information provided in other categories. When included here, such entries are of sufficient importance to warrant repetition.

Precautions for Use by Infants and Children

In addition to mandatory adjustments of drug dosage for infants and children under twelve years of age, some drugs and/or treatment situations call for special precautions. This category provides such information for selected drugs. When administering *any* drug (whether prescription or over-the-counter), it is advisable to ask the attending physician about precautions to observe or procedures to follow.

Precautions for Use by Those over 60 Years of Age

Changes in body composition and function occur naturally as part of normal aging. As would be expected, there is enormous individual variation in the speed with which such changes occur and the degree of these changes. With regard to medical management—and to drug therapy in particular—the assessment of one's "age" must be based upon the individual's mental and physical condition and never upon years alone. In general, however, it should be recognized that changes that accompany aging may affect the actions of the body on the drug, as well as the actions of the drug on the body. Appropriate precautions are outlined in this category.

Advisability of Use During Pregnancy: Pregnancy Category

Information regarding the safe use of a particular drug during pregnancy was one of the most forceful concerns that led to the formal petitioning of the Food and Drug Administration in 1975 for the provision of such guidance to the public. Most category designations are labeled "tentative" at this time in recognition of the fact that data not readily available now may be advanced by pharmaceutical manufacturers as they negotiate with the FDA to eventually determine final category assignments. The FDA definitions of the five Pregnancy Categories are listed inside the back cover of the book. It should be noted that the FDA does not make the initial category assignment; this is the responsibility of the manufacturer that markets the drug. The initial designation is then subject to review and modification by the FDA as deemed appropriate. The Pregnancy Category designations presented in each Profile were determined by the author after thorough review of pertinent literature and consultation with appropriate authorities. They are offered at this time for initial guidance only. They are in no sense "official" and do not have the endorsement of either the manufacturer or the FDA.

Advisability of Use If Breast-Feeding

Information presented here includes what could be ascertained regarding the effects of the drug on milk production, the presence of the drug in human milk and the possible effects of the drug on the nursing infant. Prudent recommendations are given where appropriate.

Suggested Periodic Examinations While Taking This Drug

This category lists those examinations your physician may recommend you undergo while taking the drug(s) he or she has prescribed, in order to monitor your reaction to them and the course of your condition. You should remember that the advisability of performing such examinations varies greatly from one situation to another, and is best left to the judgment of your physician. The selection and timing of examinations are based on many variables, including your past and present medical history, the nature of the condition under treatment, the dosage and anticipated duration of drug use and your physician's observations of your response to treatment. There may be many occasions when he or she will feel no examinations are necessary.

To assure optimal results from drug treatment, it is important that you keep your physician informed of all developments you think may be drug related.

While Taking This Drug, Observe the Following: Marijuana Smoking

The widespread "social" use of marijuana by virtually all age groups has led to inquiries regarding the possibility of interactions between the pharmacologically active chemicals in marijuana smoke and medicinal drugs in common use. Currently available literature on the health aspects of marijuana use contains very little practical information concerning the potential for drug interactions. The limited information presented in this category of selected Drug Profiles represents those *possible interactions* that are considered likely to occur in view of the known pharmacological effects of the principal components of marijuana and of the medicinal drug reviewed in the Profile. In most instances, the interaction statements are not based on documented evidence since very little is available. However, the conclusions stated—derived by logical inductive reasoning—represent the concurrence of authorities with expertise in this field.

While Taking This Drug, Observe the Following: Other Drugs

For clarification of this confusing and often controversial area of drug information, this category is divided into five subcategories of possible interactions between drugs. Observe carefully the wording of each subcategory heading (see also Interaction in Glossary). Some of the drugs listed as possible interactants do not have a representative Profile in Section Three. If you are using one of these drugs, consult your physician or pharmacist for guidance regarding potential interactions. A brand name (or names) that follows the generic name of an interacting drug is given for purposes of illustration only. It is not intended to mean that the particular brand(s) named have interactions that are different from other brands of the same generic drug. If you are taking the generic drug, *all* brand names under which it is marketed are to be considered as possible interactants.

Driving, Hazardous Activities

In addition to driving motor vehicles, the information in this category applies to any activity of a dangerous nature such as operating machinery, working on ladders, using power tools and handling weapons.

Aviation Note

Until the publication of Dr. Stanley Mohler's *Medication and Flying: A Pilot's Drug Guide* in 1982, there was no authoritative source of current drug information written specifically to serve the needs of civil aviation. The military airman enjoys the expert guidance and surveillance provided by the flight surgeon, but no tightly structured control system exists for his civilian counterpart. However, the need for practical information regarding the possible effects of medicinal drugs on flight performance is the same for pilots in all settings. This category is designed to inform the civilian pilot how a particular drug may affect his or her eligibility to fly and when it is advisable or necessary to consult a designated Aviation Medical Examiner or an FAA medical officer.

Occurrence of Unrelated Illness

This category relates to those drugs that require careful regulation of daily doses to maintain a constant drug effect within critical limits. Anticoagulants, antidiabetic medication and digitalis are examples of such drugs. Emphasis is given to those interim illnesses, separate from the condition for which the drug has been prescribed, that might affect the established schedule of drug use.

Discontinuation

This aspect of drug use is often overlooked when a plan of drug therapy is first discussed. However, for some drugs it is mandatory that the patient be fully informed on *when* to discontinue, when *not* to discontinue and precisely *how* to discontinue use of the drug.

Another consideration in discontinuation is the need to adjust the dosage schedules of other drugs being taken concurrently. The physician who is primarily responsible for your overall management must be kept informed of *all* the drugs you are taking at a given time.

The remaining information categories in the Drug Profile are self-explanatory.

Section Four is a presentation of Drug Classes arranged alphabetically according to their chemical or therapeutic class designation. The drugs within each class are listed alphabetically by their generic names. Because of their chemical composition and biological activities, some drugs will appear in two or more classes. For example, the drug product with the brand name Diuril will be represented by its generic name, chlorothiazide, in three drug classes: the Thiazide Diuretics (a chemical classification), the Diuretics (a drug action classification) and the Antihypertensives (a disease-oriented classification).

Frequently in the Drug Profiles in Section Three you are advised to "See (a particular) Drug Class." This alerts you to a possible contraindication for drug use, or to possible interactions with certain foods, alcohol or other drugs. In each case, you can determine the more readily recognized brand names for each drug listed generically within a drug class by consulting the appropriate Drug Profile. Timely use of these references will enable you to avoid many possible hazards of medication.

Section Five is a glossary of drug-related terms used throughout the book. The preferred use of each term is explained. Frequent references to the Glossary are made in the Drug Profiles. Use of the Glossary will increase your understanding of how to recognize and interpret significant drug effects.

Section Six consists of tables of drug information. The title and introductory material explain the content and purpose of each table. The information in the tables is drawn from certain information categories in the Profiles and is rearranged to emphasize pertinent aspects of drug behavior. The tables are intended to provide another source of ready reference.

The index of Brand and Generic Names in the back of the book is a single alphabetical listing that provides page references to the appropriate Drug Profile(s) for all drugs found in this book. Its usefulness will be enhanced if you read first the introductory explanation of the special features of this combined index.

2

Guidelines for Safe and Effective Drug Use

DO NOT

- pressure your physician to prescribe drugs that, in his or her judgment, you do not need.
- take prescription drugs on your own or on the advice of friends and neighbors because your symptoms are "just like theirs."
- offer drugs prescribed for you to anyone else without a physician's guidance.
- change the dose or timing of any drug without the advice of your physician (except when the drug appears to be causing adverse effects).
- continue to take a drug that you feel is causing adverse effects, until you are able to reach your physician for clarification.
- take *any* drug (prescription or nonprescription) while pregnant or nursing an infant until you are assured by your physician that no harmful effects will occur to either mother or child.
- take any more medicines than are absolutely necessary. (The greater the number of drugs taken simultaneously, the greater the likelihood of adverse effects.)
- withhold from your physician important information about previous drug experiences. He or she will want to know both beneficial and undesirable drug effects you have experienced in the past.
- take any drug in the dark. Identify every dose of medicine carefully in adequate light to be certain you are taking the drug intended.
- keep drugs on a bedside table. Drugs for emergency use, such as

nitroglycerin, are an exception. It is advisable to have only one such drug at the bedside for use during the night.

DO

- know the name (and correct spelling) of the drug(s) you are taking. It is advisable to know both the brand name and the generic name.
- read the package labels of all nonprescription drugs to become familiar with the contents of the product.
- follow your physician's instructions regarding dosage schedules as closely as possible. Notify him or her if it becomes necessary to make major changes in your treatment routine.
- thoroughly shake all liquid suspensions of drugs to ensure uniform distribution of ingredients.
- use a standardized measuring device for giving liquid medications by mouth. The household "teaspoon" varies greatly in size.
- follow your physician's instruction on dietary and other treatment measures designed to augment the actions of the drugs prescribed. This makes it possible to achieve desired drug effects with smaller doses. (A familiar example is the reduction of salt intake during drug treatment for high blood pressure.)
- keep your personal physician informed of all drugs prescribed for you by someone else. Consult him or her regarding nonprescription drugs you intend to take on your own initiative at the same time that you are taking drugs prescribed by him or her.
- inform your anesthesiologist, surgeon and dentist of *all* drugs you are taking, prior to any surgery.
- inform your physician if you become pregnant while you are taking any drugs from any source.
- keep a written record of *all* drugs (and vaccines) you take during your entire pregnancy—name, dose, dates taken and reasons for use.
- keep a written record of *all* drugs (and vaccines) to which you become allergic or experience an adverse reaction. This should be done for each member of the family, especially the elderly and infirm.
- keep a written record of *all* drugs (and vaccines) to which *your children* become allergic or experience an adverse reaction.
- inform your physician of all known or suspected allergies, especially allergies to drugs. Be certain that this information is included in your medical record. (Allergic individuals are four times more prone to drug reactions than those who are free of allergy).
- inform your physician promptly if you think you are experiencing an overdose, a side-effect or an adverse effect from a drug.

- determine if it is safe to drive a car, operate machinery or engage in other hazardous activities while taking the drug(s) prescribed.
- determine if it is safe to drink alcoholic beverages while taking the drug(s) prescribed.
- determine if any particular foods, beverages or other drugs should be avoided while taking the drug(s) prescribed.
- keep all appointments for follow-up examinations to determine the effects of the drugs and the course of your illness.
- ask for clarification of any point that is confusing or difficult to understand, at the time the drug(s) are prescribed or later if you have forgotten. Request information in writing if circumstances justify it.
- discard all outdated prescription drugs. This will prevent the use of drugs that have deteriorated with time.
- store all drugs to be retained for intermittent use out of the reach of children to prevent accidental poisoning.

PREVENTING ADVERSE DRUG REACTIONS

Our knowledge of the mechanisms of adverse reactions is very limited. For the most part, we cannot identify with certainty the person who is at greater risk of experiencing a true adverse effect. Available tests for the early detection of toxicity are of definite value, but they do not provide as full a measure of protection as we could wish.

As our understanding of drug actions and reactions expands, it becomes more apparent that there *is* a sizable proportion of adverse effects that are, to some extent, predictable and preventable. The exact percentage of preventable reactions is yet to be determined, but several contributing factors are now well recognized, and specific recommendations are available to guide both physican and patient. These fall into eleven categories of consideration.

Previous Adverse Reaction to a Drug

There is evidence to indicate that an individual who has experienced an adverse drug reaction in the past is more likely to have adverse reactions to other drugs, even though the drugs are unrelated. This suggests that some individuals may have a genetic (inborn) predisposition to unusual and abnormal drug responses. *The patient should inform the physician of any history of prior adverse drug experiences.*

Allergies

Individuals who are allergic by nature (hayfever, asthma, eczema, hives) are more likely to develop allergies to drugs than are nonallergic individuals. The allergic patient must be observed very closely for the earliest indication of a developing hypersensitivity to any drug. Known drug allergies must be noted in the medical record. The patient must inform every physician and dentist consulted that he or she is allergic by nature and is allergic to specific drugs by name. *The patient should provide this information without waiting to be asked.* The physician will then be able to avoid those drugs that could provoke an allergic reaction, as well as those related drugs to which the patient may have developed a cross-sensitivity.

Contraindications

Both patient and physician must strictly observe all known contraindications to any drug under consideration. *Absolute contraindications* include those conditions and situations that prohibit the use of the drug for any reason. *Relative contraindications* include those conditions that, in the judgment of the physician, do not preclude the use of the drug altogether, but make it essential that special considerations be given to its use to prevent the intensification of preexisting disease or the development of new disease. Such conditions and situations usually require adjustment of dosage, additional supportive measures and close supervision.

Precautions in Use

The patient should know about any special precautions to observe while taking the drug. This includes the advisability of use during pregnancy or while nursing an infant; precautions regarding exposure to the sun (or ultraviolet lamps); the avoidance of extreme heat or cold, heavy physical exertion, etc.

Dosage

The patient must adhere to the prescribed dosage schedule as closely as possible. *This is most important with those drugs that have narrow margins of safety.* Circumstances that interfere with taking the drug as prescribed (nausea, vomiting, diarrhea) must be reported to the physician so that appropriate adjustments can be made.

Interactions

Much is known today about how some drugs can interact unfavorably with certain foods, alcohol and other drugs to produce serious adverse effects. *The patient must be informed regarding all likely in-*

teractants that could alter the action of the drug he or she is using. If, during the course of treatment, the patient has reason to feel he or she has discovered a new interaction of importance, the physician should be informed so that its full significance can be determined. (It is through such observations that much of our understanding of drug interactions has come.)

Warning Symptoms

Experience has shown that many drugs will produce symptoms that are actually early indications of a developing adverse effect. Examples include the appearance of severe headaches and visual disturbances *before* the onset of a stroke in a woman taking oral contraceptives; the development of acid indigestion and stomach distress *before* the activation of a bleeding peptic ulcer in a man taking phenylbutazone (Butazolidin) for shoulder bursitis. *It is imperative that the patient be familar with those symptoms and signs that could be early indicators of impending adverse reactions.* With this knowledge he or she can act in his or her own behalf by discontinuing the drug and consulting the physician for additional guidance.

Examinations to Monitor Drug Effects

Certain drugs (less than half of those in common use) are capable of damaging vital body tissues (bone marrow, liver, kidney, eye structures, etc.)—especially when these drugs are used over an extended period. Such adverse effects are relatively rare, and many of them are not discovered until the drug has been in wide use for a long time. As our knowledge of such effects accumulates, we learn which kinds of drugs (that is, which chemical structures) are most likely to produce such tissue reactions. Hence, we know those drugs that should be monitored periodically to detect as early as possible any evidence of tissue injury resulting from their use. *The patient should cooperate fully with the physician in the performance of periodic examinations for evidence of adverse drug effects.*

Advanced Age and Debility

The altered functional capacity of vital organs that accompanies advancing age and debilitating disease can greatly influence the body's response to drugs. Such patients tend not to tolerate drugs with inherent toxic potential well; it is usually necessary for them to use smaller doses at longer intervals. *The effects of drugs on the elderly and severely ill are often unpredictable.* The frequent need for dosage adjustments or change in drug selection requires continuous observation of these patients if adverse effects are to be prevented or mini-mized.

Appropriate Drug Choice

The drug(s) selected to treat any condition should be the most appro-priate of those available. Many adverse reactions can be prevented if both physician and patient exercise good judgment and restraint. *The wise patient will not demand overtreatment.* He or she will cooperate with the physician's attempt to balance properly the seriousness of the illness and the hazard of the drug.

Polypharmacy

This term refers to the concurrent use by an individual of several drugs prescribed separately by two (or more) physicians for different disorders—often without appropriate communication between pa-tient and prescriber. This frequent practice is conducive to potentially serious drug/drug interactions. *The patient should routinely inform each physican (and dentist) consulted of all the drugs—prescription and nonprescription—that he or she may be taking at the time.* It is mandatory that each physician have this information before prescrib-ing additional drugs.

DRUGS AND THE ELDERLY

Advancing age brings changes in body structure and function that may alter significantly the action of drugs. An impaired digestive system may interfere with drug absorption. Reduced capacity of the liver and kidneys to metabolize and eliminate drugs may result in the accumulation of drugs in the body to toxic levels. By impairing the body's ability to maintain a "steady state" (homeostasis), the aging process may increase the sensitivity of many tissues to the actions of drugs, thereby altering greatly the responsiveness of the nervous and circulatory systems to standard drug doses. If aging should cause deterioration of understanding, memory, vision or physical coordina-tion, people with such impairments may not always use drugs safely and effectively.

Adverse reactions to drugs occur three times more frequently in the older population. An unwanted drug response can render a func-tioning and independent older person whose health and reserves are at marginal levels, confused, incompetent or helpless. For these rea-sons, drug treatment in the elderly must always be accompanied by the most careful consideration of the individual's health and tolerances, the selection of drugs and dosage schedules and the possible need for assistance in treatment routines.

Guidelines for the Use of Drugs by the Elderly

- Be certain that drug treatment is necessary. Many health problems of the elderly can be managed without the use of drugs.
- Avoid if possible the use of many drugs at one time. It is advisable to use not more than three drugs concurrently.
- Dosage schedules should be as uncomplicated as possible. When feasible, a single daily dose of each drug is preferable.
- In order to establish individual tolerance, treatment with most drugs is usually best begun by using smaller than standard doses. Maintenance doses should also be determined carefully. A maintenance dose is often smaller for persons over 60 years of age than for younger persons.
- Avoid large tablets and capsules if other dosage forms are available. Liquid preparations are easier for the elderly or debilitated to swallow.
- Have all drug containers labeled with the drug name and directions for use in large, easy-to-read letters.
- Ask the pharmacist to package drugs in easy-to-open containers. Avoid "child-proof" caps and stoppers.
- Do not take any drug in the dark. Identify each dose of medicine carefully in adequate light to be certain you are taking the drug intended.
- To avoid taking the wrong drug or an extra dose, do not keep drugs on a bedside table. Drugs for emergency use, such as nitroglycerin, are an exception. It is advisable to have only one such drug at the bedside for use during the night.
- Drug use by older persons may require supervision. Observe drug effects continuously to ensure safe and effective use.
- Remember the adage: "Start low, go slow and (when appropriate) learn to say no."

Drugs Best Avoided by the Elderly Because of Increased Possibility of Adverse Reactions

antacids (high sodium)*
barbiturates*
benzodiazepines (long-acting)
cyclophosphamide
diethylstilbestrol
estrogens
indomethacin
monoamine oxidase inhibitors (MAOI's)*
oxyphenbutazone

phenacetin
phenylbutazone

tetracyclines*

Drugs That Should Be Used by the Elderly in Reduced Dosages Until Full Effect Has Been Determined

anticoagulants (oral)*
antidepressants*
antidiabetic drugs*
antihistamines*
antihypertensives*
anti-inflammatory drugs*
barbiturates*
beta-blockers*
colchicine
cortisonelike drugs*
digitalis preparations*
diuretics* (all types)

ephedrine
epinephrine
haloperidol
isoetharine
nalidixic acid
narcotic drugs
prazosin
pseudoephedrine
quinidine
sleep inducers (hypnotics)*
terbutaline
thyroid preparations

Drugs That May Cause Confusion and Behavioral Disturbances in the Elderly

amantadine
antidepressants*
antidiabetic drugs*
antihistamines*
anti-inflammatory drugs*
atropine* (and drugs containing belladonna)
barbiturates*
benzodiazepines*
carbamazepine
cimetidine
digitalis preparations*
diuretics*
ergoloid mesylates

levodopa
meprobamate
methocarbamol
methyldopa
narcotic drugs
pentazocine
phenytoin
primidone
reserpine
sedatives
sleep inducers (hypnotics)*
thiothixene
tranquilizers (mild)*
trihexyphenidyl

Drugs That May Cause Orthostatic Hypotension in the Elderly

antidepressants*
antihypertensives*
diuretics* (all types)
phenothiazines*
*See Drug Class, Section Four.

sedatives
tranquilizers (mild)*
vasodilators*

Drugs That May Cause Sluggishness, Unsteadiness and Falling in the Elderly

barbiturates*
beta blockers*
chlordiazepoxide
clorazepate
diazepam

diphenhydramine
flurazepam
halazepam
prazepam
sleep inducers (hypnotics)*

Drugs That May Cause Constipation and/or Retention of Urine in the Elderly

amantadine
androgens
antidepressants*
antiparkinsonism drugs*
atropinelike drugs*
epinephrine

ergoloid mesylates
isoetharine
narcotic drugs
phenothiazines*
terbutaline

Drugs That May Cause Loss of Bladder Control (Urinary Incontinence) in the Elderly

diuretics* (all types)
sedatives

sleep inducers (hypnotics)*
tranquilizers (mild)*

THERAPEUTIC DRUG MONITORING
(Measuring Drug Levels in Blood)

The routine use of measuring drug levels in blood as an aid in managing drug therapy has evolved gradually over the past 20 years. Because individuals vary so greatly in the nature and degree of their responses to drugs, it became apparent that greater precision in determining optimal dosage for the individual was needed. For many drugs, the responses observed by the physician (clinical changes) clearly indicate that the drug is working as intended and that the dosage scheme is satisfactory. However, for some drugs—especially those with narrow safety margins—the toxic reactions closely resemble the symptoms of the disorder for which the drugs are prescribed. In many instances the patient's response is not in keeping with his or her clinical condition or program of drug therapy. By measuring the blood levels of certain drugs at appropriate times, the physician can adjust dosage schedules more accurately, predict drug

*See Drug Class, Section Four.

response more precisely, reduce the risk of toxicity and achieve greater benefit.

The timing of the blood samples is an important consideration. As a general rule, the best time for sampling is just before the next scheduled dose of the drug to be measured (the "trough" level). Sampling should be avoided during the two hours following oral administration; during this absorption period, blood levels do not represent tissue levels of the drug.

The following drugs are those most suitable for therapeutic drug monitoring. If you are using any of these on a regular basis, consult your physician regarding the advisability or need for periodic measurement of drug levels in your blood.

Generic Name	Brand Name(s)
acetaminophen	Datril, Tylenol, etc.
amikacin	Amikin
amitriptyline	Amitril, Elavil, Endep, etc.
aspirin (other salicylates)	Bufferin, Ecotrin, etc.
carbamazepine	Tegretol
chloramphenicol	Chloromycetin
chlorpromazine	Thorazine
ciprofloxacin	Cipro
clomipramine	Anafranil
clonazepam	Clonopin
cyclosporine	Sandimmune
desipramine	Norpramin, Pertofrane
digitoxin	Crystodigin
digoxin	Lanoxin
disopyramide	Norpace
doxepin	Adapin, Sinequan
dyphylline	Brophylline, Neothylline, etc.
ethosuximide	Zarontin
ethotoin	Peganone
gentamicin	Garamycin
gold salts	Auranofin, Myochrisine, etc.
imipramine	Janimine, Tofranil, etc.
isoniazid	INH, Niconyl, etc.
kanamycin	Kantrex
lidocaine	Xylocaine, etc.
lithium	Lithobid, Lithotabs, etc.
mephenytoin	Mesantoin
mephobarbital	Mebaral
methotrexate	Mexate
methsuximide	Celontin

nortriptyline	Aventyl, Pamelor
paramethadione	Paradione
phenobarbital	Luminal, etc.
phensuximide	Milontin
phenytoin	Dilantin
primidone	Mysoline
procainamide	Pronestyl
propranolol	Inderal
protriptyline	Vivactil
quinidine	Cardioquin, Quinaglute, etc.
theophylline	Aminophylline, Theo-Dur, etc.
thioridazine	Mellaril
tobramycin	Nebcin
trimethadione	Tridione
valproic acid	Depakene

THE USE
OF DRUGS IN TREATING
CHRONIC DISORDERS

Chronic Disorders Reviewed in This Section

Acne

Alzheimer's Disease

Angina Pectoris

Asthma

Cholesterol Disorders

Congestive Heart Failure

Crohn's Disease

Depression

Diabetes

Epilepsy

Glaucoma

Gout

Hypertension (High Blood Pressure)

Hypothyroidism

Lupus Erythematosus

Menopause

Migraine Headache

Myasthenia Gravis

Osteoarthritis

Osteoporosis

Parkinson's Disease

Peptic Ulcer

Psoriasis

Rheumatoid Arthritis

Schizophrenia

Ulcerative Colitis

INTRODUCTION

Of the 200 drugs prescribed most frequently by physicians in the United States in 1990, 142 (71%) are used in the treatment of chronic disorders. This section provides an overview of the management of some of the more common disorders that require drug therapy for long periods of time, some of them for life. As you read this section, you will become familiar with important principles in the use of selected drugs and will gain perspectives that can help you to understand what your physician is attempting to accomplish with the therapy recommended. Since the lack of reasonable compliance by the patient is one of the major causes of failure in today's use of drugs, your greater understanding will encourage you to cooperate fully with your physician's instructions so that together you can achieve the greatest benefit with the least risk from the drugs prescribed.

Although drugs are essential to the rational treatment of most chronic disorders, proper attention must also be given to other treatment procedures, of equal importance. Examples include adherence to the appropriate diet in the management of diabetes, cessation of smoking in the treatment of angina (coronary artery disease), weight control in the treatment of high blood pressure (hypertension) and the use of "allergy shots" (immunotherapy) in the management of asthma. The intelligent use of drugs can make a significant contribution, but it must be recognized that drugs have their limitations and should be looked upon as but one part of a comprehensive and integrated treatment program.

WARNING: Each physician develops his or her own favored approach to the use of drugs. This is based upon knowledge of the drug's characteristics plus personal experience and observation of drug performance. The treatment program recommended by your physician may vary somewhat from the guidelines provided in this book. It is important that you follow your physician's instructions precisely as given—that you comply fully. If you question any aspect of drug selection, dosage schedule, drug effects, etc., consult your physician before attempting any modification of your drug treatment program on your own. *Under no circumstances should you attempt to initiate prescription drug therapy for yourself or others without the full knowledge and guidance of a qualified physician.*

ACNE

Other Name: Acne vulgaris

Prevalence in USA: Approximately 4.6 million cases: 2.4% of the population under 18 years of age; 3% of the population 18 to 44 years of age.

Age Group: Most common in adolescents and young adults. Usually begins at puberty (9 to 12 years of age) and subsides at 18 to 20 years of age. A small percentage of cases will persist into the twenties and thirties.

Male to Female Ratio: Slightly more common in women.

Principal Features: Common acne is a disorder of the hair follicles and sebaceous (oil-producing) glands of the skin. It is characterized by the formation of open comedones (blackheads), closed comedones (whiteheads), inflammed papules (pimples) and pustules in the superficial layers of the skin. The deep form of acne includes the formation of inflammed nodules and pus-filled cysts. These skin changes occur most commonly on the face, but are also found on the neck, chest, shoulders and upper back. The degree of inflammation will vary from mild to severe throughout the course of the disorder. It is often worse in the winter and better during the summer, probably due to the beneficial effects of sun exposure.

Causes: Acne is primarily due to overactivity of the oil-producing sebaceous glands. This usually begins with the changes of puberty when the associated increase in sex hormones (principally androgens) stimulates the growth and production of the glands. The opening of the gland becomes plugged with a mixture of dead skin cells, oils and bacteria, resulting in a comedo; this progresses to the formation of fatty acids within the gland that causes inflammation, swelling and eventual rupture into the skin. Contributing causes include familial predisposition, excessive heat and humidity, poor personal hygiene, the use of oil-based cosmetics and exposure to industrial oils and tars.

Drugs That Can Cause This Disorder:
The following drugs can initiate acne or aggravate existing acne:

androgens (male hormonelike drugs)
cortisonelike drugs
cytotoxic drugs (those used to treat various types of cancer)
methotrexate
oral contraceptives that contain norethindrone or norgestrel (Brevicon, Loestrin, Lo/Ovral, Micronor, Modicon, Norinyl, Norlestrin,
Norlutin, Nor-Qd, Ortho-Novum, Ovcon, Ovral, Ovrette)
progesterone

The following drugs can cause acnelike eruptions but do not cause true
comedo formation:

bromides	phenytoin
disulfiram	quinine
iodides	thiouracil
isoniazid	trimethadione
lithium	vitamin B-12
phenobarbital	

Drugs Used to Treat This Disorder:
Locally (Topically)
- benzoyl peroxide (Benoxyl, Clearasil, Epi-Clear, Topex, etc.).
- tretinoin (retinoic acid preparations, Retin-A).
- antibiotic lotions.
- metronidazole gel (MetroGel).

Internally (Systemically)
- tetracycline (see Drug Profile).
- erythromycin (see Drug Profile).
- isotretinoin (see Drug Profile).
- prednisone (see Drug Profile).
- ibuprofen (see Drug Profile).

Goals of Drug Treatment
Improvement and control are the primary objectives; cure is not possible.
Prevention of new blemishes.
Prevention of scarring.
Note: Appropriate treatment, conscientiously followed, is beneficial in
95% of all cases.

Drug Management
Local (Topical) Drug Treatment
Often sufficient to control superficial acne with mild to moderate in-
flammation.
May be used concurrently with internal (systemic) treatment for con-
trol of deep acne with severe inflammation, nodule and cyst forma-
tion.
Start treatment slowly; determine tolerance by applying small amounts
of low-concentration products to small areas of skin.
Limit applications to once or twice daily.
Apply to *dry* skin, one-half hour after washing.

Use soap and water to remove skin oils; wash skin no more than twice daily.

Avoid abrasive preparations.

Irritation from topical drugs is common; true allergy is uncommon.

Use of Benzoyl Peroxide

1. This is the single most effective drug for the topical treatment of acne. Many preparations are available without prescription.
2. Its principal action is anti-infective; its primary use is treating superficial, inflammatory, papulo-pustular acne.
3. Start with a 5% preparation; apply once daily—in the morning.
4. This drug inactivates tretinoin (retinoic acid); do not apply these two drugs at the same time.

Use of Tretinoin (Retinoic Acid)

1. This is the only practical drug available for the topical management of comedones. It does require a prescription.
2. It is used in all forms of acne to facilitate the removal of existing comedones and to prevent the formation of new ones.
3. Start with the 0.01% gel; increase the strength of the preparation as needed and tolerated.
4. Apply once daily—in the evening or at bedtime.
5. This drug may require continual use for up to 12 weeks to obtain initial benefit; continued control will require maintenance treatment for months or years.
6. Drying and irritation of the skin are common. However, deliberate irritation and peeling are not necessary for benefit.
7. This drug may increase skin sensitivity to sunlight; use sun screen preparations if necessary, but avoid them if possible.

Use of Topical Antibiotics

1. Erythromycin is the drug of choice; tetracycline and clindamycin preparations are also used.
2. These anti-infective drugs are used primarily to treat inflammatory acne; they do not clear existing lesions but do prevent the development of new ones.
3. May be used concurrently with benzoyl peroxide or tretinoin.
4. Apply twice daily—morning and evening.
5. These drugs may require continual use for 3 to 4 weeks to obtain significant improvement.

Internal (Systemic) Drug Treatment

Required for control of moderate to severe deep acne (inflammatory nodules, cysts, abscesses) and to reduce permanent scarring.

A firm commitment to conscientious treatment for many months or years is often required to accomplish desired results.

Use of Tetracycline

1. Generally considered to be the drug of choice for long-term use. (See Drug Profile for complete description.)
2. May be used alone or concurrently with benzoyl peroxide or tretinoin.
3. Begin treatment with 500 mg to 1000 mg daily for 4 weeks or until

a satisfactory result is obtained. Then reduce gradually to the smallest effective dose for long-term maintenance; this may be as low as 250 mg every 1 to 3 days.

4. This is best taken on an empty stomach, 1 hour before or 2 hours after eating.
5. Continual use for 3 months may be required to obtain optimal benefit.
6. If tetracycline is not effective or cannot be tolerated, erythromycin is the next drug of choice.

Use of Isotretinoin

1. This drug is reserved for the treatment of severe acne that has not responded to conventional management. (See Drug Profile for complete description.)
2. Its primary action is to inhibit the production of sebum (a mix of sebaceous oils and skin cell debris). This reduces the source of fatty acids that cause inflammatory reaction.
3. ***Do not use this drug during pregnancy. Use effective birth control measures while taking it.***
4. Continual use for 20 or more weeks is usually required to produce significant benefit.
5. Monitor triglyceride blood levels during use; if level exceeds 400 mg, reduce the dose; if level exceeds 600 mg, discontinue this drug.
6. Use this drug with caution in those with type I diabetes or inflammatory bowel disease (Crohn's disease, ulcerative colitis).

Use of Prednisone

1. Cortisonelike drugs may induce acne in some individuals. However, it may be useful for some with extensive, severe inflammatory acne that is unresponsive to other treatments.
2. Initiate treatment with 30 mg to 45 mg of prednisone daily, gradually reducing this dose within 1 month. Low-dose maintenance using 2.5 mg each evening may extend control. (See Drug Profile for complete description.)

Use of Ibuprofen

1. This anti-inflammatory drug may enhance the beneficial effects of systemic tetracyline. (See Drug Profile of Ibuprofen for complete description.)
2. A trial of 600 mg 4 times per day is warranted for those with severe inflammatory acne that has shown limited benefit from standard drug therapy.

Use of Oral Contraceptives

1. High-estrogen birth control pills that contain a nonandrogenic progestin (ethynodrel, norethisterone, norethynodrel) are sometimes used to treat severe acne.
2. The beneficial action of these preparations is the reduction of sebum formation.
3. Because of the inherent risks, this use of oral contraceptives is generally not recommended. (See Drug Profile for complete description.)

Ancillary Drug Treatment (as required)

Condition	*Drug Treatment*
For candidiasis (yeast infection of genital or anal region, a complication of long-term antibiotic or oral contraceptive use):	clotrimazole (Lotrimin) nystatin (Mycostatin)

Note: Drug selection, dosage and administration schedule must be determined by the physician for each patient individually.

Resource for Additional Information and Services

Acne Research Institute
1587 Monrovia Avenue
Newport Beach, CA 92663
Phone: (714) 722-1805

Telecommunications services: 1–800-235–2263 (outside CA); 1–800-225–2263 (inside CA)
Publications available.

ALZHEIMER'S DISEASE

Other Names: Alzheimer's presenile and senile dementia, senile dementia (Alzheimer type)

Prevalence in USA: Approximately 2.5 million; more than 7% of the American population aged over 65 years; the cause of 50% of all progressive dementias.

Age Group: Occurs occasionally under 50 years of age; uncommon before 65 years; the majority occurs over 65 years: mild dementia in 5% and moderate to severe in 10–20%. Moderate to severe dementia occurs in 20% of all over 80.

Male to Female Ratio: More common in women.

Principal Features:
Insidious onset leading to progressive and permanent decline of all intellectual functions.
Mood changes: apathy, depression, irritability, anxiety, paranoia.
Loss of recent memory, inability to recall facts of common knowledge, disorientation, confusion, all worse at night.
Impaired attention, understanding, judgment. Loss of ability to think abstractly, to use language correctly, to calculate.

Eventual gait disturbances, incoordination of movements.
Social skills may be retained until late in course of disease.
Course is from 3 to 20 years, with mean duration of 7 years.

Causes: Degeneration of nerve cells in the areas of the brain that control intellectual functions. Actual cause of degeneration is unknown. Genetic predisposition appears probable; Alzheimer type dementia is four times more frequent among family members than in the general population. There is a history of previous head injury in 15% to 20% of cases. One common feature is a marked deficiency of the nerve transmitter acetylcholine.

Drugs That Can Cause This Disorder: No drugs cause true Alzheimer's dementia. However, 3% of all dementias are drug induced. The following drugs can cause symptoms in the elderly that resemble Alzheimer's disease (see Drug Classes, Section Four):

antidepressants	butyrophenones
atropinelike drugs	cortisonelike drugs
barbiturates	digitalis preparations
benzodiazepines	MAO inhibitors

Drugs Used to Treat This Disorder:
No specific or truly effective drug treatment is available at this time.
Ergoloid mesylates (Deapril-ST, Hydergine) are tried during the early stages to relieve symptoms; benefits are infrequent, negligible and fleeting.
Experimental drugs: choline, lecithin, physostigmine (none are curative or significantly beneficial).

Goals of Drug Treatment
Temporary improvement of alertness and memory.
Relief of confusion, depression and behavioral disturbances.

Drug Management
Keep all medications to a minimum.
If any drug is used, start treatment with small doses, increase the dosage cautiously and monitor the response very closely.
Avoid drugs with strong atropinelike effects and strong sedative effects.
Ergoloid mesylates may act as a mild antidepressant and may improve mood. If it is tolerated well, a trial of 6 months is justified.
Lecithin may increase the acetylcholine content of brain tissue and temporarily improve memory in some individuals. It is available in health food stores without prescription. It is safe to try. Ask your physician for guidance.
Use antipsychotics (Haldol, Mellaril, etc.) and sedatives (chloral hydrate, Benadryl, etc.) only when clearly needed. Use the smallest dose that proves to be effective.

Ancillary Drug Treatment (as required)

Condition	Drug Treatment
For agitation, confusion:	haloperidol (Haldol)
	thioridazine (Mellaril)
	thiothixene (Navane)
For insomnia:	chloral hydrate (Noctec, Somnos, etc.)
	diphenhydramine (Benadryl)
For depression:	trazodone (Desyrel)
For constipation:	docusate (Colace, Doxinate, Surfak, etc.)

Note: Drug selection, dosage and administration schedule must be determined by the physician for each patient individually.

Resource for Additional Information and Services

Alzheimer's Association
70 East Lake Street, Suite 600
Chicago, IL 60601
Phone: 1-800-621-0379; (312) 853-3060

Sends packet of information; offers information by phone. National network of 207 chapters and 1200 support groups. Publishes a Quarterly Newsletter.

ANGINA PECTORIS

Other Names: Coronary artery insufficiency, coronary artery disease, coronary heart disease, ischemic heart disease

Prevalence in USA: Approximately 6 million; coronary artery disease is the leading cause of death in the USA.

Age Group: Under 45 years—0.2% of population; 45 to 64 years—6.5% of population; over 65 years—11% of population.

Male to Female Ratio: Under 45 years—1.5 to 1; 45 to 64 years—3 to 1; 65 to 74 years—1.8 to 1; over 75 years—1 to 1.

Principal Features

Classical Angina-of-Effort (Exertional Angina): A moderate to severe discomfort (pain, pressure, tightness, fullness, squeezing or burning sensation) usually located deeply behind the breastbone (but may be felt in the jaw, neck, shoulder, arms, upper back or pit of the stomach). It is characteristically brought on by physical exertion, a large meal, emotional stress or exposure to cold; it usually lasts 1 to 3 minutes and disappears with rest.

Variant (Prinzmetal's) Angina: Usually occurs at rest, and is unpredictable and unrelated to the situations that provoke effort angina. It often occurs between midnight and 8 a.m. The two types of angina can coexist. Acute anginal pain may be accompanied by weakness, sweating, shortness of breath or nausea.

Causes

Exertional Angina: Due to atherosclerosis (thickening and hardening) of segments of coronary arteries. Contributory causes of these arterial changes include heredity (genetic susceptibility), hypertension, high blood cholesterol, diabetes and smoking.

Variant (Prinzmetal's) Angina: Due to spontaneous spasm of segments of coronary arteries; the cause of the spasm is not known. Anemia, hyperthyroidism, aortic valve disease and heart rhythm disorders predispose to angina.

Drugs That Can Cause This Disorder: The following drugs do not cause coronary artery disease per se, but they can affect heart function adversely and induce or intensify angina in susceptible individuals:

amphetamines
beta blocker drugs (abrupt
    withdrawal)
bromocriptine
cocaine
epinephrine
ergot preparations
5-fluouracil
hydralazine
indomethacin
isoetharine
isoproterenol
metaproterenol
methysergide
nifedipine (first dose)
nylidrin
oral contraceptives
phenylpropanolamine
prazosin
terbutaline
thyroid

Drugs Used to Treat This Disorder:

Nitrate Preparations
- nitroglycerin lingual aerosol (Nitrolingual Spray).
- nitroglycerin sublingual tablets (Nitrostat).
- nitroglycerin buccal tablets (Susadrin).
- nitroglycerin prolonged-action forms (Nitro-Bid, etc.).
- nitroglycerin ointment (Nitrol, etc.).
- nitroglycerin patches (Nitrodisc, Nitro-Dur, etc.).
- isosorbide dinitrate (Isordil, Sorbitrate).
- erythrityl tetranitrate (Cardilate).
- pentaerythritol tetranitrate (Peritrate).

Beta Blocker Drugs
- atenolol (Tenormin).
- labetalol (Normodyne, Trandate).
- metoprolol (Lopressor).
- nadolol (Corgard).
- propranolol (Inderal).

Other beta blockers are used but have not yet been approved by the FDA for specific use in the management of angina.

Calcium Blocker Drugs
- nicardipine (Cardene).
- nifedipine (Adalat, Procardia).
- diltiazem (Cardizem).
- verapamil (Calan, Isoptin).

Others
- aspirin (for its antiplatelet action).
- dipyridamole (Persantine). Antianginal effect is questionable and under review.

Goals of Drug Treatment

Prompt relief of acute anginal attack.

Prevention of anticipated angina by use of nitroglyerin just before physical activity.

Long-term prevention of angina; reduced frequency, severity and duration of recurrent anginal episodes.

Prevention of heart rhythm disturbances.

Prevention of heart attack (myocardial infarction).

Drug Management

For Stable Exertional Angina

Frequency and severity of angina-of-effort remain at a constant level.
Nitroglycerin spray or sublingual tablet for relief of acute attacks.
Long-acting nitrates and/or a beta blocker.
If control is not adequate, add a calcium blocker.

For Unstable Angina

Frequency and severity of angina increase over time; angina occurs with exertion and at rest, is less responsive to treatment.
Hospitalization in coronary care unit.
Mild sedation with benzodiazepines (Valium, etc.).
Combined use of nitrates, beta blocker and calcium blocker.
Aspirin, for antiplatelet effect.

For Variant (Prinzmetal's) Angina

Anginal attacks primarily at rest.
Nitroglycerin spray or sublingual tablets.
Long-acting nitrates.
Calcium blocker.
Avoid beta blockers (unless it is established that both types of angina are present).

Use of Nitroglycerin

1. Nitroglycerin is the mainstay of managing angina. Always have a supply of fresh, active tablets available. Keep them in the original dark glass bottle, tightly closed, no cotton added. Do not transfer them to a metal or plastic container.
2. The sublingual tablet will produce a mild stinging sensation under the tongue, flushing of the face and throbbing in the head. These reactions are normal and indicate that the drug is active and you are having a good response.

3. Use nitrolycerin promptly and as often as necessary, no matter how often. Unless instructed otherwise, do not consciously keep count of the tablets used.
4. If the lingual spray or sublingual tablet causes weakness, dizziness or faintness, sit down or lie down until the sensation passes.
5. Use the spray or tablet to prevent an attack by taking it just before starting a specific physical activity that is known to induce angina.
6. If anginal pain persists after taking 3 successive sublingual tablets (1 tablet at 3-to-5-minute intervals for 3 doses), consult your physician immediately or seek assistance at the nearest hospital emergency room.
7. Nitroglycerin ointment may be used at bedtime to prevent angina during sleep. Follow the instructions for application carefully. Do not use your fingers. Do not rub the ointment into the skin.
8. Nitroglycerin patches (discs) may induce tolerance to the drug and cause it to be less effective with continuous use. The intermittent use of oral dosage forms may be more effective for long-term treatment. Ask your physician for guidance.
9. If you have glaucoma, consult your physician regarding the periodic measurement of your internal eye pressures while using long-term nitrates for angina.
10. Following long-term use, nitrates should be discontinued gradually to prevent symptoms of withdrawal.

Use of Beta Blocker Drugs
1. Do not use this type of drug without your physician's knowledge and guidance.
2. Beta blockers are not recommended for mild angina that is well controlled by nitrates. Their use is generally reserved for severe and unstable angina.
3. Beta blockers are not recommended for variant (Prinzmetal's) vasospastic angina.
4. If your angina worsens with the use of a beta blocker drug, notify your physician promptly.
5. Atenolol (Tenormin) and metoprolol (Lopressor) are preferred for individuals with asthma, emphysema, diabetes or peripheral circulatory disorders.
6. Atenolol (Tenormin) and nadolol (Corgard) are effective with once-daily dosage and tend to cause less depression and insomnia.
7. Beta blocker drugs must not be discontinued suddenly. Abrupt withdrawal can cause severe angina and increase the risk of heart attack (myocardial infarction).

Use of Calcium Blocker Drugs
1. A calcium blocker is the drug of choice for treating variant (Prinzmetal's) angina.
2. Nifedipine (Adalat, Procardia) is the most potent antianginal calcium blocker. However, angina may worsen if the heart rate increases excessively.
3. Verapamil (Calan, Isoptin) can delay the excretion of digoxin and

increase the risk of digoxin toxicity. Dosage adjustments may be necessary.

4. These drugs can be used initially by individuals who should not use beta blockers.

Current Controversies in Drug Management

The nitrate drugs are well established as effective therapeutic agents for the management of angina and congestive heart failure, two conditions that require long-term drug therapy. Recent studies have shown that the "standard" practice of continuous administration of nitrates can lead to the development of tolerance (see Glossary) and loss of effectiveness. Tolerance is most likely to occur with frequent dosing and the use of prolonged-action capsules or tablets and the use of transdermal nitroglycerin patches. Continuous treatment with nitrates produces tolerance within 24 hours of the first dose and complete loss of effect when continued for one week or more. The intermittent use of nitrates ("pulse" dosing) causes only partial tolerance and is more effective for long-term protection. Intermittent rather than continuous nitrate dosing is now recommended for treating angina and congestive heart failure.

Comments: Current guidelines for the optimal use of nitrates include the following recommendations.

- Take isosorbide dinitrate (Isordil, short-acting form) 2 or 3 (but not 4) times daily; take at 8:00 a.m. and 1:00 or 3:00 p.m., or at 8:00 a.m., 1:00 p.m. and 5:00 p.m.; no dosing again until the following 8:00 a.m.
- Take the prolonged-action dosage forms of isosorbide dinitrate at 8:00 a.m., only once daily.
- Use the nitroglycerin patch for only 12 hours daily, from 8:00 a.m. to 8:00 p.m.; leave it off during the night.
- Long nitrate-free intervals appear to preserve responsiveness to the drug.

Ancillary Drug Treatment (as required)

Condition	Drug Treatment
For anxiety:	benzodiazepines (Valium, etc.) (See Drug Class, Section Four.)
For hypertension:	see Profile of Hypertension in this section
For congestive heart failure:	see Profile of Congestive Heart Failure in this section
For hyperthyroidism:	methimazole (Tapazole) propylthiouracil propranolol (Inderal)
For anemia:	iron preparations

Note: Drug selection, dosage and administration schedule must be determined by the physician for each patient individually.

Resources for Additional Information and Services

Coronary Club
9500 Euclid Avenue
Cleveland, OH 44106
Phone: (216) 444-3690

Local groups: 20.
Publications available: "Heartline" monthly, $15 per year.

Council on Arteriosclerosis of the American Heart Association
7320 Greenville Avenue
Dallas, TX 75231
Phone: (214) 373-6300

ASTHMA

Other Names: Bronchial asthma, reversible airway disease, reversible obstructive airway disease

Prevalence in USA: Approximately 7 million, 3% of population (includes 1.5 million school-age children).

Age Group: Under 18 years—2.5 million; 18 to 44 years—2.7 million; 45 to 64 years—1.6 million; 65 to 74 years—726,000; 75 years and over—308,000.

Male to Female Ratio: About equal.

Principal Features: Recurring acute attacks of shortness of breath, wheezing (labored breathing), a sensation of tightness in the chest and cough, with symptom-free intervals between attacks. Episodes of active asthma may last an hour to several days. The acute attack begins with tightening of muscles in the walls of bronchial tubes (airways), which causes constriction and reduced air flow. This is followed by swelling of the lining of bronchial tubes and the excessive production of mucus, both of which cause additional narrowing of the airways, forced breathing and coughing. Severe asthma may be accompanied by sweating, insomnia and bluish discoloration of the face and extremities (cyanosis). Asthma that begins in infancy (under 2 years of age) may persist into adulthood. With onset after 2 years, 50% of asthma cases will "outgrow" the disorder by 16 years. Asthma with onset in adulthood is often severe and persistent.

Causes
Extrinsic (Allergic) Asthma: Due to a true allergy (allergen-antibody reaction); hereditary susceptibility to the development of allergies. Com-

mon allergens are house dust (and mites in house dust), pollens, animal danders, feathers, wool, molds.

Intrinsic (Idiosyncratic) Asthma: Due to an unusual individual sensitivity (not a true allergy). Onset usually 35 to 45 years of age; 10% to 15% are sensitive to aspirin and have nasal polyps.

Exercise-induced Asthma: Usually in children and young adults; occurs alone or with other types of asthma; often worse 15 minutes after exercise.

Asthma "Triggers": Cold air, smoke, cooking odors, respiratory infections, emotional stress.

Drugs That Can Cause This Disorder:

acetaminophen

aspirin (and substitutes)

beta blocker drugs

erythromycin

griseofulvin

hydralazine

ibuprofen

indomethacin

ketoprofen

mefenamic acid

monoamine oxidase inhibitors

naproxen

nitrofurantoin

oral contraceptives

penicillin

pentazocine

phenothiazines

phenylbutazone

procainamide

propoxyphene

reserpine

tartrazine dye

Drugs Used to Treat This Disorder:

Xanthine Preparations
- aminophylline (Aminophyllin, Aminodur, etc.).
- oxtriphylline (Brondecon, Choledyl).
- theophylline (Bronkodyl, Slo-bid, Theo-Dur, etc.).

Beta-Adrenergic Drugs
- albuterol (Proventil, Ventolin).
- terbutaline (Brethine, Bricanyl).
- metaproterenol (Alupent, Metaprel).
- pirbuterol (Maxair).
- isoetharine (Bronkometer, Bronkosol).
- isoproterenol (Isuprel, Medihaler-Iso, etc.).

Cortisonelike Steroids
- beclomethasone aerosol (Beclovent, Vanceril).
- prednisolone (Delta-Cortef, Sterane, etc.).
- prednisone (Deltasone, Meticorten, etc.).

Others
- cromolyn (Intal).
- ipratropium (Atrovent).
- oxygen.

Goals of Drug Treatment

Prompt relief of acute asthmatic attacks.

Prevention of recurrent acute attacks.

Stabilization of lung function: freedom from asthma to the greatest degree possible, with a minimal use of drugs.

Prevention of later complications: bronchiectasis, emphysema, heart disease (cor pulmonale).

Drug Management

For Extrinsic (Allergic) Asthma

For occasional and predictable acute attacks, start treatment with beta-adrenergic inhalers.

For attacks of increasing frequency and duration, add albuterol or terbutaline tablets or a long-acting oral theophylline preparation.

For severe acute attacks or aggravation of chronic asthma, add beclomethasone aerosol inhaler.

If control is not adequate, use albuterol (or terbutaline) tablets and a theophylline preparation concurrently.

If control is still inadequate, add cromolyn on a regular basis.

If an adequate trial of all of the above fails to produce satisfactory relief and control, add cortisonelike steroids (tablets by mouth).

For Intrinsic (Idiosyncratic, Late-Onset) Asthma

Attacks may be less responsive to the use of the bronchodilators (beta-adrenergics and theophylline) as outlined above.

Earlier control may require the use of cromolyn and steroid preparations on a regular schedule.

For Exercise-induced Asthma

Try cromolyn on a regular schedule for prevention of attacks that follow exercise.

Use albuterol or terbutaline inhalation 5 to 10 minutes before exercise and following exercise for prevention.

Long-acting theophylline preparations may be effective in children for prevention.

Use of Theophylline Preparations

1. Theophylline elixir and uncoated tablets are used for prompt relief of acute asthma.
2. Theophylline sustained-release forms (Slo-bid, Slo-phyllin, Theo-Dur) are used for smooth maintenance therapy of chronic asthma. Theophylline blood levels are helpful in determining optimal dosage schedules.
3. Theophylline potentiates beta-adrenergic bronchodilators and increases their effectiveness.
4. See the Drug Profile of Theophylline in Section Three for important drug interactions.

Use of Beta-Adrenergic Bronchodilators

1. These presssurized inhalers are potent drugs that must be used cautiously. Avoid excessive use; follow dosage schedules precisely.
2. They are most effective at the beginning of an asthmatic attack and before exercise that induces asthma.
3. For the most effective use of aerosol bronchodilators, learn the correct procedure: exhale through the mouth to empty lungs; squirt and

inhale the first dose at the same time; hold your breath and count to 10, then exhale. If necessary, use a second inhalation in 10 to 15 minutes.
4. Limit inhalations to 1 or 2 at a time, and at least 3 to 4 hours apart.
5. Do not use isoproterenol (Isuprel) aerosol and epinephrine (Adrenalin) aerosol concurrently.

Use of Cortisonelike Steroids
1. Steroids are not bronchodilators; they will not relieve acute asthma. This includes beclomethasone.
2. Their use should be restricted to the treatment of severe acute and chronic asthma that is not controlled by conventional drugs.
3. Steroids should never be used as the sole drug for managing asthma.
4. For short-term use: when an acute attack is prolonged and fails to respond to bronchodilators; steroids are very effective when used for 7 to 10 days of a "burst and taper" schedule—high initial dose followed by gradual dose reduction and withdrawal.
5. For long-term use: when asthma becomes severe and continuous and cannot be controlled by other drugs; a trial period of 2 to 4 weeks of steroids will determine effectiveness. The optimal long-term use consists of a relatively large single dose of prednisone (or prednisolone) every other morning (alternate-day schedule). This provides adequate asthma control with minimal adverse effects of long-term steroid use.
6. The steroid beclomethasone, inhaled in aerosol form, is used to control asthma as steroid tablets are withdrawn.

Use of Cromolyn
1. Cromolyn is not a bronchodilator; it will not relieve acute asthma.
2. It is used only by inhalation; powder and liquid aerosol forms are available.
3. A trial of cromolyn (as an asthma preventive) should begin while you are free of asthma, before acute attacks occur.
4. When used on a regular schedule, cromolyn is 70% to 75% effective in preventing recurrences of acute asthma.
5. Cromolyn is most effective in preventing extrinsic (allergic) asthma, and least effective in preventing intrinsic (idiosyncratic) asthma. It may or may not prevent exercise-induced asthma but is worth a trial.
6. Cromolyn should be used on a regular basis for 8 to 10 weeks to evaluate its protective benefit.
7. For best results, a beta-adrenergic aerosol should be used 10 minutes before inhaling cromolyn.

Ancillary Drug Treatment (as required)

Condition	Drug Treatment
For anxiety:	promethazine (Phenergan)
	Note: Avoid *all* sedatives in active asthma.

For pain, mild to
moderate: acetaminophen (Tylenol, etc.)

For pain, severe: methotrimeprazine (Levoprome). This
                         does not depress respiration.

For bacterial infection of
respiratory tract
(complicating asthma):   ampicillin
                         amoxicillin
                         trimethoprim and sulfamethoxazole
                         tetracycline (avoid during pregnancy and
                         under 8 years of age)

For viral infection of
respiratory tract
(triggering asthma):   steroids: prednisone and
                         methylprednisolone

Note: Drug selection, dosage and administration schedule must be determined
by the physician for each patient individually.

Resources for Additional Information and Services

Asthma and Allergy Foundation of America
1717 Massachusetts Avenue, N.W., Suite 305
Washington, DC 20036
Phone: (202) 265-0265
Publications available.

National Jewish Center for Immunology and Respiratory Medicine
1400 Jackson Street
Denver, CO 80206
Phone: 1-800-222-LUNG
Publications available: Lung Line Letter.

National Foundation for Asthma
P.O. Box 30069
Tucson, AZ 85751
Phone: (602) 323-6046
Publications available.

CHOLESTEROL DISORDERS

Other Names: Dyslipidemia, hypercholesterolemia, hyperlipidemia, hyper-
lipoproteinemia, hypertriglyceridemia, lipid transport disorder, lipoprotein disorder

Prevalence in USA: An estimated 25% of adults are thought to have a total cholesterol level in the "too high" range: 200 to 240 mg (current standard).

0.1% of the population has congenital (familial) hypercholesterolemia.

1.0% of the population has congenital (familial) hypertriglyceridemia.

Age Group: In the USA, the low-density lipoprotein (LDL) cholesterol begins to rise after adolescence and continues to rise for 30 years. Significant elevations of LDL cholesterol levels are found in the 20-to-50-year age group.

Male to Female Ratio: 25 to 54 years of age: men show moderately higher levels of total cholesterol and LDL cholesterol; 55 years and older: women show moderately higher levels of total cholesterol and LDL cholesterol.

Principal Features

The principal blood fats (lipids)—notably cholesterol and triglycerides—are combined in the liver with proteins (to form lipoproteins) that facilitate their transport to body tissues. There are normally 3 major classes of lipoproteins: very low-density lipoproteins (VLDL), low-density lipoproteins (LDL) and high-density lipoproteins (HDL). Each class contains differing proportions of fat and protein. VLDL consists of five-sixths triglycerides and one-sixth cholesterol. While circulating in the blood, VLDL is transformed first to intermediate-density lipoprotein (IDL), which is 30% cholesterol and 40% triglyceride, and then to low-density lipoprotein (LDL), which carries from 60% to 75% of the total blood cholesterol. High levels of LDL cholesterol are associated *statistically* with an increased risk of coronary heart disease—the higher the level, the higher the risk. HDL carries less than 25% of the total blood cholesterol. It is thought to assist with the removal of LDL cholesterol from the blood and body tissues. High levels of HDL cholesterol appear to be protective against coronary heart disease—the higher the HDL level, the lower the risk.

The principal cholesterol disorders are classified into 5 major types according to the nature of the lipoprotein abnormality and associated clinical features. Types I and V are not associated with the development of atherosclerosis. Types II, III and IV are associated with the atherosclerotic process that causes coronary heart disease and peripheral vascular disorders. The lipoprotein features of these classes are as follows:

Type IIa: increased total cholesterol and LDL cholesterol; normal triglycerides.

Type IIb: increased total cholesterol, LDL cholesterol and VLDL; moderately increased triglycerides.

Type III: increased IDL cholesterol (abnormal form); increased triglycerides.

Type IV: normal total cholesterol, increased VLDL, decreased HDL cholesterol; increased triglycerides.

Causes: The major cholesterol disorders are primarily hereditary (familial) and therefore genetically determined. Secondary causes can contribute to congenital lipid disorders or can independently account for abnormalities of blood lipid metabolism. Among the secondary causes are the following conditions: Hypothyroidism, biliary cirrhosis, nephrosis, anorexia nervosa and acute intermittent porphyria can cause significant increases in blood cholesterol levels. Diabetes, chronic alcoholism, chronic kidney failure and acute hepatitis can cause significant increases in blood triglyceride levels. However, the most apparent secondary cause of lipid disorders is the high dietary cholesterol and fat content consumed by the American public.

Drugs That Can Cause This Disorder: The following drugs have been reported to cause abnormal increases in cholesterol blood levels: anabolic (male-hormonelike) steroids, chenodiol, disopyramide, thiazide diuretics (see Drug Class, Section Four), trimeprazine. The following drugs have been reported to cause abnormal increases in triglyceride blood levels: cortisonelike drugs (see Drug Class, Section Four), estrogens, isotretinoin, oral contraceptives, thiazide diuretics (see Drug Class, Section Four), timolol.

Drugs Used to Treat This Disorder:
Drugs that inhibit synthesis of cholesterol and lipoprotein: lovastatin (Mevacor), niacin (nicotinic acid, Nicobid, Nicotinex, etc.).
Drugs that hasten the clearance of lipoproteins in the bloodstream: clofibrate (Atromid-S), gemfibrozil (Lopid).
Drugs that accelerate breakdown and elimination of lipoproteins: cholestyramine (Questran), colestipol (Colestid), probucol (Lorelco).
Other drugs used less often: dextrothyroxine (Choloxin), neomycin.

New Drugs in Development for Treating This Disorder:
Drugs of the lovastatin class: mevastatin (Compactin), pravastatin (Eptastatin, Pravachol), simvastatin (Synvinolin, Zocor). These drugs, for the most part, significantly reduce total and LDL cholesterol and raise HDL cholesterol. They may prove to be effective in lower dosage and therefore less likely to cause adverse effects.
Drugs of the fibric acid class: fenofibrate. This drug (in use in Europe for several years) effectively reduces LDL cholesterol and triglycerides, raises HDL cholesterol and is well tolerated.

Goals of Drug Treatment
Normalization of blood lipid levels to currently accepted standards: total cholesterol of less than 200 mg; LDL cholesterol of less than 130 mg; triglycerides of less than 250 mg (in the absence of other significant lipid abnormalities).
Avoidance or reduction of adverse drug effects.
Prevention, retardation or reversal of atherosclerotic arterial changes throughout the body to reduce the risk of coronary heart disease, peripheral vascular disease and stroke.

Note: The following values reflect the evolving opinion regarding the "normalcy" of blood lipids over the past 15 years:

Normal Upper Limit	1975	1980	1989
Total cholesterol	300	280	200
LDL cholesterol		180	130
Triglycerides	200	165	150

A "normal" HDL cholesterol range is 40 to 80.

Drug Management
Introduction
Our present understanding of how cholesterol disorders are causally related to the development of atherosclerosis (coronary and peripheral vascular disease) is incomplete and controversial. While large population studies have demonstrated that high cholesterol blood levels are associated statistically with an increased incidence of atherosclerosis, cholesterol values alone have low predictability for the actual development of coronary heart disease on an individual basis. The somewhat exaggerated emphasis on "statistical significance" has resulted in the creation of unrealistic risk ratios based on minor changes in blood lipid levels that are meaningless in the light of wide individual variability and the unreproducibility of laboratory test results as currently obtained. Determination of isolated blood lipid levels provides at best an incomplete appraisal of an individual's status regarding an inclination to develop atherosclerosis. They represent only one aspect of a disease process in which many other causative factors are involved. An understanding of the complex interactions of the numerous cholesterol-triglyceride-apoprotein linkages (lipoprotein fractions) is the key to learning which components and what concentrations can be relied upon to predicate an increased risk for the consequent development of atherosclerosis. For example, high levels of apolipoproteins (a), AI and B are much stronger predictors than cholesterol values for identifying those at high risk for atherosclerotic heart disease. Anyone who has reason to be concerned about a possible cholesterol disorder is well advised to reduce dietary fat and cholesterol intake. The majority of individuals with elevated blood lipid values do not require drug therapy to manage their disorder. Before starting a long-term, expensive and somewhat risky program of drug treatment, the concerned individual should first seek a detailed evaluation at a reputable lipid research center, either in person or by submission of appropriate blood samples and medical information.

Determining the Need for Treatment
Observe the following procedures for the measurement of blood lipid values:
1. Do not alter your regular diet in preparation for testing. You should not be on a reducing diet.
2. You should be free of any kind of infection.

3. Avoid all alcoholic beverages for 24 hours prior to testing.
4. Fast for 12 to 16 hours prior to testing.
5. Your blood samples should be examined by a reliable laboratory that has established a record for providing accurate, precise and reproducible test results.
6. For proper evaluation, a blood lipid profile should include values for total cholesterol, LDL and HDL cholesterol fractions and triglycerides.
7. Obtain blood lipid measurements on at least 2 separate occasions (3 if in doubt) and use the average of the test results.

When to Treat
    Current recommendations regarding initiation of treatment are based on the following guidelines. Either diet therapy alone or diet plus drug therapy is recommended when the blood lipid values exceed those stated in the table.

Age Group	DIET ALONE Cholesterol	LDL	DIET AND DRUGS Cholesterol	LDL
20–29	200	140	220	160
30–39	220	155	240	175
Over 40	240	160	260	185

How to Treat
1. Diet modification is the primary treatment for all individuals with elevated blood lipid levels. The total caloric intake should be designed to achieve ideal body weight. The initial diet should restrict saturated fats to 10% of the total calories and restrict cholesterol to less than 300 mg daily. This low-fat, low-cholesterol diet should be adhered to for 4 to 6 months to fully evaluate its effectiveness. Individuals with severe blood lipid disorders may require the guidance of a registered dietitian.
2. If an adequate trial of dietary therapy fails to lower blood lipid values to acceptable levels, consideration may be given to adding a trial of drug therapy while dietary modification continues. No single drug is appropriate for treating all blood lipid disorders. The choice of the initial drug depends upon the specific nature of the lipoprotein abnormality. Begin with an adequate trial of a single drug. If the response is insufficient, substitute another drug or add a second drug as appropriate. Measure blood lipid levels 4 to 6 weeks after starting drug treatment and at 3-month intervals until a stable response is obtained.
3. To reduce LDL cholesterol (the most common form of cholesterol disorder in the USA):
   weight reduction if necessary
   diet low in saturated fats and cholesterol
   effective drugs:
       cholestyramine (Questran)

colestipol (Colestid)
lovastatin (Mevicor)
niacin (nicotinic acid)
4. To reduce VLDL triglycerides:
weight reduction
diet low in saturated fats and cholesterol
alcohol restriction
effective drugs:
niacin (nicotinic acid)
gemfibrozil (Lopid)
5. To reduce IDL (abnormal lipoprotein):
weight reduction
diet low in saturated fats and cholesterol
effective drugs:
niacin (nicotinic acid)
gemfibrozil (Lopid)
clofibrate (Atromid-S), not recommended due to serious adverse
drug effects
6. To raise HDL cholesterol:
weight reduction
smoking cessation
regular exercise
modest use of alcohol (no more than 1 to 2 drinks daily)
avoidance of progestin-containing contraceptives
no specific drug recommended currently

Notes on Specific Lipid-Lowering Drugs
(See the respective Drug Profiles in Section Three for a complete discussion.)
Lovastatin (Mevacor)
The prototype of a new and most promising class of drugs
Recent studies show it to be more effective and better tolerated than
cholestyramine.
Can reduce total cholesterol 22% to 33%
Can reduce LDL cholesterol 32% to 42%
Can reduce triglycerides 8% to 27%
Can raise HDL cholesterol slightly
More effective in women than in men
Most effective when used in combination with cholestyramine or colestipol
Infrequent adverse drug effects: indigestion, localized muscle pain
Cholestyramine (Questran) and colestipol (Colestid)
Have demonstrated effectiveness in reducing the development of coronary heart disease
Currently the drugs of choice for treating Type IIa hyperlipidemia
Can reduce total cholesterol 20%
Can reduce LDL cholesterol 23% to 27%
Can raise HDL cholesterol slightly
Triglycerides unchanged or increased

Cause severe constipation in 20% of users

Cause decreased absorption of many other drugs (due to binding)

Large doses cause deficiencies of vitamins A, D, E and K; calcium; iron

Niacin (nicotinic acid)

Used to treat Types IIa, IIb, III and IV hyperlipidemia

Can reduce total cholesterol 25%

Can reduce LDL cholesterol 35%

Can reduce triglycerides 26%

Can raise HDL cholesterol 20%

Not well tolerated by many users

Advise use of timed-release dosage form; increase dose slowly over 2 to 3 months; take with meals; take one adult aspirin tablet 30 minutes before each dose to reduce skin flushing

Significant adverse effects: liver toxicity, reduced sugar tolerance, increased blood uric acid levels, stomach irritation

Gemfibrozil (Lopid)

Used primarily to treat Types IIb, III, IV and V hyperlipidemia

Can reduce total cholesterol 10%

Can reduce LDL cholesterol 11%

Can reduce triglycerides 35%

Can raise HDL cholesterol 11%

Significant adverse effects: reduced sugar tolerance, decreased white blood cell counts, doubled risk for gall stone formation, reduced libido in 12% of men

Should be discontinued if not beneficial after 3 months of treatment

Probucol (Lorelco)

Used primarily to treat Type IIa hyperlipidemia

Can reduce total cholesterol 10% to 15%

Can reduce LDL cholesterol 8%

Can reduce HDL cholesterol 23% (possibly undesirable)

Triglycerides unchanged or raised

Significant adverse effects: anemia, diarrhea

Of limited usefulness due to reduction of HDL cholesterol

May be used in combination with more effective drugs

Current Controversies in Drug Management

1. Should individuals with "moderate" elevations of cholesterol be treated initially with diet modification alone or with combined dietary and drug treatment?

   Comments

   Dietary reduction of saturated fats and cholesterol usually reduces blood cholesterol levels by no more than 10% to 20%; no significant benefit in morbidity or mortality has been demonstrated.

   Cholestyramine drug therapy reduces blood cholesterol levels by 25% with an associated 50% reduction in the risk of developing coronary heart disease.

   Generalizations are not always appropriate or applicable when making therapeutic decisions. *Individual* assessment of benefit versus risk (and cost) must be made jointly by patient and physician. The early introduction of drug therapy is justified when there is a family history of premature coronary heart disease (before age 60), recent coronary bypass surgery or other risk factors, such as obesity, high blood pressure, diabetes or heavy use of tobacco.

2. Should individuals with "moderate" elevations of triglycerides (primarily) be treated with diet modification only or with combined dietary and drug treatment?

Comments

Not all forms of triglycerides are associated with increased risk for atherosclerosis. A detailed lipoprotein profile is necessary for specific recommendations. The triglycerides found primarily in chylomicrons (Types I and V disorders) are not atherogenic and drug therapy is not indicated. The triglycerides associated with IDL (Type III disorder) are atherogenic and require drug treatment.

Ancillary Drug Treatment (as required)

Condition	*Drug Treatment*
For constipation (due to cholestyramine or colestipol):	docusate (Colace, Dialose, Doxidan, Surfak, etc.)
	Citrucel
	Metamucil
For diarrhea (due to probucol):	diphenoxylate (Lomotil)
	loperamide (Imodium)
For associated diabetes mellitus:	see Profile of Diabetes in this section
For associated hypertension:	see Profile of Hypertension in this section
For associated hypothyroidism:	see Profile of Hypothyroidism in this section

Note: Drug selection, dosage and administration schedule must be determined by the physician for each patient individually.

Resources for Additional Information and Services

Council on Arteriosclerosis of the American Heart Association
c/o The American Heart Association
7320 Greenville Avenue
Dallas, TX 75231
Phone: (214) 373-6300
Publications available

Citizens for the Treatment of High Blood Pressure and for Public Action on Cholesterol
888 17th Street, N.W., Suite 904
Washington, DC 20006
Phone: (202) 466-4553

Publications available: Cholesterol Update bimonthly, newsletters, educational literature.

CONGESTIVE HEART FAILURE

Other Names: Chronic heart failure, cardiac decompensation, myocardial decompensation

Prevalence in USA: 2.3 million; 400,000 new cases annually.

Age Group: 45 to 54 years—2.6/1000 population; 55 to 64 years—7/1000 population; 65 to 74 years—15/1000 population.

Male to Female Ratio: 1.5 to 1.

Principal Features: The designation "congestive heart failure" refers to a condition in which the heart is unable to pump enough blood to satisfy the needs of the body. Diseased heart muscle loses its contracting power, allowing increased filling pressures inside the heart chambers (ventricles); further stretching and weakening of muscle tissue leads to muscle exhaustion and reduced pumping capacity; the forward flow of blood is impaired and excessive volumes of blood accumulate in vital areas throughout the body, producing congestion. Resulting symptoms include shortness of breath (dyspnea), first with exertion and later at rest; inability to breathe comfortably while lying down (orthopnea); fatigue and weakness, especially in the legs; a dry cough; night urination; swelling of the feet and ankles at the end of the day; and vague discomfort in the chest and abdomen.

Causes: Primary causes of heart disease that ultimately lead to congestive heart failure:

hypertension (75%)	myocarditis
coronary heart disease (10%)	diabetes (16%)
valvular heart disease (10%)	emphysema
congenital heart disease	

Precipitating causes in predisposed individuals: reduction of therapy (most common), heart rhythm disorders, severe infections, obesity, pregnancy, anemia, hyperthyroidism, excessive heat and humidity.

Drugs That Can Cause This Disorder: In individuals with borderline heart function, the following drugs can precipitate congestive heart failure:

amantadine (Symmetrel)
beta-adrenergic-blocking drugs (see Drug Class, Section Four)
cortisonelike steroids (see Drug Class, Section Four)
disopyramide (Norpace)
nonsteroidal anti-inflammatory drugs (see Drug Class, Section Four)

Drugs Used to Treat This Disorder:
- digitalis preparations: digitoxin, digoxin.
- diuretics (see Drug Class, Section Four).
- vasodilators: arterial dilators—hydralazine, prazosin; venous dilators—isosorbide dinitrate, nitroglycerin.
- calcium channel-blocking drugs: ditiazem, nifedipine, verapamil.
- ACE inhibitors: captopril, enalapril, lisinopril.
- milrinone (investigational only).
- oxygen.

New Drugs in Development for Treating This Disorder:
Xamoterol (Carwin), a new heart muscle stimulant under study in Europe and in the U.S., has been shown to be significantly better than digoxin in treating chronic heart failure. This drug is not yet available for general use.

Goals of Drug Treatment
Improvement of the heart's pumping performance by the use of digitalis.
Reduction of the heart's workload by the use of arterial and venous vasodilators.
Removal of excess salt and water from the body by the use of diuretics.
Relief of symptoms—fatigue, shortness of breath, ankle swelling, etc.—by means of the above procedures.

Drug Management
For Early, Mild Congestive Heart Failure
Two variations of initial treatment are used widely:
1. Treatment is started with digitalis (digoxin or digitoxin). This may be the only drug used if response is satisfactory. If necessary, a thiazide diuretic (or equivalent) is added.
2. Treatment is started with a thiazide diuretic (or equivalent), given alone. This may give a very adequate response, especially in the elderly. If necessary, digoxin (or digitoxin) is added.

For Moderate to Severe Congestive Heart Failure
Digoxin (or digitoxin) and thiazide diuretics are used in maximal tolerated dosage.
As necessary, a stronger diuretic, such as furosemide or ethacrynic acid, is added.
If the response is inadequate, vasodilators are started: isosorbide dinitrate or nitroglycerin patches for venous dilation; hydralazine for arterial dilation.
If additional improvement is sought, captopril (or enalapril) may be tried as a replacement for the nitrates (isosorbide dinitrate or nitroglycerin).
For long-term maintenance, a combination of hydralazine and nitrates or hydralazine and captropril may be tried.
For congestive heart failure with angina and/or hypertension, a trial of nifedipine is justified.

Use of Digitalis
1. Should be started only when there is a firm diagnosis of heart failure. Periodic reassessment is necessary to determine continued need.

Maintenance digitalis may not be necessary for life. Following correction of congestive heart failure, stable heart function may be achieved by using only diuretics and vasodilators.

2. Digoxin is the form of digitalis most frequently used. Because digoxin products vary in their absorbability, refill your prescriptions with the same brand to ensure uniform drug effects.
3. Take the exact dose at the same time each day.
4. Learn to count your pulse and check its regularity. Notify your physician if your pulse rate is below 60 beats/minute or your pulse rhythm changes significantly.
5. The elderly and individuals with hypothyroidism often have a reduced tolerance for digitalis; smaller doses are advisable.
6. Digitalis toxicity (overdosage) occurs in 20% of users; it is more common in the elderly. The earliest indications of toxicity are usually loss of appetite, nausea and vomiting; other indications include headache, facial pains, blurred vision, seeing "snowflakes" or yellowish-green halos, fatigue, weakness and disturbances of heart rhythm. The elderly may show confusion; rarely, seizures may occur.
7. Periodic blood levels can help to determine optimal dosage, especially if kidney function is impaired. The blood sample should be taken no less than 6 hours after the last dose.
8. See the Drug Profile of Digoxin in Section Three for important drug interactions.

Use of Diuretics ("Water Pills")
1. Thiazide (or equivalent) diuretics may suffice as the only drug treatment for mild heart failure in many elderly patients.
2. When possible, diuretics should be taken in the morning to minimize nighttime urination.
3. If your diuretic is one that increases the excretion of potassium in the urine, it is important that your blood level of potassium be checked periodically. An abnormally low potassium level can increase the risk of digitalis toxicity. Consult your physician regarding the advisability of omitting your diuretic every third day to minimize the loss of potassium.
4. If your diuretic is one that does not increase the excretion of potassium (amiloride, spironolactone, triamterene), you should not take a potassium supplement or eat excessive amounts of high-potassium foods.
5. If you use diuretics on a regular basis, consult your physician regarding the degree of salt restriction he or she recommends for you.
6. Many salt substitutes have a high potassium content. Ask your physician for guidance regarding the selection and use of commercially available salt substitutes.
7. In advanced congestive heart failure, you may be advised to use a thiazide diuretic concurrently with furosemide (or ethacrynic acid) and a potassium-saving diuretic; the combined actions of the three types of drugs give a maximal diuretic effect.

Use of Vasodilators
1. These are generally used when heart failure does not respond adequately to digitalis and diuretics.
2. These may be used earlier for those who cannot tolerate digitalis, and for those who need a vasodilator to treat hypertension (hydralazine) or angina (nifedipine).
3. Nitrate vasodilators (primarily venous dilators) contribute to the relief of shortness of breath.
4. Hydralazine (primarily an arterial dilator) contributes to the relief of fatigue and weakness.
5. Isosorbide dinitrate (venous) and hydralazine (arterial) vasodilators can be used concurrently to advantage; they are quite effective in the majority of cases of chronic congestive failure.
6. Prazosin (both an arterial and a venous dilator) is an alternative choice. However it causes fluid retention and requires increasing doses and additional diuretics with continued use.

Use of Oxygen
1. Oxygen must be properly humidified to prevent drying of tissues of the respiratory tract.
2. Administer by nasal prongs; avoid a mask.

Current Controversies in Drug Management

With the advent of new drugs and improved understanding of the altered physiology associated with congestive heart failure, controversy regarding drug selection for its treatment has increased. A consensus has emerged indicating that diuretics should now be considered the first-line drugs of choice, replacing digoxin.

Controversy continues, however, as to which drug should be added next if diuretics are inadequate. Some authorities favor digoxin as the second drug; others favor vasodilators (see above). Current evidence seems to favor vasodilators as the second drug, with digoxin added as a third drug when required. New studies show that angiotensin-converting enzyme (ACE) inhibitors (see above) can enhance treatment and prolong survival. Further experience and detailed analysis of drug performance are required to resolve current controversies. Drug choices at this time will remain a matter of individual physician preference.

Ancillary Drug Treatment (as required)

Condition	Drug Treatment
For anxiety:	diazepam (only as needed)
For insomnia:	chloral hydrate (Noctec, Somnos)
For anemia:	iron preparations
For hypertension:	see Profile of Hypertension in this section

Note: Drug selection, dosage and administration schedule must be determined by the physician for each patient individually.

Resource for Additional Information and Services

American Heart Association
7320 Greenville Avenue
Dallas, TX 75231
Phone: (214) 373-6300
Publications available.

CROHN'S DISEASE

Other Names: Regional enteritis, regional ileitis, granulomatous colitis, inflammatory bowel disease

Prevalence in USA: 1 million (includes 100,000 children); 15,000 new cases annually.

Age Group: Onset from infancy to 25 years of age; 15% to 30% have onset before puberty. Peak incidence is from 10 to 25 years of age.

Male to Female Ratio: Slightly more common in females.

Principal Features: An intermittent to chronic disorder of the small intestine and colon; one third of cases occur in the lower segment of the small intestine (the ileum), one third in the colon and one third in both. Less than 50% of cases involve the rectum. The onset is usually insidious, but may be rapid and resemble acute appendicitis. Symptoms include loss of appetite, fatigue, fever, loss of weight, abdominal cramps and pain after eating, nausea, vomiting, diarrhea (occasionally bloody), anal sores and retarded growth in children. There may also be inflammatory disorders in the skin, eyes, mouth and large joints. Children may experience fever and joint pains before any indications of disease in the intestine or colon. Adults may have a higher incidence of gallstones or kidney stones. This disorder often recurs throughout life.
   Caution: The early manifestations of Crohn's disease may vary. Loss of appetite and weight may lead to the mistaken diagnosis of anorexia nervosa.

Causes: The primary cause is unknown. There is a familial clustering in 15% to 20% of cases. It is thought that an inherited susceptibility may predispose to unknown environmental factors capable of inducing the disorder.

Drugs That Can Cause This Disorder: By altering the normal balance of bacteria in the intestine, several antibiotics can cause a form of enteritis that might resemble Crohn's disease. These include some of the tetracyclines, penicillin and chloramphenicol. Antibiotic-induced enteritis is transient and easily corrected; no permanent damage occurs. The vitamin A derivative etretinate (Tegison) has been reported to cause Crohn's disease.

Drugs Used to Treat This Disorder:
- sulfasalazine (Azulfidine).
- cortisonelike steroids, principally prednisone.
- azathioprine (Imuran); 6-mercaptopurine (Purinethol).
- metronidazole (Flagyl).
- antidiarrheals: diphenoxylate (Lomotil), loperamide (Imodium).
- antispasmodics: belladonna (Donnatal), dicyclomine (Bentyl).
- antibiotics: ampicillin (Amcill, etc.), tetracycline (Achromycin, etc.); used when appropriate for bacterial infections of intestine.

Goals of Drug Treatment
Induction of a remission (return to normal) during the active phase of the disease.
Relief of symptoms.
Protection of bowel, avoidance of complications.
Maintenance of general nutrition.

Drug Management
General Principles
For initial treatment of mild disease: sulfasalazine.
For moderate to severe disease: prednisone, used concurrently with sulfasalazine.
For acute recurrences: prednisone.
For long-term maintenance: sulfasalazine; avoid use of cortisonelike steroids (prednisone).
For active disease that fails to respond to combined use of sulfasalazine and prednisone: (1) a trial of metronidazole as replacement for sulfasalazine; (2) a trial of azathioprine or 6-mercaptopurine added to sulfasalazine and prednisone programs.

Use of Sulfasalazine
1. Used to initiate treatment in active disease.
2. About 50% effective when used with prednisone.
3. Most beneficial in treating Crohn's disease of the colon.
4. Usually not effective in preventing recurrences; however, it may be tried for long-term maintenance until a better treatment is developed.
5. Common adverse effects are headache, nausea and vomiting; take with or immediately following food.

Use of Cortisonelike Steroids (Prednisone, etc.)
1. Usually 60% to 70% effective during first 6 months of treatment; if use is extended to 12 months, only 20% to 30% remain in remission.
2. Good initial response in treating Crohn's disease of the colon, but the majority relapse within 1 year.
3. Long-term use for mild disease or to prevent recurrences is usually ineffective and is not advised.
4. Use primarily to control worsening symptoms and to suppress acute

flare-ups. Continue use until a sustained improvement is established. Try to use the lowest effective dose.

5. When possible, an alternate-day dosing schedule is recommended: a single morning dose every 48 hours.
6. When appropriate, taper dose very slowly over a period of 4 to 12 months.
7. Repeated intermittent short courses are preferable to continual long-term use.
8. Crohn's disease of the rectum should be treated with steroid suppositories and retention enemas.

Use of Antidiarrheals
1. Use very cautiously and as sparingly as possible.
2. Excessive use can induce two complications: (1) paralytic (adynamic) ileus, a paralysis of the small intestine that results in a functional obstruction; (2) toxic megacolon, a marked distention of the colon with air, and a danger of perforation.

Use of Adsorbents
1. Cholestyramine (Questran) and aluminum hydroxide (Amphojel) can adsorb bile in the intestine and reduce bile-induced diarrhea.
2. These adsorbents can also adsorb other drugs being used concurrently. Schedule all dosages to ensure maximal effectiveness—adequate spacing between adsorbents and other active drugs.

Use of Immunosuppressants
1. Azathioprine (Imuran) and 6-mercaptopurine (Purinethol) may be tried when sulfasalazine and prednisone have failed to control the disease after an adequate trial.
2. Either one may be tried as an adjunct to the established treatment program.
3. A trial of 4 to 6 months of treatment is often necessary to determine effectiveness.
4. These drugs make it possible to reduce the dose of steroids or withdraw them completely in some individuals.

Use of Antibiotics
1. Appropriately selected antibiotics may be used to treat a diarrhea due to specific bacterial overgrowth (superinfection).
2. Antibiotics should not be taken concurrently with sulfasalazine.

Ancillary Drug Treatment (as required)

Condition	Drug Treatment
For anemia (common):	iron preparations, vitamin B-12, folic acid (as required)
For malnutrition:	multiple vitamins and the minerals calcium, magnesium, zinc
For depression:	see Profile of Depression in this section

Note: Drug selection, dosage and administration schedule must be determined by the physician for each patient individually.

Resources for Additional Information and Services

American Digestive Disease Society
60 East 42nd Street, Room 411
New York, NY 10165

Telecommunications services: Gutline, available to the public every Tuesday evening from 7:30 to 9:00 p.m.
Publications available.

Crohn's & Colitis Foundation of America, Inc.
444 Park Avenue South, 11th Floor
New York, NY 10018
Phone: (800) 343-3637

DEPRESSION

Other Names: Depressive reaction (reactive depression, secondary depression), depressive illness (biologic depression, major depressive disorder), affective disorder: depressive phase of manic-depressive disorder

Prevalence in USA: Approximately 30 million; 5% to 8% of general population. One third of all depressions are severe enough to require medical treatment.

Age Group: Can occur at any age. Peak occurrence is between 25 and 44 years of age.

Male to Female Ratio: 1 male to 2 females; 25% of women and 10% of men will experience depression during their lifetime.

Principal Features
Depressive Reaction: A situational (exogenous) reactive depression that represents an understandable adaptive response to a significant loss or stressful life situation; a sense of despondency and distress, comparatively mild to moderate, usually self-limiting with a duration of 2 weeks to 6 months.
Depressive Illness: A spontaneous (endogenous) unexplained and seemingly unprovoked depression of moderate to severe degree; characterized by (1) a depressed mood—sadness, dejection, hopelessness, despair; (2) reduced energy level—loss of interest, fatigue, inability to function effectively; (3) negative self-image—sense of inferiority, incompetence, exaggerated guilt. Common features include loss of appetite, broken sleep, early morning awakening, constipation. Often clears spontaneously in 6 to 12 months, even without treatment.

Causes: Depressive reactions are normal mood responses to the stresses and strains of daily life. The primary cause of major depressive illness is unknown. Research indicates that in many cases there appears to be a genetic (constitutional) predisposition to depression. The actual onset of depressive illness is attributed to a deficiency of certain brain chemicals—the neurotransmitters norepinephrine, dopamine and/or serotonin. What initiates the deficiency is not known.

Drugs That Can Cause This Disorder: Drug-induced depressions are more likely to occur in those who are genetically susceptible to depression. The following drugs are known to cause depression:

benzodiazepines (in excess)	levodopa
certain beta-blocking drugs	methyldopa
clonidine	oral contraceptives
cortisonelike steroids	some phenothiazines
digitalis (toxicity)	reserpine (and related drugs)
indomethacin	

Drugs Used to Treat This Disorder:
Bicyclic Antidepressant
• fluoxetine (Prozac).
Tricyclic Antidepressants (TCA's)
• amitriptyline (Elavil, Endep).
• amoxapine (Asendin).
• desipramine (Norpramin, Pertofrane).
• doxepin (Adapin, Sinequan).
• imipramine (Imavate, Presamine, Tofranil).
• nortriptyline (Aventyl, Pamelor).
• protriptyline (Vivactil).
Tetracyclic Antidepressant
• maprotiline (Ludiomil).
Monoamine Oxidase Inhibitors (MAOI's)
• phenelzine (Nardil).
• tranylcypromine (Parnate).
Other Drugs
• alprazolam (Xanax)
• lithium (Eskalith, Lithane, Lithobid, Lithotab)
• methylphenidate (Ritalin)
• trazodone (Desyrel)

Goals of Drug Treatment
Alleviation of symptoms.
Termination of depression, restoration of normal mood.
Prevention of recurrence.
Prevention of swing from depression to manic psychosis (in manic-depressive disorder).

Drug Management
For Depressive Reactions: Reactive depressions are often mild and self-limiting; they usually respond well to supportive psychotherapy. Drug treatment is not necessary for everyone who is depressed. If this type

of depression becomes severe or is unreasonably prolonged, a tricyclic antidepressant (or a new generation equivalent) may be tried for 1 month to determine its effectiveness.

For Depressive Illness: Major endogenous depressions are usually very responsive to an appropriate and adequate trial of antidepressant drug therapy. Spontaneous remissions often occur within 6 to 12 months, but recovery can be initiated earlier and greatly accelerated by proper medication. Adequate dosage and a sufficient period of treatment are essential to a successful outcome.

Treatment is usually started with a tricyclic antidepressant or one of the newer equivalents. If response is inadequate after a reasonable trial, another tricyclic or similar antidepressant should be tried. If this fails, a monoamine oxidase inhibitor may be considered. Some cyclic depressions respond better to lithium than to tricyclic antidepressants.

Not all depressions are recurrent. For a first episode, the antidepressant drug may be gradually reduced and discontinued after 3 to 6 months of a stable mood, free of depression.

For the 50% of depressions that are recurrent, the optimal maintenance dose of the most effective drug should be determined and continued indefinitely.

Use of Tricyclic Antidepressants (TCA's)

1. These are the drugs of choice when drug treatment is deemed necessary.
2. They are 60% to 75% effective in treating major endogenous depressive illness. They may also be effective in treating severe reactive depressions.
3. Continual use on a regular schedule for 2 to 5 weeks is necessary to determine a drug's effectiveness in relieving depression.
4. Treatment with all antidepressants is necessarily empirical; a period of trial and error is unavoidable for both the selection of the best drug and the determination of optimal dosage.
5. If one TCA (or equivalent) shows no significant benefit after 3 weeks of adequate dosage, it is advisable to try another drug of the same or similar class.
6. During drug trials, and during maintenance treatment later, stay with the same brand (manufacturer) to ensure uniform results.
7. Periodic measurement of blood levels of the drug can be helpful in determining optimal dosage. (See Therapeutic Drug Monitoring in Section One.)
8. Most drugs of this class cause drowsiness, especially during the first several weeks of use. Avoid alcoholic beverages and use extreme caution in driving and engaging in all hazardous activities.
9. When the correct total daily dose has been determined, it can usually be taken as a single dose at bedtime.
10. Use these drugs cautiously if you have glaucoma, prostatism or a heart rhythm disorder.
11. Avoid rapid withdrawal of TCA's; abrupt discontinuation may cause

restlessness, headache, anxiety, insomnia, muscle aches, nausea. Withdraw gradually over a period of 10 to 14 days.
12. See the Drug Profiles of respective TCA's in Section Three for important drug interactions.

Use of Newer ("Second Generation") Antidepressants
1. Maprotiline (Ludiomil) may act more rapidly than TCA's; it is quite sedating. Avoid if you have a seizure disorder.
2. Alprazolam (Xanax) is sedating. After long-term use, withdraw gradually to avoid possible seizures.
3. Amoxapine (Asendin) is less sedating. It can cause parkinsonlike symptoms, restlessness and tardive dyskinesia (rarely). Do not use longer than 3 to 4 months.
4. Trazodone (Desyrel) is also sedating, but it has little or no atropine-like effects. It is very useful in the elderly and for those with glaucoma or prostatism.

Use of Monoamine Oxidase Inhibitors (MAOI's)
1. Used to treat biologic endogenous depressions that do not respond to TCA's.
2. Also useful for treating "atypical" and neurotic depressions that are characterized by marked anxiety, phobias, hypochondriasis, excessive eating and excessive sleeping.
3. Continual use on a regular schedule for 2 to 5 weeks is necessary to determine effectiveness in relieving depression.
4. Avoid concurrent use of over-the-counter diet pills, nose drops and cold and allergy preparations.
5. Avoid foods and beverages that contain tyramine and similar compounds. (See Tyramine in Glossary.)
6. If switching from a TCA to a MAOI, allow a "washout" period of 7 to 10 days before starting the MAOI. If switching from a MAOI to a TCA, allow a "washout" period of 14 days before starting the TCA.
7. MAOI's can cause low blood pressure, overstimulation, insomnia, confusion, nausea, vomiting, diarrhea and fluid retention.
8. MAOI's can provoke an abrupt swing from depression to manic psychosis in manic-depressive disorder.
9. MAOI's can activate psychosis in those with schizophrenia.
10. Do not discontinue these drugs suddenly. A rebound depression can follow abrupt withdrawal.
11. See the Drug Profiles of respective MAOI's in Section Three for important drug interactions.

Use of Lithium
1. Can be 70% effective in stabilizing mood, especially in bipolar manic-depressive illness; reduces the frequency and severity of attacks of both mania and depression.
2. Often effective in preventing recurrences of depression in unipolar (depression only) disorders.
3. Must be taken in divided doses to avoid stomach irritation and excessively high (toxic) blood levels.
4. When lithium proves to be effective in preventing recurrence of de-

pression, it is very important to continue maintenance treatment when feeling well and free of depression.

5. Periodic measurements of blood levels are mandatory to maintain effective concentrations and to prevent toxicity. Blood samples should be taken 12 hours after the last dose.
6. Mild side-effects (not toxicity) include loss of appetite, metallic taste, indigestion, nausea, thirst, fatigue, tremor, fluid retention, acne.
7. Early toxic effects include vomiting, dizziness, unsteadiness, weakness, slurred speech, muscle twitching, confusion.
8. While taking lithium, maintain a high liquid intake, but avoid excessive coffee, tea and cola drinks.
9. Do not restrict your salt intake.
10. Use lithium cautiously if you have heart disease, kidney disease or a thyroid disorder.
11. Check thyroid and kidney functions before and during lithium therapy.

Use of Other Antidepressant Drugs
1. Methylphenidate (Ritalin) may be tried for long-term treatment of selected elderly persons with depression.
2. Alprazolam (Xanax), a benzodiazepine tranquilizer, may be useful for short-term treatment of minor depression.

Ancillary Drug Treatment (as required)

Condition	*Drug Treatment*
For mild anxiety:	alprazolam (Xanax)
For severe anxiety and agitation:	thioridazine (Mellaril)
	thiothixene (Navane)
For psychosis:	amitriptyline and perphenazine (Etrafon, Triavil)
For constipation:	docusate (Colace, Doxinate, etc.)

Note: Drug selection, dosage and administration schedule must be determined by the physician for each patient individually.

Resources for Additional Information and Services

Depressives Anonymous: Recovery From Depression
329 East 62nd Street
New York, NY 10021
Phone: (212) 689-2600
Publications available.

Emotions Anonymous
P.O. Box 4245
St. Paul, MN 55104
Phone: (612) 647-9712

Telecommunications services: Telephone referrals to local chapters. Regional groups: 45. Local groups: 1451.
Publications available.

National Depressive and Manic Depressive Association
53 West Jackson Blvd., No. 618
Chicago, IL 60604
Phone: (312) 939-2442

Telecommunications services: Offers information, one-to-one support, referrals by telephone. Local groups: 140.

Publications, audio and video tapes available.

DIABETES

Other Names: Diabetes mellitus; insulin-dependent diabetes mellitus (IDDM), type I; non-insulin-dependent diabetes mellitus (NIDDM), type II

Prevalence in USA: Approximately 10 million: 6 million known, 4 million undiagnosed; 2% to 4% of the population, with a 6% increase (new cases) annually.

Age Group: Under 18 years—90,000; 18 to 44 years—880,000; 45 to 64 years—2.6 million; 65 to 74 years—1.6 million; 75 years and over—800,000.

Male to Female Ratio: Type I—same incidence in men and women. Type II—greater incidence in women.

Principal Features: A disorder of carbohydrate, protein and fat metabolism that renders the body unable to convert foods properly into energy for vital functions.

Type I (10% to 15% of All Diabetes): Occurs most commonly in children and adolescents, with peak onset from 11 to 14 years; can begin at any age. Individuals are usually thin or normal weight (nonobese). Requires lifelong insulin for control of blood sugar and prevention of acidosis.

Type II (85% to 90% of All Diabetes): Most common after 40 years of age, with peak onset from 45 to 64 years. Up to 90% of individuals are obese. Does not require lifelong insulin for control; not prone to development of acidosis.

Characteristic symptoms include excessive hunger and thirst, excessive urination, unexplained weight loss, blurred vision, fatigue, itching of skin, anal and vaginal yeast infections and delayed healing of wounds.

Causes: Primary causes are unknown, but a genetic (hereditary) predisposition appears certain for both types of diabetes. In addition, some individuals who develop type I diabetes may have a genetic susceptibility to viral infection of the pancreas that initiates destruction of the tissue cells that produce insulin. In type I diabetes the pancreas produces very little or no insulin. In type II diabetes insulin production may be normal or partially reduced, but not absent; the diabetes is due to insulin resistance in body tissues.

Drugs That Can Cause This Disorder: In susceptible individuals and those with latent diabetes, the following drugs may induce diabetic manifestations; these are usually mild in nature and reversible:

cortisonelike steroids	phenothiazines
ethacrynic acid	phenytoin
furosemide	propranolol
indomethacin	thiazide diuretics
lithium	tricyclic antidepressants
oral contraceptives	

Drugs Used to Treat This Disorder:
The Insulins: See Drug Profile of Insulin in Section Three.
The Sulfonylureas (Oral Hypoglycemic Drugs):
  • acetohexamide (Dymelor).
  • chlorpropamide (Diabinese).
  • glipizide (Glucotrol).
  • glyburide (Diabeta, Micronase).
  • tolazamide (Tolinase).
  • tolbutamide (Orinase).

New Drugs in Development for Treating This Disorder: Nazlin, a nasal insulin product, is now in clinical trials to evaluate its effectiveness and determine proper dosage. This dosage form will be absorbed through the nose, providing rapid absorption that more closely resembles the body's natural release of insulin.

Goals of Drug Treatment
Normalization of carbohydrate, protein and fat metabolism insofar as possible; control of blood sugar; elimination of acidosis.
Elimination of symptoms; restoration of well-being.
Prevention of hypoglycemia (insulin "shock").
Prevention of recurrent acidosis.
Promotion of normal growth and development in diabetic children.
Prevention or minimization of late complications.
Achievement of normal life expectancy.

Drug Management
General Principles
"Good control" consists of the optimal balance of properly selected foods, exercise and drugs—either insulin or a sulfonylurea in correct dosage. The degree of control is estimated by periodic measurement of blood-sugar levels or urine sugar content.
"Tight control" consists of maintaining a fasting blood sugar between 100 and 140 mg, and a 2-hour (after eating) blood sugar betweeen 100 and 200 mg. Consideration must be given to the possible benefits of "tight control" versus the possible risks of inducing hypoglycemia.
"Tight control" is appropriate for the young diabetic who is otherwise

healthy, free of coronary artery and cerebral circulatory disease, capable of excellent self-care and not living alone. It is not appropriate for the elderly, those with circulatory disorders of the brain or heart, those with established complications of long-standing diabetes and those with other serious disorders.

Although more expensive and inconvenient, the home monitoring of blood-sugar levels is the method of choice for managing diabetic control. The blood-sugar strips Chemstrip bG and Visidex II are recommended for this purpose.

The use of urine-testing strips for the detection of urine sugar and ketones is a useful and practical alternative to the use of blood-sugar strips. Regular testing of urine before meals and at bedtime provides adequate information for the proper adjustment of insulin dosage schedules and the prevention of hypoglycemia and acidosis. Accuracy is improved when the bladder is first emptied and the urine for testing is collected 30 minutes later; the sugar content of this second voiding is more representative of the current blood-sugar level.

If urine testing reveals the repeated presence of ketones, consult your physician promptly.

The following drugs can cause a *false positive* test result for urine sugar when using Clinitest: aspirin (with doses larger than 2400 mg/day), ascorbic acid (vitamin C), cephalosporins, chloral hydrate, chloramphenicol, isoniazid, levodopa, methyldopa, nalidixic acid, penicillin G, probenecid, streptomycin.

The following drugs can cause a *false negative* test result for urine sugar when using Diastix or Testape: aspirin (with doses larger than 2400 mg/day), ascorbic acid (vitamin C), levodopa, methyldopa.

The following drugs can cause a *false positive* test result for urine ketones when using Acetest or Ketostix: aspirin (in moderate to high doses), levodopa, phenazopyridine (Ketostix only).

Learn to recognize the early indications of hypoglycemia and what to do to correct it. Signs that warn of a developing insulin reaction include hunger, sweating, headache, dizziness, nervousness, trembling, blurred vision, drowsiness, confusion, inability to think, sense of inebriation. At the first indication of impending hypoglycemia, take sugar immediately: 5 small sugar cubes; or 2 teaspoonsful or 2 packets of granulated sugar; or ½ to 1 cup of fruit juice; or 1 candy bar. An alternative treatment is the injection of 1 mg of glucagon, repeated in 5 to 10 minutes if necessary. Glucagon is a pancreatic hormone that increases the level of blood sugar.

Learn to recognize the early indications of acidosis. These include the slow development of increasing thirst, excessive urination, drowsiness, fatigue, nausea, vomiting, stomach pain.

The use of beta-blocking drugs (especially in high doses) may predispose to hypoglycemia and mask its symptoms.

For Type I, IDDM

Insulin is a lifelong requirement for control. Sulfonylureas (oral hypoglycemics) are not effective and should not be used.

Insulin requirements will vary continually throughout a lifetime. Therefore, you must learn how to manage your diabetes on a day-by-day basis, modifying insulin types and dosage schedules as necessary, according to the results of regular blood- or urine sugar testing.

For the newly diagnosed diabetic who is not acutely ill and is without complications, the usual American procedure for initiating treatment is to give a single morning dose of 15 to 30 units of an intermediate-acting insulin (NPH or Lente) before breakfast; the dose is then increased by 5 units every 48 hours as required to achieve normal blood-sugar levels. The British method is to start with 6 to 10 units of an intermediate-acting insulin given twice daily, before the morning and evening meals. Either method will relieve most symptoms in 90% of cases within 4 days.

The optimal schedule of insulin injections for regulating the disordered metabolism is determined by periodic monitoring of blood-sugar levels at appropriate times during the 24-hour day. In this way individual patterns of blood-sugar fluctuation and response to insulin can be studied so that the most appropriate types and doses of insulin are given in proper relationship to eating.

A most effective and practical method of providing adequate insulin for the average diabetic is to give a mixture (1 injection) of a rapid-acting insulin (Regular) and an intermediate-acting insulin (NPH or Lente) 20 to 30 minutes before the morning and evening meals, just 2 injections daily. This scheme provides for easy modification of doses of each type of insulin as necessary to obtain smooth control throughout 24 hours.

During periods of stress—infections, injuries, surgery—insulin requirements will increase. Consult your physician for guidance if you have difficulty in making the necessary adjustments of insulin dosage, food intake, etc.

Even during periods of fasting, small amounts of insulin are necessary to control blood sugar and prevent acidosis.

For Type II, NIDDM

Diet is of primary importance and should be tried diligently before starting drugs. Dietary goals are reduction of blood sugar and correction of obesity. Seventy-five percent of cases of Type II diabetes can be controlled by diet alone.

If an adequate trial of dietary management fails, either sulfonylurea drugs (oral hypoglycemics) or insulin may be added to the treatment program. If the blood sugar is only moderately above normal, a sulfonylurea may be tried. If the blood sugar is quite high and the individual is thin, it is best to initiate drug treatment with insulin. After the blood sugar has been stabilized for 3 to 4 weeks, the insulin may be withdrawn and a sulfonylurea may be started to determine its effectiveness.

The major reaction to sulfonylureas is hypoglycemia. It is most likely to occur in the elderly, in alcoholics and in those with significant impairment of liver or kidney function. Hypoglycemic reactions occur most frequently with the use of chlorpropamide (Diabinese), the longest acting sulfonylurea.

If you experience a primary failure (on initial trial) or a secondary failure (after a temporary period of effectiveness) on attempting control with a sulfonylurea, you may need insulin to manage your diabetes successfully.

Insulin is used primarily to control the levels of blood sugar. It is not required to prevent acidosis except under stressful conditions, such as infections, trauma or surgery.

Type II diabetes is often well controlled with a single daily dose of an intermediate-acting insulin. Some individuals with a high degree of insulin resistance may require unusually high doses of insulin to achieve satisfactory control.

Use of Insulins

1. Twenty percent of all diabetics require insulin for satisfactory control.
2. Available insulins differ in their times of peak action and duration of action. An understanding of these differences is necessary for planning an insulin schedule and adjusting it to control your individual pattern of blood-sugar fluctuations during each 24-hour day. The following chart illustrates the characteristics of the three principal types of insulin.

Type of insulin	*Peak action (hours)*	*Duration (hours)*	*Hypoglycemia most likely to occur*
Short-acting			
Regular	2–4	5–7	Before lunch
Semilente	2–8	12–16	Before lunch
Actrapid	2.5–5	8	Before lunch
Semitard	7	9	Early afternoon
Velosulin	2–5	8	Before lunch
Humulin R	2–5	6–8	Before lunch
Intermediate-acting			
Lente	8–12	18–28	Late afternoon
NPH	6–12	18–28	Late afternoon
Monotard	7–15	18–24	Late afternoon
Lentard	8–12	16–24	Late afternoon
Insulatard	4–12	16–24	Mid-afternoon
Humulin N	6–12	14–24	Late afternoon
Novolin N	4–12	18–24	Mid-afternoon
Long-acting			
Protamine Zinc	14–24	24–36	During night–early morning
Ultralente	18–24	32–36	During night–early morning
Ultratard	10–28	24–36	During night–early morning

3. The peak action times and the duration of action vary greatly from person to person. Each individual will show variations of absorption

from one injection site to another and from day to day. Insulin programs must be tailored to each person individually based on response to trials. All insulin schedules need adjustment from time to time.

4. Most insulin-dependent diabetics require from 20 to 60 units of insulin daily. If the requirement reaches 200 units/day, a marked degree of insulin resistance has developed. This is best treated with highly purified pork insulin or human insulin.

5. Most of the time satisfactory control can be achieved with an intermediate-acting insulin, or with the addition of a short-acting insulin. Regular insulin can be mixed with either Lente or NPH in the same syringe and given as a single injection. The mixture retains the short and intermediate characteristics of action.

6. Long-acting insulins are rarely necessary and are seldom used.

7. Hypoglycemia that occurs during the night (excessive insulin effect) causes a "rebound" hyperglycemia that is detected by blood- or urine sugar testing the next morning. This is known as the Somogyi effect. The proper adjustment is to reduce the dose of the long-acting insulin taken in the morning or the dose of the intermediate-acting insulin taken before the evening meal; this will prevent the nocturnal hypoglycemia that causes the confusing high blood or urine sugar on arising.

8. If a true allergy to insulin develops, or if the fatty tissue under the skin at the sites of insulin injection should disappear (lipoatrophy), change to highly purified pork or human insulin.

9. If insulin use is to be intermittent (as in some cases of type II diabetes), it is best to use human insulin to reduce the possibility of developing insulin antibodies that cause insulin resistance.

10. Insulin pumps using either Regular or Ultralente insulin have been developed for use in selected individuals. While they are capable of providing excellent control, their use is quite complex and demanding. They are suitable only for the highly motivated and educated individual who needs and is dedicated to achieving "tight control."

Use of Sulfonylureas (Oral Hypoglycemic Drugs)

1. These drugs are used only for the treatment of type II, NIDDM, in those whose diabetes is not adequately controlled by diet and exercise and who cannot or will not take insulin.

2. The best candidates for a trial of sulfonylureas
   • are over 50 years old.
   • are otherwise healthy.
   • are not allergic to "sulfa" drugs.
   • have no tendency to develop acidosis.
   • have an insulin requirement of less than 30 units/day.
   • prefer tablets by mouth to injections.

3. Sulfonylureas are not suitable for treating
   • type I, insulin-dependent diabetes.
   • the acutely ill diabetic with acidosis.

- the diabetic with infection or with injury, or undergoing surgery.
- the diabetic using long-term cortisonelike steroids.
- the pregnant diabetic.
- the diabetic whose blood sugar is over 300 mg.
4. Sulfonylureas should be used with caution in treating
   - the very old.
   - alcoholics.
   - those taking multiple drugs.
   - those with significantly impaired liver or kidney function.
   - those who comply poorly with recommendations.
5. Recommended dosage schedules:

Short-acting	Duration	Doses/day
tolbutamide	6–12 hrs.	2–3
Intermediate-acting		
acetohexamide	12–24 hrs.	1–2
glipizide	18–30 hrs.	1–2
glyburide	10–30 hrs.	1–2
tolazamide	10–18 hrs.	1–2
Long-acting		
chlorpropamide	60 hrs.	1

6. All sulfonylureas can cause hypoglycemia. Because of its accumulative effects and long period of action, chlorpropamide requires the greatest caution in use; any hypoglycemic reaction is apt to be quite prolonged.
7. Sulfonylureas as a group have a high rate of primary failure (40%). A primary failure is an inability to control hyperglycemia after 3 months of continual treatment with adequate dosage. Secondary failures (25% to 30%) occur when a sulfonylurea drug loses its effectiveness after an initial period of demonstrated ability to control hyperglycemia.
8. During apparently successful long-term use of a sulfonylurea, it is prudent to periodically reduce the dosage and gradually withdraw the drug to determine if its continued use is justified. The success rate of adequate control by long-term use of sulfonylureas is no more than 20% to 30%.
9. There appears to be no general support for the concurrent use of sulfonylureas and insulin. If it is found that insulin is necessary for adequate control, the customary practice is to discontinue the sulfonylurea.

Ancillary Drug Treatment (as required)

Condition	*Drug Treatment*
For yeast infections of skin:	ciclopirox (Loprox)
	clotrimazole (Lotrimin)
	haloprogin (Halotex)

	miconazole (Micatin)
	nystatin (Mycostatin)
For yeast infections of the vagina:	
	clotrimazole (Gyne-Lotrimin, Mycelex-G)
	miconazole (Monistat)
For diabetic diarrhea:	diphenoxylate (Lomotil)
	loperamide (Imodium)
For peripheral neuritis:	carbamazepine (Tegretol) and amitriptyline (Elavil) concurrently
For neurogenic bladder:	bethanechol (Urecholine)
For high blood pressure:	see Profile of Hypertension in this section

Note: Drug selection, dosage and administration schedule must be determined by the physician for each patient individually.

Resources for Additional Information and Services

American Diabetes Association
National Service Center
P.O. Box 25757
1660 Duke Street
Alexandria, VA 22313
Phone: (703) 549-1500

State groups: 55. Local groups: 800.
Publications avilable.

Joslin Diabetes Center
One Joslin Place
Boston, MA 02215
Phone: (617) 732-2400

Publications available.

Juvenile Diabetes Foundation International
432 Park Avenue South, 16th Floor
New York, NY 10016
Phone: 1-800-223-1138; (212) 889-7575

Local groups: 150.
Publications, films, tapes available.

EPILEPSY

Other Names: Seizure disorders, convulsive disorders

Prevalence in USA: Approximately 2 million, 1% of the population.

Age Group: 24% of epileptics are under 18 years of age; 53% are 18 to 44 years; 18% are 45 to 64 years; 4% are 65 to 74 years; 1% is 75 years and older.

Male to Female Ratio: About equal.

Principal Features: True epilepsy is a chronic disorder characterized by recurring seizures lasting from a few seconds to several minutes and requiring specific medication for prevention and control. Sixty-six percent of epileptic patients require lifelong drug therapy. The principal types of epilepsy include:

Tonic-Clonic Seizures (Grand Mal): Sudden attacks that begin with an involuntary cry, followed by a loss of consciousness and falling, violent convulsive movements of the head, trunk and extremities, excessive salivation and sometimes loss of bladder and/or rectal control. The seizure lasts from 1 to 3 minutes. The individual awakens spontaneously, is dazed, confused and exhausted, and usually falls into a deep sleep that lasts several hours. The subject cannot remember the episode.

Absence Seizures (Petit Mal): These begin between 2 and 12 years of age; 90% cease by 20 years; 50% go on to develop tonic-clonic seizures by 20 years. The seizure consists of a sudden, momentary lapse of consciousness lasting several seconds (30 at the most), during which the subject has a blank stare and is oblivious of surroundings; there is no actual loss of consciousness, no fall and no convulsion; there may be a minor twitching of an eyelid or facial muscle, chewing movements or a jerk of a hand or arm. Such episodes may recur more than 100 times a day. Following each seizure, the subject resumes normal functioning as though nothing had happened; the attack is not remembered.

Complex Partial Seizures (Psychomotor or Temporal Lobe Epilepsy): This type comprises 40% of all epilepsies. It consists of sudden alterations of behavior that involve speech, hearing, memory and emotional response. Some episodes begin with an "aura" that may take the form of distorted vision, unpleasant odors, visual and auditory hallucinations and bizarre illusions; the subject may walk about aimlessly, talk irrationally, laugh, engage in purposeless and inappropriate actions, such as striking at walls in anger or fear. When the seizure ends, the subject is confused and does not recall what has happened.

Causes: The actual epileptic seizure is due to a sudden, abnormal and excessive electrical discharge within the brain. Normal electrical impulses of 80/second are suddenly increased to 500/second. In primary epilepsy the basic cause is unknown; there is usually a familial (genetic) predisposition. Secondary epilepsy can be a complication following head injuries, bacterial meningitis and malaria; it is often associated with cerebral palsy, mental retardation, brain tumors and cysts and hydrocephalus.

Drugs That Can Cause This Disorder: The following drugs have been reported to cause seizures or to aggravate existing epileptic disorders:

amphetamines
antihistamines
chloroquine
cimetidine (with large doses in
   the elderly)
cycloserine
isoniazid
metronidazole

monoamine oxidase inhibitors
   (MAOI's)
nalidixic acid
oral contraceptives
phenothiazines
tricyclic antidepressants
vincristine

Drugs Used to Treat This Disorder (in order of preference):

Generalized Tonic-Clonic Seizures (Grand Mal)
- phenytoin (Dilantin).
- phenobarbital (Luminal).
- carbamazepine (Tegretol).
- primidone (Mysoline).

Absence Seizures (Petit Mal)
- ethosuximide (Zarontin).
- valproic acid (Depakene).
- trimethadione (Tridione).
- clonazepam (Clonopin).

Complex Partial Seizures (Psychomotor, Temporal Lobe)
- carbamazepine (Tegretol).
- phenytoin (Dilantin).
- primidone (Mysoline).
- clonazepam (Clonopin).
- valproic acid (Depakene).

Goals of Drug Treatment

Complete prevention of seizures if possible (or marked reduction in frequency), with no (or minimal) adverse drug effects.

Restoration of ability to function independently.

Promotion of participation in school, employment and societal activities.

Drug Management

General Principles

Each individual who is subject to epilepsy experiences a pattern of seizures that is unique; the onset, frequency, severity and specific type (or types) of seizures are never exactly the same as those experienced by someone else.

The drugs used to control epilepsy are selected according to the specific type(s) of seizures the patient experiences.

Antiepileptic drugs are not curative; they are used to control seizures—to reduce their frequency and severity. Seizures should be prevented whenever possible; repeated, uncontrolled convulsions can cause significant brain damage.

When the drug of choice is used in adequate dosage to manage a correctly diagnosed type of epilepsy, seizures can be controlled completely in 60% of patients and substantially reduced in another 20%.

In every case a period of trial and error is necessary to find the most effective drug, the optimal dose and the correct timing of use.

Complete control of seizures with one drug is the ideal; this is possible in 85% of cases. If one drug does not give adequate control, a second drug may be added. The first drug may be continued or gradually withdrawn, depending upon individual response.

Dosage schedules are adjusted gradually to achieve the maximum of seizure control with the minimum of drug side-effects.

Because of the wide variation in drug absorption and elimination from person to person, the periodic measurement of drug levels in blood is necessary to determine the optimal dosage for each drug. An attempt is made to establish for each individual that drug level which will ensure freedom from seizures without toxic drug effects. Blood samples for measurement are usually taken just before the morning dose. (See Therapeutic Drug Monitoring in Section One.)

All antiepileptic drugs have toxic effects when taken in large doses; dosage adjustments are often necessary to prevent toxicity. However, the controllable risks of proper use do not justify withholding treatment in view of the much greater risks resulting from uncontrolled repeated seizures.

Birth defects are two to three times higher in children whose parents (father or mother) are using antiepileptic drugs, especially phenytoin, trimethadione and valproic acid. Consult your physician regarding the best course of action for you in managing your epilepsy during pregnancy.

Do not discontinue any antiepileptic drug suddenly unless advised to do so by your physician. Normally the dosage should be reduced gradually over a period of several weeks. Abrupt withdrawal can cause status epilepticus—a prolonged period of continual seizures without interruption.

Any consideration of discontinuing antiepileptic medications permanently should be made jointly with your physician. Such consideration can be made for absence seizures (petit mal) after a period of 2 to 3 years without a seizure. For other types of epilepsy, a period of 3 to 5 years is advisable. Seizures tend to return in 20% to 50% of cases after stopping medication. Any attempt to withdraw medication must be done very gradually over a period of several months.

Use of Phenytoin
1. Used to control all types of epilepsy except absence seizures.
2. A drug blood level within the therapeutic range correlates well with a decrease in seizure frequency and relative freedom from toxic effects.
3. Due to variation of absorbability among available products, it is advisable to stay with the same brand to gain and maintain control.
4. When the daily maintenance requirement has been established, it may be taken in a single dose.

5. Possible adverse effects include a measleslike rash within the first 2 weeks, excessive growth of hair (5%) and enlargement of the gums (30%).
6. Indications of early toxicity include rapid involuntary eye movements (nystagmus), dizziness, unsteadiness, lethargy and slurred speech.
7. If another drug is added for concurrent use, any significant interaction will occur within 6 weeks.

Use of Phenobarbital
1. Used to control all types of epilepsy except absence seizures.
2. Use with caution if liver or kidney function is impaired.
3. Should be taken twice a day with the largest dose at bedtime.
4. More sedative than phenytoin and carbamazepine, but relatively free of long-term adverse effects.
5. Indications of early toxicity include drowsiness, unsteadiness and impaired thinking.

Use of Primidone
1. Closely related to phenobarbital. Used to control all types of epilepsy except absence seizures.
2. Must be taken in divided doses because of its sedative effect.
3. Indications of early toxicity are the same of those for phenobarbital.

Use of Ethosuximide
1. Used to control absence seizures and some myoclonic seizures. About 75% effective in reducing the frequency of absence seizures when used in adequate dosage.
2. Indications of early toxicity include headache, drowsiness and dizziness.

Use of Valproic Acid
1. Used primarily to control both simple and complex absence seizures. Also used adjunctively to control all other types of epilepsy. It may control both absence and tonic-clonic seizures in the same individual.
2. Multiple doses are necessary to maintain 24-hour control.
3. Avoid use in presence of liver disease.
4. A possible side-effect is weight gain.
5. Monitor for indications of liver toxicity.
6. If used concurrently with other antiepileptic drugs, the periodic measurement of blood levels of all drugs being used is necessary to ensure adequate dosage and prevent toxicity.

Use of Carbamazepine
1. Used to control both tonic-clonic seizures and partial complex seizures (psychomotor epilepsy).
2. Should be taken with food to improve absorption.
3. Avoid use in presence of liver disease or impaired function.
4. Indications of early toxicity include double vision, blurred vision, dizziness, unsteadiness and tremor.
5. Routine, periodic, complete blood counts are mandatory to detect early bone marrow toxicity.

Ancillary Drug Treatment (as required)

Condition	*Drug Treatment*
For increased seizures before or after menstruation:	acetazolamide (Diamox)
For anxiety:	benzodiazepines (Tranxene, Valium, etc.)
For depression:	see Profile of Depression in this section

Note: Drug selection, dosage and administration schedule must be determined by the physician for each patient individually.

Resources for Additional Information and Services

American Epilepsy Society
179 Allyn Street, #304
Hartford, CT 06103
Phone: (203) 246-6566
Publications available.

Epilepsy Concern Service Group
1282 Wynnewood Drive
West Palm Beach, FL 33417
Phone: (407) 683-0044
Promotes formation of self-help groups.
Publications and telephone referrals available.

Epilepsy Foundation of America
4351 Garden City Drive
Landover, MD 20785
Phone: 1-800-EFA-1000 (outside MD); (301) 459-3700
Provides a low-cost pharmacy program for members.
Publications and audiovisual materials available.

GLAUCOMA

Other Names: Primary glaucoma, secondary glaucoma

Prevalence in USA: 1.7 million known, an estimated 1 million undiagnosed; 2% of the population over 40 years of age.

Age Group: Under 18 years—13,000; 18 to 44 years—124,000; 45 to 64 years—513,000; 65 to 74 years—534,000; 75 years and over—527,000.

Male to Female Ratio: Under 45 years—same incidence in men and women; 45 to 64 years—more common in men; 65 years and over—more common in women.

Principal Features: A chronic disorder characterized by abnormally high internal eye pressure that destroys the optic nerve and causes partial to complete loss of vision. Principal types include

Chronic Open-Angle (Simple, Wide-Angle) Glaucoma: The most common type, a primary glaucoma that is rare in children and young adults; usually begins after 30. The rise in intraocular pressure is gradual; the loss of vision is insidious and slowly progressive. Usually both eyes are affected. Characteristic symptoms include blurring of vision, frequent need for change of glasses, occasional headache, colored halos seen around electric lights and impaired visual adaptation to the dark.

Acute/Chronic Angle-Closure (Narrow-Angle, Closed-Angle) Glaucoma: A primary glaucoma that usually occurs after. 60. The acute glaucoma attack begins in one eye; the rise in intraocular pressure is sudden and dramatic. Within a few hours the patient experiences severe headache, throbbing eye pain, blurred vision, halos around lights, tearing, swollen eyelids, nausea and vomiting. Initially the episode may be misdiagnosed as an acute abdominal disorder, such as gallbladder disease. Attacks of lesser severity can recur in chronic fashion.

Secondary Glaucoma: The rise in intraocular pressure is a consequence of a preexistent condition, such as infection (uveitis), eye tumor, enlarged cataract or long-term treatment with cortisonelike drugs. Headache, halos and blurred vision occur in proportion to the degree and duration of increased pressure.

Causes: Increased intraocular pressure is due to an imbalance between production and drainage of the liquid (aqueous humor) in the front portion of the eye; obstruction to normal drainage is the main mechanism. The primary types of glaucoma occur in individuals with hereditary predisposition, but specific initiating causes responsible for the rise in pressure are not known. Secondary types of glaucoma are associated with other eye disorders: uveitis, tumors, cataracts, hemorrhage, injury. "Steroid responders" develop increased pressure after 1 to 8 weeks of using cortisonelike steroids.

Drugs That Can Cause This Disorder: The following drugs do not cause true, permanent glaucoma, but they can increase intraocular pressure and thereby precipitate an attack of acute angle-closure glaucoma or aggravate chronic open-angle glaucoma:

amyl nitrite
atropine and atropinelike drugs
cortisonelike drugs
epinephrine
isosorbide dinitrate

nitroglycerin
phenylephrine
tolazoline
tricyclic antidepressants

Drugs Used to Treat This Disorder:
Eye Drops/Inserts (for Local Effects)
- betaxolol (Betoptic).
- carbachol (Carbacel, Isopto Carbachol).

- demecarium (Humorsol).
- dipivefrin (DPE, Propine).
- echothiopate (Phospholine).
- epinephrine (Epifrin, Epitrate, Glaucon, Lyophrin).
- phenylephrine (Neo-Synephrine, Ocusol).
- pilocarpine solution (Almocarpine, Isoptocarpine, etc.).
- pilocarpine inserts (Ocuserts Pilo-20, Pilo-40).
- timolol (Timoptic).

Internal Medications (for Systemic Effects)
- acetazolamide (Diamox).
- glycerine (Glyrol, Osmoglyn).

Goals of Drug Treatment

Prompt reduction of intraocular pressure in acute angle-closure glaucoma; stabilization of eye status in preparation for corrective eye surgery.

Gradual reduction and long-term normalization of intraocular pressure in chronic, simple, open-angle glaucoma.

Prevention of optic nerve damage; preservation of vision.

Drug Management

General Principles

Drug treatment cannot cure but can control glaucoma.

Factors that can increase intraocular pressure and reduce the effectiveness of drugs include emotional stress (anger, fear, worry); heavy physical exertion; straining with defecation; tight collars, belts and girdles; upper respiratory infections.

Periodic measurement of intraocular pressure is most advisable during long-term use of cortisonelike steroid drugs, especially eye drops and ointments.

Soft contact lens can act as a drug reservoir for pilocarpine (when administered in eye-drop solutions).

Some individuals cannot use pilocarpine Ocuserts successfully; some cannot retain them in the eye, and the loss may be unnoticed; some cannot tolerate the foreign-body sensation.

Pilocarpine is the pupil-constricting (miotic) drug of choice for use in the elderly. The stinging sensation felt on initial use usually disappears with continued application. Some blurring of distant vision is unavoidable.

Timolol (a beta blocker) is as effective as pilocarpine in treating open-angle and secondary glaucoma; twice daily dosage (every 12 hours) is usually sufficient; it should be used very cautiously in those with asthma, slow heart rates or borderline congestive heart failure.

Epinephrine may be used concurrently with pilocarpine (or other miotic drugs) for greater effectiveness in reducing intraocular pressure; it is important that the pilocarpine be used first and be allowed to act for 5 minutes before using epinephrine. Avoid use in presence of high blood pressure (hypertension). Do not use discolored solutions of epinephrine.

Acetazolamide is usually reserved for glaucoma that is unresponsive to eye drops alone. Effectiveness is improved when both are used concurrently.

For Chronic Open-Angle Glaucoma
Eye drops: pilocarpine, timolol, carbachol, epinephrine, dipivefrin, demecarium.
Internal medications: acetazolamide.
Most cases are controlled by eye drops alone.
Treatment is started with the weakest strength; the most effective strength and dosage schedule are determined by trial and error.
Acetazolamide is not used routinely; it is added after an adequate trial of eye drops fails to maintain normal intraocular pressure.

For Acute Angle-Closure Glaucoma (Acute Attack)
Eye drops: pilocarpine, timolol.
Internal medications: glycerine and water mixture, acetazolamide.
The initial treatment is designed to lower intraocular pressure as rapidly as possible to prevent irreversible damage to the optic nerve. Eye drops and internal medications are used concurrently. The combination can reduce the pressure rapidly and abort the acute attack.
The ultimate treatment for this condition is surgical.

For Chronic, Recurrent Episodes of Subacute Angle-Closure Glaucoma
Eye drops: pilocarpine and timolol concurrently.
Internal medications: glycerine and water; acetazolamide is used only during the acute phase, not long-term.
The ultimate treatment is surgical.

For Secondary Glaucoma
Eye drops: atropine, cortisonelike steroids.
Internal medications: cortisonelike steroids, acetazolamide.
When appropriate, corrective treatment is directed at the primary eye disorder that is causing increased intraocular pressure.

For Cortisone-Induced Glaucoma
Discontinue all cortisonelike steroids if possible.
Eye drops: pilocarpine, timolol, demecarium.
Internal medications: acetazolamide.

Ancillary Drug Treatment (as required)

Condition	*Drug Treatment*
For itching, burning, redness of eyes:	naphazoline (Naphcon, Privine, Vasoclear) tetrahydralazine (Visine)

Note: Drug selection, dosage and administration schedule must be determined by the physician for each patient individually.

Resources for Additional Information and Services

Foundation for Glaucoma Research
490 Post Street, Suite 830

San Francisco, CA 94102
Phone: (415) 986-3162; 1-800-245-3005
Publications available.

National Society to Prevent Blindness
National Center for Sight
500 East Remington Road
Schaumburg, IL 60173
Phone: 1-800-221-3004; (312) 843-2020
Answers questions about vision problems.
Provides publications and films on specific problems and conditions.

GOUT

Other Names: Gouty arthritis, podagra (gouty arthritis of the big toe), hyperuricemia (abnormally high blood uric acid)

Prevalence in USA: Approximately 2.3 million, 2.8% of males in middle age. Hyperuricemia occurs in 5% to 10% of the population; 1% to 2% will have gout manifestations during a lifetime.

Age Group: Under 18 years—12,000; 18 to 44 years—316,000; 45 to 64 years—1.01 million; 65 to 74 years—494,000; 75 years and over—396,000.

Male to Female Ratio: Approximately 95% in men, 5% in women.

Principal Features: Gout consists of a group of related disorders having a single underlying feature—abnormally high blood levels of uric acid; this is referred to as hyperuricemia and implies a blood level of more than 7.0 mg of uric acid per 100 ml of blood. (The normal ranges generally recognized are 2.5 to 8.0 mg for men and 1.5 to 7.0 mg for women.) During the early years of primary (genetic) gout, hyperuricemia may exist without any symptoms to indicate its presence. During a lifetime, a small minority of these individuals will experience recurrent acute attacks of severe joint pain with tender swelling (usually one joint in an upper or lower limb), episodes of kidney stones, serious impairment of kidney function or the development of tophi—localized deposits of uric acid salts in the skin, on earlobes, on tendons and bones in and around joints (tophaceous gout).

Causes: Primary gout is due to an inherited defect in the metabolism of purines—end products of protein digestion. In approximately 10% of cases the defect results in an overproduction of uric acid; in 90% the defect is responsible for decreased excretion of uric acid by the kidneys. Either defect causes hyperuricemia. When tissue fluids cannot dissolve excessive levels of uric acid (due to saturation), uric acid crystals are deposited in joints (acute arthritis), kidneys (kidney damage and stone formation) and in soft tissue (tophi).

Drugs That Can Cause This Disorder: The following drugs can raise the blood level of uric acid and precipitate acute gouty arthritis in susceptible individuals:

acetazolamide	furosemide
alcohol	levodopa
antineoplastic drugs	nicotinic acid
aspirin (less than 2 grams/day)	pyrazinamide
ethacrynic acid	thiazide diuretics
ethambutol	triamterene

Drugs Used to Treat This Disorder:
For Reducing Blood and Tissue Levels of Uric Acid
- allopurinol (Lopurin, Zyloprim).
- probenecid (Benemid).
- sulfinpyrazone (Anturane).

For Treating and Preventing Acute Attacks of Arthritis
- colchicine.
- fenoprofen (Nalfon).
- ibuprofen (Advil, Motrin, Nuprin, Rufen).
- indomethacin (Indocin).
- naproxen (Naprosyn).
- oxyphenbutazone (Oxalid).
- phenylbutazone (Azolid, Butazolidin).
- piroxicam (Feldene).
- prednisone (Deltasone, Meticorten, Orasone, etc.).
- sulindac (Clinoril).
- tolmetin (Tolectin).

Goals of Drug Treatment
Prompt relief of symptoms of acute attack of gouty arthritis.
Maintenance of blood uric acid level below 6 mg/100 ml. (Prevention of recurrent attacks of acute arthritis, kidney stone formation, kidney damage and tophi formation.)
Dissolution of existing tophi.

Drug Management
General Principles
Only 20% of individuals with hyperuricemia will develop manifestations of gout during their lifetime. At present there is no way of identifying those who will.
Gouty arthritis is the most responsive to treatment and the most easily controlled of all types of arthritis.
The patient and physician together should determine by trial and error which drug is most effective and acceptable for treating acute attacks of gouty arthritis.

After the acute attack of arthritis has subsided, minor symptoms may persist for 2 to 3 months. If maintenance treatment with antigout drugs is started, it is advisable to use low-dose colchicine concurrently to prevent recurrent flare-ups.

Measurement of the amount of uric acid in a 24-hour collection of urine can identify the overproducer of uric acid (greater than 800 mg) and the underexcretor (less than 800 mg). The overproducer is best treated with allopurinol; the underexcretor is best treated with probenecid or sulfinpyrazone.

Authorities differ on whether and when to initiate long-term treatment for hyperuricemia. Conservative opinion: initiate drug therapy only after 2 or more episodes of gouty arthritis or kidney stone within a year. Many first attacks are not followed by recurrent episodes. Withholding long-term treatment avoids the risks of adverse drug reactions. Aggressive opinion: initiate drug therapy after the first episode of gouty arthritis or kidney stone to prevent recurrent attacks and reduce the risks of kidney damage and tophi formation. Hyperuricemia is often present for 20 years or more before the first attack; bone, cartilage and kidney damage may already have occured. The risks of untreated hyperuricemia are thought to exceed the risks of long-term drug therapy. The prudent physician will consider the pros and cons of each case individually and make the decision jointly with the patient.

Once long-term treatment is started with allopurinol and/or probenecid or sulfinpyrazone, it should be maintained for life. Start-stop treatment has no lasting benefit and may precipitate acute attacks. Low-dose colchicine should be taken preventively until the uric acid blood level is stabilized below 6.0 mg/100ml and there have been no acute attacks for 6 to 12 months.

Acute attacks of gouty arthritis can be precipitated by injury, surgery, systemic infections and severe medical illnesses. Colchicine may be used preventively to minimize acute episodes of arthritis when such events occur.

Patients with kidney stones should use allopurinol to treat hyperuricemia; probenecid and sulfinpyrazone should be avoided because they increase the uric acid content of urine.

Do not take aspirin (or other salicylates) in doses of less than 2 grams while taking probenecid or sulfinpyrazone. It abolishes the effectiveness of these drugs and raises the blood level of uric acid.

Avoid fasting to lose weight; fasting can raise the blood level of uric acid. Treat obesity by long-term reduction of food intake and gradual loss of weight.

While taking antigout drugs on a regular basis, drink 2 to 3 quarts of liquids daily to ensure a copious flow of dilute urine.

Use of Allopurinol
1. Used to lower the blood level of uric acid by reducing its formation. Of no value in treating the acute attack, and should not be started until all symptoms of acute arthritis have subsided.
2. The drug of choice for individuals who

- are overproducers of uric acid (more than 800 mg/24-hour urine excretion).
- are over 60 years of age.
- have impaired kidney function.
- are subject to kidney stones.
- have tophi formations.
- are allergic or overly sensitive to probenecid or sulfinpyrazone.

3. The total daily requirement may be taken in a single dose.
4. Once started, a commitment should be made to a lifetime of continual use.
5. May be combined with all other antigout drugs as appropriate for increased effectiveness.
6. Recommended for use prior to and during chemotherapy or irradiation therapy for selected cancers to counteract resulting hyperuricemia.
7. Serious toxicity is extremely rare.

Use of Colchicine
1. Used to treat acute attacks of gouty arthritis. It does not lower the blood level of uric acid.
2. For the quickest response and best results, treatment should be started as soon as possible after the onset of symptoms. If started within the first 12 hours, colchicine gives effective relief of acute arthritis in 90% of cases.
3. The long-term use of low-dose colchicine is very effective in preventing recurrent acute attacks of gouty arthritis.
4. Its use is recommended during the early months of maintenance therapy with allopurinol and/or probenecid or sulfinpyrazone to prevent flare-ups of acute arthritis.
5. Use with caution and reduce the dose in the presence of liver disease or impaired liver function.
6. Colchicine is destroyed by exposure to light. Be sure your supply is fresh and fully effective.

Use of Indomethacin (and Other Nonsteroidal Anti-inflammatory Drugs)
1. Now considered by many authorities to be the drug(s) of choice for treating acute attacks of gouty arthritis. They relieve pain and inflammation, but do not lower the blood level of uric acid.
2. When given promptly and in adequate dosage, these drugs usually provide relief within 6 to 12 hours and complete recovery in 3 days.
3. Take with food to prevent stomach irritation and indigestion.
4. Avoid in the presence of active peptic ulcer disease. Use with caution in hypertension and congestive heart failure.

Use of Phenylbutazone or Oxyphenbutazone
1. Used to provide prompt relief of acute gouty arthritis. It reduces pain and inflammation effectively, but does not lower the blood level of uric acid.
2. Because of its rare but very serious potential for causing bone marrow depression, this drug should never be used for long-term treatment. Treatment courses of no more than 5 to 7 days are advised.
3. This drug should not be used by the elderly (over 60 years of age).

Use of Prednisone (or Similar Cortisonelike Steroids)
1. Used to abort acute attacks of gouty arthritis. Relieves inflammation, swelling and pain, but does not lower the blood level of uric acid.
2. Should be used only after adequate trials of all other appropriate drugs have failed to relieve the acute attack.
3. "Rebound" attacks are common following withdrawal of steroid medications.
4. Not recommended for frequently repeated or long-term use.

Use of Probenecid or Sulfinpyrazone
1. Used to lower the blood level of uric acid by increasing its excretion in the urine. Of no value in treating the acute attack, and should not be started until acute arthritis has subsided.
2. Best suited for individuals who
   • are underexcretors of uric acid (less than 800 mg/24-hour urine excretion).
   • are under 60 years of age.
   • have good kidney function.
   • have no history of kidney stones.
3. Should not be used by those who
   • are overproducers of uric acid (more than 800 mg/24-hour urine excretion).
   • have impaired kidney function and low urine volume.
   • are subject to kidney stones.
4. Begin treatment with small doses to avoid precipitating an acute attack of arthritis.
5. Must be taken in 2 to 4 doses/day.
6. If the tolerance of either drug is limited, the two drugs can be taken concurrently in reduced dosage.
7. Ensure a high intake of liquids (up to 3 quarts daily). Effectiveness is improved by the concurrent use of sodium bicarbonate or potassium citrate.

Ancillary Drug Treatment (as required)

Condition	Drug Treatment
For mild pain:	acetaminophen (Tylenol, etc.). Do not use aspirin or other salicylates.
For severe pain:	codeine or meperidine (Demerol)
For diarrhea due to colchicine:	paregoric or loperimide (Imodium)
For high blood pressure:	see Profile of Hypertension in this section
For "secondary" gout due to chemotherapy for leukemia, lymphoma, multiple myeloma, polycythemia:	allopurinol (Zyloprim)

Note: Drug selection, dosage and administration schedule must be determined by the physician for each patient individually.

Resource for Additional Information and Services

Arthritis Foundation
1314 Spring Street, N.W.
Atlanta, GA 30309
Phone: (404) 872-7100

Local groups: 71.
Publications available.

HYPERTENSION

Other Names: Arterial hypertension, essential hypertension, primary hypertension, secondary hypertension high blood pressure

Prevalence in USA: 26.5 million—15% of adult white population; 25% of adult black population.

Age Group: Under 18 years—184,000; 18 to 44 years—5.6 million; 45 to 64 years—10.8 million; 65 to 74 years—6 million; 75 years and over—3.8 million.

Male to Female Ratio: Under 45 years—same incidence in men and women; 45 to 64 years—slightly more common in women; 65 years and over—more common in women (2 to 1).

Principal Features: During the early years of high blood pressure there are usually no symptoms. Brief periods of sudden elevation of blood pressure above usual levels may cause throbbing headaches and/or dizziness. After years of untreated high blood pressure, manifestations of "target organ" disease include stroke (blood clot or hemorrhage in the brain), impaired vision (retinal hemorrhage and deterioration), heart attack (myocardial infarction), congestive heart failure and kidney failure (uremia).

Causes: In primary (essential) hypertension (95% of all hypertension), no specific cause is apparent. There is a definite hereditary predisposition; 80% of hypertensive individuals have a close relative with high blood pressure. In those who are genetically susceptible, obesity and high salt intake contribute significantly to the development of hypertension. Secondary hypertension (5% of all hypertension) is due to a demonstrable (and sometimes curable) cause: narrowing of the main artery to one or both kidneys, chronic kidney disease, adrenalin or renin producing tumors, coarctation of the aorta.

Drugs That Can Cause This Disorder: The following drugs (or drug combinations) can cause significant elevations of blood pressure:

amphetamines and related drugs
carbenoxolone
ephedrine
ergot preparations
licorice
oral contraceptives
phenylephrine

phenylpropanolamine
pseudoephedrine
tricyclic antidepressants taken
concurrently with appetite
suppressants, decongestants or
antihistamines

Drugs Used to Treat This Disorder:
Diuretics
- thiazides (see Drug Class, Section Four).
- chlorthalidone (Hygroton).
- quinethazone (Hydromox).
- metolazone (Diulo, Zaroxolyn).
- indapamide (Lozol).
- bumetanide (Bumex).
- furosemide (Lasix).
- *potassium-saving diuretics:* amiloride (Midamor); spironolactone (Aldactone); triamterene (Dyrenium).

Drugs Acting on the Sympathetic Nervous System
Beta-Adrenergic-Blocking Drugs
- acebutolol (Sectral).
- atenolol (Tenormin).
- betaxolol (Kerlone).
- labetalol (Normodyne, Trandate).
- metoprolol (Lopressor).
- nadolol (Corgard).
- penbutolol (Levatol).
- pindolol (Visken).
- propranolol (Inderal).
- timolol (Blocadren).

Alpha-Adrenergic-Blocking Drugs
- doxazosin (Cardura).
- prazosin (Minipres).
- terazosin (Hytrin).

Centrally Acting Drugs (in the Brain)
- clonidine (Catapres).
- guanabenz (Wytensin).
- guanfacine (Tenex).
- methyldopa (Aldomet).

Peripherally Acting Drugs (in Peripheral Blood Vessels)
- guanadrel (Hylorel).
- guanethidine (Ismelin).
- reserpine (Serpasil).

Direct Vasodilators
- hydralazine (Apresoline).
- minoxidil (Loniten).

Calcium Channel-Blocking Drugs
- diltiazem (Cardizem).

- isradipine (DynaCirc).
- nicardipine (Cardene).
- nifedipine (Procardia).
- verapamil (Calan, Isoptin).

Angiotensin Converting Enzyme (ACE) Inhibitors
- captopril (Capoten).
- enalapril (Vasotec).
- lisinopril (Prinivil, Zestril).
- ramipril (Altace).

Goals of Drug Treatment

Maintenance of blood pressure below 140/90, or as close as possible to this level with an acceptable program of drug therapy (minimal drug side-effects and expense).

Prevention or postponement of "target organ" disease in the brain, retina (eye), heart, major blood vessels and kidneys.

Drug Management

General Principles

Although hypertension is difficult to define precisely, blood pressure is considered to be abnormally high if the systolic level is 140 or above or the diastolic level is 90 or above.

Hypertension may be classified as follows:
Diastolic pressure less than 85—normal
Diastolic pressure of 85 to 89—high normal
Diastolic pressure of 90 to 104—mild hypertension
Diastolic pressure of 105 to 114—moderate hypertension
Diastolic pressure of 115 or above—severe hypertension
Systolic pressure less than 140—normal
Systolic pressure of 140 to 159—borderline systolic hypertension
Systolic pressure of 160 or above—systolic hypertension

Most men who develop primary hypertension will have a diastolic pressure of 90 or above by age 35, most women by age 40 to 45.

An adequate program of drug therapy for hypertension will postpone serious disability and death for most hypertensive individuals.

The selection of antihypertensive drugs for initial treatment is based upon the range of the abnormally high pressures recorded on repeated measurements *and* the status of the "target organs" (brain, heart, kidneys and blood vessels) at the time hypertension is discovered.

One practical and effective approach to drug therapy for hypertension initiates treatment with a single drug and adds stronger drugs in stepwise fashion as needed to control blood pressure:

Step 1 begin treatment with   either a diuretic or a beta blocker drug.

Step 2 if necessary, add   clonidine, methyldopa or prazosin (or a diuretic or a beta blocker if not used in Step 1)

Step 3 if necessary, add	hydralazine, a calcium channel blocker or an ACE inhibitor
Step 4 if necessary, add	guanethidine or minoxidil

For most individuals, the initial drug treatment will normalize blood pressure within the first 2 months. Up to 60% of cases are controlled with a diuretic alone; 50% can be controlled with a beta blocker alone. From 70% to 80% of all hypertensive individuals will achieve satisfactory blood pressure control by compliance with Step 1 or Step 2 drug therapy. The majority of the remainder can be controlled by Steps 3 and 4.

Tranquilizers and sedatives are not effective for lowering elevated blood pressure and should not be relied upon as primary treatment for hypertension.

Obtain a blood pressure measuring instrument (preferably an aneroid manometer, arm cuff and stethoscope) and ask your physician to teach you how to take your own blood pressure. Measurements of blood pressure made at home (or at work) are far more representative of your actual day-by-day pressures than are readings made in the physician's office. By taking your own blood pressure at home, at work and at varying times and under different circumstances, you can create a record that clearly reflects your response to the antihypertensive drugs prescribed for you.

Read the Drug Profiles (Section Three) of the drugs you are taking. If you think you may be experiencing any of the side-effects or adverse effects listed in the Profile, discuss this with your physician so appropriate adjustments can be made. It is to your benefit to work along with your physician until a satisfactory selection of drugs is reached.

Avoid isometric exercises—body building, weight lifting, push-ups; these raise the blood pressure significantly. Consult your physician regarding the advisability of isotonic exercises—walking, bicycling, swimming.

Consumption of more than 2 ounces of alcohol daily can raise the blood pressure. One ounce of alcohol is present in 2 ounces of 100-proof whiskey, in 8 ounces of wine, or in 24 ounces of beer.

Five percent of oral contraceptive users will develop a diastolic blood pressure of over 90. If this occurs, the contraceptive pill should be discontinued for 6 months and the blood pressure monitored. Women with this sensitivity should use an alternative method of contraception.

The elderly individual with hypertension must approach antihypertensive drug therapy very cautiously. Goals of drug treatment are more liberal; reduction of pressures to 140–160/95–100 are usually adequate. This can usually be achieved with small doses of a diuretic. If a Step 2 drug is needed, methyldopa is better tolerated than the other choices. However, the response to all drugs must be observed closely. Drugs that cause emotional depression in the young individual can cause symptoms in the elderly that closely resemble senile dementia.

In type I diabetes, thiazides are well tolerated, but beta blockers may mask the symptoms of hypoglycemia. In type II diabetes, thiazides are best avoided; small doses of furosemide or spironolactone are preferable. Beta blockers can impair insulin release.

After blood pressure has been well controlled for a year, consideration may be given to a "step-down" reduction of both drug dosage and the number of drugs used. The blood pressure response to the gradual withdrawal of drugs must be monitored very carefully. A recent study showed that 28% of the group of hypertensives studied had normal blood pressure one year after discontinuing all antihypertensive medication. Your physician can determine if and when you meet the criteria for attempting to discontinue your program of drug treatment.

Treatment of Hypertension According to Severity
For Borderline Hypertension (120–160/90–94)
- Reduce excessive weight.
- Reduce salt intake moderately.
- Reduce stress in daily living.
- Avoid excessive consumption of alcohol.
- Stop smoking.
- Avoid isometric exercise.
- Increase isotonic exercise.
- Defer drug treatment for 3 to 6 months to determine effectiveness of above measures.

For Mild Hypertension (140–160/95–104) (80% of All Hypertensives)
- Urge all of the above measures.
- Begin Step 1 drug treatment: Use a single drug—currently a thiazide diuretic or a beta blocker. Some authorities are now advocating a trial of a calcium channel blocker or an ACE inhibitor for initiating treatment.

For Moderate Hypertension (140–180/105–114)
- Begin with Step 2 drug treatment; it is not likely that a single drug will control this degree of hypertension.
- A diuretic will enhance the effectiveness of a beta blocker, a calcium channel blocker, or a centrally acting drug.

For Severe Hypertension (160+/115+)
- Adequate control may require Step 3 or Step 4 drug treatment. When multiple drugs are used, smaller doses of individual drugs are often effective and better tolerated. A trial-and-error approach is often necessary to determine the most effective and acceptable combination of drugs.

For Isolated Systolic Hypertension (160+/85–90)
- This is usually found in the elderly. Cautious and conservative drug treatment is recommended for those under age 70.
- Calcium channel-blocking drugs may be very effective for this type of hypertension.
- If a diuretic is used, avoid dehydration and potassium loss.
- If methyldopa is used, monitor for any tendency to depression or dementia.

Use of Diuretics
1. Used as Step 1 or Step 2 drugs, diuretics are most appropriate for treating hypertensives who are black or elderly, those with congestive heart failure or kidney failure and those who cannot use a beta blocker drug.
2. A thiazide diuretic is the initial drug tried in the majority of cases. It is effective in a single dose taken in the morning.
3. While using thiazide diuretics, observe for loss of potassium (10% of users), increased blood level of uric acid (66% of users) and increased blood-sugar level.
4. Spironolactone and triamterene are as effective as thiazides in reducing blood pressure; they are used to prevent potassium loss.
5. The more potent diuretics furosemide and ethacrynic acid are no more effective than the thiazides for reducing blood pressure.
6. The most practical and reliable way to prevent a significant decline in the potassium blood level is to use a potassium-saving diuretic—amiloride, spironolactone or triamterene. The use of high-potassium foods is often unreliable. Compliance with the long-term use of oral potassium supplements is very poor.
7. It is advisable to discontinue the use of diuretics gradually to prevent fluid retention (edema) after withdrawal.

Use of Beta-Adrenergic-Blocking Drugs
1. Used as Step 1 or Step 2 drugs, beta blockers are most appropriate for treating hypertensives who are young, those who have an overactive heart (fast rate, palpitation, premature beats) and those with gout, migraine headaches and angina (coronary artery disease).
2. Avoid beta blockers if you have asthma, emphysema or a history of heart block or congestive heart failure.
3. These drugs characteristically cause fatigue and lethargy. Propranolol and metoprolol can cause emotional depression.
4. When propranolol is used alone, 10% of users can experience an increase in blood pressure. It is advisable to use a diuretic prior to starting propranolol in sensitive individuals.
5. Avoid sudden discontinuation of beta blockers, especially in the presence of coronary artery disease. Abrupt withdrawal can cause rapid heart rate, palpitation and intensification of angina; myocardial infarction has been reported.

Use of Labetalol (an Alpha- and Beta-Adrenergic Blocker)
1. This drug may be effective when the beta blockers have failed to control blood pressure.
2. Functions primarily as a vasodilator in the elderly, with no significant alteration of heart function.
3. Avoid in presence of asthma, emphysema, heart block and congestive heart failure.

Use of Clonidine
1. Characteristically causes drowsiness, fatigue and dry mouth. Is capable of causing depression.

2. Do not discontinue this drug abruptly; sudden withdrawal can cause a severe rebound hypertension with higher blood pressure than prior to treatment. Withdraw over 2 to 4 days.
3. After discontinuation of clonidine, delay the start of a beta blocker drug for 48 hours.

Use of Methyldopa

1. Usually causes lethargy and fatigue at beginning of treatment; these often subside with continued use. Is also capable of causing depression.
2. This drug causes salt and water retention; a diuretic should be taken concurrently.
3. Discontinue this drug if any of the following develop: emotional depression, drug fever, breast enlargement, milk production, indications of liver toxicity (loss of appetite, nausea, jaundice).
4. Sudden discontinuation of this drug can cause agitation, insomnia, rapid heart rate and intensification of angina.

Use of Prazosin

1. In 10% of users, this drug can provoke an idiosyncratic reaction that results in a sudden extreme drop in blood pressure following the first dose. It is advisable to begin treatment with a bedtime dose and a warning to arise cautiously the next morning in anticipation of possible orthostatic hypotension (see Glossary).
2. This drug can cause fluid retention and can aggravate angina. It is best used in conjunction with a diuretic and a beta blocker.
3. Do not use this drug concurrently with hydralazine or guanethidine because of the potential for additive postural hypotension.
4. A rapid loss of effectiveness can limit this drug's long-term usefulness.

Use of Hydralazine

1. This drug is rarely used alone. It can cause fluid retention and should be used concurrently with a diuretic.
2. This drug characteristically increases heart activity, which can be counteracted by the concurrent use of a beta blocker drug.
3. Use cautiously in the presence of angina (coronary artery disease).
4. Monitor for possible development of a lupuslike drug reaction.

Use of Reserpine

1. Limit the daily dose to 0.25 mg or less.
2. Avoid completely if you have a history of depression.
3. This drug can cause salt and water retention; a diuretic should be used concurrently.
4. Do not use this drug concurrently with methyldopa; the combination can cause marked sedation, excessive dreaming and sexual impotence.
5. Observe for the following possible adverse effects: drowsiness, lethargy, depression (can be very insidious), nightmares, nasal congestion, acid indigestion (possible ulcer), diarrhea, impotence, parkinsonlike syndrome.

Use of Guanethidine

1. This is the most potent antihypertensive drug in general use. It is

usually reserved to treat the most severe cases of hypertension and those that have been difficult to control.

2. It causes marked orthostatic hypotension. Users should avoid prolonged sitting (without moving the legs) and prolonged standing (without walking around); these are conducive to excessive drops in blood pressure and resultant fainting. Users should also arise cautiously in the morning to avoid fainting shortly after getting out of bed.

3. This drug causes salt and water retention and should be taken concurrently with a diuretic.

4. Tricyclic antidepressants can reduce this drug's antihypertensive effectiveness.

Use of Minoxidil

1. This drug is a potent, long-acting vasodilator. Its use is usually restricted to treating those whose blood pressure cannot be controlled by conventional treatment with other drugs.

2. It is generally used concurrently with a diuretic and a beta blocker drug.

3. Observe for excessive growth of hair.

Use of Calcium Channel-Blocking Drugs

1. These drugs are approved by the U.S. Food and Drug Administration only for use in the management of angina (coronary artery disease). However, they are effective antihypertensives and are being used as such by many physicians.

2. They may be used as Step 1, 2, or 3 drugs in the management of hypertension.

3. They are especially useful in treating the elderly individual with isolated systolic hypertension.

4. Use these drugs with caution if a beta blocker drug is being used concurrently.

5. A dosage of 3 to 4 times daily is required.

6. Observe for fluid retention. Effectiveness is improved if a thiazide diuretic is taken concurrently.

Use of Angiotensin Converting Enzyme (ACE) Inhibitors

1. These may be used as Step 1, 2, 3, or 4 drugs in the management of hypertension.

2. To prevent an excessive drop in blood pressure, any diuretic in use should be discontinued 5 to 7 days before starting an ACE inhibitor. After the dose is stabilized, a diuretic may be resumed if necessary.

3. Captopril should be taken 1 hour before eating, 2 to 3 times daily, for maximal effectiveness. Enalapril may be taken once or twice daily without regard to eating.

4. Full effectiveness of these drugs may not be apparent until after several weeks of continual use.

5. These drugs may increase the blood potassium level. Do not use any commercial salt substitute (most of which contain potassium) without first consulting your physician.

Current Controversies in Drug Management

The standard "stepped-care" approach to treating hypertension usually recommends the use of a thiazide diuretic as the drug of choice to initiate therapy. If an adequate trial with thiazide therapy fails to lower the blood pressure sufficiently, other drugs of the various classes listed above are *added* in a somewhat arbitrary and rigid fashion. While the guidelines provided by a standardized approach were beneficial in promoting rational therapy, new information about the older drugs and the availability of many new and more effective drugs call for a reappraisal of drug selection for managing hypertension.

Recent review of thiazide drug performance discloses that (1) while they are effective in mild hypertension, they have not decreased the incidence of heart attacks; (2) they can cause loss of potassium and/or magnesium and thereby contribute to the development of dangerous heart rhythm disorders; and (3) they cause a 10% increase in LDL cholesterol blood levels and may increase the risk of coronary artery disease. Some authorities no longer consider thiazides to be the drugs of choice for initiating treatment; they also recommend that thiazides be used in the lowest effective dose to reduce the potential risks of long-term therapy.

Current recommendations call for a greater emphasis on individualization of drug management; this includes wider flexibility in selecting drugs for starting treatment and in substituting and deleting drugs as individual monitoring dictates. Several drug classes are admirably suited for initiating treatment and provide a broad spectrum of features that permit tailoring the drug to the individual characteristics of the patient.

Ancillary Drug Treatment (as required)

Condition	Drug Treatment
For thiazide-induced gout:	allopurinol (Zyloprim)
	probenecid (Benemid)
For drug-induced fluid retention:	bumetanide (Bumex)
For guanethidine-induced diarrhea:	diphenoxylate (Lomotil)
For tension headache:	acetaminophen (Tylenol, etc.)
For migraine headache (short-term use):	ibuprofen (Motrin, Advil, Nuprin)
	oxycodone (Percodan)
	Avoid ergotamine preparations.
For musculo-skeletal pain, arthritis (long-term use):	sulindac (Clinoril)

Note: Drug selection, dosage and administration schedule must be determined by the physician for each patient individually.

Resources for Additional Information and Services

Citizens for the Treatment of High Blood Pressure
888 17th Street, N.W., Suite 904
Washington, DC 20006
Phone: (202) 466-4553

Publications available.

The Joint National Committee on Detection, Evaluation and Treatment
of High Blood Pressure
National Heart, Lung and Blood Institute
National Institutes of Health
Box 120/80
Bethesda, MD 20892
Phone: (301) 496-4000

National Institute of Hypertension Studies
Institute of Hypertension School of Research
13217 Livernois
Detroit, MI 48238
Phone: (313) 931-3427

Publications available.

HYPOTHYROIDISM

Other Names: Hypometabolism, myxedema, primary hypothyroidism, secondary hypothyroidism

Prevalence in USA: 1.9 million—0.8% of the general population; 1 in 5000 newborn infants has hypothyroidism (cretinism).

Age Group: Juvenile hypothyroidism: under 18 years—2% of total incidence. Adult hypothyroidism: percentage of total incidence by age: 18 to 44 years—34%; 45 to 64 years—40%; 65 years and over—24%.

Male to Female Ratio: More common in women—8 to 1.

Principal Features: Hypothyroidism spans a wide spectrum from very mild thyroid hormone deficiency (hypometabolism) with few nonspecific symptoms to severe deficiency (myxedema) that can be fatal if not treated adequately. The most common form of hypothyroidism is the mild to moderate hormone deficiency seen primarily in women age 20 to 65. The onset is usually insidious and the early symptoms are so vague that medical attention is rarely sought. With progression of the deficiency, the subject gradually becomes aware of lethargy, fatigability, intolerance of cold, weight gain (with no increased food intake), loss of hair, vague muscle and joint pains, and irregular menstruation. The skin may become dry and scaly, the face may appear puffy (fluid retention), the speech slows, the voice becomes hoarse and the pattern of activity becomes sluggish. Hypothyroidism in the elderly can cause mental changes, confusion, paranoia, depression and dementia.

Causes: Primary hypothyroidism can be due to (1) a congenital defect in thyroid gland development or function; (2) an "autoimmune" impairment of thyroid hormone production (45% of cases); (3) a lack of iodine in the food or water supply; or (4) intentional thyroid gland suppression by the administration of radioactive iodine or by surgical removal of thyroid tissue (35% of cases). Secondary hypothyroidism is due to inadequate stimulation of thyroid gland function from the hypothalamus (in the brain) or from the pituitary gland (the "master" gland that regulates most hormone-producing glands).

Drugs That Can Cause This Disorder: The following drugs can impair the normal production of thyroid hormones and induce varying degrees of hypothyroidism (see Drug Classes, Section Four):

amiodarone	methimazole
cyclophosphamide	pentazocine
disulfiram (?)	phenylbutazone
ethionamide	propylthiouracil
iodine compounds (iodides)	sulfonylurea antidiabetic drugs
lithium	

Drugs Used to Treat This Disorder:
- synthetic thyroxine (T-4) (Synthroid, Levothroid).
- synthetic liothyronine (T-3) (Cytomel).
- synthetic liotrix (combinations of T-4 and T-3) (Euthroid, Thyrolar).
- thyroid extract (animal origin) (Dessicated thyroid Armour).
- thyroglobulin (animal origin) (Proloid).

Goals of Drug Treatment

Adequate replacement of thyroxine; restoration of normal blood levels of T-4, T-3 and the Thyroid Stimulating Hormone (TSH).

Relief of symptoms associated with deficiency of thyroid hormones (hypothyroidism, cretinism, myxedema).

Drug Management

General Principles

Primary hypothyroidism is diagnosed by finding the blood level of the principal thyroid hormone—thyroxine (T-4)—below the normal range and the blood level of the pituitary hormone—Thyroid Stimulating Hormone (TSH)—above the normal range.

Once the diagnosis of true primary hypothyroidism is established, treatment for life is generally thought to be necessary. However, periodic evaluation is advisable to determine the need for continual thyroid hormone replacement.

Individuals taking replacement thyroid hormones should be monitored every 6 to 12 months by measurements of T-4 and TSH along with evaluation of general well-being.

Until thyroid deficiency is adequately corrected, the subject may be overly sensitive to drugs that depress brain function—sedatives, tranquilizers, hypnotics, narcotic analgesics.

In treating hypothyroidism of infancy, avoid formula feedings that contain soybean extract; they can prevent the absorption of thyroxine and perpetuate cretinism.

Anxious, thin individuals usually require smaller doses of maintenance thyroxine than lethargic, obese individuals require. Significant reduction in weight (correction of obesity) is usually followed by a reduction in the daily requirement of maintenance thyroxine.

The use of thyroid hormones for weight reduction in the presence of normal thyroid function (no hormone deficiency) is unjustified and dangerous.

Hypothyroidism causes an increase in bone mass. Thyroid replacement therapy can result in a significant loss of bone (osteoporosis) in the lumbar vertebrae (spine). Consult your physician regarding the advisability of taking supplements of calcium and vitamin D during thyroid hormone replacement. (See Profile of Osteoporosis in this section.)

Use of Thyroxine

1. Hypothyroidism is best treated with a synthetic preparation of thyroxine (see Drug Profile, Section Three). This provides replacement that approximates most closely the normal status of thyroid hormones in circulating blood.

2. Young, basically healthy individuals with hypothyroidism may take thyroxine in full dosage—1 microgram per pound of body weight daily. This usually achieves normal blood levels of T-4 and TSH.

3. Older individuals, with incipient or established heart disease, should initiate thyroxine treatment with small doses that can be increased gradually over 2 to 3 months. This reduces the risk of precipitating disturbances of heart function, such as angina and abnormal rhythm.

4. Thyroxine should be taken in the morning on an empty stomach to ensure maximal absorption and uniform effectiveness.

5. Cholestyramine and colestipol can prevent absorption of thyroxine and liothyronine; for best results, take thyroxine (and/or liothyronine) first (preferably in the morning, fasting), 2 to 3 hours before the first daily dose of either cholestyramine or colestipol.

6. Observe for possible seasonal variation in your response to thyroxine replacement therapy. Some individuals may need less in warm months and more in cold months. If the winter dose of thyroxine is somewhat excessive for summer requirements, you may develop nervousness, insomnia, headaches, intolerance of heat and loss of weight. Consult your physician if you think dosage adjustment is necessary.

7. Long-term thyroxine therapy may lead to premature bone loss in the

upper femur (thigh bone) in women. Periodic monitoring of thyroxine blood levels is advised to detect excessive dosage.

8. Do not purchase thyroxine tablets in large quantities (such as 500 to 1000). Thyroxine products can lose up to 6% of their potency per year. It is advisable to obtain a 3 to 6 months' supply (100 to 200 tablets) to ensure full-strength medication.

Ancillary Drug Treatment (as required)

Condition	Drug Treatment
For anemia:	iron preparations
	vitamin B-12 (if appropriate for type of anemia)
For constipation:	docusate (Colace, Doxinate, etc.)
	docusate with casanthranol (Peri-Colace, etc.)
For muscle or joint ache/pain:	aspirin
	acetaminophen (Tylenol, Panadol, etc.)
	ibuprofen (Advil, Nuprin, etc.)

Note: Drug selection, dosage and administration schedule must be determined by the physician for each patient individually.

Resource for Additional Information and Services

American Thyroid Association
Endocrine-Metabolic Service
Walter Reed Army Medical Center
Washington, DC 20307-5001
Phone: (202) 576-0747

Maintains professional membership directory for geographical referrals.

LUPUS ERYTHEMATOSUS

Other Names: Lupus, LE, cutaneous lupus erythematosus, CLE, systemic lupus erythematosus, SLE, disseminated lupus erythematosus

Prevalence in USA:
Approximately 500,000. 16,000 new cases are diagnosed annually.
The incidence is higher in Afro-Americans and in some Asian and North American Indian groups than in whites.

Age Group: Onset usually occurs between 15 and 45 years of age. However, lupus can occur in young children and older adults.

Male to Female Ratio: 90% of cases occur in women; 60% of these are Afro-American.

Principal Features: There are two relatively distinct forms of lupus: (1) cutaneous lupus erythematosus, a mild form that is confined primarily to the skin and tissues of the mouth; (2) systemic lupus erythematosus, a severe form that can affect virtually every organ in the body. Both forms of lupus are chronic inflammatory disorders characterized by unpredictable fluctuations in disease activity (flares and remissions).

Cutaneous lupus erythematosus (CLE) : This form of lupus can exist as the only manifestaion of this disorder or it can be an integral part of the more serious disseminated form—systemic lupus erythematosus. Only about 5% to 10% of cases that begin as the cutaneous form will eventually develop systemic lupus. Cutaneous lupus causes discrete patches of inflammation and scaling on the face, ears, neck, upper trunk and arms that can result in scarring. The skin changes are aggravated by exposure to sunlight. Mouth ulcers occur in some cases. Loss of scalp hair (balding) may be extensive and permanent. Lupus specialists now classify the varieties of skin rashes and lesions that can occur into acute, subacute and chronic cutaneous LE subgroups. With early diagnosis and prompt treatment, this form of lupus reponds well to cortisonelike creams and ointments and, if necessary, the use of antimalarial drugs by mouth (see below).

Systemic lupus erythematosus (SLE) : This more severe form of lupus can affect any organ or system in the body and mimic many other diseases. The tissues most commonly involved include joints, kidneys, brain, heart, blood vessels, lungs and blood-forming organs. Activity of this disease and resulting organ damage can range from mild to life-threatening. The early symptoms of lupus are usually vague and nonspecific: low-grade fever, weakness, fatigue, loss of appetite and weight, skin rashes, joint pains involving the hands, wrists, elbows, knees or ankles. Joints may seem stiff on arising and may ultimately become red and swollen. As the disorder progresses, involvement of the heart and lungs can cause chest pain and shortness of breath. There may be lowered resistance to infections and abnormal bleeding or bruising. Tissue damage within the nervous system can cause significant alterations of mood and behavior; seizures resembling epilepsy occur infrequently. Kidney damage is quite common in lupus, but symptoms of this may not be apparent until advanced stages are reached. Presently no curative treatment is known. However, symptom relief and acceptable stabilization of organ damage can be achieved in many cases by the skillful use of four classes of effective drugs.

Causes: While some of the mechanisms responsible for tissue damage are partially understood, the true fundamental cause of lupus is not known. Lupus is a disorder of the body's immune system, the protective system that produces antibodies designed to destroy infective agents (bacteria, viruses, etc.) that invade the body. By unknown means, the immune system is provoked to produce antibodies specifically designed to attack normal tissues of the host. For this reason, lupus is classified as an "autoimmune" disease. The destructive interaction between specific antibodies and respective tissues is responsible for the inflammatory reactions and organ damage that characterize lupus. Studies to date indicate that multiple factors contribute to the induction of lupus. Among these is genetic predisposition: approximately 30% of identical twins will develop lupus; 1 in 20 children born to a parent with lupus will develop SLE. It is well established that some cases of lupus are caused by the use of certain medicinal drugs (see below).

Drugs That Can Cause This Disorder: It has been estimated that 15,000 to 20,000 cases of drug-related lupus occur annually in the United States. More than 50 medications have been thought to be responsible for inducing lupus. A careful analysis of these reports permits their division into three groups: (1) proof of causation is definite; (2) drug causation is very possible; (3) drug causation is unlikely or rarely possible.

Group I: Drug association definite

chlorpromazine	methyldopa
hydralazine	procainamide
isoniazid	

Group II: Drug association very possible

acebutolol	metoprolol
atenolol	nitrofurantoin
captopril	oxyprenolol
carbamazepine	penicillamine
ethosuximide	phenylbutazone
hydrazine	phenytoin
labetalol	practolol
levadopa	primidone
lithium carbonate	propylthiouracil
mephytoin	quinidine
methimazole	trimethadione
methylthiouracil	

Group III: Drug association unlikely or rare

acecainide	minoxidil
allopurinol	nomifensine
aminosalicylic acid	propafenone
benzylpenicillin	psoralen
chlorthalidone	reserpine
chlorprothixene	streptomycin
estrogens	sulfasalazine
gold salts	sulfonamides
griseofulvin	tetracycline
methysergide	tolazamide

Drugs Used to Treat This Disorder:
Anti-inflammatory Drugs (Nonsteroidal Anti-inflammatory Drugs or NSAIDs)
- aspirin and other salicylates.
- antiarthritic/anti-inflammatory aspirin substitutes (see Drug Class, Section Four).

Antimalarial Drugs
- chloroquine (Aralen).
- hydroxychloroquine (Plaquenil).
- quinacrine (Atabrine).

Cortisonelike Drugs (Corticosteroids)
- cortisonelike creams and ointments for cutaneous LE
    flucinolone (Synalar).
    fluocinonide (Lidex).
    hydrocortisone.
    triamcinolone (Kenalog).
- cortisonelike drugs for oral administration
    hydrocortisone.
    prednisolone (Delta-Cortef, etc.).
    prednisone (Deltasone, Meticorten, etc.).
    methylprednisolone (Medrol).

Immunosuppressive Drugs
- azathioprine (Imuran).
- chlorambucil (Leukeran).
- cyclophosphamide (Cytoxan).
- cyclosporine (Sandimmune).
- methotrexate.

New Drugs in Development for Treating This Disorder:
A new corticosteroid derivative, deflazort, is believed to cause less bone loss than prednisone and similar drugs now commonly used. Deflazort equals prednisone as an anti-inflammatory drug for the long-term treatment of SLE; it may well provide equal therapeutic benefit but with significantly reduced risk of causing osteoporosis and osteonecrosis during extended use.

A major component of fish oil (notably salmon and mackerel) identified as eicosapentaenooic acid (EPA), a form of omega-3 fatty acid, has been shown to have significant anti-inflammatory effects. This may prove to be beneficial in treating inflammatory disorders such as lupus. Studies in mice show that EPA protects against the development of lupus nephritis and that it is relatively nontoxic.

Goals of Drug Treatment
For cutaneous LE
To improve the patient's appearance.
To prevent the development of further skin deformities.
To determine that the lupus disorder is limited to the skin and is not a manifestation of systemic LE.

For systemic LE

To achieve and maintain optimal control of disease activity.

To provide maximal symptomatic relief consistent with safe drug use.

To prevent or limit organ damage as much as possible.

To determine the selection of drugs and dosage schedules that will provide maximal benefits with minimal risks.

To monitor the course of the disorder and the response to drug therapy so that appropriate adjustments can be made as required.

Drug Management
General Principles

Currently available treatments for lupus have significantly improved the prognosis for both CLE and SLE. 80–90% of all SLE patients now live more than 10 years and very many live a normal lifespan.

Treatment programs must be planned according to the extent and severity of disease activity. Lupus characteristically fluctuates between episodes of increased activity (flares) and periods of decreased activity (remissions). This requires close monitoring by both patient and physician so that appropriate adjustments of medications can be made in a timely manner.

Approximately 25% of patients have mild lupus that can be controlled with aspirin, NSAIDs (aspirin substitutes) and/or an antimalarial drug. Another 70% have a more severe form of lupus that usually responds to prednisone or related steroid drugs. A small percent have serious multiple organ disease that requires immunosuppressant drugs for control.

Marked sensitivity of the skin to sunlight is a prominent feature of lupus. Exposure to the sun (and tanning booths) can initiate and intensify skin lesions of CLE. The regular use of sunscreen lotions or creams is mandatory; the sunscreen chosen should have a sun protective factor (SPF) of 15 or higher.

Use of local (topical) cortisonelike drugs

1. Creams and ointments containing a cortisonelike drug are beneficial but must be applied regularly to prevent atrophy, depigmentation and scarring of the skin.
2. It is advisable to use the least potent preparation that proves to be effective for each patient.
3. Lupus lesions on the face should be treated with a low- to mid-potency preparation such as hydrocortisone or desonide.
4. Lupus lesions on the trunk and extremities may be treated with a high-potency preparation such as Lidex or Synalar.
5. Lesions that do not respond to applications of creams or ointments can be injected with triamcinolone.

Use of Antimalarial Drugs

1. If lupus skin lesions are not adequately controlled by topical applications (as above), an antimalarial drug should be added to the treatment program.
2. The antimalarial drug of choice is hydroxychloroquine. (See Drug

Profile for complete description.) It is thought to be safer but less effective than chloroquine. (See Drug Profile for complete description.)

3. If hydroxychloroquine is not effective, cholorquine may be substituted for it or quinacrine may be added. (See Drug Profile for complete description.)

4. The 3 antimalarial drugs used to treat lupus can infrequently cause damage to the cornea and/or retina of the eye. A complete eye examination should be performed *before* an antimalarial drug is started and *every 3 to 6 months* during its use. The drug should be stopped if any evidence of eye damage is found.

5. Antimalarial dosage should be carefully determined on the basis of ideal body weight.

6. Antimalarial drugs are also effective in treating some features of SLE: fever, fatigue, arthritis, muscle aches, chest pains.

7. A trial of 8 to 12 weeks may be necessary to determine the effectiveness of antimalarial drugs.

8. After lupus skin lesions have responded adequately to antimalarial drugs, the dosage should be gradually reduced to the smallest effective maintenamce level. Low-dose, long-term therapy with antimalarials is considered to be quite safe.

Use of Nonsteroidal Anti-inflammatory Drugs (NSAIDs)

1. This group of drugs is the first line of treatment for the symptoms of SLE. Fever, joint and muscle pain, arthritis, and serositis (involvement of heart and lung surfaces) can often be managed by these drugs alone.

2. Aspirin (plain, buffered, sustained-release or enteric-coated) may be tried first in moderate to large doses (3 to 4 grams per day). A blood salicylate level of 20 to 30 mg/dl is recommended unless satisfactory results are obtained with lower levels.

3. If aspirin is not tolerated or is ineffective, one of the NSAID aspirin substitutes may be tried. There are now 16 different NSAIDs availble. There is no way of determining in advance which NSAID will be most effective or acceptable for any given patient. A period of trial and error is unavoidable. Physicians will favor one drug or another within the group based upon their experience. For reasons not understood, there are marked differences in response among patients to all NSAIDs. The selected NSAID should be tried for at least 2 weeks at maximal dose in order to judge effectiveness and acceptance.

4. Indomethacin (Indocin) is considered by many to be the drug of choice for treating serositis.

5. Like aspirin, all NSAIDs may cause gastrointestinal irritation, microscopic ulceration and bleeding in susceptible individuals. Patients with a history of peptic ulcer disease should consult their physicians regarding the need for medications to prevent gastrointestinal ulceration. (See the Drug Profiles of misoprostol, omeprazole, sucralfate, and the Glossary listing of Histamine H-2 Blocking drugs used to prevent ulcer recurrence.)

6. Patients with a history of liver disease or pancreatitis are well advised to avoid the use of sulindac.
7. The long-term use of NSAIDs requires periodic evaluation of kidney function for evidence of drug-induced kidney damage. This is especially true in the presence of SLE.

Use of Cortisonelike Drugs (Corticosteroids) Systemically

1. The drugs of this class possess the most potent anti-inflammatory action available, hence their value in treating the more serious manifestations of SLE.
2. Corticosteroids are the first drugs used to treat SLE organ involvement: pleurisy and pericarditis (serositis unresponsive to indomethacin), interstitial pneumonia, hemolytic anemia, blood platelet destruction, lupus nephritis (kidney damage), brain and peripheral nervous system tissues.
3. Prednisone is the drug most commonly used. (See Drug Profile for complete description.) It is the drug of choice among the short-acting steroids, which are preferable for most severe SLE involvements. Long-acting steroids are best avoided in treating SLE.
4. Prednisone is usually started with high doses to achieve rapid suppression of disease activity. As improvement occurs, the dose is gradually reduced until the lowest maintenance dose is determined. In some instances it is possible to use alternate-day dosing. However, activity "flares" on the off days may require return to daily dosing.
5. The risks of significant adverse effects that accompany long-term use of prednisone require that maintenance doses be kept as low as possible.

Use of Immunosuppressive Drugs

1. When SLE disease activity reaches life-threatening proportions and corticosteroids in maximal doses are inadequate for control, drugs that are capable of suppressing the abnormal "autoimmune" mechanisms are used. In addition to reducing the degree of disease activity, they also permit the continued use of corticosteroids in smaller (less risky) dosage.
2. Because of the serious toxicities associated with these drugs, their use is restricted to the following situations:
   - life-threatening disease that is unresponsive to optimal trials of prednisone.
   - active major organ disease that is unresponsive to optimal trials of prednisone.
   - active major organ disease that recurs when prednisone dosage is reduced and requires unacceptably high maintenance doses of prednisone.
   - intolerable prednisone toxicity in a patient that requires prednisone to suppress disease activity.
   - active major organ disease in a patient who has significant contraindications to the use of high-dose prednisone.
   - certain active organ disease that has been shown to respond more

satisfactorily to the combined use of immunosuppressive drugs and prednisone.

3. Cyclophosphamide appears to reduce the degree of deterioration of kidney function in the patient with lupus nephritis; however, this drug has marked potential for serious toxic effects. (See Drug Profile for complete description.)

4. Cyclophosphamide also has potential for suppressing SLE activity in the lung, the brain and peripheral nervous system, and blood-forming organs.

5. Azathioprine has been used to treat SLE for over 20 years. (See Drug Profile for complete description.) It is thought to be effective in treating resistant CLE (discoid lupus) that failed to respond to antimalarial drugs. It is also beneficial in some cases of lupus nephritis. It is not recommended as the first immunosuppressive drug to be tried in life-threatening disease or in organ damage involving the brain, lung or blood-forming tissues.

6. Methotrexate has been used less frequently in treating SLE, but some dramatic improvements have been reported. (See Drug Profile for complete description.) In patients who become resistant to azathioprine after 10 to 15 months of treatment, a plan of alternate use of azathioprine and methotrexate has proved to be effective in some cases.

Current Controversies in Drug Management

Lupus nephritis, the kidney disease associated with SLE, is the major cause of morbidity and mortality in this disorder. It is also one of the more difficult aspects of SLE to manage satisfactorily. One prominent disagreement has focused on the relative merits of high-dose versus low-dose prednisone treatment, with or without other drugs. The consensus that seems to have emerged from several studies in diverse settings is that long-term high-dose prednisone modifies the disease course more favorably than low-dose prednisone treatment regimens.

Ancillary Drug Treatment (as required)

Condition	*Drug Treatment*
For intercurrent infections:	specific anti-infectives based on culture and sensitivity testing as appropriate
For organic brain syndrome with psychosis:	neuroleptics: haloperidol (Haldol), thiothixene (Navane)
For organic brain syndrome with seizures:	anticonvulsants; see Profile of Epilepsy in this section

For migraine headache:	beta blockers; see Profile of Migraine Headache in this section
For hypertension:	see Profile of Hypertension in this section
For Raynaud's phenomenon:	calcium channel blockers: diltiazem (Cardizem), nifedipine (Procardia)
For hemolytic anemia or blood platelet destruction:	danazol (Danocrine), as adjunct to prednisone

Note: Drug selection, dosage and administration schedule must be determined by the physician for each patient individually.

Resources for Additional Information and Services

The American Lupus Society
East 2617 Columbia Avenue
Spokane, WA 99207
Phone: 1-800-331-1802
Publications available.

Lupus Foundation of America, Inc.
1717 Massachusetts Avenue, N.W., Suite 203
Washington, DC 20036
Phone: (202) 328-4550; 1-800-558-0121
Local groups: 108 chapters in 48 states; 38 international associates in 18 countries.
Publications available: "Lupus News" official newsletter.

National Lupus Erythematosus Foundation
5430 Van Nuys Blvd., Suite 206
Van Nuys, CA 91401
Phone: (818) 885-8787
Publications available.

MENOPAUSE

Other Names: Menopausal syndrome, estrogen withdrawal syndrome, female climacteric, change of life

Prevalence in USA: 12.8 million women (candidates for menopause).

Age Group: 45 to 55 years; the mean age of natural menopause is 50 years.

Principal Features: The term "menopause" refers to the permanent cessation of menstruation. This occurs naturally in most women between 45

and 55 years of age. The characteristic indication of the "change"—altered menstrual pattern with eventual cessation of menstrual periods—usually lasts from 6 to 18 months. The majority of women (85%) experience some physical effects of progressive estrogen withdrawal: recurring hot flushes, episodic sweating, shrinkage of breast tissue, reduction of vaginal secretions and a variety of nervous and emotional symptoms—anxiety, depression, insomnia, headaches, dizziness, nausea. For approximately 25%, the symptoms are of sufficient intensity to warrant a trial of estrogen replacement therapy. Up to 35% of menopausal women experience hot flushes for 5 or more years.

Causes: Natural menopause occurs spontaneously to terminate reproductive capability. Therapeutic menopause follows surgical removal of the uterus or ovaries and irradiation or removal of the pituitary gland.

Drugs That Can Cause This Disorder: The following drugs can cause cessation of menstruation for varying periods of time, sometimes permanently: busulfan, chlorambucil, cyclophosphamide, mechlorethamine, oral contraceptives and vincristine. The antiestrogen drug tamoxifen, used for the treatment of breast cancer, can cause hot flushes, dizziness and menstrual irregularities typical of the menopausal syndrome.

Drugs Used to Treat This Disorder:
"Natural-type" estrogens are preferred:
- conjugated estrogens (Genisis, Premarin).
- esterified estrogens (Evex, Menest).
- estradiol cypionate (Depo-Estradiol, injection).
- estradiol valerate (Delestrogen, injection).
- estriol (Hormonin, a mixture of estriol, estradiol, and estrone).
- piperazine estrone sulfate (Ogen).
- micronized 17-B estradiol (Estrace).
- transdermal estradiol skin patch (Estraderm-50 and 100).

Goals of Drug Treatment
Reduction in the frequency and severity of hot flushes and night sweats with attendant insomnia.
Relief of nervous and emotional symptoms.
Prevention or relief of atrophic changes of the vulva, vagina and urethra.
Prevention of thinning of the skin.
Prevention of osteoporosis (long-term treatment).

Drug Management
General Principles
It is now generally held that for the well-informed menopausal woman who has obvious symptoms of estrogen deficiency and does not have any contraindications to its use, the benefits of estrogen replacement therapy outweigh the possible risks. The use of estrogen is considered effective and safe when prescribed appropriately and monitored properly.

As each women reaches the menopausal years (45 to 55), she should assess her own status and perceived needs. Next she should familiarize herself with the benefits and possible risks of estrogen replacement therapy. (See the Drug Profile of Estrogen, Section Three.) If she thinks she needs medical guidance and/or treatment, she should discuss all aspects of her situation with her physician and share in the decision regarding the use of hormones.

A clear indication for the use of estrogen should exist. It should not be given routinely to the menopausal woman, but should be reserved to treat those with symptoms of estrogen deficiency. Estrogen does not retard the natural progression of general aging; it should not be used for the sole purpose of "preserving femininity."

Before estrogen therapy is started, appropriate examinations should be performed and due consideration given to the following possible contraindications to the use of estrogen:

1. Pregnancy
2. History of deep venous thrombosis or pulmonary embolism
3. Present or previous cancer of the breast
4. Cancer of the uterus
5. Strong family history of breast or uterine cancer
6. Current liver disease or previous drug-induced jaundice
7. Chronic gallbladder disease, with or without stones
8. Abnormal elevation of blood fats (cholesterol, triglycerides, etc.)
9. History of porphyria
10. Large uterine fibroid tumors
11. Any estrogen-dependent tumor
12. Combination of obesity, varicose veins and cigarette smoking
13. Diabetes mellitus
14. Severe hypertension

In the young woman experiencing premature menopause (destruction or removal of both ovaries), the *long-term* use of estrogen replacement is justified, provided appropriate precautions are observed (see Guidelines below).

In the menopausal woman experiencing hot flushes and/or atrophic vaginitis, the *short-term* use of estrogen therapy is generally felt to be acceptable with appropriate supervision and guidance. Estrogen replacement therapy provides symptomatic relief; it is not a permanent cure for hot flushes.

Long-term estrogen therapy for *all* women after the menopause cannot be justified. Treatment must be carefully individualized (see Guidelines below).

It is generally recommended that estrogens be taken cyclically. The customary schedule is from the 1st through the 25th day of each month, with no estrogen during the remaining days of the month. After 6 to 12 months of continuous use, the estrogen dose should be gradually reduced over a period of 2 to 3 months and then discontinued to assess the individual's need for resumption of use.

The lowest effective daily dose of estrogen should be determined and maintained for the duration of the treatment.

Vaginal cream preparations of estrogen may be considered instead of orally administered estrogen if the only indication is atrophic vaginitis. However, it should be noted that these preparations allow rapid absorption of estrogen into the systemic circulation, and do not permit accurate control of dosage. They should be used intermittently and only as needed to correct the symptoms of atrophic vaginitis. (Note: The estrogen in vaginal creams can be absorbed through the skin of the penis and cause tenderness of the breast in men.)

The unnecessary prolongation of estrogen therapy should be avoided. It is advisable to use estrogens in the lowest effective dose and for only as long as necessary to relieve symptoms.

Guidelines for the Use of Estrogens in Specific Deficiency States

I. The young woman (under 45 years of age) with both ovaries and uterus removed:
  1. Choice of estrogen: a conjugated "natural" estrogen (see list of estrogen preparations).
     The lowest effective dose should be used.*
  2. Dosage schedule: once daily from the 1st through the 25th day of each month.
     Note: If the uterus is present, it is advisable to add a progestin (medroxyprogesterone), 4 to 10 mg daily during the last 7 to 10 days of the estrogen course.**
  3. Duration of use: if well tolerated, until 50 years of age, when assessment of continued need is made individually.
  4. Periodic examinations:
     Base-line mammogram (low-radiation-dose xeroradiography); mammogram should be repeated only as necessary to evaluate possible breast tumor (American Cancer Society guideline).
     Self-examination of breasts monthly.
     Physician examination of breasts (and uterus if present) every 6 to 12 months.
     Measurement of blood pressure.
II. The woman experiencing the "menopausal syndrome" of hot flushes and sweating (usually 45 to 55 years of age):
  A. Uterus not removed
    1. Choice of hormones and recommended dosage range:
       Estrogen: conjugated equine estrogens—0.3 to 0.625 mg daily. (See list of alternative estrogen preparations.)

*The lowest effective dose is determined by keeping a daily "flush count" to ascertain the lowest daily dose that will reduce the frequency and severity of flushes to an acceptable level.
**The use of a supplemental progestin during the last 7 to 10 days of estrogen administration is still controversial. A possible benefit is the reduced potential for uterine cancer; a possible risk is the increased potential for coronary artery disease; a possible inconvenience is withdrawal bleeding (induced menstruation). The risks of this form of long-term progestin therapy are not known.

Progestin: medroxyprogesterone—5 to 10 mg daily.

The lowest effective dose of estrogen should be used.*

2. Dosage schedule:

Estrogen: once daily from the 1st through the 25th day of each month.

Progestin: once daily during the last 7 to 10 days of the estrogen course.**

3. Duration of use: 6 to 12 months, followed by gradual reduction of dose over a period of 2 to 3 months, and then discontinuation to assess the need for continued use. Treatment should be resumed only if symptoms require it. An attempt should be made to discontinue all hormones after 2 to 3 years of continual use, unless a clear need for continuation is apparent.

4. Periodic examinations:

Base-line mammogram (low-radiation-dose xeroradiography).

Low-dose mammogram annually (over 50 years of age) during continuous use of estrogen (American Cancer Society guideline).

Self-examination of breasts monthly.

Physician examination of breasts every 6 to 12 months.

Cervical cytology and endometrial biopsy (aspiration curettage) annually.

Blood pressure measurement every 3 to 6 months.

Two-hour blood sugar assay annually.

B. Uterus removed

1. Choice of estrogen and dose: conjugated equine estrogens—0.3 to 0.625 mg daily.

The lowest effective dose should be used.*

2. Dosage schedule: once daily from the 1st through the 25th day of each month.

3. Duration of use: 6 to 12 months, followed by gradual reduction of dose over a period of 2 to 3 months, and then discontinuation to assess the need for continued use. Treatment should be resumed only if symptoms require it. An attempt should be made to discontinue all hormones after 2 to 3 years of continual use.

4. Periodic examinations:

Base-line mammogram (low-radiation-dose xeroradiography).

Low-dose mammogram annually (over 50 years of age) during continuous use of estrogen (American Cancer Society guideline).

Self-examination of breasts monthly.

Physician examination of breasts every 6 to 12 months.

Blood pressure measurement every 3 to 6 months.

Two-hour blood sugar assay annually.

III. The woman in the "post-menopausal" period (usually over 55 years of age): treatment should be individualized as follows:

1. If there are no specific symptoms of estrogen deficiency (hot flushes or atrophic vaginitis), estrogen should not be given.

2. If specific symptoms of estrogen deficiency persist to a degree requiring subjective relief, the recommendations in category II

apply. However, in addition to limiting courses of estrogen to 6 to 12 months followed by gradual withdrawal, dosage might be limited to 3 times weekly on a trial basis. Estrogen should be discontinued altogether as soon as possible. If only flushes persist beyond 60 years of age, all estrogen should be discontinued. Nonhormonal drugs such as clonidine, ergot preparations and certain sedatives may be substituted for the relief of hot flushes.

3. Although we do not yet have accurate and reliable predictive indicators, an attempt should be made to identify the woman who may be at high risk for the development of osteoporosis. The following features suggest the possibility of increased risk:
    (1) slender build, light-boned, white or Oriental race
    (2) a sedentary life style or restricted physical activity
    (3) a family history (mother or sister) of osteoporosis (reported by some investigators)
    (4) a low-sodium diet (also likely to be a low-calcium diet)
    (5) heavy smoking
    (6) excessive use of antacids that contain aluminum
    (7) long-term use of cortisone-related drugs
    (8) habitual use of carbonated beverages (reported by some investigators)
    (9) excessive consumption of alcohol
    (10) increased urinary excretion of calcium

For the woman thought to be at increased risk for the development of osteoporosis, estrogen treatment should be started within 3 years after menstruation ceases. The following schedule of estrogen therapy may be recommended for prevention: conjugated equine estrogens—0.625 mg daily or 3 times weekly, for the first 3 weeks of each month. Periodic examinations as outlined in category II above should be performed. Estrogen replacement therapy may continue indefinitely, always with appropriate supervision.

In addition to the prudent use of estrogen, regular exercise and a daily intake of 1500 mg of calcium and 400 units of vitamin D are generally thought to be beneficial in slowing the development of osteoporosis.

Ancillary Drug Treatment (as required)

Condition	Drug Treatment
For anxiety and/or depression:	alprazolam (Xanax), for intermittent, short-term use
For insomnia:	doxylamine (Unisom), available OTC diphenhydramine (Benadryl)
For headache:	aspirin acetaminophen (Tylenol, Panadol, etc.) ibuprofen (Advil, Nuprin, etc.)

For atrophic vaginitis
and painful
intercourse: estrogen creams (Dienestrol, Estrace,
                                              Premarin)

Note: Drug selection, dosage and administration schedule must be determined
by the physician for each patient individually.

Resource for Additional Information and Services

A Friend Indeed Publications, Inc.
P. O. Box 515
Place du Parc Station
Montreal, Canada H2W 2P1
Monthly newsletter "A Friend Indeed."

MIGRAINE HEADACHE

Other Names: Classic migraine, common migraine

Prevalence in USA: Approximately 30 million cases, 15% of the general
population under 40 years of age.

Age Group: Under 18 years—0.8% of population; 18 to 44 years—4.7% of
population; 45 to 64 years—5% of population; over 65 years—1.9% of
population.

Male to Female Ratio
With onset at puberty, boys and girls are affected equally.
By age 40 there is a 3 to 2 predominance in women.

Principal Features: Migraine headaches may first appear in childhood but
usually begin in the late teens or early twenties; they often cease after
menopause. The migraine attack occurs in one of two patterns:
(1) Classic migraine (15% of the total) begins with an "aura" of symptoms that may precede the onset of headache by 15 to 20 minutes; these
usually consist of visual manifestations described as blind spots, zig-
zag effects or flashing lights. The attack may begin at any time of the
day or night; the headache is usually (70% of attacks) located on one
side of the head, but may spread to both sides before terminating. The
pain is usually pulsating or throbbing in nature and varies in intensity
from mild to severe. The migraine attack commonly (90% of attacks)
includes nausea, vomiting and increased sensitivity to light and noise.
Other associated features are scalp tenderness, dizziness, dry mouth,
tremors, sweating and chilliness.
(2) Common migraine (85% of the total) begins as a headache without
a warning "aura." Otherwise the pattern is essentially the same. Attacks

may occur rarely (1 or 2 a year) or every few days; the average frequency is 2 to 4 per month. Individual episodes usually last from 12 to 48 hours.

Causes: The exact complex of mechanisms responsible for the migraine attack is not known. It is basically a disturbance in the autonomic nervous system that causes instability in the control of cerebral arteries. There is a positive family history in 70% of those who experience migraine attacks. The majority of women who experience migraine find frequent association of the episode with menstruation. Other factors that are reported to trigger migraine attacks include emotional stress, excessive fatigue, erratic patterns of eating and sleeping, bright sunlight, loud noises, and the use of alcohol. The following foods are thought to be responsible for migraine attacks in sensitive individuals: aged cheese, bananas, chicken livers, chocolate, citrus fruits, monosodium glutamate, onions, pickled herring, pork, red wine, excessive salt, shell fish, sodium nitrite, vinegar, yogurt.

Drugs That Can Cause This Disorder: The following drugs may induce migrainelike headaches or aggravate existing migraine syndromes:
aminophylline
analgesics (chronic use of acetaminophen or aspirin)
antihypertensive drugs that cause vasodilation
caffeine (chronic use may cause vascular headache)
estrogens (can worsen migraine in 50% of women)
hydralazine
indomethacin
nifedipine
nitrates
oral contraceptives
prazosin
reserpine

Drugs Used to Treat This Disorder:
For Prevention of Migraine Attacks
   Beta-Adrenergic-Blocking Drugs (Beta Blockers)
       • propranolol (Inderal).
       • nadolol (Corgard).
       • atenolol (Tenormin).
       • timolol (Blocadren).
       • metoprolol (Lopressor).
   Calcium Channel-Blocking Drugs (Calcium Blockers)
       • nifedipine (Procardia).
       • verapamil (Calan, Isoptin).
   Anti-inflammatory Drugs (Aspirin Substitutes)
       • naproxen (Naprosyn).
       • ibuprofen (Motrin, Rufen, Advil, etc.).
       • fenoprofen (Nalfon).

Antidepressants
- amitriptyline (Elavil, Endep).
- doxepin (Sinequan, Adapin).

methysergide (Sansert)

lithium (Lithane, Lithobid, etc.)

For Abortion and Relief of Migraine Attacks

Vasoconstrictor Drugs
- ergotamine: oral (Cafergot, Wigraine); rectal (Cafergot, Wigraine suppositories); sublingual (Ergostat, Ergomar, Wigrettes); inhalant (Medihaler ergotamine).
- isometheptene (Midrin).

Anti-inflammatory Drugs
- aspirin.
- meclofenamate (Meclomen).
- ibuprofen (Motrin, Rufen, Advil, etc.).
- naproxen (Naprosyn).
- diflunisal (Dolobid).

Opioid Analgesics
- codeine.
- meperidine (Demerol).

Goals of Drug Treatment

Prompt abortion and relief of the acute migraine attack.

Reduction in the frequency and severity of recurrent migraine attacks.

A permanent cure is not available.

Drug Management

Important note: Not every drug is effective with every patient. Trial and experimentation may be necessary to determine the most effective treatment for each individual.

For fewer than 3 attacks per month of mild to moderate migraine, use abortive medications at the onset of symptoms. Ergotamine and anti-inflammatory drugs are the medications of choice.

For 3 or more attacks per month and for severe, prolonged migraine, use preventive medications on a continual basis. Beta blockers are the drugs of choice to reduce the frequency and severity of recurrent migraine attacks.

Always try to take your medication as soon as possible after the first indications of a developing migraine attack.

Isometheptene (Midrin) is a mild, well-tolerated and safer drug than ergotamine; use it first to determine its effectiveness. Go to stronger drugs only as needed.

Metoclopramide (Reglan) is an effective addition to the treatment of migraine attacks; it often controls nausea and vomiting, and it enhances the effectiveness of other oral migraine drugs.

Antidepressants may be used concurrently with other preventive drugs. They may be very effective *even in the absence of depression*.

For best results, start the preventive treatment of menstrual migraine 3

days before the onset of menstruation and continue it until all spotting
has ceased.

Use of Beta Blockers
1. These are the drugs of choice for long-term prevention of migraine
   attacks. Propranolol (Inderal) is the most widely used; nadolol (Corgard) is a good second choice.
2. The preventive dose varies greatly and must be determined by individual trial. Effective dosage ranges from 80 mg to 320 mg daily.
3. After a period of 6 to 12 months of good headache control, the dose
   may be reduced gradually and the drug eventually discontinued.

Use of Calcium Blockers
1. The preventive use of this class of drugs is still experimental in this
   country; they have been highly effective in Europe.
2. Verapamil (Calan, Isoptin) is the most effective of this class currently
   available in the USA. Nifedipine (Procardia) has been found to intensify migraine attacks in some individuals. Its use is not recommended.
3. A trial of 6 to 8 weeks is usually required to determine the preventive
   effectiveness of these drugs.
4. Observe for the development of fluid retention and constipation.

Use of Anti-inflammatory Drugs
1. These drugs are useful in both preventing and relieving migraine
   attacks. They are usually well tolerated and are not habit-forming.
2. Meclofenamate (Meclomen) is the fastest acting of the class and is
   very effective in aborting acute migraine.
3. Naproxen (Naprosyn) and fenoprofen (Nalfon) are also effective and
   widely used for intermittent prevention (as in menstrual migraine).
4. The prolonged-action forms of these drugs should be used cautiously,
   especially in the elderly, because of their potential for reducing kidney blood flow.

Use of Antidepressants
1. The long-term use of amitriptyline (Elavil, Endep, etc.) is effective in
   preventing all types of chronic headaches: tension headaches, migraine attacks and mixed forms.
2. Effectiveness is not dependent upon the drug's antidepressant action;
   the dose required for headache control is less than the antidepressant
   dose.
3. For migraine patients with sleep problems, the antidepressants of
   choice are amitriptyline, doxepin and trazodone because of their
   sedative effects. The total daily requirement is best given as a single
   dose at bedtime.
4. Desipramine (Norpramin, Pertofrane) is usually considered to have
   the fewest side-effects.

Use of Methysergide
1. While very effective as a migraine preventive, this drug is inherently
   dangerous. It can cause serious and life-threatening adverse effects
   with long-term use: formation of scar tissue (fibrosis) involving the
   heart, lungs, blood vessels and kidneys.

2. It is usually reserved to treat severe migraine that has not responded to safer drugs.
3. Its use should be limited to courses of no more than 4 to 6 months followed by drug-free intervals of 4 to 6 weeks.
4. This drug should not be used in the presence of valvular heart disease or serious blood vessel disorders.
5. The smallest effective dose should be determined; the total daily dosage should not exceed 8 mg.

Use of Ergotamine

1. This is the most effective abortive drug if taken early in the migraine attack; it can relieve the headache in 1 to 2 hours. It tends to be less effective if taken later.
2. It may be taken orally or sublingually in tablet form, rectally in the form of suppositories, by inhalation or by injection.
3. Dosage should be limited to no more than 6 mg/24 hours or 10 mg/week to prevent serious adverse effects. (See Drug Profile.)
4. Avoid concurrent use with dopamine, erythromycins, troleandomycin and beta blockers.
5. Avoid frequent and regular use; this drug can cause dependence (see Glossary). Long-term use on a daily basis can *cause* chronic migrainelike headaches.
6. Ergotamine "rebound" (return and intensification of headache) can be prevented by allowing 48 hours between courses.

Ancillary Drug Treatment (as required)

Condition	Drug Treatment
For nausea and vomiting:	metoclopramide (Reglan)
For preheadache visual disturbances:	nitroglycerin, sublingual isoproterenol (Isuprel), inhalation

Note: Drug selection, dosage and administration schedule must be determined by the physician for each patient individually.

Resource for Additional Information and Services

National Headache Foundation
5252 North Western Avenue
Chicago, IL 60625
Phone: 1-800-843-2256 (outside IL); 1-800-523-8858 (inside IL); (312) 878-5558

Publications available.

MYASTHENIA GRAVIS

Other Names: MG, autoimmune myasthenia gravis, myasthenia gravis pseudoparalytica

Prevalence in USA: Estimated to be 1 in 25,000. Approximately 24,000 documented cases. (Because many mild forms of this disorder are not recognized or reported, it is estimated that the prevalence may approach 100,000.)

Age Group: The autoimmune form of myasthenia gravis (over 90% of all forms of MG) can have its onset at any age from birth to 90 years. 30% of all cases begin in women between puberty and 40 years of age, with the highest incidence in the twenties. 30% of all cases begin in men after the age of 40, with the highest incidence in the fifties.

Male to Female Ratio
   Age of onset under 40 years—1 to 3
   Age of onset 30–50 years—1 to 1
   Age of onset over 40 years—3 to 1

Principal Features: Myasthenia gravis is a chronic disorder of neuromuscular function attributed to the presence of antibodies in the blood that impair the transmission of nerve impulses across the junction of nerve and muscle tissue. The characteristic symptoms are periods of fluctuating fatigue and early exhaustion of affected muscles. Involvement may be restricted to a single muscle group or may gradually expand to affect major muscle groups throughout the body. The first muscles to show abnormal fatigability in 50% of all cases are those of the eye, resulting in drooping eyelids and blurred or double vision; 25% of cases first become aware of weakness while speaking, chewing or swallowing; 20% first notice unusual weakness and fatigue in the arms or legs. The course of the disorder varies greatly from one person to another, but the point of maximal involvement is usually reached within 3 years. Stage 1, the "active" stage, is characterized by increasing disability and fluctuation of symptoms; it may last from 5 to 10 years. Stage 2, the "inactive" stage, is marked by less variation and greater stability. Stage 3, the "burned out" stage, is usually reached 14 to 20 years after the initial onset of symptoms; it generally represents the residual pattern of the disorder that must be managed for the remaining life of the individual. Spontaneous remissions occur in fewer than 10% of cases, and these may last only 2 to 3 years.

Causes: The current belief is that myasthenia gravis is an autoimmune disorder characterized by the formation of antibodies that impair acetylcholine receptors of the nerve-muscle junctions in affected voluntary muscles. Such antibodies are present in 80% to 90% of all MG patients. Their presence implies damage or destruction of receptors by autoimmune complexes. The resulting reduction of available receptors for nerve impulse transmission is responsible for the muscle weakness and easy fatigability that characterize this disorder. The mechanisms responsible for the formation of destructive antibodies are not understood. There is no clear pattern of heredity to account for the development of MG.

Drugs That Can Cause This Disorder: The drug penicillamine (Cuprimine, Depen), used to treat rheumatoid arthritis and Wilson's disease, can cause true myasthenia gravis in about 1% of users.

The following drugs may impair neuromuscular impulse transmission and should be avoided or used with great caution in patients with myasthenia gravis:

antihistamines	morphine
barbiturates	neomycin
beta blocker drugs	opioid analgesics
calcium channel blocker drugs	phenytoin
clindamycin	polymyxin A and B
colistimethate	procainamide
colistin	quinidine
gentamycin	quinine
kanamycin	streptomycin
lidocaine	tranquilizers
lithium	trimethadione
magnesium sulfate	tubocurarine

Drugs Used to Treat This Disorder:
Cholinesterase Inhibitors
* ambenonium (Mytelase).
* neostigmine (Prostigmin).
* pyridostigmine (Mestinon).
Cortisonelike Drug (Corticosteroid)
* prednisone
azathioprine (Imuran)

Goals of Drug Treatment
The primary aim is to minimize disability; cure is not possible.
Prompt determination of the optimal drug regimen for each patient individually.
Smooth control of fluctuating muscle weakness and fatigability; restoration of sustained strength and endurance.
Prevention of both myasthenic crisis and cholinergic crisis.
Achievement of remission of the disease process.

Drug Management
Dosage requirements may vary from day to day, according to the course of the disorder, the physical demands of daily routines, the emotional state of the patient, etc. Doses should be adjusted according to need,

larger doses being taken at times of greatest fatigue—as just before meals, to facilitate eating.

Restoration of muscle strength and endurance beyond 80% of normal status (before MG) is usually not possible. Learn by experience the limit of your response to the drugs that work best for you and do not exceed the optimal dose.

Cholinesterase inhibitors provide only transient symptomatic relief and are of limited usefulness in most cases of moderate to severe MG. They are most useful for nonprogressive eye muscle weakness and mild limb muscle weakness.

Use caution when taking drugs concurrently that can cause low blood potassium levels (hypokalemia). Many diuretics in wide use can cause potassium loss and thereby increase muscle weakness and fatigue.

Use of Cholinesterase Inhibitors

1. These drugs are generally used first to treat the newly diagnosed case of MG. A trial of 1 to 3 months is usually sufficient to determine their effectiveness.
2. The drug of choice must be determined for each patient individually by trial and error, as must the optimal dose and administration schedule.
3. Pyridostigmine (Mestinon) is usually preferred by most patients with ocular or mild nonprogressive MG.
4. These drugs are prone to irregular absorption and consequent variation in therapeutic effect. They are best taken with food to reduce stomach upset.
5. Careful dosage adjustment is mandatory. Underdosage can result in myasthenic crisis. Overdosage can result in cholinergic crisis. Both reactions can cause sudden muscle weakness and be life-threatening if respiration is seriously impaired. Sudden weakness occurring 1 hour after taking medication usually indicates overdosage (cholinergic crisis).
6. After prolonged use, these drugs may lose their effectiveness. Your ability to respond to them can be restored by reducing the dose or withdrawing them for several days. *However, this must be done under the supervision of your physician.*
7. Long-term treatment with high doses of these drugs may itself cause permanent changes in the motor end-plates and adversely affect neuromuscular transmission.

Use of Cortisonelike Drugs (Corticosteroids)

1. These drugs have become more widely used within the past 5 years for treating MG. Some physicians initiate treatment with prednisone if there are no contraindications. The usual course of treatment is 2 years, to minimize the possibility of relapse.
2. Prednisone is given initially in high doses daily until improvement begins, then changed to an alternate-day schedule. With sustained improvement and stabilization of function, the dose is gradually reduced to the smallest effective maintenance level.
3. A trial period of 60 days is usually necessary to determine the effec-

tiveness of prednisone therapy for MG. For those who respond favorably, marked improvement occurs within 3 months and maximal improvement is usually attained within 9 months. Favorable results are reported in 80% of patients, with remissions in 25% to 35%.

4. Significant worsening of symptoms can occur in 48% of patients during the early phase of high-dose prednisone treatment. For this reason a trial of prednisone is best initiated in the hospital.

5. Approximately 90% of patients remain dependent upon long-term prednisone treatment for sustained improvement. Only 10% can withdraw successfully and remain in remission.

6. Observe carefully for the possible development of adverse effects that often accompany long-term use of cortisonelike drugs. See the Drug Profile of Prednisone in Section Three.

7. Some experts now recommend that thymectomy be done in serious cases *before* corticosteroids are used. A consensus is emerging that long-term corticosteroid therapy should be avoided if possible.

Use of Azathioprine (Imuran)

1. It is now felt that azathioprine is significantly less toxic than long-term steroid therapy. It is useful in reducing steroid requirement, and can produce improvement or remission when used alone.

2. It may be used alone or in conjunction with cortisonelike drugs to treat advanced stages of MG with severe disability.

3. For those who respond favorably, improvement usually begins within 3 to 12 months; maximal improvement may require continual treatment for 12 to 36 months. Approximately 53% of patients show some improvement using azathioprine alone, with 40% achieving temporary remission. However, continued improvement usually requires high doses.

4. Only 10% of patients show sustained improvement following discontinuation of this drug.

5. Observe carefully for the development of serious adverse effects. See the Drug Profile of Azathioprine in Section Three.

Ancillary Drug Treatment (as required)

Condition	Drug Treatment
For apathy, lethargy:	ephedrine
For hypokalemia:	potassium supplements (see Drug Profile)
For diarrhea:	diphenoxylate (Imodium)

Note: Drug selection, dosage and administration schedule must be determined by the physician for each patient individually.

Resource for Additional Information and Services

Myasthenia Gravis Foundation
53 West Jackson Boulevard, Suite 1352
Chicago, IL 60604
Phone: (312) 427-6252; 1-800-541-5454

Sponsors 54 state groups and low-cost pharmacy service.

Publications: physicians' and nurses' manuals, patient handbooks, brochures, pamphlets.

OSTEOARTHRITIS

Other Names: Osteoarthrosis, degenerative arthritis, degenerative joint disease, hypertrophic arthritis

Prevalence in USA: 16 million—8.7% of the adult population; 10% of the elderly population.

Age Group: 55 years and over.

Male to Female Ratio: Same incidence in men and women.

Principal Features: Osteoarthritis is the most common joint disease and the major cause of disability of our older population. It is an insidious, slowly progressive deterioration of the surface cartilage on the ends of bones where they come together to form joints. During the early phases of change, there are no symptoms. With progressive destruction of protective cartilage, bone surface becomes exposed and irritated; this results in pain, stiffness and muscle spasm. As the central area of cartilage is destroyed, new bone and cartilage begin to form on the edges of the joint (spur formation). These degenerative changes can start as early as the fourth decade of life; they usually begin to cause symptoms in sixth and seventh decades; by age 75, all individuals have some degree of osteoarthritis in one or more joints. The most commonly involved joints are: fingers, thumb, shoulders, hips, knees, base of the first toe, neck and lower (lumbar) spine. Progressive changes in the weight-bearing joints, principally the lower spine, hips and knees, eventually give rise to pain, deep ache and muscle spasm. Discomfort grows worse after prolonged activity that involves diseased joints.

Causes: There is no apparent initiating cause for primary osteoarthritis. The disorder does have a familial pattern, and it is thought that genetic biochemical defects in cartilage structure predispose some individuals to excessive "wear and tear" deterioration of vulnerable joints. Secondary osteoarthritis is due to congenital joint malformations, joint injuries and infections and other infrequent causes of bone and cartilage deterioration.

Drugs That Can Cause This Disorder: Although some drugs are capable of causing joint aches and pains (e.g., barbiturates, "sulfa" drugs, oral contraceptives, isoniazid, pyrazinamide), no drugs cause the bone and cartilage destruction characteristic of osteoarthritis. Rarely the systemic (internal) use of cortisonelike steroid drugs can cause aseptic necrosis of bone (destruction without infection); this can initiate a secondary form of osteoarthritis.

Drugs Used to Treat This Disorder: There are no drugs that can prevent, halt the progression of or reverse the degenerative changes of osteoarthritis. The following drugs are used to relieve pain, stiffness and muscle spasm.

Nonsteroidal Anti-inflammatory Drugs (NSAIDs)
Salicylates
  • aspirin (Bufferin, Ascriptin, Cama, etc.).
  • aspirin, enteric-coated (Easprin, Ecotrin, etc.).
  • aspirin, zero-order-release (Zorpin).
  • magnesium salicylate (Magan, Mobidin).
  • choline magnesium salicylate (Trisilate).
  • salsalate (Disalcid).
  • diflunisal (Dolobid).
  • sodium salicylate.
Indole Derivatives
  • indomethacin (Indocin).
  • sulindac (Clinoril).
  • tolmetin (Tolectin).
Propionic Acid Derivatives
  • fenoprofen (Nalfon).
  • flurbiprofen (Ansaid).
  • ibuprofen (Motrin, Rufen, Advil, etc.).
  • ketoprofen (Orudis).
  • naproxen (Naprosyn).
  • suprofen (Suprol).
Fenamic Acid Derivatives
  • meclofenamate (Meclomen).
  • mefenamic acid (Ponstel).
Oxicam Derivative
  • piroxicam (Feldene).
Phenylacetic Acid Derivative
  • diclofenac (Voltaren).
Simple Analgesics
  • acetaminophen (Tylenol, Panadol, etc.).
  • propoxyphene (Darvon, etc.).
  • codeine (Tylenol with codeine, etc.).
  • hydrocodone (Vicodin, etc.).
  • oxycodone (Percodan, Percocet, Tylox).
Muscle Relaxants
  • carisoprodol (Soma).
  • cyclobenzaprine (Flexeril).
  • diazepam (Valium).
  • methocarbamol (Robaxin).
  • orphenadrine (Norflex).

Goals of Drug Treatment
Relief of pain and stiffness sufficient to permit continued activity, therapeutic exercise and physiotherapy.

Relief of associated anxiety and/or depression.

Drug Management
General Principles
Osteoarthritis is a chronic but slowly progressive disorder; although there is no curative treatment available, the symptoms are generally mild for long periods of time and can usually be relieved satisfactorily with available drugs.

Nonsteroidal anti-inflammatory drugs (NSAIDs) are the primary drugs of choice for managing osteoarthritis. Their principal actions are within the tissues of the diseased joint.

Simple analgesics, such as propoxyphene, codeine, oxycodone, etc., suppress pain perception in the brain; they are used to supplement the analgesic effects of NSAIDs.

Cortisonelike steroids by mouth should not be used in the management of osteoarthritis. They may be helpful when injected directly into osteoarthritis joints, sometimes providing prompt and lasting relief of pain and swelling. If effective, steroid injections may be repeated at intervals of 4 to 6 months for a limited number of times.

Symptomatic drug treatment will be more effective if it is supplemented by appropriate physiotherapy and the use of physical aids, such as canes, crutches, walkers, railings, etc.

Avoid prolonged and repeated overuse of diseased joints to (1) slow the progression of joint destruction and (2) minimize requirements for analgesic drugs.

Excessive body weight (obesity) can accelerate deterioration of weight-bearing joints. Prudent weight reduction programs are a most important part of treatment for osteoarthritis of the lower spine, hips and knees.

Use of Nonsteroidal Anti-inflammatory Drugs (NSAIDs)
1. These drugs are not thought to be able to favorably influence the natural course of osteoarthritis, but they can relieve pain and inflammation and thereby improve joint function and mobility.

2. Treatment is usually initiated with aspirin (lowest cost). Unfortunately, large doses (2 to 4 tablets of 325 mg each, 3 to 4 times daily) are often necessary to achieve satisfactory relief. The high blood levels required can cause ringing in the ears (tinnitus) and loss of hearing, especially in the elderly. Measurements of salicylate blood levels can be most helpful in establishing correct dosage. (See Therapeutic Drug Monitoring in Section One.)

3. Soluble aspirin preparations (regular aspirin, Bufferin, Ascriptin, etc.) often cause stomach ulceration and bleeding; they should be taken with food to minimize this effect.

4. The preferred forms of aspirin for continual use in large doses in-

clude (1) enteric-coated preparations and (2) zero-order-release tablets. (See list above.)

5. Salicylates other than aspirin can also be used. (See list above.) These cause significantly less stomach irritation; some are effective with twice daily dosage.

6. All NSAID aspirin substitutes are better tolerated than aspirin. However, they may share a cross-sensitivity in individuals who are allergic to aspirin and may induce asthmatic reactions.

7. An NSAID should be used on a regular schedule for a trial period of 3 to 4 weeks; if it is not effective, another one should be tried in sequence (selecting one from a different chemical group). An attempt is made to find the NSAID that provides the best relief with the fewest side-effects.

8. Authorities do not recommend the use of NSAIDs in combination with each other. A small dose of aspirin taken along with an NSAID may provide additional relief of pain.

9. NSAIDs have a potential for injuring the kidney and impairing kidney function. They should be used with caution in individuals over 50 years old, in those with hypertension, diabetes, congestive heart failure and especially in those taking diuretics.

10. NSAIDs can increase the effects of oral antidiabetic drugs (sulfonylureas) and anticoagulants. Dosage adjustments may be necessary.

Use of Narcoticlike Analgesics

1. In advanced cases of osteoarthritis, mild analgesics such as acetaminophen or propoxyphene may not provide adequate pain relief. Codeine, hydrocodone and oxycodone may be tried cautiously on an intermittent schedule to avoid tolerance and dependence.

2. The use of stronger narcotic (opioid) analgesics (morphine, meperidine, etc.) should be avoided completely. Their potential for causing dependence (addiction) precludes repetitious, long-term use in chronically painful disorders like osteoarthritis.

Use of Muscle Relaxants

1. Muscle spasm prevents exercise and use of affected joints. The cautious use of muscle relaxants in conjunction with physiotherapy may be beneficial in preserving joint mobility and muscle strength.

2. Muscle relaxants are most useful in managing osteoarthritis of the lower spine with associated lumbo-sacral muscle spasm.

Ancillary Drug Treatment (as required)

Condition	*Drug Treatment*
For anxiety and/or mild depression:	alprazolam (Xanax), for intermittent, short-term use
For moderate or severe depression:	trazodone (Desyrel) (see Profile of Depression in this section)

For drug-induced
   constipation: docusate with casanthranol (Peri-Colace)

Note: Drug selection, dosage and administration schedule must be determined by the physician for each patient individually.

Resource for Additional Information and Services

Arthritis Foundation
1314 Spring Street, N.W.
Atlanta, GA 30309
Phone: (404) 872-7100
Publications available.

OSTEOPOROSIS

Other Names: Osteopenia, type I postmenopausal or spinal osteoporosis (95% of all cases), type II senile osteoporosis

Prevalence in USA: 24 million—approximately 25% of white women over 60 years of age have osteoporosis; 1.3 million fractures due to osteoporosis occur annually.

Age Group: Type I osteoporosis—50 to 65 years. Type II osteoporosis—65 years and over.

Male to Female Ratio: Much higher incidence in women: 8 to 1.

Principal Features: Osteoporosis is a major disorder of bone in the elderly, occurring most often in postmenopausal women. As ovarian function declines and estrogen is withdrawn, the natural loss of bone mass is accelerated. This eventually weakens bone structure and predisposes to fractures that can result from minimal trauma. Osteoporosis can be localized in a single bone (a leg immobilized in a cast), but it is usually more widely distributed, with most fractures occurring in the spine, wrist and hip. The basic defect is a relative increase in the rate of bone destruction without a compensating increase in the reformation of new bone. There are usually no symptoms prior to the occurrence of a spontaneous or traumatic fracture. A sudden compression fracture of a vertebra in the middle or lower section of the spine can result from such minor strains as bending, lifting or sneezing; it causes immediate pain and disability lasting several weeks. Gradual compression of the vertebrae (usually painless) causes loss of height and the development of a stooped, rounded back ("dowager's hump"). A spontaneous fracture of a hip (femur) can occur on arising from a chair or while walking. Untreated osteoporosis can cause a loss of 30% to 60% of bone mass.

Causes: Primary osteoporosis is a normal consequence of aging. A woman loses approximately 50% of bone mass, and a man approximately 25%, during a normal life span. Type I primary osteoporosis refers to the estrogen withdrawal syndrome following menopause. Type II primary osteoporosis occurs later as a feature of senility. Secondary osteoporosis refers to the bone loss that is associated with other diseases and disorders: hyperthyroidism, hyperparathyroidism, adrenal cortical hormone excess (Cushing's syndrome or drug-induced), multiple myeloma, diabetes, and alcoholism.

Drugs That Can Cause This Disorder:
- Cortisonelike steroids, especially in immobilized women over 50 years of age receiving large doses.
- Heparin, when used in long-term therapy.
- Methotrexate, when used in prepubertal children for long-term therapy.

Drugs Used to Treat This Disorder:
Estrogens ("Natural-type" Estrogens Are Preferred)
- conjugated estrogens (Genisis, Premarin).
- esterified estrogens (Evex, Menest).
- estradiol cypionate (Depo-Estradiol, injection).
- estradiol valerate (Delestrogen, injection).
- estriol (Hormonin, a mixture of estriol, estradiol and estrone).
- piperazine estrone sulfate (Ogen).
- micronized 17-B estadiol (Estrace).
- transdermal estradiol skin patch (Estraderm-50 and 100).

Calcium Preparations
- calcium carbonate (40% calcium) (generic tablets, Alka-2, Biocal, Caltrate, OsCal-500, Tums).
- calcium gluconate (9% calcium) (generic tablets).
- calcium lactate (13% calcium) (generic tablets).
- dibasic calcium phosphate (31% calcium) (generic tablets).

Vitamin D Analogs
- calcifediol (Calderol).
- calcitriol (Rocaltrol).

Other Drugs
- calcitonin (Calcimar).
- fluorides (investigational).

Goals of Drug Treatment
Primary prevention: early initiation of estrogen therapy—during or immediately after menopause—to prevent acceleration of natural bone loss.

Secondary prevention: initiation of estrogen therapy 3 or more years following menopause (after some degree of osteoporosis is present) to arrest or retard progressive bone loss.

Prevention of osteoporosis-related fractures.

Relief of pain and muscle spasm associated with fracture of osteoporotic bone.

Drug Management
General Principles
It is now firmly established that excessive bone loss (osteoporosis) following menopause can be prevented or significantly reduced by the timely
administration of low-dose estrogen.

Accurate assessment of bone mass for the detection of osteoporosis can
be made by quantitative CAT scan of vertebrae and by photon absorpti-
ometry of wrist bones. However, these procedures are expensive and
not generally available.

Currently it is not feasible to screen all postmenopausal women for osteoporosis. To identify those who may benefit from estrogen used preventively, the following "risk factors" characterize the candidates for post-
menopausal osteoporosis:
1. slender build, light-boned, white or Oriental race
2. a sedentary life style or restricted physical activity
3. a family history of osteoporosis (grandmother, mother, aunt or
   sister)
4. a high-protein diet
5. a low-sodium diet (also likely to be a low-calcium diet)
6. lifelong avoidance of dairy products
7. heavy smoking
8. excessive use of antacids that contain aluminum
9. long-term use of cortisonelike steroid drugs
10. habitual use of carbonated beverages
11. excessive consumption of alcohol
12. increased urinary excretion of calcium

Thyroid replacement therapy (in appropriate dosage) may increase bone
loss and predispose to the development of osteoporosis in the vertebrae
of the lower spine. If you are taking a thyroid preparation to correct
hypothyroidism, consult your physician regarding a possible need for
calcium and vitamin D supplements to prevent potential bone loss.

Use of Estrogens
1. Estrogen increases the absorption of dietary calcium and reduces the
   rate of calcium loss from bone. Recent studies have shown that
   estrogen can reduce the risk of hip fractures by as much as 66%.
2. Estrogen does not substantially increase bone mass; it does not enhance restoration of bone following loss.
3. To be effective in preventing significant osteoporosis, estrogen therapy must begin within 3 years after menopause. Available evidence
   seems to indicate that continued protection against the development
   of osteoporosis requires ongoing use of estrogen—probably for life
   by those at risk.
4. Fifty percent of women are protected by 0.3 mg of conjugated estrogens daily; close to 100% are protected by 0.625 mg daily. Your
   physician can advise the dose most appropriate for you.
5. For detailed information regarding the use of estrogen, see the Profile of Menopause in this section and the Drug Profile of Estrogen in
   Section Three.

Use of Calcium Preparations
1. Calcium supplementation of the diet is appropriate for preventing or treating osteoporosis because the calcium content of the diet is usually less than the ongoing requirement for the maintenance of normal bone density. The average dietary intake of calcium by women is 500 to 600 mg daily. The daily requirement for the postmenopausal woman is 1500 to 2000 mg (all sources).
2. There is some evidence that calcium supplements (taken alone) may reduce the rate of bone loss and the incidence of fracture, but further proof is needed. Calcium is most effective when taken in conjunction with vitamin D and estrogen.
3. Supplemental calcium must not be taken in excessive doses. The recommended daily intake of calcium is approximately 1000 mg if taking estrogen and 1500 mg if not taking estrogen.
4. Excessive intake of supplemental calcium (more than 2000 mg daily) can cause abnormal increases in the blood and urine levels of calcium and predispose to kidney stone formation.
5. The most appropriate calcium preparations to use for supplementation are listed above.
6. Calcium supplements made from bone meal or mineral clay (dolomite, montmorillomite) may contain lead or other toxic metals and should be avoided.
7. Calcium supplements may be more effective if taken as a single late-evening dose to suppress the normal nocturnal rise in parathyroid hormone that increases bone loss.
8. Calcium may decrease the effects of aspirin (and other salicylates), calcium channel-blocking drugs, iron and tetracyclines. Do not take calcium preparations within 2 hours of taking other drugs.

Use of Vitamin D Analogs
1. Elderly individuals with osteoporosis who have a normal life style are not likely to a have a vitamin D deficiency; they usually have an adequate supply from their diet and exposure to sunlight.
2. Shut-ins (those confined to home, nursing home or hospital) probably need a supplement of vitamin D. Currently recommended sources include Calderol and Rocaltrol.
3. When vitamin D is used, limit calcium intake to 600 to 700 mg daily to prevent excessive absorption and abnormally high calcium levels in blood and urine.

Use of Calcitonin (a Thyroid Hormone That Reduces Bone Loss)
1. Studies to date show that calcitonin in doses of 100 units daily can produce an increase in total body calcium (99% in bone) after 2 years of treatment. A favorable response was achieved in 70% of users.
2. Calcitonin is given by injection and is used in conjunction with calcium and vitamin D.
3. Studies using other dosage forms of calcitonin—oral, buccal (cheek), intranasal—are under way.

Use of Fluoride
1. The use of fluoride in the prevention and treatment of osteoporosis

is still investigational. Directions for its optimal use have not been established.

2. A dose of 40 to 65 mg/day is required to stimulate bone formation. Adverse effects occur in over 30% of users; these include nausea, stomach pain, gastrointestinal bleeding, bone and joint pain and severe foot discomfort, often intense enought to preclude compliance with treatment.

3. Calcium must always be used concurrently with fluoride to avoid the development of osteomalacia (abnormal mineral composition of bone).

Ancillary Drug Treatment (as required)

Condition	*Drug Treatment*
For calcium-induced constipation:	docusate (Colace, etc.)
	docusate with casanthranol (Peri-Colace, etc.)
For fracture pain:	acetaminaphen with codeine (Tylenol with codeine)
	acetaminophen with propoxyphene (Darvocet-N 100)
	Avoid opiate analgesics stronger than codeine.
For muscle spasm:	diazepam (Valium)
For mild depression:	alprazolam (Xanax), for intermittent, short-term use
For marked depression:	trazodone (Desyrel)

Note: Drug selection, dosage and administration schedule must be determined by the physician for each patient individually.

Resources for Additional Information and Services

National Institute of Arthritis and Musculoskeletal and Skin Diseases
Information Office: Building 31, Room 4C32B
9000 Rockville Pike
Bethesda, MD 20892
Phone: Information Specialist, (301) 496-8188

Handles inquiries on arthritis, bone diseases (including osteoporosis), and skin diseases.

National Osteoporosis Foundation
2100 M Street, N.W., Suite 602
Washington, DC 20037
Phone: (202) 223-2226

Publications available.

A Friend Indeed Publications, Inc.
P. O. Box 515

Place du Parc Station
Montreal, Canada H2W 2P1
Monthly newsletter "A Friend Indeed."

PARKINSON'S DISEASE

Other Names: Paralysis agitans, parkinsonism, parkinsonian syndrome

Prevalence in USA: Approximately 1.5 million—50,000 new cases annually; 1% of the population over 50 years old.

Age Group: 10% of cases under 40 years old; 20% of cases 40 to 50 years old; 70% of cases 50 years old and over. The mean age at onset is 58 to 62 years.

Male to Female Ratio: More common in men, 3 to 2.

Principal Features: Parkinson's disease is a slowly progressive, debilitating disorder of certain brain centers that contribute to the control and regulation of body movement. The earliest symptoms begin very insidiously; one arm or one leg (or the arm and leg on one side) will gradually develop a sense of weakness, retarded movement and stiffness. A fine tremor in a hand or foot will appear in 70% of cases; this occurs at rest and disappears with intentional use of the affected limb and while asleep. Symptoms may remain mild for years or they may progress steadily. Eventually the principal features of the disorder become generalized; the tremor spreads, most of the body musculature becomes rigid, the posture is stooped, movement is slow and jerky, the gait is shuffling and unsteady. Facial expression is lost; the voice grows weak and speech indistinct. Withdrawal and depression may occur as disability advances. Loss of mental acuity occurs in 30% of cases within 7 to 10 years. Currently available drug therapy can slow the progress of the disorder significantly for many, and life expectancy has been extended to equal the norms.

Causes: Primary Parkinson's disease is due to degeneration of the nerve cells in the brain that produce dopamine, one of the major nerve impulse transmitters. In most instances, the initiating cause of the cellular degeneration is unknown. Infrequently a virus infection of the brain (encephalitis) can initiate the degenerative process. Secondary parkinsonism can be caused by hardening of brain arteries, strokes, brain tumors, trauma, carbon monoxide or manganese poisoning and a few rare degenerative disorders of brain tissue.

Drugs That Can Cause This Disorder: The following drugs can block the action of dopamine and cause a form of secondary parkinsonism with features that are indistinguishable from primary Parkinson's disease:

phenothiazines, droperidol, haloperidol, reserpine, chlorprothixene, thiothixene, methyldopa, metoclopromanide, lithium. (See respective Drug Profiles in Section Three or Drug Classes in Section Four.)

Drugs Used to Treat This Disorder:
- levodopa (Dopar, Larodopa).
- levodopa carbidopa (Sinemet).
- levodopa bensarazide (Prolopa in Canada).
- amantadine (Symmetrel).
- anticholinergics (atropinelike drugs): benztropine (Cogentin), diphenhydramine (Benadryl), trihexyphenidyl (Artane).
- bromocriptine (Parlodel).
- pergolide (Permax).
- selegiline (Eldepryl).

New Drugs in Development for Treating This Disorder: Sinemet CR-4, a new slow-release formulation of Sinemet, is now being tested in clinical trials. It is designed to reduce or eliminate the wearing-off phenomenon or end-of-dose failure that some individuals experience with standard Sinemet. Dosing frequency can be reduced by 25% to 50% and fluctuations in drug response minimized or eliminated throughout the day.

Goals of Drug Treatment
Improvement of overall function and mobility.
Reduction of muscular rigidity and tremor.
Reversal of slowed movement.
Improvement of posture, balance, gait, speech and writing.

Drug Management
General Principles
The symptoms of Parkinson's disease are due to a relative increase in the effects of acetylcholine in the brain centers that regulate body movement. The exaggerated acetylcholine effects are the result of a reduced supply of dopamine (primary Parkinson's disease) or to a blocking of dopamine action (drug-induced parkinsonism).
Drugs used to manage parkinsonism utilize three distinct mechanisms of action: (1) anticholinergic drugs reduce the excessive effects of acetylcholine; (2) levodopa is converted to dopamine in the brain, increasing its supply to restore a balance closer to normal; (3) bromocriptine serves as a substitute for dopamine by stimulating its receptor cells directly. Amantadine is thought to have both anticholinergic and direct-stimulating effects.
Appropriate drugs, properly used, can improve function and mobility for significant periods of time; up to 50% of those treated have no major disabilities after 10 years of disease.
The optimal drug program—either one drug used alone or two or more used in combination—is that which provides satisfactory relief of symptoms or the most acceptable compromise between symptom relief

and drug side-effects. (Complete relief of symptoms may not be possible.)

Drug selection and dosage schedules *must be carefully individualized;* adjustments will be necessary throughout the course of this disorder. Daily fluctuations in symptoms and drug responses occur in almost every individual and vary greatly from person to person. A "trial-and-error" process is unavoidable in determining the best drug(s) and the best dosage schedule. For the best treatment results, keep your physician informed regarding all aspects of your response to the drugs prescribed.

Combinations of several drugs taken in small doses are often more beneficial than a single drug taken in large doses.

Use of Levodopa

1. Only 25% of levodopa taken alone by mouth enters the brain. The large doses required to be effective often cause unacceptable side-effects. To prevent this, levodopa is combined with carbidopa; the combination (marketed as Sinemet) permits a 75% dosage reduction of levodopa.

2. Levodopa is the most effective drug available in the USA and has been the drug of choice for managing primary parkinsonism for the past 15 years. Approximately 80% of users achieve 80% improvement in muscular rigidity and retarded movement.

3. Levodopa may be tried at any time during the course of this disorder. It is most effective during the first 2 to 5 years of use. However, authorities differ in their opinions as to the best time to use levodopa. Some advise early use—within the first year of symptoms—to obtain the fullest benefit possible. Others advise later use to delay the onset of side-effects and adverse effects that develop with long-term use of levodopa.

4. Levodopa is more completely absorbed when taken on an empty stomach. However, it may be necessary to take it following food to prevent nausea. If so, avoid meat when possible; proteins can interfere with absorption of levodopa.

5. After a year or more of continual use of levodopa, 80% of users will develop abnormal involuntary movements (dyskinesias) of various muscle groups—jerks and twitches of the head and face or purpose-like movement of the extremities. In 30% of the users these may be severe enough to interfere with normal functioning. They last for a few minutes to several hours and seem to coincide with the times of both high and low blood levels of levodopa.

6. Another 20% of users will experience "on-off" episodes—changes from relatively good function and mobility (drug effects "on") to marked loss of function and mobility (drug effects "off"). To minimize these periods of fluctuating effectiveness, levodopa may be taken in small doses every 1 to 3 hours throughout the day to maintain a more constant blood level.

7. Levodopa can cause a variety of mental disturbances: euphoria, hypomania, depression, confusion, nightmares, vivid hallucinations.

8. Levodopa should not be used concurrently with those antipsychotic drugs that block the action of dopamine; or with monoamine oxidase (MAO) inhibitors that increase the risk of a hypertensive crisis.
9. Some authorities advocate the use of "drug holidays" to reduce the toxic manifestations of levodopa. The very gradual withdrawal and reintroduction of the drug are essential to success.

Use of Amantadine
1. This drug probably releases dopamine from nerve cells and increases its availability. It may also seve as a dopamine substitute and stimulate receptor cells directly. It has anticholinergic effects that contribute to its effectiveness.
2. Amantadine may be tried first in all patients. It can produce a 15% to 25% improvement in 60% of users. A trial period of 1 week is usually adequate; if not beneficial or if mentality is adversely affected, discontinue use.
3. Amantadine may also be used in conjunction with anticholinergics and levodopa. It is usually well tolerated by the elderly.
4. This drug has a low incidence of side-effects. Ankle swelling and a reddish-blue mottling of the arms or legs may occur after 1 month to 1 year of use. These are not serious and are reversible.
5. Doses over 200 mg can cause excitement, increased tremor, jerkiness, insomnia and nightmares in sensitive individuals.
6. Amantadine may lose some of its effectiveness after 6 to 12 weeks of continual use.
7. In very rare cases the long-term use of this drug is associated with the unexpected development of congestive heart failure. If shortness of breath appears during exertion or while lying down or rouses you from sleep, report this promptly.
8. Recent reports indicate that this drug should not be stopped abruptly in the elderly patient (over 70 years of age). Sudden withdrawal can result in the prompt return of parkinsonian features and rapid deterioration.

Use of Anticholinergic Drugs
1. These atropinelike drugs are often used to initiate treatment when symptoms are mild. They can produce a 20% to 30% improvement by suppressing effects due to overactivity of acetylcholine: tremor, excessive salivation, rigidity and slow movement.
2. They may be used alone as long as symptoms remain mild. They may be combined with any of the other drugs used and at any stage of the disorder.
3. These drugs are not well tolerated by individuals over 70 years old. They can provoke latent glaucoma and can aggravate urinary retention in men with prostatism (see Glossary).
4. Unavoidable side-effects include blurring of near vision, dry mouth, constipation and urinary hesitancy. High doses may cause drowsiness, confusion, impaired memory, hallucinations and nightmares.
5. Following long-term use, these drugs must be discontinued very gradually to avoid a dangerous withdrawal syndrome.

Use of Bromocriptine
1. This drug may be used alone but is usually added to the treatment program at a later stage. It is the drug of choice for alleviating the abnormal involuntary movements associated with long-term levodopa use. It can also have a stabilizing effect when the "on-off" effects of levodopa therapy become apparent.
2. Bromocriptine is initiated with very small doses, and the dose is increased very slowly. Some individuals develop extreme hypotension (low blood pressure) with the first doses. It is advisable to try a test dose at bedtime for several days to determine individual blood pressure response.
3. This drug may not be effective in severe Parkinson's disease or in those with a poor response to levodopa.
4. High doses can cause acute personality changes, mood swings and other intolerable adverse effects; 40% of users discontinue this drug because of undesirable reactions.
5. This drug is an ergot derivative; it should be used with caution in the presence of angina, hypertension or any form of peripheral vascular disease.

Current Controversies in Drug Management

The difference of opinion among authorities regarding the best time to begin treatment with levodopa (Sinemet) has not been resolved to date. Those advocating early use—when symptoms are causing only mild disability—argue that the individual's quality of life is significantly improved and that his or her period of productive functioning is prolonged. Those advocating late introduction of levodopa—when symptoms are causing moderate to severe disability—argue that the early use of levodopa hastens the onset of adverse levodopa effects (abnormal involuntary movements, "wearing-off" effects, "on-off" effects). They propose the use of amantadine and/or anticholinergic drugs to manage the early period of mild disability and the later use of levodopa only if and when progression of symptoms requires greater relief. Studies to date have not been sufficiently conclusive to resolve the controversy.

One recently published study, however, does show that levodopa treatment started early (1 to 3 years after the onset of symptoms) significantly reduces mortality rates, especially those related to the disease itself.

Comment: The decision as to when levodopa therapy is to be started must be made jointly by the patient and the physician on an individual, case-by-case basis. The patient should be informed of the issues involved in making the decision and should share the resposibility for making the best decision for all concerned.

Ancillary Drug Treatment (as required)

Condition	*Drug Treatment*
For levodopa-induced drowsiness:	methylphenidate (Ritalin)
For levodopa-induced nausea:	diphenidol (Vontrol)

For action tremor:	propranolol (Inderal)
For muscle spasm and rigidity:	diazepam (Valium)
For nocturnal leg cramps:	quinine (Quinamm) at bedtime
For constipation:	docusate (Colace)
	docusate with casanthranol (Peri-Colace)
For insomnia:	chloral hydrate (Noctec, Somnos)
For ankle swelling:	hydrochlorothiazide (generic)
For depression:	amitriptyline (Elavil)
	desipramine (Norpramin)
	imipramine (Tofranil)
	trazodone (Desyrel)
	fluoxetine (Prozac)
For action tremor (that accompanies resting tremor):	propranolol (Inderal)

Note: Drug selection, dosage and administration schedule must be determined by the physician for each patient individually.

Resources for Additional Information and Services

American Parkinson Disease Association
116 John Street, Suite 417
New York, NY 10038
Phone: 1-800-223-APDA; (212) 732-9550

Available 8:30 a.m.–5:00 p.m. EST, M–F.
Sponsors 35 information and referral centers.
Provides publications, referrals, references and answers to inquiries regarding research and treatment.

Parkinson's Disease Foundation
Columbia Presbyterian Medical Center
640 West 168th Street
New York, NY 10032
Phone: (212) 923-4700; 1-800-457-6676

Local groups: 400.
Serves as a source of information to patients and physicians on all aspects of Parkinson's disease.

United Parkinson Foundation
360 West Superior Street
Chicago, IL 60610
Phone: (312) 664-2344

Serves 38,000 members (patients, family members, medical personnel); publishes reliable information on all aspects of Parkinson's disease.

National Parkinson Foundation
1501 N.W. Ninth Avenue
Miami, FL 33136

Phones: (305) 547-6666
1-800-327-4545
1-800-544-4882 in California
1-800-433-7022 in Florida

Publishes "The Parkinson Handbook: How to Start and Run a Support Group".

PEPTIC ULCER

Other Names: Peptic ulcer disease, duodenal ulcer, gastric ulcer

Prevalence in USA: Approximately 20 million; 10% of the general population will have a symptomatic peptic ulcer sometime during life; 25% of men and 16% of women have scars of peptic ulcer disease on autopsy examination.

Age Group: Duodenal ulcer occurs most commonly between 25 and 40 years. Gastric ulcer occurs most commonly between 40 and 55 years. Of all ulcers, 1.9% occur under 18 years; 43% occur between 18 and 44 years; 36% occur between 45 and 64 years; 12.8% occur between 65 and 74 years; 6.3% occur at 75 years and over.

Male to Female Ratio: Duodenal ulcer: higher incidence in men—2 to 1. Gastric ulcer: same incidence in men and women.

Principal Features: Peptic ulcer disease refers to an intermittent disorder of the stomach and first portion of the small intestine (duodenum) that is characterized by the formation of ulcers in the lining of these organs. The tissues subject to ulceration are constantly bathed in digestive juices produced in the stomach; the principal components of these juices include hydrochloric acid and the digestive enzyme pepsin (hence "peptic" ulcer). Most individuals with peptic ulcer disease produce excessive amounts of acid and pepsin, which overwhelm the normal protection of the lining tissues and cause erosion (ulceration). The singular feature of an active duodenal ulcer is a gnawing or burning pain in the upper mid-abdomen that usually occurs between meals and in the early morning hours—when acid secretion is high. The pain is characteristically relieved by food or antacids. The pattern of pain-food-relief typifies active duodenal ulcer. Episodes of ulcer activation occur unpredictably, but are often more frequent and troublesome in the spring and fall of the year. By nature, peptic ulcer disease is a chronically recurrent disorder. The recurrence rate of duodenal ulcer is approximately 70% within 1 year and 90% within 2 years. Frequent recurrence predisposes to serious complications in 30% of ulcer patients, 10% to 15% will experience bleeding, 5% to 10% will suffer perforation of the duodenal wall and 5% will develop obstruction at the stomach outlet (pylorus) due to the extensive scarring that follows ulcer healing.

Causes: A predisposition to develop peptic ulcer disease appears to be hereditary. The primary initiating cause of ulceration is not known. Those individuals who produce excessive amounts of stomach acid and pepsin are often prone to the development of duodenal ulcer. Others with normal amounts of acid and pepsin develop ulceration because the protective mechanisms in the lining tissues are defective and inadequate. Certain states of physical stress (burns, trauma, surgery) can increase the incidence of peptic ulcer.

Drugs That Can Cause This Disorder: The following drugs can initiate ulceration of the stomach or duodenum in susceptible individuals or aggravate existing ulcers:

alcohol	cortisonelike steroids
aminophylline	phenylbutazone
aspirin and other nonsteroidal anti-inflammatory drugs	reserpine (?)

Drugs Used to Treat This Disorder:
- antacids (Delcid, Maalox TC, Mylanta II, etc.).
- cimetidine (Tagamet).
- famotidine (Pepcid).
- misoprostol (Cytotec). Used for prevention and treatment.
- nizatidine (Axid).
- omepraole (Prilosec).
- ranitidine (Zantac).
- sucralfate (Carafate).
- anticholinergic drugs (Darbid, Pro-Banthine, Robinul) for adjunctive use.

Goals of Drug Treatment
Short-term control of stomach acidity sufficient to relieve pain and promote ulcer healing.
Long-term control of stomach acidity to prevent ulcer recurrence.
Prevention of complications.

Drug Management
General Principles
Most cases of peptic ulcer disease can be managed successfully by appropriate drug therapy. A treatment program of 4 to 6 weeks will heal up to 90% of duodenal ulcers. Surgery is needed only for the management of ulcer complications: uncontrolled bleeding, perforation, obstruction, persistent pain.
The four principal drugs used to promote healing of duodenal ulcer are all equally effective when taken in adequate dosage for 4 to 6 weeks. However, some individuals may respond more favorably to 2 (or more)

drugs used concurrently. In the treatment of gastric ulcer, antacids are less effective than cimetidine, ranitidine, or sucralfate.

Anticholinergic (atropinelike) drugs are used only when ulcer symptoms are not adequately controlled by antacids and/or cimetidine or ranitidine.

Tranquilizers and sedatives should not be used routinely but only as necessary to relieve significant anxiety and nervous tension that could possibly contribute to hyperacidity.

If possible, it is advisable to avoid cortisonelike steroid therapy in the presence of active peptic ulcer or in those individuals who are subject to recurrently active peptic ulcer disease. If steroid treatment is necessary, antacids and/or cimetidine (or ranitidine) should be used protectively.

The chronic use of aspirin (and substitute nonsteroidal anti-inflammatory drugs) increases the chance of developing active peptic ulcer.

Cigarette smoking doubles the chance of developing peptic ulcer disease; it also delays healing significantly.

Caffeine-containing beverages (coffee, tea, cola) can stimulate stomach acid production and aggravate an existing ulcer.

Alcohol (in excess) can aggravate gastric ulcer and increase the risk of bleeding.

Use of Antacids

1. These drugs are used to neutralize stomach acids and thereby (1) relieve pain, heartburn and acid indigestion; and (2) correct hyperacidity and promote ulcer healing.

2. The antacids of choice are composed of magnesium aluminum hydroxide (Delcid, Maalox TC, Mylanta II). The optimal treatment schedule is 1 ounce taken 1 hour and 3 hours after meals and at bedtime until free of pain for 2 weeks; then 1 hour after meals and at bedtime for an additional 4 weeks.

3. Avoid long-term use of aluminum hydroxide and magnesium trisilicate preparations; they may cause depletion of phosphate and increase the risk of osteomalacia (softening of bones).

4. Avoid calcium-containing antacids (Alka-2, Titralac, Tums); these stimulate secretion of gastrin, a stomach hormone that in turn stimulates production of hydrochloric acid and pepsin, referred to as rebound hyperacidity.

5. When practical, antacid liquids (suspensions) are more effective than tablets.

6. Antacids can interfere with the absorption of cimetidine (but not ranitidine), digoxin, iron, isoniazid and tetracyclines.

Use of Histamine (H-2)-Blocking Drugs

1. These drugs reduce the production of hydrochloric acid by blocking the stomach's response to stimulation by histamine. They promote healing of peptic ulcer in 70% to 80% of cases when taken for 4 to 6 weeks.

2. Treatment with one of these drugs alone is a reasonable alternative to high-dose antacid therapy.

3. Cimetidine may cause confusion and unsteadiness in the elderly, especially those with impaired kidney function; infrequently it can cause breast enlargement and impotence in men; it increases the effects of warfarin when taken concurrently.

4. Ranitidine taken in a single dose at bedtime is as effective as other multidose drug regimens for healing peptic ulcer.

5. Ranitidine is less likely to cause confusion, unsteadiness, breast changes or altered sexual functions; in addition, it does not appear to be involved in any significant drug-drug interactions.

6. In the presence of liver disease or impaired liver function, avoid the concurrent use of ranitidine and acetaminophen to reduce the risk of liver toxicity.

7. Drugs of this class taken once daily at bedtime, can reduce the recurrence rate (in 1 year) for duodenal ulcer from 70% to 10%, and for gastric ulcer from 56% to 20%.

Use of Sucralfate

1. This drug is used for short-term (8 weeks') treatment of active duodenal ulcer. It promotes ulcer healing by forming a dense coating over the ulcer that protects it from the erosive action of hydrochloric acid. Its effectiveness is comparable to antacids and histamine blockers (cimetidine and ranitidine) when used alone.

2. Sucralfate should not be used in conjunction with antacids or histamine blockers.

3. Food may impair the effectivemess of sucralfate. The recommended schedule is as follows:

    (1) If other drugs are being used concurrently, take these 1 hour before sucralfate.

    (2) Take sucralfate on an empty stomach, 1 hour before meals and at bedtime.

    (3) Food may be taken 1 hour after sucralfate.

4. This drug is very safe; it has no contraindications and minimal side-effects—constipation (2%).

5. It can interfere with the absorption of tetracyclines and phenytoin.

Current Controversies in Drug Management

Should histamine (H-2)-blocking drugs (see above) be used intermittently or continuously in treating peptic ulcer disease?

Recently completed studies (219 patients followed for 5 years) have shown that continuous treatment with cimetidine (Tagamet) is significantly more effective than intermittent treatment in preventing recurrence of ulcer activity. Current recommendations call for continuous treatment (daily bedtime maintenance dosing) of anyone who has two or more relapses within two years.

Comments: Such long-term treatment must be individualized; consult your physician regarding its advisability for you. The optimal duration of such treatment and the long-term effects of chronic histamine (H-2)-blocking drug use have not been determined.

Ancillary Drug Treatment (as required)

Condition	*Drug Treatment*
For persistant nocturnal ulcer pain:	isopropamide (Combid, Darbid) taken at bedtime
For constipation:	docusate (Colace, etc.)
	docusate with casanthranol (Peri-Colace, etc.)
For anxiety or nervous tension:	buspirone (Buspar)
	diazepam (Valium)
For headache, minor aches and pains:	acetaminophen (Tylenol, etc.)
	propoxyphene (Darvon)
	Avoid aspirin.

Note: Drug selection, dosage and administration schedule must be determined by the physician for each patient individually.

Resources for Additional Information and Services

American Digestive Disease Society
60 East 42nd Street, Room 411
New York, NY 10165

Telecommunications services: Gutline, available to the public every Tuesday evening from 7:30 to 9:00 p.m., EST.
Publications available.

National Ulcer Foundation
675 Main Street
Melrose, MA 02176
Phone: (617) 665-6210
Publication: newsletter concerning peptic ulcer disease.

PSORIASIS

Other Name: Psoriasis vulgaris

Prevalence in USA: 2% to 4% of the white population; less than 1% of the black population. 6% to 7% of individuals with psoriasis have associated arthritis (psoriatic arthritis).

Age Group: The usual onset is between 10 and 40 years of age. However, psoriasis may begin at any age.

Male to Female Ratio: Slightly more common in men in all age groups.

Principal Features: Psoriasis is the most common type of chronic, recurrent scaling dermatitis. It begins gradually, often with one or two small patches, and follows a course of irregular and unpredictable remissions and recurrences throughout life. The characteristic skin change consists of a well-demarcated pink to reddish patch (plaque), one to three inches in size, which is covered almost completely by dry, silvery scales. Removal of the scales exposes numerous small, red bleeding points. Itching, if present at all, is usually mild. The size, number and distribution of the patches varies greatly. They may remain localized to a few small areas or they may spread to involve the entire body surface. The areas most commonly involved include the scalp, back of the neck and the outer surfaces of the arms and legs, especially the elbows, knees and shins. Less commonly psoriasis may involve the eyebrows, armpits, palms of the hands, soles of the feet, finger nails, umbilicus and the anal and genital areas. A rare form may involve the back, hips and thighs. Very rarely patches may occur in the mouth or on the tongue. During remission the patches fade and clear, the skin heals without scarring and there is no alteration of hair in involved areas. Permanent remission is rare. Currently there is no curative treatment, but most cases can be controlled satisfactorily.

Usually the general health is not affected. Infrequently a more serious and extensive form of psoriasis may develop. An acute, generalized, pustular form with fever, weakness and systemic debility can occur. Another unusual type causes extensive inflammation and peeling of the skin. Approximately 7% of cases will develop a form of arthritis that resembles rheumatoid arthritis; this varies in severity from relatively mild to permanently disabling.

Causes: The primary, fundamental cause is unknown. Psoriasis is a genetically determined, hereditary defect of the factors that regulate skin growth. The characteristic scaly patch is caused by a ten-fold increase in the turnover rate of the surface cells of the skin. Precipitating factors that can "trigger" the development of psoriasis plaques include excessive sunburn, acute respiratory infections (such as "strep" throat), local injury to the skin, surgical incisions and vaccination.

Drugs That Can Cause This Disorder: Drugs cannot cause or initiate psoriasis in an individual with normal skin (hereditary defect absent). However, a few drugs can exacerbate existing psoriasis. These include beta blockers, chloroquine, hydroxychloroquine, lithium, quinidine and the withdrawal of cortisonelike drugs.

Drugs Used to Treat This Disorder: Lubricants: lotions, creams, ointments; used to reduce water loss from psoriasis plaques. Examples: Lac-Hydrin, Moisturel lotion, Eucerin Creme, Aquaphor Creme, Vaseline Petroleum Jelly.

Keratolytic agents: used to remove scale. Examples: 6% salicylic acid (Keralyt Gel), 10% to 20% urea in petrolatum.

Coal tar preparations: used with and without ultraviolet light. Examples: Aquatar, Estar, Fototar, psoriGel, P&S Plus.

Anthralin preparations: used with and without ultraviolet light. Examples: Dithroceme, Lasan.

Cortisonelike preparations: topical creams, gels and ointments for local use. Examples: Aristocort, Cyclocort, Diprolene, Kenalog, Lidex, Topicort, Valisone, others.

Psoralen preparations: used with ultraviolet light. Example: methoxsalen, topical and oral forms.

Methotrexate: see Drug Profile, Section Three.

Etretinate: see Drug Profile, Section Three.

Fish oil containing eicosapentanoic acid (EPA): for relief of itching and inflammation.

New Drugs in Development for Treating This Disorder:

Vitamin A derivatives similar to etretinate and isotretinoin are currently under investigation.

Cyclosporine, a drug in current use to prevent rejection in organ transplant surgery, appears to be effective for psoriasis when used in small doses; this use is currently under investigation. It can cause dramatic clearing of generalized psoriasis, but its long-term adverse effects preclude its use except in very severe and resistant cases.

Goals of Drug Treatment

Acceleration of clearing of active plaques; this can usually be achieved in close to 90% of cases.

Prevention of recurrence of plaques; while remissions of several months can be achieved, permanent remission is not possible with currently available drugs.

Drug Management

Topical Use of Drugs

1. Coal tar preparations: method of action is not fully known. Available in solutions, bath oils, shampoos, lotions and ointments.

   When used in conjunction with ultraviolet light (UVL), they can produce remissions lasting 6 to 12 months.

   Can cause burning, stinging reactions ("tar smarts") in skin on exposure to sun or large doses of UVL.

2. Anthralin preparations: interfere with DNA synthesis and skin cell reproduction.

   Available in creams, ointments and paste.

   Apply only to psoriasis plaques; can irritate normal skin and stain it brown.

   More effective when used in conjunction with UVL.

3. Cortisonelike preparations for local use: reduce inflammation, swelling and itching of psoriasis plaques.

   These are the drugs most commonly used in the current management of mild to moderate psoriasis.

   Available in lotions, creams and ointments. Lotions are preferred for treating the scalp; creams are preferred for treating the armpits and groin; ointments are preferred for remaining skin areas. The ointment is more effective when used under occlusive dressings.

These drugs are used primarily when (1) the skin is "sore" and vulnerable to the irritant effects of other drugs; (2) other drugs are unacceptable for cosmetic reasons; (3) results with coal tar or anthralin preparations alone are unsatisfactory.

Prolonged use without interruption can cause skin atrophy and loss of drug effectiveness.

Possible side-effects: rosacealike skin changes, excessive hair growth (at point of application), lowered resistance to infection, systemic absorption, glaucoma (when applied around eyes).

Systemic Use of Drugs
1. Psoralens: inhibit DNA synthesis and suppress skin cell reproduction.

   Available as methoxsalen and trioxsalen for both local and systemic use.

   These are photosensitizing drugs and are used in conjunction with ultraviolet light in the A range; the combined treatment program is referred to as PUVA. The drug is taken orally 2 hours before UVL exposure; food impairs absorption and should be avoided. Treatments are given 2 to 4 times per week until the skin is clear. Maintenance treatment is given every 1 to 3 weeks to prevent recurrence. Protective glasses should be worn during treatment and for 8 hours following treatment to prevent cataracts.

   Side-effects include itching, nausea and accelerated aging of the skin.

   When properly used, this form of treatment produces improvement in 2 to 3 weeks and clearance of plaques within 1 to 3 months in 75% to 80% of cases.
2. Methotrexate: reduces the turnover rate of superficial skin cells.

   This drug is reserved for use in treating severe, resistant cases of psoriasis, especially the generalized pustular forms and those with chronic extensive plaque formation that have not responded to safer treatment measures. It may also be beneficial in cases of psoriatic arthritis.

   This drug can be highly effective. However, it has very serious potential toxicity. It can depress bone marrow function, damage liver tissue and impair kidney function.

   Avoid alcohol, aspirin and aspirin substitutes while taking this drug.

   See the Drug Profile in Section Three for a complete discussion.
3. Etretinate:

   This vitamin A derivative may be used alone or in conjunction with other appropriate treatments, especially PUVA. It provides excellent relief in severe pustular psoriasis and when there is involvement of the palms and soles.

   This drug should be used only to treat severe, resistant forms of psoriasis that have failed to respond to standard treatments. It can cause major birth defects, significant elevations of blood triglycerides and toxic effects on bone marrow, liver and kidney tissue.

See the Drug Profile in Section Three for a complete discussion.

Current Controversies in Drug Management

Should doses of psoralen and ultraviolet light (PUVA) and the duration of treatment be reduced to lessen the long-term risk of developing skin cancer?

Comments: PUVA treatment is an established, highly effective therapy for severe psoriasis. The best results are obtained when relatively high doses and extended treatment periods are used. Two recently published research reports demonstrate a significantly increased risk of developing two types of skin cancer five years after initial treatment with PUVA. The risk for squamous cell skin cancer was 12 times greater for those who received over 260 PUVA treatments than for those who received 160 or fewer treatments. The risk for basal cell skin cancer was moderately increased and also dose-related. It is recommended that PUVA treatment dosage be reduced by alternating it with other treatment methods, even if this means less than complete clearing of the skin.

Ancillary Drug Treatment (as required)

Condition	Drug Treatment
For itching:	hydroxyzine (Atarax, Vistaril)

Note: Drug selection, dosage and administration schedule must be determined by the physician for each patient individually.

Resources for Additional Information and Services

National Institute of Arthritis and Musculoskeletal and Skin Diseases
Information Office: Building 31, Room 4C32B
9000 Rockville Pike
Bethesda, MD 20892
Phone: Information Specialist, (301) 496-8188

Handles inquiries on arthritis, bone diseases, and skin diseases (including psoriasis).

National Psoriasis Foundation
6443 S.W. Beaverton Hwy, Suite 210
Portland, OR 97221
Phone: (503) 297-1545

Patient-oriented publications and services.

Psoriasis Research Association
107 Vista del Grande
San Carlos, CA 94070
Phone: (415) 593-1394

Publications available.

Psoriasis Research Institute
600 Town and Country Village
Palo Alto, CA 94301
Phone: (415) 326-1848

Maintains Psoriasis Medical Center providing advanced treatment programs.

Publications available.

RHEUMATOID ARTHRITIS

Other Names: Atrophic arthritis, chronic inflammatory arthritis, proliferative arthritis

Prevalence in USA: Approximately 7 million—2% to 3% of the general population.

Age Group: Affects all ages—infancy to senescence. Usual onset is between 20 and 50 years. Mean age at onset is 30 to 40 years.

Male to Female Ratio: In 20-to-50-year age group—more common in women, 3 to 1. Over 50 years—same incidence in men and women.

Principal Features: Rheumatoid arthritis is a highly complex inflammatory disorder that can affect several systems of the body simultaneously. It is quite variable in its manifestations: it may last a few days or up to 50 years; it may affect a single joint or up to 60 joints; it may involve the skin, the eyes, the nervous system, the lungs, the heart and blood vessels and the spleen; it can be mild, moderately severe or life-threatening in its most virulent forms. It usually begins with fatigue, poor appetite, loss of weight, morning stiffness and joint pains. Initially the small joints of the hands, wrists and feet are affected; larger joints may be affected later. The painful and destructive disease of the joints is the major feature of this disorder. The disease process begins with a severe inflammation of the joint lining (synovial membrane). This is followed by the formation of thick granulation tissue that ultimately destroys joint cartilage, bone and adjacent ligaments. The affected joints are swollen, warm, tender, stiff and painful to use; after a sustained period of active disease, joint destruction results in irreversible deformity. All of the joints that are affected will show evidence of disease within the first 2 years. Ten percent of cases will have a spontaneous complete remission (recovery) within 6 to 24 months after the onset of symptoms.

Causes: A specific definitive cause for rheumatoid arthritis has not been established. However, there is evidence to support the theory that the disease process is initiated by a virus that infects the joints of individuals who are genetically susceptible because of a defective immune system.

Drugs That Can Cause This Disorder: There are no drugs that induce true rheumatoid arthritis. The following drugs may aggravate an active or latent arthritis: iron dextran, isoniazid and pyrazinamide (in combination), oral contraceptives (?).

Drugs Used to Treat This Disorder: There are no drugs that can cure rheumatoid arthritis. The drugs currently available for use in managing this form of arthritis fall into 2 groups: (1) those that relieve symptoms but do not alter the basic disease process—do not produce remission; (2) those that may retard or arrest the disease and initiate remission.

Drugs Used to Relieve Symptoms
  Salicylates
- aspirin (Bufferin, Ascriptin, Cama, etc.).
- aspirin, enteric-coated (Easprin, Ecotrin, etc.).
- aspirin, zero-order-release (Zorprin).
- magnesium salicylate (Magan, Mobidin).
- choline magnesium salicylate (Trisilate).
- salsalate (Disalcid).
- diflunisal (Dolobid).
- sodium salicylate (Pabalate).

  Other Nonsteroidal Anti-inflammatory Drugs (NSAIDs)
  Indole derivatives:
- indomethacin (Indocin).
- sulindac (Clinoril).
- tolmetin (Tolectin).

  Propionic acid derivatives:
- fenoprofen (Nalfon).
- flurbiprofen (Ansaid)
- ibuprofen (Motrin, Rufen, etc.).
- ketoprofen (Orudis).
- naproxen (Naprosyn).
- suprofen (Suprol).

  Fenamic acid derivative: meclofenamate (Meclomen).
  Oxicam derivative: piroxicam (Feldene).
  Phenylacetic acid derivative: diclofenac (Voltaren).

  Cortisonelike Steroid Drugs
- prednisone.
- triamcinolone (Aristocort).
- dexamethasone (Decadron).
- methylprednisolone (Medrol).

  Immunosuppressive Drugs
- azathioprine (Imuran).
- chlorambucil (Leukeran).
- cyclophosphamide (Cytoxan).
- methotrexate (Mexate).

Drugs Used to Produce Remission
  Gold Preparations
- auranofin (Ridaura).

- aurothioglucose (Solganal).
- gold sodium thiomalate (Myochrysine).

hydroxychloroquine (Plaquenil)

penicillamine (Cuprimine, Depen)

Goals of Drug Treatment

Relief of pain, tenderness and stiffness.

Control of inflammation in joint tissues.

Production of remission; arrest of active disease.

Prevention of joint destruction; preservation of joint function.

Drug Management

General Principles

Rheumatoid arthritis can be the most difficult of all arthritic disorders to control; in its more severe forms, it is the most damaging to joint tissues. Its course is usually intermittent to chronic. No cure is known.

If the diagnosis is made early, and if adequate treatment is started promptly, severe crippling can often be prevented or minimized.

Every case of rheumatoid arthritis is a unique, individual problem; successful management depends upon a treatment program that is carefully individualized.

Many drugs are available to treat rheumatoid arthritis. None is curative, and none is effective in all cases. Drugs that control inflammation can provide symptomatic relief but do not modify the underlying disease process; they cannot induce a remission. Disease-altering drugs are used in an attempt to modify the actual disease process and thereby initiate a remission. If successful, maintenance drug treatment may be continued for months or years.

Treatment is usually started with the safest and best tolerated drugs. There is marked individual variation in response to most drugs; this is very apparent with the use of the nonsteroidal anti-inflammatory drugs (aspirin substitutes). Trial-and-error experimentation is necessary to find the most effective and acceptable anti-inflammatory drug for each person.

Drug treatment of rheumatoid arthritis often requires a combination of drugs. The more severe forms of this arthritis respond more favorably when a disease-modifying drug is added to an established program of salicylates or NSAIDs. (See drugs listed above.)

Use of Salicylates

1. Aspirin is often the first drug used to provide adequate anti-inflammatory effects; it must be taken in large doses. A trial of salicylates is indicated in all cases of rheumatoid arthritis. (Avoid if there is a history of aspirin allergy, peptic ulcer disease, gastritis or gastrointestinal bleeding.)
2. Aspirin preparations that are designed for absorption in the small intestine (instead of in the stomach) are preferred: Disalcid, Easprin, Ecotrin, Zorprin.
3. The measurement of salicylate blood levels is advisable to determine

the optimal dose of the salicylate used and to avoid serious toxicity.
4. Warning symptoms of early salicylate toxicity are ringing in the ears (tinnitus) and loss of hearing. However, these may not occur in the very young or in the elderly.
5. Approximately 50% of patients cannot tolerate the large doses of aspirin required to achieve adequate anti-inflammatory effects. Other salicylates may be tried or a nonsteroidal anti-inflammatory drug may be substituted.

Use of Other Nonsteroidal Anti-inflammatory Drugs (NSAIDs)
1. These may be used as substitutes for aspirin by those who cannot tolerate (or should not take) salicylates; or they may be used to initiate treatment at the outset.
2. As a group, the NSAIDs are not superior to salicylates in anti-inflammatory effect, but they are generally better tolerated.
3. These drugs produce significant decrease in morning stiffness, improve comfort and function and may be more effective than aspirin for some.
4. Fenoprofen and naproxen are among the more active NSAIDs; a trial of 2 weeks will identify those who can respond favorably.
5. Response to NSAIDs is highly variable from person to person. If an NSAID from one chemical class proves to be ineffective or unacceptable, a drug from another class within the NSAID group should be tried. A trial of 2 weeks is usually adequate to determine effectiveness and tolerance. (See drugs listed above.)

Use of Cortisonelike Steroid Drugs
1. Steroids are used infrequently and for short periods of time in both acute and chronic stages of rheumatoid arthritis. They are always added to existing drug programs as needed. Their use is justified, in small doses, to control acute "flares" of inflammation that prevent any degree of mobility in severly diseased joints.
2. Steroids provide a powerful anti-inflammatory effect, but they do not alter the underlying disease process or induce remission. They should be used to provide short-term comfort as necessary but not to abolish all symptoms.
3. Long-term maintenance use of steroids—even in small doses—must be avoided. Risks of excessive use include cataracts, osteoporosis, muscle wasting, atherosclerosis.

Use of Immunosuppressive Drugs
1. These highly toxic and hazardous drugs are used only when arthritis activity persists in spite of combined treatment with NSAIDs and disease-modifying agents. They are used in an attempt to prevent further joint destruction, deformity and disability.
2. Cyclophosphamide is the most effective drug of this group. Its use is reserved for patients with disabling systemic complications of rheumatoid arthritis.
3. Methotrexate is often the first choice of this group to try in the treatment of severe rheumatoid arthritis that has not responded to

conventional therapy. In low dosage it can be very effective in approximately 50% of patients. Potential risks include severe depression of the bone marrow, liver damage, ulceration of the mouth and intestine and birth defects. Avoid alcohol and salicylates during methotrexate therapy.

Use of Gold Preparations
1. Based upon long experience with its use, gold is the standard disease-modifying drug for treating rheumatoid arthritis. It is often the first choice to add to an established program of NSAID therapy.
2. Gold is used only when arthritis cannot be controlled with safer drugs. A trial of 6 months or longer is necessary to determine its ability to induce remission. Approximately 50% of patients respond favorably.
3. Risks of gold therapy include dermatitis, kidney damage and blood cell and bone marrow toxicity. Treatment should be stopped immediately if any of the following develop: skin rash, mouth ulcers, fever, sore throat, abnormal bleeding or bruising.

Use of Hydroxychloroquine
1. This drug is used to treat mild or moderately severe rheumatoid arthritis. It can be very effective in some cases, relieving symptoms and retarding disease activity.
2. A trial of 6 months is necessary to determine this drug's ability to induce remission.
3. After 1 year of continual use, this drug can (rarely) damage eye structures and impair vision. Corneal deposits, retinal pigmentation and optic neuritis have been reported. The estimated incidence is 1 in 1000 to 1 in 2000 patients.
4. Other possible adverse drug effects include skin rash, abnormally low white blood cell count and peripheral neuritis (see Glossary).
5. This drug can aggravate existing psoriasis.

Use of Penicillamine
1. This drug is an effective substitute for gold therapy when a disease-modifying drug is needed.
2. A trial of 6 to 12 months is necessary to determine its ability to induce remission.
3. For maximal effectiveness, this drug should be taken on an empty stomach.
4. This is a potent drug; it can cause the following adverse effects: dermatitis, kidney damage, blood cell and bone marrow toxicity, bronchiolitis (dry cough and shortness of breath) and a pattern of muscular weakness similar to myasthenia gravis.

Ancillary Drug Treatment (as required)

Condition	*Drug Treatment*
For additional analgesia:	propoxyphene (Darvon)
	hydrocodone (Vicodin) (for short-term, intermittent use only)

For night pain:	indomethacin (Indocin) (taken with food at bedtime)
For anemia:	iron preparations folic acid (if appropriate for type of anemia)
For anxiety and tension:	diazepam (Valium)
For depression:	tricyclic antidepressants (see Profile of Depression in this section)
For drug-induced peptic ulcer:	cimetidine (Tagamet) famotidine (Pepcid) nizatidine (Axid) ranitidine (Zantac) (see Profile of Peptic Ulcer in this section)

Note: Drug selection, dosage and administration schedule must be determined by the physician for each patient individually.

Resources for Additional Information and Services

American Juvenile Arthritis Organization
1314 Spring Street
Atlanta, GA 30309
Phone: (404) 872-7100
Publications available.

Arthritis Foundation (parent organization)
1314 Spring Street
Atlanta, GA 30309
Phone: (404) 872-7100
Publications available.

SCHIZOPHRENIA

Other Name: Dementia praecox

Prevalence in USA: Approximately 2.4 million—1% of the general population; 100,000 new cases annually.

Age Group: Onset most common between 16 and 25 years of age. Onset uncommon after 30 and rare after 40 years of age.

Male to Female Ratio: Equal incidence in men and women.

Principal Features: Schizophrenia refers to a group of disorders of the brain manifested by severe disturbances of the mind and personality. Cardinal features are abnormal thinking, behavior and mood; the schizophrenic pattern is characterized by misinterpretation of reality, withdrawal, delusions, hallucinations (usually auditory), bizarre or regressive behavior. It usually begins early in life, may be mild and transient in nature or may develop into a psychosis of major dimension that is intermittent or chronic for life. The first group—referred to as schizophreniform—experiences one episode of varying severity (often in response to stress), responds well to treatment and has no relapse after treatment is stopped. The second group—classical chronic schizophrenia—experiences recurrent episodes of disabling symptoms that require long-term antipsychotic drug therapy for control. Most of this group will relapse if maintenance treatment is stopped. A variety of subtypes are identified according to their dominant features: delusions of persecution and grandeur (paranoid type); primitive mentality, markedly disorganized thought and behavior (hebephrenic type); withdrawn, negativistic, uncommunicative, apathetic behavior pattern (catatonic); disorganized thinking, delusions, hallucinations accompanied by either mania or depression (schizo-affective); insidious loss of motivation and ambition, avoidance of interpersonal relationships (simple type); mixed or indefinite symptom complex (undifferentiated type). Though the presentations may vary according to type, the same group of antipsychotic drugs is used to treat all types without distinction.

Causes: The fundamental cause of schizophrenia is unknown. No anatomical or biochemical abnormality of the brain has been identified. Studies suggest that a genetic predisposition is necessary for the development of schizophrenia, rendering the subject vulnerable to disturbances of neurochemical transmission of nerve impulses or to alterations of brain circuitry. Effective antipsychotic drugs block dopamine receptors in certain brain cells; this suggests that increased dopamine activity is somehow responsible for the schizophrenic syndrome.

Drugs That Can Cause This Disorder: The following drugs may aggravate existing schizophrenia or produce schizophrenialike symptoms in normal individuals:

albuterol
alcohol (intoxication)
amantadine
amphetamines (abuse)
anticonvulsants
apomorphine
atropinelike drugs
bromides
bromocriptine
cimetidine
cocaine

cortisonelike steroids
digitalis
disopyramide
disulfiram (toxicity)
indomethacin
isoniazid
levodopa
methyldopa
propranolol
tocainide
triazolam

Drugs Used to Treat This Disorder:
Phenothiazines

Aliphatic type:
- chlorpromazine (Thorazine)

Piperidine type:
- thioridazine (Mellaril)
- mesoridazine (Serentil)

Piperazine type:
- perphenazine (Trilafon)
- trifluoperazine (Stelazine)
- fluphenazine (Prolixin, Permitil)

Thioxanthenes
- thiothixene (Navane).

Butyrophenones
- haloperidol (Haldol).

Dibenzoxazepines
- loxapine (Loxitane).

Dihydroindolones
- molindone (Moban).

Goals of Drug Treatment

Good control of symptoms with the lowest possible dose of antipsychotic drug.

Determination of the most effective drug and dosage schedule for each individual: intermittent dosage (as needed) versus continual long-term dosage.

Prevention of relapse (recurrent psychotic episode).

Improvement of capacity to function in society as normally as possible.

Drug Management

General Principles

The primary management of schizophrenia is based upon the rational use of antipsychotic drugs. Psychotherapy and drug therapy are considered to be complementary; psychotherapy can improve the patient's social adjustment; drug therapy can control disabling symptoms and make the situation somewhat manageable. Drug therapy is not curative.

If appropriate drug treatment is started early, 30% to 50% of patients will have a satisfactory remission; another 30% will improve sufficiently to live outside of a hospital. Drug therapy can abolish delusions, hallucinations, hyperactivity and combative behavior. Approximately 10% to 20% of patients do not respond to any drugs currently available.

The initial treatment of an acute psychotic episode consists of a course of carefully selected antipsychotic drugs taken for 6 to 12 months. Many individuals will respond favorably to one drug and not at all to another. History of previous drug use and response can be very helpful in selecting a drug for the management of recurrent episodes.

Current practice is to attempt withdrawal of antipsychotic drugs from all patients who have had a good response to drug treatment during their first episode of schizophrenia. This allows identification of those who will have a self-limited type of schizophrenia (schizophreniform disorder) and will do well without maintenance drug therapy. From 15% to 30% of patients will recover spontaneously following the initial episode and drug withdrawal. Antipsychotic drugs should be discontinued gradually over a period of 1 to 2 weeks.

The majority of schizophrenic patients will require continual drug therapy for long periods of time—possibly for life. Many will relapse rapidly and severely after drugs are discontinued. The nature of the drug maintenance program is determined by the type and frequency of continuing psychotic symptoms and the pattern of relapses experienced by each individual. When the patient complies well, maintenance drug therapy is successful in 85% of cases.

The principal action of antipsychotic drugs is to block dopamine receptors in the brain. By blocking dopamine action in the mesolimbic system, the drugs control the abnormal manifestations of schizophrenia; by blocking dopamine action in the nigrostriatal system, the drugs cause parkinsonism (and related adverse effects). Thus parkinsonism is now recognized as an *unavoidable* side-effect of most antipsychotic drugs. It is usually very responsive to the anticholinergic drugs used to treat Parkinson's disease, but not to levodopa. (See Profile of Parkinson's Disease in this section.)

It is generally recommended that antiparkinsonism drugs *not* be used routinely while taking antipsychotic drugs. Reasons given are: (1) antiparkinsonism drugs can produce toxic brain syndromes; (2) they can interfere with the effectiveness of antipsychotic drugs; (3) they may increase the risk of developing tardive dyskinesia.

Tardive dyskinesia (see Glossary) is one of the most serious adverse effects of long-term antipsychotic drug use. The reported incidence ranges from 3% after 1 year of medication to 21% after 7 years of medication. It appears to occur more frequently in elderly women.

"Drug holidays" of 4 to 6 weeks without medication are being used by some physicians treating chronic schizophrenia to reduce the risk of developing tardive dyskinesia. Among those who have been on maintenance therapy for 1 year without relapsing, 66% will not relapse within 6 months after stopping medication. For this group of patients, a "drug holiday" is feasible and possibly beneficial.

Antipsychotic drugs usually improve behavior. However, excessively high doses can cause a toxic state that worsens behavior. Drug response and tolerance vary greatly from person to person and must be monitored carefully in each individual.

Patients with schizo-affective disorders will probably require an antipsychotic drug and an additional drug for the affective component; this could be either lithium or an antidepressant.

Lithium may aggravate the neurological complications of antipsychotic drug therapy. The concurrent use of these two drugs requires caution and careful monitoring.

Use of Phenothiazines

1. Because of its numerous side-effects, chlorpromazine (the first phenothiazine) is used less frequently.
2. Because of its relatively greater sedative effects, thioridazine is fa-

vored for treatment of acute psychotic episodes. It causes parkinsonism (and possibly tardive dyskinesia) less frequently.
3. Fluphenazine is less sedating but is thought to have a higher risk for
causing parkinsonism and tardive dyskinesia.
4. Trifluoperazine is thought to be preferable for the elderly schizophrenic because it has less sedative and atropinelike side-effects.

Use of Thiothixene
1. This antipsychotic drug is thought to be more effective for the retarded and regressed schizophrenic.
2. Because of its mild antidepressant effect, this drug is preferred for
the schizo-affective patient who has features of depression.
3. This drug has less sedative and atropinelike side-effects, but a higher
risk for causing parkinsonism.

Use of Haloperidol
1. This drug is reported to be effective in patients who are not responsive to chlorpromazine.
2. It can control aggressive behavior without causing significant sedation.
3. Although it has a relatively high potential for causing parkinsonism
(and related effects), it is useful in the elderly because it is less sedating and has fewer atropinelike side-effects.

Use of Loxapine
1. This drug is especially useful in treating the paranoid schizophrenic.
2. It is less sedating than chlorpromazine and equal to haloperidol in
effectiveness.

Use of Molindone
1. This is the only antipsychotic drug that appears to contribute to
weight loss; many antipsychotic drugs tend to promote weight gain.
2. This drug is as effective as other major antipsychotics and is less
sedating than many.

Current Controversies in Drug Management

Is "low-dose" antipsychotic drug therapy feasible for maintenance following release from the hospital?

The vast majority of schizophrenic individuals will experience a return
of symptoms shortly after discontinuing a stabilizing maintenance
dose of effective medication. Conventional practice has not favored
reduction of dosage that proved effective for long-term maintenance.
Recent studies have shown that many responsive and stabilized schizophrenic patients can be maintained satisfactorily at home (following
hospital discharge) with one-fifth of the usually prescribed dose of
injectable, long-acting fluphenazine: 5 mg every 2 weeks instead of the
standard 25 mg dose. Patients on low-dose maintenane therapy adjusted better to family and work situations, were less apathetic and
experienced fewer adverse drug effects. The lower dosage may also
reduce the potential for the development of tardive dyskinesia (see
Glossary).

Ancillary Drug Treatment (as required)

Condition	*Drug Treatment*
For anxiety:	buspirone (Buspar)
For depression:	see Profile of Depression in this section
For insomnia:	chloral hydrate (Noctec, etc.)
	temazepam (Restoril)
For constipation:	docusate (Colace, etc.)
	docusate with casanthranol (Peri-Colace)
For parkinsonism:	benztropine (Cogentin)
	trihexyphenidyl (Artane)
For akathisia (marked restlessness):	propranolol (Inderal)
	diphenhydramine (Benadryl)

Note: Drug selection, dosage and administration schedule must be determined by the physician for each patient individually.

Resources for Additional Information and Services

American Schizophrenia Association
900 North Federal Highway, Suite 330
Boca Raton, FL 33432
Phone: 1-800-847-3802; (407) 393-6167

State groups: 35. Publications available.

National Mental Health Association
1021 Prince Street
Alexandria, VA 22314
Phone: (703) 684-7722

State groups: 650
Publications: *FOCUS*; also provides pamphlets and films.

National Mental Health Consumers' Association
213 Monroe Street
Rockville, MD 20850

Publications available.

Schizophrenics Anonymous
1209 California Road
Eastchester, NY 10709
Phone: (914) 337-2252

Twenty-five local groups. A self-help organization sponsored by the American Schizophrenia Association. Conduct meetings for discussion of all aspects of managing and coping with schizophrenia.

ULCERATIVE COLITIS

Other Names: Idiopathic proctocolitis, inflammatory bowel disease

Prevalence in USA: 1 million (includes 100,000 children); 15,000 new cases annually.

Age Group: Peak incidence occurs between 19 and 49 years of age; 75% of cases develop before the age of 40.

Male to Female Ratio: Same incidence in men and women.

Principal Features: Ulcerative colitis is a chronically recurrent disorder of the colon (large intestine) and rectum characterized by inflammation and ulceration. Its course follows a pattern of frequent spontaneous remissions and recurrences without apparent cause. It may be associated with disease in other organs of the body, notably the skin, joints, eye, liver and blood vessels, making it a multiple system disorder. The principle symptoms of the diseased colon are abdominal cramping and bloody diarrhea; associated symptoms include fatigue, weakness, occasional low-grade fever, weight loss, anemia and dehydration. The more severe forms of ulcerative colitis can be very difficult to control.

Causes: The basic cause of ulcerative colitis is not known. Theories of possible causes include infection, environmental toxins, psychological stress, sensitivities to foods and "autoimmunity"—a disorder of the immune system that results in the selective destruction of body tissues. There is some evidence that indicates a familial pattern, suggesting a hereditary susceptibility to a causative agent.

Drugs That Can Cause This Disorder: No drugs initiate true ulcerative colitis. However, the following anti-infective drugs can cause pseudomembranous colitis, a disorder that closely resembles an acute attack of ulcerative colitis:

amoxicillin
ampicillin
cephalosporins
chloramphenicol
clindamycin
lincomycin

penicillin
tetracycline
trimethoprim and
   sulfamethoxsazole in
   combination

Drugs Used to Treat This Disorder:
Anti-inflammatory Drugs
 • 5-aminosalicylic acid (5-ASA)
 • mesalamine (Rowasa) rectal suspension
 • sulfasalazine (Azulfidine)
Cortisonelike Steroids
 • prednisone, prednisolone (generic).

- hydrocortisone enemas (Cortenema).
- methylprednisolone enema (Medrol Enpak).

Antidiarrheals
- diphenoxylate (Lomotil).
- loperamide (Imodium).

Antispasmodics
- dicyclomine (Bentyl).
- propantheline (Pro-Banthine).

Immunosuppressive Drugs
- azathioprine (Imuran).
- 6-mercatopurine (Purinethol).

Goals of Drug Treatment

Control of pain and diarrhea.

Prompt control of acute attacks; surppression of inflammation and ulceration.

Induction of a remission.

Prevention of recurrence of acute attacks.

Drug Management

General Principles

The majority (up to 90%) of cases of active ulcerative colitis respond well to medical treatment or have a spontaneous remission. Approximately 20% have a prolonged remission after the first acute attack.

Studies indicate that 55% of individuals who experience ulcerative colitis remain in remission at any given time during the course of the disorder. To minimize the risks of long-term drug use, the smallest dose of maintenance drugs (azulfidine and steroids) that prevents recurrence should be determined.

It is essential that every recurrence of acute colitis (relapse) be treated promptly and vigorously. Chronically active ulcerative colitis predisposes to a higher than normal incidence of cancer of the colon and rectum. Estimates are 3% after the first 10 years of disease, increasing to 20% per decade thereafter. Everyone subject to ulcerative colitis should have a thorough examination of the colon and rectum annually regardless of the status of the disorder.

Antidiarrheal drugs should be used with extreme caution. Excessive use can induce a paralysis of colon activity and increase the risk of developing toxic megacolon—a massive distention of the colon with air; perforation constitutes a surgical emergency.

Iron preparations for anemia should not be taken during a period of acute inflammation or active ulceration. Withhold iron therapy until a remission is established.

Use of Sulfasalazine
1. This effective and reliable drug is used to treat acute attacks of active colitis and to prevent relapse during periods of remission.
2. It is used concurrently with cortisonelike steroids during acute at-

tacks to control inflammation and ulceration and to induce remission.

3. During the quiescent phase of colitis, it is used in small doses (up to 2 grams/day) for the long-term maintenance of remission. It may be taken indefinitely.
4. This drug is best taken with or following food to reduce stomach irritation.
5. The long-term use of this drug can impair folic acid absorption and may cause a folic acid deficiency. Consult your physician regarding the need for a supplement.
6. During long-term use, it is advisable to monitor blood cell counts to detect the development of anemia or abnormally low white blood cells.
7. Mesalamine, the active derivative of sulfasalazine, is used in the form of a rectal suspension (retention enema), taken at bedtime for night-long action. The initial course of treatment is from 3 to 6 weeks. Carefully read and follow the printed instructions that are provided with this drug.

Use of Cortisonelike Steroids

1. These drugs are the mainstay of treatment for acute, active ulcerative colitis. They can induce remission in 70% to 80% of cases.
2. Steroids should be used when there are obvious symptoms of disease activity: diarrhea, bloody stools, nocturnal bowel movements, anemia, weight loss, etc. They are also of value in treating the systemic manifestations of this disorder: dermatitis, arthritis, iritis, etc.
3. To ensure prompt and adequate control of acute inflammation, initial dosage should be high. Response usually occurs within 10 to 14 days.
4. After a remission has been induced, steroid dosage is reduced to a minimum that will stabilize the colon and prevent relapse. The long-term maintenance use of steroids is controversial. If individual circumstances warrant the continual use of low-dose steroids, it is preferable to use alternate-day dosage—a single morning dose every 48 hours. This is effective in preventing recurrence for some patients and it carries a lower risk of causing adverse effects.
5. When the inflammation and ulceration are limited to the rectum, steroids can be administered in the form of enemas, foams and suppositories for local application. This minimizes systemic effects.
6. The long-term use of steroids (even in small doses) can cause significant adverse effects:
   • susceptibility to infection.
   • mineral and water imbalance.
   • reduced tolerance for sugar, potential for diabetes.
   • cataracts.
   • hypertension.
   • acne, excessive hair growth.
   • muscle wasting.
   • mental disturbances.

- osteoporosis.
- peptic ulcer activation.
- retarded growth in children.

Ancillary Drug Treatment (as required)

Condition	*Drug Treatment*
For abdominal cramps:	dicyclomine (Bentyl) propantheline (Pro-Banthine) Use these sparingly.
For diarrhea:	diphenoxylate (Lomotil) loperamide (Imodium) Use these sparingly.
For anxiety:	buspirone (Buspar), nonsedating diazepam (Valium), sedating
For depression:	see Profile of Depression in this section
For anemia:	iron preparations (not during acute stage of colitis) folic acid (if appropriate for type of anemia)

Note: Drug selection, dosage and administration schedule must be determined by the physician for each patient individually.

Resources for Additional Information and Services

American Digestive Disease Society
60 East 42nd Street, Room 411
New York, NY 10165

Telecommunications services: Gutline, available to the public every Tuesday evening from 7:30 to 9:00 p.m.
Publications available.

Crohn's & Colitis Foundation of America, Inc.
444 Park Avenue South, 11th Floor
New York, NY 10018
Phone: (800) 343-3637

DRUG PROFILES

ACEBUTOLOL
(a se BYU toh lohl)

Introduced: 1973

Class: Antihypertensive, heart rhythm regulator, beta-adrenergic blocker

Prescription: USA: Yes

Controlled Drug: USA: No

Available as Generic: No

Brand Name: Sectral

BENEFITS versus RISKS

Possible Benefits	*Possible Risks*
EFFECTIVE ANTIHYPERTENSIVE in mild to moderate high blood pressure	CONGESTIVE HEART FAILURE in advanced heart disease Worsening of angina in coronary heart disease (abrupt withdrawal) Masking of low blood sugar (hypoglycemia) in drug-treated diabetes

---

▷ **Principal Uses**

As a Single Drug Product: The treatment of mild to moderately severe high blood pressure. May be used alone or concurrently with other antihypertensive drugs, such as diuretics. Also used to prevent premature ventricular heartbeats.

How This Drug Works: By blocking certain actions of the sympathetic nervous system, this drug
- reduces the rate and contraction force of the heart, thus lowering the ejection pressure of the blood leaving the heart.
- reduces the degree of contraction of blood vessel walls, resulting in their relaxation and expansion and consequent lowering of the blood pressure.
- prolongs the conduction time of nerve impulses through the heart, of benefit in the management of certain heart rhythm disorders.

Available Dosage Forms and Strengths
Capsules — 200 mg, 400 mg

▷ **Usual Adult Dosage Range:** Initially 400 mg daily, either as a single dose in the morning or as 200 mg taken morning and evening (12 hours apart). The usual maintenance dose is 400 to 800 mg/24 hours. The total dose should not exceed 1200 mg/24 hours, given as 600 mg twice daily. **Note: Actual dosage and administration schedule must be determined by the physician for each patient individually.**

▷ **Dosing Instructions:**   May be taken without regard to eating. Capsule may be opened for administration. Do not discontinue this drug abruptly.

Usual Duration of Use: Continual use on a regular schedule for 10 to 14 days is usually necessary to determine this drug's effectiveness in lowering the blood pressure or abolishing premature heartbeats. The long-term use of this drug will be determined by the course of your blood pressure over time and your response to the overall treatment program (weight reduction, salt restriction, smoking cessation, etc.). Consult your physician on a regular basis.

Possible Advantages of This Drug

Causes less slowing of the heart rate than most other beta blocker drugs. Less likely to cause asthma (in susceptible individuals) when used in low doses.

Currently a "Drug of Choice"

for initiating treatment of hypertension with a single drug, especially for those subject to bronchial asthma or diabetes.

▷ **This Drug Should Not Be Taken If**

- you have had an allergic reaction to it previously.
- you have congestive heart failure.
- you have an abnormally slow heart rate or a serious form of heart block.
- you are taking, or have taken within the past 14 days, any monoamine oxidase (MAO) type A inhibitor drug (see Drug Class, Section Four).

▷ **Inform Your Physician Before Taking This Drug If**

- you have had an adverse reaction to any beta blocker drug in the past (see Drug Class, Section Four).
- you have a history of serious heart disease, with or without episodes of heart failure.
- you have a history of hay fever (allergic rhinitis), asthma, chronic bronchitis or emphysema.
- you have a history of overactive thyroid function (hyperthyroidism).
- you have a history of low blood sugar (hypoglycemia).
- you have impaired liver or kidney function.
- you have diabetes or myasthenia gravis.
- you are currently taking any form of digitalis, quinidine or reserpine, or any calcium blocker drug (see Drug Class, Section Four).
- you plan to have surgery under general anesthesia in the near future.

Possible Side-Effects (natural, expected and unavoidable drug actions)

Lethargy and fatigability (11%), cold extremities (0.2%), slow heart rate, light-headedness in upright position (see Orthostatic Hypotension in Glossary).

▷ **Possible Adverse Effects** (unusual, unexpected and infrequent reactions)
If any of the following develop, consult your physician promptly for guidance.

Mild Adverse Effects
Allergic Reactions: Skin rash, itching.
Headache, dizziness, insomnia, abnormal dreams.
Indigestion, nausea, constipation, diarrhea.
Joint and muscle discomfort, fluid retention (edema).

Serious Adverse Effects
Mental depression (2%), anxiety.
Chest pain, shortness of breath, precipitation of congestive heart failure.
Induction of bronchial asthma (in asthmatic individuals).

▷ **Possible Effects on Sexual Function:** Impotence (2%), decreased libido, Peyronie's disease (see Glossary).

Possible Effects on Laboratory Tests
Antinuclear Antibodies (ANA) and LE cells: frequently positive after 3 to 6 months of use.
Free fatty acids (FFA): decreased.
Glucose tolerance test (GTT): decreased; increased blood sugar levels at 60 and 120 minutes.

CAUTION
1. *Do not discontinue this drug suddenly* without the knowledge and guidance of your physician. Carry a notation on your person that you are taking this drug.
2. Consult your physician or pharmacist before using nasal decongestants usually present in over-the-counter cold preparations and nose drops. These can cause sudden increases in blood pressure when taken concurrently with beta blocker drugs.
3. Report the development of any tendency to emotional depression.

Precautions for Use
By Infants and Children: Safety and effectiveness for use by those under 12 years of age have not been established. However, if this drug is used, observe for the development of low blood sugar (hypoglycemia) during periods of reduced food intake.
By Those over 60 Years of Age: Proceed *cautiously* with all antihypertensive drugs. Unacceptably high blood pressure should be reduced without creating the risks associated with excessively low blood pressure. Start treatment with small doses, and monitor the blood pressure response frequently. Sudden, rapid and excessive reduction of blood pressure can predispose to stroke or heart attack. Total daily dosage should not exceed 800 mg. Observe for dizziness, unsteadiness, tendency to fall, confusion, hallucinations, depression or urinary frequency.

▷ **Advisability of Use During Pregnancy**
Pregnancy Category: B (tentative). See Pregnancy Code inside back cover.
Animal studies: No significant increase in birth defects found in rats or rabbits.
Human studies: Information from adequate studies of pregnant women is not available.
Use this drug only if clearly needed. Ask physician for guidance.

Advisability of Use if Breast-Feeding
Presence of this drug in breast milk: Yes.
Avoid drug or refrain from nursing.

Habit-Forming Potential: None.

Effects of Overdosage: Weakness, slow pulse, low blood pressure, fainting, cold and sweaty skin, congestive heart failure, possible coma and convulsions.

Possible Effects of Long-Term Use: Reduced heart reserve and eventual heart failure in susceptible individuals with advanced heart disease.

Suggested Periodic Examinations While Taking This Drug
(at physician's discretion)
Measurements of blood pressure, evaluation of heart function.

▷ **While Taking This Drug, Observe the Following**
Foods: No restrictions. Avoid excessive salt intake.
Beverages: No restrictions. May be taken with milk.
▷ *Alcohol:* Use with caution until the combined effect has been determined. Alcohol may exaggerate this drug's ability to lower the blood pressure and may increase its mild sedative effect.
Tobacco Smoking: Nicotine may reduce this drug's effectiveness in treating high blood pressure. In addition, high doses of this drug may potentiate the constriction of the bronchial tubes caused by regular smoking.
▷ *Other Drugs*
Acebutolol may *increase* the effects of
• other antihypertensive drugs and cause excessive lowering of the blood pressure. Dosage adjustments may be necessary.
• reserpine (Ser-Ap-Es, etc.) and cause sedation, depression, slowing of the heart rate and lowering of the blood pressure.
Acebutolol *taken concurrently* with
• clonidine (Catapres) requires close monitoring for rebound high blood pressure if clonidine is withdrawn while acebutolol is still being taken.
• insulin requires close monitoring to avoid undetected hypoglycemia (see Glossary).
The following drugs may *decrease* the effects of acebutolol
• indomethacin (Indocin), and possibly other "aspirin substitutes," may impair acebutolol's antihypertensive effect.
▷ *Driving, Hazardous Activities:* Use caution until the full extent of drowsiness, lethargy and blood pressure change has been determined.

Aviation Note: The use of this drug *is a disqualification* for piloting. Consult a designated Aviation Medical Examiner.

Exposure to Sun: No restrictions.

Exposure to Heat: Caution advised. Hot environments can lower the blood pressure and exaggerate the effects of this drug.

Exposure to Cold: Caution advised. Cold environments can enhance the circulatory deficiency in the extremities that may occur with this drug. The elderly should take precautions to prevent hypothermia (see Glossary).

Heavy Exercise or Exertion: It is advisable to avoid exertion that produces light-headedness, excessive fatigue or muscle cramping. The use of this drug may intensify the hypertensive response to isometric exercise.

Occurrence of Unrelated Illness: The fever that accompanies systemic infections can lower the blood pressure and require adjustment of dosage. Illnesses that cause nausea or vomiting may interrupt the regular dosage schedule. Ask your physician for guidance.

Discontinuation: It is advisable to avoid sudden discontinuation of this drug in all situations. If possible, gradual reduction of dose over a period of 2 to 3 weeks is recommended. Ask your physician for specific guidance.

ACETAZOLAMIDE
(a set a ZOHL a mide)

Introduced: 1953

Class: Anticonvulsant, anti-glaucoma, diuretic, sulfonamides

Prescription: USA: Yes
Canada: Yes

Controlled Drug: USA: No
Canada: No

Available as Generic: USA: Yes
Canada: No

Brand Names: ✦Acetazolam, Ak-Zol, ✦Apo-Acetazolamide, Dazamide, Diamox, Diamox Sequles, Storzolamide

---

BENEFITS versus RISKS

Possible Benefits	*Possible Risks*
REDUCTION OF INTERNAL EYE PRESSURE in selected cases of glaucoma CONTROL OF ABSENCE (PETIT MAL) SEIZURES TREATMENT OF PERIODIC PARALYSIS	Acidosis with long-term use Increased risk of kidney stone Rare bone marrow, liver or kidney injury

▷ **Principal Uses**

As a Single Drug Product: Primarily to treat certain types of glaucoma. Also used with other anticonvulsant drugs to manage petit mal epilepsy. Used less frequently to treat familial periodic paralysis and to prevent altitude sickness.

How This Drug Works: By inhibiting the action of the enzyme carbonic anhydrase, it decreases the formation of fluid (the aqueous humor) in the eye and increases the volume of urine.

Available Dosage Forms and Strengths

Capsules, prolonged-action — 500 mg

Injections — 500 mg per vial

Tablets — 125 mg, 250 mg

▷ **Usual Adult Dosage Range:**   For glaucoma: 250 to 1000 mg/24 hours, in 2 or 3 doses. For epilepsy: 250 to 1000 mg/24 hours. As a diuretic: 250 to 375 mg/24 hours, in one morning dose. **Note: Actual dosage and administration schedule must be determined by the physician for each patient individually.**

▷ **Dosing Instructions:**   Best taken with food or milk to prevent stomach irritation. Tablet may be crushed. Diamox Sequels may be opened, but do not chew or crush contents for administration.

Usual Duration of Use: Treatment of glaucoma and epilepsy require long-term use. If taken to control seizures, do not stop this drug abruptly. Consult your physician on a regular basis.

▷ **This Drug Should Not Be Taken If**

• you have had an allergic reaction to any dosage form of it previously.
• you have serious liver or kidney disease.
• you have Addison's disease.

▷ **Inform Your Physician Before Taking This Drug If**

• you have had an allergic reaction to any "sulfa" drug in the past.
• you have gout or lupus erythematosus.

Possible Side-Effects (natural, expected and unavoidable drug actions)

Drowsiness, temporary nearsightedness.

▷ **Possible Adverse Effects** (unusual, unexpected and infrequent reactions)

If any of the following develop, consult your physician promptly for guidance.

Mild Adverse Effects

Allergic Reactions: Skin rash, hives, drug fever.

Reduced appetite, indigestion, nausea.

Fatigue; weakness; dizziness; tingling of face, arms or legs.

Serious Adverse Effects

Allergic Reactions: Hemolytic anemia (see Glossary), spontaneous bruising (reduced blood platelet count, see Glossary).

Bone marrow depression (see Glossary)—fatigue, weakness, fever, sore throat, abnormal bleeding or bruising.

Hepatitis with jaundice (see Glossary)—yellow eyes and skin, dark-colored urine, light-colored stools.

▷ **Possible Effects on Sexual Function:** Decreased libido (male and female), impotence (both infrequent). Effects may begin after 2 weeks of use and subside when drug is discontinued.

▷ **Adverse Effects That May Mimic Natural Diseases or Disorders**
Toxic liver reaction may suggest viral hepatitis.
Lupus erythematosuslike syndrome.

Natural Diseases or Disorders That May Be Activated by This Drug
Gout, acidosis secondary to chronic obstructive lung disease—asthma, bronchitis, emphysema.

Possible Effects on Laboratory Tests
Complete blood cell counts: decreased red cells, hemoglobin, white cells and platelets.
Blood chloride level: increased.
Blood glucose level: increased in prediabetics and with use of oral antidiabetic drugs (see Drug Class, Section Four).
Blood lupus erythematosus (LE) cells: positive.
Blood uric acid level: increased.

CAUTION
1. Observe for possible loss of drug effectiveness when used as a diuretic or to control seizures.
2. Emotional depression may occur and not be recognized as an adverse effect of this drug.
3. This drug may cause an excessive loss of potassium from the body. Consult your physician regarding the need for a high-potassium diet or potassium supplements.

Precautions for Use
By Infants and Children: Excessive dosage may cause drowsiness and numbness of the face and extremities. Not recommended for use as a diuretic in children.
By Those over 60 Years of Age: Do not exceed recommended doses. Increased dosage may cause excessive loss of sodium and potassium, with resultant weakness, confusion, numbness in the extremities and nausea. If taking a digitalis preparation (digitoxin, digoxin), consult your physician regarding the need for a high-potassium diet or potassium supplements.

▷ **Advisability of Use During Pregnancy**
Pregnancy Category: C (tentative). See Pregnancy Code inside back cover.
Animal studies: Limb and skeletal defects reported in mice and rats.
Human studies: Information from adequate studies of pregnant women is not available.

Avoid completely during the first 3 months and during labor and delivery.

Advisability of Use if Breast-Feeding
Presence of this drug in breast milk: Yes.
Diuretic effect of drug may temporarily impair milk production. Monitor nursing infant closely and discontinue drug or nursing if adverse effects develop.

Habit-Forming Potential: None.

Effects of Overdosage: Drowsiness, numbness and tingling, thirst, nausea, vomiting, confusion, excitement, convulsions, coma.

Possible Effects of Long-Term Use: The development of low blood potassium and/or acidosis.

Suggested Periodic Examinations While Taking This Drug (at physician's discretion)
Complete blood cell counts, measurements of blood sodium, potassium and uric acid levels, liver and kidney function tests.

▷ **While Taking This Drug, Observe the Following**
Foods: Consult your physician regarding the advisability of eating a high-potassium diet. See Section Six for the Table of High Potassium Foods.
Beverages: No restrictions. May be taken with milk.
▷ *Alcohol:* Use with caution until the combined effect has been determined. Alcohol may impair the anticonvulsant effect of this drug and reduce its control of seizures.
Tobacco Smoking: No interactions expected.
▷ *Other Drugs*
Acetazolamide may *increase* the effects of
• quinidine.
Acetazolamide may *decrease* the effects of
• lithium.
▷ *Driving, Hazardous Activities:* Usually no restrictions. Be alert to the possible occurrence of drowsiness or dizziness.
Aviation Note: The use of this drug *may be a disqualification* for piloting. Consult a designated Aviation Medical Examiner.
Exposure to Sun: No restrictions.

ACYCLOVIR
(ay SI kloh ver)

Introduced: 1979

Prescription: USA: Yes
 Canada: Yes

Available as Generic: No

Brand Name: Zovirax

Class: Antiviral

Controlled Drug: USA: No
 Canada: No

BENEFITS versus RISKS

Possible Benefits	*Possible Risks*
HASTENED RECOVERY FROM INITIAL EPISODE OF GENITAL HERPES PREVENTION OF RECURRENCE OF GENITAL HERPES	Nausea, vomiting, diarrhea (8% in long-term use) Nervousness, depression (less than 3%) Joint and muscle pain (3%)

▷ **Principal Uses**

As a Single Drug Product: Used primarily for the treatment of initial episodes and prevention of recurrent episodes of genital herpes in selected
 individuals.

In addition to its primary use, this drug is proving to be beneficial in the
 treatment of herpes simplex infections of skin, brain, eye and rectum;
 infectious mononucleosis; shingles; and pneumonia caused by the
 chicken pox virus. It is also in trial for the treatment of AIDS.

How This Drug Works: By inhibiting DNA replication of the herpes simplex
 virus, this drug arrests the multiplication and spread of the infecting
 virus and thus reduces the severity and duration of the herpes infection.

Available Dosage Forms and Strengths
 Capsules — 200 mg
 Ointment — 5%

▷ **Usual Adult Dosage Range:** For initial episode of genital herpes—200 mg/4
 hours for a total of 5 capsules daily for 10 consecutive days (total dose
 of 50 capsules). For intermittent recurrence—200 mg/4 hours for a
 total of 5 capsules daily for 5 consecutive days (total dose of 25 capsules). Begin treatment at the earliest indication of recurrence. For
 prevention of frequent recurrence—400 mg taken 2 times daily for up
 to 12 months. For the ointment form—cover all infected areas every 3
 hours for a total of 6 times daily for 7 consecutive days. Begin treatment at the earliest indication of infection. **Note: Actual dosage and
 administration schedule must be determined by the physician for
 each patient individually.**

▷ **Dosing Instructions:**   May be taken without regard to eating. Capsule may be opened for administration. Take the full course of the exact dose prescribed. Use a finger cot or rubber glove to apply the ointment.

Usual Duration of Use: Continual use on a regular schedule for 10 days is usually necessary to determine this drug's effectiveness in reducing the severity and duration of the initial infection. Continual use for 6 months to 3 years may be necessary to prevent frequent recurrence of herpes eruptions.

▷ **This Drug Should Not Be Taken If**
  • you have had an allergic reaction to any dosage form of it previously.

▷ **Inform Your Physician Before Taking This Drug If**
  • you have impaired liver or kidney function.
  • you are taking any other drugs at this time.

Possible Side-Effects (natural, expected and unavoidable drug actions)
  With use of capsules—none.
  With use of ointment—mild pain, burning or stinging at site of application (28%).

▷ **Possible Adverse Effects** (unusual, unexpected and infrequent reactions)
  If any of the following develop, consult your physician promptly for guidance.
  Mild Adverse Effects
  Allergic Reaction: Skin rash.
  Headache, dizziness, nervousness, insomnia, depression, fatigue.
  Nausea, vomiting, diarrhea.
  Joint pains, muscle cramps.
  Acne, hair loss.
  Serious Adverse Effects
  Superficial thrombophlebitis, enlarged lymph glands.

▷ **Possible Effects on Sexual Function:**   Altered timing and pattern of menstruation.

Possible Effects on Laboratory Tests
  Complete blood cell counts: decreased red cells and hemoglobin.
  Blood urea nitrogen (BUN): increased.

CAUTION
  1. This drug does not eliminate all herpes virus and is not a permanent cure. Observe for possible recurrence and resume treatment at the earliest indication of active infection.
  2. Avoid sexual intercourse while herpes blisters and inflammation are visible.
  3. Do not exceed the prescribed dosage.
  4. Inform physician if the frequency and severity of recurrent infections do not improve.

Precautions for Use
   By Infants and Children: Safety and effectiveness for use by those under 12 years of age have not been established.
   By Those over 60 Years of Age: Avoid dehydration. Drink 2 to 3 quarts of liquids daily.

▷ **Advisability of Use During Pregnancy**
   Pregnancy Category: C (tentative). See Pregnancy Code inside back cover.
   Animal studies: No birth defects found in mouse, rat or rabbit studies.
   Human studies: Information from adequate studies of pregnant women is not available.
   Avoid use if possible. Use only if clearly needed.

Advisability of Use if Breast-Feeding
   Presence of this drug in breast milk: Unknown.
   Avoid drug or refrain from nursing.

Habit-Forming Potential: None.

Effects of Overdosage: Possible impairment of kidney function.

Possible Effects of Long-Term Use: Development of strains of herpes virus that are resistant to this drug.

Suggested Periodic Examinations While Taking This Drug (at physician's discretion)
   Kidney function tests.

▷ **While Taking This Drug, Observe the Following**
   Foods: No restrictions.
   Beverages: No restrictions. May be taken with milk. Drink 2 to 3 quarts of liquids daily.
▷   *Alcohol:* Use caution until the combined effects have been determined. Dizziness or fatigue may be accentuated.
   Tobacco Smoking: No interactions expected.
▷   *Other Drugs*
       The following drugs may *increase* the effects of acyclovir
       • probenecid (Benemid) may delay its elimination.
▷   *Driving, Hazardous Activities:* Use caution if dizziness or fatigue occurs.
   Aviation Note: The use of this drug *may be a disqualification* for piloting. Consult a designated Aviation Medical Examiner.
   Exposure to Sun: No restrictions.

ALBUTEROL
(al BYU ter ohl)

Other Name: Salbutamol

Introduced: 1968

Class: Antiasthmatic, bronchodilator

Prescription: USA: Yes
Canada: Yes

Controlled Drug: USA: No
Canada: No

Available as Generic: Yes

Brand Names: ♦Novosalmol, Proventil Inhaler, Proventil Repetabs, Proventil Tablets, Ventolin Inhaler, Ventolin Rotacaps, Ventolin Tablets

---

BENEFITS versus RISKS

Possible Benefits	*Possible Risks*
VERY EFFECTIVE RELIEF OF BRONCHOSPASM	Increased blood pressure Fine hand tremor Irregular heart rhythm (with excessive use)

▷ **Principal Uses**

As a Single Drug Product: To relieve acute bronchial asthma and to reduce
the frequency and severity of chronic, recurrent asthmatic attacks.

How This Drug Works: It is thought that by increasing the production of
cyclic AMP, this drug relaxes constricted bronchial muscles to relieve
asthmatic wheezing.

Available Dosage Forms and Strengths

Aerosol — 90 mcg per actuation
Capsules for inhalation — 200 mcg
Solution for inhalation — 0.83 mg per ml, 5 mg per ml
Syrup — 2 mg per 5-ml teaspoonful
Tablets — 2 mg, 4 mg
Tablets, prolonged-action — 4 mg

▷ **Usual Adult Dosage Range:** Inhaler—1 to 2 inhalations (90 to 180 mcg) up
to 4 times daily, every 4 to 6 hours. Tablets—2 to 4 mg 3 to 4 times daily,
every 4 to 6 hours. **Do not exceed** 8 inhalations (720 mcg)/24 hours,
or 32 mg (tablet form)/24 hours. **Note: Actual dosage and administration schedule must be determined by the physician for each patient
individually.**

▷ **Dosing Instructions:** May be taken on empty stomach or with food or milk.
Tablet may be crushed. For inhaler, follow the written instructions
carefully. Do not overuse.

Usual Duration of Use: According to individual requirements. Do not use beyond the time necessary to terminate episodes of asthma.

▷ **This Drug Should Not Be Taken If**
- you have had an allergic reaction to any dosage form of it previously.
- you currently have an irregular heart rhythm.
- you are taking, or have taken within the past 2 weeks, any monoamine oxidase (MAO) type A inhibitor drug (see Drug Class, Section Four).

▷ **Inform Your Physician Before Taking This Drug If**
- you have any type of heart or circulatory disorder, especially high blood pressure or coronary heart disease.
- you have diabetes.
- you are taking any form of digitalis or any stimulant drug.

Possible Side-Effects (natural, expected and unavoidable drug actions)
Aerosol—dryness or irritation of mouth or throat, altered taste.
Tablet—nervousness, palpitation.

▷ **Possible Adverse Effects** (unusual, unexpected and infrequent reactions)
If any of the following develop, consult your physician promptly for guidance.
Mild Adverse Effects
Headache (7%), dizziness (2%), restlessness, insomnia, fine tremor of hands (20%).
Nausea (2%), heartburn, vomiting.
Leg cramps (3%), flushing of skin.
Serious Adverse Effects
Rapid or irregular heart rhythm, increased blood pressure, difficult urination.

▷ **Possible Effects on Sexual Function:** None reported.

Natural Diseases or Disorders That May Be Activated By This Drug
Latent coronary artery disease, diabetes or high blood pressure.

Possible Effects on Laboratory Tests
Blood HDL Cholesterol level: increased.
Blood glucose level: increased.

CAUTION
1. Concurrent use of this drug by inhalation with beclomethasone aerosol (Beclovent, Vanceril) may increase the risk of toxicity due to fluorocarbon propellants. It is advisable to use albuterol aerosol 20 to 30 minutes *before* beclomethasone aerosol. This will reduce the risk of toxicity and will enhance the penetration of beclomethasone.
2. The excessive or prolonged use of this drug by inhalation can reduce its effectiveness and cause serious heart rhythm disturbances, including cardiac arrest.

Precautions for Use
By Infants and Children: Safety and effectiveness of use in children under 12 years of age have not been established.

By Those over 60 Years of Age: Avoid excessive and continual use. If acute asthma is not relieved promptly, other drugs will have to be tried. Observe for the development of nervousness, palpitations, irregular heart rhythm and muscle tremors.

▷ **Advisability of Use During Pregnancy**
Pregnancy Category: C (tentative). See Pregnancy Code inside back cover.

Animal studies: Cleft palate reported in mice.

Human studies: Information from adequate studies of pregnant women is not available.

Avoid use during first 3 months if possible.

Advisability of Use if Breast-Feeding
Presence of this drug in breast milk: Unknown.

Avoid drug or refrain from nursing.

Habit-Forming Potential: None.

Effects of Overdosage: Nervousness, palpitation, rapid heart rate, sweating, headache, tremor, vomiting, chest pain.

Possible Effects of Long-Term Use: Loss of effectiveness.

Suggested Periodic Examinations While Taking This Drug (at physician's discretion)

Blood pressure measurements, evaluation of heart status.

▷ **While Taking This Drug, Observe the Following**
Foods: No restrictions.

Beverages: Avoid excessive use of caffeine-containing beverages—coffee, tea, cola, chocolate.

▷   *Alcohol:* No interactions expected.

Tobacco Smoking: No interactions expected.

▷   *Other Drugs*
Albuterol *taken concurrently* with

• monoamine oxidase (MAO) type A inhibitor drugs may cause excessive increase in blood pressure and undesirable heart stimulation.

▷   *Driving, Hazardous Activities:* Use caution if excessive nervousness or dizziness occurs.

Aviation Note: The use of this drug *is a disqualification* for piloting. Consult a designated Aviation Medical Examiner.

Exposure to Sun: No restrictions.

Heavy Exercise or Exertion: Use caution. Excessive exercise can induce asthma in sensitive individuals.

ALLOPURINOL
(al oh PURE i nohl)

Introduced: 1963

Prescription: USA: Yes
Canada: Yes

Available as Generic: USA: Yes
Canada: No

Brand Names: ✦Alloprin, ✦Apo-Allopurinol, Lopurin, ✦Novopurol, ✦Purinol, Zurinol, Zyloprim

Class: Antigout

Controlled Drug: USA: No
Canada: No

BENEFITS versus RISKS

Possible Benefits

EFFECTIVE CONTROL OF GOUT
CONTROL OF HIGH BLOOD
 URIC ACID due to
 polycythemia, leukemia, cancer
 and chemotherapy

Possible Risks

Increased frequency of acute gout
 initially
Peripheral neuritis
Allergic reactions in skin, blood
 vessels and liver
Bone marrow depression
 (questionable)

▷ **Principal Uses**

As a Single Drug Product: Used primarily in the long-term management of gout to *prevent* episodes of acute gout. (It does not relieve the symptoms of acute gout attacks.) Also used to prevent abnormally high blood levels of uric acid in individuals who have recurrent uric acid kidney stones, and in those receiving chemotherapy or radiation therapy for cancer.

How This Drug Works: By inhibiting the action of the tissue enzyme xanthine oxidase, this drug decreases the conversion of purines (protein nutrients) to uric acid.

Available Dosage Forms and Strengths

Tablets — 100 mg, 300 mg (and 200 mg in Canada)

▷ **Usual Adult Dosage Range:** Initially 100 mg/24 hours. Increase by 100 mg/24 hours at intervals of 1 week until uric acid blood level is 6 mg/dl or less. Usual dose is 200 to 300 mg/24 hours for mild gout, and 400 to 600 mg/24 hours for moderate to severe gout. Daily doses of 300 mg or less may be taken as a single dose. Doses exceeding 300 mg daily should be divided into 2 or 3 equal portions; for the high uric acid levels associated with cancer, 600 to 800 mg/24 hours, divided into 3 equal portions. **Note: Actual dosage and administration schedule must be determined by the physician for each patient individually.**

▷ **Dosing Instructions:**   Best taken with food or milk to reduce stomach irritation. Tablet may be crushed. Drink 2 to 3 quarts of liquids daily.

Usual Duration of Use: According to individual requirements. Blood uric acid levels usually begin to decrease in 48 to 72 hours and may reach a normal range in 1 to 3 weeks. Regular use for several months may be required to prevent attacks of acute gout. Continual use for many years may be necessary for adequate control. Consult your physician on a regular basis.

▷ **This Drug Should Not Be Taken If**
  • you have had an allergic reaction to any dosage form of it previously.
  • you are experiencing an acute attack of gout at the present time.

▷ **Inform Your Physician Before Taking This Drug If**
  • you have a personal or family history of hemochromatosis.
  • you have a history of liver or kidney disease.
  • you have had a blood cell or bone marrow disorder.
  • you have any type of convulsive disorder (epilepsy).

Possible Side-Effects (natural, expected and unavoidable drug actions)
  An increase in the frequency and severity of episodes of acute gout may occur during the first several weeks of drug use. Consult your physician regarding the need for other drugs during this period.

▷ **Possible Adverse Effects** (unusual, unexpected and infrequent reactions)
  If any of the following develop, consult your physician promptly for guidance.
  Mild Adverse Effects
  Allergic Reactions: Skin rash, hives, itching, drug fever.
  Headache, dizziness, drowsiness.
  Nausea, vomiting, diarrhea, stomach cramps.
  Loss of scalp hair.
  Serious Adverse Effects
  Allergic Reactions: Severe skin reactions, high fever, chills, joint pains, swollen glands, kidney damage.
  Hepatitis with or without jaundice (see Glossary)—yellow eyes and skin, dark-colored urine, light-colored stools.
  Bone marrow depression (see Glossary)—questionable.
  Seizures, peripheral neuritis.
  Macular eye damage, cataract formation—questionable.

▷ **Possible Effects on Sexual Function:**   Less than 1% and causal relationship not established: male infertility, male breast enlargement, impotence.

▷ **Adverse Effects That May Mimic Natural Diseases or Disorders**
Toxic liver reaction may suggest viral hepatitis.
Severe skin reactions may resemble the Stevens-Johnson syndrome (erythema multiforme).

Possible Effects on Laboratory Tests
Complete blood cell counts: decreased red cells, hemoglobin and platelets; increased eosinophils.
Liver function tests: increased liver enzymes (ALT/GPT, AST/GOT, alkaline phosphatase).

CAUTION
1. During the early weeks of treatment, the frequency of acute attacks of gout may increase. These subside with continuation of treatment.
2. This drug will not relieve the symptoms of acute gout. It should not be started during the presence of acute gout symptoms.
3. Vitamin C in doses of 2 grams or more daily may acidify the urine and increase the risk of kidney stone formation during the use of allopurinol.
4. The concurrent use of thiazide diuretics (see Drug Class, Section Four) is reported to cause a possible allergic-type kidney damage. Avoid this drug combination.

Precautions for Use
By Infants and Children: Monitor closely for allergic skin reactions and blood cell disorders. This drug may increase the toxicity of azathioprine (Imuran) or mercaptopurine (Purinethol) in children receiving chemotherapy for cancer.
By Those over 60 Years of Age: The natural decline in kidney function makes it advisable to use smaller initial and maintenance doses of this drug.

▷ **Advisability of Use During Pregnancy**
Pregnancy Category: C (tentative). See Pregnancy Code inside back cover.
Animal studies: Results are conflicting and inconclusive.
Human studies: Information from adequate studies of pregnant women is not available.
Avoid use of drug during the first 3 months. Use during the last 6 months only if clearly needed.

Advisability of Use if Breast-Feeding
Presence of this drug in breast milk: Yes.
Avoid drug or refrain from nursing.

Habit-Forming Potential: None.

Effects of Overdosage: Nausea, vomiting or diarrhea may occur as a result of individual sensitivity. No serious toxic effects expected.

Possible Effects of Long-Term Use: None identified.

Suggested Periodic Examinations While Taking This Drug (at physician's discretion)

Blood uric acid levels, complete blood cell counts, liver and kidney function tests. If appropriate, eye examinations for possible cataract formation or macular damage. A cause-and-effect relationship (see Glossary) between this drug and eye changes has not been established.

▷ **While Taking This Drug, Observe the Following**

Foods: Follow physician's advice regarding the need for a low-purine diet.

Beverages: No restrictions. May be taken with milk.

▷ *Alcohol:* No interactions expected.

Tobacco Smoking: No interactions expected.

▷ *Other Drugs*

Allopurinol may *increase* the effects of

• azathioprine (Imuran) and mercaptopurine (Purinethol), making it necessary to reduce their dosages.
• oral anticoagulants (see Drug Class, Section Four) in *some* individuals.
• theophylline (aminophylline, Elixophyllin, Theo-Dur, etc.)

Allopurinol *taken concurrently* with

• ampicillin may increase the incidence of skin rash.

▷ *Driving, Hazardous Activities:* Drowsiness may occur in some individuals. Determine sensitivity before engaging in hazardous activities.

Aviation Note: The use of this drug *may be a disqualification* for piloting. Consult a designated Aviation Medical Examiner.

Exposure to Sun: No restrictions.

ALPRAZOLAM
(al PRAY zoh lam)

Introduced: 1973

Class: Mild tranquilizer, benzodiazepines

Prescription: USA: Yes
Canada: Yes

Controlled Drug: USA: C-IV*
Canada: No

Available as Generic: No

Brand Name: Xanax

Warning: The brand names Xanax and Zantac are similar and can be mistaken for each other; this can lead to serious medication errors. These names represent very different drugs. Xanax (white, yellow, blue oval tablets) is the generic drug alprazolam; it is a mild tranquilizer. Zantac (a large white tablet) is the generic drug ranitidine; it is used to treat peptic ulcer disease. Verify that you are taking the correct drug.

*See Schedules of Controlled Drugs inside back cover.

BENEFITS versus RISKS

Possible Benefits	*Possible Risks*
RELIEF OF ANXIETY AND NERVOUS TENSION in 75% of users	Habit-forming potential with prolonged use
EFFECTIVE TREATMENT OF PANIC DISORDER in 47% of users	Minor impairment of mental functions with therapeutic doses
Wide margin of safety with therapeutic doses	

▷ **Principal Uses**

As a Single Drug Product: Used primarily as a mild tranquilizer for the short-term relief of mild to moderate anxiety and nervous tension. It is also used to relieve anxiety associated with depression and to prevent or relieve panic attacks.

How This Drug Works: It is thought that this drug produces a calming effect by enhancing the action of the nerve transmitter gamma-aminobutyric acid (GABA), which in turn blocks the arousal of higher brain centers.

Available Dosage Forms and Strengths
Tablets — 0.25 mg, 0.5 mg, 1 mg, 2 mg

▷ **Usual Adult Dosage Range:**   For anxiety and nervous tension: 0.25 mg to 0.5 mg 3 times daily. The maximal dose is 4 mg/24 hours, taken in divided doses. For panic disorder: Initially 0.5 mg 3 times daily; increase dose by 1 mg every 3 to 4 days as needed and tolerated. The maximal daily dosage is 10 mg. **Note: Actual dosage and administration schedule must be determined by the physician for each patient individually.**

▷ **Dosing Instructions:**   May be taken on empty stomach or with food or milk. Tablet may be crushed for administration. Do not discontinue this drug abruptly if taken for more than 4 weeks.

Usual Duration of Use: Several days to several weeks. Avoid prolonged and uninterrupted use. Continual use should not exceed 8 weeks without evaluation by your physician.

▷ **This Drug Should Not Be Taken If**
- you have had an allergic reaction to it previously.
- you are pregnant (first 3 months).
- you have acute narrow-angle glaucoma.
- you have myasthenia gravis.

▷ **Inform Your Physician Before Taking This Drug If**
- you are allergic to other benzodiazepine drugs (see Drug Class, Section Four).
- you are pregnant (last 6 months) or planning pregnancy.

- you are breast-feeding.
- you have a history of depression or serious mental illness (psychosis).
- you have a history of alcoholism or drug abuse.
- you have impaired liver or kidney function.
- you have open-angle glaucoma.
- you have a seizure disorder (epilepsy).
- you have severe chronic lung disease.

Possible Side-Effects (natural, expected and unavoidable drug actions)
Drowsiness, light-headedness.

▷ **Possible Adverse Effects** (unusual, unexpected and infrequent reactions)
If any of the following develop, consult your physician promptly for guidance.
Mild Adverse Effects
Allergic Reactions: Skin rash, hives.
Headache, dizziness, fatigue, blurred vision, dry mouth.
Nausea, vomiting, constipation.
Serious Adverse Effects
Confusion, hallucinations, depression, unexpected excitement, agitation (paradoxical reaction).

▷ **Possible Effects on Sexual Function:** Rare but documented: inhibited female orgasm (5 mg/day); impaired ejaculation (3.5 mg/day); decreased libido, impaired erection (4.5 mg/day); altered timing and pattern of menstruation (0.75 to 4 mg/day).

Possible Effects on Laboratory Tests
Liver function tests: increased liver enzymes (ALT/GPT, AST/GOT), rare and insignificant.
Urine screening tests for drug abuse: may be **positive.** (Test results depend upon amount of drug taken and testing method used.)

CAUTION
1. This drug should not be discontinued abruptly if it has been taken continually for more than 4 weeks.
2. The concurrent use of some over-the-counter drug products that contain antihistamines (allergy and cold preparations, sleep aids) can cause excessive sedation in sensitive individuals.

Precautions for Use
By Infants and Children: Safety and effectiveness for use by those under 18 years of age have not been established.
By Those over 60 Years of Age: The starting dose should be 0.25 mg 2 or 3 times daily. Monitor for excessive drowsiness, dizziness, unsteadiness and incoordination (possible low blood pressure).

▷ **Advisability of Use During Pregnancy**
Pregnancy Category: D (tentative). See Pregnancy Code inside back cover.
Animal studies: Diazepam (a closely related benzodiazepine) can cause

cleft palate in mice and skeletal defects in rats. No information available for alprazolam.

Human studies: Some studies suggest a possible association between the use of diazepam and defects such as cleft lip and heart deformities. Information from adequate studies on the use of alprazolam by pregnant women is not available.

Avoid use during entire pregnancy if possible.

Advisability of Use if Breast-Feeding
Presence of this drug in breast milk: Probably yes.
Avoid drug or refrain from nursing.

Habit-Forming Potential: This drug can produce psychological and/or physical dependence (see Glossary) if used in large doses for an extended period of time.

Effects of Overdosage: Marked drowsiness, weakness, feeling of drunkenness, staggering gait, tremor, stupor progressing to deep sleep or coma.

Possible Effects of Long-Term Use: Psychological and/or physical dependence.

Suggested Periodic Examinations While Taking This Drug (at physician's discretion)
None required for short-term use.

▷ **While Taking This Drug, Observe the Following**
Foods: No restrictions.
Beverages: Avoid excessive intake of caffeine-containing beverages: coffee, tea, cola. This drug may be taken with milk.
▷ *Alcohol:* Use with extreme caution and in very small amounts until the combined effect is determined. Alcohol may increase the sedative effects of alprazolam. Alprazolam may increase the intoxicating effects of alcohol. Avoid alcohol completely—throughout the day and night— if you find it necessary to drive or to engage in *any* hazardous activity.
Tobacco Smoking: Heavy smoking may reduce the calming action of alprazolam.
Marijuana Smoking
  Occasional (once or twice weekly): Mild increase in the sedative effect of this drug. *Daily:* Marked increase in the sedative effect of this drug.
▷ *Other Drugs*
  Alprazolam may *increase* the effects of
  • digoxin (Lanoxin), and cause digoxin toxicity.
  Alprazolam may *decrease* the effects of
  • levodopa (Sinemet, etc.), and reduce its effectiveness in treating Parkinson's disease.
  The following drugs may *increase* the effects of alprazolam
  • cimetidine (Tagamet).
  • disulfiram (Antabuse).
  • isoniazid (INH, Rifamate, etc.).

- oral contraceptives.
- valproic acid (Depakene).

The following drugs may *decrease* the effects of alprazolam

- rifampin (Rimactane, etc.).
- theophylline (aminophylline, Theo-Dur, etc.).

▷ *Driving, Hazardous Activities:* This drug can impair mental alertness, judgment, physical coordination and reaction time. Avoid hazardous activities accordingly.

Aviation Note: The use of this drug *is a disqualification* for piloting. Consult a designated Aviation Medical Examiner.

Exposure to Sun: No restrictions.

Discontinuation: If it has been necessary to use this drug for an extended period of time, do not discontinue it abruptly. Reduce dose gradually at the rate of 1 mg per week until a total daily dose of 4 mg is reached; by 0.5 mg per week until a total daily dose of 2 mg is reached; then by 0.25 mg per week thereafter. Ask physician for guidance.

AMANTADINE
(a MAN ta deen)

Introduced: 1966

Class: Antiparkinsonism, antiviral

Prescription: USA: Yes
Canada: Yes

Controlled Drug: USA: No
Canada: No

Available as Generic: USA: Yes
Canada: No

Brand Names: Symadine, Symmetrel

BENEFITS versus RISKS

Possible Benefits	*Possible Risks*
PARTIAL RELIEF OF RIGIDITY, TREMOR AND IMPAIRED MOTION in all forms of parkinsonism (in 60% of users) PREVENTION AND TREATMENT OF REPIRATORY TRACT INFECTIONS CAUSED BY INFLUENZA TYPE A VIRUSES*	Skin rashes, mild to severe Confusion, hallucinations Congestive heart failure Increased prostatism (see Glossary) Abnormally low white blood cell counts

---

*This drug is not effective for the prevention or treatment of viral infections other than those caused by influenza type A viruses.

▷ **Principal Uses**

As a Single Drug Product: This drug has two primary uses: (1) to treat all forms of parkinsonism, and (2) to prevent and treat respiratory tract infections caused by strains of influenza type A virus.

How This Drug Works: Not completely known. It is thought that by increasing the availability of the nerve impulse transmitter known as dopamine in certain nerve centers, this drug reduces the muscular rigidity, tremor and impaired movement associated with all forms of parkinsonism. By blocking the penetration of infectious material from virus particles into tissue cells, this drug prevents the development of influenza type A.

Available Dosage Forms and Strengths
Capsules — 100 mg
  Syrup — 50 mg per 5-ml teaspoonful

▷ **Usual Adult Dosage Range:** Antiparkinsonism: 100 mg once or twice daily. The total daily dose should not exceed 400 mg. Antiviral: 200 mg once daily; or 100 mg/12 hours. **Note: Actual dosage and administration schedule must be determined by the physician for each patient individually.**

▷ **Dosing Instructions:** May be taken with or following meals. The capsule may be opened for administration.

Usual Duration of Use: Continual use on a regular schedule for up to 2 weeks is usually necessary to determine this drug's effectiveness in relieving the symptoms of parkinsonism. Long-term use (months to years) requires periodic evaluation of response and dosage adjustment. Consult your physician on a regular basis.

Following exposure to influenza type A, maximal protection requires continual daily dosage for at least 10 days. During influenza epidemics, this drug may be given for 6 to 8 weeks.

Currently a "Drug of Choice"
for prevention of influenza Type A infection (70% to 90% effective), and for treatment of such infections (50% reduction of severity and length of illness).

▷ **This Drug Should Not Be Taken If**
• you have had an allergic reaction to it previously.

▷ **Inform Your Physician Before Taking This Drug If**
• you have any type of seizure disorder.
• you have a history of serious emotional or mental disorder.
• you have a history of heart disease, especially previous heart failure.
• you have impaired liver or kidney function.
• you have a history of peptic ulcer disease.
• you have eczema or recurring eczemalike skin rashes.
• you are taking any drugs for emotional or mental disorders.

Possible Side-Effects (natural, expected and unavoidable drug actions)
Light-headedness, dizziness, weakness, feeling of impending faint in up-right position (see Orthostatic Hypotension in Glossary). Dry mouth, constipation. Reddish-blue network pattern or patchy discoloration of the skin of the legs and feet (livedo reticularis); this is transient and unimportant.

▷ **Possible Adverse Effects** (unusual, unexpected and infrequent reactions)
If any of the following develop, consult your physician promptly for guidance.
Mild Adverse Effects
Allergic Reaction: Skin rash.
Headache, nervousness, irritability, inability to concentrate, insomnia, nightmares.
Unsteadiness, visual disturbances, slurred speech.
Loss of appetite, nausea, vomiting.
Serious Adverse Effects
Allergic Reaction: Severe eczemalike skin rashes.
Idiosyncratic Reactions: Confusion, depression, hallucinations.
Increased seizure activity in presence of epilepsy.
Swelling (fluid retention) of the arms, feet or ankles.
Development of congestive heart failure (rare).
Aggravation of prostatism (see Glossary).
Abnormally low white blood cell counts: fever, sore throat, infections.

▷ **Possible Effects on Sexual Function:**   None reported.

▷ **Adverse Effects That May Mimic Natural Diseases or Disorders**
Mood or mental changes, confusion or hallucinations may suggest a psychotic disorder.
Swelling of the legs and feet may suggest (but not necessarily be indicative of) heart, liver or kidney disorder.

Natural Diseases or Disorders That May Be Activated by This Drug
Latent epilepsy, incipient congestive heart failure.

Possible Effects on Laboratory Tests
Liver function tests: increased liver enzymes (AST/GOT, alkaline phosphatase), mild and transient.
Kidney function tests: increased blood urea nitrogen (BUN), mild and transient.

CAUTION
1. This drug has a narrow margin of safety. Do not exceed a total dose of 400 mg/24 hours. Observe closely for indications of adverse effects with doses over 200 mg/24 hours.
2. After an initial period of benefit lasting 3 to 6 months, this drug may lose its effectiveness in the treatment of parkinsonism. If this occurs, consult your physician regarding dosage adjustment or drug replacement.

3. This drug is reported to increase susceptibility to German measles. Avoid exposure to anyone with active German measles infection.
4. Observe for early indications of congestive heart failure: shortness of breath on exertion or during the night while sleeping, mild cough, swelling of the feet and ankles. Report these developments promptly to your physician.

Precautions for Use
By Infants and Children: Safety and effectiveness for use by those under 1 year of age have not been established.

By Those over 60 Years of Age: Observe for the possible development of confusion, delirium, hallucinations and disorderly conduct. Prostatism may be aggravated by this drug.

▷ **Advisability of Use During Pregnancy**
Pregnancy Category: C (tentative). See Pregnancy Code inside back cover.
Animal studies: Birth defects reported in rat studies; no defects reported in rabbit studies.
Human studies: Information from adequate studies of pregnant women is not available. Avoid this drug during the first 3 months if possible. Ask your physician for guidance.

Advisability of Use if Breast-Feeding
Presence of this drug in breast milk: Yes.
The nursing infant may develop skin rash, vomiting or retention of urine. Avoid drug or refrain from nursing.

Habit-Forming Potential: While not habituating, this drug does have a potential for abuse because of its ability to cause euphoria, hallucinations and feelings of detachment.

Effects of Overdosage: Hyperactivity, disorientation, confusion, visual hallucinations, aggressive behavior, severe toxic psychosis, seizures, heart rhythm disturbances, drop in blood pressure.

Possible Effects of Long-Term Use: Livedo reticularis (see Possible Side-Effects above). Congestive heart failure in predisposed individuals.

Suggested Periodic Examinations While Taking This Drug (at physician's discretion)
White blood cell counts, liver and kidney function tests.
Evaluation of heart function.

▷ **While Taking This Drug, Observe the Following**
Foods: No restrictions.
Beverages: No restrictions. May be taken with milk.
▷   *Alcohol:* Use caution until combined effects have been determined. This combination may impair mental function and lower blood pressure excessively.

Tobacco Smoking: No interactions expected.
Marijuana Smoking: No interactions expected.
▷ *Other Drugs*
Amantadine may *increase* the effects of
- those atropinelike drugs that are used to treat parkinsonism, especially benztropine (Cogentin), orphenadrine (Disipal) and trihexyphenidyl (Artane). Amantadine can increase their therapeutic effectiveness. However, if doses are too large, these drugs taken concurrently with amantadine may cause mental confusion, delirium, hallucinations and nightmares.
- levodopa (Dopar, Larodopa, Sinemet, etc.), and enhance its therapeutic effectiveness. However, this combination may cause acute mental disturbances.

The following drugs may *increase* the effects of amantadine
- amphetamine and amphetaminelike stimulant drugs may cause excessive stimulation and adverse behavioral effects.
- hydrochlorothiazide triamterene may increase the blood level of amantadine.

▷ *Driving, Hazardous Activities:* This drug may cause drowsiness, dizziness, blurred vision or confusion. If these drug effects occur, avoid all hazardous activities.
Aviation Note: The use of this drug *may be a disqualification* for piloting. Consult a designated Aviation Medical Examiner.
Exposure to Sun: No restrictions.
Exposure to Heat: No restrictions.
Exposure to Cold: Use caution. Excessive chilling may enhance the development of livedo reticularis (see Possible Side-Effects above).
Discontinuation: When used to treat parkinsonism, this drug should not be stopped abruptly. Sudden discontinuation may cause an acute parkinsonian crisis. When used to treat influenza A infections, this drug should be continued for 48 hours after the disappearance of all symptoms.

AMBENONIUM
(am bee NOH ni um)

Introduced: 1956

Class: Antimyasthenic

Prescription: USA: Yes
Canada: No

Controlled Drug: USA: No
Canada: No

Available as Generic: USA: No
Canada: No

Brand Name: Mytelase Caplets

BENEFITS versus RISKS

Possible Benefits	*Possible Risks*
MODERATELY EFFECTIVE TREATMENT OF OCULAR AND MILD FORMS OF MYASTHENIA GRAVIS (symptomatic relief of muscle weakness)	Cholinergic crisis (overdose): excessive salivation, nausea, vomiting, stomach cramps, diarrhea, shortness of breath (asthmalike wheezing), excessive weakness

▷ **Principal Uses**

As a Single Drug Product: Used primarily to treat the ocular and milder forms of myasthenia gravis by providing temporary relief of muscle weakness and fatigability. Because of its potential for serious adverse effects, its use is generally reserved for treating those individuals who cannot use neostigmine (Prostigmin) or pyridostigmine (Mestinon).

How This Drug Works: This drug inhibits cholinesterase, the enzyme that destroys acetylcholine. This results in higher levels of acetylcholine, the nerve transmitter that facilitates the stimulation of muscular activity. The net effects are increased muscle strength and endurance.

Available Dosage Forms and Strengths

Tablets — 10 mg

▷ **Usual Adult Dosage Range:** Initially: 2.5 to 5 mg 3 or 4 times daily; adjust dosage as needed and tolerated at intervals of 48 hours. Maintenance: up to 300 mg/24 hours; the average dose is 15 to 100 mg/24 hours. It is advisable to try to determine the smallest dose that will provide the greatest strength. **Note: Actual dosage and administration schedule must be determined by the physician for each patient individually.**

▷ **Dosing Instructions:** Take with food or milk to reduce the intensity of side-effects. Larger portions of the daily maintenance dosage should be timed according to the pattern of fatigue and weakness. The tablet may be crushed for administration.

Usual Duration of Use: Continual use on a regular schedule (with dosage adjustment) for 10 to 14 days is usually necessary to determine this drug's effectiveness in relieving the symptoms of myasthenia gravis. Long-term use (months to years) requires periodic evaluation of response and dosage adjustment. Consult your physician on a regular basis.

▷ **This Drug Should Not Be Taken If**
- you have had an allergic reaction to it previously.

▷ **Inform Your Physician Before Taking This Drug If**
- you have any type of seizure disorder.
- you are subject to heart rhythm disorders or bronchial asthma.

- you have recurrent urinary tract infections.
- you have prostatism (see Glossary).
- you plan to have surgery under general anesthesia in the near future.

Possible Side-Effects (natural, expected and unavoidable drug actions)
Small pupils, watering of eyes, slow pulse, low blood pressure, excessive salivation, nausea, vomiting, stomach cramps, diarrhea, urge to urinate, increased sweating.

▷ **Possible Adverse Effects** (unusual, unexpected and infrequent reactions)
If any of the following develop, consult your physician promptly for guidance.
Mild Adverse Effects
Allergic Reaction: Skin rash.
Nervousness, anxiety, unsteadiness, muscle cramps or twitching.
Serious Adverse Effects
Confusion, slurred speech, seizures, difficult breathing (asthmatic wheezing).
Increased muscle weakness or paralysis.
Excessive vomiting or diarrhea may induce abnormally low blood potassium levels (hypokalemia). This will accentuate muscle weakness.

▷ **Possible Effects on Sexual Function:**   None reported.

▷ **Adverse Effects That May Mimic Natural Diseases or Disorders**
Seizures may suggest the possibility of epilepsy.

Natural Diseases or Disorders That May Be Activated by This Drug
Latent bronchial asthma.

Possible Effects on Laboratory Tests
None reported.

CAUTION
1. Certain drugs can block the action of this drug and reduce its effectiveness in treating myasthenia gravis. (See *Other Drugs* below.) Consult your physician before starting any new drug, prescription or over-the-counter.
2. The dosage schedule of this drug must be carefully individualized for each patient. Variations in response may occur from time to time. Because generalized muscle weakness is a major symptom of both myasthenia crisis (underdosage) and cholinergic crisis (overdosage), it may be difficult to recognize the correct cause. As a rule, weakness that begins within 1 hour after taking this drug probably represents overdosage; weakness that begins 3 or more hours after taking this drug is probably due to underdosage. Observe these time relationships and inform your physician.
3. During long-term use of this drug, observe for the possible development of resistance to the drug's therapeutic action (loss of effectiveness). Consult your physician regarding the advisability of discon-

tinuing this drug for a few days to see if responsiveness can be restored.

Precautions for Use
By Infants and Children: Dosage and administration schedule should be determined by a qualified pediatric neurologist.
By Those over 60 Years of Age: Avoid high doses that are more likely to cause serious adverse effects.

▷ **Advisability of Use During Pregnancy**
Pregnancy Category: C (tentative). See Pregnancy Code inside back cover.
Animal studies: No information available.
Human studies: Information from adequate studies of pregnant women is not available.
There are no reports of birth defects due to the use of this drug during pregnancy. However, there are reports of significant muscular weakness in 10% to 20% of newborn infants whose mothers had taken this class of drugs during pregnancy. Ask your physician for guidance.

Advisability of Use if Breast-Feeding
Presence of this drug in breast milk: Probably not.
Monitor nursing infant closely and discontinue drug or nursing if adverse effects develop.

Habit-Forming Potential: None.

Effects of Overdosage: Generalized muscular weakness, blurred vision, very small pupils, slow heart rate, difficult breathing (wheezing), excessive salivation, nausea, vomiting, stomach cramps, diarrhea, muscle cramps or twitching. This syndrome constitutes the cholinergic crisis.

Possible Effects of Long-Term Use: Development of tolerance (see Glossary) with loss of therapeutic effectiveness.

Suggested Periodic Examinations While Taking This Drug (at physician's discretion)
Assessment of drug effectiveness and dosage schedule for optimal therapeutic results.

▷ **While Taking This Drug, Observe the Following**
Foods: No restrictions.
Beverages: No restrictions. May be taken with milk.
▷ *Alcohol:* Use caution until the combined effects are determined. Weakness and unsteadiness may be accentuated.
Tobacco Smoking: No interactions expected.
▷ *Other Drugs*
The following drugs may *decrease* the effects of ambenonium
- atropine (belladonna).
- clindamycin (Cleocin).
- guanadrel (Hylorel).

- guanethidine (Esimil, Ismelin).
- procainamide (Procan SR, Pronestyl).
- quinidine (Cardioquin, Duraquin, etc.).
- quinine (Quinamm).

▷ *Driving, Hazardous Activities:* This drug may cause blurred vision, confusion or generalized weakness. Restrict activities as necessary.

Aviation Note: The use of this drug *is a disqualification* for piloting. Consult a designated Aviation Medical Examiner.

Exposure to Sun: No restrictions.

Exposure to Heat: Use caution. This may cause excessive sweating and increased weakness.

Exposure to Environmental Chemicals: Avoid excessive exposure (inhalation, skin contamination) to the insecticides Baygon, Diazinon and Sevin. These can accentuate the potential toxicity of this drug.

Discontinuation: Do not discontinue this drug abruptly without your physician's knowledge and guidance.

AMILORIDE
(a MIL oh ride)

Introduced: 1967

Class: Diuretic

Prescription: USA: Yes
Canada: Yes

Controlled Drug: USA: No
Canada: No

Available as Generic: Yes

Brand Names: Midamor, ✦Moduret [CD], Moduretic [CD]

BENEFITS versus RISKS	
Possible Benefits	*Possible Risks*
EFFECTIVE DIURETIC WITHOUT LOSS OF POTASSIUM	ABNORMALLY HIGH BLOOD POTASSIUM with excessive use Rare bone marrow depression

▷ **Principal Uses**

As a Single Drug Product: To eliminate excessive fluid retention (edema).

As a Combination Drug Product

[CD]: It is combined with other diuretics of the thiazide class primarily to prevent the loss of potassium from the body.

How This Drug Works: It is thought that this drug promotes the loss of sodium and water from the body and the retention of potassium by altering the enzyme systems of the kidney that control the formation of urine.

Available Dosage Forms and Strengths
Tablets — 5 mg

▷ **Usual Adult Dosage Range:** Initially 5 mg once daily, preferably in the morning. May increase up to 15 mg daily as needed and tolerated. Should not exceed 20 mg/24 hours. **Note: Actual dosage and administration schedule must be determined by the physician for each patient individually.**

▷ **Dosing Instructions:** Preferably taken on arising, with the stomach empty. For best results, withhold food for 4 hours. May be taken with food if necessary to reduce stomach irritation. Tablet may be crushed for administration.

Usual Duration of Use: As needed for elimination of edema or maintenance of normal blood pressure. Intermittent or alternate-day use is recommended to minimize imbalance of sodium and potassium. Consult your physician on a regular basis.

▷ **This Drug Should Not Be Taken If**
• you have had an allergic reaction to any dosage form of it previously.
• your blood potassium level is above the normal range.
• your kidneys are not producing urine.

▷ **Inform Your Physician Before Taking This Drug If**
• you have diabetes or glaucoma.
• you have a history of kidney disease or impaired kidney function.
• you are taking any other diuretic, blood pressure drug, any form of digitalis or lithium.

Possible Side-Effects (natural, expected and unavoidable drug actions)
Abnormally high blood potassium level (10% of users), abnormally low blood sodium level, dehydration, constipation.

▷ **Possible Adverse Effects** (unusual, unexpected and infrequent reactions)
If any of the following develop, consult your physician promptly for guidance.
Mild Adverse Effects
Allergic Reactions: Skin rash, itching.
Headache, dizziness, weakness, fatigue, numbness and tingling.
Dry mouth, nausea, vomiting, stomach pains, diarrhea.
Loss of scalp hair.
Serious Adverse Effects
Idiosyncratic Reactions: Joint and muscle pains.
Excessively high blood potassium level—marked fatigue and weakness, confusion, numbness and tingling of lips and extremities, slow and irregular heartbeats.
Increased internal eye pressure (of concern in glaucoma).
Mental depression, visual disturbances, ringing in ears, tremors.
Aplastic anemia (see Glossary)—unusual fatigue or weakness, fever, sore throat, abnormal bleeding or bruising.

▷ **Possible Effects on Sexual Function:**   More than 1%: decreased libido and impotence (5 to 10 mg/day).

▷ **Adverse Effects That May Mimic Natural Diseases or Disorders**
Nervousness, confusion and/or depression may resemble spontaneous mental disorder.

Natural Diseases or Disorders That May Be Activated by This Drug
Preexisting peptic ulcer, latent glaucoma.

Possible Effects on Laboratory Tests
Blood cholesterol level: decreased.
Blood creatinine level: increased with long-term use.
Blood potassium level: increased.
Blood uric acid level: may increase with long-term use, especially if taken with thiazide diuretics.

CAUTION
1. Do not take potassium supplements, and do not increase your intake of high-potassium foods.
2. If taking any form of digitalis, report as directed for periodic measurements of your blood potassium level.
3. Do not discontinue this drug abruptly unless directed to do so by your physician.

Precautions for Use
By Infants and Children: Safety and effectiveness for use by those under 12 years of age have not been established.
By Those over 60 Years of Age: The natural decline in kidney function may predispose to excessive retention of potassium in the body. It is advisable to limit use of this drug to periods of 2 to 3 weeks if possible. Overdosage and extended use can cause excessive loss of body water, increased viscosity of the blood and an increased tendency to abnormal blood clotting (thrombosis, heart attack, stroke).

▷ **Advisability of Use During Pregnancy**
Pregnancy Category: B (tentative). See Pregnancy Code inside back cover.
Animal studies: No birth defects reported.
Human studies: Information from adequate studies of pregnant women is not available.
Use only if clearly needed.

Advisability of Use if Breast-Feeding
Presence of this drug in breast milk: Unknown, but probably present. This drug may suppress milk production.
Avoid drug if possible. If use is necessary, monitor nursing infant closely and discontinue drug or nursing if adverse effects develop.

Habit-Forming Potential: None.

Effects of Overdosage: Thirst, drowsiness, fatigue, weakness, nausea, vomiting, confusion, numbness and tingling of face and extremities, irregular heart rhythm, shortness of breath.

Suggested Periodic Examinations While Taking This Drug (at physician's discretion)
  Complete blood cell counts; measurements of blood levels of sodium, potassium and chloride; kidney function tests; and assessment of water balance (state of hydration).

▷ **While Taking This Drug, Observe the Following**
  Foods: No restrictions. Avoid excessive restriction of salt. Avoid excessive amounts of high-potassium foods.
  Beverages: No restrictions. May be taken with milk.
▷ *Alcohol:* Use with caution until the combined effect has been determined. Alcohol can exaggerate the blood-pressure-lowering effect of this drug and cause orthostatic hypotension (see Glossary).
  Tobacco Smoking: No interactions expected.
▷ *Other Drugs*
  Amiloride may *increase* the effects of
  • other blood-pressure-lowering drugs. Dosage adjustments may be necessary.
  Amiloride may *decrease* the effects of
  • digoxin (Lanoxin, etc.), and reduce its effectiveness in treating heart failure.
  Amiloride *taken concurrently* with
  • spironolactone (Aldactone, Aldactazide) or triamterene (Dyrenium, Dyazide) may cause excessive (dangerous) increase in blood potassium levels. Avoid the concurrent use of these drugs.
  • lithium may cause lithium accumulation to toxic levels.
▷ *Driving, Hazardous Activities:* This drug may cause drowsiness, dizziness and orthostatic hypotension in sensitive individuals. If these drug effects occur, avoid hazardous activities.
  Aviation Note: The use of this drug *may be a disqualification* for piloting. Consult a designated Aviation Medical Examiner.
  Exposure to Sun: No restrictions.
  Exposure to Heat: Caution advised. Excessive perspiration can cause water, sodium and potassium imbalance. Hot environments can cause lowering of blood pressure.
  Occurrence of Unrelated Illness: Consult your physician if you contract an illness that causes vomiting or diarrhea.
  Discontinuation: With high dosage or prolonged use, withdraw this drug gradually. Sudden withdrawal can cause excessive loss of potassium from the body.

AMITRIPTYLINE
(a mee TRIP ti leen)

Introduced: 1961

Class: Antidepressant

Prescription: USA: Yes
Canada: Yes

Controlled Drug: USA: No
Canada: No

Available as Generic: Yes

Brand Names: Amitril, ✦Apo-Amitriptyline, Elavil, ✦Elavil Plus [CD], Emitrip, Endep, Etrafon [CD], Etrafon-A [CD], Etrafon-Forte [CD], ✦Levate, Limbitrol [CD], ✦Novotriptyn, Triavil [CD]

BENEFITS versus RISKS

Possible Benefits	*Possible Risks*
EFFECTIVE RELIEF OF ENDOGENOUS DEPRESSION in 60% to 75% of users	ADVERSE BEHAVIORAL EFFECTS: Confusion, disorientation, hallucinations CONVERSION OF DEPRESSION TO MANIA in manic-depressive disorders Irregular heart rhythms Rare blood cell abnormalities

---

▷ **Principal Uses**

As a Single Drug Product: To relieve the symptoms associated with spontaneous (endogenous) depression, and to initiate the restoration of normal mood. This drug should be used only when a diagnosis of a true, primary depression of significant degree has been established. It should not be used to treat the symptoms of mild and transient (reactive) depression that may be associated with many life situations in the absence of a bona fide affective illness.

As a Combination Drug Product [CD]: This drug is available in combination with chlordiazepoxide, a mild tranquilizer of the benzodiazepine class. This combination is used to relieve anxiety that may accompany depression. This drug is also available in combination with perphenazine, a strong tranquilizer of the phenothiazine class. This combination is used to relieve severe agitation that may accompany depression.

How This Drug Works: It is thought that this drug relieves depression by slowly restoring to normal levels certain constituents of brain tissue (norepinephrine and serotonin) that transmit nerve impulses.

Available Dosage Forms and Strengths

Tablets — 10 mg, 25 mg, 50 mg, 75 mg, 100 mg, 150 mg

▷ **Usual Adult Dosage Range:**   Initially 25 mg 2 to 4 times daily. Dose may be increased cautiously as needed and tolerated by 10 to 25 mg daily at intervals of 1 week. Usual maintenance dose is 50 to 100 mg/24 hours. Total dose should not exceed 150 mg/24 hours. When the optimal requirement is determined, it may be taken at bedtime as one dose. **Note: Actual dosage and administration schedule must be determined by the physician for each patient individually.**

▷ **Dosing Instructions:**   May be taken without regard to meals. Tablet may be crushed for administration.

Usual Duration of Use: Some benefit may be apparent within 1 to 2 weeks, but adequate response may require continual use for 4 to 6 weeks or longer. Long-term use should not exceed 6 months without evaluation regarding the need for continuation of the drug. Consult your physician on a regular basis.

▷ **This Drug Should Not Be Taken If**
  • you are allergic to any of the drugs bearing the brand names listed above.
  • you are taking or have taken within the past 14 days any monoamine oxidase (MAO) type A inhibitor drug (see Drug Class, Section Four).
  • you are recovering from a recent heart attack.
  • you have narrow-angle glaucoma.

▷ **Inform Your Physician Before Taking This Drug If**
  • you are allergic or sensitive to any other tricyclic antidepressant (see Drug Class, Section Four).
  • you have a history of any of the following: diabetes, epilepsy, glaucoma, heart disease, prostate gland enlargement or overactive thyroid function.
  • you plan to have surgery under general anesthesia in the near future.

Possible Side-Effects (natural, expected and unavoidable drug actions)
Drowsiness, blurred vision, dry mouth, constipation, impaired urination.

▷ **Possible Adverse Effects** (unusual, unexpected and infrequent reactions)
If any of the following develop, consult your physician promptly for guidance.
Mild Adverse Effects
Allergic Reactions: Skin rash, hives, swelling of face or tongue, drug fever (see Glossary).
Headache, dizziness, weakness, fainting, unsteady gait, tremors.
Peculiar taste, irritation of tongue or mouth, nausea, indigestion.
Fluctuation of blood sugar levels.
Serious Adverse Effects
Allergic Reactions: Hepatitis, with or without jaundice (see Glossary).
Idiosyncratic Reactions: Neuroleptic malignant syndrome (see Glossary).
Confusion, hallucinations, agitation, restlessness, nightmares.

Heart palpitation and irregular rhythm.

Bone marrow depression (see Glossary)—fatigue, weakness, fever, sore throat, abnormal bleeding or bruising.

Peripheral neuritis (see Glossary)—numbness, tingling, pain, loss of strength in arms and legs.

Parkinson-like disorders (see Glossary)—usually mild and infrequent; more likely to occur in the elderly.

▷ **Possible Effects on Sexual Function:**   Decreased libido (8%), increased libido (antidepressant effect), impotence (19%), inhibited female orgasm, inhibited ejaculation, male and female breast enlargement, milk production, swelling of testicles. These effects usually disappear within 2 to 10 days after discontinuation of the drug.

▷ **Adverse Effects That May Mimic Natural Diseases or Disorders**
Liver toxicity may suggest viral hepatitis.

Natural Diseases or Disorders That May Be Activated by This Drug
Latent diabetes, epilepsy, glaucoma, impaired urination due to prostate gland enlargement.

Possible Effects on Laboratory Tests
Complete blood cell counts: decreased white cells and platelets; increased eosinophils.

Liver function tests: increased liver enzymes (ALT/GPT, AST/GOT, alkaline phosphatase), increased bilirubin.

Blood glucose levels: increased and decreased (fluctuations).

CAUTION
1. Dosage must be adjusted for each person individually. Report for follow-up evaluation and laboratory tests as directed by your physician.
2. It is advisable to withhold this drug if electroconvulsive therapy (ECT, "shock" treatment) is to be used to treat your depression.

Precautions for Use
By Infants and Children: Safety and effectiveness for use by those under 12 years of age have not been established.

By Those over 60 Years of Age: During the first 2 weeks of treatment, observe for the development of confusion, agitation, forgetfulness, disorientation, delusions and hallucinations. Reduction of dosage or discontinuation may be necessary. Unsteadiness may predispose to falling and injury. This drug can increase the degree of impaired urination associated with prostate gland enlargement (prostatism).

▷ **Advisability of Use During Pregnancy**
Pregnancy Category: C (tentative). See Pregnancy Code inside back cover.
Animal studies: Skull deformities reported in rabbits.
Human studies: No defects reported in 21 exposures. Information from adequate studies of pregnant women is not available.

Avoid use of drug during first 3 months. Use during last 6 months only if clearly needed.

Advisability of Use if Breast-Feeding
Presence of this drug in breast milk: Yes, in small amounts.
Monitor nursing infant closely and discontinue drug or nursing if adverse effects develop.

Habit-Forming Potential: Psychological or physical dependence is rare and unexpected.

Effects of Overdosage: Confusion, hallucinations, marked drowsiness, heart palpitations, dilated pupils, tremors, stupor, deep sleep, coma, convulsions.

Suggested Periodic Examinations While Taking This Drug (at physician's discretion)
Complete blood cell counts, liver function tests, serial blood pressure readings and electrocardiograms.

▷ **While Taking This Drug, Observe the Following**
Foods: No restrictions. This drug may increase the appetite and cause excessive weight gain.
Beverages: No restrictions. May be taken with milk.
▷   *Alcohol:* Avoid completely. This drug can markedly increase the intoxicating effects of alcohol and accentuate its depressant action on brain function.
Tobacco Smoking: May hasten the elimination of this drug. Higher doses may be necessary.
▷   *Other Drugs*
Amitriptyline may *increase* the effects of
• atropinelike drugs (see Drug Class, Section Four).
Amitriptyline may *decrease* the effects of
• clonidine (Catapres).
• guanethidine (Ismelin).
Amitriptyline *taken concurrently* with
• monoamine oxidase (MAO) type A inhibitor drugs may cause high fever, delirium and convulsions (see Drug Class, Section Four).
• thyroid preparations may impair heart rhythm and function. Ask physician for guidance regarding adjustment of thyroid dose.
▷   *Driving, Hazardous Activities:* This drug may impair mental alertness, judgment, physical coordination and reaction time. Avoid hazardous activities.
Aviation Note: The use of this drug *is a disqualification* for piloting. Consult a designated Aviation Medical Examiner.
Exposure to Sun: Use caution until sensitivity to sun has been determined. This drug may cause photosensitivity (see Glossary).
Exposure to Heat: This drug can inhibit sweating and impair the body's adaptation to hot environments, increasing the risk of heat stroke. Avoid saunas.

Exposure to Cold: The elderly should use caution and avoid conditions conducive to hypothermia (see Glossary).

Discontinuation: It is advisable to discontinue this drug gradually. Abrupt withdrawal after long-term use can cause headache, malaise and nausea.

AMOXAPINE
(a MOX a peen)

Introduced: 1970

Class: Antidepressant

Prescription: USA: Yes
   Canada: Yes

Controlled Drug: USA: No
   Canada: No

Available as Generic: No

Brand Name: Asendin

BENEFITS versus RISKS

Possible Benefits	*Possible Risks*
EFFECTIVE RELIEF OF PRIMARY DEPRESSIONS: Endogenous, neurotic, reactive	ADVERSE BEHAVIORAL EFFECTS: Confusion, delusions, disorientation, hallucinations
Well tolerated by most persons	CONVERSION OF DEPRESSION TO MANIA in manic-depressive disorders
	Rare blood cell abnormalities

▷ **Principal Uses**

As a Single Drug Product: To provide symptomatic relief in all types of depression, and to initiate the restoration of normal mood.

How This Drug Works: It is thought that by increasing the availability of certain nerve impulse transmitters (norepinephrine and serotonin) in brain tissue, this drug relieves the symptoms associated with depression.

Available Dosage Forms and Strengths

Tablets — 25 mg, 50 mg, 100 mg, 150 mg

▷ **Usual Adult Dosage Range:** Initially 50 mg 3 times daily. Dose may be increased cautiously on the third day as needed and tolerated to 100 mg 3 times daily. Usual maintenance dose is 200 to 300 mg/24 hours. Total dosage should not exceed 400 mg/24 hours. When determined, the optimal requirement may be taken at bedtime as one dose, not to exceed 300 mg. **Note: Actual dosage and administration schedule must be determined by the physician for each patient individually.**

▷ **Dosing Instructions:**   May be taken without regard to meals. Tablet may be crushed for administration.

Usual Duration of Use: Benefit may be apparent within 4 to 7 days in some individuals, but continual use on a regular schedule for 2 to 3 weeks is usually necessary to determine this drug's effectiveness. Long-term use should not exceed 6 months without evaluation regarding the need for continuation. Consult your physician on a regular basis.

▷ **This Drug Should Not Be Taken If**
   • you have had an allergic reaction to it previously.
   • you are taking or have taken within the past 14 days any monoamine oxidase (MAO) type A inhibitor drug (see Drug Class, Section Four).
   • you are recovering from a recent heart attack.

▷ **Inform Your Physician Before Taking This Drug If**
   • you are allergic or overly sensitive to other antidepressant drugs.
   • you have a history of any of the following: diabetes, epilepsy, glaucoma, heart disease, paranoia, prostate gland enlargement, schizophrenia or overactive thyroid function.
   • you plan to have surgery under general anesthesia in the near future.

Possible Side-Effects (natural, expected and unavoidable drug actions)
   Drowsiness, blurred vision, dry mouth, constipation, impaired urination.

▷ **Possible Adverse Effects** (unusual, unexpected and infrequent reactions)
   If any of the following develop, consult your physician promptly for guidance.
   Mild Adverse Effects
   Allergic Reactions: Skin rash, hives, swellings, drug fever (see Glossary).
   Insomnia, nervousness, palpitations, dizziness, unsteadiness, tremors, fainting.
   Peculiar taste, indigestion, nausea, vomiting.
   Serious Adverse Effects
   Idiosyncratic Reactions: Neuroleptic malignant syndrome (see Glossary).
   Behavioral effects: anxiety, confusion, excitement, disorientation, hallucinations, delusions.
   Aggravation of paranoid psychosis and schizophrenia.
   Aggravation of epilepsy (seizures).
   Parkinson-like disorders (see Glossary).
   Peripheral neuritis (see Glossary)—numbness, tingling, pain, loss of strength in arms and legs.
   Reduced white blood cell count—fever, sore throat.

▷ **Possible Effects on Sexual Function:**   Decreased libido (150 mg/day), increased libido (antidepressant effect), inhibited ejaculation (75 to 150 mg/day), painful ejaculation (75 mg/day), inhibited female orgasm (100 mg/day), female breast enlargement/milk production (300 mg/day), altered menstrual timing and pattern (300 mg/day), swelling of testicles. These effects usually disappear within 2 to 10 days after discontinuation of the drug.

Natural Diseases or Disorders That May Be Activated by This Drug
Latent epilepsy, glaucoma, prostatism.

Possible Effects on Laboratory Tests
White blood cell counts: decreased.

CAUTION
1. The dosage of this drug must be adjusted carefully for each person individually. This requires observation of symptom improvement and, in some instances, the measurement of drug levels in the blood.
2. Observe for early indications of toxicity: confusion, agitation, rapid heartbeat.
3. It is advisable to withhold this drug if electroconvulsive therapy (ECT, "shock" treatment) is to be used.

Precautions for Use
By Infants and Children: Safety and effectiveness for use by those under 16 years of age have not been established.
By Those over 60 Years of Age: During the first 2 weeks of treatment, observe for the development of confusion, restlessness, agitation, forgetfulness, disorientation, delusions and hallucinations. Reduction of dosage or discontinuation may be necessary. Observe for unsteadiness that may predispose to falling and injury. This drug can increase the degree of impaired urination associated with prostate gland enlargement (prostatism). It is advisable to take the total dose at bedtime to reduce the risk of postural hypotension (see Glossary).

▷ **Advisability of Use During Pregnancy**
Pregnancy Category: C (tentative). See Pregnancy Code inside back cover.
Animal studies: Reveal toxic effects on the embryo in rats and rabbits but no birth defects in the newborn.
Human studies: Information from adequate studies of pregnant women is not available.
Avoid drug during first 3 months. Use during the last 6 months only if clearly needed.

Advisability of Use if Breast-Feeding
Presence of this drug in breast milk: Yes, in small amounts.
Monitor nursing infant closely and discontinue drug or nursing if adverse effects develop.

Habit-Forming Potential: None.

Effects of Overdosage: Confusion, hallucinations, marked drowsiness, tremors, dilated pupils, cold skin, stupor, coma, convulsions, rapid heartbeat, low blood pressure.

Suggested Periodic Examinations While Taking This Drug (at physician's discretion)

   Complete blood cell counts, serial blood pressure readings and electrocardiograms.

▷ **While Taking This Drug, Observe the Following**

   Foods: No restrictions. Drug may increase appetite and cause excessive weight gain.

   Beverages: No restrictions. May be taken with milk.

▷ *Alcohol:* Avoid completely. This drug can markedly increase the intoxicating effects of alcohol and accentuate its depressant action on brain function.

   Tobacco Smoking: May hasten the elimination of this drug. Higher doses may be necessary.

▷ *Other Drugs*

   Amoxapine may *increase* the effects of
   • atropinelike drugs (see Drug Class, Section Four).

   Amoxapine may *decrease* the effects of
   • clonidine (Catapres).
   • guanethidine (Ismelin).

   Amoxapine *taken concurrently* with
   • monoamine oxidase (MAO) type A inhibitor drugs may cause high fever, delirium and convulsions (see Drug Class, Section Four).
   • thyroid preparations may impair heart rhythm and function. Ask physician for guidance regarding adjustment of thyroid dose.

▷ *Driving, Hazardous Activities:* This drug may impair mental alertness, judgment, physical coordination and reaction time. Avoid hazardous activities.

   Aviation Note: The use of this drug *is a disqualification* for piloting. Consult a designated Aviation Medical Examiner.

   Exposure to Sun: Use caution until sensitivity to sun has been determined. This drug may cause photosensitivity (see Glossary).

   Exposure to Heat: This drug can inhibit sweating and impair the body's adaptation to hot environments, increasing the risk of heat stroke. Avoid saunas.

   Exposure to Cold: The elderly should use caution and avoid conditions conducive to hypothermia (see Glossary).

   Discontinuation: It is advisable to discontinue this drug gradually. Abrupt withdrawal after long-term use can cause headache, malaise and nausea.

AMOXICILLIN
(a mox i SIL in)

Introduced: 1969

Class: Antibiotic, penicillins

Prescription: USA: Yes
    Canada: Yes

Controlled Drug: USA: No
    Canada: No

Available as Generic: USA: Yes
    Canada: No

Brand Names: Amoxil, ✦Apo-Amoxi, Augmentin [CD], ✦Clavulin [CD], Larotid, ✦Novamoxin, Polymox, Trimox, Utimox, Wymox

---

BENEFITS versus RISKS

Possible Benefits	*Possible Risks*
EFFECTIVE TREATMENT OF INFECTIONS due to susceptible microorganisms	ALLERGIC REACTIONS, mild to severe, in 3% of the general population and 15% of allergic individuals Superinfections (yeast) Drug-induced colitis

---

▷ **Principal Uses**
    As a Single Drug Product: To treat certain infections of the skin and soft tissues; of the ear, nose and throat; and of the genitourinary tract, including gonorrhea.

How This Drug Works: This drug destroys susceptible infecting bacteria by interfering with their ability to produce new protective cell walls as they multiply and grow.

Available Dosage Forms and Strengths
    Capsules — 250 mg, 500 mg
    Chewable tablets — 125 mg, 250 mg
    Oral suspension — 125 mg, 250 mg per 5-ml teaspoonful
    Pediatric drops — 50 mg per ml

▷ **Usual Adult Dosage Range:**   250 to 500 mg/8 hours. The usual maximal dose is 4500 mg/24 hours. **Note: Actual dosage and administration schedule must be determined by the physician for each patient individually.**

▷ **Dosing Instructions:**   May be taken on an empty stomach or with food, milk, fruit juice, ginger ale or other cold drinks. Capsule may be opened for administration.

Usual Duration of Use: For all streptococcal infections—not less than 10 consecutive days (without interruption) to reduce the possibility of developing rheumatic fever or glomerulonephritis. For all other infections—as long as necessary to eradicate the infection.

▷ **This Drug Should Not Be Taken If**
- you have had an allergic reaction to any dosage form of it previously.
- you are certain you are allergic to *any* form of penicillin.

▷ **Inform Your Physician Before Taking This Drug If**
- you suspect you may be allergic to penicillin or you have a history of a previous "reaction" to penicillin.
- you are allergic to cephalosporin antibiotics (Ancef, Ceporan, Ceporex, Kafocin, Keflex, Keflin, Kefzol, Loridine).
- you are allergic by nature (hay fever, asthma, hives, eczema).

Possible Side-Effects (natural, expected and unavoidable drug actions)
Superinfections (see Glossary), often due to yeast organisms.

▷ **Possible Adverse Effects** (unusual, unexpected and infrequent reactions)
If any of the following develop, consult your physician promptly for guidance.
Mild Adverse Effects
Allergic Reactions: Skin rashes, hives, itching.
Irritations of mouth and tongue, "black tongue," nausea, vomiting, mild diarrhea, dizziness (rare).
Serious Adverse Effects
Allergic Reactions: Anaphylactic reaction (see Glossary), severe skin reactions, drug fever, swollen painful joints, sore throat, abnormal bleeding or bruising.

▷ **Possible Effects on Sexual Function:** None reported.

Possible Effects on Laboratory Tests
White blood cell counts: decreased.

CAUTION
1. Take the exact dose and the full course prescribed.
2. This drug should not be used concurrently with antibiotics like erythromycin or tetracycline.

Precautions for Use
By Infants and Children: A generalized rash occurs in approximately 90% of individuals who take this drug during an episode of infectious mononucleosis. This drug may cause diarrhea, which sometimes necessitates discontinuation.
By Those over 60 Years of Age: Natural changes in the skin may predispose to prolonged itching reactions in the genital and anal regions. Report such reactions promptly.

▷ **Advisability of Use During Pregnancy**
Pregnancy Category: B (tentative). See Pregnancy Code inside back cover.
Animal studies: No information available.

Human studies: Information from adequate studies of pregnant women indicates no increased risk of birth defects in 3546 pregnancies exposed to penicillin derivatives.
Ask physician for guidance.

Advisability of Use if Breast-Feeding
Presence of this drug in breast milk: Yes.
The nursing infant may be sensitized to penicillin and may be at risk for developing diarrhea or yeast infections.
Avoid drug if possible or refrain from nursing.

Habit-Forming Potential: None.

Effects of Overdosage: Possible nausea, vomiting and/or diarrhea.

Possible Effects of Long-Term Use: Superinfections, often due to yeast organisms.

Suggested Periodic Examinations While Taking This Drug (at physician's discretion)
Complete blood cell counts.

▷ **While Taking This Drug, Observe the Following**
Foods: No restrictions.
Beverages: No restrictions. May be taken with milk, fruit juices or carbonated drinks.
▷   *Alcohol:* No interactions expected.
Tobacco Smoking: No interactions expected.
▷   *Other Drugs*
Amoxicillin may *decrease* the effects of
• oral contraceptives in some women, and impair their effectiveness in preventing pregnancy.
The following drugs may *decrease* the effects of amoxicillin
• antacids reduce the absorption of amoxicillin.
• chloramphenicol (Chloromycetin).
• erythromycin (Erythrocin, E-Mycin, etc.).
• tetracyclines (Achromycin, Declomycin, Minocin, etc.). (See Drug Class, Section Four.)
▷   *Driving, Hazardous Activities:* Usually no restrictions. Be alert to the rare occurrence of dizziness and/or nausea, and restrict activities accordingly.
Aviation Note: The use of this drug *may be a disqualification* for piloting. Consult a designated Aviation Medical Examiner.
Exposure to Sun: No restrictions.
Special Storage Instructions: Oral suspension and pediatric drops should be refrigerated.
Observe the Following Expiration Times: Do not take the oral suspension or drops of this drug if older than 7 days when kept at room temperature or 14 days when kept refrigerated.

AMPICILLIN
(am pi SIL in)

Introduced: 1961

Class: Antibiotic, penicillins

Prescription: USA: Yes
Canada: Yes

Controlled Drug: USA: No
Canada: No

Available as Generic: Yes

Brand Names: Amcill, ✚Ampicin, ✚Ampicin PRB [CD], ✚Ampilean, ✚Apo-Ampi, 500 Kit [CD], ✚Novo-Ampicillin, Omnipen, Omnipen Pediatric Drops, ✚Penbritin, Polycillin, Polycillin Pediatric Drops, Polycillin-PRB [CD], Principen, Probampacin [CD], ✚Pro-Biosan, Totacillin

---

BENEFITS versus RISKS

Possible Benefits	*Possible Risks*
EFFECTIVE TREATMENT OF INFECTIONS due to susceptible microorganisms	ALLERGIC REACTIONS, mild to severe, in 3% of the general population and 15% of allergic individuals Superinfections (yeast) Drug-induced colitis

---

▷ **Principal Uses**

As a Single Drug Product: To treat certain infections of the skin and soft tissues, of the respiratory tract, of the gastrointestinal tract, and of the genitourinary tract (including gonorrhea in females). Also used to treat certain types of septicemia and meningitis.

As a Combination Drug Product [CD]: May be combined with probenecid (Benemid) to delay the elimination of ampicillin by the kidney and thereby increase its level in the blood. This combination drug is designed primarily for the treatment of gonorrhea in males and females.

How This Drug Works: This drug destroys susceptible infecting bacteria by interfering with their ability to produce new protective cell walls as they multiply and grow.

Available Dosage Forms and Strengths

Capsules — 250 mg, 500 mg
Oral suspension — 100 mg per ml, 125 mg, 250 mg, 500 mg per 5-ml teaspoonful
Pediatric drops — 100 mg per ml

▷ **Usual Adult Dosage Range:** 250 to 500 mg/6 hours. The usual maximal dose is 6000 mg/24 hours. **Note: Actual dosage and administration schedule must be determined by the physician for each patient individually.**

▷ **Dosing Instructions:**   Best taken on an empty stomach, 1 hour before or 2 hours after eating. Capsule may be opened for administration.

Usual Duration of Use: For all streptococcal infections—not less than 10 consecutive days (without interruption) to reduce the possibility of developing rheumatic fever or glomerulonephritis. For all other infections—as long as necessary to eradicate the infection.

▷ **This Drug Should Not Be Taken If**
  • you have had an allergic reaction to any dosage form of it previously.
  • you are certain you are allergic to *any* form of penicillin.

▷ **Inform Your Physician Before Taking This Drug If**
  • you suspect you may be allergic to penicillin or you have a history of a previous "reaction" to penicillin.
  • you are allergic to cephalosporin antibiotics (Ancef, Ceporan, Ceporex, Kafocin, Keflex, Keflin, Kefzol, Loridine).
  • you are allergic by nature (hay fever, asthma, hives, eczema).

Possible Side-Effects (natural, expected and unavoidable drug actions)
Superinfections (see Glossary), often due to yeast organisms.

▷ **Possible Adverse Effects** (unusual, unexpected and infrequent reactions)
  If any of the following develop, consult your physician promptly for guidance.
  Mild Adverse Effects
  Allergic Reactions: Skin rashes, hives, itching.
  Irritations of mouth and tongue, "black tongue," nausea, vomiting, mild diarrhea, dizziness (rare).
  Serious Adverse Effects
  Allergic Reactions: Anaphylactic reaction (see Glossary), severe skin reactions, drug fever, swollen painful joints, sore throat, abnormal bleeding or bruising.

▷ **Possible Effects on Sexual Function:**   None reported.

Possible Effects on Laboratory Tests
  Complete blood cell counts: decreased red cells, white cells and platelets; increased eosinophils.
  Bleeding time: may be prolonged, related to dose of drug.
  Coombs' antiglobulin test: may be positive, indicating drug-induced hemolytic anemia.
  Urine analysis: positive for red blood cells and casts, indicating kidney damage.
  Urine sugar tests: using Tes-Tape—no drug effect; using Clinistix or Diastix—false low or negative; using Clinitest—false positive.

CAUTION
  1. Take the exact dose and the full course prescribed.
  2. This drug should not be used concurrently with antibiotics like erythromycin or tetracycline.

Precautions for Use
By Infants and Children: A generalized rash occurs in approximately 90% of individuals who take this drug during an episode of infectious mononucleosis. This drug may cause diarrhea, which sometimes necessitates discontinuation.
By Those over 60 Years of Age: Natural changes in the skin may predispose to prolonged itching reactions in the genital and anal regions. Report such reactions promptly.

▷ **Advisability of Use During Pregnancy**
Pregnancy Category: B (tentative). See Pregnancy Code inside back cover.
Animal studies: No birth defects due to this drug found in mice or rats.
Human studies: Information from adequate studies of pregnant women indicates no increased risk of birth defects in 3546 pregnancies exposed to penicillin derivatives.
Ask physician for guidance.

Advisability of Use if Breast-Feeding
Presence of this drug in breast milk: Yes, in small amounts.
The nursing infant may be sensitized to penicillin and may be at risk for developing diarrhea or yeast infections.
Avoid drug if possible or refrain from nursing.

Habit-Forming Potential: None.

Effects of Overdosage: Possible nausea, vomiting and/or diarrhea.

Possible Effects of Long-Term Use: Superinfections, often due to yeast organisms.

Suggested Periodic Examinations While Taking This Drug (at physician's discretion)
Complete blood cell counts.

▷ **While Taking This Drug, Observe the Following**
Foods: No restrictions.
Beverages: No restrictions. May be taken with milk.
▷ *Alcohol:* No interactions expected.
Tobacco Smoking: No interactions expected.
▷ *Other Drugs*
Ampicillin may *decrease* the effects of
• oral contraceptives in some women, and impair their effectiveness in preventing pregnancy.
The following drugs may *decrease* the effects of ampicillin
• antacids reduce the absorption of amoxicillin.
• chloramphenicol (Chloromycetin).
• erythromycin (Erythrocin, E-Mycin, etc.).
• tetracyclines (Achromycin, Declomycin, Minocin, etc.). (See Drug Class, Section Four.)
▷ *Driving, Hazardous Activities:* Usually no restrictions. Be alert to the rare occurrence of dizziness and/or nausea, and restrict activities accordingly.

Aviation Note: The use of this drug *may be a disqualification* for piloting. Consult a designated Aviation Medical Examiner.

Exposure to Sun: No restrictions.

Special Storage Instructions: Oral suspension and pediatric drops should be refrigerated.

Observe the Following Expiration Times: Do not take the oral suspension or drops of this drug if older than 7 days when kept at room temperature or 14 days when kept refrigerated.

ASPIRIN*
(AS pir in)

Other Names: ASA, acetylsalicylic acid

Introduced: 1899

Class: Mild analgesic, anti-inflammatory, antiplatelet, antipyretic, salicylates

Prescription: USA: No
Canada: No

Controlled Drug: USA: No
Canada: No

Available as Generic: Yes

Brand Names: Alka-Seltzer Effervescent Pain Reliever & Antacid [CD], Alka-Seltzer Plus [CD], Anacin [CD], Anacin Maximum Strength [CD], ✦Anacin w/Codeine [CD], ✦Ancasal, A.S.A. Enseals, ✦Asasantine [CD], Ascriptin [CD], Ascriptin A/D [CD], Aspergum, ✦Aspirin*, ✦Astrin, Axotal [CD], Azdone [CD], Bayer Aspirin, Bayer Children's Chewable Aspirin, Bufferin [CD], Bufferin Arthritis Strength [CD], Bufferin Extra Strength [CD], Bufferin w/Codeine [CD], Cama Arthritis Pain Reliever [CD], Cope [CD], ✦Coryphen, ✦Coryphen-Codeine [CD], Darvon Compound [CD], Darvon Compound-65 [CD], Darvon w/ASA [CD], ✦Darvon-N Compound [CD], Darvon-N w/ASA [CD], Dolene Compound-65 [CD], Easprin, Ecotrin Preparations, 8-Hour Bayer, Empirin, Empirin w/Codeine No. 2, 4 [CD], ✦Entrophen, Excedrin [CD], Fiorinal [CD], Fiorinal w/Codeine [CD], ✦Fiorinal-C 1/4, -C 1/2 [CD], 4-Way Cold Tablets [CD], Lortab ASA [CD], Maximum Bayer Aspirin, Measurin, Midol Caplets [CD], Norgesic [CD], Norgesic Forte [CD], ✦Novasen, ✦Novopropoxyn Compound [CD], ✦Oxycodan [CD], Percodan [CD], Percodan-Demi [CD], ✦Phenaphen [CD], ✦Phenaphen No. 2, 3, 4 [CD], ✦Riphen-10, Robaxisal [CD], ✦Robaxisal-C [CD], Roxiprin [CD], ✦Sal-Adult, ✦Sal-Infant, Sine-Off Tablets [CD], St. Joseph Children's Aspirin, ✦Supasa, Synalgos [CD], Synalgos-DC [CD], Talwin Compound [CD], Talwin Compound-50 [CD], ✦Triaphen-10, Trigesic [CD]

*In the United States *aspirin* is an official generic designation. In Canada *Aspirin* is the Registered Trade Mark of the Bayer Company Division of Sterling Drug Limited.

BENEFITS versus RISKS

Possible Benefits	*Possible Risks*
EFFECTIVE RELIEF OF MILD TO MODERATE PAIN and INFLAMMATION	Stomach irritation, bleeding, and/or ulceration
REDUCTION OF FEVER	Hearing loss
PREVENTION OF BLOOD CLOTS (as in heart attack, phlebitis and stroke)	Decreased numbers of white blood cells and platelets
	Hemolytic anemia

▷ **Principal Uses**

As a Single Drug Product: To relieve mild to moderate pain from any cause, to provide symptomatic relief in conditions characterized by inflammation and to reduce high fever. A major use is to treat musculoskeletal disorders, especially acute and chronic arthritis. It is also used selectively in low dosage to prevent platelet embolism to the brain (in men) and to reduce the risk of thromboembolism in patients recovering from a recent heart attack, in those with artificial heart valves and in those undergoing hip surgery. (See Blood Platelets in the Glossary.)

As a Combination Drug Product [CD]: Frequently combined with other mild or strong analgesic drugs to enhance pain relief. Also combined with antihistamines and decongestants in many cold preparations to relieve the headache and general discomfort that often accompany respiratory infections.

How This Drug Works: Aspirin reduces the tissue concentrations of prostaglandins, chemicals involved in the production of inflammation and pain. By modifying the temperature-regulating center in the brain, dilating blood vessels in the skin, and increasing sweating, aspirin hastens the loss of body heat and reduces fever. By preventing the production of thromboxane in blood platelets, aspirin inhibits the aggregation of platelets and the initiation of blood clots.

Available Dosage Forms and Strengths

Capsules, enteric-coated — 500 mg
Capsules, enteric-coated granules — 325 mg
Gum tablets — 227.5 mg
Suppositories — 60 mg, 120 mg, 125 mg, 130 mg, 195 mg, 200 mg, 300 mg, 325 mg, 600 mg, 650 mg, 1.2 grams
Tablets — 65 mg, 81 mg, 325 mg, 500 mg
Tablets, chewable — 81 mg
Tablets, enteric-coated — 325 mg, 500 mg, 650 mg, 975 mg
Tablets, prolonged-action — 650 mg, 800 mg

▷ **Usual Adult Dosage Range:**   For pain or fever—325 to 650 mg/4 hours as needed. For arthritis (and related conditions)—3600 to 5400 mg daily in divided doses. For the prevention of blood clots—80 to 150 mg/24 to 48 hours. **Note: For long-term use, actual dosage and administration schedule must be determined by the physician for each patient individually.**

▷ **Dosing Instructions:**   Take with food, milk, or a full glass of water to reduce stomach irritation. Regular tablets may be crushed and capsules opened for administration. Enteric-coated tablets, prolonged-action tablets, A.S.A. Enseals, Cama tablets and Ecotrin tablets should not be crushed.

Usual Duration of Use: Short-term use is recommended—3 to 5 days. Daily use should not exceed 10 days without physician supervision. Continual use on a regular schedule for 1 week is usually necessary to determine this drug's effectiveness in relieving the symptoms of chronic arthritis. Long-term use requires periodic evaluation of response and dosage adjustment. Consult your physician on a regular basis.

▷ **This Drug Should Not Be Taken If**
- you have had an allergic reaction or unfavorable response to any form of aspirin previously.
- you have any type of bleeding disorder (such as hemophilia).
- you have active peptic ulcer disease.
- you are in the last 3 months of pregnancy.
- it has an odor resembling vinegar. This is due to the presence of acetic acid and indicates the decomposition of aspirin.

▷ **Inform Your Physician Before Taking This Drug If**
- you are taking any anticoagulant drug.
- you are taking oral antidiabetic drugs.
- you have a history of peptic ulcer disease or gout.
- you have lupus erythematosus.
- you are pregnant or planning pregnancy.
- you plan to have surgery of any kind in the near future.

Possible Side-Effects (natural, expected and unavoidable drug actions)
Mild drowsiness in sensitive individuals.

▷ **Possible Adverse Effects** (unusual, unexpected and infrequent reactions)
If any of the following develop, consult your physician promptly for guidance.
Mild Adverse Effects
Allergic Reactions: Skin rash, hives, nasal discharge (resembling hay fever), nasal polyps.
Stomach irritation, heartburn, nausea, vomiting, constipation.
Serious Adverse Effects
Allergic Reactions: Acute anaphylactic reaction (see Glossary), asthma, unusual bruising due to allergic destruction of blood platelets (see Glossary).
Idiosyncratic Reactions: Hemolytic anemia (see Glossary).

Erosion of stomach lining, with silent bleeding.

Activation of peptic ulcer, with or without hemorrhage.

Bone marrow depression (see Glossary)—fatigue, weakness, fever, sore throat, abnormal bleeding or bruising.

Hepatitis with jaundice (see Glossary)—yellow skin and eyes, dark-colored urine, light-colored stool (very rare).

Kidney damage, if used in large doses or for a prolonged period of time.

▷ **Possible Effects on Sexual Function:** None reported.

▷ **Adverse Effects That May Mimic Natural Diseases or Disorders**

Liver damage may suggest viral hepatitis.

Possible Effects on Laboratory Tests

Complete blood cell counts: decreased red cells, hemoglobin, white cells and platelets.

Bleeding time: prolonged.

Prothrombin time: increased by large doses; decreased by small doses.

Blood glucose level: decreased in diabetics.

Blood uric acid level: increased by small doses; decreased by large doses.

Liver function tests: increased liver enzymes (ALT/GPT, AST/GOT, alkaline phosphatase).

Kidney function tests: increased blood creatinine and urea nitrogen levels with long-term use; increased protein and kidney cells in urine.

Thyroid function tests: increased T^3 uptake, free T^3 and free T^4; decreased TSH, T^3, T^4, and free thyroxine index (FTI).

Pregnancy tests: large doses of aspirin may cause a false positive urine test (mouse and rabbit tests).

Urine sugar tests: false positive with Clinitest or Benedict's solution.

Fecal occult blood test: positive with large doses of aspirin.

CAUTION

1. It is most important to understand that aspirin is a drug. While it is one of our most useful drugs, we have an unrealistic sense of safety and unconcern regarding its action within the body and its potential for adverse effects.

2. In order to know if you are taking aspirin, make it a point to learn the contents of all drugs you take—those prescribed by your physician and those you purchase over-the-counter (OTC) without prescription.

3. Limit the dose of aspirin to no more than 3 tablets (975 mg) at one time, allow at least 4 hours between doses and take no more than 10 tablets (3250 mg) in 24 hours without physician supervision.

4. Remember that aspirin can
   • cause new illnesses.
   • complicate existing illnesses.
   • complicate pregnancy.
   • complicate surgery.
   • interact unfavorably with other drugs.

5. When your physician asks "Are you taking any drugs?" the answer is yes if you are taking aspirin. This also applies to *any* nonprescription drug you may be taking. (See OTC Drugs in the Glossary.)

Precautions for Use

By Infants and Children: Reye syndrome (brain and liver damage in children, often fatal) can follow flu or chicken pox in children and teenagers. While the exact cause and nature of the syndrome are not known, some reports suggest that the use of aspirin by children with flu or chicken pox can increase the risk of developing this complication. Consult your physician before giving aspirin to a child or teenager with chicken pox, flu or similar infection.

Usual dosage schedule for children:

Up to 2 years of age—consult physician.

2 to 4 years of age—160 mg/4 hours, up to 5 doses/24 hours.

4 to 6 years of age—240 mg/4 hours, up to 5 doses/24 hours.

6 to 9 years of age—320 mg/4 hours, up to 5 doses/24 hours.

9 to 11 years of age—400 mg/4 hours, up to 5 doses/24 hours.

11 to 12 years of age—480 mg/4 hours, up to 5 doses/24 hours.

Do not exceed 5 days of continual use without consulting your physician.

Give all doses with food, milk or a full glass of water.

By Those over 60 Years of Age: The natural decline in kidney function can reduce your tolerance for aspirin. Observe for indications of excessive dosage: nervous irritabilty, confusion, ringing in the ears, deafness, loss of appetite, nausea and stomach irritation. Aspirin can cause excessive bleeding from the stomach in sensitive individuals. This can occur as "silent" bleeding of small amounts over an extended period of time, resulting in anemia. In addition, sudden hemorrhage can occur, even without a history of stomach ulcer. Observe stools for gray to black discoloration—an indication of stomach bleeding.

▷ Advisability of Use During Pregnancy

Pregnancy Category: D (tentative). See Pregnancy Code inside back cover.

Animal studies: Significant birth defects due to this drug have been reported.

Human studies: Information from studies of pregnant women indicates no increased risk of birth defects in 32,164 pregnancies exposed to aspirin. However, studies show that the regular use of salicylates during pregnancy is often detrimental to the health of the mother and to the welfare of the fetus. Excessive use of salicylate drugs can cause anemia, hemorrhage before and after delivery and an increased incidence of stillbirths and newborn deaths. It is advisable to limit the use of aspirin during pregnancy to small doses and for brief periods of time, and to avoid aspirin altogether during the last 3 months.

Advisability of Use if Breast-Feeding

Presence of this drug in breast milk: Yes.

Avoid drug or refrain from nursing.

Habit-Forming Potential: Use of this drug in large doses for a prolonged period of time may cause a form of psychological dependence (see Glossary).

Effects of Overdosage: Stomach distress, nausea, vomiting, ringing in the ears, dizziness, impaired hearing, sweating, stupor, fever, deep and rapid breathing, muscular twitching, delirium, hallucinations, convulsions.

Possible Effects of Long-Term Use
A form of psychological dependence (see Glossary).
Anemia due to chronic blood loss from erosion of stomach lining.
The development of stomach ulcer.
The development of "aspirin allergy"—nasal discharge, nasal polyps, asthma.
Kidney damage.
Excessive prolongation of bleeding time, of major importance in the event of injury or surgery.

Suggested Periodic Examinations While Taking This Drug (at physician's discretion)
Complete blood cell counts.
Kidney function tests and urine analyses.
Liver function tests.

▷ **While Taking This Drug, Observe the Following**
Foods: No restrictions.
Nutritional Support: If supplementing the diet with vitamin C, take no more than the recommended daily allowance. Do not take large doses of vitamin C while taking aspirin on a regular basis.
Beverages: No restrictions. May be taken with milk.
▷ *Alcohol:* No interactions expected. However, the concurrent use of alcohol and aspirin may significantly increase the possibility of erosion and ulceration of the stomach lining and may result in bleeding.
Tobacco Smoking: No interactions expected.
▷ *Other Drugs*
Aspirin may *increase* the effects of
• oral anticoagulants, and cause abnormal bleeding.
• Dosage adjustment is often necessary.
• oral antidiabetic drugs and insulin, and cause hypoglycemia (see Glossary). Dosage adjustment is often necessary.
• heparin, and cause abnormal bleeding.
• methotrexate, and increase its toxic effects.
• valproic acid (Depakene).
Aspirin may *decrease* the effects of
• beta-adrenergic-blocking drugs (see Drug Class, Section Four).
• captopril (Capoten).
• probenecid (Benemid), and reduce its effectiveness in the treatment of gout—with aspirin doses of less than 2 grams/24 hours.

- spironolactone (Aldactone), and reduce its diuretic effect.
- sulfinpyrazone (Anturane), and reduce its effectiveness in the treatment of gout—with aspirin doses of less than 2 grams/24 hours.

The following drugs may *increase* the effects of aspirin
- acetazolamide (Diamox).
- para-aminobenzoic acid (Pabalate).
- vitamin C, taken as ascorbic acid and in large doses, may acidify the urine in some individuals and cause aspirin accumulation and toxicity.

The following drugs may *decrease* the effects of aspirin
- antacids, in regular continual use.
- cortisonelike drugs (see Drug Class, Section Four).
- urinary alkalizers (sodium bicarbonate, sodium citrate).

▷ *Driving, Hazardous Activities:* No restrictions or precautions.

Aviation Note: Usually no restrictions. However, it is advisable to observe for the possible occurrence of mild drowsiness and to restrict activities accordingly.

Exposure to Sun: No restrictions.

Discontinuation: The use of aspirin should be discontinued completely at least 1 week before surgery of any kind.

ASTEMIZOLE
(a STEM i zohl)

Introduced: 1982

Class: Antihistamines

Prescription: USA: Yes
  Canada: No

Controlled Drug: USA: No
  Canada: No

Available as Generic: No

Brand Name: Hismanal

BENEFITS versus RISKS

Possible Benefits	*Possible Risks*
EFFECTIVE, LONG-LASTING RELIEF OF ALLERGIC RHINITIS AND ALLERGIC SKIN DISORDERS	Mild fatigue (infrequent)

▷ **Principal Uses**

As a Single Drug Product: Used primarily to provide symptomatic relief in allergic and related disorders: seasonal and perennial allergic rhinitis (hay fever), allergic conjunctivitis and vasomotor rhinitis; also in hives and localized swellings (angioedema) of allergic origin.

How This Drug Works: Antihistamines reduce the intensity of the allergic response by blocking the action of histamine after it has been released from sensitized tissue cells in the eyes, nose and skin.

Available Dosage Forms and Strengths
   Suspension — 10 mg per 5-ml teaspoonful (Canada)
   Tablets — 10 mg

▷ **Usual Adult Dosage Range:**   10 mg once daily. The total daily dosage should not exceed 30 mg. **Note: Actual dosage and administration schedule must be determined by the physician for each patient individually.**

▷ **Dosing Instructions:**   Take on an empty stomach, 1 hour before eating or 2 hours after eating. The tablet may be crushed for administration.

Usual Duration of Use: Continual use on a regular schedule for 3 days is usually necessary to determine this drug's effectiveness in relieving the symptoms of allergic rhinitis and dermatosis. It may be necessary to take this drug throughout the entire pollen season, depending upon individual sensitivity. However, antihistamines should not be taken continually (without interruption) for long-term use. Limit their use to periods that require symptomatic relief. Consult your physician on a regular basis.

Possible Advantages of This Drug
   Effective relief with once-a-day dosage.
   No loss of effectiveness with continual use.
   No drowsiness or impaired mental function that is so characteristic of many other antihistamines.
   No or very slight atropinelike effects.
   No interaction with alcohol or other drugs.
   No significant toxicity.

▷ **This Drug Should Not Be Taken If**
   • you have had an allergic reaction to any dosage form of it previously.
   • you are currently undergoing allergy skin tests.

▷ **Inform Your Physician Before Taking This Drug If**
   • you have had any allergic reactions or unfavorable responses to the previous use of antihistamines.
   • you have impaired liver or kidney function.

Possible Side-Effects (natural, expected and unavoidable drug actions)
   Dry nose, mouth or throat.

▷ **Possible Adverse Effects** (unusual, unexpected and infrequent reactions)
   If any of the following develop, consult your physician promptly for guidance.
   Mild Adverse Effects
   Allergic Reactions: Skin rash, itching.

Headache, nervousness, fatigue.

Increased appetite and weight (3.6%), indigestion, nausea, diarrhea.

Serious Adverse Effects
None reported.

▷ **Possible Effects on Sexual Function**
None reported.

Possible Effects on Laboratory Tests
None reported.

CAUTION
1. Discontinue this drug 4 days before diagnostic skin testing procedures in order to prevent false negative test results.
2. Do not use this drug if you have active bronchial asthma, bronchitis or pneumonia. It may thicken bronchial mucus and make it more difficult to remove (by absorption or coughing).

Precautions for Use
By Infants and Children: Safety and effectiveness for use by those under 12 years of age have not been established.
By Those over 60 Years of Age: You may be more susceptible to the development of headache and fatigue. Use smaller doses at longer intervals if necessary.

▷ **Advisability of Use During Pregnancy**
Pregnancy Category: C (tentative). See Pregnancy Code inside back cover.
Animal studies: No birth defects due to this drug reported.
Human studies: Information from adequate studies of pregnant women is not available.
Use this drug only if clearly needed. Ask your physician for guidance.

Advisability of Use if Breast-Feeding
Presence of this drug in breast milk: Unknown.
Avoid drug or refrain from nursing.

Habit-Forming Potential: None.

Effects of Overdosage: Serious heart rhythm abnormalities.

Possible Effects of Long-Term Use: None reported.

Suggested Periodic Examinations While Taking This Drug (at physician's discretion)
None required.

▷ **While Taking This Drug, Observe the Following**
Foods: No restrictions.
Beverages: No restrictions. May be taken with milk.
▷   *Alcohol:* No interactions expected.
Tobacco Smoking: No interactions expected.

▷ *Other Drugs:* No significant interactions reported to date.
Hazardous Activities: No restrictions.
Aviation Note: The use of this drug *is probably not a disqualification* for piloting. Consult a designated Aviation Medical Examiner.
Exposure to Sun: Use caution until sensitivity has been determined. Rare cases of photosensitivity have been reported (see Glossary).

ATENOLOL
(a TEN oh lohl)

Introduced: 1973

Class: Antianginal, antihypertensive, beta-adrenergic blocker

Prescription: USA: Yes
Canada: Yes

Controlled Drug: USA: No
Canada: No

Available as Generic: No

Brand Names: Tenoretic [CD], Tenormin

BENEFITS versus RISKS

Possible Benefits	*Possible Risks*
EFFECTIVE ANTIANGINAL DRUG in the management of effort-induced angina EFFECTIVE, WELL-TOLERATED ANTIHYPERTENSIVE in mild to moderate high blood pressure	CONGESTIVE HEART FAILURE in advanced heart disease Worsening of angina in coronary heart disease (abrupt withdrawal) Masking of low blood sugar (hypoglycemia) in drug-treated diabetes Provocation of bronchial asthma (with high doses)

▷ **Principal Uses**
As a Single Drug Product: Used primarily to treat (1) classical, effort-induced angina pectoris; (2) mild to moderately severe high blood pressure. May be used alone or concurrently with other antihypertensive drugs, such as diuretics.

How This Drug Works: By blocking certain actions of the sympathetic nervous system, this drug
- reduces the rate and contraction force of the heart, thus lowering the ejection pressure of the blood leaving the heart and reducing the oxygen requirement for heart function.
- reduces the degree of contraction of blood vessel walls, resulting in

their relaxation and expansion and consequent lowering of blood pressure.

Available Dosage Forms and Strengths
Tablets — 50 mg, 100 mg

▷ **Usual Adult Dosage Range:**   Initially 50 mg once daily. Dose may be increased gradually at intervals of 7 to 10 days as needed and tolerated up to 100 mg/24 hours. The usual maintenance dose is 50 to 100 mg/24 hours. The total dose should not exceed 100 mg/24 hours. **Note: Actual dosage and administration schedule must be determined by the physician for each patient individually.**

▷ **Dosing Instructions:**   May be taken without regard to eating. Tablet may be crushed for administration. Do not discontinue this drug abruptly.

Usual Duration of Use: Continual use on a regular schedule for 10 to 14 days is usually necessary to determine this drug's effectiveness in lowering blood pressure. The long-term use of this drug will be determined by the course of your blood pressure over time and your response to the overall treatment program (weight reduction, salt restriction, smoking cessation, etc.) Consult your physician on a regular basis.

Possible Advantages of This Drug: The least likely of all beta blocker drugs to cause central nervous system adverse effects: confusion, hallucinations, nervousness, nightmares.

Currently a "Drug of Choice"
for initiating treatment of hypertension with a single drug, especially for those subject to bronchial asthma or diabetes.

▷ **This Drug Should Not Be Taken If**
- you have had an allergic reaction to it previously.
- you have congestive heart failure.
- you have an abnormally slow heart rate or a serious form of heart block.
- you are taking, or have taken within the past 14 days, any monoamine oxidase (MAO) type A inhibitor drug (see Drug Class, Section Four).

▷ **Inform Your Physician Before Taking This Drug If**
- you have had an adverse reaction to any beta blocker drug in the past (see Drug Class, Section Four).
- you have a history of serious heart disease, with or without episodes of heart failure.
- you have a history of hay fever (allergic rhinitis), asthma, chronic bronchitis or emphysema.
- you have a history of overactive thyroid function (hyperthyroidism).
- you have a history of low blood sugar (hypoglycemia).
- you have impaired liver or kidney function.
- you have diabetes or myasthenia gravis.

- you are currently taking any form of digitalis, quinidine or reserpine, or any calcium blocker drug (see Drug Class, Section Four).
- you plan to have surgery under general anesthesia in the near future.

Possible Side-Effects (natural, expected and unavoidable drug actions)
Lethargy, fatigability, cold extremities, slow heart rate, light-headedness in upright position (see Orthostatic Hypotension in Glossary).

▷ **Possible Adverse Effects** (unusual, unexpected and infrequent reactions)
If any of the following develop, consult your physician promptly for guidance.
Mild Adverse Effects
Allergic Reactions: Skin rash, itching.
Headache, dizziness, drowsiness, abnormal dreams.
Indigestion, nausea, diarrhea.
Joint and muscle discomfort, fluid retention (edema).
Serious Adverse Effects
Mental depression, anxiety.
Chest pain, shortness of breath, precipitation of congestive heart failure.
Induction of bronchial asthma (in asthmatic individuals).

▷ **Possible Effects on Sexual Function:** Decreased libido and impaired potency (50 to 100 mg/day). This beta blocker is less likely to cause reduced erectile capacity than most other drugs of this class.

Possible Effects on Laboratory Tests
Blood cholesterol levels: no effect with doses of 50 mg/day; increased with doses of 100 mg/day.
Blood HDL cholesterol levels: no effect with doses of 50 mg/day; decreased with doses of 100 mg/day.
Blood LDL cholesterol levels: no effect with doses of 50 mg/day; increased with doses of 100 mg/day.
Blood VLDL cholesterol levels: no effect with doses of 50 mg/day; increased with doses of 100 mg/day.
Blood triglyceride levels: no effect with doses of 50 mg/day; increased with doses of 100 mg/day.

CAUTION
1. ***Do not discontinue this drug suddenly*** without the knowledge and guidance of your physician. Carry a notation on your person that you are taking this drug.
2. Consult your physician or pharmacist before using nasal decongestants usually present in over-the-counter cold preparations and nose drops. These can cause sudden increases in blood pressure when taken concurrently with beta blocker drugs.
3. Report the development of any tendency to emotional depression.

Precautions for Use
By Infants and Children: Safety and effectiveness for use by those under 12 years of age have not been established. However, if this drug is used,

observe for the development of low blood sugar (hypoglycemia) during periods of reduced food intake.

By Those over 60 Years of Age: Proceed **cautiously** with all antihypertensive drugs. Unacceptably high blood pressure should be reduced without creating the risks associated with excessively low blood pressure. Start treatment with small doses, and monitor the blood pressure response frequently. Sudden, rapid and excessive reduction of blood pressure can predispose to stroke or heart attack. Total daily dosage should not exceed 100 mg. Observe for dizziness, unsteadiness, tendency to fall, confusion, hallucinations, depression or urinary frequency.

▷ **Advisability of Use During Pregnancy**
Pregnancy Category: C (tentative). See Pregnancy Code inside back cover.
  Animal studies: Increased resorptions of embryo and fetus reported in rats, but no birth defects.
  Human studies: Information from adequate studies of pregnant women is not available.
  Avoid use of drug during the first 3 months if possible. Avoid use during labor and delivery because of the possible effects on the newborn infant.

Advisability of Use if Breast-Feeding
Presence of this drug in breast milk: Yes.
  Avoid drug if possible. If drug is necessary, observe nursing infant for slow heart rate and indications of low blood sugar.

Habit-Forming Potential: None.

Effects of Overdosage: Weakness, slow pulse, low blood pressure, fainting, cold and sweaty skin, congestive heart failure, possible coma and convulsions.

Possible Effects of Long-Term Use: Reduced heart reserve and eventual heart failure in susceptible individuals with advanced heart disease.

Suggested Periodic Examinations While Taking This Drug (at physician's discretion)
  Measurements of blood pressure, evaluation of heart function.

▷ **While Taking This Drug, Observe the Following**
Foods: No restrictions. Avoid excessive salt intake.
Beverages: No restrictions. May be taken with milk.
▷ *Alcohol:* Use with caution until the combined effect has been determined. Alcohol may exaggerate this drug's ability to lower blood pressure and may increase its mild sedative effect.
Tobacco Smoking: Nicotine may reduce this drug's effectiveness in treating high blood pressure. In addition, high doses of this drug may potentiate the constriction of the bronchial tubes caused by regular smoking.
▷ *Other Drugs*
  Atenolol may **increase** the effects of

- other antihypertensive drugs and cause excessive lowering of blood pressure. Dosage adjustments may be necessary.
- reserpine (Ser-Ap-Es, etc.) and cause sedation, depression, slowing of heart rate and lowering of blood pressure.

Atenolol *taken concurrently* with
- clonidine (Catapres) requires close monitoring for rebound high blood pressure if clonidine is withdrawn while atenolol is still being taken.
- insulin requires close monitoring to avoid undetected hypoglycemia (see Glossary).

The following drugs may *decrease* the effects of atenolol
- indomethacin (Indocin), and possibly other "aspirin substitutes," may impair atenolol's antihypertensive effect.

▷ *Driving, Hazardous Activities:* Use caution until the full extent of drowsiness, lethargy, and blood pressure change has been determined.

Aviation Note: The use of this drug *is a disqualification* for piloting. Consult a designated Aviation Medical Examiner.

Exposure to Sun: No restrictions.

Exposure to Heat: Caution advised. Hot environments can lower blood pressure and exaggerate the effects of this drug.

Exposure to Cold: Caution advised. Cold environments can enhance the circulatory deficiency in the extremities that may occur with this drug. The elderly should take precautions to prevent hypothermia (see Glossary).

Heavy Exercise or Exertion: It is advisable to avoid exertion that produces light-headedness, excessive fatigue, or muscle cramping. The use of this drug may intensify the hypertensive response to isometric exercise.

Occurrence of Unrelated Illness: The fever that accompanies systemic infections can lower blood pressure and require adjustment of dosage. Illnesses that cause nausea or vomiting may interrupt the regular dosage schedule. Ask your physician for guidance.

Discontinuation: It is advisable to avoid sudden discontinuation of this drug in all situations. If possible, gradual reduction of dose over a period of 2 to 3 weeks is recommended. Ask your physician for specific guidance.

ATROPINE*
(A troh peen)

Other Names: Belladonna alkaloids, hyoscyamine, scopolamine

Introduced: 1831

Class: Antispasmodic, atropinelike drugs, anticholinergics

Prescription: USA: Yes
Canada: No

Controlled Drug: USA: No
Canada: No

Available as Generic: Yes

Brand Names: Barbidonna [CD], Barbidonna Elixir [CD], Belladenal [CD], Belladenal-S [CD], ✦Belladenal Spacetabs [CD], ✦Bellergal [CD], Bellergal-S [CD], ✦Bellergal Spacetabs [CD], Butibel [CD], Cafergot P-B [CD], Chardonna-2 [CD], Donnagel [CD], ✦Donnagel w/Neomycin [CD], Donnagel-PG [CD], Donnatal [CD], Donnazyme [CD], Kinesed [CD], Lomotil [CD], Levsin/SL , Pyridium Plus [CD], Transderm Scop, Urised [CD], ✦Wigraine [CD]

BENEFITS versus RISKS

Possible Benefits	*Possible Risks*
EFFECTIVE ANTISPASMODIC ACTION in spastic disorders of the stomach and intestine (for atropine)	Increased internal eye pressure (important in glaucoma)
	Constipation (may be quite marked)
EFFECTIVE PREVENTION OF MOTION SICKNESS (for scopolamine)	Urinary retention (in predisposed persons)
	Mouth dryness

▷ **Principal Uses**

As a Single Drug Product: Atropine is used primarily for its antispasmodic effect in the treatment of spastic disorders of the digestive tract and lower urinary tract.

Scopolamine is used primarily to prevent motion sickness.

As a Combination Drug Product [CD]: Frequently combined with mild sedatives (especially barbiturates) to utilize their calming effects in the management of functional disorders associated with anxiety and nervous tension. The combination of a mild tranquilizer and an antispasmodic medication is more effective than either drug used alone.

How This Drug Works: By blocking the action of the chemical (acetylcholine) that transmits impulses at parasympathetic nerve endings, this drug prevents stimulation of muscular contraction and glandular se-

---

*Atropine, hyoscyamine and scopolamine are the principal belladonna alkaloids. The characteristics of atropine are representative of the group.

crection within the organs involved. This results in reduced overall activity, including the prevention or relief of muscle spasm.

Available Dosage Forms and Strengths
> Injection — 0.05 mg, 0.1 mg, 0.3 mg, 0.4 mg, 0.5 mg, 0.8 mg, 1 mg, 1.2 mg, all per ml
> Tablets — 0.4 mg
> Tablets, soluble — 0.3 mg, 0.4 mg, 0.6 mg
> Tablets, sublingual — 0.125 mg
> Transdermal disc — 0.5 mg

▷ **Usual Adult Dosage Range:** For atropine: 0.3 to 1.2 mg/4 to 6 hours. For scopolamine disc: one application every 72 hours as needed. **Note: Actual dosage and administration schedule must be determined by the physician for each patient individually.**

▷ **Dosing Instructions:** For maximal absorption and effect, this drug should be taken 30 to 60 minutes before eating. Regular tablets may be crushed and regular capsules may be opened for administration. Prolonged-action and sustained-release dosage forms should be taken whole (neither crushed nor opened).

For scopolamine transdermal disc: Apply to the hairless area behind one ear 4 hours before travel. The disc is designed to deliver 0.5 mg of scopolamine over 3 days. Apply only one disc at any time. If travel time requires application of another disc, this should be applied behind the other ear.

Usual Duration of Use: Continual use on a regular schedule for 2 to 5 days is usually necessary to determine this drug's effectiveness in relieving the symptoms of spastic disorders of the digestive system. Limit use to the relief of symptoms as necessary. Ask physician for guidance regarding long-term use.

▷ **This Drug Should Not Be Taken If**
- you have had an allergic reaction or unfavorable response to any atropine or belladonna preparation in the past.
- your stomach cannot empty properly into the intestine (pyloric obstruction).
- you are unable to empty the urinary bladder completely.
- you have glaucoma (narrow-angle type).
- you have severe ulcerative colitis.

▷ **Inform Your Physician Before Taking This Drug If**
- you have glaucoma (open-angle type).
- you have angina or coronary heart disease.
- you have chronic bronchitis.
- you have a hiatal hernia or peptic ulcer disease.
- you have enlargement of the prostate gland.

- you have myasthenia gravis.
- you plan to have surgery under general anesthesia in the near future.

Possible Side-Effects (natural, expected and unavoidable drug actions)
Blurring of near vision (impairment of focus), dryness of mouth and throat, constipation, hesitancy in urination.

▷ **Possible Adverse Effects** (unusual, unexpected and infrequent reactions)
If any of the following develop, consult your physician promptly for guidance.
Mild Adverse Effects
Allergic Reactions: Skin rash, hives.
Light-headedness, dizziness, unsteadiness.
Dilation of pupils, causing sensitivity to light.
Flushing and dryness of skin, reduced sweating.
Serious Adverse Effects
Allergic Reactions: Severe skin reactions—exfoliative dermatitis.
Idiosyncratic Reactions: Paradoxical excitement, nervousness, confusion, delirium.
Increased internal eye pressure, development of glaucoma in susceptible individuals.

▷ **Possible Effects on Sexual Function:** Inhibited female orgasm, reduced male fertility (0.4 to 0.6 mg/dose).

Natural Diseases or Disorders That May Be Activated by This Drug
Latent glaucoma (narrow-angle type), latent myasthenia gravis.

Possible Effects on Laboratory Tests
White blood cell counts: increased in children.

CAUTION
1. Use cautiously in the presence of asthma and chronic bronchitis. This drug can thicken bronchial secretions and promote retention of mucous plugs.
2. Many over-the-counter medications (see OTC Drugs in the Glossary) for allergies, colds and coughs contain antihistamines that can augment this drug's drying effects. Ask your physician or pharmacist for guidance before using such preparations.

Precautions for Use
By Infants and Children: Children are particularly vulnerable to atropine toxicity. Start with low doses and increase cautiously as needed and tolerated. Observe for idiosyncratic reactions consisting of flushing, high fever, agitation, rapid pulse and breathing. Children with Down's syndrome or brain damage are more susceptible to this type of reaction.
The scopolamine transdermal disc should not be used on children.

By Those over 60 Years of Age: Observe for agitation, confusion, loss of short-term memory, disorientation, visual and auditory hallucinations, delirium. This drug can increase the degree of impaired urination associated with prostate gland enlargement (prostatism).

The scopolamine transdermal disc should be avoided or used very cautiously in this age group.

▷ **Advisability of Use During Pregnancy**

Pregnancy Category: C (tentative). See Pregnancy Code inside back cover.

Animal studies: Birth defects reported in mouse studies.

Human studies: No increase in birth defects reported in 1198 exposures to this drug. Information from adequate studies of pregnant women is not available.

Avoid drug completely during first 3 months.

Advisability of Use if Breast-Feeding

Presence of this drug in breast milk: Yes, in very small amounts.

Monitor nursing infant closely and discontinue drug or nursing if adverse effects develop.

Habit-Forming Potential: None.

Effects of Overdosage: Dilated pupils, blurring of near vision, dryness of mouth and throat, heart palpitation, impaired urination, high fever, hot skin, excitement, confusion, hallucinations, delirium, convulsions, coma.

Possible Effects of Long-Term Use: Chronic constipation, severe enough to result in fecal impaction. (Constipation should be treated promptly with effective laxatives.)

Suggested Periodic Examinations While Taking This Drug (at physician's discretion)

Measurement of internal eye pressure to detect any significant increase that could indicate developing glaucoma.

▷ **While Taking This Drug, Observe the Following**

Foods: Avoid constipating foods, such as cheeses. Follow the diet prescribed by your physician.

Beverages: Avoid large amounts of tea (may be constipating).

▷ *Alcohol:* No interactions expected.

Tobacco Smoking: No interactions expected.

▷ *Other Drugs*

Atropine may *increase* the effects of

• all other drugs having atropinelike actions (see Drug Class, Section Four).

Atropine may *decrease* the effects of

• haloperidol (Haldol), and reduce its effectiveness.

• phenothiazines (Thorazine, etc.), and reduce their effectiveness.

- pilocarpine eye drops, and reduce their effectiveness in lowering internal eye pressure in the treatment of glaucoma.

▷ *Driving, Hazardous Activities:* This drug may cause drowsiness, dizziness or blurred vision. Avoid hazardous activities if these drug effects occur.

Aviation Note: The use of this drug *is a disqualification* for piloting. Consult a designated Aviation Medical Examiner.

Exposure to Sun: No restrictions.

Exposure to Heat: Use extreme caution. The use of this drug in hot environments may significantly increase the risk of heat stroke.

Heavy Exercise or Exertion: Use caution in warm or hot environments. This drug may impair normal perspiration (heat loss) and interfere with the regulation of body temperature.

Discontinuation: Avoid prolonged and unnecessary use of this drug. When symptoms have been controlled for an adequate period of time, and discontinuation appears possible, reduce the dose gradually over a period of several days.

AURANOFIN
(aw RAY noh fin)

Introduced: 1976

Class: Antiarthritic, gold compounds

Prescription: USA: Yes
Canada: Yes

Controlled Drug: USA: No
Canada: No

Available as Generic: No

Brand Name: Ridaura

BENEFITS versus RISKS	
Possible Benefits	*Possible Risks*
REDUCTION OF JOINT PAIN, TENDERNESS AND SWELLING in active, severe RHEUMATOID ARTHRITIS	SIGNIFICANTLY REDUCED LEVELS OF RED AND WHITE BLOOD CELLS AND BLOOD PLATELETS (1% to 3%)
Medication effective when taken by mouth	LIVER DAMAGE WITH JAUNDICE (less than 0.1%)
	Diarrhea (47%), ulcerative colitis (less than 0.1%)
	Skin rash (24%)
	Mouth sores (13%)

▷ **Principal Uses**

As a Single Drug Product: Used *only* for the treatment of adults with active, severe rheumatoid arthritis who have had an inadequate and disappointing response to aspirin, aspirin substitutes and other antiarthritic drugs and treatment programs. It is usually added to a well-established program of antiarthritic drugs of the aspirin-substitute class.

How This Drug Works: Its method of action is unknown. It suppresses but does not cure arthritis and associated synovitis.

Available Dosage Forms and Strengths
Capsules — 3 mg

▷ **Usual Adult Dosage Range:** 6 mg daily, taken either as one dose every 24 hours or as two doses of 3 mg each every 12 hours. If response is inadequate after 6 months of regular continual use, the dose may be increased to 9 mg daily, taken as 3 doses of 3 mg each. If response remains inadequate after 3 months of 9 mg daily, this drug should be discontinued. **Note: Actual dosage and administration schedule must be determined by the physician for each patient individually.**

▷ **Dosing Instructions:** Take with or following food to reduce stomach irritation. Take the capsule whole with milk or a full glass of water.

Usual Duration of Use: Continual use on a regular schedule for 3 to 4 months is usually necessary to determine this drug's effectiveness in reducing the joint pain, tenderness and swelling associated with rheumatoid arthritis. The extent of long-term use will be determined by the degree of benefit and the pattern of adverse effects experienced by the individual patient. Consult your physician on a regular basis.

▷ **This Drug Should Not Be Taken If**
- you have had an allergic reaction or serious adverse effect from previous use of gold.
- you have active ulcerative colitis.
- you have a current blood cell or bone marrow disorder.
- you have active liver or kidney disease.
- you are pregnant or breast-feeding.
- you are taking penicillamine or antimalarial drugs for your arthritis.

▷ **Inform Your Physician Before Taking This Drug If**
- you are allergic by nature, or have a history of allergic reactions to drugs.
- you have diabetes.
- you have a history of heart disease, high blood pressure, circulatory disorders, liver or kidney disease, or ulcerative colitis.
- you are taking any other drugs at this time.
- you are planning pregnancy in the near future.

Possible Side-Effects (natural, expected and unavoidable drug actions)
Metallic taste.

▷ **Possible Adverse Effects** (unusual, unexpected and infrequent reactions)
If any of the following develop, consult your physician promptly for guidance.
Mild Adverse Effects
Allergic Reactions: Itching, skin rash.
Sores in mouth and throat and on tongue, loss of appetite, nausea, vomiting, stomach cramps, diarrhea.
Headache, partial or complete hair loss.
Serious Adverse Effects
Allergic Reactions: Severe skin reactions, exfoliative dermatitis.
Fever, cough, shortness of breath, drug-induced pneumonia and lung damage.
Liver damage with jaundice, ulcerative colitis.
Kidney damage.
Blood cell and bone marrow toxicity—fatigue, weakness, sore throat, abnormal bleeding or bruising.
Peripheral neuritis—pain, numbness, weakness of arms and legs.

▷ **Possible Effects on Sexual Function:**   None reported.

Possible Delayed Adverse Effects: Adverse effects from gold may occur many months after treatment has been discontinued. This is due to accumulation of gold in body tissues and its slow elimination. Report any indications of possible toxicity to your physician promptly.

▷ **Adverse Effects That May Mimic Natural Diseases or Disorders**
Fever, cough and chest discomfort may suggest respiratory tract infections such as bronchitis or pneumonia.
Liver damage may suggest viral hepatitis.

Possible Effects on Laboratory Tests
Complete blood cell counts: decreased red cells, hemoglobin and white cells; increased eosinophils and platelets; these effects occur in about 13% of users.

CAUTION
1. Periodic examinations (blood and urine tests) are mandatory during the use of this drug. Keep all appointments as directed by your physician.
2. Inform your physician promptly of any indications of possible toxic reactions. If there is a delay in reaching your physician, discontinue this drug until you obtain medical guidance.

Precautions for Use
By Infants and Children: Safety and effectiveness for use by those under 12 years of age have not been established.
By Those over 60 Years of Age: Tolerance to gold usually decreases with advancing age. Use small doses initially and observe closely for indications of adverse effects.

▷ **Advisability of Use During Pregnancy**
Pregnancy Category: C (tentative). See Pregnancy Code inside back cover.
Animal studies: Rabbit studies revealed an increase in resorptions, abortions and birth defects.
Human studies: Information from adequate studies of pregnant women is not available.
The manufacturer does not recommend the use of this drug during pregnancy.

Advisability of Use if Breast-Feeding
Presence of this drug in breast milk: Yes.
Avoid drug or refrain from nursing.

Habit-Forming Potential: None.

Effects of Overdosage: Nausea, vomiting, diarrhea, confusion, delirium, peripheral neuritis.

Suggested Periodic Examinations While Taking This Drug (at physician's discretion)
Complete blood cell counts, urine analyses, liver and kidney function tests.

▷ **While Taking This Drug, Observe the Following**
Foods: No restrictions.
Beverages: No restrictions. May be taken with milk.
▷ *Alcohol:* Use caution until the combined effects have been determined. Alcohol may intensify the irritant effect of this drug on the gastrointestinal tract.
Tobacco Smoking: No interactions expected.
▷ *Other Drugs*
Auranofin may *increase* the effects of
• phenytoin (Dilantin), by increasing its blood level. Monitor closely for indications of phenytoin toxicity.
▷ *Driving, Hazardous Activities:* Usually no restrictions.
Aviation Note: The use of this drug *may be a disqualification* for piloting. Consult a designated Aviation Medical Examiner.
Exposure to Sun: Use caution. This drug may cause photosensitivity (see Glossary). Avoid sun and sun lamps if a drug-induced rash occurs.

AZATHIOPRINE
(ay za THI oh preen)

Introduced: 1965

Class: Antiarthritic, immunosuppressive

Prescription: USA: Yes
Canada: Yes

Controlled Drug: USA: No
Canada: No

Available as Generic: Yes

Brand Name: Imuran

BENEFITS versus RISKS

Possible Benefits	*Possible Risks*
REDUCTION OF JOINT PAIN, TENDERNESS AND SWELLING in active, severe RHEUMATOID ARTHRITIS (66% of users)	UNACCEPTABLE ADVERSE EFFECTS IN 15% OF USERS
PREVENTION OF REJECTION IN ORGAN TRANSPLANTATION	REDUCED LEVELS OF WHITE BLOOD CELLS (28% in rheumatoid arthritis, 50% in kidney transplants)
	REDUCED LEVELS OF RED BLOOD CELLS AND PLATELETS
	LIVER DAMAGE WITH JAUNDICE (less than 1%)
	POSSIBLE INCREASED RISK OF MALIGNANCY (3%)

▷ **Principal Uses**

As a Single Drug Product: Used primarily as an immunosuppressant to prevent rejection in organ transplantation (mainly kidney transplants). Also used to manage active, severe rheumatoid arthritis (in adults) that has failed to respond adequately to conventional treatment. Progression of the arthritic process may be slowed or even stopped. Lesser uses include treatment of lupus erythematosus, ulcerative colitis, chronic active hepatitis and other "autoimmune" disorders.

How This Drug Works: Not fully known. It is thought that by impairing purine metabolism, blocking production of DNA and RNA, and inhibiting cell multiplication, this drug suppresses the immune reaction that is responsible for such "autoimmune" disorders as rheumatoid arthritis, lupus erythematosus, etc.

Available Dosage Forms and Strengths
Injection — 100 mg per 20-ml vial
Tablets — 50 mg

▷ **Usual Adult Dosage Range:** As immunosuppressant—3 to 5 mg/kilogram of body weight daily, 1 to 3 days before transplantation surgery; for postoperative maintenance—1 to 2 mg/kilogram of body weight daily. As antiarthritic—1 mg/kilogram of body weight daily for 6 to 8 weeks; increase dose by 0.5 mg/kilogram of body weight every 4 weeks as needed and tolerated. Maximal daily dose is 2.5 mg/kilogram of body weight. Total dose may be taken once daily or divided into 2 equal doses taken 12 hours apart. **Note: Actual dosage and administration schedule must be determined by the physician for each patient individually.**

▷ **Dosing Instructions:** Take with or following food to reduce stomach irritation. Tablet may be crushed for administration.

Usual Duration of Use: Continual use on a regular schedule for 12 weeks is usually necessary to determine this drug's effectiveness in favorably modifying the course of rheumatoid arthritis. This drug has been used successfully for periods of up to 11 years. Consult your physician on a regular basis.

▷ **This Drug Should Not Be Taken If**
- you have had an allergic reaction to it previously.
- you are pregnant, and this drug is prescribed to treat rheumatoid arthritis.
- you have an active blood cell or bone marrow disorder.
- you are taking, or have recently taken, any form of chlorambucil (Leukeran), cyclophosphamide (Cytoxan) or melphalan (Alkeran).

▷ **Inform Your Physician Before Taking This Drug If**
- you have any kind of active infection.
- you have any form of cancer.
- you have gout or are taking allopurinol (Zyloprim).
- you have a history of blood cell or bone marrow disorders.
- you have impaired liver or kidney function.
- you are taking any form of gold, penicillamine or an antimalarial drug for arthritis.
- you plan pregnancy in the near future.

Possible Side-Effects (natural, expected and unavoidable drug actions)
Development of infection (2.4%).

▷ **Possible Adverse Effects** (unusual, unexpected and infrequent reactions)
If any of the following develop, consult your physician promptly for guidance.
Mild Adverse Effects
Allergic Reaction: Skin rash (2%).
Loss of appetite, nausea, vomiting, diarrhea (19%).
Sores on lips and in mouth.
Serious Adverse Effects
Allergic Reactions: Drug fever (see Glossary), joint and muscle pain.

Pancreatitis—severe stomach pain with nausea and vomiting (0.18%).
Bone marrow depression (see Glossary)—fatigue, weakness, fever, sore throat, abnormal bleeding or bruising.
Liver damage—yellow eyes and skin, dark-colored urine, light-colored stools (0.37%). (See Hepatitis and Jaundice in Glossary.)
Drug-induced pneumonia—cough, shortness of breath.
Development of cancer—skin cancer, reticulum-cell sarcoma, lymphoma, leukemia (3.3%).

▷ **Possible Effects on Sexual Function:**   Reversal of male infertility that is due to the body's production of autoantibodies to sperm; this drug suppresses the formation of autoantibodies and permits the normal accumulation of sperm as they are produced.

Possible Delayed Adverse Effects: Bone marrow depression may become apparent many weeks after discontinuing this drug.

▷ **Adverse Effects That May Mimic Natural Diseases or Disorders**
Liver damage may suggest viral hepatitis.

Possible Effects on Laboratory Tests
Complete blood cell counts: decreased red cells, hemoglobin, white cells and platelets.
Blood amylase and lipase levels: increased—possible pancreatitis.
Blood uric acid levels: increased with rapid tissue destruction; decreased in patients with gout.
Liver function tests: increased liver enzymes (ALT/GPT, AST/GOT and alkaline phosphatase); increased bilirubin.
Sperm counts: decreased.

CAUTION
1. Report promptly any indications of a developing infection—fever, chills, lip or mouth sores, etc.
2. Inform your physician promptly if you become pregnant.
3. Periodic blood counts are mandatory for the safe use of this drug. Report for examinations as directed.

Precautions for Use
By Infants and Children: Safety and effectiveness for use by those under 12 years of age have not been established.
By Those over 60 Years of Age: To reduce the risk of possible toxic reactions, the minimal effective dose should be determined and maintained.

▷ **Advisability of Use During Pregnancy**
Pregnancy Category: D (tentative). See Pregnancy Code inside back cover.
Animal studies: Birth defects reported in rodent studies.
Human studies: Two incidents of birth defects reported.
Information from adequate studies of pregnant women is not available.
Avoid completely during entire pregnancy if possible.

Advisability of Use if Breast-Feeding
Presence of this drug in breast milk: Unknown.
Avoid drug or refrain from nursing.

Habit-Forming Potential: None.

Effects of Overdosage: Immediate—nausea, vomiting, diarrhea. Delayed—lowered white blood cell and platelet counts.

Possible Effects of Long-Term Use: Susceptibility to infection, bone marrow depression, development of malignancies.

Suggested Periodic Examinations While Taking This Drug (at physician's discretion)
Complete blood cell counts, liver function tests.

▷ **While Taking This Drug, Observe the Following**
Foods: No restrictions.
Beverages: No restrictions. May be taken with milk.
▷ *Alcohol:* No interactions expected.
Tobacco Smoking: No interactions expected.
▷ *Other Drugs*
Azathioprine may *decrease* the effects of
- oral anticoagulants (warfarin, etc.), and make it necessary to increase their dosage.
- certain muscle relaxants (gallamine, pancuronium, tubocurarine), and make it necessary to increase their dosage.

The following drugs may *increase* the effects of azathioprine
- allopurinol (Zyloprim) may increase its activity and toxicity and make it necessary to reduce its dosage.

▷ *Driving, Hazardous Activities:* No restrictions.
Aviation Note: The use of this drug *may be a disqualification* for piloting. Consult a designated Aviation Medical Examiner.
Exposure to Sun: No restrictions.
Discontinuation: If possible, do not discontinue this drug suddenly. A gradual reduction in dosage is preferable. Consult your physician for a withdrawal schedule.

BACAMPICILLIN
(bak am pi SIL in)

Introduced: 1979

Class: Antibiotic, penicillins

Prescription: USA: Yes
Canada: Yes

Controlled Drug: USA: No
Canada: No

Available as Generic: No

Brand Names: ✤Penglobe, Spectrobid

BENEFITS versus RISKS

Possible Benefits

EFFECTIVE TREATMENT OF
INFECTIONS due to susceptible
microorganisms

Possible Risks

ALLERGIC REACTIONS, mild to
severe, in 3% of the general
population and 15% of allergic
individuals
Superinfections (yeast)
Drug-induced colitis

▷ **Principal Uses**

As a Single Drug Product: To treat certain infections of the skin and skin
structures, of the upper and lower respiratory tract, and of the genitourinary tract, including gonorrhea.

How This Drug Works: During its absorption from the gastrointestinal
tract, bacampicillin is converted to ampicillin. The unique chemical
modification that characterizes bacampicillin permits its more rapid
and complete absorption than ampicillin. When given in equivalent
doses, bacampicillin provides peak blood levels that are 3 times higher
than the levels provided by unmodified ampicillin. Thus bacampicillin
can be effective when given every 12 hours; ampicillin requires a dosage schedule of every 6 hours. (See the Drug Profile of ampicillin.)

Available Dosage Forms and Strengths

Oral suspension — 125 mg per 5-ml teaspoonful
Tablets — 400 mg

▷ **Usual Adult Dosage Range:**   400 to 800 mg/12 hours. **Note: Actual dosage
and administration schedule must be determined by the physician
for each patient individually.**

▷ **Dosing Instructions:** Tablets may be taken without regard to eating. The
oral suspension should be taken on an empty stomach, 1 hour before
or 2 hours after eating. The tablet may be crushed for administration.

Usual Duration of Use: Continual use on a regular schedule for 5 to 7 days
is usually necessary to determine this drug's effectiveness in eradicating the infection. Treatment is usually continued for 2 to 3 days after
all indications of infection are gone. Treatment for all streptococcal
infections should be for no less than 10 consecutive days (without
interruption) to reduce the possibility of developing rheumatic fever or
glomerulonephritis.

▷ **While Taking This Drug, Observe the Following**
▷ *Other Drugs*

Bacampicillin *taken concurrently* with
• allopurinol (Zyloprim) substantially increases the incidence of skin
rash.

- disulfiram (Antabuse) can cause a disulfiramlike reaction (see Glossary). Avoid the concurrent use of these 2 drugs.

The following drugs may **decrease** the effects of bacampicillin
- chloramphenicol (Chloromycetin).
- erythromycins (E-Mycin, Erythrocin, etc.).
- sulfonamides ("Sulfa" drugs, see Drug Class, Section Four).
- tetracyclines (see Drug Class, Section Four).

Note: The information categories provided in this Profile are appropriate for bacampicillin. For specific information that is normally found in those categories that have been omitted from this Profile, the reader is referred to the Drug Profile of ampicillin.

BECLOMETHASONE
(be kloh METH a sohn)

Introduced: 1976

Class: Antiallergic, antiasthmatic, cortisonelike drugs

Prescription: USA: Yes
Canada: Yes

Controlled Drug: USA: No
Canada: No

Available as Generic: No

Brand Names: Beclovent, ✦Beclovent Rotacaps, ✦Beclovent Rotahaler, Beconase AQ Nasal Spray, Beconase Nasal Inhaler, ✦Propaderm, Vancenase AQ Nasal Spray, Vancenase Nasal Inhaler, Vanceril

BENEFITS versus RISKS	
Possible Benefits	*Possible Risks*
EFFECTIVE RELIEF OF ALLERGIC RHINITIS	FUNGUS INFECTIONS OF THE MOUTH AND THROAT
EFFECTIVE CONTROL OF SEVERE, CHRONIC ASTHMA	Localized areas of "allergic" pneumonia

▷ **Principal Uses**

As a Single Drug Product: Used primarily to treat bronchial asthma in those individuals who do not respond to bronchodilators and who require cortisonelike drugs for asthma control. This inhalation dosage form is significantly more advantageous than cortisone taken by mouth (swallowed) or by injection in that it works locally on the tissues of the respiratory tract and does not require absorption and systemic distribution. This prevents the more serious adverse effects that usually result from the long-term use of cortisone taken for systemic effects.

How This Drug Works: Not established. One possibility is that by increasing the amount of cyclic AMP in appropriate tissues, this drug may thereby increase the concentration of epinephrine, which is an effective bronchodilator and antiasthmatic. Additional benefit may be due to the drug's ability to reduce local inflammation in the lining tissues of the respiratory tract.

Available Dosage Forms and Strengths
Nasal inhaler — 16.8 grams (200 doses of 42 mcg each)
Nasal spray — 0.042%
Oral inhaler — 16.8 grams (200 doses of 42 mcg each)

▷ **Usual Adult Dosage Range:**   Nasal inhaler—1 inhalation (42 mcg) 2 to 4 times daily. Oral inhaler—2 inhalations (84 mcg) 3 or 4 times daily. For severe asthma—12 to 16 inhalations daily. The maximal daily dose should not exceed 20 inhalations. **Note: Actual dosage and administration schedule must be determined by the physician for each patient individually.**

▷ **Dosing Instructions:**   May be used as needed without regard to eating. Rinse the mouth and throat (gargle) with water thoroughly after each inhalation.

Usual Duration of Use: Continual use on a regular schedule for 1 to 4 weeks is usually necessary to determine this drug's effectiveness in relieving severe, chronic allergic rhinitis and in controlling severe, chronic asthma. Long-term use requires the supervision and guidance of the physician. Consult your physician on a regular basis.

▷ **This Drug Should Not Be Taken If**
• you have had an allergic reaction to any of the drugs bearing the brand names listed above.
• you are experiencing severe acute asthma or status asthmaticus that requires more intense treatment for prompt relief.
• your asthma can be controlled by bronchodilators and other antiasthmatic drugs that are not related to cortisone.
• your asthma requires cortisonelike drugs infrequently for control.
• you have a form of nonallergic bronchitis with asthmatic features.

▷ **Inform Your Physician Before Taking This Drug If**
• you are now taking or have recently taken any cortisone-related drug (including ACTH by injection) for any reason (see Drug Class, Section Four).
• you have a history of tuberculosis of the lungs.
• you have chronic bronchitis or bronchiectasis.
• you think you may have an active infection of any kind, especially a respiratory infection.

Possible Side-Effects (natural, expected and unavoidable drug actions)
Fungus infections (thrush) of the mouth and throat.

▷ **Possible Adverse Effects** (unusual, unexpected and infrequent reactions)
  If any of the following develop, consult your physician promptly for guidance.
  Mild Adverse Effects
  Allergic Reaction: Skin rash (rare).
  Dryness of mouth, hoarseness, sore throat.
  Serious Adverse Effects
  Allergic Reaction: Localized areas of "allergic" pneumonitis (lung inflammation).
  Bronchospasm, asthmatic wheezing (rare).

▷ **Possible Effects on Sexual Function:** None reported.

Natural Diseases or Disorders That May Be Activated by This Drug
  Cortisone-related drugs that have systemic effects can impair immunity and lead to reactivation of "healed" or quiescent tuberculosis of the lungs. Individuals with a history of tuberculosis must be observed closely during use of this drug by inhalation.

Possible Effects on Laboratory Tests
  Blood cortisol levels: decreased.

CAUTION
  1. This drug does not act primarily as a brochodilator and should not be relied upon for the immediate relief of acute asthma.
  2. If you were using any cortisone-related drugs for treatment of your asthma *before* transferring to this inhaler drug, it may be necessary to resume the former cortisone-related drug if you experience injury or infection of any kind, or if you require surgery. Be sure to notify your attending physician of your prior use of cortisone-related drugs taken either by mouth or by injection.
  3. If you experience a return of severe asthma while using this drug, notify your physician immediately so that additional supportive treatment with cortisone-related drugs by mouth or injection can be provided as needed.
  4. It is advisable to carry a card of personal identification with a notation (if applicable) that you have used cortisone-related drugs within the past year. During periods of stress it may be necessary to resume cortisone treatment in adequate dosage.
  5. An interval of approximately 5 to 10 minutes should separate the inhalation of bronchodilators such as epinephrine, isoetharine, or isoproterenol (which should be used first) and the inhalation of this drug. This sequence will permit greater penetration of beclomethasone into the bronchial tubes. The delay between inhalations will also reduce the possibility of adverse effects from the propellants used in the two inhalers.

Precautions for Use
  By Infants and Children: Safety and effectiveness for use of the nasal inhaler

by those under 12 years of age have not been established. Safety and effectiveness for use of the oral inhaler by those under 6 years of age have not been established. The maximal daily dose in children 6 to 12 years of age should not exceed 10 inhalations.

By Those over 60 Years of Age: Individuals with bronchiectasis should be observed closely for the development of lung infections.

▷ **Advisability of Use During Pregnancy**
Pregnancy Category: C (tentative). See Pregnancy Code inside back cover.
Animal studies: Mouse, rat and rabbit studies reveal significant birth defects due to this drug.
Human studies: Information from adequate studies of pregnant women is not available.
Avoid drug during the first 3 months. Use infrequently and only as clearly needed during the last 6 months.

Advisability of Use if Breast-Feeding
Presence of this drug in breast milk: Probably yes.
Avoid drug or refrain from nursing.

Habit-Forming Potential: With recommended dosage, a state of functional dependence (see Glossary) is not likely to develop.

Effects of Overdosage: Indications of cortisone excess (due to systemic absorption)—fluid retention, flushing of the face, stomach irritation, nervousness.

Suggested Periodic Examinations While Taking This Drug (at physician's discretion)
Inspection of nose, mouth and throat for evidence of fungus infection.
Assessment of the status of adrenal function in individuals who have used cortisone-related drugs over an extended period of time prior to using this drug.
X-ray examination of the lungs of individuals with a prior history of tuberculosis.

▷ **While Taking This Drug, Observe the Following**
Foods: No specific restrictions beyond those advised by your physician.
Beverages: No specific restrictions.
▷ *Alcohol:* No interactions expected.
Tobacco Smoking: No interactions expected. However, smoking can affect the condition under treatment and reduce the effectiveness of this drug. Follow your physician's advice.
▷ *Other Drugs*
The following drugs may *increase* the effects of beclomethasone
• inhalant bronchodilators—epinephrine, isoetharine, isoproterenol.
• oral bronchodilators—aminophylline, ephedrine, terbutaline, theophylline, etc.
▷ *Driving, Hazardous Activities:* No restrictions.
Aviation Note: The use of this drug and the disorder for which this drug is

prescribed *may be disqualifications* for piloting. Consult a designated Aviation Medical Examiner.

Exposure to Sun: No restrictions.

Occurrence of Unrelated Illness: Acute infections, serious injuries, and surgical procedures can create an urgent need for the administration of additional supportive cortisone-related drugs given by mouth and/or injection. Notify your physician immediately in the event of new illness or injury of any kind.

Discontinuation: If the regular use of this drug has made it possible to reduce or discontinue maintenance doses of cortisonelike drugs by mouth, *do not* discontinue this drug abruptly. If you find it necessary to discontinue this drug for any reason, consult your physician promptly. It may be necessary to resume cortisone preparations and to institute other measures for satisfactory management.

Special Storage Instructions : Store at room temperature. Avoid exposure to temperatures above 120 degrees F (49 degrees C). Do not store or use this inhaler near heat or open flame. Protect from light.

BENZTROPINE
(BENZ troh peen)

Introduced: 1954

Class: Antiparkinsonism, atropinelike drugs

Prescription: USA: Yes
Canada: No

Controlled Drug: USA: No
Canada: No

Available as Generic: USA: No
Canada: Yes

Brand Names: ✦Apo-Benztropine, ✦Bensylate, Cogentin, ✦PMS Benztropine

BENEFITS versus RISKS	
Possible Benefits	*Possible Risks*
PARTIAL RELIEF OF SYMPTOMS OF PARKINSON'S DISEASE	Atropinelike side-effects: blurred vision, dry mouth, constipation, impaired urination

▷ **Principal Uses**

As a Single Drug Product: Used adjunctively in the management of all types of parkinsonism to relieve the characteristic rigidity, tremor and sluggish movement. Should it fail to provide adequate relief, it may be supplemented with more potent drugs such as levodopa and bromocriptine. This drug is also used to control the parkinsonian reactions that can result from the use of certain antipsychotic drugs, such as the phenothiazines and related compounds.

How This Drug Works: By restoring a more normal balance of the chemical activities responsible for the transmission of nerve impulses within the basal ganglia of the brain, this drug relieves the symptoms of parkinsonism.

Available Dosage Forms and Strengths
Injection — 1 mg per ml
Tablets — 0.5 mg, 1 mg, 2 mg

▷ **Usual Adult Dosage Range:** For Parkinson's disease—0.5 to 2 mg daily, taken in a single dose at bedtime. For drug-induced parkinsonian reactions—1 to 4 mg daily, either in a single dose or in 2 to 3 divided doses. The total daily dose should not exceed 6 mg. **Note: Actual dosage and administration schedule must be determined by the physician for each patient individually.**

▷ **Dosing Instructions:** May be taken with or following food to reduce stomach irritation. Tablet may be crushed for administration.

Usual Duration of Use: Continual use on a regular schedule for 2 to 4 weeks is usually necessary to determine this drug's effectiveness in relieving the symptoms of parkinsonism and to determine the optimal dosage schedule. Long-term use (months to years) requires physician supervision and guidance. Consult your physician on a regular basis.

▷ **This Drug Should Not Be Taken If**
- you have had an allergic reaction to any dosage form of it previously.
- it is prescribed for a child under 3 years of age.

▷ **Inform Your Physician Before Taking This Drug If**
- you have experienced an unfavorable reaction to atropine or atropine-like drugs in the past.
- you have glaucoma or myasthenia gravis.
- you have heart disease or high blood pressure.
- you have a history of liver or kidney disease.
- you have difficulty emptying the urinary bladder, especially if due to an enlarged prostate gland.
- you are taking, or have taken within the past 2 weeks, any monoamine oxidase (MAO) type A inhibitor drug (see Drug Class, Section Four).

Possible Side-Effects (natural, expected and unavoidable drug actions)
Nervousness, blurring of vision, dryness of mouth, constipation, impaired urination. (These often subside as drug use continues.)

▷ **Possible Adverse Effects** (unusual, unexpected and infrequent reactions)
If any of the following develop, consult your physician promptly for guidance.
Mild Adverse Effects
Allergic Reaction: Skin rashes.

Headache, dizziness, drowsiness, muscle cramps.

Indigestion, nausea, vomiting.

Serious Adverse Effects

Idiosyncratic Reactions: Abnormal behavior, confusion, delusions, hallucinations, agitation.

▷ **Possible Effects on Sexual Function**

Reversal of male impotence due to the use of fluphenazine (a phenothiazine antipsychotic drug).

Male infertility (0.5 to 6 mg/day).

Natural Diseases or Disorders That May Be Activated by This Drug

Latent glaucoma, latent myasthenia gravis.

Possible Effects on Laboratory Tests

None reported.

CAUTION

1. Many over-the-counter (OTC) medications for allergies, colds and coughs contain drugs that can interact unfavorably with this drug. Ask your physician or pharmacist for guidance before using such preparations.
2. This drug may aggravate tardive dyskinesia (see Glossary). Ask physician for guidance.

Precautions for Use

By Infants and Children: Safety and effectiveness for use by those under 3 years of age have not been established. Children are especially susceptible to the atropinelike effects of this drug.

By Those over 60 Years of Age: Small doses are advisable until your response has been determined. You may be more susceptible to the development of impaired thinking, confusion, nightmares, hallucinations, increased internal eye pressure (glaucoma) and impaired urination associated with prostate gland enlargement (prostatism).

▷ **Advisability of Use During Pregnancy**

Pregnancy Category: C (tentative). See Pregnancy Code inside back cover.

Animal studies: No data available.

Human studies: Information from adequate studies of pregnant women is not available.

Avoid use if possible, especially close to delivery. This drug can impair the proper functioning of the infant's intestinal tract following birth.

Advisability of Use if Breast-Feeding

Presence of this drug in breast milk: Unknown.

Avoid drug or refrain from nursing.

Habit-Forming Potential: None with recommended doses. At higher doses it may cause euphoria and hallucinations, creating a potential for abuse.

Effects of Overdosage: Weakness; drowsiness; stupor; impaired vision; rapid pulse; excitement; confusion; hallucinations; dry, hot skin; skin rash; dilated pupils.

Possible Effects of Long-Term Use: Increased internal eye pressure—possible glaucoma, especially in the elderly.

Suggested Periodic Examinations While Taking This Drug (at physician's discretion)
Measurement of internal eye pressure at regular intervals.

▷ **While Taking This Drug, Observe the Following**
Foods: No restrictions.
Beverages: No restrictions.
▷ *Alcohol:* Use caution until the combined effects have been determined. Alcohol may increase the sedative effects of this drug.
Tobacco Smoking: No interactions expected.
▷ *Other Drugs*
Benztropine may *decrease* the effects of
• haloperidol (Haldol), and reduce its effectiveness.
• phenothiazines (Thorazine, etc.), and reduce their effectiveness.
The following drugs may *increase* the effects of benztropine
• antihistamines may add to the dryness of mouth and throat.
• tricyclic antidepressants (Elavil, etc.) may add to the effects on the eye and further increase internal eye pressure (dangerous in glaucoma).
• monoamine oxidase (MAO) type A inhibitor drugs may intensify all effects of this drug (see Drug Class, Section Four).
▷ *Driving, Hazardous Activities:* Drowsiness and dizziness may occur in sensitive individuals. Avoid hazardous activities until full effects and tolerance have been determined.
Aviation Note: The use of this drug *is a disqualification* for piloting. Consult a designated Aviation Medical Examiner.
Exposure to Sun: No restrictions.
Exposure to Heat: Use caution. This drug may reduce sweating, cause an increase in body temperature, and contribute to the development of heat stroke.
Heavy Exercise or Exertion: Use caution. Avoid in hot environments.
Discontinuation: Do not discontinue this drug abruptly. Ask physician for guidance in reducing the dose gradually.

BETAXOLOL
(be TAX oh lohl)

Introduced: 1983

Class: Antihypertensive, beta-adrenergic blocker

Prescription: USA: Yes

Controlled Drug: USA: No

Available as Generic: No

Brand Names: Betoptic, Kerlone

BENEFITS versus RISKS

Possible Benefits	*Possible Risks*
EFFECTIVE, WELL-TOLERATED ANTIHYPERTENSIVE in mild to moderate high blood pressure	CONGESTIVE HEART FAILURE in advanced heart disease
EFFECTIVE TREATMENT OF CHRONIC, OPEN-ANGLE GLAUCOMA	Worsening of angina in coronary heart disease (abrupt withdrawal)
	Masking of low blood sugar (hypoglycemia) in drug-treated diabetes
	Provocation of bronchial asthma (with high doses)

▷ **Principal Uses**

As a Single Drug Product: Used primarily to treat (1) mild to moderately severe high blood pressure; (2) chronic open-angle glaucoma (eye drops). May be used alone or concurrently with other antihypertensive drugs, such as diuretics.

How This Drug Works: By blocking certain actions of the sympathetic nervous system, this drug

- reduces the rate and contraction force of the heart, thus lowering the ejection pressure of the blood leaving the heart and reducing the oxygen requirement for heart function.
- reduces the degree of contraction of blood vessel walls, resulting in their relaxation and expansion and consequent lowering of blood pressure.
- reduces the internal pressure of the eye.

Available Dosage Forms and Strengths

Eye drops — 0.5%

Tablets — 10 mg, 20 mg

▷ **Usual Adult Dosage Range:** Initially 10 mg once daily. Dose may be increased gradually at intervals of 7 to 14 days as needed and tolerated up to 20 mg/24 hours. The usual maintenance dose is 10 to 15 mg/24 hours. The total dose should not exceed 20 mg/24 hours. **Note: Actual**

dosage and administration schedule must be determined by the physician for each patient individually.

▷ **Dosing Instructions:**   May be taken without regard to eating. The tablet may
be crushed for administration. Do not discontinue this drug abruptly.

Usual Duration of Use: Continual use on a regular schedule for 10 to 14
days is usually necessary to determine this drug's effectiveness in lowering blood pressure. The long-term use of this drug will be determined
by the course of your blood pressure over time and your response to
the overall treatment program (weight reduction, salt restriction,
smoking cessation, etc.) Consult your physician on a regular basis.

Possible Advantages of This Drug: Usually effective and well tolerated with
a single dose daily.

Currently a "Drug of Choice"
for initiating treatment of hypertension with a single drug, especially for
those subject to bronchial asthma or diabetes.

▷ **This Drug Should Not Be Taken If**
  • you have had an allergic reaction to it previously.
  • you have congestive heart failure.
  • you have an abnormally slow heart rate or a serious form of heart
    block.
  • you are taking, or have taken within the past 14 days, any monoamine
    oxidase (MAO) type A inhibitor drug (see Drug Class, Section Four).

▷ **Inform Your Physician Before Taking This Drug If**
  • you have had an adverse reaction to any beta blocker drug in the past
    (see Drug Class, Section Four).
  • you have a history of serious heart disease, with or without episodes
    of heart failure.
  • you have a history of hay fever (allergic rhinitis), asthma, chronic
    bronchitis or emphysema.
  • you have a history of overactive thyroid function (hyperthyroidism).
  • you have a history of low blood sugar (hypoglycemia).
  • you have impaired liver or kidney function.
  • you have diabetes or myasthenia gravis.
  • you are currently taking any form of digitalis, quinidine or reserpine,
    or any calcium blocker drug (see Drug Class, Section Four).
  • you plan to have surgery under general anesthesia in the near future.

Possible Side-Effects (natural, expected and unavoidable drug actions)
Lethargy (2.8%), fatigability (2.9%), cold extremities (1.9%), slow heart
rate (8.1%), light-headedness in upright position (see Orthostatic Hypotension in Glossary).

▷ **Possible Adverse Effects** (unusual, unexpected and infrequent reactions)
**If any of the following develop, consult your physician promptly for
guidance.**

Mild Adverse Effects

Allergic Reactions: Skin rash (1.2%), itching.

Headache (6.5%), dizziness (4.5%), drowsiness, insomnia (1.2%), abnormal dreams (1.0%).

Indigestion (4.7%), nausea (1.6%), diarrhea (2.0%).

Joint and muscle discomfort (3.1%), fluid retention (edema) (1.8%).

Serious Adverse Effects

Mental depression (0.8%), anxiety (0.8%).

Chest pain (2.4%), shortness of breath (2.4%), precipitation of congestive heart failure.

Induction of bronchial asthma (in asthmatic individuals).

▷ **Possible Effects on Sexual Function:**   Decreased libido, impotence (1.2%). Altered menstrual patterns.

▷ **Adverse Effects That May Mimic Natural Diseases or Disorders**

Reduced blood flow to extremities may resemble Raynaud's phenomenon (see Glossary).

Possible Effects on Laboratory Tests

Glaucoma-screening test (measurement of internal eye pressure): pressure is decreased (false low or normal value).

Antinuclear antibodies (ANA) test: positive in 5.3% of users.

Blood platelet counts: decreased (rarely).

CAUTION

1. *Do not discontinue this drug suddenly* without the knowledge and guidance of your physician. Carry a notation on your person that you are taking this drug.
2. Consult your physician or pharmacist before using nasal decongestants usually present in over-the-counter cold preparations and nose drops. These can cause sudden increases in blood pressure when taken concurrently with beta blocker drugs.
3. Report the development of any tendency to emotional depression.

Precautions for Use

By Infants and Children: Safety and effectiveness for use by those under 12 years of age have not been established. However, if this drug is used, observe for the development of low blood sugar (hypoglycemia) during periods of reduced food intake.

By Those over 60 Years of Age: Proceed *cautiously* with all antihypertensive drugs. Unacceptably high blood pressure should be reduced without creating the risks associated with excessively low blood pressure. Start treatment with 5 mg daily and monitor the blood pressure response frequently. Sudden, rapid and excessive reduction of blood pressure can predispose to stroke or heart attack. Total daily dosage should not exceed 10 to 15 mg. Observe for dizziness, unsteadiness, tendency to fall, confusion, hallucinations, depression or urinary frequency. This age group is more prone to develop excessively slow heart rates and hypothermia.

▷ **Advisability of Use During Pregnancy**
   Pregnancy Category: C (tentative). See Pregnancy Code inside back cover.
     Animal studies: Rat studies reveal increased resorptions of embryo and fetus, retarded growth and development of newborn and mild skeletal defects.
     Human studies: Information from adequate studies of pregnant women is not available.
     Avoid use of drug during the first 3 months if possible. Avoid use during labor and delivery because of the possible effects on the newborn infant.

Advisability of Use if Breast-Feeding
   Presence of this drug in breast milk: Yes.
     Avoid drug if possible. If drug is necessary, observe nursing infant for slow heart rate and indications of low blood sugar.

Habit-Forming Potential: None.

Effects of Overdosage: Weakness, slow pulse, low blood pressure, fainting, cold and sweaty skin, congestive heart failure, possible coma and convulsions.

Possible Effects of Long-Term Use: Reduced heart reserve and eventual heart failure in susceptible individuals with advanced heart disease.

Suggested Periodic Examinations While Taking This Drug (at physician's discretion)
   Measurements of blood pressure, evaluation of heart function.

▷ **While Taking This Drug, Observe the Following**
   Foods: No restrictions. Avoid excessive salt intake.
   Beverages: No restrictions. May be taken with milk.
▷   *Alcohol:* Use with caution until the combined effect has been determined. Alcohol may exaggerate this drug's ability to lower blood pressure and may increase its mild sedative effect.
   Tobacco Smoking: Nicotine may reduce this drug's effectiveness in treating high blood pressure. In addition, high doses of this drug may potentiate the constriction of the bronchial tubes caused by regular smoking.
▷   *Other Drugs*
   Betaxolol may *increase* the effects of
   • other antihypertensive drugs and cause excessive lowering of blood pressure. Dosage adjustments may be necessary.
   • reserpine (Ser-Ap-Es, etc.) and cause sedation, depression, slowing of heart rate and lowering of blood pressure (light-headedness, fainting).
   Betaxolol *taken concurrently* with
   • clonidine (Catapres) requires close monitoring for rebound high blood pressure if clonidine is withdrawn while betaxolol is still being taken.
   • insulin requires close monitoring to avoid undetected hypoglycemia (see Glossary).
   The following drugs may *decrease* the effects of betaxolol

- indomethacin (Indocin), and possibly other "aspirin substitutes," may impair betaxolol's antihypertensive effect.

▷ *Driving, Hazardous Activities:* Use caution until the full extent of drowsiness, lethargy, and blood pressure change has been determined.

Aviation Note: The use of this drug *is a disqualification* for piloting. Consult a designated Aviation Medical Examiner.

Exposure to Sun: No restrictions.

Exposure to Heat: Caution advised. Hot environments can lower blood pressure and exaggerate the effects of this drug.

Exposure to Cold: Caution advised. Cold environments can enhance the circulatory deficiency in the extremities that may occur with this drug. The elderly should take precautions to prevent hypothermia (see Glossary).

Heavy Exercise or Exertion: It is advisable to avoid exertion that produces light-headedness, excessive fatigue, or muscle cramping. The use of this drug may intensify the hypertensive response to isometric exercise.

Occurrence of Unrelated Illness: The fever that accompanies systemic infections can lower blood pressure and require adjustment of dosage. Illnesses that cause nausea or vomiting may interrupt the regular dosage schedule. Ask your physician for guidance.

Discontinuation: It is advisable to avoid sudden discontinuation of this drug in all situations. If possible, gradual reduction of dose over a period of 2 to 3 weeks is recommended. Ask your physician for specific guidance.

BITOLTEROL
(bi TOHL ter ohl)

Introduced: 1985

Class: Antiasthmatic, bronchodilator

Prescription: Yes

Controlled Drug: No

Available as Generic: No

Brand Name: Tornalate

BENEFITS versus RISKS	
Possible Benefits	*Possible Risks*
EFFECTIVE PREVENTION AND RELIEF OF ASTHMA for 5 to 8 hours	Fine hand tremor (14%) Nervousness (5%) Throat irritation (5%) Irregular heart rhythm (with excessive use)

▷ **Principal Uses**

As a Single Drug Product: To relieve acute bronchial asthma and to reduce the frequency and severity of chronic, recurrent asthmatic attacks.

How This Drug Works: It is thought that by increasing the production of cyclic AMP, this drug relaxes constricted bronchial muscles to relieve asthmatic wheezing.

Available Dosage Forms and Strengths

Aerosol inhaler — 15 ml (300 inhalations of 0.37 mg each)

▷ **Usual Adult Dosage Range:**   For acute bronchospasm—2 inhalations at intervals of 1 to 3 minutes, followed by a third inhalation in 3 to 4 minutes if needed. For prevention of bronchospasm—2 inhalations/8 hours. **Note: Actual dosage and administration schedule must be determined by the physician for each patient individually.**

▷ **Dosing Instructions:**   May be used without regard to eating. Follow the written directions for use carefully. Do not overuse.

Usual Duration of Use: According to individual requirements. Do not use beyond the time necessary to terminate episodes of acute asthma. Ask physician for guidance regarding duration of use for prevention of asthma attacks.

▷ **This Drug Should Not Be Taken If**
- you have had an allergic reaction to it previously.
- you currently have an irregular heart rhythm.
- you are taking, or have taken within the past 2 weeks, any monoamine oxidase (MAO) type A inhibitor drug (see Drug Class, Section Four).

▷ **Inform Your Physician Before Taking This Drug If**
- you have any type of heart or circulatory disorder, especially high blood pressure or coronary heart disease.
- you have diabetes, epilepsy or an overactive thyroid gland.
- you are taking any form of digitalis or any stimulant drug.

Possible Side-Effects (natural, expected and unavoidable drug actions)

Dryness or irritation of mouth or throat (5%).

▷ **Possible Adverse Effects** (unusual, unexpected and infrequent reactions)
If any of the following develop, consult your physician promptly for guidance.
Mild Adverse Effects

Headache (4%), dizziness (3%), nervousness (5%), insomnia (less than 1%), fine tremor of hands (14%).
Nausea (3%), indigestion.
Serious Adverse Effects

Rapid or irregular heart rhythm or increased blood pressure can occur with excessive use.

▷ **Possible Effects on Sexual Function:**   None reported.

Natural Diseases or Disorders That May Be Activated by This Drug
Latent coronary artery disease, diabetes or high blood pressure.

Possible Effects on Laboratory Tests
None reported.

CAUTION
1. Concurrent use of this drug by inhalation with beclomethasone aerosol (Beclovent, Vanceril) may increase the risk of toxicity due to fluorocarbon propellants. It is advisable to use bitolterol aerosol 20 to 30 minutes *before* beclomethasone aerosol. This will reduce the risk of toxicity and will enhance the penetration of beclomethasone.
2. The excessive or prolonged use of this drug by inhalation can reduce its effectiveness and cause serious heart rhythm disturbances.

Precautions for Use
By Infants and Children: Safety and effectiveness for use by children under 12 years of age have not been established.
By Those over 60 Years of Age: Avoid excessive and continual use. If acute asthma is not relieved promptly, other drugs will have to be tried. Observe for the development of nervousness, palpitations, irregular heart rhythm and muscle tremors.

▷ **Advisability of Use During Pregnancy**
Pregnancy Category: C (tentative). See Pregnancy Code inside back cover.
Animal studies: Cleft palate reported in mice.
Human studies: Information from adequate studies of pregnant women is not available.
Avoid use during first 3 months if possible.

Advisability of Use if Breast-Feeding
Presence of this drug in breast milk: Unknown.
Avoid drug or refrain from nursing.

Habit-Forming Potential: None.

Effects of Overdosage: Nervousness, palpitation, rapid heart rate, sweating, headache, tremor, vomiting, chest pain.

Possible Effects of Long-Term Use: Loss of effectiveness.

Suggested Periodic Examinations While Taking This Drug (at physician's discretion)
Blood pressure measurements, evaluation of heart status.

▷ **While Taking This Drug, Observe the Following**
Foods: No restrictions.
Beverages: Avoid excessive use of caffeine-containing beverages—coffee, tea, cola, chocolate.

▷ *Alcohol:* No interactions expected.
  Tobacco Smoking: No interactions expected.
▷ *Other Drugs*
  Bitolterol **taken concurrently** with
  • monoamine oxidase (MAO) type A inhibitor drugs (see Drug Class, Section Four) may cause excessive increase in blood pressure and undesirable heart stimulation.
▷ *Driving, Hazardous Activities:* Use caution if excessive nervousness or dizziness occurs.
  Aviation Note: The use of this drug **is a disqualification** for piloting. Consult a designated Aviation Medical Examiner.
  Exposure to Sun: No restrictions.
  Heavy Exercise or Exertion: Use caution. Excessive exercise can induce asthma in sensitive individuals.

BROMOCRIPTINE
(broh moh KRIP teen)

Introduced: 1975

Class: Antiparkinsonism, dopamine agonist, ergot derivative

Prescription: USA: Yes
Canada: Yes

Controlled Drug: USA: No
Canada: No

Available as Generic: No

Brand Name: Parlodel

BENEFITS versus RISKS

Possible Benefits	*Possible Risks*
PARTIAL RELIEF OF SYMPTOMS OF PARKINSON'S DISEASE	ABNORMAL INVOLUNTARY MOVEMENTS AND ALTERED BEHAVIOR IN 20% to 35% of users taking high doses
PREVENTION OF LACTATION following childbirth	Raynaud's phenomenon (see Glossary) in 30% to 60% of users taking high doses
CORRECTION OF INFERTILITY AND ABSENT MENSTRUATION in women with high prolactin levels	

▷ **Principal Uses**
  As a Single Drug Product: This drug is used primarily to
  1. Treat the manifestations of Parkinson's disease. It may be used as the initial drug in treating those with early-stage symptoms. More often it is used in conjunction with levodopa when it is found that levodopa is losing its effectiveness, or the patient cannot tolerate the adverse

effects of levodopa and dosage adjustment or withdrawal is necessary.

2. Suppress the production of milk and thereby prevent the breast congestion and engorgement that normally follow childbirth.
3. Treat those disorders that are due to excessive production of prolactin by the pituitary gland: absence of menstruation, infertility, and inappropriate production of milk.

How This Drug Works: By directly stimulating the dopamine receptor sites in the corpus striatum of the brain, this drug helps to offset the deficiency of dopamine that is responsible for the rigidity, tremor, and sluggish movement characteristic of Parkinson's disease. By inhibiting the production of the hormone prolactin by the anterior pituitary gland, this drug

- reduces the amount of prolactin in the blood to below the level required to stimulate the breast glands to produce milk.
- reduces abnormally high levels of prolactin in the blood, restoring it to normal levels that permit menstrual regularity and fertility.

Available Dosage Forms and Strengths
Capsules — 5 mg
Tablets — 2.5 mg

▷ **Usual Adult Dosage Range:**   For Parkinson's disease—initially 1.25 to 2.5 mg once daily; for maintenance, 2.5 to 100 mg daily in divided doses. Increase dose by no more than 2.5 to 5 mg on alternate days. The usual dosage range is 10 to 40 mg daily. Do not exceed 300 mg daily. For suppression of lactation—2.5 mg 2 times a day for 14 days; may extend to 21 days if needed. For absent menstruation and infertility—initially 1.25 to 2.5 mg daily; for maintenance, 2.5 mg 2 or 3 times a day. **Note: Actual dosage and administration schedule must be determined by the physician for each patient individually.**

▷ **Dosing Instructions:**   Take with food or milk to reduce stomach irritation. Capsule may be opened and tablet may be crushed for administration.

Usual Duration of Use: Continual use on a regular schedule for 3 to 4 months is usually necessary to determine this drug's effectiveness in controlling the symptoms of Parkinson's disease. Treatment for 4 to 12 weeks restores fertility and normal menstruation in most women; however, treatment may be necessary for 6 to 12 months. Long-term use (up to 3 years or more) must be under physician supervision and guidance. Consult your physician on a regular basis.

▷ **This Drug Should Not Be Taken If**
- you have had an allergic reaction to it previously.
- you have had a serious adverse effect from any ergot preparation in the past.
- you have severe coronary artery disease or peripheral vascular disease.
- you are pregnant.

▷ **Inform Your Physician Before Taking This Drug If**
- you have constitutionally low blood pressure.
- you are taking any antihypertensive drugs or phenothiazines (see Drug Classes, Section Four).
- you have any degree of coronary artery disease, especially with a history of a "heart attack" (myocardial infarction).
- you have a history of heart rhythm abnormalities.
- you have impaired liver function.
- you have a seizure disorder (epilepsy).

Possible Side-Effects (natural, expected and unavoidable drug actions)
Fatigue, lethargy, light-headedness in upright position (see Orthostatic Hypotension in Glossary).

▷ **Possible Adverse Effects** (unusual, unexpected and infrequent reactions)
If any of the following develop, consult your physician promptly for guidance.
Mild Adverse Effects
Allergic Reaction: Skin rash.
Headache, drowsiness, dizziness, fainting, nervousness, nightmares.
Nasal congestion, dry mouth, loss of appetite, nausea, vomiting, stomach cramps, constipation, diarrhea.
Serious Adverse Effects
Abnormal involuntary movements, confusion, hallucinations, incoordination, visual disturbances, depression, seizures.
Swelling of feet and ankles (edema).
Loss of urinary bladder control, inability to empty bladder.
Indications of "ergotism": numbness and tingling of fingers, cold hands and feet, muscle cramps of legs and feet.
Vomiting blood, bloody or black stools (gastrointestinal bleeding).

▷ **Possible Effects on Sexual Function:**   Rare occurrence of impotence. However, this drug can correct impotence and reduced libido when these conditions are due to increased blood levels of prolactin (a pituitary hormone).

▷ **Adverse Effects That May Mimic Natural Diseases or Disorders**
Effects on mental function and behavior may resemble psychotic disorders.

Natural Diseases or Disorders That May Be Activated by This Drug
Coronary artery disease with anginal syndrome, Raynaud's syndrome.

Possible Effects on Laboratory Tests
Blood alkaline phosphatase level: increased.

CAUTION
1. During treatment of parkinsonism, avoid excessive and hurried activity as improvement occurs; this will reduce the risk of falls and injury.

2. The neurological and psychiatric disturbances due to this drug may last for 2 to 6 weeks after stopping it.
3. During treatment to reduce the blood level of prolactin and restore normal menstruation and fertility, it is mandatory that you use a barrier method of contraception to prevent pregnancy. Oral contraceptives should not be used while taking bromocriptine.
4. If pregnancy occurs, notify your physician immediately.

Precautions for Use
By Infants and Children: Safety and effectiveness for use by those under 15 years of age have not been established.
By Those over 60 Years of Age: Your initial test dose should be 1.25 mg. Observe closely for any tendency to light-headedness or faintness on attempting to stand after this first dose. You may be more susceptible to the development of impaired thinking, confusion, agitation, nightmares, hallucinations, nausea or vomiting. Close monitoring and careful dosage adjustments are mandatory.

▷ Advisability of Use During Pregnancy
Pregnancy Category: X (tentative). See Pregnancy Code inside back cover.
Animal studies: Rabbit studies reveal an increase in cleft lip.
Human studies: Serious birth defects have been reported in infants whose mothers took this drug during early pregnancy. Because the incidence of these defects (3.3%) does not exceed that reported for the general population, a cause-and-effect relationship is uncertain. Information from adequate studies of pregnant women is not available.
Pending further studies, it is recommended that this drug not be taken during the entire pregnancy.

Advisability of Use if Breast-Feeding
This drug prevents the production of milk and makes nursing impossible.

Habit-Forming Potential: None.

Effects of Overdosage: Weakness, low blood pressure, nausea, vomiting, diarrhea, confusion, agitation, hallucinations, loss of consciousness.

Possible Effects of Long-Term Use: Drug-induced changes in the lung tissue, thickening of the pleura and pleural effusion (fluid formation within the chest cage). These effects appear to be reversible after discontinuation of the drug. Fibrosis (scar tissue formation) in the back wall of the abdominal cavity and contractures of the extremities have also been reported.

Suggested Periodic Examinations While Taking This Drug (at physician's discretion)
Blood pressure measurements; CAT scan of the pituitary gland for enlargement due to tumor; pregnancy test; blood tests for anemia; evaluation of heart, lung and liver functions.

▷ **While Taking This Drug, Observe the Following**
Foods: No restrictions.
Beverages: No restrictions. May be taken with milk.
▷ *Alcohol:* Use caution until the combined effects have been determined. Alcohol can exaggerate the blood-pressure-lowering effects and sedative effects of this drug.
▷ *Other Drugs*
Bromocriptine ***taken concurrently*** with
• antihypertensive drugs (and other drugs that can lower blood pressure) requires careful monitoring for excessive drops in pressure. Dosage adjustments may be necessary.
The following drugs may ***decrease*** the effects of bromocriptine
• phenothiazines (see Drug Class, Section Four). Theoretically, bromocriptine and phenothiazines have opposite effects on the utilization of dopamine in the brain. It is probably best to avoid the concurrent use of these drugs until the results of further studies are available.
▷ *Driving, Hazardous Activities:* Be alert to the possible occurrence of orthostatic hypotension, dizziness, drowsiness or impaired coordination.
Aviation Note: Parkinsonism ***is a disqualification*** for piloting. The use of this drug otherwise ***may be a disqualification*** for piloting. Consult a designated Aviation Medical Examiner.
Exposure to Sun: No restrictions.

BUMETANIDE
(byu MET a nide)

Introduced: 1983

Prescription: USA: Yes

Available as Generic: No

Brand Name: Bumex

Class: Diuretic

Controlled Drug: USA: No

BENEFITS versus RISKS	
Possible Benefits	*Possible Risks*
POTENT, EFFECTIVE DIURETIC BY MOUTH OR INJECTION	ABNORMALLY LOW BLOOD POTASSIUM with excessive use Impaired sexual function

▷ **Principal Uses**
As a Single Drug Product: To relieve edema (fluid retention) associated with congestive heart failure, liver disease or kidney disease.

How This Drug Works: By increasing the elimination of salt and water from the body (through increased urine production), this drug reduces the volume of fluid in the blood and body tissues and lowers the sodium content throughout the body.

Available Dosage Forms and Strengths
Injection — 0.25 mg per ml (2-ml ampules)
Tablets — 0.5 mg, 1 mg, 2 mg

▷ **Usual Adult Dosage Range:**　0.5 to 2 mg daily, usually taken in the morning as a single dose. If needed, an additional second or third dose may be taken later in the day at 4- to 5-hour intervals. The total daily dose should not exceed 10 mg. Alternate-day dosage (taken every other day) may be adequate for some individuals. **Note: Actual dosage and administration schedule must be determined by the physician for each patient individually.**

▷ **Dosing Instructions:**　May be taken with or following food to reduce stomach irritation. Tablet may be crushed for administration.

Usual Duration of Use:　Continual use on a regular schedule for 2 to 3 days is usually necessary to determine this drug's effectiveness in relieving edema. After maximal benefit has been achieved, intermittent use will reduce the risk of sodium, potassium and water imbalance. Long-term use requires the supervision and guidance of the physician. Consult your physician on a regular basis.

Possible Advantages of This Drug
Diuretic effect is usually complete in 4 hours; diuretic effect of furosemide usually lasts from 6 to 8 hours.

▷ **This Drug Should Not Be Taken If**
- you have had an allergic reaction to either dosage form previously.
- your kidneys are unable to produce urine.

▷ **Inform Your Physician Before Taking This Drug If**
- you are allergic to any form of "sulfa" drug.
- you are pregnant or planning pregnancy.
- you have impaired liver or kidney function.
- you have diabetes or a tendency to diabetes.
- you have a history of gout.
- you have impaired hearing.
- you are taking any form of cortisone, digitalis, oral antidiabetic drugs, insulin, probenecid (Benemid), indomethacin (Indocin), lithium or drugs for high blood pressure.
- you plan to have surgery under general anesthesia in the near future.

Possible Side-Effects (natural, expected and unavoidable drug actions)
Light-headedness on arising from sitting or lying position (see Orthostatic Hypotension in Glossary).
Increase in level of blood sugar, affecting control of diabetes.
Increase in level of blood uric acid, affecting control of gout.

Decrease in levels of blood potassium and sodium, resulting in muscle weakness and cramping.

▷ **Possible Adverse Effects** (unusual, unexpected and infrequent reactions)
If any of the following develop, consult your physician promptly for guidance.
Mild Adverse Effects
Allergic Reactions: Skin rashes, hives, itching.
Headache, dizziness, vertigo, fatigue, weakness, sweating, earache.
Nausea, vomiting, stomach pain, diarrhea.
Breast nipple tenderness, joint and muscle pains.
Serious Adverse Effects
Impaired hearing, precipitation of liver coma (in preexisting liver disease).

▷ **Possible Effects on Sexual Function:**   Difficulty maintaining an erection; premature ejaculation (0.5 to 2 mg/day).

Natural Diseases or Disorders That May Be Activated by This Drug
Latent diabetes, gout.

Possible Effects on Laboratory Tests
White blood cell counts: increased (usual); decreased (rare).
Blood lithium levels: increased.
Blood uric acid levels: increased.

CAUTION
1. Do not exceed recommended doses. Increased dosage can cause excessive excretion of water, sodium and potassium, with resultant loss of appetite, nausea, weakness, confusion and profound drop in blood pressure (circulatory collapse).
2. If you are also taking a digitalis preparation (digitoxin, digoxin), ensure an adequate intake of high-potassium foods to prevent potassium deficiency—a potential cause of digitalis toxicity.
3. If you are being treated for cirrhosis of the liver, do not increase your dose without consulting your physician. Excessive dosage can alter blood chemistry significantly and induce liver coma.

Precautions for Use
By Infants and Children: Safety and effectiveness for use by those under 18 years of age have not been established.
By Those over 60 Years of Age: Small doses are advisable until your individual response has been determined. You may be more susceptible to the development of impaired thinking, orthostatic hypotension, potassium loss and elevation of blood sugar. Overdosage and prolonged use of this drug can cause excessive loss of body water, thickening of the blood, and an increased tendency of the blood to clot, predisposing to stroke, heart attack or thrombophlebitis.

▷ **Advisability of Use During Pregnancy**
Pregnancy Category: C (tentative). See Pregnancy Code inside back cover.
Animal studies: High-dose studies of rats and rabbits reveal defects in bone development.
Human studies: Information from adequate studies of pregnant women is not available.
This drug should not be used during pregnancy unless a very serious complication of pregnancy occurs for which this drug is significantly beneficial.

Advisability of Use if Breast-Feeding
Presence of this drug in breast milk: Unknown.
Avoid drug or refrain from nursing.

Habit-Forming Potential: None.

Effects of Overdosage: Weakness, lethargy, dizziness, confusion, nausea, vomiting, muscle cramps, thirst, drowsiness progressing to deep sleep or coma, weak and rapid pulse.

Possible Effects of Long-Term Use: Impaired balance of water, salt, and potassium in blood and body tissues. Dehydration with resultant increase in blood viscosity and potential for abnormal clotting. Development of diabetes in predisposed individuals.

Suggested Periodic Examinations While Taking This Drug (at physician's discretion)
Complete blood cell counts; measurements of blood levels of sodium, potassium, chloride, sugar, uric acid; liver and kidney function tests.

▷ **While Taking This Drug, Observe the Following**
Foods: Consult your physician regarding the advisability of eating a high-potassium diet. See Section Six for the Table of High Potassium Foods. Follow your physician's instructions regarding the use of salt.
Beverages: No restrictions unless directed by your physician. May be taken with milk.
▷ *Alcohol:* Use with caution until the combined effect has been determined. Alcohol can exaggerate the blood-pressure-lowering effect of this drug and cause orthostatic hypotension (see Glossary).
Tobacco Smoking: No interactions expected. Follow your physician's advice regarding smoking.
▷ *Other Drugs*
Bumetanide may *increase* the effects of
• antihypertensive drugs. Careful adjustment of dosages is necessary to prevent excessive lowering of the blood pressure.
Bumetanide *taken concurrently* with
• aminoglycoside antibiotics (amikacin, gentamicin, kanamycin, neomycin, streptomycin, tobramycin, viomycin) may increase the risk of hearing loss.

- cortisone-related drugs may cause excessive loss of potassium from the body.
- digitalis-related drugs requires very careful monitoring and dosage adjustments to prevent serious disturbances of heart rhythm.
- lithium may increase the risk of lithium toxicity.

The following drugs may *decrease* the effects of bumetanide
- indomethacin (Indocin) may reduce its diuretic effect.

▷ *Driving, Hazardous Activities:* Use caution until the possible occurrence of dizziness, weakness or orthostatic hypotension (see Glossary) has been determined.

Aviation Note: The use of this drug *may be a disqualification* for piloting. Consult a designated Aviation Medical Examiner.

Exposure to Sun: No restrictions.

Occurrence of Unrelated Illness: Illnesses that cause vomiting or diarrhea can produce a serious imbalance of important body chemistry. Report such illnesses promptly.

Discontinuation: It may be advisable to discontinue this drug 5 to 7 days before major surgery. Consult your physician, surgeon, or anesthesiologist for guidance regarding dosage reduction or withdrawal.

BUSPIRONE
(byu SPI rohn)

Introduced: 1979

Class: Mild tranquilizer

Prescription: USA: Yes

Controlled Drug: USA: No

Available as Generic: No

Brand Name: Buspar

BENEFITS versus RISKS	
Possible Benefits	*Possible Risks*
EFFECTIVE RELIEF OF MILD TO MODERATE ANXIETY without significant sedation or risk of dependence	Mild dizziness, faintness or headache (uncommon) Rare restlessness, tremor and rigidity (with high doses)

▷ **Principal Uses**

As a Single Drug Product: Used to relieve anxiety and nervous tension states of mild to moderate severity. Because of its lack of significant sedative effects and of abuse potential, it is particularly useful in the elderly, the alcoholic and the addiction-prone individual.

How This Drug Works: Not completely established. This drug is thought to be a "mid-brain modulator" with effects on dopamine, norepinephrine and serotonin transmission activities. Its exact method of action is not understood.

Available Dosage Forms and Strengths
Tablets — 5 mg, 10 mg

▷ **Usual Adult Dosage Range:**   20 to 30 mg/day, in divided doses. Initially, 5 mg three times/day; if needed, increase dose by 5 to 10 mg/day every 3 to 4 days, with individual doses every 6 to 8 hours. The total daily dose should not exceed 60 mg. **Note: Actual dosage and administration schedule must be determined by the physician for each patient individually.**

▷ **Dosing Instructions:**   May be taken without regard to food. The tablet may be crushed for administration.

Usual Duration of Use: Continual use on a regular schedule for 7 to 10 days is usually necessary to determine this drug's effectiveness in relieving anxiety and nervous tension. Use intermittently and only as necessary; avoid prolonged and uninterrupted use.

Possible Advantages of This Drug
Relieves anxiety and nervous tension without causing significant sedation or impairing mental function.
Does not cause withdrawal symptoms upon discontinuation..

▷ **This Drug Should Not Be Taken If**
• you have had an allergic reaction to it previously.

▷ **Inform Your Physician Before Taking This Drug If**
• you are taking other drugs that affect the function of the brain and nervous system: tranquilizers, sedatives, hypnotics, analgesics, narcotics, antidepressants, antipsychotic drugs, anticonvulsants or drugs for parkinsonism.
• you have impaired liver or kidney function.

Possible Side-Effects (natural, expected and unavoidable drug actions)
Infrequent and mild drowsiness (less than with benzodiazepines), lethargy, fatigue.

▷ **Possible Adverse Effects** (unusual, unexpected and infrequent reactions)
If any of the following develop, consult your physician promptly for guidance.
Mild Adverse Effects
Headache, dizziness, faintness, excitement, nausea.
Serious Adverse Effects
Depression (3%).
With high doses: restlessness, rigidity, tremors.

▷ **Possible Effects on Sexual Function:**   Increased or decreased libido, inhibited ejaculation, impotence, breast milk production, altered timing and pattern of menstruation (10 to 40 mg/day).

Possible Effects on Laboratory Tests
None reported.

CAUTION
Although this drug is reported to have no significant (or very mild) sedative effects and no potential for causing dependence, it should be used with caution and only when clearly needed. It has not been used by large numbers of people for long periods of time; some unexpected side-effects or adverse effects may become apparent after general use for several years.

Precautions for Use
By Infants and Children: Safety and effectiveness for use by those under 18 years of age have not been established.
By Those over 60 Years of Age: This drug should be tolerated much better than benzodiazepines and barbiturates when used by this age group. Observe for some possible increase in dizziness and/or weakness; use caution to avoid falls.

▷ **Advisability of Use During Pregnancy**
Pregnancy Category: B (tentative). See Pregnancy Code inside back cover.
Animal studies: No birth defects found in rat and rabbit studies.
Human studies: Information from adequate studies of pregnant women is not available.
Use this drug during pregnancy only when clearly needed. Until more experience has been gained from wider use, it is advisable to avoid this drug during the first 3 months of pregnancy.

Advisability of Use if Breast-Feeding
Presence of this drug in breast milk: Unknown; probably yes.
Avoid drug or refrain from nursing.

Habit-Forming Potential: None demonstrated in premarketing trials.

Effects of Overdosage: No experience reported. Probable effects would be increased dizziness, weakness and lethargy.

Possible Effects of Long-Term Use: None reported.

Suggested Periodic Examinations While Taking This Drug (at physician's discretion)
None required or recommended at the time of this writing.

▷ **While Taking This Drug, Observe the Following**
Foods: No restrictions.
Beverages: No restrictions.
▷ *Alcohol:* No interactions expected.
Tobacco Smoking: No interactions expected.
▷ *Other Drugs:* No significant drug interactions have been reported at the time of this writing.

▷   *Driving, Hazardous Activities:* This drug may cause dizziness, faintness or fatigue. Restrict activities as necessary.

   Aviation Note: The use of this drug *may be a disqualification* for piloting. Consult a designated Aviation Medical Examiner.

   Exposure to Sun: No restrictions.

CAPTOPRIL
(KAP toh pril)

Introduced: 1979

Class: Antihypertensive, ACE inhibitor

Prescription: USA: Yes
        Canada: Yes

Controlled Drug: USA: No
        Canada: No

Available as Generic: No

Brand Names: Capoten, Capozide [CD]

BENEFITS versus RISKS

Possible Benefits	*Possible Risks*
EFFECTIVE CONTROL OF MILD TO SEVERE HIGH BLOOD PRESSURE	Rash, itching, fever (10%)
	Lost or altered taste (7%)
USEFUL ADJUNCTIVE TREATMENT FOR CONGESTIVE HEART FAILURE	Impaired white blood cell production (0.3%)
	Bone marrow depression (rare)
	Kidney damage (rare)
	Liver damage (rare)

▷ **Principal Uses**

   As a Single Drug Product: Used primarily to treat all degrees of high blood pressure. Mild to moderate high blood pressure usually responds to low doses; severe high blood pressure requires higher doses, with greater risk of serious adverse effects. Also used to treat selected cases of advanced heart failure that have not responded to conventional treatment with digitalis and diuretics.

How This Drug Works: Not completely known. It is thought that by blocking certain enzyme systems that influence arterial function, this drug contributes to the relaxation of arterial walls throughout the body and thus lowers the resistance to blood flow that causes high blood pressure. This, in turn, reduces the workload of the heart and improves its performance.

Available Dosage Forms and Strengths
   Tablets — 12.5 mg, 25 mg, 50 mg, 100 mg

▷ **Usual Adult Dosage Range:** Initially 12.5 to 25 mg 2 or 3 times daily for 2 weeks. If necessary, dose may be increased to 50 mg 3 times daily. Usual maintenance dose is 50 to 100 mg 3 times daily. Total daily dose should not exceed 450 mg. **Note: Actual dosage and administration schedule must be determined by the physician for each patient individually.**

▷ **Dosing Instructions:** Take on empty stomach, 1 hour before meals, at same time each day. Tablet may be crushed for administration.

Usual Duration of Use: Continual use on a regular schedule for several weeks is usually necessary to determine this drug's effectiveness in controlling high blood pressure. The proper treatment of high blood pressure usually requires the long-term use of effective medications. Consult your physician on a regular basis.

▷ **This Drug Should Not Be Taken If**
• you have had an allergic reaction to it previously.
• you currently have a blood cell or bone marrow disorder.
• you have active liver disease.
• you have an abnormally high level of blood potassium.

▷ **Inform Your Physician Before Taking This Drug If**
• you have a history of kidney disease or impaired kidney function.
• you have scleroderma or systemic lupus erythematosus.
• you have any form of heart disease.
• you have diabetes.
• you are taking any of the following drugs: other antihypertensives, diuretics, nitrates, allopurinol (Zyloprim), Indocin or potassium supplements.
• you plan to have surgery under general anesthesia in the near future.

Possible Side-Effects (natural, expected and unavoidable drug actions)
Dizziness, light-headedness, fainting (excessive drop in blood pressure).

▷ **Possible Adverse Effects** (unusual, unexpected and infrequent reactions)
If any of the following develop, consult your physician promptly for guidance.
Mild Adverse Effects
Allergic Reactions: Skin rash; swelling of face, hands or feet; fever.
Lost or altered taste, mouth or tongue sores.
Rapid heart rate, palpitation.
Serious Adverse Effects
Bone marrow depression—fatigue, weakness, fever, sore throat, abnormal bleeding or bruising.
Kidney damage—water retention (edema).
Liver damage—with or without jaundice.

▷ **Possible Effects on Sexual Function:** Decreased male libido (20% to 30%) with recommended dosage.

Possible Effects on Laboratory Tests
Complete blood cell counts: decreased red cells, hemoglobin, white cells and platelets; increased eosinophils.
Blood antinuclear antibodies (ANA): increased.
Blood cholesterol and triglycerides: no effects.
Blood sodium level: decreased.
Blood urea nitrogen level (BUN): increased.
Liver function tests: increased liver enzymes (alkaline phosphatase, AST/GOT, LDH), increased bilirubin.
Urine ketone tests: false positive results with Keto-diastix and Chemstrip-6.

CAUTION
1. If possible, it is advisable to discontinue all other antihypertensive drugs (especially diuretics) for 1 week before starting captopril.
2. **Report promptly** any indications of infection (fever, sore throat), and any indications of water retention (weight gain, puffiness, swollen feet or ankles).
3. Do not use a salt substitute without your physician's knowledge and approval. (Many salt substitutes contain potassium.)
4. It is advisable to obtain blood cell counts and urine analyses **before** starting this drug.

Precautions for Use
By Infants and Children: Safety and effectiveness for use by those in this age group have not been established.
By Those over 60 Years of Age: Small doses are advisable until tolerance has been determined. Sudden and excessive lowering of blood pressure can predispose to stroke or heart attack in those with impaired brain circulation or coronary artery heart disease.

▷ **Advisability of Use During Pregnancy**
Pregnancy Category: C (tentative). See Pregnancy Code inside back cover.
Animal studies: No birth defects found in rat, rabbit or hamster studies. However, this drug was shown to be toxic to the embryo and newborn.
Human studies: Information from adequate studies of pregnant women is not available.
Avoid during first 3 months if possible. Use only if clearly needed during last 6 months.

Advisability of Use if Breast-Feeding
Presence of this drug in breast milk: Yes, in small amounts.
Monitor nursing infant closely and discontinue drug or nursing if adverse effects develop.

Habit-Forming Potential: None.

Effects of Overdosage: Excessive drop in blood pressure—light-headedness, dizziness, fainting.

Possible Effects of Long-Term Use: Gradual increase in blood potassium level.

Suggested Periodic Examinations While Taking This Drug (at physician's discretion)
Before starting drug: Complete blood cell counts; urine analysis with measurement of protein content, blood potassium level. During use of drug: Blood cell counts every 2 weeks during the first 3 months of treatment, then periodically for duration of use. Urine protein measurements every month during the first 9 months of treatment, then periodically for duration of use. Periodic measurements of blood potassium.

▷ **While Taking This Drug, Observe the Following**
Foods: Consult physician regarding salt intake.
Nutritional Support: **Do not take** potassium supplements unless directed by your physician.
Beverages: No restrictions. May be taken with milk.
▷ *Alcohol:* Use caution until combined effect has been determined. Alcohol may enhance the blood-pressure-lowering effect of this drug.
Tobacco Smoking: No interactions expected.
▷ *Other Drugs*
Captopril *taken concurrently* with
• potassium preparations (K-Lyte, Slow-K, etc.) may cause increased blood levels of potassium with risk of serious heart rhythm disturbances.
• potassium-sparing diuretics: amiloride (Moduretic), spironolactone (Aldactazide), triamterene (Dyazide) may cause increased blood levels of potassium with risk of serious heart rhythm disturbances.
The following drugs may *decrease* the effects of captopril
• indomethacin (Indocin).
• salicylates (aspirin, etc.).
▷ *Driving, Hazardous Activities:* Usually no restrictions. Be aware of possible drops in blood pressure with resultant dizziness or faintness.
Aviation Note: The use of this drug *may be a disqualification* for piloting. Consult a designated Aviation Medical Examiner.
Exposure to Sun: Caution advised. This drug can cause photosensitivity.
Exposure to Heat: Caution advised. Avoid excessive perspiring with resultant loss of body water and drop in blood pressure.
Occurrence of Unrelated Illness: Report promptly any disorder that causes nausea, vomiting or diarrhea. Fluid and chemical imbalances must be corrected as soon as possible.

CARBAMAZEPINE
(kar ba MAZ e peen)

Introduced: 1962

Class: Anticonvulsant, antineural-
gic

Prescription: USA: Yes
Canada: Yes

Controlled Drug: USA: No
Canada: No

Available as Generic: Yes

Brand Names: ✦Apo-Carbamazepine, Epitol, ✦Mazepine, ✦PMS-Car-
bamazepine, Tegretol

BENEFITS versus RISKS

Possible Benefits	*Possible Risks*
RELIEF OF PAIN IN TRIGEMINAL NEURALGIA	RARE BONE MARROW DEPRESSION (reduced formation of all blood cells)
EFFECTIVE CONTROL OF CERTAIN TYPES OF EPILEPTIC SEIZURES	Liver damage with jaundice
Relief of pain in some rare forms of neuralgia	

▷ **Principal Uses**

As a Single Drug Product: This drug is used primarily in the management
of two uncommon but serious disorders: (1) for relief of pain in true
trigeminal neuralgia (tic douloureux) and glossopharyngeal neuralgia;
(2) for control of several types of epilepsy, namely grand mal, psychomotor or temporal lobe, and mixed seizure patterns. Because of its
potential for serious toxic effects, precise diagnosis and careful management are mandatory for its proper use.

In addition to it primary uses, this drug has also proved to be beneficial
in the treatment of bipolar affective disorders, schizoaffective disorders, resistant schizophrenia and alcohol withdrawal.

How This Drug Works: Not completely known. It is thought that by reducing the transmission of impulses at certain nerve terminals, this drug
relieves or reduces pain (of trigeminal neuralgia) and also reduces the
excitability of certain nerve fibers in the brain and thereby inhibits the
repetitive spread of electrical impulses along nerve pathways. This
action may prevent seizures altogether or reduce their frequency and
severity.

Available Dosage Forms and Strengths

Oral suspension — 100 mg per 5-ml teaspoonful
Tablets — 200 mg
Tablets, chewable — 100 mg

▷ **Usual Adult Dosage Range:** Initially 200 mg/12 hours. Dose may be increased at weekly intervals by 200 mg/24 hours as needed and tolerated. Total daily dosage should not exceed 1200 mg. **Note: Actual dosage and administration schedule must be determined by the physician for each patient individually.**

▷ **Dosing Instructions:** Take at same time each day, with or following food to reduce stomach irritation. Tablet may be crushed for administration.

Usual Duration of Use: Continual use on a regular schedule for 3 months is usually necessary to determine this drug's effectiveness in relieving the pain of trigeminal neuralgia. Longer periods, with dosage adjustment, may be required to determine its ability to control epileptic seizures. Careful evaluation of each individual's tolerance and response should be made every 3 months during long-term treatment. Consult your physician on a regular basis.

▷ **This Drug Should Not Be Taken If**
   • you have had an allergic reaction to it previously.
   • you have active liver disease.
   • you currently have a blood cell or bone marrow disorder.
   • you are currently taking, or have taken within the past 14 days, any monoamine oxidase (MAO) type A inhibitor drug (see Drug Class, Section Four).

▷ **Inform Your Physician Before Taking This Drug If**
   • you have had an allergic reaction to any tricyclic antidepressant drug (see Drug Class, Section Four).
   • you have taken this drug in the past.
   • you have a history of any kind of blood cell or bone marrow disorder, especially one due to a drug.
   • you have a history of liver or kidney disease.
   • you have had serious mental depression or other mental disorder.
   • you have had thrombophlebitis.
   • you have high blood pressure, heart disease or glaucoma.
   • you take more than 2 alcoholic drinks a day.

Possible Side-Effects (natural, expected and unavoidable drug actions)
   Dry mouth and throat, constipation, impaired urination.

▷ **Possible Adverse Effects** (unusual, unexpected and infrequent reactions)
   If any of the following develop, consult your physician promptly for guidance.
   Mild Adverse Effects
   Allergic Reactions: Skin rash, hives, itching, drug fever.
   Headache, dizziness, drowsiness, unsteadiness, fatigue, blurred vision, confusion.
   Exaggerated hearing, ringing in ears.
   Loss of appetite, nausea, vomiting, indigestion, diarrhea.
   Water retention (edema), frequent urination.

Changes in skin pigmentation, hair loss.

Aching of muscles and joints, leg cramps.

Serious Adverse Effects

Allergic Reactions: Severe dermatitis with peeling of skin, irritation of mouth and tongue, swelling of lymph glands.

Idiosyncratic Reactions: Lung inflammation (pneumonitis): cough, shortness of breath.

Bone marrow depression (see Glossary)—fatigue, weakness, fever, sore throat, abnormal bleeding or bruising.

Liver damage with jaundice (see Glossary)—yellow eyes and skin, dark-colored urine, light-colored stools.

Kidney damage—reduced urine volume, uremic poisoning.

Mental depression and agitation.

Double vision, visual hallucinations, speech disturbances, peripheral neuritis (see Glossary).

Thrombophlebitis.

▷ **Possible Effects on Sexual Function**

Decreased libido and/or impotence (13%), male infertility.

This drug is used to control hypersexuality (exaggerated sexual behavior) that can result from injury to the temporal lobe of the brain.

▷ **Adverse Effects That May Mimic Natural Diseases or Disorders**

Liver reactions may suggest viral hepatitis.

Rare lung reactions may suggest interstitial pneumonitis.

Natural Diseases or Disorders That May Be Activated by This Drug

Latent psychosis, systemic lupus erythematosus.

Possible Effects on Laboratory Tests

Complete blood cell counts: decreased red cells, hemoglobin, white cells and platelets; increased eosinophils.

Blood calcium level: decreased.

Blood prothrombin time: decreased.

Blood urea nitrogen level (BUN): increased.

Liver function tests: increased liver enzymes (ALT/GPT, AST/GOT and alkaline phosphatase), increased bilirubin.

Urine pregnancy tests: false negative or inconclusive results with Preputex, Predictor, Gonavislide, Pregnosticon.

CAUTION

1. Because this drug can cause serious adverse effects, it should be used only after a trial of less hazardous drugs has been ineffective.
2. *Before* the first dose is taken, pretreatment blood cell counts, liver function tests and kidney function tests should be performed.
3. Careful periodic testing for early indications of blood cell or bone marrow toxicity is *mandatory.*
4. During periods of spontaneous remission from trigeminal neuralgia, this drug *should not be used* to prevent recurrence.

5. If used to control epileptic seizures, ***do not discontinue this drug suddenly.***

6. This drug may lose up to one third of its effectiveness if stored in humid conditions. When exposed to humidity, the tablet form of this drug hardens; this results in poor absorption from the gastrointestinal tract and erratic control of seizures. Store this drug in a cool, dry place; avoid bathrooms and other humidified areas.

Precautions for Use

By Infants and Children: Safety and effectiveness for use by those under 6 years of age have not been established. Because of the high frequency of adverse effects (up to 25%), careful testing of blood cell production, liver function and kidney function must be performed regularly. This drug can reduce the effectiveness of other anticonvulsant drugs. Blood levels of all anticonvulsant drugs should be monitored when this drug is added to the treatment program.

By Those over 60 Years of Age: This drug can cause confusion and agitation. Observe for the possible aggravation of glaucoma, coronary artery disease (angina) or prostatism (see Glossary).

▷ **Advisability of Use During Pregnancy**

Pregnancy Category: C (tentative). See Pregnancy Code inside back cover.
Animal studies: Rat studies reveal significant birth defects.
Human studies: Information from adequate studies of pregnant women is not available.
Avoid completely during the first 3 months. Use during the last 6 months only if clearly needed.

Advisability of Use if Breast-Feeding

Presence of this drug in breast milk: Yes.
Avoid drug or refrain from nursing.

Habit-Forming Potential: None.

Effects of Overdosage: Dizziness, unsteadiness, drowsiness, disorientation, tremor, involuntary movements, nausea, vomiting, flushed skin, dilated pupils, stupor progressing to coma.

Possible Effects of Long-Term Use: Water retention (edema), impaired liver function, possible liver damage with jaundice.

Suggested Periodic Examinations While Taking This Drug (at physician's discretion)
Complete blood cell counts weekly during the first 3 months of treatment, and monthly thereafter until the drug is discontinued. Liver and kidney function tests. Complete eye examinations.

▷ **While Taking This Drug, Observe the Following**

Foods: No restrictions.

Beverages: No restrictions. May be taken with milk.

▷ *Alcohol:* Use caution until the combined effect has been determined. This drug may increase the sedative effect of alcohol.

Tobacco Smoking: No interactions expected.

▷ *Other Drugs*

Carbamazepine may *increase* the effects of
- sedatives, tranquilizers, hypnotics, narcotics, and enhance their sedative effects.

Carbamazepine may *decrease* the effects of
- doxycycline (Doxy-II, Vibramycin, etc.).
- haloperidol (Haldol).
- valproic acid (Depakene, etc.).
- warfarin (Coumadin, Panwarfin, etc.).

Carbamazepine *taken concurrently* with
- lithium may cause serious neurological disturbances: confusion, drowsiness, weakness, unsteadiness, tremors, muscle twitching.
- monoamine oxidase (MAO) type A inhibitor drugs (see Drug Class, Section Four) may cause severe toxic reactions.
- phenytoin (Dilantin, etc.) may cause unpredictable fluctuations of blood levels of both drugs and impair seizure control.
- theophylline (Slo-bid, Theo-Dur, etc.) may reduce the effects of both drugs.

The following drugs may *increase* the effects of carbamazepine
- cimetidine (Tagamet).
- danazol (Danocrine).
- diltiazem (Cardizem).
- erythromycin (E.E.S., E-Mycin, etc.).
- isoniazid (INH).
- nicotinamide (nicotinic acid amide).
- propoxyphene (Darvon, Darvocet, etc.).
- troleandomycin (Tao).
- verapamil (Calan, Isoptin).

▷ *Driving, Hazardous Activities:* This drug can cause dizziness, drowsiness or blurred vision. Adjust activities accordingly.

Aviation Note: The use of this drug *is a disqualification* for piloting. Consult a designated Aviation Medical Examiner.

Exposure to Sun: This drug can cause photosensitivity (see Glossary). Use caution until sensitivity to sun has been determined.

Heavy Exercise or Exertion: Use caution if you have coronary artery disease. This drug can intensify angina and reduce tolerance for physical activity.

Occurrence of Unrelated Illness: Because of this drug's potential for serious adverse effects, it is mandatory that you inform each physician and dentist you consult that you are taking carbamazepine.

Discontinuation: If used to treat trigeminal neuralgia, attempt should be made every 3 months to reduce the maintenance dose or to discontinue this drug altogether. If used to control epilepsy, this drug *must not be discontinued abruptly.*

Special Storage Instructions
> Store the tablet form of this drug in a cool, dry place. Protect it from exposure to humid conditions.

CARBENICILLIN
(kar ben i SIL in)

Introduced: 1964

Class: Antibiotic, penicillins

Prescription: USA: Yes
Canada: Yes

Controlled Drug: USA: No
Canada: No

Available as Generic: No

Brand Names: Geocillin, Geopen, ✦Geopen Oral, Pyopen

BENEFITS versus RISKS

Possible Benefits	*Possible Risks*
EFFECTIVE TREATMENT OF INFECTIONS due to susceptible microorganisms	ALLERGIC REACTIONS, mild to severe Superinfections (yeast) Drug-induced colitis Rare blood cell disorders

---

▷ **Principal Uses**
> *As a Single Drug Product:* Oral tablets are used to treat certain infections of the urinary tract and prostate gland. Injections are used to treat a wider variety of more serious infections.

How This Drug Works: This drug destroys susceptible infecting bacteria by interfering with their ability to produce new protective cell walls as they multiply and grow.

Available Dosage Forms and Strengths
> Injections — Vials of 1 gram, 2 grams, 5 grams
> Tablets, film-coated — 382 mg

▷ **Usual Adult Dosage Range:** 382 to 764 mg/6 hours (4 doses/24 hours). **Note: Actual dosage and administration schedule must be determined by the physician for each patient individually.**

▷ **Dosing Instructions:** Take on an empty stomach, 1 hour before or 2 hours after eating, at same times each day. Tablet be crushed for administration, but drug has a bitter taste.

Usual Duration of Use: For urinary tract infections—10 days.
> For prostate gland infections—2 to 4 weeks. Recurrent and chronic infections require longer periods of treatment.

▷ **This Drug Should Not Be Taken If**
- you have had an allergic reaction to any dosage form of it previously.
- you are certain you are allergic to *any* form of penicillin.

▷ **Inform Your Physician Before Taking This Drug If**
- you suspect you may be allergic to penicillin or you have a history of a previous "reaction" to penicillin.
- you are allergic to cephalosporin antibiotics (Ancef, Ceporan, Ceporex, Kafocin, Keflex, Keflin, Kefzol, Loridine).
- you are allergic by nature—hay fever, asthma, hives, eczema.
- you have a history of a bleeding disorder, kidney disease, regional enteritis or ulcerative colitis.

Possible Side-Effects (natural, expected and unavoidable drug actions)
Superinfections (see Glossary), often due to yeast organisms.

▷ **Possible Adverse Effects** (unusual, unexpected and infrequent reactions)
If any of the following develop, consult your physician promptly for guidance.
Mild Adverse Effects
Allergic Reactions: Skin rashes, hives, itching.
Irritations of mouth and tongue, unpleasant taste, nausea, vomiting, mild diarrhea.
Serious Adverse Effects
Allergic Reactions: Anaphylactic reaction (see Glossary), severe skin reactions, drug fever, swollen painful joints, sore throat, abnormal bleeding or bruising.
Hemolytic anemia (see Glossary).
Pseudomembranous colitis—severe diarrhea.

▷ **Possible Effects on Sexual Function:** None reported.

Possible Effects on Laboratory Tests
Complete blood cell counts: decreased red cells, hemoglobin, white cells and platelets; increased eosinophils.
Blood potassium level: decreased.
Prothrombin time: increased, especially in uremia.
Liver function tests: increased liver enzymes (ALT/GPT, AST/GOT, alkaline phosphatase).
Urine sugar tests: normal results with Diastix and TesTape; false positive and false negative results with Clinitest;

CAUTION
1. Take the exact dose and the full course prescribed.
2. This drug should not be used concurrently with antibiotics like erythromycin or tetracycline.

Precautions for Use
By Infants and Children: Safety and effectiveness for use by those under 12 years of age have not been established.
By Those over 60 Years of Age: It is advisable to evaluate kidney function

before and during use of this drug to determine the need for dosage adjustment. Natural changes in the skin may predispose to prolonged itching reactions in the genital and anal regions. Report such reactions promptly.

▷ **Advisability of Use During Pregnancy**
Pregnancy Category: B (tentative). See Pregnancy Code inside back cover.
Animal studies: No information available.
Human studies: Information from adequate studies of pregnant women indicates no increased risk of birth defects in 3546 pregnancies exposed to penicillin derivatives.
Ask physician for guidance.

Advisability of Use if Breast-Feeding
Presence of this drug in breast milk: Probably yes.
The nursing infant may be sensitized to penicillin and be at risk for developing diarrhea or yeast infections.
Avoid drug if possible or refrain from nursing.

Habit-Forming Potential: None.

Effects of Overdosage: Possible nausea, vomiting and/or diarrhea.

Possible Effects of Long-Term Use: Superinfections, often due to yeast organisms.

Suggested Periodic Examinations While Taking This Drug (at physician's discretion)
Complete blood cell counts. Liver and kidney function tests with long-term use.

▷ **While Taking This Drug, Observe the Following**
Foods: No restrictions.
Beverages: No restrictions.
▷ *Alcohol:* No interactions expected.
Tobacco Smoking: No interactions expected.
▷ *Other Drugs*
Carbenicillin may *decrease* the effects of
• oral contraceptives in some women, and impair their effectiveness in preventing pregnancy.
The following drugs may *decrease* the effects of carbenicillin
• antacids may reduce the absorption of carbenicillin.
• chloramphenicol (Chloromycetin).
• erythromycin (Erythrocin, E-Mycin, etc.).
• tetracyclines (Achromycin, Declomycin, Minocin, etc.). (See Drug Class, Section Four.)
▷ *Driving, Hazardous Activities:* Usually no restrictions.
Aviation Note: The use of this drug *may be a disqualification* for piloting. Consult a designated Aviation Medical Examiner.
Exposure to Sun: No restrictions.

CARTEOLOL
(KAR tee oh lohl)

Introduced: 1983

Class: Antihypertensive, beta-adrenergic blocker

Prescription: USA: Yes

Controlled Drug: USA: No

Available as Generic: No

Brand Name: Cartrol

BENEFITS versus RISKS

Possible Benefits	*Possible Risks*
EFFECTIVE, WELL-TOLERATED ANTIHYPERTENSIVE in mild to moderate high blood pressure	CONGESTIVE HEART FAILURE in advanced heart disease
	Worsening of angina in coronary heart disease (abrupt withdrawal)
	Masking of low blood sugar (hypoglycemia) in drug-treated diabetes
	Provocation of asthma

▷ **Principal Uses**

As a Single Drug Product: The treatment of mild to moderately severe high blood pressure. May be used alone or concurrently with other antihypertensive drugs, such as diuretics. It is also being used to treat classical effort-induced angina.

How This Drug Works: By blocking certain actions of the sympathetic nervous system, this drug
- reduces the rate and contraction force of the heart, thus lowering the ejection pressure of the blood leaving the heart.
- reduces the degree of contraction of blood vessel walls, resulting in their relaxation and expansion and consequent lowering of blood pressure.

Available Dosage Forms and Strengths
Tablets — 2.5 mg, 5 mg

▷ **Usual Adult Dosage Range:** Initially 2.5 mg once daily. The dose may be increased gradually by 2.5 mg/day at intervals of 2 weeks as needed and tolerated up to 10 mg/day. For maintenance, 2.5 to 7.5 mg once daily is usually adequate. The total daily dose should not exceed 10 mg. **Note: Actual dosage and administration schedule must be determined by the physician for each patient individually.**

▷ **Dosing Instructions:**   May be taken without regard to eating. The tablet may be crushed for administration. Do not discontinue this drug abruptly.

Usual Duration of Use: Continual use on a regular schedule for 2 to 3 weeks is usually necessary to determine this drug's effectiveness in lowering blood pressure. The long-term use of this drug (months to years) will be determined by the course of your blood pressure over time and your response to the overall treatment program (weight reduction, salt restriction, smoking cessation, etc.). Consult your physician on a regular basis.

Possible Advantages of This Drug
Adequate control of blood pressure with a single daily dose.
Causes less slowing of the heart rate than most other beta blocker drugs.

Currently a "Drug of Choice"
for initiating treatment of hypertension with a single drug.

▷ **This Drug Should Not Be Taken If**
• you have had an allergic reaction to it previously.
• you have congestive heart failure.
• you have an abnormally slow heart rate or a serious form of heart block.
• you are subject to bronchial asthma.

▷ **Inform Your Physician Before Taking This Drug If**
• you have had an adverse reaction to any beta blocker drug in the past (see Drug Class, Section Four).
• you have a history of serious heart disease, with or without episodes of heart failure.
• you have a history of hay fever (allergic rhinitis), asthma, chronic bronchitis or emphysema.
• you have a history of overactive thyroid function (hyperthyroidism).
• you have a history of low blood sugar (hypoglycemia).
• you have impaired liver or kidney function.
• you have diabetes or myasthenia gravis.
• you have impaired circulation in the extremities (Raynaud's disorder, claudication pains in legs).
• you are currently taking any form of digitalis, quinidine or reserpine, or any calcium blocker drug (see Drug Class, Section Four).
• you plan to have surgery under general anesthesia in the near future.

Possible Side-Effects (natural, expected and unavoidable drug actions)
Lethargy and fatigability, cold extremities, slow heart rate, light-headedness in upright position (see Orthostatic Hypotension in Glossary).

▷ **Possible Adverse Effects** (unusual, unexpected and infrequent reactions)
If any of the following develop, consult your physician promptly for guidance.

Mild Adverse Effects
  Allergic Reactions: Skin rash.
  Dizziness, nervousness, drowsiness, insomnia, abnormal dreams.
  Indigestion, nausea, vomiting, constipation, diarrhea.
  Joint and muscle discomfort, numbness of fingers or toes.
Serious Adverse Effects
  Mental depression, anxiety.
  Chest pain, irregular heartbeat, shortness of breath, precipitation of congestive heart failure.
  Induction of bronchial asthma (in asthmatic individuals).
  Aggravation of myasthenia gravis.

▷ **Possible Effects on Sexual Function:**   Decreased libido, impotence.

▷ **Adverse Effects That May Mimic Natural Diseases or Disorders**
  Reduced blood flow to extremities may resemble Raynaud's phenomenon (see Glossary).

Natural Diseases or Disorders That May Be Activated by This Drug
  Raynaud's disease, intermittent claudication, myasthenia gravis.

Possible Effects on Laboratory Tests
  Blood creatine kinase level: increased.

CAUTION
  1. ***Do not discontinue this drug suddenly*** without the knowledge and guidance of your physician. Carry a notation on your person that you are taking this drug.
  2. Consult your physician or pharmacist before using nasal decongestants usually present in over-the-counter cold preparations and nose drops. These can cause sudden increases in blood pressure when taken concurrently with beta blocker drugs.
  3. Report the development of any tendency to emotional depression.

Precautions for Use
  By Infants and Children: Safety and effectiveness for use by those under 12 years of age have not been established. However, if this drug is used, observe for the development of low blood sugar (hypoglycemia) during periods of reduced food intake.
  By Those over 60 Years of Age: Proceed *cautiously* with all antihypertensive drugs. Unacceptably high blood pressure should be reduced without creating the risks associated with excessively low blood pressure. Start treatment with small doses, and monitor the blood pressure response frequently. Sudden, rapid and excessive reduction of blood pressure can predispose to stroke or heart attack. Observe for dizziness, unsteadiness, tendency to fall, confusion, hallucinations, depression or urinary frequency.

▷ **Advisability of Use During Pregnancy**
Pregnancy Category: C (tentative). See Pregnancy Code inside back cover.
Animal studies: No birth defects due to this drug found in rat or rabbit studies.
Human studies: Information from adequate studies of pregnant women is not available.
Use this drug only if clearly needed. Ask physician for guidance.

Advisability of Use if Breast-Feeding
Presence of this drug in breast milk: Unknown.
Avoid drug or refrain from nursing.

Habit-Forming Potential: None.

Effects of Overdosage: Weakness, slow pulse, low blood pressure, fainting, cold and sweaty skin, congestive heart failure, possible coma and convulsions.

Possible Effects of Long-Term Use: Reduced heart reserve and eventual heart failure in susceptible individuals with advanced heart disease.

Suggested Periodic Examinations While Taking This Drug (at physician's discretion)
Measurements of blood pressure, evaluation of heart function.

▷ **While Taking This Drug, Observe the Following**
Foods: No restrictions. Avoid excessive salt intake.
Beverages: No restrictions. May be taken with milk.
▷ *Alcohol:* Use with caution until the combined effect has been determined. Alcohol may exaggerate this drug's ability to lower the blood pressure and may increase its mild sedative effect.
Tobacco Smoking: Nicotine may reduce this drug's effectiveness in treating high blood pressure. In addition, high doses of this drug may potentiate the constriction of the bronchial tubes caused by regular smoking.
▷ *Other Drugs*
Carteolol may *increase* the effects of
• other antihypertensive drugs, and cause excessive lowering of the blood pressure. Dosage adjustments may be necessary.
• reserpine (Ser-Ap-Es, etc.), and cause sedation, depression, slowing of the heart rate and lowering of the blood pressure. This combination is best avoided.
• theophyllines (aminophylline, dyphylline, oxtriphylline, etc.).
• verapamil (Calan, Isoptin), and cause excessive depression of heart function; monitor this combination closely.
Carteolol *taken concurrently* with
• clonidine (Catapres) requires close monitoring for rebound high blood pressure if clonidine is withdrawn while carteolol is still being taken.
• epinephrine (Adrenalin, etc.) may cause sudden and excessive rise in

blood pressure followed by slowing of the heart rate. Avoid the concurrent use of beta blockers and epinephrine.

- ergot preparations (ergotamine, methysergide, etc.) may enhance ergot-induced constriction of peripheral circulation to a dangerous degree.
- insulin requires close monitoring to avoid undetected hypoglycemia (see Glossary).

The following drugs may *decrease* the effects of carteolol

- indomethacin (Indocin), and possibly other "aspirin substitutes," may impair carteolol's antihypertensive effect.

▷ *Driving, Hazardous Activities:* Use caution until the full extent of fatigue, dizziness and blood pressure change have been determined.

Aviation Note: The use of this drug *is a disqualification* for piloting. Consult a designated Aviation Medical Examiner.

Exposure to Sun: No restrictions.

Exposure to Heat: Caution advised. Hot environments can lower the blood pressure and exaggerate the effects of this drug.

Exposure to Cold: Caution advised. Cold environments can enhance the circulatory deficiency in the extremities that may occur with this drug. The elderly should take precautions to prevent hypothermia (see Glossary).

Heavy Exercise or Exertion: It is advisable to avoid exertion that produces light-headedness, excessive fatigue or muscle cramping. The use of this drug may intensify the hypertensive response to isometric exercise.

Occurrence of Unrelated Illness: The fever that accompanies systemic infections can lower the blood pressure and require adjustment of dosage. Illnesses that cause nausea or vomiting may interrupt the regular dosage schedule. Ask your physician for guidance.

Discontinuation: It is advisable to avoid sudden discontinuation of this drug in all situations. If possible, gradual reduction of dose over a period of 2 to 3 weeks is recommended. Ask your physician for specific guidance.

CEFACLOR
(SEF a klor)

Introduced: 1979

Class: Antibiotic, cephalosporins

Prescription: USA: Yes
Canada: Yes

Controlled Drug: USA: No
Canada: No

Available as Generic: No

Brand Name: Ceclor

BENEFITS versus RISKS

Possible Benefits
EFFECTIVE TREATMENT OF
INFECTIONS due to susceptible
microorganisms

Possible Risks
ALLERGIC REACTIONS mild to
severe (up to 5% of general
population, up to 16% of those
allergic to penicillin)
Drug-induced colitis (rare)
Superinfections (see Glossary)

▷ **Principal Uses**

As a Single Drug Product: To treat certain infections of the skin and skin structures, the upper and lower respiratory tract (including middle ear infections and "strep" throat) and certain infections of the urinary tract.

How This Drug Works: This drug destroys susceptible infecting bacteria by interfering with their ability to produce new protective cell walls as they multiply and grow.

Available Dosage Forms and Strengths
Capsules — 250 mg, 500 mg
Oral suspension — 125 mg, 250 mg per 5-ml teaspoonful

▷ **Usual Adult Dosage Range:** 250 to 500 mg/8 hours. Total daily dose should not exceed 4 grams. **Note: Actual dosage and administration schedule must be determined by the physician for each patient individually.**

▷ **Dosing Instructions:** May be taken on an empty stomach or with food if stomach irritation occurs. Capsule may be opened for administration. Shake suspension well before measuring dose. Take the full course prescribed.

Usual Duration of Use: Continual use on a regular schedule for 3 to 5 days is usually necessary to determine this drug's effectiveness in controlling the infection under treatment. Response varies with the nature of the infection. Total treatment time will vary from 1 to 4 weeks. Certain infections require that this drug be taken for 10 consecutive days to prevent the development of rheumatic fever. Follow your physician's instructions regarding duration of use.

▷ **This Drug Should Not Be Taken If**
• you are allergic to any cephalosporin antibiotic (see Drug Class, Section Four).

▷ **Inform Your Physician Before Taking This Drug If**
• you have a history of allergy to any form of penicillin (see Drug Class, Section Four).

- you have a history of regional enteritis or ulcerative colitis.
- you have impaired kidney function.

Possible Side-Effects (natural, expected and unavoidable drug actions)
   Superinfections (see Glossary).

▷ **Possible Adverse Effects** (unusual, unexpected and infrequent reactions)
   If any of the following develop, consult your physician promptly for guidance.
   Mild Adverse Effects
   Allergic Reactions: Skin rash, itching, hives.
   Nausea and vomiting (1 in 90), mild diarrhea (1 in 70), sore mouth or tongue.
   Serious Adverse Effects
   Allergic Reactions: Drug fever (see Glossary), joint aches and pains, anaphylactic reaction (see Glossary).
   Idiosyncratic Reactions: Minor and temporary changes in white blood cell counts and liver function tests (infrequent).
   Genital itching (may represent a fungus superinfection).
   Severe diarrhea, possibly indicating a drug-induced form of colitis (rare).

▷ **Possible Effects on Sexual Function:**   None reported.

▷ **Adverse Effects That May Mimic Natural Diseases or Disorders**
   Skin rash and fever may resemble measles.

Possible Effects on Laboratory Tests
   Blood platelet counts: decreased (rare).

CAUTION
   In the management of diabetes it should be noted that this drug can cause a false positive test result for urine sugar when using Clinitest tablets, Benedict's solution or Fehling's solution, but not with Tes-Tape.

Precautions for Use
   By Infants and Children: Not recommended for use in infants less than 1 month old. The maximal dose in children should not exceed 1 gram/24 hours.
   By Those over 60 Years of Age: Dosage must be carefully individualized and based upon evaluation of kidney function. Natural changes in the skin may predispose to severe and prolonged itching reactions in the genital and anal regions. Such reactions should be reported promptly.

▷ **Advisability of Use During Pregnancy**
   Pregnancy Category: B (tentative). See Pregnancy Code inside back cover.
   Animal studies: No birth defects reported.

Human studies: Information from adequate studies of pregnant women is not available.
Generally considered to be safe. Ask physician for guidance.

Advisability of Use if Breast-Feeding
Presence of this drug in breast milk: Yes, in small amounts.
Avoid drug or refrain from nursing.

Habit-Forming Potential: None.

Effects of Overdosage: Nausea, vomiting, stomach cramps and/or diarrhea.

Possible Effects of Long-Term Use: Superinfections (see Glossary).

Suggested Periodic Examinations While Taking This Drug (at physician's discretion)
Complete blood cell counts.

▷ **While Taking This Drug, Observe the Following**
Foods: No restrictions.
Beverages: No restrictions. May be taken with milk.
▷ *Alcohol:* No interactions expected.
Tobacco Smoking: No interactions expected.
▷ *Other Drugs*
Cefaclor *taken concurrently* with
• probenecid (Benemid) will slow the elimination of cefaclor, resulting in higher blood levels and prolonged effect.
▷ *Driving, Hazardous Activities:* Usually no restrictions.
Aviation Note: The use of this drug *may be a disqualification* for piloting. Consult a designated Aviation Medical Examiner.
Exposure to Sun: No restrictions.
Special Storage Instructions: Oral suspension should be refrigerated.
Observe the Following Expiration Times: Do not take the oral suspension of this drug if it is older than 14 days.

CEFADROXIL
(sef a DROX il)

Introduced: 1977

Class: Antibiotic, cephalosporins

Prescription: USA: Yes
Canada: Yes

Controlled Drug: USA: No
Canada: No

Available as Generic: Yes

Brand Names: Duricef, Ultracef

```
┌─────────────────────────────────────────────────────────────────┐
│                    BENEFITS versus RISKS                          │
│                                                                   │
│      Possible Benefits              Possible Risks                │
│  EFFECTIVE TREATMENT OF         ALLERGIC REACTIONS mild to        │
│   INFECTIONS due to susceptible    severe (up to 5% of general    │
│   microorganisms                   population, up to 16% of those │
│                                    allergic to penicillin)        │
│                                 Drug-induced colitis (rare)       │
│                                 Superinfections (see Glossary)    │
└─────────────────────────────────────────────────────────────────┘
```

▷ **Principal Uses**

As a Single Drug Product: To treat certain infections of the skin and skin structures, the upper respiratory tract (including tonsillitis and "strep" throat) and certain infections of the urinary tract.

How This Drug Works: This drug destroys susceptible infecting bacteria by interfering with their ability to produce new protective cell walls as they multiply and grow.

Available Dosage Forms and Strengths

Capsules — 500 mg

Oral suspension — 125 mg, 250 mg, 500 mg per 5-ml teaspoonful

Tablets — 1000 mg (1 gram)

▷ **Usual Adult Dosage Range:**   Skin infections—500 mg/12 hours, or 1 gram daily. "Strep" throat—500 mg/12 hours for 10 days. Urinary tract infections—500 mg to 1 gram/12 hours, or 1 to 2 grams daily. Total daily dosage should not exceed 6 grams. **Note: Actual dosage and administration schedule must be determined by the physician for each patient individually.**

▷ **Dosing Instructions:**   May be taken on an empty stomach or with food if stomach irritation occurs. Capsule may be opened for administration. Shake suspension well before measuring dose. Take the full course prescribed.

Usual Duration of Use: Continual use on a regular schedule for 3 to 5 days is usually necessary to determine this drug's effectiveness in controlling the infection under treatment. Response varies with the nature of the infection. Total treatment time will vary from 1 to 4 weeks. Certain infections require that this drug be taken for 10 consecutive days to prevent the development of rheumatic fever. Follow your physician's instructions regarding duration of use.

Possible Advantages of This Drug

Higher cure rate (90%) than penicillin V (76%) in treating streptococcal infections of the throat; also, lower recurrence rate (7%) than penicillin V (15%).

▷ **This Drug Should Not Be Taken If**

• you are allergic to any cephalosporin antibiotic (see Drug Class, Section Four).

▷ **Inform Your Physician Before Taking This Drug If**
- you have a history of allergy to any form of penicillin (see Drug Class, Section Four).
- you have a history of regional enteritis or ulcerative colitis.
- you have impaired kidney function.

Possible Side-Effects (natural, expected and unavoidable drug actions)
Superinfections (see Glossary).

▷ **Possible Adverse Effects** (unusual, unexpected and infrequent reactions)
If any of the following develop, consult your physician promptly for guidance.
Mild Adverse Effects
Allergic Reactions: Skin rash, itching, hives, localized swellings.
Headache, drowsiness, dizziness.
Indigestion, stomach cramping, nausea, vomiting, mild diarrhea, sore mouth or tongue.
Serious Adverse Effects
Allergic Reactions: Drug fever (see Glossary), joint aches and pains, anaphylactic reaction (see Glossary).
Idiosyncratic Reactions: Minor and temporary changes in white blood cell counts and liver function tests (infrequent).
Genital itching (may represent a fungus superinfection).
Severe diarrhea, possibly indicating a drug-induced form of colitis (rare).

▷ **Possible Effects on Sexual Function:** None reported.

▷ **Adverse Effects That May Mimic Natural Diseases or Disorders**
Skin rash and fever may resemble measles.

Possible Effects on Laboratory Tests
No significant effects reported.

CAUTION
In the management of diabetes it should be noted that this drug can cause a false positive test result for urine sugar when using Clinitest tablets, Benedict's solution or Fehling's solution, but not with Tes-Tape.

Precautions for Use
By Infants and Children: Dosage is based upon weight, and must be determined by the physician for each individual. Follow your physician's instructions exactly.
By Those over 60 Years of Age: Dosage must be carefully individualized and based upon evaluation of kidney function. Natural changes in the skin may predispose to severe and prolonged itching reactions in the genital and anal regions. Such reactions should be reported promptly.

▷ **Advisability of Use During Pregnancy**
Pregnancy Category: B (tentative). See Pregnancy Code inside back cover.
Animal studies: No birth defects reported.

Human studies: Information from adequate studies of pregnant women is not available.
Generally considered to be safe. Ask physician for guidance.

Advisability of Use if Breast-Feeding
Presence of this drug in breast milk: Yes, in small amounts.
Avoid drug or refrain from nursing.

Habit-Forming Potential: None.

Effects of Overdosage: Nausea, vomiting, stomach cramps and/or diarrhea.

Possible Effects of Long-Term Use: Superinfections (see Glossary).

Suggested Periodic Examinations While Taking This Drug (at physician's discretion)
Complete blood cell counts. Liver and kidney function tests.

▷ **While Taking This Drug, Observe the Following**
Foods: No restrictions.
Beverages: No restrictions. May be taken with milk.
▷ *Alcohol:* No interactions expected.
Tobacco Smoking: No interactions expected.
▷ *Other Drugs*
Cefadroxil *taken concurrently* with
• probenecid (Benemid) will slow the elimination of cefadroxil, resulting in higher blood levels and prolonged effect.
▷ *Driving, Hazardous Activities:* Usually no restrictions. If drowsiness or dizziness occurs, restrict activities accordingly.
Aviation Note: The use of this drug *may be a disqualification* for piloting. Consult a designated Aviation Medical Examiner.
Exposure to Sun: No restrictions.
Special Storage Instructions: Oral suspension should be refrigerated.
Observe the Following Expiration Times: Do not take the oral suspension of this drug if it is older than 14 days.

CEFIXIME
(sef IX eem)

Introduced: 1986

Class: Antibiotic, cephalosporins

Prescription: USA: Yes

Controlled Drug: USA: No

Available as Generic: No

Brand Name: Suprax

BENEFITS versus RISKS

Possible Benefits	*Possible Risks*
EFFECTIVE TREATMENT OF INFECTIONS due to susceptible microorganisms	ALLERGIC REACTIONS mild to severe (up to 1% of general population, up to 2% of those allergic to penicillin) Drug-induced colitis (rare) Superinfections (see Glossary)

▷ **Principal Uses**

As a Single Drug Product: Used primarily to treat certain infections of the middle ear, tonsils, throat, bronchial tubes and urinary tract.

How This Drug Works: This drug destroys susceptible infecting bacteria by interfering with their ability to produce new protective cell walls as they multiply and grow.

Available Dosage Forms and Strengths

Oral suspension — 100 mg per 5 ml teaspoonful
Tablets — 200 mg, 400 mg

▷ **Usual Adult Dosage Range:** 400 mg daily, taken as a single dose or as 200 mg every 12 hours. **Note: Actual dosage and administration schedule must be determined by the physician for each patient individually.**

▷ **Dosing Instructions:** May be taken on an empty stomach or with food if stomach irritation occurs. The tablet may be crushed and mixed with food (such as applesauce or ice cream) if necessary to facilitate swallowing. Take the full course prescribed.

Usual Duration of Use: Continual use on a regular schedule for 3 to 5 days is usually necessary to determine this drug's effectiveness in controlling the infection under treatment. Response varies with the nature of the infection. Total treatment time will vary from 1 to 4 weeks. Certain infections require that this drug be taken for 10 consecutive days to prevent the development of rheumatic fever. Follow your physician's instructions regarding duration of use.

▷ **This Drug Should Not Be Taken If**
- you are allergic to any cephalosporin antibiotic (see Drug Class, Section Four).
- you have active colitis of any type.

▷ **Inform Your Physician Before Taking This Drug If**
- you have a history of allergy to any form of penicillin (see Drug Class, Section Four).
- you have a history of regional enteritis or ulcerative colitis.
- you have impaired kidney function.

Possible Side-Effects (natural, expected and unavoidable drug actions)
Superinfections (see Glossary): vaginitis (yeast infection).

▷ **Possible Adverse Effects** (unusual, unexpected and infrequent reactions)
If any of the following develop, consult your physician promptly for guidance.
Mild Adverse Effects
Allergic Reactions: Skin rash, hives, itching, drug fever (see Glossary).
Nausea (7%), indigestion (3%), loose stools (6%), diarrhea (16%), abdominal pain (3%).
Headache, dizziness.
Serious Adverse Effects
Severe diarrhea, possibly indicating a drug-induced form of colitis (rare). This may begin during use of the drug or after discontinuation of the drug.

▷ **Possible Effects on Sexual Function:** None reported.

▷ **Adverse Effects That May Mimic Natural Diseases or Disorders**
Skin rash may resemble measles.

Possible Effects on Laboratory Tests
Complete blood cell counts: transient decreases in white blood cells and platelets; no serious consequences reported.

CAUTION
1. Otitis media (middle ear infection) should be treated with the oral suspension; this produces higher blood levels of the drug. Tablets should not be substituted for the suspension.
2. In the management of diabetes it should be noted that this drug can cause a false positive test result for urine sugar when using Clinitest tablets, Benedict's solution or Fehling's solution, but not with Clinistix or Tes-Tape. This drug can also cause a false positive reaction for urine ketones with tests using nitroprusside but not with tests using nitroferricyanide.

Precautions for Use
By Infants and Children: Safety and effectiveness for use by those under 6 months of age have not been established. For those over 6 months of age, the recommended dose is 8 mg/kg/day of the oral suspension. This may be given as a single daily dose or as 4 mg/kg every 12 hours.
By Those over 60 Years of Age: Dosage must be carefully individualized and based upon evaluation of kidney function. Natural changes in the skin may predispose to severe and prolonged itching reactions in the genital and anal regions. Such reactions should be reported promptly.

▷ **Advisability of Use During Pregnancy**
Pregnancy Category: B (tentative). See Pregnancy Code inside back cover.
Animal studies: No birth defects due to this drug reported in mouse and rat studies.

Human studies: Information from adequate studies of pregnant women is not available.
Generally considered to be safe. Ask physician for guidance.

Advisability of Use if Breast-Feeding
Presence of this drug in breast milk: Unknown.
Avoid drug or refrain from nursing.

Habit-Forming Potential: None.

Effects of Overdosage: Nausea, vomiting, stomach cramps and/or diarrhea.

Possible Effects of Long-Term Use: Superinfections (see Glossary).

Suggested Periodic Examinations While Taking This Drug (at physician's discretion)
Complete blood cell counts.

▷ **While Taking This Drug, Observe the Following**
Foods: No restrictions.
Beverages: No restrictions. May be taken with milk.
▷ *Alcohol:* No interactions expected.
Tobacco Smoking: No interactions expected.
▷ *Other Drugs*
No interactions reported to date.
▷ *Driving, Hazardous Activities:* Usually no restrictions. Observe for the rare occurrence of dizziness.
Aviation Note: The use of this drug *may be a disqualification* for piloting. Consult a designated Aviation Medical Examiner.
Exposure to Sun: No restrictions
Special Storage Instructions: Keep the oral suspension at room temperature. Do not refrigerate. Shake well before measuring dose.
Observe the Following Expiration Time: Do not take the oral suspension of this drug it older than 14 days.

CEFUROXIME
(sef yur OX eem)

Introduced: 1976

Class: Antibiotic, cephalosporins

Prescription: USA: Yes

Controlled Drug: USA: No

Available as Generic: No

Brand Name: Ceftin

BENEFITS versus RISKS

Possible Benefits	*Possible Risks*
EFFECTIVE TREATMENT OF INFECTIONS due to susceptible microorganisms	ALLERGIC REACTIONS mild to severe (up to 1% of general population, up to 2.9% of those allergic to penicillin)
	Drug-induced colitis (rare)
	Superinfections (see Glossary)

▷ **Principal Uses**

As a Single Drug Product: Used primarily to treat certain infections of the middle ear, tonsils, throat, bronchial tubes, urinary tract and skin.

How This Drug Works: This drug destroys susceptible infecting bacteria by interfering with their ability to produce new protective cell walls as they multiply and grow.

Available Dosage Forms and Strengths

Tablets — 125 mg, 250 mg, 500 mg

▷ **Usual Adult Dosage Range:**   250 to 500 mg/12 hrs. Total daily dosage should not exceed 4 grams. **Note: Actual dosage and administration schedule must be determined by the physician for each patient individually.**

▷ **Dosing Instructions:**   May be taken on an empty stomach or with food if stomach irritation occurs. The tablet may be crushed and mixed with food (such as applesauce or ice cream) if necessary to facilitate swallowing. (Note: The crushed tablet has a persistent, bitter taste.) Take the full course prescribed.

Usual Duration of Use: Continual use on a regular schedule for 3 to 5 days is usually necessary to determine this drug's effectiveness in controlling the infection under treatment. Response varies with the nature of the infection. Total treatment time will vary from 1 to 4 weeks. Certain infecti ns require that this drug be taken for 10 consecutive days to prevent the development of rheumatic fever. Follow your physician's instructions regarding duration of use.

▷ **This Drug Should Not Be Taken If**
- you are allergic to any cephalosporin antibiotic (see Drug Class, Section Four).

▷ **Inform Your Physician Before Taking This Drug If**
- you have a history of allergy to any form of penicillin (see Drug Class, Section Four).
- you have a history of regional enteritis or ulcerative colitis.
- you have impaired kidney function.

Possible Side-Effects (natural, expected and unavoidable drug actions)
Superinfections (see Glossary): vaginitis (1.9%).

▷ **Possible Adverse Effects** (unusual, unexpected and infrequent reactions)
If any of the following develop, consult your physician promptly for guidance.
Mild Adverse Effects
Allergic Reactions: Skin rash (0.6%), hives (0.2%), itching (0.3%).
Nausea (2.4%), vomiting (2.0%), loose stools (1.3%), mild diarrhea (3.5%).
Headache (0.7%), dizziness (0.2%).
Serious Adverse Effects
Severe diarrhea, possibly indicating a drug-induced form of colitis (rare).

▷ **Possible Effects on Sexual Function:**   None reported.

▷ **Adverse Effects That May Mimic Natural Diseases or Disorders**
Skin rash may resemble measles.

Possible Effects on Laboratory Tests
White blood cell counts: decreased (very rare).
Liver function tests: increased liver enzymes (ALT/GPT, AST/GOT) in individuals with impaired liver function.

CAUTION
In the management of diabetes it should be noted that this drug can cause a false positive test result for urine sugar when using Clinitest tablets, Benedict's solution or Fehling's solution, but not with Clinistix or Tes-Tape.

Precautions for Use
By Infants and Children: The usual dose is 125 mg/12 hours. For middle ear infection, the recommended dose for those under 2 years of age is 125 mg/12 hours, and 250 mg/12 hours for those over 2 years of age.
By Those over 60 Years of Age: Dosage must be carefully individualized and based upon evaluation of kidney function. Natural changes in the skin may predispose to severe and prolonged itching reactions in the genital and anal regions. Such reactions should be reported promptly.

▷ **Advisability of Use During Pregnancy**
Pregnancy Category: B (tentative). See Pregnancy Code inside back cover.
Animal studies: No birth defects due to this drug reported in mouse and rat studies.
Human studies: Information from adequate studies of pregnant women is not available.
Generally considered to be safe. Ask physician for guidance.

Advisability of Use if Breast-Feeding
Presence of this drug in breast milk: Yes, in small amounts.
Avoid drug or refrain from nursing.

Habit-Forming Potential: None.

Effects of Overdosage: Nausea, vomiting, stomach cramps and/or diarrhea.

Possible Effects of Long-Term Use: Superinfections (see Glossary).

Suggested Periodic Examinations While Taking This Drug (at physician's discretion)
None.

▷ **While Taking This Drug, Observe the Following**
Foods: No restrictions. Food enhances the absorption of this drug.
Beverages: No restrictions. May be taken with milk.
▷ *Alcohol:* No interactions expected.
Tobacco Smoking: No interactions expected.
▷ *Other Drugs*
Cefuroxime *taken concurrently* with
• probenecid (Benemid) will slow the elimination of cefuroxime, resulting in higher blood levels and prolonged effect.
▷ *Driving, Hazardous Activities:* Usually no restrictions. Observe for the rare occurrence of dizziness.
Aviation Note: The use of this drug *may be a disqualification* for piloting. Consult a designated Aviation Medical Examiner.
Exposure to Sun: No restrictions.

CEPHALEXIN
(sef a LEX in)

Introduced: 1969

Class: Antibiotic, cephalosporins

Prescription: USA: Yes
Canada: Yes

Controlled Drug: USA: No
Canada: No

Available as Generic: Yes

Brand Names: Cefanex, ✦Ceporex, Keflet, Keflex, Keftab, ✦Novolexin

BENEFITS versus RISKS	
Possible Benefits	*Possible Risks*
EFFECTIVE TREATMENT OF INFECTIONS due to susceptible microorganisms	ALLERGIC REACTIONS mild to severe (up to 5% of general population, up to 16% of those allergic to penicillin) Drug-induced colitis (rare) Superinfections (see Glossary)

▷ **Principal Uses**

As a Single Drug Product: To treat certain infections of the skin and skin structures, the upper respiratory tract (including middle ear infections and "strep" throat), the genitourinary tract and certain infections involving bones and joints.

How This Drug Works: This drug destroys susceptible infecting bacteria by interfering with their ability to produce new protective cell walls as they multiply and grow.

Available Dosage Forms and Strengths

Capsules — 250 mg, 500 mg
Oral suspension — 125 mg, 250 mg per 5-ml teaspoonful
Pediatric oral suspension — 100 mg per ml
Tablets — 250 mg, 500 mg, 1000 mg (1 gram)

▷ **Usual Adult Dosage Range:** 250 to 500 mg/6 hours. Total daily dose should not exceed 4 grams. **Note: Actual dosage and administration schedule must be determined by the physician for each patient individually.**

▷ **Dosing Instructions:** May be taken on an empty stomach or with food if stomach irritation occurs. Capsule may be opened and tablet may be crushed for administration. Shake suspension well before measuring dose. Take the full course prescribed.

Usual Duration of Use: Continual use on a regular schedule for 3 to 5 days is usually necessary to determine this drug's effectiveness in controlling the infection under treatment. Response varies with the nature of the infection. Total treatment time will vary from 1 to 4 weeks. Certain infections require that this drug be taken for 10 consecutive days to prevent the development of rheumatic fever. Follow your physician's instructions regarding duration of use.

▷ **This Drug Should Not Be Taken If**
• you are allergic to any cephalosporin antibiotic (see Drug Class, Section Four).

▷ **Inform Your Physician Before Taking This Drug If**
• you have a history of allergy to any form of penicillin (see Drug Class, Section Four).
• you have a history of regional enteritis or ulcerative colitis.
• you have impaired kidney function.

Possible Side-Effects (natural, expected and unavoidable drug actions)
Superinfections (see Glossary).

▷ **Possible Adverse Effects** (unusual, unexpected and infrequent reactions)
If any of the following develop, consult your physician promptly for guidance.

Mild Adverse Effects
   Allergic Reactions: Skin rash (0.8%), itching, hives (0.3%).
   Headache, drowsiness, dizziness.
   Irritation of mouth or tongue, indigestion, stomach cramping, nausea, vomiting (1.8%), diarrhea (1.1%).

Serious Adverse Effects
   Allergic Reactions: Drug fever (see Glossary), joint aches and pains, anaphylactic reaction (see Glossary).
   Idiosyncratic Reactions: Minor and temporary changes in white blood cell counts and liver function tests (infrequent).
   Genital itching (may represent a fungus superinfection).
   Severe diarrhea, possibly indicating a drug-induced form of colitis (rare).

▷ **Possible Effects on Sexual Function:**   None reported.

▷ **Adverse Effects That May Mimic Natural Diseases or Disorders**
   Skin rash and fever may resemble measles.

Possible Effects on Laboratory Tests
   Complete blood cell counts: decreased white blood cells, increased eosinophils.
   Urine sugar tests: false positive results with Benedict's solution, Fehling's solution and Clinitest.

CAUTION
   1. In the management of diabetes it should be noted that this drug can cause a false positive test result for urine sugar when using Clinitest tablets, Benedict's solution or Fehling's solution, but not with Tes-Tape.
   2. Do not use this drug concurrently with other antibiotics such as erythromycin or tetracyclines.

Precautions for Use
   By Infants and Children: Not recommended for use in infants less than 1 year old. Monitor allergic children closely for evidence of developing allergy to this drug.
   By Those over 60 Years of Age: Dosage must be carefully individualized and based upon evaluation of kidney function. Natural changes in the skin may predispose to severe and prolonged itching reactions in the genital and anal regions. Such reactions should be reported promptly.

▷ **Advisability of Use During Pregnancy**
   Pregnancy Category: B (tentative). See Pregnancy Code inside back cover.
   Animal studies: No birth defects reported.
   Human studies: Information from adequate studies of pregnant women is not available.
   Generally considered to be safe. Ask physician for guidance.

Advisability of Use if Breast-Feeding
　　Presence of this drug in breast milk: Yes, in small amounts.
　　Avoid drug or refrain from nursing.

Habit-Forming Potential:　None.

Effects of Overdosage:　Nausea, vomiting, stomach cramps and/or diarrhea.

Possible Effects of Long-Term Use:　Superinfections (see Glossary).

Suggested Periodic Examinations While Taking This Drug (at physician's discretion)
　　Complete blood cell counts. Liver and kidney function tests.

▷ **While Taking This Drug, Observe the Following**
　　Foods: No restrictions.
　　Beverages: No restrictions. May be taken with milk.
▷ 　*Alcohol:* No interactions expected.
　　Tobacco Smoking: No interactions expected.
▷ 　*Other Drugs*
　　　Cephalexin *taken concurrently* with
　　　　• probenecid (Benemid) will slow the elimination of cephalexin, resulting in higher blood levels and prolonged effect.
▷ 　*Driving, Hazardous Activities:* Usually no restrictions. Use caution if drowsiness or dizziness occurs.
　　Aviation Note: The use of this drug *may be a disqualification* for piloting. Consult a designated Aviation Medical Examiner.
　　Exposure to Sun: No restrictions.
　　Special Storage Instructions: Oral suspension should be refrigerated.
　　Observe the Following Expiration Times: Do not take the oral suspension of this drug if it is older than 14 days.

CHLORAL HYDRATE
(klor al HI drayt)

Introduced: 1832　　　　**Class:** Sedative, hypnotic

Prescription: USA: Yes　　**Controlled Drug:** USA: C-IV*
　Canada: Yes　　　　　　　　Canada: No

Available as Generic: Yes

Brand Names: Aquachloral Supprettes, Noctec, ✦Novochlorhydrate

*See Schedules of Controlled Drugs inside back cover.

▷ **Principal Uses**

As a Single Drug Product: Used primarily as a bedtime sedative in sufficient dosage to induce sleep. It is the drug of choice for use in the elderly because it produces less "hangover" effect and is less likely to cause the confusion so commonly seen with use of barbiturates.

How This Drug Works: Not completely known. It is converted into an alcohol, which is thought to have a sedative effect on the wake-sleep centers of the brain.

Available Dosage Forms and Strengths

Capsules — 250 mg, 500 mg

Suppositories — 324 mg, 500 mg, 648 mg

Syrup — 250 mg, 500 mg per 5-ml teaspoonful

▷ **Usual Adult Dosage Range:** As sedative—250 mg 3 times daily. As hypnotic—500 to 1000 mg, 15 to 30 minutes before bedtime. Total daily dosage should not exceed 2000 mg (2 grams). **Note: Actual dosage and administration schedule must be determined by the physician for each patient individually.**

▷ **Dosing Instructions:** Take capsules whole (unopened) with a full glass of water, fruit juice or ginger ale to prevent stomach irritation. Mix the elixir or syrup in half a glass of water, fruit juice or ginger ale. Daytime doses are best taken after meals.

Usual Duration of Use: As sedative, use intermittently and not on a regular basis. As hypnotic, limit use to periods of 7 to 10 days. Avoid continual and prolonged use. Duration of use should not exceed 14 days without drug-free periods of several days, and reappraisal of continued need.

▷ **This Drug Should Not Be Taken If**
- you have had an allergic or unfavorable reaction to it previously.
- you have severely impaired liver or kidney function.
- you have severe heart disease.
- you have active gastritis or peptic ulcer disease.
- you have a history of intermittent porphyria.

▷ **Inform Your Physician Before Taking This Drug If**
- you have a history of heart disease or peptic ulcer disease.

- you are taking other sedatives, hypnotics, tranquilizers or narcotic drugs of any kind.
- you plan to have surgery under general anesthesia in the near future.

Possible Side-Effects (natural, expected and unavoidable drug actions)
Light-headedness in upright position, unsteadiness, weakness.
"Hangover" effect following nighttime use as hypnotic.

▷ **Possible Adverse Effects** (unusual, unexpected and infrequent reactions)
If any of the following develop, consult your physician promptly for guidance.
Mild Adverse Effects
Allergic Reactions: Skin rashes, hives, conjunctivitis.
Dizziness, confusion, hallucinations, nightmares.
Unpleasant taste, stomach irritation, nausea, vomiting, diarrhea.
Serious Adverse Effects
Allergic Reactions: Severe forms of dermatitis.
Idiosyncratic Reactions: Sleepwalking, delirium, disorientation, paranoid behavior.
Double vision, temporary blindness.

▷ **Possible Effects on Sexual Function:**   None reported.

Possible Delayed Adverse Effects: Allergic skin reactions may occur up to 10 days following the last dose.

▷ **Adverse Effects That May Mimic Natural Diseases or Disorders**
Paradoxical excitement or delirium may suggest latent psychosis.

Natural Diseases or Disorders That May Be Activated by This Drug
Intermittent porphyria.

Possible Effects on Laboratory Tests
Liver function tests: increased liver enzymes (ALT/GPT, AST/GOT)—liver damage.
Urine sugar tests: normal results with TesTape; false low results with Clinistix and Diastix; false positive results with Benedict's solution.

CAUTION
1. Use with caution in the presence of bronchial asthma. Avoid high and frequent doses.
2. Take all doses well diluted with water, milk, fruit juice or ginger ale to prevent stomach irritation.

Precautions for Use
By Infants and Children: Avoid concurrent use with other drugs that have a sedative effect. Use very cautiously in asthmatic children.
By Those over 60 Years of Age: Small doses are advisable until your individual response has been determined. You may be more susceptible to the development of "hangover" effect, dizziness, confused thinking, impaired memory, unsteadiness, loss of bladder control or constipation.

▷ **Advisability of Use During Pregnancy**
Pregnancy Category: C (tentative). See Pregnancy Code inside back cover.
Animal studies: No information available.
Human studies: Information from adequate studies of pregnant women
is not available.
Use this drug only if clearly needed. Continual use during pregnancy can
cause withdrawal symptoms in the newborn infant.

Advisability of Use if Breast-Feeding
Presence of this drug in breast milk: Yes.
Monitor nursing infant closely and discontinue drug or nursing if ad-
verse effects develop.

Habit-Forming Potential: This drug can cause psychological and/or physical dependence (see Glossary). Avoid large doses and continual use.

Effects of Overdosage: Marked drowsiness, confusion, incoordination,
slurred speech, staggering gait, weakness, vomiting, stupor, deep sleep.

Possible Effects of Long-Term Use: Psychological and/or physical dependence, toxic psychosis, liver and kidney damage.

Suggested Periodic Examinations While Taking This Drug (at physician's
discretion)
Complete blood cell counts. Liver and kidney function tests.

▷ **While Taking This Drug, Observe the Following**
Foods: No restrictions.
Beverages: No restrictions. May be taken with milk.
▷ *Alcohol:* Avoid completely for at least 6 hours before taking this drug.
Alcohol can greatly increase the sedative and depressant actions of this
drug on brain function.
Tobacco Smoking: No interactions expected.
Marijuana Smoking: Increased drowsiness, impaired mental and physical
performance.
▷ *Other Drugs*
Chloral hydrate may *increase* the effects of
• oral anticoagulants (Coumadin, etc.), and cause abnormal bleeding or
hemorrhage. Consult physician regarding prothrombin time testing
and dosage adjustment.
▷ *Driving, Hazardous Activities:* This drug can impair mental alertness, judgment, physical coordination and reaction time. Avoid hazardous activities until all sensation of drowsiness has disappeared.
Aviation Note: The use of this drug *is a disqualification* for piloting.
Consult a designated Aviation Medical Examiner.
Exposure to Sun: No restrictions.
Discontinuation: If this drug has been used continually over an extended
period of time, it should be discontinued gradually under physician
supervision.

CHLORAMBUCIL
(klor AM byu sil)

Introduced: 1974

Class: Anticancer, immunosuppressant

Prescription: USA: Yes
Canada: Yes

Controlled Drug: USA: No
Canada: No

Available as Generic: USA: No
Canada: No

Brand Name: Leukeran,

BENEFITS versus RISKS

Possible Benefits	*Possible Risks*
EFFECTIVE PALLIATIVE TREATMENT FOR CHRONIC LYMPHOCYTIC LEUKEMIA	BONE MARROW DEPRESSION (see Glossary)
EFFECTIVE PALLIATIVE TREATMENT FOR HODGKIN'S DISEASE AND OTHER LYMPHOMAS	INCREASED SUSCEPTIBILITY TO INFECTIONS
	CENTRAL NERVOUS SYSTEM TOXICITY
Immunosuppression of nephrotic syndrome	Male and female sterility
	Drug-induced liver damage
Immunosuppression of systemic lupus erythematosus	Drug-induced lung damage
	Development of secondary cancers

▷ **Principal Uses**

As a Single Drug Product: Used primarily to treat (1) chronic lymphocytic leukemia; (2) Hodgkin's lymphoma and other malignant lymphomas; (3) hairy cell leukemia; (4) cancer of the ovary and testicle; (5) polycythemia vera; (6) nephrotic syndrome; (7) systemic lupus erythematosus.

How This Drug Works: The primary actions of this drug are to combine with many structures within target cells, impair the functions of DNA and RNA, and inhibit the production of essential proteins. This reduces the population of cancerous cells.

Available Dosage Forms and Strengths

Tablets — 2 mg

▷ **Usual Adult Dosage Range:** For leukemia and lymphoma: Initially 0.1 to 0.2 mg per kilogram of body weight daily, or 3 to 6 mg per square meter of body surface daily (usually 4 to 10 mg daily) as a single dose or in divided doses.

For immunosuppression: 0.1 to 0.2 mg per kilogram of body weight daily, in a single dose, for 8 to 12 weeks. **Note: Actual dosage and administration schedule must be determined by the physician for each patient individually.**

▷ **Dosing Instructions:** Take with food or milk to reduce stomach irritation. The tablet may be crushed for administration. Consult physician if vomiting prevents adherence to dosage schedule.

Usual Duration of Use:
Continual use on a regular schedule for 3 to 4 weeks is usually necessary to determine this drug's effectiveness in controlling leukemia or lymphoma; several months of treatment may be required to assess the effects of immunosuppression. Long-term use requires periodic evaluation of response and dosage adjustment. Consult your physician on a regular basis.

Currently a "Drug of Choice"
for treating chronic lymphocytic leukemia and primary macroglobulinemia.

▷ **This Drug Should Not Be Taken If**
- you have had an allergic reaction to it previously.
- you currently have any degree of bone marrow depression.
- you have recently had or been exposed to chicken pox or herpes zoster.
- you currently have an uncontrolled infection.

▷ **Inform Your Physician Before Taking This Drug If**
- you are allergic to melphalan (Alkeran).
- you are pregnant, planning pregnancy, or breast-feeding.
- you have a history of bone marrow depression or a blood cell disorder.
- you have a history of gout or urate kidney stones.
- you have a seizure disorder of any kind.
- you have a history of porphyria.
- you have impaired liver or kidney function.
- you have had cancer chemotherapy or radiation therapy previously.
- you are currently taking prednisone or other drugs than can impair your immunity.

Possible Side-Effects (natural, expected and unavoidable drug actions)
Decreased white blood cell and platelet counts.
Decreased immunity, susceptibility to infections.
Increased blood levels of uric acid, formation of urate kidney stones.

▷ **Possible Adverse Effects**
(unusual, unexpected and infrequent reactions)
If any of the following develop, consult your physician promptly for guidance.
Mild Adverse Effects
Allergic Reactions: Skin rash, itching, drug fever (see Glossary).
Mouth and lip sores, nausea, vomiting.

Serious Adverse Effects
Allergic Reactions: Drug-induced hepatitis with jaundice.
Cataract formation with high-dose usage.
Central nervous system toxicity: agitation, confusion, hallucinations, seizures, tremors, paralysis.
Peripheral neuritis (see Glossary).
Lung damage: cough, shortness of breath.
Bone marrow damage, aplastic anemia (see Glossary).

▷ **Possible Effects on Sexual Function:**   Suppression of testicular and ovarian function: Cessation of sperm production (male sterility); altered menstrual patterns, cessation of ovulation and menstruation (female sterility).

Possible Delayed Adverse Effects: Evidence of severe bone marrow depression may occur after cessation of drug use.
Secondary cancers (especially leukemia) have been reported.
Lung damage (pulmonary fibrosis).

▷ **Adverse Effects That May Mimic Natural Diseases or Disorders**
Drug-induced seizures may suggest epilepsy.
Drug-induced jaundice may suggest viral hepatitis.

Natural Diseases or Disorders That May Be Activated by This Drug
Gout, urate kidney stones, porphyria, latent epilepsy.

Possible Effects on Laboratory Tests
Complete blood cell counts: decreased red cells, hemoglobin, white cells and platelets.
Blood uric acid level: increased.
Liver function tests: increased liver enzymes (ALT/GPT, AST/GOT), increased bilirubin, increased icterus index.
Sperm counts: decreased or absent.

CAUTION
1. The long-term use of this drug (as for immunosuppression) in non-cancerous conditions requires extreme caution. The risks include permanent sterility, lung damage, and the development of secondary cancers. Its use is recommended only for conditions that have not responded satisfactorily to conventional use of less toxic drugs.
2. It is advisable to complete necessary dental procedures prior to using this drug. The bone marrow depressant effects of this drug could predispose to gum infection, excessive bleeding and delayed healing.
3. In treating individuals with gout, allopurinol is the drug of choice to control the increased blood levels of uric acid caused by chlorambucil.
4. This drug impairs the body's immune system by decreasing its ability to produce protective antibodies. For this reason, both killed virus vaccines and live virus vaccines will be ineffective. In addition, there is an increased risk that a live virus vaccine may actually induce

infection and cause significant adverse effects. It is estimated that a period of 3 months to 1 year is required for the immune system to recover its ability to repond appropriately to vaccination after discontinuation of this and similar drugs. Persons in close contact with anyone taking this drug should not receive oral poliovirus vaccine; this will eliminate the risk of accidental exposure to live polio virus.

5. Report immediately any indications of the following: onset of infection, unusual bruising or bleeding, excessive fatigue or weakness, tremors or muscle twitching, difficulty walking, loss of appetite with nausea or vomiting.

6. It is advisable to avoid pregnancy while taking this drug. A nonhormonal method of contraception is recommended. Notify your physician promptly if you think pregnancy has occurred.

Precautions for Use

By Infants and Children: Dosage schedules and treatment monitoring should be supervised by a qualified pediatrician.

Children with nephrotic syndrome may be more prone to seizures induced by this drug.

By Those over 60 Years of Age: Observe closely for greater susceptibility to central nervous system toxicity.

▷ ## Advisability of Use During Pregnancy

Pregnancy Category: D (tentative). See Pregnancy Code inside back cover.

Animal studies: Rat studies reveal drug associated defects of the nervous system, palate, skeleton and urogenital system.

Human studies: Information from adequate studies of pregnant women is not available. There are two known cases of an infant born with an absent kidney and ureter following exposure to this drug during early pregnancy.

If possible, this drug should be avoided during pregnancy, especially the first 3 months.

It is generally recommended that a nonhormonal contraceptive be used during treatment with this and similar drugs.

Advisability of Use if Breast-Feeding

Presence of this drug in breast milk: Unknown.

Avoid drug or refrain from nursing.

Habit-Forming Potential: None.

Effects of Overdosage: Fatigue, weakness, fever, sore throat, bruising, agitation, unstable gait, seizures.

Possible Effects of Long-Term Use: Permanent sterility; secondary cancers (leukemia); lung damage (pulmonary fibrosis).

Suggested Periodic Examinations While Taking This Drug

(atphysician's discretion)*Before* drug treatment is started and *periodically* during drug use: complete blood cell counts, blood uric acid levels, liver function tests, sperm counts.

▷ **While Taking This Drug, Observe the Following**
 Foods: No restrictions.
 Beverages: No restrictions. May be taken with milk. It is advisable to drink 2 to 3 quarts of liquids daily to reduce the risk of kidney stone formation.
▷ *Alcohol:* Use with caution. Avoid if platelet counts are low and there is a risk of stomach bleeding.
 Tobacco Smoking: No interactions expected.
 Marijuana Smoking
  : Best avoided. This could increase the risk of central nervous system toxicity.
▷ *Other Drugs*
  Chlorambucil *taken concurrently* with
  • aspirin may increase the risk of bruising or bleeding; the platelet-reduction effects of chlorambucil and the antiplatelet action of aspirin are additive; avoid aspirin while taking chlorambucil.
  • antidepressant or antipsychotic (neuroleptic) drugs requires careful monitoring; these drugs can lower the threshold for the occurrence of seizures and increase the risk of chlorambucil induced seizures.
  • other immunosuppressant drugs can increase the risk of infection and the development of secondary cancers.
▷ *Driving, Hazardous Activities:* This drug may cause nervous agitation, confusion, hallucinations or seizures. Restrict activities as necessary.
 Aviation Note: The use of this drug **may be a disqualification** for piloting. Consult a designated Aviation Medical Examiner.
 Exposure to Sun: No restrictions.
 Discontinuation: Whether used as an anticancer drug or as an immunosuppressant, many factors will determine when and how this drug should be discontinued. To obtain maximal benefit, comply with your physician's guidance as closely as possible.

CHLORAMPHENICOL
(klor am FEN i kohl)

Introduced: 1947

Class: Antibiotic

Prescription: USA: Yes
 Canada: Yes

Controlled Drug: USA: No
 Canada: No

Available as Generic: USA: Yes
 Canada: No

Brand Names: Ak-Chlor, Chloromycetin, Chloroptic, ✦Fenicol, ✦Isopto Fenicol, ✦Minims, ✦Nova-Phenicol, ✦Novochlorocap, Ophthochlor, ✦Pentamycetin

```
┌─────────────────────────────────────────────────────────────┐
│                   BENEFITS versus RISKS                        │
│                                                                │
│      Possible Benefits              Possible Risks            │
│   VERY EFFECTIVE TREATMENT      BONE MARROW DEPRESSION        │
│      OF INFECTIONS due to          APLASTIC ANEMIA (see        │
│      susceptible microorganisms       Glossary)               │
│                                    Peripheral neuritis (see Glossary) │
│                                    Liver damage, jaundice     │
└─────────────────────────────────────────────────────────────┘
```

▷ **Principal Uses**

As a Single Drug Product: This drug is quite effective in a broad spectrum of serious infections. However, because of its potential for serious toxicity (fatal aplastic anemia), its use is now reserved for life-threatening infections caused by organisms that are resistant to safer antibiotics, and for infections in individuals who, for one reason or another, cannot take other appropriate anti-infective drugs.

How This Drug Works: This drug prevents the growth and multiplication of susceptible microorganisms by interfering with their formation of essential proteins.

Available Dosage Forms and Strengths

>   Capsules — 250 mg, 500 mg
>   Cream — 1%
> Eye/ear solutions — 0.5%
>   Eye ointment — 1%
>   Injection — 100 mg per ml
> Oral suspension — 150 mg per 5-ml teaspoonful

▷ **Usual Adult Dosage Range:**   Total daily dose is 250 mg for each 10 pounds of body weight, given in 4 equally divided doses, 6 hours apart. Total daily dose should not exceed 500 mg for each 10 pounds of body weight. **Note: Actual dosage and administration schedule must be determined by the physician for each patient individually.**

▷ **Dosing Instructions:**   Take with a full glass of water on an empty stomach, 1 hour before or 2 hours after eating. Capsule may be opened for administration. Shake oral suspension well before measuring dose.

Usual Duration of Use: Continual use on a regular schedule for 3 to 5 days is usually necessary to determine this drug's effectiveness in controlling the infection. Limit use to the time required to eradicate the infection. Avoid repeated courses of treatment if possible.

▷ **This Drug Should Not Be Taken If**
- you have had an allergic reaction to it previously.
- you have an active blood cell or bone marrow disorder.
- it is prescribed for a mild or trivial infection such as a cold, sore throat or "flulike" illness.

  • it is prescribed for a premature or newborn infant (under 2 weeks of age).

▷ **Inform Your Physician Before Taking This Drug If**
  • you have a history of a blood cell or bone marrow disorder.
  • you have impaired liver or kidney function.
  • you are taking anticoagulants.

Possible Side-Effects (natural, expected and unavoidable drug actions)
Superinfections (see Glossary).

▷ **Possible Adverse Effects** (unusual, unexpected and infrequent reactions)
If any of the following develop, consult your physician promptly for guidance.
Mild Adverse Effects
Allergic Reactions: Skin rashes, hives, swelling of face or extremities, fever.
Headache, confusion, peripheral neuritis (see Glossary)—numbness, pain, weakness in hands and/or feet.
Sore mouth or tongue, "black tongue," nausea, vomiting, diarrhea.
Serious Adverse Effects
Allergic Reactions: Anaphylactic reaction (see Glossary), liver damage with jaundice (rare).
Bone marrow depression (see Glossary)—fatigue, weakness, fever, sore throat, abnormal bleeding or bruising.

▷ **Possible Effects on Sexual Function:**   None reported.

▷ **Adverse Effects That May Mimic Natural Diseases or Disorders**
Liver reaction with jaundice may suggest viral hepatitis.

Possible Effects on Laboratory Tests
Complete blood cell counts: decreased red cells, hemoglobin, white cells and platelets (bone marrow depression); increased white cells (possible leukemia following bone marrow depression); increased eosinophils (allergic reaction).
Prothrombin time: increased.
Blood glucose level: decreased.
Liver function tests: increased liver enzymes (ALT/GPT, AST/GOT, alkaline phosphatase), increased bilirubin.
Fecal occult blood: positive (intestinal bleeding or drug-induced colitis).

CAUTION
  1. This drug can cause serious bone marrow depression and aplastic anemia (see Glossary). It must not be used to treat trivial infections or as a preventive medication under any circumstances. Its use must be restricted to the treatment of serious or life-threatening infections that fail to respond to other anti-infective drugs.
  2. Troublesome and persistent diarrhea can develop in sensitive in-

dividuals. If diarrhea persists for more than 24 hours, discontinue this drug and consult your physician.

Precautions for Use

By Infants and Children: Follow prescribed dosage exactly. Blood cell counts should be monitored twice a week. Long-term use of this drug can cause optic neuritis. This may be prevented by taking supplemental vitamin B complex during treatment. Idiosyncratic aplastic anemia is rare (1 in 40,000 users), but may occur weeks or months after discontinuation of this drug.

By Those over 60 Years of Age: The natural decline in liver and kidney function after 60 may require reduction in dosage and adjustment of dosage interval. Natural changes in the skin after 60 may predispose to severe and prolonged itching reactions in the genital and anal regions. Report such reactions promptly.

▷ **Advisability of Use During Pregnancy**

Pregnancy Category: C (tentative). See Pregnancy Code inside back cover. Animal studies: Results are inconclusive.

Human studies: Information from adequate studies of pregnant women is not available. Limited studies (348 exposures) indicate that this drug does not cause birth defects. However, it has been shown to be potentially toxic for the fetus and newborn. Ask physician for guidance.

Advisability of Use if Breast-Feeding

Presence of this drug in breast milk: Yes.
Avoid drug or refrain from nursing.

Habit-Forming Potential: None.

Effects of Overdosage: Possible nausea, vomiting, diarrhea.

Possible Effects of Long-Term Use: Superinfections, impaired vision, bone marrow depression.

Suggested Periodic Examinations While Taking This Drug (at physician's discretion)

Complete blood cell counts—before treatment is started and every 2 to 3 days during administration of drug.
Liver and kidney function tests.

▷ **While Taking This Drug, Observe the Following**

Foods: No restrictions.
Nutritional Support: Supplemental vitamins B-2, B-6 and B-12 are recommended.
Beverages: No restrictions. May be taken with milk.

▷ *Alcohol:* Avoid completely if you have liver disease. Use cautiously until the combined effect has been determined. Some sensitive individuals may develop a disulfiramlike reaction (see Glossary).

Tobacco Smoking: No interactions expected.

▷ *Other Drugs*

Chloramphenicol may *increase* the effects of
- oral anticoagulants (Coumadin, dicumarol, etc.), and increase the risk of bleeding.
- barbiturates (phenobarbital, etc.), and cause excessive sedation.
- phenytoin (Dilantin), and cause phenytoin toxicity.
- sulfonylureas (Diabinese, Dymelor, Orinase, Tolinase), and cause hypoglycemia (see Glossary).

Chloramphenicol may *decrease* the effects of
- iron preparations, used to treat anemia.
- penicillins.
- vitamin B-12.

The following drugs may *decrease* the effects of chloramphenicol
- barbiturates (phenobarbital, etc.).
- rifampin (Rifadin, Rimactane, etc.).

▷ *Driving, Hazardous Activities:* Usually no restrictions. Be alert to the rare occurrence of confusion, and restrict activities accordingly.

Aviation Note: The use of this drug *may be a disqualification* for piloting. Consult a designated Aviation Medical Examiner.

Exposure to Sun: No restrictions.

CHLORDIAZEPOXIDE
(klor di az e POX ide)

Introduced: 1960

Class: Mild tranquilizer, benzodiazepines

Prescription: USA: Yes
Canada: Yes

Controlled Drug: USA: C-IV*
Canada: No

Available as Generic: Yes

Brand Names: ✦Apo-Chlorax [CD], ✦Apo-Chlordiazepoxide, ✦Corium [CD], Librax [CD], Libritabs, Librium, Lidox [CD], Limbitrol [CD], Lipoxide, Menrium [CD], ✦Novopoxide, ✦Pentrium [CD], ✦Solium

---

BENEFITS versus RISKS

Possible Benefits	*Possible Risks*
RELIEF OF ANXIETY AND NERVOUS TENSION in 70% to 80% of users	Habit-forming potential with prolonged use
Wide margin of safety with therapeutic doses	Minor impairment of mental functions
Very few drug interactions	Very rare jaundice
	Very rare blood cell disorders

---

*See Schedules of Controlled Drugs inside back cover.

▷ **Principal Uses**

  As a Single Drug Product: Used primarily to (1) provide short-term relief of mild to moderate anxiety, and (2) relieve the symptoms of acute alcohol withdrawal: agitation, tremors, hallucinations, incipient delirium tremens.

  As a Combination Drug Product [CD]: Used in combination with amitriptyline (an antidepressant) to allay the anxiety that is often a troublesome feature in the agitated and depressed individual. Also used in combination with clidinium (a synthetic atropinelike antispasmodic) to treat peptic ulcer disease and irritable bowel syndrome.

How This Drug Works: It is thought that this drug produces a calming effect by enhancing the action of the nerve transmitter gamma-aminobutyric acid (GABA), which in turn blocks the arousal of higher brain centers.

Available Dosage Forms and Strengths

  Capsules — 5 mg, 10 mg, 25 mg
  Injection — 100 mg/ampul
  Tablets — 5 mg, 10 mg, 25 mg

▷ **Usual Adult Dosage Range:** 5 to 25 mg, 3 or 4 times daily. Dose may be increased cautiously as needed and tolerated. After 1 week of continual use, the total daily dose may be taken at bedtime. Total daily dose should not exceed 150 mg for anxiety and tension, or 300 mg for alcohol withdrawal. **Note: Actual dosage and administration schedule must be determined by the physician for each patient individually.**

▷ **Dosing Instructions:** May be taken on empty stomach or with food or milk. Capsule may be opened and tablet may be crushed for administration. Do not discontinue this drug abruptly if taken for more than 4 weeks.

Usual Duration of Use: Continual use on a regular schedule for 3 to 5 days is usually necessary to determine this drug's effectiveness in relieving moderate anxiety. Limit continual use to 1 to 3 weeks. Avoid uninterrupted and prolonged use.

▷ **This Drug Should Not Be Taken If**

  • you have had an allergic reaction to any dosage form of it previously.
  • you have acute narrow-angle glaucoma.
  • it is prescribed for a child under 6 years of age.

▷ **Inform Your Physician Before Taking This Drug If**

  • you are allergic to any benzodiazepine drug (see Drug Class, Section Four).
  • you have a history of alcoholism or drug abuse.
  • you are pregnant or planning pregnancy.
  • you have impaired liver or kidney function.
  • you have a history of serious depression or mental disorder.

- you have any of the following: asthma, emphysema, epilepsy, myasthenia gravis, porphyria.

Possible Side-Effects (natural, expected and unavoidable drug actions)
Drowsiness (3.9%), lethargy, unsteadiness; "hangover" effects on the day following bedtime use.

▷ **Possible Adverse Effects** (unusual, unexpected and infrequent reactions)
If any of the following develop, consult your physician promptly for guidance.
Mild Adverse Effects
Allergic Reactions: Rashes, fixed skin eruptions, bruising.
Dizziness, fainting, blurred vision, double vision, slurred speech, sweating, nausea.
Serious Adverse Effects
Allergic Reactions: Liver damage with jaundice (see Glossary), abnormally low blood platelet count.
Idiosyncratic Reactions: Inappropriate female breast enlargement and milk production (rare). Acute hepatic porphyria.
Bone marrow depression—impaired production of red and white blood cells.
Paradoxical responses of excitement, agitation, anger, rage.

▷ **Possible Effects on Sexual Function**
Decreased libido with high doses, increased libido with low doses (antianxiety effect); rare report of inhibited ejaculation.
Altered timing and pattern of menstruation; female breast enlargement and milk production.

▷ **Adverse Effects That May Mimic Natural Diseases or Disorders**
Liver reaction with jaundice may suggest viral hepatitis.

Natural Diseases or Disorders That May Be Activated by This Drug
Acute intermittent hepatic porphyria, systemic lupus erythematoslike syndrome.

Possible Effects on Laboratory Tests
Complete blood cell counts: decreased red cells, hemoglobin, white cells and platelets.
Prothrombin time: conflicting reports—this drug may have no effect or it may increase or decrease prothrombin times.
Liver function tests: increased liver enzymes (ALT/GPT, AST/GOT, alkaline phosphatase), increased bilirubin.
Urine pregnancy tests: false positive results with Gravindex.
Urine screening tests for drug abuse: may be **positive**. (Test results depend upon amount of drug taken and testing method used.)

CAUTION
1. This drug should not be discontinued abruptly if it has been taken continually for more than 4 weeks.

2. The concurrent use of some over-the-counter drug products that contain antihistamines (allergy and cold preparations, sleep aids) can cause excessive sedation in sensitive individuals.

Precautions for Use
By Infants and Children: Safety and effectiveness for use by those under 6 years of age have not been established. This drug should not be used in the hyperactive or psychotic child of any age.

By Those over 60 Years of Age: It is advisable to use smaller doses at longer intervals to avoid overdosage. Observe for the possible development of lethargy, indifference, fatigue, weakness, unsteadiness, disturbing dreams, nightmares and paradoxical reactions of excitement, agitation, anger, hostility and rage.

▷ ### Advisability of Use During Pregnancy
Pregnancy Category: D (tentative). See Pregnancy Code inside back cover.
Animal studies: Cleft palate reported in mice.
Human studies: Available information is conflicting and inconclusive. Some studies found a fourfold increase in serious birth defects associated with the use of this drug. Other studies have found no significant increase in birth defects.
Frequent use in late pregnancy can cause the "floppy infant" syndrome in the newborn: weakness, lethargy, unresponsiveness, depressed breathing, low body temperature.
Avoid use during entire pregnancy if possible.

Advisability of Use if Breast-Feeding
Presence of this drug in breast milk: Yes, in small amounts.
Monitor nursing infant closely and discontinue drug or nursing if adverse effects develop.

Habit-Forming Potential:
This drug can produce psychological and/or physical dependence (see Glossary) if used in large doses for an extended period of time.

Effects of Overdosage:
Marked drowsiness, weakness, feeling of drunkenness, staggering gait, tremor, stupor progressing to deep sleep or coma.

Possible Effects of Long-Term Use:
Psychological and/or physical dependence, rare blood cell disorders.

Suggested Periodic Examinations While Taking This Drug (at physician's discretion)
Complete blood cell counts during long-term use.

▷ ### While Taking This Drug, Observe the Following
Foods: No restrictions.
Beverages: Avoid excessive intake of caffeine-containing beverages: coffee, tea, cola. May be taken with milk.
▷ *Alcohol:* Use with extreme caution until the combined effect is determined.

Alcohol may increase the absorption of this drug and add to its depressant effects on the brain. It is advisable to avoid alcohol completely—throughout the day and night—if it is necessary to drive or to engage in any hazardous activity.

Tobacco Smoking: Heavy smoking may reduce the calming action of this drug.

Marijuana Smoking: Increased sedation and significant impairment of intellectual and physical performance.

▷ *Other Drugs*

Chlordiazepoxide may *increase* the effects of
• digoxin (Lanoxin), and cause digoxin toxicity.

Chlordiazepoxide may *decrease* the effects of
• levodopa (Sinemet, etc.), and reduce its effectiveness in treating Parkinson's disease.

The following drugs may *increase* the effects of chlordiazepoxide
• cimetidine (Tagamet).
• disulfiram (Antabuse).
• isoniazid (INH, Rifamate, etc.).
• oral contraceptives.
• valproic acid (Depakene).

The following drugs may *decrease* the effects of chlordiazepoxide
• rifampin (Rimactane, etc.).
• theophylline (aminophylline, Theo-Dur, etc.).

▷ *Driving, Hazardous Activities:* This drug can impair mental alertness, judgment, physical coordination and reaction time. Avoid hazardous activities accordingly.

Aviation Note: The use of this drug *is a disqualification* for piloting. Consult a designated Aviation Medical Examiner.

Exposure to Sun: Use caution until sensitivity is determined. A photoallergic skin reaction may occur rarely.

Discontinuation: Avoid sudden discontinuation if this drug has been taken for over 4 weeks. Dosage should be tapered gradually to prevent a withdrawal syndrome that could include depression, confusion, hallucinations, tremor, seizures, muscle cramping, sweating and vomiting.

CHLOROQUINE
(KLOR oh kwin)

Introduced: 1964

Class: Antiamebic, antimalarial, lupus suppressant, rheumatoid arthritis suppressant

Prescription: USA: Yes
Canada: Yes

Controlled Drug: USA: No
Canada: No

Available as Generic: USA: Yes
Canada: No

Brand Name: Aralen,

Warning: The brand names Aralen and Arlidin are similar and can be mistaken for each other; this can lead to serious medication errors. These names represent very different drugs. Aralen (a purple tablet imprinted with " W" in a square) is the generic drug chloroquine (see above). Arlidin (a white round tablet imprinted with "A" in a shield) is the generic drug nylidrin, a vasodilator. Verify that you are taking the correct drug.

BENEFITS versus RISKS

Possible Benefits	*Possible Risks*
EFFECTIVE PREVENTION AND TREATMENT OF CERTAIN FORMS OF MALARIA	INFREQUENT BUT SERIOUS DAMAGE OF CORNEAL AND RETINAL EYE TISSUES
EFFECTIVE TREATMENT OF CERTAIN FORMS OF AMEBIC INFECTION in conjunction with other drugs	RARE BUT SERIOUS BONE MARROW DEPRESSION: aplastic anemia, deficient white blood cells and platelets
Possibly effective in the management of acute and chronic rheumatoid arthritis and juvenile arthritis	Rare heart muscle damage
Possibly effective in the management of chronic discoid and systemic lupus erythematosus	Rare ear damage: hearing loss, ringing in ears

---

▷ **Principal Uses**

As a Single Drug Product: Used primarily to (1) suppress the development of and to treat acute attacks of certain types of malarial infection; (2) provide adjunctive treatment for certain forms of amebic infection; (3) reduce disease activity in rheumatoid and juvenile arthritis; (4) suppress disease activity in certain types of lupus erythematosus. It is also used in the treatment of sarcoidosis, polymorphous light eruption, porphyria, solar urticaria and chronic vasculitis.

How This Drug Works: Not completely established. As an anti-infective in treating malaria and amebiasis, it is thought that this drug binds to and impairs the function of DNA in the protozoa that cause these diseases. As an antiarthritic and antilupus drug, it is thought to act as a mild immunosuppressant. It accumulates in white blood cells and inhibits many enzymes involved in tissue destruction.

Available Dosage Forms and Strengths
Injection — 50 mg per ml
Tablets — 250 mg, 500 mg

▷ **Usual Adult Dosage Range:**   For malaria suppression: 500 mg once every 7 days.
For malaria treatment: Initially 1 gram, followed by 500 mg in 6 to 8 hours; then 500 mg once a day on the second and third days.
For amebiasis (other than intestinal): Initially 250 mg 4 times daily for 2 days; then 250 mg 2 times daily for 2 to 3 weeks.
For rheumatoid arthritis: Up to 4 mg per kilogram of lean body weight daily.
For lupus erythematosus: Up to 4 mg per kilogram of lean body weight daily. **Note: Actual dosage and administration schedule must be determined by the physician for each patient individually.**

▷ **Dosing Instructions:**   Take with food or milk to reduce stomach irritation. The tablet may be crushed for administration. Take full course of treatment as prescribed. Note: For malaria prevention, begin medication 2 weeks before entering malarious area; continue medication while in the area and for 4 weeks after leaving the area. For treating arthritis and lupus, take medication on a regular schedule daily; continual use for 6 months may be necessary to determine maximal benefit.

Usual Duration of Use:
Continual use on a regular schedule for 2 weeks before exposure, during period of exposure, and 4 weeks after exposure is usually necessary to determine this drug's effectiveness in preventing attacks of malaria. Continual use on a regular schedule for periods up to 6 months may be required to evaluate the potential benefits in reducing the activity of rheumatoid arthritis and lupus erythematosus. If significant improvement is not achieved within this time, this drug should be discontinued. Long-term use (months to years) requires periodic evaluation of response and dosage adjustment. Consult your physician on a regular basis.

Possible Advantages of This Drug
May be more effective than hydroxychloroquine in some cases of lupus.

▷ **This Drug Should Not Be Taken If**
  • you have had an allergic reaction to either chloroquine or hydroxy-chloroquine previously.
  • you have an active bone marrow or blood cell disorder.

▷ **Inform Your Physician Before Taking This Drug If**
  • you are pregnant or planning pregnancy.
  • you have a history of bone marrow depression or a blood cell disorder previously.
  • you have a deficiency of glucose-6-phosphate dehydrogenase.
  • you have any disorder of the eyes, especially disease of the cornea or retina, or visual field changes.
  • you have impaired hearing or ringing in the ears.
  • you have a seizure disorder of any kind.
  • you have a history of peripheral neuritis.
  • you have low blood pressure or a heart rhythm disorder.
  • you have a history of peptic ulcer disease, Crohn's disease or ulcerative colitis.
  • you have impaired liver or kidney function.
  • you have a history of porphyria.
  • you have any form of psoriasis.
  • you are taking antacids, cimetidine or penicillamine.

Possible Side-Effects
  (natural, expected and unavoidable drug actions)
  Light-headedness (low blood pressure); blue-black discoloration of skin, fingernails, or mouth lining with long-term use.

▷ **Possible Adverse Effects**
  (unusual, unexpected and infrequent reactions)
  If any of the following develop, consult your physician promptly for guidance.
  Mild Adverse Effects
  Allergic Reactions: Skin rash, itching (more common in Afro-Americans).
  Loss of hair color, loss of hair.
  Headache, blurring of near vision (reading), ringing in ears.
  Loss of appetite, nausea, vomiting, stomach cramps, diarrhea.
  Serious Adverse Effects
  Allergic Reactions: Severe skin rash (erythema multiforme).
  Idiosyncratic Reactions: Hemolytic anemia in those with glucose-6-phosphate dehydrogenase deficiency in red blood cells.
  Emotional or psychotic mental changes; seizures.
  Loss of hearing.
  Excessive muscle weakness.
  Eye tissue damage, specifically cornea and retina, with significant impairment of vision.
  Heart rhythm abnormalities.
  Aplastic anemia (see Glossary): abnormally low red blood cell counts

(fatigue and weakness), abnormally low white blood cell counts (fever, sore throat, infections), abnormally low platelet counts (abnormal bruising or bleeding).

▷ **Possible Effects on Sexual Function:**   None reported.

Possible Delayed Adverse Effects: Irreversible retinal damage has developed 7 years after discontinuation of this drug. Retinal damage is more likely to occur following high-dose and/or long-term use.

▷ **Adverse Effects That May Mimic Natural Diseases or Disorders**
Central nervous system toxicity may suggest unrelated neuropsychiatric disorder. Seizures may suggest the onset of epilepsy.

Natural Diseases or Disorders That May Be Activated by This Drug
Porphyria, psoriasis.

Possible Effects on Laboratory Tests
Complete blood cell counts: decreased red cells, hemoglobin, white cells and platelets.
Liver function tests: increased liver enzymes (AST/GOT) and bilirubin.
Urine screening tests for drug abuse: *initial* test result may be falsely **positive**; *confirmatory* test result will be **negative**. (Test results depend upon amount of drug taken and testing method used.)
Electrocardiogram: conduction abnormalities, prolonged QRS interval, T wave changes, heart block.

CAUTION
1. This drug does not prevent relapses in certain types of malaria. Consult your physician regarding this.
2. This drug is not effective in treating acute amebic dysentery (intestinal infection) or asymptomatic carriers of this disease.
3. High-dose and/or long-term use of this drug may cause irreversible retinal damage and significant impairment of vision; such use may also cause hearing loss due to nerve damage. Report promptly any changes in vision or hearing so appropriate evaluation can be made.

Precautions for Use
By Infants and Children: This age group is very sensitive to the effects of this drug. Dosages should be determined and therapy should be monitored by a qualified pediatrician.
By Those over 60 Years of Age: Tolerance for this drug during high-dose and/or long-term use may be reduced. Observe for behavioral changes, low blood pressure, heart rhythm disturbances, muscle weakness and changes in vision or hearing.

▷ **Advisability of Use During Pregnancy**
Pregnancy Category: D (tentative). See Pregnancy Code inside back cover.
Animal studies: 47% of rat fetuses revealed undeveloped or partially developed eyes.

Human studies: Information from adequate studies of pregnant women is not available. A 1964 report includes drug-induced congenital deafness, retinal damage, gait instability and asymmetric body growth.
Avoid use during pregnancy except for the suppression or treatment of malaria or amebic infection of the liver.

Advisability of Use if Breast-Feeding
Presence of this drug in breast milk: Yes.
Avoid drug or refrain from nursing.

Habit-Forming Potential: None.

Effects of Overdosage: Drowsiness, headache, blurred vision, excitability, low blood pressure, seizures, coma.

Possible Effects of Long-Term Use: Irreversible eye damage (cornea and retina), hearing loss, myocarditis, muscle weakness, aplastic anemia.

Suggested Periodic Examinations While Taking This Drug
(atphysician's discretion)
Complete blood cell counts; liver and kidney function tests.
Serial blood pressure readings and electrocardiograms.
Neurological examinations for significant muscle weakness.
Complete eye examinations before starting high-dose and/or long-term treatment and every 3 to 6 months during drug use.
Hearing tests as indicated.

▷ **While Taking This Drug, Observe the Following**
Foods: No restrictions.
Beverages: No restrictions. May be taken with milk.
▷ *Alcohol:* Use sparingly to minimize stomach irritation.
Tobacco Smoking: No interactions expected.
▷ *Other Drugs*
Chloroquine may *increase* the effects of
• penicillamine (Cuprimine, Depen), and increase its toxic potential.
The following drug may *increase* the effects of chloroquine
• cimetidine (Tagamet).
The following drugs may *decrease* the effects of chloroquine
• magnesium salts and antacids.
▷ *Driving, Hazardous Activities:* This drug may cause light-headedness, blurred vision or impaired hearing. Restrict activities as necessary.
Aviation Note: The use of this drug **may be a disqualification** for piloting. Consult a designated Aviation Medical Examiner.
Exposure to Sun: Use caution until sensitivity has been determined. This drug may cause photosensitivity (see Glossary).
Discontinuation: This drug should be discontinued and prompt evaluation made if any of the following develop: any changes in vision or hearing, seizures, unusual muscle weakness, indications of infection (fever, sore throat, etc.), abnormal bruising or bleeding.

CHLOROTHIAZIDE
(klor oh THI a zide)

Introduced: 1957

Class: Antihypertensive, diuretic, thiazides

Prescription: USA: Yes

Controlled Drug: USA: No

Available as Generic: USA: Yes

Brand Names: Aldoclor [CD], Diachlor, Diupres [CD], Diurigen, Diuril

---

BENEFITS versus RISKS

Possible Benefits	*Possible Risks*
EFFECTIVE, WELL-TOLERATED DIURETIC	Loss of body potassium
	Increased blood sugar
POSSIBLY EFFECTIVE IN MILD HYPERTENSION	Increased blood uric acid
	Increased blood calcium
ENHANCES EFFECTIVENESS OF OTHER ANTIHYPERTENSIVES	Rare blood cell disorders
Beneficial in treatment of diabetes insipidus	

▷ **Principal Uses**

As a Single Drug Product: Thiazide diuretics are used primarily to (1) increase the volume of urine (diuresis) to correct the excessive fluid retention associated with congestive heart failure and certain types of liver and kidney disease; and (2) initiate treatment for high blood pressure (hypertension). They are often the first drugs tried in treating mild to moderate hypertension. Less frequent uses include the treatment of diabetes insipidus and the prevention of kidney stones that contain calcium.

As a Combination Drug Product [CD]: When this drug is used alone to treat hypertension, it is referred to as a "step 1" antihypertensive. Should it fail to reduce the blood pressure adequately, a "step 2" antihypertensive drug is added to be taken concurrently with the "step 1" drug. These drugs may be combined into one drug product. Thiazides are available in combination with beta blockers, hydralazine, methyldopa, reserpine and other diuretics to increase their effectiveness in treating hypertension.

How This Drug Works: By increasing the elimination of salt and water from the body (through increased urine production), this drug reduces the volume of fluid in the blood and body tissues and lowers the sodium content throughout the body. By relaxing the walls of smaller arteries and allowing them to expand, this drug increases the total capacity of the arterial system. The combined effect of these two actions (reduced blood volume in expanded space) results in lowering of the blood pressure.

Available Dosage Forms and Strengths
Injection — 500 mg per 20 ml
Oral suspension — 250 mg per 5-ml teaspoonful
Tablets — 250 mg, 500 mg

▷ **Usual Adult Dosage Range:** As antihypertensive: 500 to 1000 mg/day initially; 500 to 2000 mg/day for maintenance. As diuretic: 500 to 2000 mg/day initially; the smallest effective dose should be determined. The total daily dose should not exceed 2000 mg. **Note: Actual dosage and administration schedule must be determined by the physician for each patient individually.**

▷ **Dosing Instructions:** May be taken with or following meals to reduce stomach irritation. Best taken in the morning to avoid nighttime urination. The tablet may be crushed for administration.

Usual Duration of Use: Continual use on a regular schedule for 2 to 3 weeks is usually necessary to determine this drug's effectiveness in lowering high blood pressure. Long-term use (months to years) requires periodic evaluation of response and possible dosage adjustment. Use as a diuretic should be intermittent with "drug holidays" (no drug taken) to reduce the risk of sodium and potassium imbalance. Consult your physician on a regular basis.

▷ **This Drug Should Not Be Taken If**
- you have had an allergic reaction to any dosage form of it previously.

▷ **Inform Your Physician Before Taking This Drug If**
- you are allergic to any form of "sulfa" drug.
- you are pregnant or planning pregnancy.
- you have a history of kidney or liver disease.
- you have diabetes, gout or lupus erythematosus.
- you are taking any form of cortisone, digitalis, oral antidiabetic drug or insulin.
- you plan to have surgery under general anesthesia in the near future.

Possible Side-Effects (natural, expected and unavoidable drug actions)
Light-headedness on arising from sitting or lying position (see Orthostatic Hypotension in Glossary).
Increase in blood sugar level, affecting control of diabetes.
Increase in blood uric acid level, affecting control of gout.
Decrease in blood potassium level, causing muscle weakness and cramping.

▷ **Possible Adverse Effects** (unusual, unexpected and infrequent reactions)
If any of the following develop, consult your physician promptly for guidance.

Mild Adverse Effects
   Allergic Reactions: Skin rashes, hives, drug fever.
   Headache, dizziness, blurred or yellow vision.
   Reduced appetite, indigestion, nausea, vomiting, diarrhea.
Serious Adverse Effects
   Allergic Reactions: Hepatitis with jaundice (see Glossary), anaphylactic
      reaction (see Glossary), severe skin reactions.
   Inflammation of the pancreas—severe abdominal pain.
   Bone marrow depression (see Glossary)—fatigue, weakness, fever, sore
      throat, abnormal bleeding or bruising.

▷ **Possible Effects on Sexual Function:**   Impotence (500 to 2000 mg/day).

▷ **Adverse Effects That May Mimic Natural Diseases or Disorders**
   Liver reaction may suggest viral hepatitis.

Natural Diseases or Disorders That May Be Activated by This Drug
   Diabetes, gout, systemic lupus erythematosus.

Possible Effects on Laboratory Tests
   Complete blood cell counts: decreased red cells, hemoglobin, white cells
      and platelets.
   Blood amylase level: increased soon after starting drug.
   Blood calcium level: increased with long-term use.
   Blood chloride level: increased with long-term use.
   Blood glucose level: increased; drug induces diabetes.
   Glucose tolerance test (GTT): decreased; drug induces diabetes.
   Blood potassium level: decreased.
   Blood sodium level: decreased.
   Blood uric acid level: increased; drug may induce gout.
   Blood LE cells: positive; drug may cause a lupus erythematosuslike reac-
      tion.
   Liver function tests: increased liver enzymes (ALT/GPT, AST/GOT and
      alkaline phosphatase), increased bilirubin.

CAUTION
   1. Do not exceed recommended doses. Increased dosage can cause ex-
      cessive loss of sodium and potassium, with resultant loss of appetite,
      nausea, fatigue, weakness, confusion and tingling in the extremities.
   2. If you are also taking a digitalis preparation (digitoxin, digoxin),
      ensure an adequate intake of high-potassium foods to prevent potas-
      sium deficiency—a potential cause of digitalis toxicity. (See Table of
      High Potassium Foods in Section Six.)

Precautions for Use
   By Infants and Children: Avoid overdosage that could cause serious dehy-
      dration. Significant potassium loss can occur within the first 2 weeks
      of drug use.
   By Those over 60 Years of Age: Small doses are advisable until your individ-
      ual response has been determined. You may be more susceptible to the

development of impaired thinking, orthostatic hypotension, potassium loss and blood sugar increase. Overdosage and extended use of this drug can cause excessive loss of body water, thickening (increased viscosity) of the blood and an increased tendency for the blood to clot—predisposing to stroke, heart attack or thrombophlebitis (vein inflammation with blood clot).

▷ **Advisability of Use During Pregnancy**
Pregnancy Category: D (tentative). See Pregnancy Code inside back cover.
Animal studies: No birth defects found in rat studies.
Human studies: Reports are conflicting and inconclusive. This drug does not seem to carry the risk of birth defects that has been found with other related diuretics. However, other types of fetal injury are possible with this drug. It should not be used during pregnancy unless a very serious complication occurs for which this drug is significantly beneficial. Ask physician for guidance.

Advisability of Use if Breast-Feeding
Presence of this drug in breast milk: Yes, in small amounts.
Avoid drug or refrain from nursing.

Habit-Forming Potential: None.

Effects of Overdosage: Dry mouth, thirst, lethargy, weakness, muscle cramping, nausea, vomiting, drowsiness progressing to stupor or coma.

Possible Effects of Long-Term Use: Impaired balance of water, salt and potassium in blood and body tissues. Development of diabetes in predisposed individuals. Pathological changes in parathyroid glands with increased blood calcium levels and decreased blood phosphate levels.

Suggested Periodic Examinations While Taking This Drug (at physician's discretion)
Complete blood cell counts, measurements of blood levels of sodium, potassium, chloride, sugar and uric acid.
Kidney and liver function tests.

▷ **While Taking This Drug, Observe the Following**
Foods: Consult your physician regarding the advisability of eating foods rich in potassium. If so advised, see the Table of High Potassium Foods in Section Six. Follow physician's advice regarding the use of salt.
Beverages: No restrictions. This drug may be taken with milk.
▷ *Alcohol:* Use with caution until the combined effects have been determined. Alcohol may exaggerate the blood-pressure-lowering effects of this drug and cause orthostatic hypotension.
Tobacco Smoking: No interactions expected. Follow physician's advice.
▷ *Other Drugs*
Chlorothiazide may *increase* the effects of

- other antihypertensive drugs; dosage adjustments may be necessary to prevent excessive lowering of blood pressure.
- lithium, and cause lithium toxicity.

Chlorothiazide may *decrease* the effects of
- oral antidiabetic drugs (sulfonylureas); dosage adjustments may be necessary for proper control of blood sugar.

Chlorothiazide *taken concurrently* with
- digitalis preparations (digitoxin, digoxin) requires very careful monitoring and dosage adjustments to prevent fluctuations of blood potassium levels and serious disturbances of heart rhythm.

The following drugs may *decrease* the effects of chlorothiazide
- cholestyramine (Cuemid, Questran) may interfere with its absorption.
- colestipol (Colestid) may interfere with its absorption.

Take cholestyramine and colestipol 1 hour before any oral diuretic.

▷ *Driving, Hazardous Activities:* Use caution until the possible occurrence of orthostatic hypotension, dizziness or impaired vision has been determined.

Aviation Note: The use of this drug *may be a disqualification* for piloting. Consult a designated Aviation Medical Examiner.

Exposure to Sun: Use caution until sensitivity has been determined. This drug can cause photosensitivity (see Glossary).

Exposure to Heat: Avoid excessive perspiring, which could cause additional loss of salt and water from the body.

Heavy Exercise or Exertion: Avoid exertion that produces light-headedness, excessive fatigue or muscle cramping. Isometric exercises—the "overload" technique for strengthening individual muscles—can raise blood pressure significantly. Ask physician for guidance regarding participation in this form of exercise.

Occurrence of Unrelated Illness: Illnesses that cause vomiting or diarrhea can produce a serious imbalance of important body chemistry. Consult your physician for guidance.

Discontinuation: This drug should not be stopped abruptly following long-term use; serious thiazide-withdrawal fluid retention (edema) can develop after sudden withdrawal. The dose should be reduced gradually. It may be advisable to discontinue this drug 5 to 7 days before major surgery. Ask your physician, surgeon and/or anesthesiologist for guidance regarding dosage adjustment or drug withdrawal.

CHLORPROMAZINE
(klor PROH ma zeen)

Introduced: 1952

Class: Strong tranquilizer, pheno-thiazines

Prescription: USA: Yes
Canada: Yes

Controlled Drug: USA: No
Canada: No

Available as Generic: Yes

Brand Names: ✦Chlorpromanyl, ✦Largactil, ✦Novochlorpromazine, Promapar, Sonazine, Thorazine

---

BENEFITS versus RISKS

Possible Benefits	*Possible Risks*
EFFECTIVE CONTROL OF ACUTE MENTAL DISORDERS in the majority of patients	SERIOUS TOXIC EFFECTS ON BRAIN with long-term use
Beneficial effects on thinking, mood and behavior	Liver damage with jaundice (less than 0.5%)
Moderately effective control of nausea and vomiting	Rare blood cell disorders: hemolytic anemia, abnormally low white blood cell count

---

▷ **Principal Uses**

As a Single Drug Product: This antipsychotic drug is used primarily to treat acute and chronic psychotic disorders such as agitated depression, schizophrenia and similar states of mental dysfunction. It may be used as a tranquilizer in the management of agitated and disruptive behavior in the absence of true psychosis. Less frequently it may be used to relieve severe nausea or vomiting.

How This Drug Works: Not completely established. Present theory is that by inhibiting the action of dopamine, this drug acts to correct an imbalance of nerve impulse transmissions that is thought to be responsible for certain mental disorders.

Available Dosage Forms and Strengths
Capsules, prolonged-action — 30 mg, 75 mg, 150 mg, 200 mg, 300 mg
Concentrate — 30 mg per ml, 100 mg per ml
Injection — 25 mg per ml
Suppositories — 25 mg, 100 mg
Syrup — 10 mg per 5-ml teaspoonful
Tablets — 10 mg, 25 mg, 50 mg, 100 mg, 200 mg

▷ **Usual Adult Dosage Range:**   Initially 10 to 25 mg 3 or 4 times daily. Dose may be increased by 20 to 50 mg at 3- to 4-day intervals as needed and tolerated. Usual dosage range is 300 to 800 mg daily. Extreme range is 25 to 2000 mg daily. Total daily dosage should not exceed 2000 mg.

Note: Actual dosage and administration schedule must be determined by the physician for each patient individually.

▷ **Dosing Instructions:**   May be taken with or following meals to reduce stomach irritation. Tablets may be crushed for administration. Prolonged-action capsules may be opened, but do not crush or chew contents.

Usual Duration of Use: Continual use on a regular schedule for several weeks is usually necessary to determine this drug's effectiveness in controlling psychotic disorders. If not significantly beneficial within 6 weeks, it should be discontinued. Long-term use (months to years) requires periodic evaluation of response, appropriate dosage adjustment and consideration of continued need. Consult your physician on a regular basis.

▷ **This Drug Should Not Be Taken If**
  • you are allergic to any of the drugs bearing the brand names listed above.
  • you have active liver disease.
  • you have cancer of the breast.
  • you have a current blood cell or bone marrow disorder.

▷ **Inform Your Physician Before Taking This Drug If**
  • you are allergic or abnormally sensitive to any phenothiazine drug (see Drug Class, Section Four).
  • you have impaired liver or kidney function.
  • you have any type of seizure disorder.
  • you have diabetes, glaucoma or heart disease.
  • you have a history of lupus erythematosus.
  • you are taking any drug with sedative effects.
  • you plan to have surgery under general or spinal anesthesia in the near future.

Possible Side-Effects (natural, expected and unavoidable drug actions)
  Drowsiness (usually during the first 2 weeks), orthostatic hypotension (see Glossary), blurred vision, dry mouth, nasal congestion, constipation, impaired urination.
  Pink or purple coloration of urine, of no significance.

▷ **Possible Adverse Effects** (unusual, unexpected and infrequent reactions)
  If any of the following develop, consult your physician promptly for guidance.
  Mild Adverse Effects
  Allergic Reactions: Skin rash, hives, low-grade fever.
  Lowering of body temperature, especially in the elderly.
  Increased appetite and weight gain.
  Weakness, agitation, insomnia, impaired day and night vision.
  Chronic constipation, fecal impaction.
  Serious Adverse Effects
  Allergic Reactions: Hepatitis with jaundice (see Glossary), usually be-

tween second and fourth week; high fever; asthma; anaphylactic reaction (see Glossary).

Idiosyncratic Reactions: Neuroleptic malignant syndrome (see Glossary).

Depression, disorientation, seizures.

Disturbances of heart rhythm, rapid heart rate.

Hemolytic anemia (see Glossary), impaired production of white blood cells—fever, sore throat, infections.

Parkinson-like disorders (see Glossary); muscle spasms of face, jaw, neck, back, extremities.

Prolonged drop in blood pressure with weakness, perspiration and fainting.

▷ **Possible Effects on Sexual Function**

Decreased libido and impotence (1200 mg/day); inhibited ejaculation (400 mg/day); priapism (see Glossary) (250 mg/day); male infertility (30 to 800 mg/day); enlargement of male breasts, enlargement of female breasts with milk production, cessation of menstruation (30 to 800 mg/day).

This drug may also cause a false positive pregnancy test.

▷ **Adverse Effects That May Mimic Natural Diseases or Disorders**

Nervous system reactions may suggest Parkinson's disease.

Liver reactions may suggest viral hepatitis.

Reactions resembling systemic lupus erythematosus can occur.

Natural Diseases or Disorders That May Be Activated by This Drug

Latent epilepsy, glaucoma, diabetes mellitus (25%), prostatism (see Glossary).

Possible Effects on Laboratory Tests

Complete blood cell counts: decreased red cells, hemoglobin, white cells and platelets; increased eosinophils (often a precursor of jaundice).

Antinuclear antibodies (ANA): positive in 63% of long-term users.

Blood cholesterol level: increased (with liver damage).

Blood glucose level: increased with long-term use.

Glucose tolerance test (GTT): decreased; abnormal results in 40% of chronic users.

Prothrombin time: increased.

Blood uric acid level: decreased.

Liver function tests: increased liver enzymes (ALT/GPT, AST/GOT and alkaline phosphatase; increased bilirubin.

Urine pregnancy tests: false positive results with frog, rabbit and immunological tests.

CAUTION

1. Many over-the-counter medications (see OTC Drugs in Glossary) for allergies, colds and coughs contain drugs that can interact unfavorably with this drug. Ask your physician or pharmacist for guidance before using any such medications.

2. Antacids that contain aluminum and/or magnesium can prevent the absorption of this drug and reduce its effectiveness.
3. Obtain prompt evaluation of any change or disturbance of vision.
4. This drug can cause false positive pregnancy tests.

Precautions for Use

By Infants and Children: Do not use this drug in infants under 6 months of age, or in children of any age with symptoms suggestive of Reye syndrome (see Glossary). Monitor carefully for blood cell changes.

By Those over 60 Years of Age: Small doses are advisable until individual response has been determined. You may be more susceptible to the development of drowsiness, lethargy, constipation, lowering of body temperature (hypothermia) and orthostatic hypotension (see Glossary). This drug can enhance existing prostatism (see Glossary). You may also be more susceptible to the development of Parkinson-like reactions and/or tardive dyskinesia (see discussion of these terms in Glossary). These reactions must be recognized early since they may become unresponsive to treatment and irreversible.

▷ Advisability of Use During Pregnancy

Pregnancy Category: C (tentative). See Pregnancy Code inside back cover.

Animal studies: No birth defects reported in rodent studies. However, rodent studies suggest possible permanent neurological damage to the fetus.

Human studies: No increase in birth defects reported in 284 exposures. Information from adequate studies of pregnant women is not available.

Limit use to small and infrequent doses only when clearly needed. Avoid drug during the last month because of possible adverse effects on the newborn infant.

Advisability of Use if Breast-Feeding

Presence of this drug in breast milk: Yes, in small amounts.
Avoid drug or refrain from nursing.

Habit-Forming Potential: None.

Effects of Overdosage: Marked drowsiness, weakness, tremor, agitation, unsteadiness, deep sleep, coma, convulsions.

Possible Effects of Long-Term Use: Tardive dyskinesia in 10% to 20% (see Glossary); eye changes—cataracts and pigmentation of retina; gray to violet pigmentation of skin in exposed areas, more common in women; severe ulcerative colitis.

Suggested Periodic Examinations While Taking This Drug (at physician's discretion)

Complete blood cell counts, especially between the fourth and tenth weeks of treatment.
Liver function tests, electrocardiograms.
Complete eye examinations—eye structures and vision.

Careful inspection of the tongue for early evidence of fine, involuntary, wavelike movements that could indicate the beginning of tardive dyskinesia.

▷ **While Taking This Drug, Observe the Following**

Foods: No restrictions.

Nutritional Support: A riboflavin (vitamin B-2) supplement should be taken with long-term use.

Beverages: No restrictions. May be taken with milk.

▷ *Alcohol:* Avoid completely. Alcohol can increase the sedative action of phenothiazines and accentuate their depressant effects on brain function and blood pressure. Phenothiazines can increase the intoxicating effects of alcohol.

Tobacco Smoking: Possible reduction of drowsiness from drug.

Marijuana Smoking: Moderate increase in drowsiness; accentuation of orthostatic hypotension; increased risk of precipitating latent psychoses, confusing the interpretation of mental status and drug responses.

▷ *Other Drugs*

Chlorpromazine may *increase* the effects of

• all sedative drugs, especially meperidine (Demerol), and cause excessive sedation.

• all atropinelike drugs, and cause nervous system toxicity.

Chlorpromazine may *decrease* the effects of

• guanethidine (Ismelin, Esimil), and reduce its effectiveness in lowering blood pressure.

Chlorpromazine *taken concurrently* with

• propranolol (Inderal) may cause increased effects of both drugs; monitor drug effects closely and adjust dosages as necessary.

The following drugs may *decrease* the effects of chlorpromazine

• antacids containing aluminum and/or magnesium.

• benztropine (Cogentin).

• trihexyphenidyl (Artane).

▷ *Driving, Hazardous Activities:* This drug can impair mental alertness, judgment and physical coordination. Avoid hazardous activities.

Aviation Note: The use of this drug *is a disqualification* for piloting. Consult a designated Aviation Medical Examiner.

Exposure to Sun: Use caution until sensitivity has been determined. Some phenothiazines can cause photosensitivity (see Glossary).

Exposure to Heat: Use caution and avoid excessive heat as much as possible. This drug may impair the regulation of body temperature and increase the risk of heat stroke.

Exposure to Cold: Use caution and dress warmly. This drug can increase the risk of hypothermia in the elderly.

Discontinuation: After a period of long-term use, do not discontinue this drug suddenly. Gradual withdrawal over 2 to 3 weeks under physician supervision is recommended. Do not discontinue this drug without your physician's knowledge and approval. The relapse rate of schizophrenia after discontinuation is 50% to 60%.

CHLORPROPAMIDE
(klor PROH pa mide)

Introduced: 1958

Class: Antidiabetic, sulfonylureas

Prescription: USA: Yes
Canada: Yes

Controlled Drug: USA: No
Canada: No

Available as Generic: Yes

Brand Names: ✦Apo-Chlorpropamide, ✦Chloronase, Diabinese, ✦Novo-propamide

---

BENEFITS versus RISKS

Possible Benefits	*Possible Risks*
Assistance in regulating blood sugar in noninsulin-dependent diabetes (adjunctive to appropriate diet and weight control)	HYPOGLYCEMIA, severe and prolonged Allergic skin reactions (some severe) Water retention Liver damage Rare blood cell and bone marrow disorders

---

▷ **Principal Uses**

As a Single Drug Product: To assist in the control of mild to moderately severe type II diabetes mellitus (adult, maturity-onset) that does not require insulin, but that cannot be adequately controlled by diet alone.

How This Drug Works: It is thought that this drug (1) stimulates the secretion of insulin (by a pancreas that is capable of responding to stimulation), and (2) enhances the utilization of insulin by appropriate tissues.

Available Dosage Forms and Strengths
Tablets — 100 mg, 250 mg

▷ **Usual Adult Dosage Range:** Initially 250 mg daily with breakfast. After 5 to 7 days, dose may be increased to 500 mg daily if needed and tolerated. Total daily dosage should not exceed 750 mg. A "loading" or priming dose is not necessary and should not be given. **Note: Actual dosage and administration schedule must be determined by the physician for each patient individually.**

▷ **Dosing Instructions:** May be taken with food to reduce stomach irritation. Tablet may be crushed for administration.

Usual Duration of Use: Continual use on a regular schedule for 1 to 2 weeks is usually necessary to determine this drug's effectiveness in controlling diabetes. Failure to respond to maximal doses within 1 month constitutes a primary failure. Up to 15% of those who respond initially may develop secondary failure of the drug within the first year of use. The duration of effective use can only be determined by periodic measurement of the blood sugar. Consult your physician on a regular basis.

▷ **This Drug Should Not Be Taken If**
- you have had an allergic reaction to it previously.
- you have severe impairment of liver or kidney function.
- you are pregnant.

▷ **Inform Your Physician Before Taking This Drug If**
- you are allergic to other sulfonylurea drugs or to "sulfa" drugs.
- your diabetes has been unstable or "brittle" in the past.
- you do not know how to recognize or treat hypoglycemia (see Glossary).
- you have a history of congestive heart failure, peptic ulcer disease, cirrhosis of the liver, hypothyroidism or porphyria.

Possible Side-Effects (natural, expected and unavoidable drug actions)
If drug dosage is excessive or food intake is delayed or inadequate, abnormally low blood sugar (hypoglycemia) will occur as a predictable drug effect.

▷ **Possible Adverse Effects** (unusual, unexpected and infrequent reactions)
If any of the following develop, consult your physician promptly for guidance.
Mild Adverse Effects
Allergic Reactions: Skin rash, hives, itching, drug fever.
Headache, ringing in ears, weakness, numbness and tingling.
Indigestion, nausea, vomiting, diarrhea (may be severe).
Serious Adverse Effects
Allergic Reactions: Hepatitis with jaundice (see Glossary), severe skin reactions.
Idiosyncratic Reaction: Hemolytic anemia (see Glossary).
Disulfiramlike reaction with concurrent use of alcohol (see Glossary).
Water retention (edema), weight gain.
Bone marrow depression (see Glossary)—fatigue, weakness, fever, sore throat, abnormal bleeding or bruising.

▷ **Possible Effects on Sexual Function:** None reported.

▷ **Adverse Effects That May Mimic Natural Diseases or Disorders**
Liver reactions may suggest viral hepatitis.

Natural Diseases or Disorders That May Be Activated by This Drug
Acute intermittent porphyria, congestive heart failure (in predisposed individuals), peptic ulcer disease.

Possible Effects on Laboratory Tests
Complete blood cell counts: decreased red cells, hemoglobin, white cells and platelets; increased eosinophils (allergic reaction).
Prothrombin time: increased (with liver damage).

Blood thyroxine (T^4) level: decreased.

Liver function tests: increased liver enzymes (ALT/GPT, AST/GOT and alkaline phosphatase), increased bilirubin.

CAUTION

1. This drug must be regarded as only one part of the total program for the management of your diabetes. It is not a substitute for a properly prescribed diet and regular exercise.
2. Over a period of time (usually several months), this drug may lose its effectiveness in controlling blood sugar levels. Periodic follow-up examinations are necessary to monitor all aspects of response to drug treatment.
3. This drug has a long duration of action (up to 60 hours) and therefore can be cumulative in its effects. It can produce severe and prolonged hypoglycemia in some individuals, especially the elderly.

Precautions for Use

By Infants and Children: This drug is not effective in type I (juvenile, growth-onset) insulin-dependent diabetes.

By Those over 60 Years of Age: This drug is best avoided in this age group. Due to its long duration of action it can accumulate and cause marked and prolonged hypoglycemia. Repeated episodes of hypoglycemia in the elderly can cause brain damage.

▷ **Advisability of Use During Pregnancy**

Pregnancy Category: X (tentative). See Pregnancy Code inside back cover.
Animal studies: This class of drugs has been shown to cause birth defects in animals.
Human studies: Information from adequate studies of pregnant women is not available.
The manufacturer states that this drug is contraindicated during entire pregnancy.

Advisability of Use if Breast-Feeding

Presence of this drug in breast milk: Yes.
Avoid drug or refrain from nursing.

Habit-Forming Potential: None.

Effects of Overdosage: Symptoms of mild to severe hypoglycemia: headache, light-headedness, faintness, nervousness, confusion, tremor, sweating, heart palpitation, weakness, hunger, nausea, vomiting, stupor progressing to coma.

Possible Effects of Long-Term Use: Reduced function of the thyroid gland (hypothyroidism). Reports of increased frequency and severity of heart and blood vessel diseases associated with long-term use of this class of drugs are highly controversial and inconclusive. A direct cause-and-effect relationship (see Glossary) is tenuous. Ask your physician for guidance.

Suggested Periodic Examinations While Taking This Drug (at physician's discretion)

Complete blood cell counts, liver function tests, thyroid function tests, periodic evaluation of heart and circulatory system.

▷ **While Taking This Drug, Observe the Following**

Foods: Follow the diabetic diet prescribed by your physician.

Beverages: As directed in the diabetic diet. May be taken with milk.

▷ *Alcohol:* Use with extreme caution until the combined effect has been determined. Alcohol can exaggerate this drug's hypoglycemic effect. This drug can cause a marked intolerance of alcohol resulting in a disulfiramlike reaction (see Glossary): facial flushing, sweating, palpitation.

Tobacco Smoking: No interactions expected.

▷ *Other Drugs*

The following drugs may *increase* the effects of chlorpropamide
- ammonium chloride.
- aspirin, and other salicylates.
- chloramphenicol (Chloromycetin).
- clofibrate (Atromid S).
- dicumarol.
- fenfluramine (Pondimin).
- monoamine oxidase (MAO) type A inhibitor drugs (see Drug Class, Section Four).
- phenylbutazone (Butazolidin).
- some "sulfa" drugs: sulfamethoxazole (Gantanol), sulfisoxazole (Gantrisin).

The following drugs may *decrease* the effects of chlorpropamide
- diazoxide (Proglycem).
- propranolol (Inderal).
- rifampin (Rifidin, Rimactane).
- sodium bicarbonate.
- thiazide diuretics (see Drug Class, Section Four).

▷ *Driving, Hazardous Activities:* Regulate your dosage schedule, eating schedule and physical activities very carefully to prevent hypoglycemia. Be able to recognize the early symptoms of hypoglycemia so you can avoid hazardous activities and take corrective measures.

Aviation Note: Diabetes *is a disqualification* for piloting. Consult a designated Aviation Medical Examiner.

Exposure to Sun: Use caution until sensitivity has been determined. Some drugs of this class can cause photosensitivity (see Glossary).

Occurrence of Unrelated Illness: Acute infections, illnesses causing vomiting or diarrhea, serious injuries and surgical procedures can interfere with diabetic control and may require the use of insulin. If any of these conditions occur, consult your physician promptly.

Discontinuation: It is estimated that no more than 12% of patients remain well controlled by this drug for more than 6 to 7 years. Because of the high incidence of secondary failures, it is advisable to evaluate the continued benefit of this drug every 6 months.

CHLORTHALIDONE
(klor THAL i dohn)

Introduced: 1960

Class: Antihypertensive, diuretic

Prescription: USA: Yes
Canada: Yes

Controlled Drug: USA: No
Canada: No

Available as Generic: USA: Yes
Canada: Yes

Brand Names: ✦Apo-Chlorthalidone, Combipres [CD], Demi-Regroton [CD], Hygroton, ✦Hygroton-Reserpine [CD], Hylidone, ✦Novothalidone, Regroton [CD], Tenoretic [CD], Thalitone, ✦Uridon

---

BENEFITS versus RISKS

Possible Benefits	*Possible Risks*
EFFECTIVE, WELL-TOLERATED DIURETIC	Loss of body potassium
POSSIBLY EFFECTIVE IN MILD HYPERTENSION	Increased blood sugar
ENHANCES EFFECTIVENESS OF OTHER ANTIHYPERTENSIVES	Increased blood uric acid
Beneficial in treatment of diabetes insipidus	Increased blood calcium
	Rare blood cell disorders

▷ **Principal Uses**

As a Single Drug Product: Thiazidelike diuretics are used primarily to (1) increase the volume of urine (diuresis) to correct the excessive fluid retention associated with congestive heart failure and certain types of liver and kidney disease; and (2) initiate treatment for high blood pressure (hypertension). They are often the first drugs tried in treating mild to moderate hypertension. Less frequent uses include the treatment of diabetes insipidus and the prevention of kidney stones that contain calcium.

As a Combination Drug Product [CD]: When this drug is used alone to treat hypertension, it is referred to as a "step 1" antihypertensive. Should it fail to reduce the blood pressure adequately, a "step 2" antihypertensive drug is added to be taken concurrently with the "step 1" drug. These drugs may be combined into one drug product. This drug is available in combination with atenolol, clonidine and reserpine to increase their effectiveness in treating hypertension.

How This Drug Works: By increasing the elimination of salt and water from the body (through increased urine production), this drug reduces the volume of fluid in the blood and body tissues and lowers the sodium content throughout the body. By relaxing the walls of smaller arteries and allowing them to expand, this drug increases the total capacity of the arterial system. The combined effect of these two actions (reduced blood volume in expanded space) results in lowering of blood pressure.

Available Dosage Forms and Strengths
Tablets — 25 mg, 50 mg, 100 mg

▷ **Usual Adult Dosage Range:**   As antihypertensive: 25 to 50 mg/day initially; 50 to 100 mg/day for maintenance. As diuretic: 50 to 100 mg/day initially; the smallest effective dose should be determined. The total daily dose should not exceed 200 mg. **Note: Actual dosage and administration schedule must be determined by the physician for each patient individually.**

▷ **Dosing Instructions:**   May be taken with or following meals to reduce stomach irritation. Best taken in the morning to avoid nighttime urination. The tablet may be crushed for administration.

Usual Duration of Use: Continual use on a regular schedule for 2 to 3 weeks is usually necessary to determine this drug's effectiveness in lowering high blood pressure. Long-term use (months to years) requires periodic evaluation of response and possible dosage adjustment. Use as a diuretic should be intermittent with "drug holidays" (no drug taken) to reduce the risk of sodium and potassium imbalance. Consult your physician on a regular basis.

▷ **This Drug Should Not Be Taken If**
- you have had an allergic reaction to it previously.

▷ **Inform Your Physician Before Taking This Drug If**
- you are allergic to any form of "sulfa" drug.
- you are pregnant or planning pregnancy.
- you have a history of kidney or liver disease.
- you have diabetes, gout or lupus erythematosus.
- you are taking any form of cortisone, digitalis, oral antidiabetic drug or insulin.
- you plan to have surgery under general anesthesia in the near future.

Possible Side-Effects (natural, expected and unavoidable drug actions)
Light-headedness on arising from sitting or lying position (see Orthostatic Hypotension in Glossary).
Increase in blood sugar level, affecting control of diabetes.
Increase in blood uric acid level, affecting control of gout.
Decrease in blood potassium level, causing muscle weakness and cramping.

▷ **Possible Adverse Effects** (unusual, unexpected and infrequent reactions)
If any of the following develop, consult your physician promptly for guidance.
Mild Adverse Effects
Allergic Reactions: Skin rashes, hives, drug fever.

Headache, dizziness, blurred or yellow vision.

Reduced appetite, indigestion, nausea, vomiting, diarrhea.

Serious Adverse Effects

Allergic Reactions: Hepatitis with jaundice (see Glossary), anaphylactic reaction (see Glossary), severe skin reactions.

Inflammation of the pancreas—severe abdominal pain.

Bone marrow depression (see Glossary)—fatigue, weakness, fever, sore throat, abnormal bleeding or bruising.

▷ **Possible Effects on Sexual Function:**   Decreased libido and impotence, beginning from 2 weeks to several months after starting drug (100 mg/day).

▷ **Adverse Effects That May Mimic Natural Diseases or Disorders**

Liver reaction may suggest viral hepatitis.

Natural Diseases or Disorders That May Be Activated by This Drug

Diabetes, gout, systemic lupus erythematosus (questionable).

Possible Effects on Laboratory Tests

Complete blood cell counts: decreased red cells, hemoglobin, white cells and platelets.

Prothrombin time: increased (with concurrent use of warfarin).

Blood amylase level: increased (possible pancreatitis).

Blood calcium level: increased.

Blood cholesterol and triglyceride levels: effects vary from no drug effect to drug-induced increases.

Blood glucose level: increased in prediabetic and diabetic individuals.

Glucose tolerance test (GTT): decreased (drug is diabetogenic in predisposed individuals).

Blood potassium level: decreased.

Blood uric acid level: increased (may induce gout).

Kidney function tests: increased creatinine and blood urea nitrogen levels (kidney damage).

CAUTION

1. Do not exceed recommended doses. Increased dosage can cause excessive loss of sodium and potassium, with resultant loss of appetite, nausea, fatigue, weakness, confusion and tingling in the extremities.

2. If you are also taking a digitalis preparation (digitoxin, digoxin), ensure an adequate intake of high-potassium foods to prevent potassium deficiency, a potential cause of digitalis toxicity. (See Table of High Potassium Foods in Section Six.)

Precautions for Use

By Infants and Children: Avoid overdosage that could cause serious dehydration. Significant potassium loss can occur within the first 2 weeks of drug use.

By Those over 60 Years of Age: Small doses are advisable until your individual response has been determined. You may be more susceptible to the development of fatigue (40%), low blood potassium (10%), elevated blood uric acid (30%), impaired thinking, orthostatic hypotension and blood sugar increase. Overdosage and extended use of this drug can cause excessive loss of body water, thickening (increased viscosity) of the blood, and an increased tendency for the blood to clot—predisposing to stroke, heart attack, or thrombophlebitis (vein inflammation with blood clot). Report promptly any type of skin reaction.

▷ **Advisability of Use During Pregnancy**
Pregnancy Category: D (tentative). See Pregnancy Code inside back cover.
Animal studies: No birth defects reported.
Human studies: Information from adequate studies of pregnant women is not available.
It should not be used during pregnancy unless a very serious complication occurs for which this drug is significantly beneficial. This drug can cause serious adverse effects in the newborn infant. Ask physician for guidance.

Advisability of Use if Breast-Feeding
Presence of this drug in breast milk: Yes.
Avoid drug or refrain from nursing.

Habit-Forming Potential: None.

Effects of Overdosage: Dry mouth, thirst, lethargy, weakness, muscle cramping, nausea, vomiting, drowsiness progressing to stupor or coma.

Possible Effects of Long-Term Use: Impaired balance of water, salt and potassium in blood and body tissues. Development of diabetes in predisposed individuals. Pathological changes in parathyroid glands with increased blood calcium levels and decreased blood phosphate levels.

Suggested Periodic Examinations While Taking This Drug (at physician's discretion)
Complete blood cell counts; measurements of blood levels of sodium, potassium, chloride, sugar and uric acid.
Kidney and liver function tests.

▷ **While Taking This Drug, Observe the Following**
Foods: Consult your physician regarding the advisability of eating foods rich in potassium. If so advised, see the Table of High Potassium Foods in Section Six. Follow physician's advice regarding the use of salt.
Beverages: No restrictions. This drug may be taken with milk.
▷ *Alcohol:* Use with caution until the combined effects have been determined. Alcohol may exaggerate the blood-pressure-lowering effects of this drug and cause orthostatic hypotension (see Glossary).
Tobacco Smoking: No interactions expected. Follow physician's advice.
▷ *Other Drugs*
Chlorthalidone may **increase** the effects of
• other antihypertensive drugs; dosage adjustments may be necessary to prevent excessive lowering of blood pressure.

- lithium, and cause lithium toxicity.

Chlorthalidone may *decrease* the effects of

- oral antidiabetic drugs (sulfonylureas); dosage adjustments may be necessary for proper control of blood sugar.

Chlorthalidone *taken concurrently* with

- digitalis preparations (digitoxin, digoxin) requires very careful monitoring and dosage adjustments to prevent fluctuations of blood potassium levels and serious disturbances of heart rhythm.

The following drugs may *decrease* the effects of chlorthalidone

- cholestyramine (Cuemid, Questran) may interfere with its absorption.
- colestipol (Colestid) may interfere with its absorption.

Take cholestyramine and colestipol 1 hour before any oral diuretic.

▷ *Driving, Hazardous Activities:* Use caution until the possible occurrence of orthostatic hypotension, dizziness or impaired vision has been determined.

Aviation Note: The use of this drug *may be a disqualification* for piloting. Consult a designated Aviation Medical Examiner.

Exposure to Sun: Use caution until sensitivity has been determined. This drug can cause photosensitivity (see Glossary).

Exposure to Heat: Avoid excessive perspiring which could cause additional loss of salt and water from the body.

Heavy Exercise or Exertion: Avoid exertion that produces light-headedness, excessive fatigue or muscle cramping. Isometric exercises—the "overload" technique for strengthening individual muscles—can raise the blood pressure significantly. Ask physician for guidance regarding participation in this form of exercise.

Occurrence of Unrelated Illness: Illnesses that cause vomiting or diarrhea can produce a serious imbalance of important body chemistry. Consult your physician for guidance.

Discontinuation: It may be advisable to discontinue this drug 5 to 7 days before major surgery. Ask your physician, surgeon and/or anesthesiologist for guidance regarding dosage adjustment or drug withdrawal. Following long-term use, this drug should be withdrawn gradually to prevent the occurrence of rebound edema.

CHLORZOXAZONE
(klor ZOX a zohn)

Introduced: 1958   **Class:** Muscle relaxant

Prescription: USA: Yes   **Controlled Drug:** USA: No
    Canada: No   Canada: No

Available as Generic: USA: Yes
    Canada: No

Brand Names: Paraflex, Parafon Forte [CD]

BENEFITS versus RISKS

Possible Benefits
Mild to moderate relief of
discomfort due to spasm of
voluntary muscles

Possible Risks
Red and white blood cell
disorders
Gastrointestinal bleeding
Liver damage, jaundice
(questionable)
(All rare)

▷ **Principal Uses**

As a Single Drug Product: Used primarily to relieve the pain and stiffness associated with spasm of voluntary muscles, such as that resulting from accidental injury of musculoskeletal structures. It is often necessary to supplement the use of this drug with other treatment measures, such as rest, support and physiotherapy.

As a Combination Drug Product [CD]: It is combined with acetaminophen to enhance its effectiveness in relieving discomfort. Acetaminophen is an effective analgesic and may be necessary to control the pain that is not relieved by chlorzoxazone alone.

How This Drug Works: Not completely established. It is thought that this drug may relieve muscle spasm and pain by blocking the transmission of nerve impulses over reflex pathways and/or by producing a sedative effect that decreases the perception of pain.

Available Dosage Forms and Strengths
Caplets — 500 mg
Tablets — 250 mg

▷ **Usual Adult Dosage Range:**   250 to 750 mg, 3 or 4 times daily; adjust dosage as needed and tolerated. **Note: Actual dosage and administration schedule must be determined by the physician for each patient individually.**

▷ **Dosing Instructions:**   Take either on empty stomach or with food to prevent stomach irritation. Tablet may be crushed for administration.

Usual Duration of Use: Continual use on a regular schedule for 2 to 3 days is usually necessary to determine this drug's effectiveness in relieving the discomfort of muscle spasm. Evaluate need for continued use after periods of 7 to 10 days.

▷ **This Drug Should Not Be Taken If**
• you have had an allergic reaction to it previously.
• you have active liver disease.

▷ **Inform Your Physician Before Taking This Drug If**
• you have experienced any unfavorable reactions to muscle relaxants in the past.
• you have a history of liver or kidney disease.

Possible Side-Effects (natural, expected and unavoidable drug actions)
Drowsiness, orange or reddish purple discoloration of the urine (of no significance).

▷ **Possible Adverse Effects** (unusual, unexpected and infrequent reactions)
If any of the following develop, consult your physician promptly for guidance.
Mild Adverse Effects
Allergic Reactions: Skin rash, hives, itching, spontaneous bruising.
Light-headedness, dizziness, lethargy.
Indigestion, heartburn, nausea.
Serious Adverse Effects
Idiosyncratic Reactions: Nervousness, excitement, irritability.
Anemia, abnormally low white blood cell count—weakness, fever, sore throat.
Gastrointestinal bleeding—black- or dark-colored stools.
Liver reaction with or without jaundice (see Glossary)—yellow eyes and skin, dark-colored urine, light-colored stools.

▷ **Possible Effects on Sexual Function:**   None reported.

▷ **Adverse Effects That May Mimic Natural Diseases or Disorders**
Liver reaction may suggest viral hepatitis.

Possible Effects on Laboratory Tests
Complete blood cell counts: reduced red cells, hemoglobin and white cells.
Liver function tests: increased liver enzymes (ALT/GPT, AST/GOT and alkaline phosphatase), increased bilirubin.

Precautions for Use
By Infants and Children: Dosage is based on the child's age and weight. Consult your physician for exact dosage schedule.
By Those over 60 Years of Age: Small doses are advisable initially. You may be more susceptible to the development of drowsiness, dizziness, weakness, unsteadiness and falling.

▷ **Advisability of Use During Pregnancy**
Pregnancy Category: C (tentative). See Pregnancy Code inside back cover.
Animal studies: No data available.
Human studies: Information from adequate studies of pregnant women is not available.
Avoid drug if possible; use only if clearly needed.

Advisability of Use if Breast-Feeding
Presence of this drug in breast milk: Yes.
Avoid drug or refrain from nursing.

Habit-Forming Potential: None.

Effects of Overdosage: Nausea, vomiting, diarrhea, headache, drowsiness, dizziness, marked weakness, sense of paralysis of arms and legs, rapid and irregular breathing.

Possible Effects of Long-Term Use: None reported.

Suggested Periodic Examinations While Taking This Drug (at physician's discretion)
Complete blood cell counts. Liver function tests.

▷ **While Taking This Drug, Observe the Following**
Foods: No restrictions.
Beverages: No restrictions. May be taken with milk.
▷ *Alcohol:* Use with caution until the combined effect has been determined. This drug may add to the depressant action of alcohol on the brain.
Tobacco Smoking: No interactions expected.
Marijuana Smoking: Moderate to marked drowsiness, muscle weakness, incoordination, accentuation of orthostatic hypotension (see Glossary).
▷ *Other Drugs*
The following drugs may ***decrease*** the effects of chlorzoxazone
• testosterone is reported to reduce its ability to relax muscles in spasm.
▷ *Driving, Hazardous Activities:* This drug can cause drowsiness, light-headedness or dizziness in susceptible individuals. Avoid hazardous activities if these drug effects occur.
Aviation Note: The use of this drug ***is a disqualification*** for piloting. Consult a designated Aviation Medical Examiner.
Exposure to Sun: No restrictions.

CHOLESTYRAMINE
(koh LES tir a meen)

Introduced: 1959   **Class:** Anticholesterol

Prescription: USA: Yes   **Controlled Drug:** USA: No
    Canada: No   Canada: No

Available as Generic: USA: No
    Canada: No

Brand Names: Cholybar, Questran, Questran Light

```
┌─────────────────────────────────────────────────────────────────┐
│                    BENEFITS versus RISKS                          │
│                                                                   │
│        Possible Benefits              Possible Risks              │
│  EFFECTIVE REDUCTION OF         Constipation (may be severe)      │
│    TOTAL CHOLESTEROL AND        Reduced absorption of fat,        │
│    LOW DENSITY CHOLESTEROL        fat-soluble vitamins (A, D, E    │
│    IN TYPE IIa CHOLESTEROL        and K) and folic acid           │
│    DISORDERS (15% to 25%        Reduced formation of              │
│    reduction of total cholesterol,  prothrombin with resultant    │
│    25% to 35% reduction of LDL    bleeding                        │
│    cholesterol)                                                   │
│  EFFECTIVE RELIEF OF                                              │
│    ITCHING associated with                                        │
│    biliary obstruction                                            │
└─────────────────────────────────────────────────────────────────┘
```

▷ **Principal Uses**

  As a Single Drug Product: Used primarily to (1) reduce abnormally high blood levels of total cholesterol and low density (LDL) cholesterol in Type IIa cholesterol disorders; (2) relieve the itching due to the deposit of bile acids in the skin associated with partial biliary obstruction.

  How This Drug Works: By combining with bile acids and bile salts in the intestinal tract, this drug forms insoluble complexes that are excreted in the feces. This removal of bile acids (which are necessary for food digestion) stimulates the conversion of cholesterol to bile acids to replace the loss; this in turn reduces the blood levels of cholesterol. By reducing the blood levels of bile acids, this drug hastens the absorption and clearance of bile acids deposited in the skin and thus relieves itching.

  Available Dosage Forms and Strengths
      Bars — 4 grams
      Cans — 378 grams
    Packets — 4 grams, 9 grams

▷ **Usual Adult Dosage Range:** 9 grams of powder (equivalent to 4 grams of cholestyramine) 3 times daily. Dose may be increased slowly as needed and tolerated. The total daily dosage should not exceed 72 grams of powder (32 grams of cholestyramine). **Note: Actual dosage and administration schedule must be determined by the physician for each patient individually.**

▷ **Dosing Instructions:** Always take just before or with a meal; this drug is ineffective when taken without food. Mix the powder thoroughly in 4 to 6 ounces of water, fruit juice, milk, thin soup or a soft food like applesauce; do not use carbonated beverages. **Do not take it in its dry form.**

Usual Duration of Use: Continual use on a regular schedule for 4 to 6 weeks is usually necessary to determine this drug's effectiveness in lowering excessively high blood levels of cholesterol. Duration of use should not exceed 3 months if an adequate response does not occur. Long-term use (months to years) requires periodic evaluation of response and dosage adjustment. Consult your physician on a regular basis.

Currently a "Drug of Choice"
for initiating treatment of elevated LDL cholesterol. See Cholesterol Disorders in Section Two.

▷ **This Drug Should Not Be Taken If**
- you have had an allergic reaction to it previously.
- you have complete biliary obstruction.

▷ **Inform Your Physician Before Taking This Drug If**
- you are prone to constipation.
- you have peptic ulcer disease.
- you have a bleeding disorder of any kind.
- you have impaired kidney function.

Possible Side-Effects (natural, expected and unavoidable drug actions)
Constipation (25%); interference with normal fat digestion and absorption; reduced absorption of vitamins A, D, E and K and folic acid.

▷ **Possible Adverse Effects** (unusual, unexpected and infrequent reactions)
If any of the following develop, consult your physician promptly for guidance.
Mild Adverse Effects
Allergic Reactions: Skin rash, hives, tongue irritation, anal itching.
Loss of appetite, indigestion, heartburn, abdominal discomfort, excessive gas, nausea, vomiting, diarrhea.
Serious Adverse Effects
Allergic Reaction: Asthmalike wheezing.
Vitamin K deficiency with resultant deficiency of prothrombin and increased bleeding tendency.
Impaired absorption of calcium; predisposition to osteoporosis.
Gallbladder colic.

▷ **Possible Effects on Sexual Function:** Increased libido (questionable).

Natural Diseases or Disorders That May Be Activated by This Drug
Peptic ulcer disease; steatorrhea (excessive fat in stools) with large doses.

Possible Effects on Laboratory Tests
Blood cholesterol and triglyceride levels: decreased (therapeutic effect).
Blood hemoglobin and iron levels: decreased (drug impairs absorption of iron).
Prothrombin time: increased (drug impairs absorption of vitamin K).

Liver function tests: increased liver enzymes (ALT/GPT, AST/GOT) in a few cases; not thought to be liver damage.

Urine calcium: increased (drug impairs absorption of calcium from intestine).

CAUTION

1. The powder should never be taken in its dry form; always mix it thoroughly with a suitable liquid before swallowing.
2. Observe carefully for the development of constipation; use stool softeners and laxatives as needed.
3. This drug may bind other drugs taken concurrently and impair their absorption. It is advisable to take *all other drugs* 1 to 2 hours before or 4 to 6 hours after taking this drug.

Precautions for Use

By Infants and Children: Safety and effectiveness for use by those under 6 years of age have not been established. Observe carefully for the possible development of acidosis and vitamin A or folic acid deficiency. (Ask your physician for guidance.)

By Those over 60 Years of Age: There may be increased risk of developing severe constipation. Impaired kidney function may predispose to the development of acidosis.

▷ **Advisability of Use During Pregnancy**

Pregnancy Category: C (tentative). See Pregnancy Code inside back cover.

Animal studies: No information available.

Human studies: Information from adequate studies of pregnant women is not available.

Use this drug only if clearly needed. Ensure adequate intake of vitamins and minerals since this drug can reduce their availability to both mother and fetus. Ask physician for guidance.

Advisability of Use if Breast-Feeding

Presence of this drug in breast milk: No.

Breast-feeding is permitted.

Habit-Forming Potential: None.

Effects of Overdosage: Progressive constipation.

Possible Effects of Long-Term Use

Deficiencies of vitamins A, D, E and K and folic acid.

Calcium deficiency, osteoporosis.

Acidosis due to excessive retention of chloride.

Suggested Periodic Examinations While Taking This Drug (at physician's discretion)

Measurements of blood levels of total cholesterol, low density (LDL) cholesterol and high density (HDL) cholesterol.

Hemoglobin and red blood cell studies for possible anemia.

▷ **While Taking This Drug, Observe the Following**
   Foods: Avoid foods that tend to constipate (cheeses, etc.).
   Nutritional Support: Consult your physician regarding the need for supplements of vitamins A, D, E and K, folic acid and calcium.
   Beverages: Avoid carbonated beverages. Ensure adequate liquid intake (up to 2 quarts daily). This drug may be taken with milk.
▷ *Alcohol:* No interactions expected.
   Tobacco Smoking: No interactions expected.
▷ *Other Drugs*
   Cholestyramine may ***decrease*** the effects of
   • acetaminophen; give 2 hours before cholestyramine.
   • digitoxin and digoxin; give 2 hours before.
   • iron preparations; give 2 to 3 hours before.
   • phenobarbital; give 2 hours before.
   • thiazide diuretics (see Drug Class, Section Four); give 2 hours before.
   • thyroxin; give 5 hours before.
   • warfarin; give 6 hours after.
▷ *Driving, Hazardous Activities:* No restrictions.
   Aviation Note: The use of this drug ***is usually not a disqualification*** for piloting. Consult a designated Aviation Medical Examiner.
   Exposure to Sun: No restrictions.
   Discontinuation: The dose of any potentially toxic drug taken concurrently must be reduced appropriately when this drug is discontinued.

CIMETIDINE
(si MET i deen)

Introduced: 1976

Class: Antiulcer, H-2 receptor blocker

Prescription: USA: Yes
Canada: Yes

Controlled Drug: USA: No
Canada: No

Available as Generic: No

Brand Names: ✦Apo-Cimetidine, ✦Novocimetine, ✦Peptol, Tagamet

---

BENEFITS versus RISKS

Possible Benefits	*Possible Risks*
EFFECTIVE TREATMENT OF PEPTIC ULCER DISEASE: relief of symptoms, acceleration of healing, prevention of recurrence	CONFUSIONAL STATES in the elderly and debilitated
	Rare blood cell and bone marrow disorders
CONTROL OF HYPERSECRETORY STOMACH DISORDERS	Rare pancreatitis
	Rare liver damage
	Rare kidney damage
EFFECTIVE TREATMENT OF EROSIVE REFLUX DISEASE OF ESOPHAGUS	

▷ **Principal Uses**

As a Single Drug Product: Used primarily in the treatment of peptic ulcer disease, specifically to hasten the healing of duodenal ulcer and to prevent its recurrence. Also used to control the excessive production of stomach acid in Zollinger-Ellison syndrome. This drug is also effective in the management of stomach (gastric) ulcer, esophagitis (as with hiatal hernia) and upper gastrointestinal bleeding.

How This Drug Works: By blocking the action of histamine, this drug effectively inhibits the secretion of stomach acid and thus creates a more favorable environment for the healing of peptic ulcers of the duodenum, esophagus and stomach.

Available Dosage Forms and Strengths

Injection — 300 mg per 2 ml
Liquid — 300 mg per 5-ml teaspoonful (2.8% alcohol)
Tablets — 200 mg, 300 mg, 400 mg, 800 mg

▷ **Usual Adult Dosage Range:** For active peptic ulcer and hypersecretory states—300 mg, 4 times daily, taken with meals and at bedtime. For prevention of recurrent ulcer—400 mg at bedtime. For erosive reflux disease of the esophagus—800 mg twice daily. Total daily dosage should not exceed 1600 mg. **Note: Actual dosage and administration schedule must be determined by the physician for each patient individually.**

▷ **Dosing Instructions:**   To obtain the longest period of stomach acid reduction, this drug should be taken with or immediately following meals. The tablet may be crushed for administration.

Usual Duration of Use: Continual use on a regular schedule for 4 to 6 weeks is usually necessary to determine this drug's effectiveness in healing active peptic ulcer. Continual use for 1 year or more is recommended for prevention of ulcer recurrence. Continual use for 6 to 12 weeks is usually necessary to accomplish healing of the esophagus. Consult your physician on a regular basis.

▷ **This Drug Should Not Be Taken If**
  • you have had an allergic reaction to any dosage form of it previously.

▷ **Inform Your Physician Before Taking This Drug If**
  • you have impaired liver or kidney function.
  • you have a low sperm count.
  • you are taking any oral anticoagulant, propranolol or quinidine.

Possible Side-Effects (natural, expected and unavoidable drug actions)
  None reported.

▷ **Possible Adverse Effects** (unusual, unexpected and infrequent reactions)
  If any of the following develop, consult your physician promptly for guidance.
  Mild Adverse Effects
  Allergic Reactions: Skin rash, hives, drug fever (see Glossary).
  Headache, dizziness, double vision, fatigue, muscular pains, diarrhea.
  Serious Adverse Effects
  Allergic Reactions: Pancreatitis, kidney damage.
  Idiosyncratic Reactions: Nervous agitation, confusion, delirium, hallucinations, coma.
  Slowed heart rate, liver damage.
  Bone marrow depression (see Glossary)—weakness, fever, sore throat, abnormal bleeding or bruising.

▷ **Possible Effects on Sexual Function:**   Decreased libido (600 mg/day); impaired erection and impotence (1000 mg/day); decreased male fertility (1200 mg/day); male breast enlargement (1000 mg/day); female breast enlargement with milk production (1600 mg/day).

▷ **Adverse Effects That May Mimic Natural Diseases or Disorders**
  Liver reactions may suggest viral hepatitis.

Natural Diseases or Disorders That May Be Activated by This Drug
  Psoriasis (questionable).

Possible Effects on Laboratory Tests

Complete blood cell counts: decreased white cells and platelets (very rare).

Blood HDL cholesterol level: varies from no drug effect to significant increase.

Blood LDL and VLDL cholesterol level: no drug effect.

Liver function tests: increased liver enzymes (ALT/GPT, AST/GOT and alkaline phosphatase), increased bilirubin (all in one isolated case).

Sperm counts: decreased.

CAUTION

1. Do not discontinue this drug abruptly. Ulcer activation and perforation have occurred following abrupt cessation.
2. Hemodialysis can remove from 8% to 14% of this drug. Schedule the dosage to follow completion of each dialysis treatment.

Precautions for Use

By Infants and Children: Safety and effectiveness for use by those under 16 years of age have not been established. If use of this drug is deemed necessary, observe for sedation, confusion, breast enlargement, milk secretion and possible kidney damage.

By Those over 60 Years of Age: Initiate treatment with one-half the usual dose. Observe for the development of nervous agitation, depression, confusion, slurred speech or excessive drowsiness. This drug can contribute to the formation of stomach phytobezoars (masses of undigested vegetable fibers). Individuals with poor chewing ability (missing teeth) and those who have had partial gastrectomy or vagotomy (stomach surgery) are most susceptible. Observe for loss of appetite, stomach fullness, nausea and vomiting.

▷ **Advisability of Use During Pregnancy**

Pregnancy Category: B (tentative). See Pregnancy Code inside back cover.

Animal studies: No birth defects reported.

Human studies: Information from adequate studies of pregnant women is not available.

Use this drug only if clearly needed. Ask physician for guidance.

Advisability of Use if Breast-Feeding

Presence of this drug in breast milk: Yes, in large amounts.

Avoid drug or refrain from nursing.

Habit-Forming Potential: None.

Effects of Overdosage: Confusion, delirium, slurred speech, flushing, sweating, drowsiness, muscle twitching, seizures, coma.

Possible Effects of Long-Term Use: Liver damage (reversible), swelling and tenderness of breast tissue in men.

Suggested Periodic Examinations While Taking This Drug (at physician's discretion)

Complete blood cell counts, liver and kidney function tests, sperm counts, prothrombin times if an anticoagulant is taken concurrently.

▷ **While Taking This Drug, Observe the Following**

Foods: Protein-rich foods produce maximal stomach acid secretion. Follow the diet prescribed to derive optimal benefit from this drug.

Nutritional Support: This drug may inhibit the absorption of vitamin B-12. Consult physician regarding the need for B-12 supplement.

Beverages: No restrictions. May be taken with milk.

▷ *Alcohol:* No interactions with drug. However, alcoholic beverages increase stomach acidity and can reduce the effectiveness of this drug.

Marijuana Smoking: Possible accentuation of reduced sperm production due to this drug.

▷ *Other Drugs*

Cimetidine may *increase* the effects of

- oral anticoagulants, and increase the risk of bleeding.
- benzodiazepines (Librium, Valium, etc.), see Drug Class, Section Four.
- phenytoin (Dilantin).
- procainamide (Procan, Pronestyl).
- propranolol (Inderal).
- quinidine (Quinaglute, etc.).
- theophylline (Theo-Dur, Bronkodyl, Slo-bid, etc.).

Cimetidine *taken concurrently* with

- carmustine (BCNU) may cause severe bone marrow depression. Do not use these drugs concurrently.

▷ *Driving, Hazardous Activities:* This drug can cause erratic driving behavior. Use caution until it has been determined that dizziness, confusion or double vision does not occur.

Aviation Note: The use of this drug *may be a disqualification* for piloting. Consult a designated Aviation Medical Examiner.

Exposure to Sun: No restrictions.

Discontinuation: Do not discontinue this drug suddenly if taken for peptic ulcer disease. Consult physician for withdrawal instructions. This drug does not provide an extended protective effect. Be alert to the possibility of ulcer recurrence anytime after discontinuation.

CIPROFLOXACIN
(sip roh FLOX a sin)

Introduced: 1984   **Class:** Anti-infective

Prescription: USA: Yes   **Controlled Drug:** USA: No

Available as Generic: USA: No

Brand Name: Cipro

BENEFITS versus RISKS

Possible Benefits	*Possible Risks*
HIGHLY EFFECTIVE TREATMENT FOR INFECTIONS OF THE LOWER RESPIRATORY TRACT, URINARY TRACT, BONES, JOINTS AND SKIN TISSUES due to susceptible organisms	Nausea (1.6%), diarrhea (1.5%), very rare drug-induced colitis
	Mild allergic reactions (1.4%)
	Very rare hallucination or seizure
Effective treatment for some forms of bacterial gastroenteritis (diarrhea)	

▷ **Principal Uses**

As a Single Drug Product: Used primarily to treat responsive infections (in adults) of: (1) the lower respiratory tract (lungs and bronchial tubes); (2) the urinary tract (kidneys, bladder, urethra and prostate gland); (3) the digestive tract (small intestine and colon); (4) bones and joints; (5) skin and related tissues.

How This Drug Works: By interfering with the bacterial enzyme DNA gyrase (which is required for DNA synthesis and cell reproduction), this drug arrests bacterial growth (in low concentrations) and destroys bacteria (in high concentrations).

Available Dosage Forms and Strengths
Tablets — 250 mg, 500 mg, 750 mg

▷ **Usual Adult Dosage Range:** 250 mg to 750 mg/12 hours, depending upon the nature and severity of the infection. The total daily dosage should not exceed 1500 mg. **Note: Actual dosage and administration schedule must be determined by the physician for each patient individually.**

▷ **Dosing Instructions:** May be taken with or without food. Preferably it should be taken 2 hours after eating. Drink fluids liberally during the entire course of treatment. Avoid antacids containing aluminum or magnesium for 2 hours before and after dosing. The tablet may be crushed for administration.

Usual Duration of Use: Continual use on a regular schedule for 7 to 14 days is usually necessary to determine this drug's effectiveness in eradicating the infection. The drug should be continued for at least 2 days after all indications of infection have disappeared. Bone and joint infections may require treatment for 6 weeks or longer. Long-term use requires periodic evaluation of response and dosage adjustment. Consult your physician on a regular basis.

Possible Advantages of This Drug

The broadest spectrum of antibacterial activity of all currently available oral antimicrobial drugs.

The most potent anti-infective action of the drugs in this class (quinolones).

Highly effective in treating numerous types of infection caused by a wide spectrum of bacteria (overall clinical response rate of 96%).

Capable of establishing effective drug levels throughout the prostate gland (clinical response rate of 83% in treating prostatitis).

Effective one-dose treatment for uncomplicated gonorrheal infection of the urethra.

No significant effect on kidney function.

Currently a "Drug of Choice"

for (1) starting treatment of urinary tract infections prior to obtaining the results of urine bacterial culture and sensitivity tests; (2) treating infections due to *Pseudomonas aeruginosa*, a bacterial strain often resistant to other anti-infective drugs.

▷ **This Drug Should Not Be Taken If**

• you have had an allergic reaction to it previously.
• you are pregnant or breast-feeding.
• you have a seizure disorder that is not adequately controlled.
• it is prescribed for a person under 18 years of age.

▷ **Inform Your Physician Before Taking This Drug If**

• you are allergic to cinoxacin (Cinobac), nalidixic acid (NegGram) or norfloxacin (Noroxin).
• you have a history of a seizure disorder or a circulatory disorder of the brain.
• you have impaired liver or kidney function.
• you are taking any form of probenecid or theophylline.

Possible Side-Effects (natural, expected and unavoidable drug actions)
Superinfections (5%). (See Superinfection in the Glossary.)

▷ **Possible Adverse Effects** (unusual, unexpected and infrequent reactions)
If any of the following develop, consult your physician promptly for guidance.
Mild Adverse Effects
Allergic Reactions: Rash (0.83%), itching (0.47%), localized swelling (0.12%).

Dizziness (0.53%), headache (0.30%), weakness (0.36%), migraine (0.06%), anxiety (0.06%), abnormal vision (0.06%).
Nausea (1.6%), diarrhea (1.5%), vomiting (0.7%), indigestion (0.36%).
Serious Adverse Effects
Allergic Reactions: None reported.
Idiosyncratic Reactions: None reported.
Central nervous system stimulation: restlessness, tremor, confusion, hallucinations, seizures (all very rare).

▷ **Possible Effects on Sexual Function:**   None reported.

▷ **Natural Diseases or Disorders That May Be Activated by This Drug**
Latent epilepsy, latent gout.

Possible Effects on Laboratory Tests
Kidney function tests: increased blood creatinine and urea nitrogen (BUN) in very rare cases.

CAUTION
1. With high doses or prolonged use, crystal formation in the kidney may occur. This can be prevented by drinking copious amounts of water, up to 2 quarts/24 hours.
2. Drugs of this class may decrease the formation of saliva and predispose to the development of dental cavities or gum disease. Consult your dentist if dry mouth persists.

Precautions for Use
By Infants and Children: Avoid the use of this drug completely. It can impair normal bone growth and development.
By Those over 60 Years of Age: Impaired kidney function may require dosage reduction.
If you are taking theophylline concurrently with this drug, observe closely for possible theophylline accumulation and toxicity.

▷ **Advisability of Use During Pregnancy**
Pregnancy Category: C (tentative). See Pregnancy Code inside back cover.
Animal studies: No birth defects due to this drug found in mouse, rat or rabbit studies. However, this drug can impair normal bone development in immature dogs.
Human studies: Information from adequate studies of pregnant women is not available. However, the potential for adverse effects on fetal bone development contraindicates the use of this drug during entire pregnancy.

Advisability of Use if Breast-Feeding
Presence of this drug in breast milk: Probably yes.
Avoid drug or refrain from nursing.

Habit-Forming Potential: None.

Effects of Overdosage: No information available.

Possible Effects of Long-Term Use: Superinfections (see Glossary); crystal formation in kidneys.

Suggested Periodic Examinations While Taking This Drug (at physician's discretion)
Liver function tests, urine analysis.

▷ **While Taking This Drug, Observe the Following**
Foods: No restrictions.
Beverages: No restrictions. May be taken with milk.
▷ *Alcohol:* No interactions expected.
Tobacco Smoking: No interactions expected.
▷ *Other Drugs*
Ciprofloxacin may *increase* the effects of
• theophylline, and cause theophylline toxicity.
The following drug may *increase* the effects of ciprofloxacin
• probenecid (Benemid).
The following drugs may *decrease* the effects of ciprofloxacin
• antacids containing aluminum or magnesium can reduce the absorption of ciprofloxacin and lessen its effectiveness.
▷ *Driving, Hazardous Activities:* This drug may cause dizziness and impair vision. Restrict activities as necessary.
Aviation Note: The use of this drug *may be a disqualification* for piloting. Consult a designated Aviation Medical Examiner.
Exposure to Sun: This drug may rarely cause photosensitivity (see Glossary). Sunglasses are advised if eyes are overly sensitive to bright light.
Discontinuation: If you experience no adverse effects from this drug, take the full course prescribed for maximal results. Consult your physician regarding termination of treatment.

CLINDAMYCIN
(klin da MI sin)

Introduced: 1973

Class: Antibiotic

Prescription: USA: Yes
Canada: Yes

Controlled Drug: USA: No
Canada: No

Available as Generic: USA: Yes
Canada: No

Brand Names: Cleocin, Cleocin T, ✦Dalacin C

```
┌─────────────────────────────────────────────────────────────┐
│                   BENEFITS versus RISKS                       │
│                                                               │
│      Possible Benefits              Possible Risks            │
│  EFFECTIVE TREATMENT FOR        SEVERE DRUG-INDUCED           │
│    SERIOUS INFECTIONS OF          COLITIS (fatalities reported)│
│    THE LOWER RESPIRATORY        Rare liver injury with jaundice│
│    TRACT, ABDOMINAL CAVITY,     Rare reduction in white blood cell│
│    GENITAL TRACT IN WOMEN,        and platelet counts         │
│    BLOOD STREAM                                               │
│    (SEPTICEMIA), SKIN AND                                     │
│    RELATED TISSUES caused by                                  │
│    susceptible organisms                                      │
│  SPECIFIC PREVENTION AND                                      │
│    TREATMENT FOR                                              │
│    PNEUMOCYSTIS CARINII                                       │
│    PNEUMONIA (PCP)                                            │
│    ASSOCIATED WITH AIDS                                       │
│  Possibly effective for the local                             │
│    treatment of acne                                          │
└─────────────────────────────────────────────────────────────┘
```

▷ **Principal Uses**

As a Single Drug Product

Used primarily to treat serious and unusual infections of the lungs and bronchial tubes, organs and tissues within the abdominal cavity, the genital tract and pelvic organs in women, the skin and soft tissue structures and generalized infections involving the bloodstream.

A more recent use has been the prevention and treatment of pneumocystis carinii pneumonia, a frequent infection associated with AIDS.

How This Drug Works: By interfering with the formation of proteins necessary for cell growth and reproduction, this drug (in low concentrations) arrests the multiplication of bacteria and (in high concentrations) destroys bacteria.

Available Dosage Forms and Strengths

Capsules — 75 mg, 150 mg, 300 mg
Injection — 150 mg per ml
Oral solution — 75 mg per 5-ml teaspoonful
Topical solution — 10 mg per ml

▷ **Usual Adult Dosage Range:** For infections of average severity: 150 to 300 mg/6 hours; for more severe infections: 300 to 450 mg/6 hours. The total daily dosage should not exceed 1800 mg. **Note: Actual dosage and administration schedule must be determined by the physician for each patient individually.**

▷ **Dosing Instructions:** Take the capsule with a full glass of water or with food to prevent irritation of the esophagus. The capsule may be opened and the contents mixed with food for administration. Shake the oral solution well before measuring the dose. Do not refrigerate the oral solution; chilling can cause it to thicken, making administration difficult.

Usual Duration of Use: Continual use on a regular schedule for 3 to 5 days is usually necessary to determine this drug's effectiveness in controlling responsive infections. The duration of use should not exceed the time required to eliminate the infection.

Possible Advantages of This Drug: Bacterial sensitivity testing may show this drug to be more effective than commonly used antibiotics in treating some severe and unusual infections.

Currently a "Drug of Choice"
for preventing and treating pneumonia due to pneumocystis carinii, a frequent complication of AIDS.

▷ **This Drug Should Not Be Taken If**
- you are allergic to either clindamycin or lincomycin.
- it is prescribed for a mild or trivial infection such as a cold, sore throat or "flu-like" illness.
- you have a history of Crohn's disease or ulcerative colitis.

▷ **Inform Your Physician Before Taking This Drug If**
- you have a history of allergy to any drug.
- you have a history of drug-induced colitis.
- you are allergic by nature: hay fever, asthma, hives, eczema.
- you have a history of previous yeast infections.
- you have myasthenia gravis.
- you have impaired liver or kidney function.
- you plan to have surgery under general anesthesia in the near future.

Possible Side-Effects (natural, expected and unavoidable drug actions)
Superinfections (see Glossary).

▷ **Possible Adverse Effects** (unusual, unexpected and infrequent reactions)
If any of the following develop, consult your physician promptly for guidance.
Mild Adverse Effects
Allergic Reactions: Skin rashes (3% to 5%), hives.
Nausea, vomiting, mild diarrhea (3% to 30%), stomach pain.
Multiple joint pains (rare).
Serious Adverse Effects
Allergic Reactions: Severe skin reactions: erythema multiforme (Stevens-Johnson syndrome).
Toxic liver reaction with jaundice (see Glossary).
Severe colitis with persistent diarrhea (0.01% to 10%); stools may contain blood and/or mucus.
Rare reduction of white blood cell and platelet counts.

▷ **Possible Effects on Sexual Function:**   None reported.

Possible Delayed Adverse Effects: Severe colitis with diarrhea (pseudomembranous colitis) may begin several weeks after discontinuing this drug.

▷ **Adverse Effects That May Mimic Natural Diseases or Disorders**
Liver reactions may suggest viral hepatitis.
Multiple joint pains may suggest the onset of arthritis.

▷ **Natural Diseases or Disorders That May Be Activated by This Drug**
Crohn's disease, ulcerative colitis, myasthenia gravis.

Possible Effects on Laboratory Tests
Complete blood cell counts: decreased white cells and platelets; increased
eosinophils (allergic reaction).
Liver function tests: uncommon, mild and transient increases in liver
enzymes (ALT/GPT, AST/GOT, alkaline phosphatase).

CAUTION
1. Troublesome and persistent diarrhea can develop in sensitive individuals. If diarrhea persists longer than 24 hours, discontinue this
drug and consult your physician for guidance.
2. If surgery under general anesthesia is planned while taking this drug,
the choice of anesthetic must be considered carefully to prevent
excessive muscle relaxation and associated impairment of breathing.

Precautions for Use
By Infants and Children: Safety and effectiveness for use by those under 1
month of age have not been established. Use with caution.
By Those over 60 Years of Age: Observe closely for the possible development
of diarrhea (more common in this age group). Also observe for the
possible development of yeast infection of the skin in the genital and
anal regions, a form of superinfection (see Glossary). Report such
developments promptly to your physician.

▷ **Advisability of Use During Pregnancy**
Pregnancy Category: B (tentative). See Pregnancy Code inside back cover.
Animal studies: No birth defects due to this drug found in mouse or rat
studies.
Human studies: Information from adequate studies of pregnant women
is not available. Use this drug only if clearly needed. Ask your physician
for guidance.

Advisability of Use if Breast-Feeding
Presence of this drug in breast milk: Yes.
Avoid drug or refrain from nursing.

Habit-Forming Potential: None.

Effects of Overdosage: Nausea, vomiting, cramping, diarrhea.

Possible Effects of Long-Term Use
Superinfections, especially from yeast organisms.
Severe colitis with persistent diarrhea.

Suggested Periodic Examinations While Taking This Drug (at physician's
discretion)
Complete blood cell counts, liver function tests.

▷ **While Taking This Drug, Observe the Following**
  Foods: No restrictions.
  Beverages: No restrictions. May be taken with milk.
▷ *Alcohol:* No interactions expected.
  Tobacco Smoking: No interactions expected.
▷ *Other Drugs*
  Clindamycin *taken concurrently* with
  • antidiarrheal drugs (diphenoxylate, loperamide, paregoric) may result in worsening of the underlying colitis because of impaired elimination of causative toxins.
  • antimyasthenic drugs (ambenonium, neostigmine, pyridostigmine) may reduce their effectiveness in relieving the muscle weakness of myasthenia gravis.
  The following drugs may *decrease* the effects of clindamycin
  • chloramphenicol (Chloromycetin).
  • erythromycin (E.E.S., E-Mycin, etc.).
▷ *Driving, Hazardous Activities:* This drug may cause nausea and diarrhea. Restrict activities as necessary.
  Aviation Note: The use of this drug *may be a disqualification* for piloting. Consult a designated Aviation Medical Examiner.
  Exposure to Sun: Use caution until sensitivity is determined.
  Discontinuation: If tolerated satisfactorily, take the full course prescribed. When used to treat infections that may predispose to rheumatic fever or nephritis, take continually in full dosage for no less than 10 days.
  Special Storage Instructions: Oral solution should be kept at room temperature; do not refrigerate.
  Observe the Following Expiration Times: Do not take the oral solution if it is older than 14 days.

CLOMIPRAMINE
(kloh MI pra meen)

Introduced: 1970

Class: Antiobsessive-compulsive, Antidepressant

Prescription: USA: Yes
Canada: Yes

Controlled Drug: USA: No
Canada: No

Available as Generic: USA: No
Canada: No

Brand Name: Anafranil

BENEFITS versus RISKS

Possible Benefits	*Possible Risks*
EFFECTIVE TREATMENT OF SEVERE OBSESSIVE-COMPULSIVE NEUROSIS	DRUG-INDUCED SEIZURES (appoximately 1%)
Effective relief of symptoms in the management of some types of endogenous depression	ADVERSE BEHAVIORAL EFFECTS: confusion, delirium, disorientation, hallucinations, delusions, paranoia
	Conversion of depression to mania in manic-depressive disorders
	Aggravation of schizophrenia
	Rare liver toxicity
	Rare bone marrow depression and blood cell disorders

▷ **Principal Uses**

As a Single Drug Product: In the U.S., used primarily to relieve the manifestations of severe, disabling obsessive-compulsive disorder.

In other countries, used primarily to relieve severe endogenous emotional depression and to initiate gradual restoration of normal mood.

How This Drug Works: Not completely established. It is thought that by increasing brain tissue concentrations of certain nerve impulse transmitters, principally serotonin, this drug reduces the frequency and intensity of obsessive and compulsive behavior patterns.

Available Dosage Forms and Strengths

Capsules — 25 mg, 50 mg, 75 mg

▷ **Usual Adult Dosage Range:**   Initially 25 mg daily, taken in the evening. Dose may be increased cautiously as needed and tolerated by 25 mg daily at intervals of 3 to 4 days until a dose of 100 mg daily is reached in 2 weeks. This larger dose should be divided and taken after meals. The usual maintenance dose is 50 mg to 150 mg/24 hours. The total daily dosage should not exceed 250 mg. (When determined, the optimal daily requirement may be given at bedtime as a single dose.) **Note: Actual dosage and administration schedule must be determined by the physician for each patient individually.**

▷ **Dosing Instructions:**   May be taken without regard to meals. If necessary, may be taken with or following food to reduce stomach irritation. The capsule may be opened for administration.

Usual Duration of Use:

Continual use on a regular schedule for 3 to 4 weeks is usually necessary to determine this drug's effectiveness in controlling obsessive-compulsive behavior; optimal response may require 3 or more months of use.

Long-term use (months to years) requires periodic evaluation of response and dosage adjustment. Consult your physician on a regular basis.

Currently a "Drug of Choice"
for the management of obsessive-compulsive disorder.

▷ **This Drug Should Not Be Taken If**
- you have had an allergic reaction to it previously.
- you are taking, or have taken within the past 14 days, any monoamine oxidase (MAO) type A inhibitor drug (see Drug Class, Section Four).
- you have active bone marrow depression or a current blood cell disorder.
- you have had a recent heart attack (myocardial infarction).
- you have narrow-angle glaucoma.

▷ **Inform Your Physician Before Taking This Drug If**
- you have had an adverse reaction to any other antidepressant drug, especially one of the tricyclic class.
- you have a history of bone marrow or blood cell disorder.
- you have any type of seizure disorder.
- you have increased internal eye pressure.
- you have any type of heart disease, especially coronary artery disease or a heart rhythm disorder.
- you are subject to bronchial asthma.
- you have impaired liver or kidney function.
- you have any type of thyroid disorder or are taking thyroid medication.
- you have an adrenalin-producing tumor.
- you have prostatism (see Glossary).
- you have a history of alcoholism.
- you plan to have surgery under general anesthesia in the near future.

Possible Side-Effects
(natural, expected and unavoidable drug actions)
Drowsiness (54%), increased sweating (29%), light-headedness (6%), blurred vision (18%), dry mouth (84%), constipation (47%), impaired urination (14%).

▷ **Possible Adverse Effects**
(unusual, unexpected and infrequent reactions)
If any of the following develop, consult your physician promptly for guidance.
Mild Adverse Effects
Allergic Reactions: Skin rash (8%), itching (6%), drug fever (4%), (see Glossary).
Headache (52%), dizziness (54%), nervousness (18%), impaired memory (9%), weakness (39%), tremors (54%), insomnia (25%), muscle cramps (13%), flushing (8%).
Increased appetite (32%), weight gain (18%).

Altered taste (8%), indigestion (22%), nausea (33%), vomiting (7%), diarrhea (13%).

Serious Adverse Effects

Allergic Reactions: Drug-induced hepatitis, with or without jaundice.

Idiosyncratic Reactions: Neuroleptic malignant syndrome (see Glossary).

Adverse behavioral effects: confusion (3%), delirium, disorientation, delusions, hallucinations, paranoia.

Seizures; reduced control of epilepsy.

Aggravation of paranoid psychoses and schizophrenia.

Heart rhythm disturbances.

Bone marrow depression (see Glossary): fatigue, weakness, fever, sorethroat, infections, abnormal bleeding or bruising.

▷ **Possible Effects on Sexual Function**

Altered libido (21%), impaired ejaculation (42%), impotence (20%), inhibited male orgasm, inhibited female orgasm, female breast enlargement with milk production (4%).

▷ **Adverse Effects That May Mimic Natural Diseases or Disorders**

Liver toxicity may suggest viral hepatitis.

Natural Diseases or Disorders That May Be Activated by This Drug

Latent epilepsy, glaucoma, prostatism, schizophrenia.

Possible Effects on Laboratory Tests

Complete blood cell counts: decreased red cells, hemoglobin, white cells and platelets.

Liver function tests: increased liver enzymes (ALT/GPT, AST/GOT)—liver damage.

CAUTION

1. Observe for early indications of toxicity or overdosage: confusion, agitation, rapid heart rate, heart irregularity. Measurement of the blood level of the drug will clarify the situation.
2. Use with caution in the presence of schizophrenia. Observe closely for any deterioration of thinking or behavior.
3. Use with caution in the presence of epilepsy. Observe for any change in the frequency or severity of seizures.

Precautions for Use

By Infants and Children: Safety and effectiveness for use by those under 10 years of age have not been established. Dosage and management should be supervised by a properly trained pediatrician. Total daily dosage should not exceed 200 mg.

By Those over 60 Years of Age: Initiate treatment with 10 mg at bedtime. Dosage may be increased gradually as needed and tolerated to 75 mg daily in divided doses. During the first 2 weeks of treatment, observe for behavioral reactions: restlessness, agitation, forgetfulness, disorientation, delusions or hallucinations. Also observe for unsteadiness and instability that may predispose to falling. This drug may aggravate prostatism.

▷ **Advisability of Use During Pregnancy**
Pregnancy Category: C (tentative). See Pregnancy Code inside back cover.
Animal studies: No drug-induced birth defects reported in mouse or rat studies.
Human studies: Information from adequate studies of pregnant women is not available.
Use only if clearly needed. Avoid use during the last 3 months, if possible, to prevent withdrawal symptoms in the newborn infant: irritability, tremors, seizures.

Advisability of Use if Breast-Feeding
Presence of this drug in breast milk: Yes.
Avoid drug or refrain from nursing.

Habit-Forming Potential: Psychological or physical dependence is rare and unexpected. This drug is not liable to abuse.

Effects of Overdosage: Confusion, delirium, hallucinations, drowsiness, tremors, unsteadiness, heart irregularity, seizures, stupor, sweating, fever.

Possible Effects of Long-Term Use: Neuroleptic malignant syndrome (see Glossary): fever, fast or irregular heartbeat, fast breathing, sweating, weakness, muscle stiffness, seizures, loss of bladder control.

Suggested Periodic Examinations While Taking This Drug
(at physician's discretion)
Monitoring of blood drug levels as appropriate.
Complete blood cell counts; liver and kidney function tests.
Serial blood pressure readings and electrocardiograms.
Measurement of internal eye pressure.

▷ **While Taking This Drug, Observe the Following**
Foods: No specific restrictions. May need to limit food intake to avoid excessive weight gain.
Beverages: No restrictions. May be taken with milk.
▷ *Alcohol:* Avoid completely. This drug can markedly increase the intoxicating effects of alcohol; the combination can depress brain function significantly.
Tobacco Smoking: May delay the elimination of this drug and require dosage adjustment.
Marijuana Smoking: Increased drowsiness and mouth dryness; possible reduced effectiveness of this drug.
▷ *Other Drugs*
Clomipramine may *increase* the effects of
• all drugs with sedative effects; observe for excessive sedation.
• all drugs with atropinelike effects (see Drug Class, Section Four).

Clomipramine may *decrease* the effects of
- clonidine (Catapres).
- guanadrel (Hylorel).
- guanethidine (Ismelin, Esimil).

Clomipramine *taken concurrently* with
- anticonvulsants requires careful monitoring for changes in seizure patterns and need to adjust anticonvulsant dosage.
- monoamine oxidase (MAO) type A inhibitor drugs (see Drug Class, Section Four) may cause high fever, seizures and excessive rise in blood pressure; avoid concurrent use of these drugs and provide periods of 14 days between administration of either.
- stimulant drugs (amphetamine, cocaine, epinephrine, phenylpropanolamine, etc.) may cause severe high blood pressure and/or high fever.
- thyroid preparations may increase the risk of heart rhythm disorders.

The following drugs may *increase* the effects of clomipramine
- cimetidine (Tagamet).
- estrogens.
- fluoxetine (Prozac).
- haloperidol (Haldol).
- methylphenidate (Ritalin).
- oral contraceptives.
- phenothiazines (see Drug Class, Section Four).
- ranitidine (Zantac).

The following drugs may *decrease* the effects of clomipramine
- barbiturates (see Drug Class, Section Four).
- carbamazepine (Tegretol).
- chloral hydrate (Noctec, Somnos, etc.).
- lithium (Lithobid, Lithotab, etc.).
- reserpine (Serpasil, Ser-Ap-Es, etc.).

▷ *Driving, Hazardous Activities:* This drug may cause seizures and may impair mental alertness, judgment, physical coordination and reaction time. Restrict activities as necessary.

Aviation Note: The use of this drug **is a disqualification** for piloting. Consult a designated Aviation Medical Examiner.

Exposure to Sun: No restrictions.

Exposure to Heat: Use caution. This drug may impair the body's adaptation to hot environments, increasing the risk of heat stroke. Avoid saunas.

Exposure to Environmental Chemicals: This drug may mask the symptoms of poisoning due to handling certain insecticides (organophosphorus types). Read their labels carefully.

Discontinuation: It is advisable to discontinue this drug gradually over a period of 3 to 4 weeks. Abrupt withdrawal after prolonged use may cause nausea, vomiting, diarrhea, headache, dizziness, malaise, disturbed sleep and irritability. Obsessive-compulsive behavior may worsen when this drug is stopped. It may be necessary to adjust the dosages of other drugs taken concurrently when this drug is discontinued.

CLONAZEPAM
(kloh NA ze pam)

Introduced: 1977

Class: Anticonvulsant, benzodiaze-pines

Prescription: USA: Yes
Canada: Yes

Controlled Drug: USA: C-IV*
Canada: No

Available as Generic: No

Brand Names: Klonopin, ✦Rivotril

Warning: The brand name Klonopin and the generic name clonidine are similar and can be mistaken for each other; this can lead to serious medication errors. These names represent very different drugs. Klono-pin (small round tablets colored according to strength: yellow, blue or white) is the generic drug clonazepam; it is used to treat epilepsy. Clonidine (also available in small white tablets) is a genereic drug used to treat high blood pressure. Verify that you are taking the correct drug.

BENEFITS versus RISKS

Possible Benefits	*Possible Risks*
EFFECTIVE CONTROL OF SOME TYPES OF PETIT MAL, AKINETIC AND MYOCLONIC SEIZURES	Paradoxical reactions: excitement, agitation, hallucinations
Possibly effective in the nanagement of panic disorders	Minor impairment of mental functions
	Rare blood cell disorders: anemia, abnormally low white blood cell and platelet counts

---

▷ **Principal Uses**

As a Single Drug Product: Used primarily to (1) treat several types of epi-lepsy: petit mal variations, akinetic, myoclonic, simple and complex partial seizure patterns; (2) control panic disorders.

How This Drug Works: It is thought that this drug produces an anticonvul-sant effect by enhancing the action of the nerve transmitter gamma-aminobutyric acid (GABA), which in turn blocks the spread of seizure activity that originates in higher brain centers.

Available Dosage Forms and Strengths
Tablets — 0.5 mg, 1 mg, 2 mg

▷ **Usual Adult Dosage Range:** Initially 0.5 mg three times daily. The dose may be increased by 0.5 mg to 1.0 mg every three days, as needed and tolerated, until seizures are controlled. Total daily dose should not

*See Schedules of Controlled Drugs inside back cover.

exceed 20 mg. **Note: Actual dosage and administration schedule must be determined by the physician for each patient individually.**

▷ **Dosing Instructions:**   May be taken on empty stomach or with food or milk. The tablet may be crushed for administration. Do not discontinue this drug abruptly if taken for control of seizures, or if taken for more than 4 weeks to control panic attacks.

Usual Duration of Use: Continual use on a regular schedule for 2 to 3 weeks is usually necessary to determine this drug's effectiveness in reducing the frequency and severity of seizures. Optimal control will require careful dosage adjustments over a period of several months. Long-term use (months to years) requires ongoing supervision and periodic evaluation by your physician. Consult your physician on a regular basis.

▷ **This Drug Should Not Be Taken If**
  • you have had an allergic reaction to it previously.
  • you have acute narrow-angle glaucoma.
  • you have active liver disease.

▷ **Inform Your Physician Before Taking This Drug If**
  • you are allergic to any benzodiazepine drug (see Drug Class, Section Four).
  • you have a history of alcoholism or drug abuse.
  • you are pregnant or planning pregnancy.
  • you have impaired liver or kidney function.
  • you have a history of serious depression or mental disorder.
  • you have any of the following: asthma, emphysema, chronic bronchitis, myasthenia gravis.

Possible Side-Effects (natural, expected and unavoidable drug actions)
  Drowsiness (50%), lethargy, unsteadiness (30%), increased salivation (7%).

▷ **Possible Adverse Effects** (unusual, unexpected and infrequent reactions)
  If any of the following develop, consult your physician promptly for guidance.
  Mild Adverse Effects
  Allergic Reactions: Skin rash, hives, itching.
  Headache, dizziness, blurred vision, double vision, slurred speech, impaired memory, confusion, mental depression.
  Muscle weakness, trembling, uncontrolled body movements.
  Nausea, vomiting, constipation, diarrhea, impaired urination.
  Serious Adverse Effects
  Idiosyncratic Reactions: Paradoxical responses of excitement, hyperactivity, agitation, anger, hostility.
  Rare blood cell disorders: abnormally low red blood cell, white blood cell and platelet counts.

▷ **Possible Effects on Sexual Function:** Increased libido, enlargement of male breasts.

Possible Effects on Laboratory Tests

Complete blood cell counts: decreased red cells, hemoglobin, white cells and platelets.

Urine screening tests for drug abuse: may be **positive.** (Test results depend upon amount of drug taken and testing method used.)

CAUTION

1. This drug should not be discontinued abruptly if it is being used to control seizures.
2. The concurrent use of some over-the-counter drug products that contain antihistamines (allergy and cold preparations, sleep aids) can cause excessive sedation in sensitive individuals.
3. Adverse behavioral reactions are more common in individuals with brain damage, mental retardation or a history of psychiatric disorders.
4. A decreased therapeutic response to this drug occurs in approximately 30% of users within 3 months after initiating treatment. Dosage adjustment may be necessary to restore seizure control.

Precautions for Use

By Infants and Children: This drug is used to treat infants and children of all ages. Careful dosage adjustment based on weight and age is mandatory. Abnormal behavioral responses are more common in children.

By Those over 60 Years of Age: It is advisable to use smaller doses at longer intervals to avoid overdosage. Observe for the possible development of lethargy, indifference, fatigue, weakness, unsteadiness, disturbing dreams, nightmares and paradoxical reactions of excitement, agitation, anger, hostility and rage.

▷ **Advisability of Use During Pregnancy**

Pregnancy Category: D (tentative). See Pregnancy Code inside back cover.

Animal studies: This drug causes cleft palates, open eyelids, fused rib structures and limb defects in rabbits.

Human studies: Information from adequate studies of pregnant women is not available.

It is advisable to avoid this drug during the first 3 months if possible. Frequent use in late pregnancy may cause the "floppy infant" syndrome in the newborn: weakness, lethargy, unresponsiveness, depressed breathing, low body temperature.

Advisability of Use if Breast-Feeding

Presence of this drug in breast milk: Probably yes.

Avoid drug or refrain from nursing.

Habit-Forming Potential: This drug can produce psychological and/or physical dependence (see Glossary) if used in large doses for an extended period of time. However, it is not liable to abuse.

Effects of Overdosage: Marked drowsiness, weakness, confusion, slurred speech, staggering gait, tremor, stupor progressing to deep sleep or coma.

Possible Effects of Long-Term Use: Benefits versus risks must be considered carefully during the extended use of this drug in children. Possible adverse effects on physical or mental development may not be apparent for many years.

Suggested Periodic Examinations While Taking This Drug (at physician's discretion)
During long-term use: Complete blood cell counts; liver function tests.

▷ **While Taking This Drug, Observe the Following**
Foods: No restrictions.
Beverages: No restrictions. May be taken with milk.
▷   *Alcohol:* Use with extreme caution until the combined effect is determined. Alcohol may increase the depressant effects of this drug on the brain. It is advisable to avoid alcohol completely—throughout the day and night—if it is necessary to drive or to engage in any hazardous activity.
Tobacco Smoking: No interactions expected.
Marijuana Smoking: Increased sedation and significant impairment of intellectual and physical performance.
▷   *Other Drugs*
Clonazepam *taken concurrently* with
• valproic acid (Depakene, etc.) may cause continuous absence seizures.
The following drugs may *increase* the effects of clonazepam
• cimetidine (Tagamet).
• disulfiram (Antabuse).
• omeprazole (Losec).
• oral contraceptives.
The following drugs may *decrease* the effects of clonazepam
• theophylline (aminophylline, Theo-Dur, etc.).
▷   *Driving, Hazardous Activities:* This drug can impair mental alertness, judgment, physical coordination and reaction time. Avoid hazardous activities accordingly.
Aviation Note: The use of this drug *is a disqualification* for piloting. Consult a designated Aviation Medical Examiner.
Exposure to Sun: No restrictions.
Discontinuation: Avoid sudden discontinuation if this drug is being used to control any type of seizure, or if it has been taken for more than 4 weeks to treat other conditions. Dosage should be tapered gradually to prevent a withdrawal syndrome that could include depression, confusion, hallucinations, tremor, seizures, muscle cramping, sweating and vomiting.

CLONIDINE
(KLOH ni deen)

Introduced: 1969

Class: Antihypertensive

Prescription: USA: Yes
Canada: Yes

Controlled Drug: USA: No
Canada: No

Available as Generic: USA: Yes
Canada: No

Brand Names: Catapres, Catapres-TTS, Combipres [CD], ✦Dixarit

---

BENEFITS versus RISKS

Possible Benefits	*Possible Risks*
EFFECTIVE ANTIHYPERTENSIVE in mild to moderate high blood pressure Effective control of menopausal hot flashes (in selected cases)	ACUTE WITHDRAWAL SYNDROME and hypertensive "overshoot" with abrupt discontinuation Raynaud's phenomenon (cold fingers or toes)

▷ **Principal Uses**

As a Single Drug Product: This antihypertensive drug is often used as a "step 2" drug in the treatment of mild to moderate high blood pressure. It is generally not used to initiate treatment, but is added when a "step 1" drug proves to be inadequate. It may also be used as a "step 3 or 4" drug in place of drugs that cause marked orthostatic hypotension (see Glossary). It is sometimes used to prevent migraine headache, to prevent hot flashes of the menopause and to treat menstrual cramps.

As a Combination Drug Product [CD]: This "step 2" antihypertensive is available in combination with the "step 1" antihypertensive drug chlorthalidone, a diuretic. The differing methods of action complement each other to make the combination a more effective antihypertensive.

How This Drug Works: By decreasing the activity of the vasomotor center in the brain, this drug reduces the ability of the sympathetic nervous system to maintain the degree of blood vessel constriction responsible for the elevation of blood pressure. This change results in relaxation of blood vessel walls and lowering of blood pressure.

Available Dosage Forms and Strengths
Patches — 0.1 mg, 0.2 mg, 0.3 mg
Tablets — 0.1 mg, 0.2 mg, 0.3 mg

▷ **Usual Adult Dosage Range:** Tablets—initially 0.1 mg twice daily. Increase by 0.1 to 0.2 mg daily as needed and tolerated. Usual range is 0.2 to 0.8 mg daily, taken in 2 doses. Total daily dosage should not exceed 2.4 mg.

Medicated patches are applied once a week. **Note: Actual dosage and administration schedule must be determined by the physician for each patient individually.**

▷ **Dosing Instructions:**   Tablets may be taken without regard to eating. The tablet may be crushed for administration.

Usual Duration of Use: Continual use on a regular schedule for 2 to 3 weeks is usually necessary to determine this drug's effectiveness in controlling high blood pressure. Long-term use (months to years) requires supervision and guidance by the physician. Consult your physician on a regular basis.

▷ **This Drug Should Not Be Taken If**
• you have had an allergic reaction to it previously.

▷ **Inform Your Physician Before Taking This Drug If**
• you have a circulatory disorder of the brain.
• you have angina or coronary artery disease.
• you have or have had serious emotional depression.
• you have Buerger's disease or Raynaud's phenomenon.
• you are taking any sedative or hypnotic drugs or an antidepressant.
• you plan to have surgery under general anesthesia in the near future.

Possible Side-Effects (natural, expected and unavoidable drug actions)
Drowsiness (35%), dry nose and mouth (40%), constipation (common), decreased heart rate, mild orthostatic hypotension (see Glossary).

▷ **Possible Adverse Effects** (unusual, unexpected and infrequent reactions)
If any of the following develop, consult your physician promptly for guidance.
Mild Adverse Effects
Allergic Reactions: Skin rash, hives, localized swellings, itching.
Headache, dizziness, fatigue, anxiety, nervousness, dryness and burning of eyes.
Painful parotid (salivary) gland, nausea, vomiting.
Weight gain, urinary retention.
Serious Adverse Effects
Idiosyncratic Reaction: Raynaud's phenomenon (see Glossary).
Aggravation of congestive heart failure, heart rhythm disorders, vivid dreaming, nightmares, depression, hallucinations.
Corneal ulcers (rare). Acute pancreatitis (rare).

▷ **Possible Effects on Sexual Function:**   Decreased libido in 10% (0.2 to 0.8 mg/day); impotence in 8% to 24% (0.5 to 3.6 mg/day); impaired ejaculation (rare); enlargement of male breasts (0.2 to 0.8 mg/day).

Possible Effects on Laboratory Tests
Blood cholesterol and triglyceride levels: no consistent or significant effects.

Blood sodium level: increased.

Liver function tests: one case of increased liver enzymes (ALT/GPT, AST/GOT, alkaline phosphatase).

CAUTION
1. ***Do not discontinue this drug suddenly.*** Sudden withdrawal can produce a severe and possibly fatal reaction.
2. Hot weather and the fever associated with infection can reduce blood pressure significantly. Dosage adjustments may be necessary.
3. Report the development of any tendency to emotional depression.

Precautions for Use
By Infants and Children: Safety and effectiveness for use by those under 12 years of age have not been established.

*By Those over 60 Years of Age: **Proceed cautiously*** with the use of any antihypertensive drug. Unacceptably high blood pressure should be reduced without creating the risks associated with excessively low blood pressure. Start treatment with small doses and monitor the blood pressure response frequently. Observe for the development of lightheadedness, dizziness, unsteadiness, fainting and falling. Sedation and dry mouth occur in 50% of elderly users. Report promptly any changes in mood or behavior: depression, delusions, hallucinations.

▷ Advisability of Use During Pregnancy
Pregnancy Category: C (tentative). See Pregnancy Code inside back cover.

Animal studies: No birth defects reported. However, this drug is toxic to the embryo in low dosage.

Human studies: Information from adequate studies of pregnant women is not available.

The manufacturer recommends that this drug be avoided by women who are or who may become pregnant. Ask physician for guidance.

Advisability of Use if Breast-Feeding
Presence of this drug in breast milk: Yes.

This drug may impair milk production. Monitor nursing infant closely and discontinue drug or nursing if adverse effects develop.

Habit-Forming Potential: None.

Effects of Overdosage: Marked drowsiness, weakness, dry mouth, slow pulse, low blood pressure, vomiting, stupor progressing to coma.

Possible Effects of Long-Term Use: Development of tolerance (see Glossary) with loss of drug effectiveness; weight gain due to salt and water retention; temporary sexual impotence.

Suggested Periodic Examinations While Taking This Drug (at physician's discretion)
Blood pressure measurements, monitoring of body weight.

▷ **While Taking This Drug, Observe the Following**

Foods: Avoid excessive salt. Ask physician for guidance regarding degree of salt restriction.

Beverages: No restrictions. May be taken with milk.

▷ *Alcohol:* Use with extreme caution. The combined effects can cause marked drowsiness and exaggerated reduction of blood pressure.

Tobacco Smoking: No interactions expected. Follow your physician's advice regarding use of tobacco.

▷ *Other Drugs*

Clonidine may *decrease* the effects of

- levodopa (Larodopa, Sinemet, etc.), causing an increase in parkinsonism symptoms.

Clonidine *taken concurrently* with

- beta-adrenergic-blocking drugs (Inderal, Lopressor, etc.) may increase the risk of serious rebound hypertension if clonidine is discontinued first. It is advisable to discontinue the beta blocker first and then withdraw clonidine gradually.

The following drugs may *decrease* the effects of clonidine

- tricyclic antidepressants (Elavil, Sinequan, etc.) may reduce its effectiveness in lowering blood pressure.

▷ *Driving, Hazardous Activities:* Use caution. This drug can cause drowsiness and can impair mental alertness, judgment and coordination.

Aviation Note: Hypertension (high blood pressure) *is a disqualification* for piloting. Consult a designated Aviation Medical Examiner.

Exposure to Sun: No restrictions.

Exposure to Heat: Use caution. Hot environments may reduce the blood pressure significantly; be alert to the possibility of orthostatic hypotension (see Glossary).

Exposure to Cold: Use caution. This drug may cause painful blanching and numbness of the hands and feet on exposure to cold air or water (Raynaud's phenomenon).

Heavy Exercise or Exertion: Use caution. Isometric exercises—the "overload" technique for strengthening individual muscles—can raise blood pressure significantly. The use of this drug may intensify the hypertensive response to isometric exercise. Ask physician for guidance.

Occurrence of Unrelated Illness: Fever associated with infections may lower the blood pressure significantly. Repeated vomiting may prevent the regular use of this drug and result in an acute withdrawal reaction. Consult your physician.

Discontinuation: Do not discontinue this drug suddenly. A severe withdrawal reaction can occur within 12 to 48 hours after the last dose. The dose should be reduced gradually over 3 to 4 days, with periodic monitoring of the blood pressure.

CLORAZEPATE
(klor AZ e payt)

Introduced: 1968

Class: Mild tranquilizer, benzodiazepines

Prescription: USA: Yes
Canada: Yes

Controlled Drug: USA: C-IV*
Canada: No

Available as Generic: Yes

Brand Names: Gen-Xene, ✦Novoclopate, Tranxene, Tranxene-SD, Tranxene-SD Half Strength

---

BENEFITS versus RISKS

Possible Benefits	*Possible Risks*
RELIEF OF ANXIETY AND NERVOUS TENSION in 70% to 80% of users	Habit-forming potential with prolonged use
Wide margin of safety with therapeutic doses	Minor impairment of mental functions
Very few drug interactions	

▷ **Principal Uses**

As a Single Drug Product: Used primarily to (1) provide short-term relief of
mild to moderate anxiety, and (2) provide adjunctive treatment in
controlling "partial" seizures, a type of epilepsy.

How This Drug Works: It is thought that this drug produces a calming effect
by enhancing the action of the nerve transmitter gamma-aminobutyric
acid (GABA), which in turn blocks the arousal of higher brain centers.

Available Dosage Forms and Strengths
Capsules — 3.75 mg, 7.5 mg, 15 mg
Tablets — 3.75 mg, 7.5 mg, 15 mg
Tablets, single dose — 11.25 mg, 22.5 mg

▷ **Usual Adult Dosage Range:** 15 to 60 mg/24 hours, in 2 to 4 divided doses
or as a single dose at bedtime. The usual dose is 30 mg/24 hours. Total
daily dose should not exceed 90 mg. **Note: Actual dosage and administration schedule must be determined by the physician for each patient individually.**

▷ **Dosing Instructions:** May be taken on empty stomach or with food or milk.
Capsule may be opened and regular tablet may be crushed for administration; the single-dose tablet should not be crushed. Do not discontinue this drug abruptly if taken for more than 4 weeks.

*See Schedules of Controlled Drugs inside back cover.

Usual Duration of Use: Continual use on a regular schedule for 5 to 7 days is usually necessary to determine this drug's effectiveness in relieving moderate anxiety. Limit continual use to 1 to 3 weeks. Avoid uninterrupted and prolonged use.

▷ **This Drug Should Not Be Taken If**
- you have had an allergic reaction to any dosage form of it previously.
- you have acute narrow-angle glaucoma.

▷ **Inform Your Physician Before Taking This Drug If**
- you are allergic to any benzodiazepine drug (see Drug Class, Section Four).
- you have a history of alcoholism or drug abuse.
- you are pregnant or planning pregnancy.
- you have impaired liver or kidney function.
- you have a history of serious depression or mental disorder.
- you have any of the following: asthma, emphysema, epilepsy, myasthenia gravis.

Possible Side-Effects (natural, expected and unavoidable drug actions)
Drowsiness, lethargy, unsteadiness; "hangover" effects on the day following bedtime use.

▷ **Possible Adverse Effects** (unusual, unexpected and infrequent reactions)
If any of the following develop, consult your physician promptly for guidance.
Mild Adverse Effects
Allergic Reactions: Skin rash, hives.
Dizziness, fainting, blurred vision, double vision, slurred speech, sweating, nausea.
Serious Adverse Effects
Idiosyncratic Reactions: Paradoxical responses of excitement, agitation, anger, rage.

▷ **Possible Effects on Sexual Function:**   Altered timing and pattern of menstruation.

Possible Effects on Laboratory Tests
Urine screening tests for drug abuse: may be **positive.** (Test results depend upon amount of drug taken and testing method used.)

CAUTION
1. This drug should not be discontinued abruptly if it has been taken continually for more than 4 weeks.
2. The concurrent use of some over-the-counter drug products that contain antihistamines (allergy and cold preparations, sleep aids) can cause excessive sedation in sensitive individuals.
3. If this drug is taken at bedtime as a hypnotic (see Glossary), significant impairment of intellectual and physical skills may persist into

the following day; avoid alcohol and hazardous activities (driving, etc.).

Precautions for Use

By Infants and Children: Safety and effectiveness for use by those under 9 years of age have not been established. This drug should not be used in the hyperactive or psychotic child of any age.

By Those over 60 Years of Age: It is advisable to use smaller doses at longer intervals to avoid overdosage. Observe for the possible development of lethargy, indifference, fatigue, weakness, unsteadiness, disturbing dreams, nightmares and paradoxical reactions of excitement, agitation, anger, hostility and rage.

▷ **Advisability of Use During Pregnancy**

Pregnancy Category: D (tentative). See Pregnancy Code inside back cover.

Animal studies: No birth defects reported in mouse, rat and rabbit studies.

Human studies: Information from adequate studies of pregnant women is not available.

There has been one report of multiple birth defects in a fetus exposed to this drug during the first 3 months. Frequent use in late pregnancy can cause the "floppy infant" syndrome in the newborn: weakness, lethargy, unresponsiveness, depressed breathing, low body temperature. Avoid use during entire pregnancy.

Advisability of Use if Breast-Feeding

Presence of this drug in breast milk: Yes, in small amounts.

Avoid drug or refrain from nursing.

Habit-Forming Potential: This drug can produce psychological and/or physical dependence (see Glossary) if used in large doses for an extended period of time.

Effects of Overdosage: Marked drowsiness, weakness, feeling of drunkenness, staggering gait, tremor, stupor progressing to deep sleep or coma.

Possible Effects of Long-Term Use: Psychological and/or physical dependence.

Suggested Periodic Examinations While Taking This Drug (at physician's discretion)

During long-term use: Complete blood cell counts.

▷ **While Taking This Drug, Observe the Following**

Foods: No restrictions.

Beverages: Avoid excessive intake of caffeine-containing beverages: coffee, tea, cola. May be taken with milk.

▷ *Alcohol:* Use with extreme caution until the combined effect is determined. Alcohol may increase the absorption of this drug and add to its depressant effects on the brain. It is advisable to avoid alcohol completely—throughout the day and night—if it is necessary to drive or to engage in any hazardous activity.

Tobacco Smoking: Heavy smoking may reduce the calming action of this drug.

Marijuana Smoking: Increased sedation and significant impairment of intellectual and physical performance.

▷ *Other Drugs*

Clorazepate may *increase* the effects of
- digoxin (Lanoxin), and cause digoxin toxicity.

Clorazepate may *decrease* the effects of
- levodopa (Sinemet, etc.), and reduce its effectiveness in treating Parkinson's disease.

The following drugs may *increase* the effects of clorazepate
- cimetidine (Tagamet).
- disulfiram (Antabuse).
- isoniazid (INH, Rifamate, etc.).
- oral contraceptives.
- valproic acid (Depakene).

The following drugs may *decrease* the effects of clorazepate
- rifampin (Rimactane, etc.).
- theophylline (aminophylline, Theo-Dur, etc.).

▷ *Driving, Hazardous Activities:* This drug can impair mental alertness, judgment, physical coordination and reaction time. Avoid hazardous activities accordingly.

Aviation Note: The use of this drug *is a disqualification* for piloting. Consult a designated Aviation Medical Examiner.

Exposure to Sun: No restrictions.

Discontinuation: Avoid sudden discontinuation if this drug has been taken for more than 4 weeks. Dosage should be tapered gradually to prevent a withdrawal syndrome that could include depression, confusion, hallucinations, tremor, seizures, muscle cramping, sweating and vomiting.

CLOXACILLIN
(klox a SIL in)

Introduced: 1962

Class: Antibiotic, penicillins

Prescription: USA: Yes
Canada: Yes

Controlled Drug: USA: No
Canada: No

Available as Generic: USA: Yes
Canada: No

Brand Names: ✦Apo-Cloxi, ✦Bactopen, Cloxapen, ✦Novocloxin, ✦Orbenin, Tegopen

---

BENEFITS versus RISKS

Possible Benefits	*Possible Risks*
EFFECTIVE TREATMENT OF INFECTIONS due to susceptible microorganisms	ALLERGIC REACTIONS, mild to severe Superinfections (yeast) Drug-induced colitis Rare blood cell disorders

---

▷ **Principal Uses**

As a Single Drug Product: Used primarily to treat infections that are caused by bacteria (principally staphylococcus) that have developed resistance to the original types of penicillin. It is of value in treating infections of the skin and skin structures, the upper and lower respiratory tract (including "strep" throat) and infections that are widely scattered throughout the body.

How This Drug Works: This drug destroys susceptible infecting bacteria by interfering with their ability to produce new protective cell walls as they multiply and grow.

Available Dosage Forms and Strengths

Capsules — 250 mg, 500 mg
Oral solution — 125 mg per 5-ml teaspoonful

▷ **Usual Adult Dosage Range:**   250 to 500 mg/6 hours (4 doses/24 hours). The maximal dose is 6000 mg/24 hours. **Note: Actual dosage and administration schedule must be determined by the physician for each patient individually.**

▷ **Dosing Instructions:**   Take on empty stomach, 1 hour before or 2 hours after eating, at same times each day. Capsule may be opened for administration.

Usual Duration of Use: As long as necessary to eradicate the infection. For all streptococcal infections: not less than 10 consecutive days (without interruption) to reduce the possibility of developing rheumatic fever or glomerulonephritis.

▷ **This Drug Should Not Be Taken If**
   • you have had an allergic reaction to any dosage form of it previously.
   • you are certain you are allergic to *any* form of penicillin.

▷ **Inform Your Physician Before Taking This Drug If**
   • you suspect you may be allergic to penicillin or you have a history of a previous "reaction" to penicillin.
   • you are allergic to cephalosporin antibiotics (Ancef, Ceporan, Ceporex, Duricef, Kafocin, Keflex, Keflin, Kefzol, Loridine).
   • you are allergic by nature—hay fever, asthma, hives, eczema.

- you have a history of kidney disease, regional enteritis or ulcerative colitis.

Possible Side-Effects (natural, expected and unavoidable drug actions)
Superinfections (see Glossary), often due to yeast organisms.

▷ **Possible Adverse Effects** (unusual, unexpected and infrequent reactions)
If any of the following develop, consult your physician promptly for guidance.
Mild Adverse Effects
Allergic Reactions: Skin rashes, hives, itching.
Irritations of mouth and tongue, unpleasant taste, nausea, vomiting, mild diarrhea.
Serious Adverse Effects
Allergic Reactions: Anaphylactic reaction (see Glossary), severe skin reactions, drug fever, swollen painful joints, sore throat.
Pseudomembranous colitis—severe diarrhea.

▷ **Possible Effects on Sexual Function:**   None reported.

Possible Effects on Laboratory Tests
Complete blood cell counts: decreased white cells; increased eosinophils (allergic reaction).

CAUTION
1. Take the exact dose and the full course prescribed.
2. This drug should not be used concurrently with antibiotics like erythromycin or tetracycline.

Precautions for Use
By Infants and Children: Dosage is based on age and weight. Consult your physician for precise dosage schedule.
By Those over 60 Years of Age: It is advisable to evaluate kidney function before and during use of this drug to determine the need for dosage adjustment. Natural changes in the skin may predispose to prolonged itching reactions in the genital and anal regions. Report such reactions promptly.

▷ **Advisability of Use During Pregnancy**
Pregnancy Category: B (tentative). See Pregnancy Code inside back cover.
Animal studies: No birth defects reported in rabbit studies.
Human studies: Information from adequate studies of pregnant women indicates no increased risk of birth defects in 3546 pregnancies exposed to penicillin derivatives.
Use only if clearly needed. Ask physician for guidance.

Advisability of Use if Breast-Feeding
Presence of this drug in breast milk: Probably yes.
The nursing infant may be sensitized to penicillin and may be at risk for diarrhea or yeast infections. Avoid drug if possible or refrain from nursing.

Habit-Forming Potential: None.

Effects of Overdosage: Possible nausea, vomiting and/or diarrhea.

Possible Effects of Long-Term Use: Superinfections, often due to yeast organisms.

Suggested Periodic Examinations While Taking This Drug (at physician's discretion)
Complete blood cell counts. Liver and kidney function tests with long-term use.

▷ **While Taking This Drug, Observe the Following**
Foods: No restrictions.
Beverages: No restrictions.
▷ *Alcohol:* No interactions expected.
Tobacco Smoking: No interactions expected.
▷ *Other Drugs*
Cloxacillin may *decrease* the effects of
• oral contraceptives in some women, and impair their effectiveness in preventing pregnancy.
The following drugs may *decrease* the effects of cloxacillin
• antacids may reduce the absorption of cloxacillin.
• chloramphenicol (Chloromycetin).
• erythromycin (Erythrocin, E-Mycin, etc.).
• tetracyclines (Achromycin, Declomycin, Minocin, etc.). (See Drug Class, Section Four.)
▷ *Driving, Hazardous Activities:* Usually no restrictions.
Aviation Note: The use of this drug *may be a disqualification* for piloting. Consult a designated Aviation Medical Examiner.
Exposure to Sun: No restrictions.
Special Storage Instructions: Keep capsules in a tightly closed container at room temperature. Keep oral solution in the refrigerator.
Observe the Following Expiration Times: Oral solution kept refrigerated is good for 14 days; when kept at room temperature, it is good for only 3 days.

CLOZAPINE
(KLOH za peen)

Introduced: 1975
(Antipsychotic)

Class: Strong tranquilizer

Prescription: USA: Yes

Controlled Drug: USA: No

Available as Generic: USA: No

Brand Name: Clozaril

Note: In the U.S., this drug is available only by special arrangement through the Clozaril Patient Management System, administered by Caremark Homecare Corporation (telephone: (800–237-CPMS). Consult your physician for details.

BENEFITS versus RISKS

Possible Benefits	*Possible Risks*
EFFECTIVE CONTROL OF SEVERE SCHIZOPHRENIA that has failed to respond adequately to other appropriate drugs	SERIOUS BLOOD CELL DISORDERS: abnormally low white blood cell and platelet counts (3%)
Improvement in 30% of refractory cases	DRUG-INDUCED SEIZURES (1% to 5%, depending upon size of dose)

▷ **Principal Uses**

As a Single Drug Product: This atypical antipsychotic drug is used solely in the management of severe schizophrenia that has failed to respond to adequate trials of at least two standard antipsychotic medications. Because of its potential for causing serious blood cell disorders and seizures, its use is reserved for the severely ill schizophrenic patient.

How This Drug Works: Not completely established. It is thought that by inhibiting the action of dopamine in certain brain areas, this drug acts to correct an imbalance of nerve impulse transmissions that is thought to be responsible for schizophrenic thought disorders.

Available Dosage Forms and Strengths
Tablets — 25 mg, 100 mg

▷ **Usual Adult Dosage Range:** Initially 25 mg one or two times a day; the dose is gradually increased by 25 mg to 50 mg daily, as tolerated, to reach a dose of 300 mg to 450 mg daily by the end of two weeks. Subsequent increases should be limited to 100 mg one or two times a week. Average dosage requirements are 600 mg daily. Total daily dosage should not exceed 900 mg. **Note: Actual dosage and administration schedule must be determined by the physician for each patient individually.**

▷ **Dosing Instructions:** May be taken without regard to meals or with food if necessary to reduce stomach irritation. The tablet may be crushed for administration.

Usual Duration of Use:
Continual use on a regular schedule for several weeks is usually necessary to determine this drug's effectiveness in controlling schizophrenic manifestations. If not significantly beneficial within 6 to 8 weeks, consideration should be given to discontinuing this drug. Long-term use (months to years) requires periodic evaluation of response and dosage adjustment. Consult your physician on a regular basis.

Possible Advantages of This Drug
Rarely causes significant sexual dysfunction.
Low incidence of Parkinson-like reactions (see Glossary).
Does not cause tardive dyskinesia (see Glossary).

Currently a "Drug of Choice"
for treatment of severe schizophrenia in patients who have not responded satisfactorily to other standard antipsychotic drugs or have experienced unacceptable adverse effects from them.

▷ **This Drug Should Not Be Taken If**
- you have had an allergic reaction to it previously.
- you have experienced severe bone marrow depression (impaired white blood cell production) with previous use of this drug.
- you presently have any type of bone marrow or blood cell disorder.
- you are currently taking any other drug that can cause bone marrow depression (see Glossary).

▷ **Inform Your Physician Before Taking This Drug If**
- you have a history of any type of seizure disorder.
- you have a history of narrow-angle glaucoma.
- you have any type of heart or circulatory disorder, especially heart rhythm abnormalities or hypertension.
- you have impaired liver or kidney function.
- you have prostatism (see Glossary).

Possible Side-Effects
(natural, expected and unavoidable drug actions)
Drowsiness (39%), dizziness (19%), light-headedness, orthostatic hypotension (9%) (see Glossary).
Blurred vision (5%), salivation (31%), dry mouth (6%), impaired urination (2%), constipation (14%).

▷ **Possible Adverse Effects**
(unusual, unexpected and infrequent reactions)
If any of the following develop, consult your physician promptly for guidance.

Mild Adverse Effects

Allergic Reactions: Skin rash (2%); drug fever (see Glossary) which usually occurs within the first 3 weeks of treatment and is self-limiting (5%).

Headache (7%), tremor (6%), fainting (6%), nightmares (4%), restlessness (4%), confusion (3%), depression (1%).

Rapid heartbeat (25%), hypertension (4%), chest pain (1%).

Nausea (5%), indigestion (4%), vomiting (3%), diarrhea (2%).

Serious Adverse Effects

Bone marrow depression: specific impairment of white blood cell production with potential for serious infection (3%).

Drug-induced seizures, dose-related (1% to 5%).

▷ **Possible Effects on Sexual Function:** Impotence (rare), abnormal ejaculation (1%).

▷ **Adverse Effects That May Mimic Natural Diseases or Disorders**

Drug-induced fever (usually benign) may suggest the possibility of systemic infection. Because of the risk of bone marrow depression and secondary infection, any occurrence of fever must be carefully evaluated.

Drug-induced seizures may suggest the possibility of epilepsy.

Natural Diseases or Disorders That May Be Activated by This Drug

Latent glaucoma, prostatism.

Possible Effects on Laboratory Tests

White blood cell counts: decreased.

CAUTION

1. The early detection of any tendency to drug-induced bone marrow depression is mandatory. Baseline white blood cell counts must be determined before clozapine treatment is started; followup counts must be made every week during the entire course of treatment and for 4 weeks after discontinuation of clozapine.
2. Report promptly any indications of a possible infection: fever, sore throat, flulike symptoms, skin infections, painful urination, etc.
3. Report promptly any tendency to light-headedness or dizziness on rising from a sitting or lying position; this could be an indication of orthostatic hypotension (see Glossary).
4. Consult your physician before taking any other medication while taking clozapine. This includes all prescription and over-the-counter drugs.

Precautions for Use

By Infants and Children: Safety and effectiveness for use by those under 16 years of age have not been established.

By Those over 60 Years of Age: You may be more susceptible to the development of orthostatic hypotension, confusion, excitement and prostatism. Report related symptoms promptly.

▷ **Advisability of Use During Pregnancy**
  Pregnancy Category: B (tentative). See Pregnancy Code inside back cover.
  Animal studies: No birth defects due to this drug reported.
  Human studies: Information from adequate studies of pregnant women
    is not available.
  Use this drug only if clearly needed.

Advisability of Use if Breast-Feeding
  Presence of this drug in breast milk: Unknown.
  Avoid drug or refrain from nursing.

Habit-Forming Potential: None.

Effects of Overdosage: Marked drowsiness, delirium, hallucinations, rapid
    and irregular heartbeat, irregular breathing, fainting.

Possible Effects of Long-Term Use: None reported to date.

Suggested Periodic Examinations While Taking This Drug
  (at physician's discretion)
  White blood cell and differential counts prior to starting therapy, every
    week during therapy and for 4 weeks after termination of therapy.
  Serial blood pressure measurements and electrocardiograms.

▷ **While Taking This Drug, Observe the Following**
  Foods: No restrictions.
  Beverages: No restrictions. May be taken with milk.
▷ *Alcohol:* Avoid completely. Alcohol can increase the sedative action of this
    drug and accentuate its depressant effects of brain function and blood
    pressure. This drug can increase the intoxicating effects of alcohol.
  Tobacco Smoking: May accelerate the elimination of this drug and require
    increased dosage.
  Marijuana Smoking: Moderate increase in drowsiness; accentuation of or-
    thostatic hypotension; increased risk of aggravating psychosis.
▷ *Other Drugs*
  Clozapine may ***increase*** the effects of
    • drugs with sedative actions; observe for excessive sedation.
    • drugs with atropinelike actions (see Drug Class, Section Four).
    • antihypertensive drugs; observe for excessive reduction of blood pres-
      sure.
  Clozapine ***taken concurrently*** with
    • other bone marrow depressant drugs may increase the risk of impaired
      white blood cell production.
    • warfarin (Coumadin, etc.) may increase the anticoagulant effect and
      cause abnormal bleeding.
    • lithium (Lithobid, Lithotab, etc.) may increase the risk of confusional
      states, seizures and neuroleptic malignant syndrome (see Glossary).
▷ *Driving, Hazardous Activities:* This drug may cause drowsiness, dizziness,
    blurred vision, confusion and seizures. Restrict activities as necessary.
  Aviation Note: The use of this drug **is a disqualification** for piloting. Consult
    a designated Aviation Medical Examiner.

Exposure to Sun: No restrictions.

Exposure to Heat: Use caution until tolerance to environmental heat is determined. This drug can cause fever and can impair the body's adaptation to heat.

Occurrence of Unrelated Illness: Monitor all intercurrent infections very carefully and provide vigorous treatment. Observe white blood cell response to infection closely.

Discontinuation: If possible, this drug should be discontinued gradually over a period of 1 to 2 weeks. If abrupt withdrawal is necessary, observe carefully for recurrence of psychotic symptoms.

CODEINE
(KOH deen)

Introduced: 1886

Class: Analgesic, narcotic

Prescription: USA: Yes
Canada: Yes

Controlled Drug: USA: C-II*
Canada: <N>

Available as Generic: Yes

Brand Names: Actifed w/Codeine [CD], Ambenyl Expectorant [CD], Ambenyl Syrup [CD], Atasol-8, -15, -30 [CD], Benylin Syrup w/Codeine [CD], Bufferin w/Codeine [CD], ✦Coryphen-Codeine [CD], Dimetane Cough Syrup-DC [CD], Dimetane Expectorant-C [CD], Dimetapp-C [CD], Dimetapp w/Codeine [CD], Empirin w/Codeine No. 2, 4 [CD], Empracet w/Codeine No. 3, 4 [CD], ✦Empracet-30, -60 [CD], ✦Emtec-30 [CD], ✦Exdol [CD], ✦Exdol-8, -15, -30 [CD], ✦Fiorinal-C 1/4, -C 1/2 [CD], Fiorinal w/Codeine No. 1, 2, 3 [CD], Isoclor Expectorant [CD], ✦Lenoltec w/Codeine No. 1, 2, 3, 4 [CD], Naldecon-CX [CD], ✦Novahistex C [CD], ✦Paveral, Penntuss [CD], ✦Phenaphen No. 2, 3, 4 [CD], Phenaphen w/Codeine No. 2, 3, 4 [CD], Phenergan w/Codeine [CD], Robaxisal-C [CD], ✦Rounox w/Codeine [CD], Triaminic Expectorant w/Codeine [CD], ✦Tylenol w/Codeine [CD], Tylenol w/Codeine No. 1, 2, 3, 4 [CD], ✦Tylenol w/Codeine Elixir [CD]

BENEFITS versus RISKS

Possible Benefits	*Possible Risks*
EFFECTIVE RELIEF OF MODERATE TO SEVERE PAIN	Low potential for habit formation (dependence)
EFFECTIVE CONTROL OF COUGH	Mild allergic reactions (infrequent)
	Nausea, constipation

*See Schedules of Controlled Drugs inside back cover.

▷ **Principal Uses**

As a Single Drug Product: Used primarily to (1) relieve moderate to severe pain; (2) control cough; (3) control diarrhea. Its widest use is as an ingredient in analgesic preparations and cough remedies. Its constipating effect is sometimes used to treat diarrhea, though better drugs are now available for this purpose.

As a Combination Drug Product [CD]: Codeine is commonly combined with other milder analgesics to enhance their effectiveness, notably aspirin and acetaminophen. It is frequently added to cough mixtures containing antihistamines, decongestants and expectorants to make these "shotgun" preparations more effective in reducing the frequency and severity of cough.

How This Drug Works: Acting primarily as a depressant of certain brain functions, this drug suppresses the perception of pain, calms the emotional response to pain, reduces the sensitivity of the cough reflex and inhibits the activity of brain centers that regulate the intestinal tract.

Available Dosage Forms and Strengths
Injection — 30 mg per ml, 60 mg per ml
Tablets — 15 mg, 30 mg, 60 mg
Tablets, soluble — 15 mg, 30 mg, 60 mg

▷ **Usual Adult Dosage Range:**   As analgesic—15 to 60 mg/3 to 6 hours as needed. For cough—10 to 20 mg/4 to 6 hours as needed. For diarrhea—30 mg/6 hours as needed. Total daily dosage should not exceed 200 mg for pain or 120 mg for cough or diarrhea. **Note: Actual dosage and administration schedule must be determined by the physician for each patient individually.**

▷ **Dosing Instructions:**   May be taken with or following food to reduce stomach irritation or nausea. Tablet may be crushed for administration.

Usual Duration of Use: As required to control pain, cough or diarrhea. Continual use should not exceed 5 to 7 days without interruption and reassessment of need.

▷ **This Drug Should Not Be Taken If**
• you have had an allergic reaction to any dosage form of it previously.
• you are having an acute attack of asthma.

▷ **Inform Your Physician Before Taking This Drug If**
• you have a history of drug abuse or alcoholism.
• you have impaired liver or kidney function.
• you have gall-bladder disease, a seizure disorder or an underactive thyroid gland.
• you are taking any other drugs that have a sedative effect.
• you plan to have surgery under general anesthesia in the near future.

Possible Side-Effects (natural, expected and unavoidable drug actions)
Drowsiness, light-headedness, dry mouth, urinary retention, constipation.

▷ **Possible Adverse Effects** (unusual, unexpected and infrequent reactions)
If any of the following develop, consult your physician promptly for guidance.
Mild Adverse Effects
Allergic Reactions: Skin rash, hives, itching.
Dizziness, impaired concentration, sensation of drunkenness, confusion, depression, blurred or double vision.
Nausea, vomiting.
Serious Adverse Effects
Allergic Reactions: Anaphylaxis (rare), severe skin reactions.
Idiosyncratic Reactions: Delirium, hallucinations, excitement, increased sensitivity to pain after the analgesic effect has worn off.
Seizures (rare), impaired breathing.

▷ **Possible Effects on Sexual Function:**   None reported.

▷ **Adverse Effects That May Mimic Natural Diseases or Disorders**
Paradoxical behavioral disturbances may suggest psychotic disorder.

Possible Effects on Laboratory Tests
Blood platelet counts: decreased.
Blood amylase and lipase levels: increased (natural side-effect).
Urine screening tests for drug abuse: may be **positive**. (Test results depend upon amount of drug taken and testing method used.)

CAUTION
1. If you have asthma, chronic bronchitis or emphysema, excessive use of this drug may cause significant respiratory difficulty, thickening of bronchial secretions and suppression of coughing.
2. The concurrent use of this drug with atropinelike drugs can increase the risk of urinary retention and reduced intestinal function.
3. Do not take this drug following acute head injury.

Precautions for Use
By Infants and Children: Do not use this drug in children under 2 years of age because of their vulnerability to life-threatening respiratory depression.
By Those over 60 Years of Age: Use small doses initially and increase dosage as needed and tolerated. Limit use to short-term treatment only. There may be increased susceptibility to the development of drowsiness, dizziness, unsteadiness, falling, urinary retention and constipation (often leading to fecal impaction).

▷ **Advisability of Use During Pregnancy**
Pregnancy Category: C (tentative). See Pregnancy Code inside back cover.
Animal studies: Skull defects reported in hamster studies.

Human studies: Information from adequate studies of pregnant women is not available. Some studies suggest a possible increase in significant birth defects when this drug is taken during the first 6 months of pregnancy. Codeine taken during the last few weeks before delivery can cause withdrawal symptoms in the newborn infant.

Use this drug only if clearly needed and in small, infrequent doses.

Advisability of Use if Breast-Feeding
Presence of this drug in breast milk: Yes, in small amounts.
Avoid drug or refrain from nursing.

Habit-Forming Potential: Psychological and/or physical dependence can develop with use of large doses for an extended period of time. However, true dependence is infrequent and unlikely with prudent use.

Effects of Overdosage: Drowsiness, restlessness, agitation, nausea, vomiting, dry mouth, vertigo, weakness, lethargy, stupor, coma, seizures.

Possible Effects of Long-Term Use: Psychological and physical dependence, chronic constipation.

Suggested Periodic Examinations While Taking This Drug (at physician's discretion)
None.

▷ **While Taking This Drug, Observe the Following**
Foods: No restrictions.
Beverages: No restrictions. May be taken with milk.
▷ *Alcohol:* Use extreme caution until the combined effects have been determined. Codeine can intensify the intoxicating effects of alcohol, and alcohol can intensify the depressant effects of codeine on brain function, breathing and circulation.
Tobacco Smoking: No interactions expected.
Marijuana Smoking: Increase in drowsiness and pain relief; impairment of mental and physical performance.
▷ *Other Drugs*
Codeine may *increase* the effects of
• other drugs with sedative effects.
• atropinelike drugs, and increase the risk of constipation and urinary retention.
▷ *Driving, Hazardous Activities:* This drug can impair mental alertness, judgment, reaction time and physical coordination. Avoid hazardous activities accordingly.
Aviation Note: The use of this drug *is a disqualification* for piloting. Consult a designated Aviation Medical Examiner.
Exposure to Sun: No restrictions.
Discontinuation: It is advisable to limit this drug to short-term use. If it is necessary to use it for extended periods of time, discontinuation should be gradual to minimize possible effects of withdrawal (usually mild with codeine).

COLCHICINE
(KOL chi seen)

Introduced: 1763

Class: Antigout

Prescription: USA: Yes
Canada: No

Controlled Drug: USA: No
Canada: No

Available as Generic: Yes

Brand Names: Colabid [CD], ColBENEMID [CD], Proben-C [CD], ✦Verban [CD]

BENEFITS versus RISKS	
Possible Benefits	*Possible Risks*
EFFECTIVE RELIEF OF ACUTE GOUT SYMPTOMS	Loss of hair
Prevention of recurrent gout attacks	Rare bone marrow depression (see Glossary)
Prevention of attacks of Mediterranean fever	Rare peripheral neuritis (see Glossary)
	Rare liver damage

▷ **Principal Uses**
   As a Single Drug Product: Used primarily to reduce the pain, swelling and inflammation associated with acute attacks of gout. It is also used in smaller doses to prevent recurrent gout attacks. An infrequent use is the prevention and control of attacks of familial Mediterranean fever.
   As a Combination Drug Product [CD]: Colchicine is combined with probenecid to enhance its ability to prevent recurrent attacks of gout. While colchicine is most effective in relieving the symptoms of acute gout, it has some effect in preventing recurrent and chronic discomfort. Probenecid increases the elimination of uric acid by the kidneys and thereby reduces the blood level of uric acid to a point at which acute episodes of gout will not occur. This dual action is more effective than either drug used alone in the long-term management of gout.

How This Drug Works: It is thought that by decreasing the acidity of joint tissues, this drug reduces the deposit of uric acid crystals that cause acute inflammation and pain. (Colchicine does not lower the level of uric acid in the blood or increase the level of uric acid in the urine.)

Available Dosage Forms and Strengths
   Injection — 1 mg per 2 ml
   Tablets — 0.5 mg, 0.6 mg

▷ **Usual Adult Dosage Range:** For acute attack—0.5 to 1.3 mg initially, followed by 0.5 to 0.65 mg/1 to 2 hours until pain is relieved or nausea, vomiting or diarrhea occurs. The total dose should not exceed 10 mg.

For prevention of recurrent attacks—0.5 to 0.65 mg, 1 to 3 times/day.
Note: Actual dosage and administration schedule must be determined by the physician for each patient individually.

▷ **Dosing Instructions:**   May be taken either on an empty stomach or with food to reduce nausea or stomach irritation. Start treatment at the earliest indication of an acute attack. Take the exact dose prescribed. The tablet may be crushed for administration.

Usual Duration of Use: For acute attack—discontinue when pain is relieved or when nausea, vomiting or diarrhea occurs; do not resume this drug for 3 days without consulting your physician. For prevention—use the smallest effective dose for long-term management; consult your physician regarding dosage schedule and duration.

▷ **This Drug Should Not Be Taken If**
  • you have had an allergic reaction to it previously.
  • you have an active stomach or duodenal ulcer.
  • you have active ulcerative colitis.

▷ **Inform Your Physician Before Taking This Drug If**
  • you have a history of peptic ulcer disease or ulcerative colitis.
  • you have any type of heart disease.
  • you have impaired liver or kidney function.
  • you plan to have surgery in the near future.

Possible Side-Effects (natural, expected and unavoidable drug actions)
  Nausea, vomiting, abdominal cramping, diarrhea.

▷ **Possible Adverse Effects** (unusual, unexpected and infrequent reactions)
  If any of the following develop, consult your physician promptly for guidance.
  Mild Adverse Effects
  Allergic Reactions: Skin rash, hives, fever.
  Serious Adverse Effects
  Allergic Reaction: Anaphylactic reaction (see Glossary).
  Loss of hair.
  Bone marrow depression (see Glossary)—fatigue, weakness, fever, sore throat, abnormal bleeding or bruising.
  Peripheral neuritis (see Glossary)—numbness, tingling, pain, weakness in hands and/or feet.
  Inflammation of colon with bloody diarrhea.
  Liver damage.

▷ **Possible Effects on Sexual Function:**   None reported.

Possible Delayed Adverse Effects: Impaired production of sperm, possibly resulting in birth defects of child that was conceived while father was taking this drug.

Natural Diseases or Disorders That May Be Activated by This Drug
Peptic ulcer disease, ulcerative colitis.

Possible Effects on Laboratory Tests
Complete blood cell counts: decreased red cells, hemoglobin, white cells and platelets; increased white cells (follows initial decrease).

Prothrombin time: decreased (with concurrent use of warfarin).

Blood vitamin B^{12} level: decreased.

Liver function tests: increased liver enzymes (ALT/GPT, AST/GOT and alkaline phosphatase), increased bilirubin.

Fecal occult blood test: positive.

Sperm counts: decreased (may be marked).

CAUTION
1. If this drug causes vomiting and/or diarrhea before relief of joint pain, discontinue it and inform your physician.
2. Try to limit each course of treatment for acute gout to 4 to 8 mg. Do not exceed 3 mg/24 hours or a total of 10 mg/course.
3. Omit drug for 3 days between courses to avoid toxicity.
4. Carry this drug with you while traveling if you are subject to attacks of acute gout.
5. It is advisable to take colchicine preventively prior to and following surgery if you have recurrent gout. (Surgery often precipitates acute attacks of gout.) Ask your physician for proper dosage schedule.

Precautions for Use
By Infants and Children: Dosage has not been established. Ask physician for guidance.

By Those over 60 Years of Age: This drug has a very narrow margin of safety. Because the total dosage required to relieve the pain of acute gout often causes vomiting and/or diarrhea, extreme caution is advised when this drug is used by anyone with heart or circulatory disorders, reduced liver or kidney function or general debility.

▷ Advisability of Use During Pregnancy
Pregnancy Category: D (tentative). See Pregnancy Code inside back cover.

Animal studies: This drug causes significant birth defects in hamsters and rabbits.

Human studies: Information from adequate studies of pregnant women is not available. However, it is reported that colchicine can cause harm to the fetus.

Avoid during entire pregnancy if possible. Ask physician for guidance.

Advisability of Use if Breast-Feeding
Presence of this drug in breast milk: Unknown.

Avoid drug or refrain from nursing.

Habit-Forming Potential: None.

Effects of Overdosage: Nausea, vomiting, abdominal cramping, diarrhea (may be bloody), burning sensation in throat and skin, weak and rapid pulse, progressive paralysis, inability to breathe.

Possible Effects of Long-Term Use: Hair loss, aplastic anemia (see Glossary), peripheral neuritis (see Glossary).

Suggested Periodic Examinations While Taking This Drug (at physician's discretion)
Complete blood cell counts, uric acid blood levels to monitor status of gout, sperm analysis for quantity and condition, liver function tests.

▷ **While Taking This Drug, Observe the Following**
Foods: Follow physician's advice regarding the need for a low-purine diet.
Beverages: It is advisable to drink no less than 3 quarts of liquids/24 hours. This drug may be taken with milk. Some "herbal teas" (promoted as being beneficial for arthritis) contain phenylbutazone and other potentially toxic ingredients. Avoid herbal teas if you are not certain of their source, content and medicinal effects.
▷ *Alcohol:* No interactions expected. However, alcohol may increase the risk of gastrointestinal irritation or bleeding. It also raises uric acid blood levels and could interfere with gout management.
Tobacco Smoking: No interactions expected.
▷ *Other Drugs*
Colchicine *taken concurrently* with
  • allopurinol (Zyloprim), probenecid (Benemid) or sulfinpyrazone (Anturane) can prevent attacks of acute gout that often occur when treatment with these drugs is first started.
▷ *Driving, Hazardous Activities:* Usually no restrictions when taken continually in small (preventive) doses. Be alert to the possible occurrence of nausea, vomiting and/or diarrhea when taken in larger (treatment) doses.
Aviation Note: The use of this drug *may be a disqualification* for piloting. Consult a designated Aviation Medical Examiner.
Exposure to Sun: No restrictions.
Exposure to Cold: This drug can lower body temperature. Use caution to prevent excessive lowering (hypothermia), especially if you are over 60 years of age.
Occurrence of Unrelated Illness: Inform your physician if you are injured or if you develop any new illness or disorder. During periods of such stress you may be subject to acute attacks of gout, and it may be necessary to adjust your medication schedule.

COLESTIPOL
(koh LES ti pohl)

Introduced: 1974

Prescription: USA: Yes
Canada: Yes

Available as Generic: USA: No
Canada: No

Brand Name: Colestid

Class: Anticholesterol

Controlled Drug: USA: No
Canada: No

BENEFITS versus RISKS

Possible Benefits	*Possible Risks*
EFFECTIVE REDUCTION OF TOTAL CHOLESTEROL AND LOW DENSITY CHOLESTEROL IN TYPE IIa CHOLESTEROL DISORDERS (15% to 25% reduction of total cholesterol, 25% to 35% reduction of LDL cholesterol)	Constipation (may be severe)
	Reduced absorption of fat, fat-soluble vitamins (A, D, E and K) and folic acid
	Reduced formation of prothrombin with resultant bleeding
EFFECTIVE RELIEF OF ITCHING associated with biliary obstruction	

▷ **Principal Uses**

As a Single Drug Product: Used primarily to (1) reduce abnormally high blood levels of total cholesterol and low density (LDL) cholesterol in Type IIa cholesterol disorders; (2) relieve the itching due to the deposit of bile acids in the skin associated with partial biliary obstruction.

How This Drug Works: By combining with bile acids and bile salts in the intestinal tract, this drug forms insoluble complexes that are excreted in the feces. This removal of bile acids (which are necessary for food digestion) stimulates the conversion of cholesterol to bile acids to replace the loss; this in turn reduces the blood levels of cholesterol. By reducing the blood levels of bile acids, this drug hastens the absorption and clearance of bile acids deposited in the skin and thus relieves itching.

Available Dosage Forms and Strengths

Bottles — 250 grams, 500 grams
Packets — 5 grams

▷ **Usual Adult Dosage Range:** Initially 5 grams of powder 3 times daily. Dose may be increased slowly as needed and tolerated to 30 grams daily in

2 to 4 divided doses. **Note: Actual dosage and administration schedule must be determined by the physician for each patient individually.**

▷ **Dosing Instructions:** Always take just before or with a meal; this drug is ineffective when taken without food. Mix the powder thoroughly in 4 to 6 ounces of water, fruit juice, tomato juice, milk, thin soup or a soft food like applesauce. **Do not take it in its dry form.**

Usual Duration of Use: Continual use on a regular schedule for 4 to 6 weeks is usually necessary to determine this drug's effectiveness in lowering excessively high blood levels of cholesterol. Duration of use should not exceed 3 months if an adequate response does not occur. Long-term use (months to years) requires periodic evaluation of response and dosage adjustment. Consult your physician on a regular basis.

Currently a "Drug of Choice"
for initiating treatment of elevated LDL cholesterol. See Cholesterol Disorders in Section Two.

▷ **This Drug Should Not Be Taken If**
- you have had an allergic reaction to it previously.
- you have complete biliary obstruction.

▷ **Inform Your Physician Before Taking This Drug If**
- you are prone to constipation.
- you have peptic ulcer disease.
- you have a bleeding disorder of any kind.
- you have impaired kidney function.

Possible Side-Effects (natural, expected and unavoidable drug actions)
Constipation (10%); interference with normal fat digestion and absorption; reduced absorption of vitamins A, D, E and K and folic acid.

▷ **Possible Adverse Effects** (unusual, unexpected and infrequent reactions)
If any of the following develop, consult your physician promptly for guidance.
Mild Adverse Effects
Allergic Reactions: Skin rash (0.1%), hives, tongue irritation, anal itching.
Headache, dizziness, weakness, muscle and joint pains.
Loss of appetite, indigestion, heartburn, abdominal discomfort, excessive gas, nausea, vomiting, diarrhea.
Serious Adverse Effects
Vitamin K deficiency with resultant deficiency of prothrombin and increased bleeding tendency.
Impaired absorption of calcium; predisposition to osteoporosis.
Gallbladder colic (questionable).

▷ **Possible Effects on Sexual Function:** None reported.

Natural Diseases or Disorders That May Be Activated by This Drug
Peptic ulcer disease; steatorrhea (excessive fat in stools) with large doses.

Possible Effects on Laboratory Tests
Blood cholesterol and triglyceride levels: decreased (therapeutic effect).
Blood thyroxine (T^4) level: decreased when colestipol and niacin are
taken concurrently (in presence of normal thyroid function).

CAUTION
1. The powder should never be taken in its dry form; always mix it thoroughly with a suitable liquid before swallowing.
2. Observe carefully for the development of constipation; use stool softeners and laxatives as needed.
3. This drug may bind other drugs taken concurrently and impair their absorption. It is advisable to take *all other drugs* 1 to 2 hours before or 4 to 6 hours after taking this drug.

Precautions for Use
By Infants and Children: Safety and effectiveness for use by those under 12 years of age have not been established. Observe carefully for the possible development of acidosis and vitamin A or folic acid deficiency. (Ask your physician for guidance.)
By Those over 60 Years of Age: There may be increased risk of developing severe constipation. Impaired kidney function may predispose to the development of acidosis.

▷ **Advisability of Use During Pregnancy**
Pregnancy Category: C (tentative). See Pregnancy Code inside back cover.
Animal studies: No information available.
Human studies: Information from adequate studies of pregnant women is not available.
Use this drug only if clearly needed. Ensure adequate intake of vitamins and minerals to satisfy needs of mother and fetus.

Advisability of Use if Breast-Feeding
Presence of this drug in breast milk: No.
Breast-feeding is permitted.

Habit-Forming Potential: None.

Effects of Overdosage: Progressive constipation.

Possible Effects of Long-Term Use: Deficiencies of vitamins A, D, E and K and folic acid. Calcium deficiency, osteoporosis. Acidosis due to excessive retention of chloride.

Suggested Periodic Examinations While Taking This Drug (at physician's discretion)
Measurements of blood levels of total cholesterol, low density (LDL) cholesterol and high density (HDL) cholesterol.
Hemoglobin and red blood cell studies for possible anemia.

▷ **While Taking This Drug, Observe the Following**

Foods: Avoid foods that tend to constipate (cheeses, etc.).

Nutritional Support: Consult your physician regarding the need for supplements of vitamins A, D, E and K, folic acid and calcium.

Beverages: Ensure adequate liquid intake (up to 2 quarts daily). This drug may be taken with milk.

▷ *Alcohol:* No interactions expected.

Tobacco Smoking: No interactions expected.

▷ *Other Drugs*

Colestipol may *decrease* the effects of
- acetaminophen; give 2 hours before colestipol.
- aspirin; give 2 hours before.
- digitoxin and digoxin; give 2 hours before.
- iron preparations; give 2 to 3 hours before.
- penicillin G; give 2 hours before.
- phenobarbital; give 2 hours before.
- tetracycline; give 2 hours before.
- thiazide diuretics (see Drug Class, Section Four); give 2 hours before.
- thyroxin; give 5 hours before.
- warfarin; give 6 hours after.

▷ *Driving, Hazardous Activities:* No restrictions.

Aviation Note: The use of this drug *is usually not a disqualification* for piloting. Consult a designated Aviation Medical Examiner.

Exposure to Sun: No restrictions.

Discontinuation: The dose of any potentially toxic drug taken concurrently must be reduced appropriately when this drug is discontinued. Following discontinuation of this drug, cholesterol blood levels usually return to pretreatment levels in approximately 1 month.

CROMOLYN
(KROH moh lin)

Other Names: Cromolyn sodium, sodium cromoglycate

Introduced: 1968

Class: Asthma preventive, rhinitis preventive

Prescription: USA: Yes
Canada: Yes

Controlled Drug: USA: No
Canada: No

Available as Generic: USA: No
Canada: No

Brand Names: ✦Fivent, Gastrocrom, Intal, ✦Nalcrom, Nasalcrom, Opticrom, ✦Rynacrom, ✦Vistacrom

BENEFITS versus RISKS

Possible Benefits	*Possible Risks*
LONG-TERM PREVENTION OF RECURRENT ASTHMA ATTACKS (70% to 75% effective)	Rare anaphylactic reaction (see Glossary)
Prevention of acute asthma due to allergens or exercise	Rare spasm of bronchial tubes, increased wheezing
Prevention and treatment of allergic rhinitis	Rare allergic pneumonitis (allergic reaction in lung tissue)
Relief of allergic conjunctivitis	

▷ **Principal Uses**

As a Single Drug Product: Used primarily to *prevent* allergic reactions in the nose (allergic rhinitis, hay fever) and allergic reactions in the bronchial tubes (bronchial asthma). (It is of no value in relieving asthma after the attack has begun.) It is also used to treat the symptoms of allergic rhinitis (70% effective) and conjunctivitis.

Additional uses include prevention of exercise-induced asthma, treatment of mastocytosis, and management of food allergies and several allergy-related skin disorders.

How This Drug Works: By blocking the release of histamine (and other substances) that normally occurs in allergic reactions, this drug acts to prevent the sequence of tissue changes that leads to swelling and itching of nasal membranes (allergic rhinitis) and to constriction of bronchial tubes (asthma).

Available Dosage Forms and Strengths

Capsules, oral — 100 mg
Eye drops — 2%, 4%
Inhalation aerosol — 0.8 mg per metered spray
Inhalation capsules (powder) — 20 mg
Inhalation solution — 20 mg per ampul
Nasal insufflation (powder) — 10 mg per cartridge
Nasal solution — 40 mg per ml

▷ **Usual Adult Dosage Range**

Eye drops: 1 drop 4 to 6 times daily at regular intervals.

Inhalation aerosol: 1.6 mg (2 inhalations) 4 times daily at regular intervals for long-term prevention of asthma, or as a single dose 10 to 15 minutes before exposure to prevent acute allergen-induced or exercise-induced asthma.

Inhalation powder: 20 mg (1 capsule) 4 times daily at regular intervals for long-term prevention of asthma; 20 mg (1 capsule) as a single dose 10 to 15 minutes before exposure to prevent acute allergen-induced or exercise-induced asthma. Total daily dosage should not exceed 160 mg (8 capsules).

Inhalation solution: Same as inhalation powder.

Nasal insufflation: Initially 10 mg in each nostril every 4 to 6 hours as needed; reduce to every 8 to 12 hours for maintenance.

Nasal solution: 2.6 mg to 5.2 mg in each nostril 3 to 6 times daily as needed. **Note: Actual dosage and administration schedule must be determined by the physician for each patient individually.**

▷ **Dosing Instructions:** Follow carefully the dosing instructions provided with each of the above dosage forms, especially the inhalers. Do not swallow the capsules; the powder is intended for inhalation into the air passages of the lungs. (If the capsule is swallowed inadvertently, the drug will cause no beneficial or adverse effects.)

Usual Duration of Use: Continual use on a regular schedule for 4 to 6 weeks is usually necessary to determine this drug's effectiveness in preventing recurrent attacks of asthma or allergic rhinitis. Long-term use (months to years) requires periodic evaluation of response and dosage adjustment. Consult your physician on a regular basis.

Possible Advantages of This Drug
May be quite effective in the young asthmatic.
Usually well tolerated.
Serious adverse effects are very rare.

▷ **This Drug Should Not Be Taken If**
• you have had an allergic reaction to any dosage form of it previously.

▷ **Inform Your Physician Before Taking This Drug If**
• you are allergic to milk, milk products or lactose. (The inhalation powder contains lactose.)
• you have impaired liver or kidney function.
• you have angina or a heart rhythm disorder. (The inhalation aerosol contains propellants that could be hazardous.)

Possible Side-Effects (natural, expected and unavoidable drug actions)
Unpleasant taste with use of inhalation aerosol.
Mild throat irritation, hoarseness, cough. (These can be minimized by a few swallows of water after each inhalation of powder.)

▷ **Possible Adverse Effects** (unusual, unexpected and infrequent reactions)
If any of the following develop, consult your physician promptly for guidance.
Mild Adverse Effects
Allergic Reactions: Skin rash, hives, itching.
Headache, dizziness.
Nausea, vomiting, urinary urgency and pain, joint and muscle pain.
Serious Adverse Effects
Allergic Reactions: Rare anaphylactic reaction (see Glossary). Allergic pneumonitis (allergic reaction in lung tissue).

▷ **Possible Effects on Sexual Function:**   None reported.

Possible Effects on Laboratory Tests
None reported.

CAUTION
1. Remember that this drug acts solely as a *preventive* in the management of bronchial asthma; its effectiveness is limited to the pretreatment phase of asthma—*before* the onset of acute bronchial constriction (asthmatic wheezing).
2. *Do not* use this drug during an acute attack of asthma; it could worsen and prolong asthmatic wheezing.
3. This drug does *not* interfere with the actions of those drugs used to relieve the acute asthma attack after it has begun. Cromolyn is used *before and between* acute attacks to prevent their development; bronchodilators are used *during* acute attacks to relieve them.
4. If you are also using a bronchodilator drug by inhalation, it is advisable to take it about 5 minutes before inhaling cromolyn.

Precautions for Use
By Infants and Children: Safety and effectiveness for use by those under 5 years of age have not been established. Young children may find it easier to use the nebulized solution than the powder.
By Those over 60 Years of Age: This drug is not effective in the management of chronic bronchitis or emphysema.

▷ **Advisability of Use During Pregnancy**
Pregnancy Category: B (tentative). See Pregnancy Code inside back cover.
Animal studies: Mouse, rat and rabbit studies revealed no birth defects due to this drug.
Human studies: Information from adequate studies of pregnant women is not available.
Use this drug only if clearly needed.

Advisability of Use if Breast-Feeding
Presence of this drug in breast milk: Unknown.
Avoid drug or refrain from nursing.

Habit-Forming Potential: None.

Effects of Overdosage: No significant effects reported.

Possible Effects of Long-Term Use: Allergic reaction of lung tissue (allergic pneumonitis, very rare).

Suggested Periodic Examinations While Taking This Drug (at physician's discretion)
Examination of lungs by sputum analysis and X-ray if symptoms suggest allergic pneumonitis.

▷ **While Taking This Drug, Observe the Following**
Foods: Follow diet prescribed by your physician. Avoid all foods to which you may be allergic.
Beverages: Avoid all beverages to which you may be allergic.
▷ *Alcohol:* No interactions expected.
Tobacco Smoking: Follow your physician's advice regarding smoking.
▷ *Other Drugs:* Cromolyn may make it possible to reduce the dosage of cortisonelike drugs in the management of chronic asthma. Consult your physician regarding dosage adjustment.
▷ *Driving, Hazardous Activities:* This drug may cause dizziness. Restrict activities as necessary.
Aviation Note: The use of this drug *may be a disqualification* for piloting. Consult a designated Aviation Medical Examiner.
Exposure to Sun: No restrictions.
Heavy Exercise or Exertion: This drug may be effective in preventing exercise-induced asthma if taken 10 to 15 minutes before exertion. It is most effective in young individuals.
Discontinuation: If the regular use of cromolyn has made it possible to reduce or discontinue maintenance doses of cortisonelike drugs, and you find it necessary to discontinue cromolyn for any reason, observe closely for a sudden return of asthma. It may be necessary to resume a cortisonelike drug and to institute other measures for satisfactory control of asthma.
Special Storage Instructions: Keep the powder cartridges in a dry, tightly closed container. Store in a cool place but not in the refrigerator. Do not handle the cartridges or the inhaler when hands are wet.

CYCLOBENZAPRINE
(si kloh BENZ a preen)

Introduced: 1977

Class: Muscle relaxant

Prescription: USA: Yes
Canada: Yes

Controlled Drug: USA: No
Canada: No

Available as Generic: USA: Yes
Canada: No

Brand Name: Flexeril

BENEFITS versus RISKS	
Possible Benefits	*Possible Risks*
Mild to moderate relief of discomfort due to spasm of voluntary muscles	Confusion, depression Impaired urination Allergic reactions: skin rash, hives, swelling of face or tongue

▷ **Principal Uses**
As a Single Drug Product: Used primarily to relieve the pain and stiffness associated with spasm of voluntary muscles, such as that resulting from accidental injury of musculoskeletal structures. It is often necessary to supplement the use of this drug with other treatment measures, such as rest, support and physiotherapy.

How This Drug Works: Not completely established. It is thought that this drug may relieve muscle spasm and pain by blocking the transmission of nerve impulses over reflex pathways and/or by producing a sedative effect that decreases the perception of pain.

Available Dosage Forms and Strengths
Tablets — 10 mg

▷ **Usual Adult Dosage Range:**   10 mg, 2 to 4 times daily; adjust dosage as needed and tolerated. Total daily dosage should not exceed 60 mg. **Note: Actual dosage and administration schedule must be determined by the physician for each patient individually.**

▷ **Dosing Instructions:**   Take either on empty stomach or with food to prevent stomach irritation. Tablet may be crushed for administration.

Usual Duration of Use: Continual use on a regular schedule for 7 to 10 days is usually necessary to determine this drug's effectiveness in relieving the discomfort of muscle spasm. Evaluate need for continued use after periods of 2 to 3 weeks.

▷ **This Drug Should Not Be Taken If**
• you have had an allergic reaction to it previously.
• you have taken any monoamine oxidase (MAO) type A inhibitor drug within the past 14 days (see Drug Class, Section Four).
• you are recovering from a recent heart attack.
• you have congestive heart failure or a serious heart rhythm disorder.
• you have uncorrected hyperthyroidism (overactive thyroid function).

▷ **Inform Your Physician Before Taking This Drug If**
• you have experienced any unfavorable reactions to other muscle relaxants or to tricyclic antidepressants (see Drug Class, Section Four) in the past.
• you have a history of heart disease or heart rhythm disorder.
• you have glaucoma or prostatism (see Glossary).
• you are currently taking any drugs with atropinelike effects or sedative effects.

Possible Side-Effects (natural, expected and unavoidable drug actions)
Drowsiness (40%), dizziness (11%), dry mouth (28%), constipation (3%).

▷ **Possible Adverse Effects** (unusual, unexpected and infrequent reactions)
   If any of the following develop, consult your physician promptly for guidance.
   Mild Adverse Effects
   Allergic Reactions: Skin rash, hives, swelling of face and tongue.
   Headache, fatigue, weakness, numbness, blurred vision, slurred speech, unsteadiness.
   Unpleasant taste, indigestion, nausea.
   Serious Adverse Effects
   Idiosyncratic Reactions: Euphoria, confusion, disorientation, hallucinations, depression.
   Impaired urination (urine retention).

▷ **Possible Effects on Sexual Function:** Increased or decreased libido, impotence, swelling of testicles, enlargement of male breasts, enlargement of female breasts with milk production. (Any effect may occur with dosage of 30 to 60 mg/day.)

▷ **Adverse Effects That May Mimic Natural Diseases or Disorders**
   Mental and behavioral reactions may suggest acute psychosis.

Possible Effects on Laboratory Tests
   None reported.

Precautions for Use
   By Infants and Children: Safety and effectiveness for use by those under 15 years of age have not been established.
   By Those over 60 Years of Age: Small doses are advisable initially. You may be more susceptible to the development of drowsiness, dizziness, weakness, unsteadiness and falling. This drug can aggravate existing prostatism (see Glossary).

▷ **Advisability of Use During Pregnancy**
   Pregnancy Category: B (tentative). See Pregnancy Code inside back cover.
   Animal studies: No birth defects reported in mice, rats or rabbits.
   Human studies: Information from adequate studies of pregnant women is not available.
   Avoid drug if possible; use only if clearly needed.

Advisability of Use if Breast-Feeding
   Presence of this drug in breast milk: Probably yes.
   Avoid drug or refrain from nursing.

Habit-Forming Potential: None.

Effects of Overdosage: Excessive drowsiness, confusion, impaired concentration, visual disturbances, vomiting, stupor progressing to coma, seizures, weak and rapid pulse.

Possible Effects of Long-Term Use: None reported.

Suggested Periodic Examinations While Taking This Drug (at physician's discretion)

Measurements of internal eye pressure (if any predisposition to glaucoma).

▷ **While Taking This Drug, Observe the Following**

Foods: No restrictions.

Beverages: No restrictions. May be taken with milk.

▷ *Alcohol:* Use with caution until the combined effect has been determined. This drug may add to the depressant action of alcohol on the brain.

Tobacco Smoking: No interactions expected.

Marijuana Smoking: Moderate to marked drowsiness, muscle weakness, incoordination, impairment of intellectual and physical performance. All hazardous activities should be avoided.

▷ *Other Drugs*

Cyclobenzaprine may ***increase*** the effects of

• atropinelike drugs (see Drug Class, Section Four).

• all drugs with sedative effects, and cause excessive sedation.

Cyclobenzaprine ***taken concurrently*** with

• monoamine oxidase (MAO) type A inhibitor drugs may cause high fever, seizures and life-threatening reactions (theoretical).

▷ *Driving, Hazardous Activities:* This drug may cause drowsiness, dizziness and incoordination in susceptible individuals. Avoid hazardous activities if these drug effects occur.

Aviation Note: The use of this drug ***is a disqualification*** for piloting. Consult a designated Aviation Medical Examiner.

Exposure to Sun: Use caution until sensitivity to sun has been determined. Other drugs closely related to this drug can cause photosensitivity (see Glossary).

Exposure to Heat: Use caution in hot environments. This drug may increase the risk of heat stroke.

CYCLOPHOSPHAMIDE
(si kloh FOSS fa mide)

Introduced: 1959

Class: Anticancer, immunosuppressive

Prescription: USA: Yes
Canada: Yes

Controlled Drug: USA: No
Canada: No

Available as Generic: No

Brand Names: Cytoxan, Neosar, ✦Procytox

```
┌─────────────────────────────────────────────────────────────┐
│                   BENEFITS versus RISKS                       │
│                                                               │
│      Possible Benefits                Possible Risks          │
│   CURE OR CONTROL OF            REDUCED WHITE BLOOD CELL       │
│     CERTAIN TYPES OF CANCER       COUNT                        │
│   PREVENTION OF REJECTION IN    SECONDARY INFECTION           │
│     ORGAN TRANSPLANTATION       URINARY BLADDER BLEEDING      │
│   Possibly beneficial in the    HEART, LUNG, LIVER OR          │
│     treatment of rheumatoid       KIDNEY DAMAGE               │
│     arthritis and lupus         Loss of hair                  │
│     erythematosus                                             │
│   Possibly beneficial in selected                             │
│     cases of nephrotic syndrome in                            │
│     children                                                  │
└─────────────────────────────────────────────────────────────┘
```

▷ **Principal Uses**

As a Single Drug Product: Used primarily in the treatment of various forms of cancer, notably malignant lymphomas, multiple myeloma, leukemias and cancers of the breast and ovary. Because this drug exerts a suppressant effect on the immune system, it is also used to prevent rejection in organ transplantation and to treat certain autoimmune disorders. It is also approved for treating certain resistant forms of nephrotic syndrome in children.

How This Drug Works: Not completely known. Because of its ability to kill cancer cells during all phases of their development and reproduction, this drug suppresses the primary growth and secondary spread (metastasis) of certain types of cancer.

Available Dosage Forms and Strengths

Injection — vials of 100 mg, 200 mg, 500 mg, 1 gram, 2 grams
Tablets — 25 mg, 50 mg

▷ **Usual Adult Dosage Range:** 1 to 5 mg per kg of body weight daily. **Note: Actual dosage and administration schedule must be determined by the physician for each patient individually.**

▷ **Dosing Instructions:**   It is preferable to take the tablet on an empty stomach. However, if nausea or indigestion occurs, this drug may be taken with or following food. The total liquid intake should be no less than 3 quarts/24 hours to reduce the risk of bladder irritation. Tablets may be crushed for administration.

Usual Duration of Use: Continual use on a regular schedule is required to achieve and maintain a significant remission of the cancer under treatment. Actual duration of use depends upon the response of the cancer and the tolerance of the patient to the effects of the drug. Consult your physician on a regular basis.

▷ **This Drug Should Not Be Taken If**
  • you have had an allergic reaction to any dosage form of it previously.
  • you have an active infection of any kind.
  • you have bloody urine for any reason.

▷ **Inform Your Physician Before Taking This Drug If**
  • you have impaired liver or kidney function.
  • you have a blood cell or bone marrow disorder.
  • you have had previous chemotherapy or X-ray therapy for any type of cancer.
  • you are now taking, or have taken within the past year, any cortisone-like drug (adrenal corticosteroids).
  • you have diabetes.
  • you plan to have surgery under general anesthesia in the near future.

Possible Side-Effects (natural, expected and unavoidable drug actions)
  Bone marrow depression (see Glossary)—impaired production of primarily white blood cells and, to a lesser degree, red blood cells and blood platelets (see Glossary). Possible effects include fever, chills, sore throat, fatigue, weakness, abnormal bleeding or bruising.
  Impairment of natural resistance (immunity) to infection.

▷ **Possible Adverse Effects** (unusual, unexpected and infrequent reactions)
  If any of the following develop, consult your physician promptly for guidance.
  Mild Adverse Effects
  Allergic Reaction: Skin rash (rare).
  Headache, dizziness.
  Loss of scalp hair (50% of users), darkening of skin and fingernails, transverse ridging of nails.
  Loss of appetite, nausea (30%), vomiting (25%), ulceration of mouth, diarrhea (may be bloody).
  Serious Adverse Effects
  Idiosyncratic Reaction: Hemolytic anemia (see Glossary).
  Liver damage with jaundice—yellow eyes and skin, dark-colored urine, light-colored stools.
  Kidney damage—impaired kidney function, reduced urine volume, bloody urine.
  Severe inflammation of bladder (10%)—painful urination, bloody urine.
  Drug-induced damage of heart and lung tissue.

▷ **Possible Effects on Sexual Function**
  Suppression of ovarian function—irregular menstrual pattern or cessation of menstruation (18% to 57% of users depending upon dosage and duration of use).
  Suppression of testicular function—reduction or cessation of sperm production (100% of users).

Possible Delayed Adverse Effects
> Development of other types of cancer (secondary malignancies).
> Development of severe cystitis with bleeding from the bladder wall. (This may occur many months after the last dose.)

Possible Effects on Laboratory Tests
> Complete blood cell counts: decreased red cells, hemoglobin, white cells and platelets.
> Prothrombin time: increased.
> Liver function tests: increased liver enzymes (ALT/GPT, AST/GOT and alkaline phosphatase), increased bilirubin.

CAUTION
> 1. This drug may interfere with the normal healing of wounds.
> 2. This drug can cause significant changes (mutations) in the chromosome structure of both sperm and eggs (ova). Any man or woman taking this drug should understand its potential for causing serious defects in children that are conceived during or following the course of medication.
> 3. This drug can suppress natural resistance (immunity) to infection, resulting in life-threatening illness.
> 4. Avoid live-virus vaccines while taking this drug.

Precautions for Use
> *By Infants and Children:* This drug should not be given if the child is dehydrated. Provide adequate fluid intake to ensure a copious urine volume for 4 hours following each dose. Prevent exposure of child to anyone with active chicken pox or shingles. This drug may cause ovarian or testicular sterility.
> *By Those over 60 Years of Age:* To reduce the risk of developing serious chemical cystitis, it is necessary to maintain a copious volume of urine. This may increase the risk of urinary retention in the man with prostatism (see Glossary).

▷ **Advisability of Use During Pregnancy**
> *Pregnancy Category:* D (tentative). See Pregnancy Code inside back cover.
> Animal studies: Significant birth defects reported in mice, rat and rabbit studies.
> Human studies: Information from studies of pregnant women indicates that this drug can cause serious birth defects or fetal death.
> Avoid completely during the first 3 months. Use of this drug during the last 6 months must be carefully individualized.

Advisability of Use if Breast-Feeding
> Presence of this drug in breast milk: Yes.
> Avoid drug or refrain from nursing.

Habit-Forming Potential: None.

Effects of Overdosage: Nausea, vomiting, diarrhea, bloody urine, water retention, weight gain, severe bone marrow depression, severe infections.

Possible Effects of Long-Term Use: Development of fibrous tissue in lungs; secondary malignancies.

Suggested Periodic Examinations While Taking This Drug (at physician's discretion)
Complete blood cell counts, every 2 to 4 days during initial treatment; then every 3 to 4 weeks during maintenance treatment.
Liver and kidney function tests.
Thyroid function tests (if symptoms warrant).

▷ **While Taking This Drug, Observe the Following**
Foods: No restrictions.
Beverages: No restrictions. May be taken with milk.
▷ *Alcohol:* No interactions expected.
Tobacco Smoking: No interactions expected.
▷ *Other Drugs*
Cyclophosphamide *taken concurrently* with
• allopurinol (Zyloprim) may increase the degree of bone marrow depression.
▷ *Driving, Hazardous Activities:* Use caution if dizziness occurs.
Aviation Note: The use of this drug *may be a disqualification* for piloting. Consult a designated Aviation Medical Examiner.
Exposure to Sun: No restrictions.
Occurrence of Unrelated Illness: Report promptly the development of any indications of infection—fever, chills, sore throat, cough, flulike symptoms. It may be necessary to discontinue this drug until the infection is controlled. Consult your physician.

CYCLOSPORINE
(SI kloh spor een)

Other Names: Ciclosporin, cyclosporin A

Introduced: 1983   **Class:** Immunosuppressant

Prescription: USA: Yes   **Controlled Drug:** USA: No
        Canada: Yes   Canada: No

Available as Generic: USA: No
        Canada: No

Brand Name: Sandimmune

BENEFITS versus RISKS

Possible Benefits	*Possible Risks*
EFFECTIVE PREVENTION AND TREATMENT OF REJECTION IN ORGAN TRANSPLANTATION	MARKED KIDNEY TOXICITY (25% to 38%)
	DEVELOPMENT OF HYPERTENSION (13% TO 53%)
Limited effectiveness in the treatment of Crohn's disease, myasthenia gravis, severe psoriasis, rheumatoid arthritis	Excessive hair growth (21% to 45%)
	Overgrowth of gums (5% to 16%)
	Liver toxicity (4% to 7%)
	Development of lymphoma (0.2%)

▷ **Principal Uses**

As a Single Drug Product: Used primarily (in conjunction with cortisonelike drugs) to prevent organ rejection in kidney, liver and heart transplantation; also used to treat chronic rejection of transplanted organs in patients treated previously with other immunosuppressive drugs.

Used increasingly in transplantation of the pancreas, bone marrow and heart/lung combinations.

Used on an investigational basis in the management of several autoimmune disorders: Crohn's disease, Graves' disease, psoriasis, myasthenia gravis, insulin-dependent diabetes, rheumatoid arthritis and others.

How This Drug Works: Not completely established. It is thought that by inhibiting the immune function of certain lymphocytes (white blood cells) and their growth factors, this drug suppresses the antigen-antibody reaction which is responsible for organ rejection and graft-versus-host disease.

Available Dosage Forms and Strengths

Capsules, soft gelatin — 25 mg, 100 mg
Injection, intravenous — 50 mg per ml
Oral solution — 100 mg per ml

▷ **Usual Adult Dosage Range:**   Initially 15 mg/kg/day taken 4 to 12 hours prior to transplantation surgery. This dose is continued following surgery for 1 to 2 weeks; then gradually reduce the dose by 5% per week to a maintenance dose of 5 to 10 mg/kg/day. **Note: Actual dosage and administration schedule must be determined by the physician for each patient individually.**

▷ **Dosing Instructions:**   Preferably taken with or immediately following food to reduce stomach irritation. The capsule should be swallowed whole; do not open, crush or chew. The oral solution should be mixed with milk, chocolate milk or orange juice (at room temperature) in a glass or ceramic cup; do not use a wax-lined or plastic container. Stir well and drink immediately. It is advisable to take this drug at the same time each day to maintain steady blood levels.

Usual Duration of Use:
Continual use on a regular schedule for several weeks is usually necessary to determine this drug's effectiveness in preventing organ rejection or arresting rejection that is already underway. Long-term use (months to years) requires periodic evaluation of response and dosage adjustment. Consult your physician on a regular basis as directed for mandatory blood tests and evaluation of your overall status.

▷ **This Drug Should Not Be Taken If**
- you have had an allergic reaction to it previously.
- you are taking any immunosuppressant drug other than cortisonelike preparations.
- you have an active lymphoma of any type.
- you have an active, uncontrolled infection, especially chicken pox or shingles.

▷ **Inform Your Physician Before Taking This Drug If**
- you are pregnant or breast-feeding.
- you have a history of liver or kidney disease, or impaired liver or kidney function.
- you have a history of hypertension or gout.
- you have a chronic gastrointestinal disorder.
- you are taking a potassium supplement or drugs that can raise the blood level of potassium.

Possible Side-Effects
(natural, expected and unavoidable drug actions)
Predisposition to infections (74%).

▷ **Possible Adverse Effects** (unusual, unexpected and infrequent reactions)
If any of the following develop, consult your physician promptly for guidance.
Mild Adverse Effects
Allergic Reactions: Skin rash (15%), itching (3%).
Excessive hair growth (21 to 45%), acne (1 to 2%).
Headache (2 to 15%), confusion (2%), tremors (21 to 55%).
Mouth sores (2%), gum overgrowth (5 to 16%), nausea/vomiting (4 to 10%), diarrhea (3 to 8%).
Serious Adverse Effects
Allergic Reactions: Anaphylactoid reaction (see Glossary) to intravenous solution (0.1%).
Severe kidney injury (25 to 38%).
Hypertension, mild to severe (13 to 53%).
Seizures (1 to 5%).
Liver injury (4 to 7%).
Pancreatitis (rare).

Lymphoma (0.2 to 0.7%), possibly drug-induced.
Elevation of blood potassium and uric acid levels.

▷ **Possible Effects on Sexual Function**
Enlargement and tenderness of male breast (1 to 4 %).

▷ **Adverse Effects That May Mimic Natural Diseases or Disorders**
Liver toxicity may suggest viral hepatitis.

Natural Diseases or Disorders That May Be Activated by This Drug
Latent infections, hypertension, gout.

Possible Effects on Laboratory Tests
Complete blood cell counts: decreased red cells, hemoglobin and white
cells.
Blood potassium level: increased.
Blood uric acid level: increased.
Liver function tests: increased liver enzymes (ALT/GPT, AST/GOT and
alkaline phosphatase), increased bilirubin.
Kidney function tests: blood creatinine and urea nitrogen levels (BUN)
increased; urine casts present.

CAUTION
1. Report promptly any indications of infection of any kind.
2. Report promptly any indication of swollen glands, sores or lumps in
   the skin, abnormal bleeding or bruising.
3. Inform your physician promptly if you become pregnant.
4. Comply fully with all instructions regarding periodic laboratory
   tests. These are mandatory to ensure safe and effective drug treatment.
5. It is advisable to avoid immunizations while taking this drug. Also,
   avoid contact with individuals who have recently taken oral poliovirus vaccine.

Precautions for Use
By Infants and Children: This drug has been used successfully and safely in
children of all ages.
By Those over 60 Years of Age: Reduced kidney function that accompanies
normal aging may require adjustment of dosage. Kidney function tests
and measurement of cyclosporine blood levels will provide guidance.

▷ **Advisability of Use During Pregnancy**
Pregnancy Category: C (tentative). See Pregnancy Code inside back cover.
Animal studies: Rat and rabbit studies reveal that this drug is toxic to the
embryo and fetus. No drug-induced birth defects were found.
Human studies: Information from adequate studies of pregnant women
is not available.
Avoid this drug during entire pregnancy unless it is clearly needed.

Advisability of Use if Breast-Feeding
  Presence of this drug in breast milk: Yes.
  Avoid drug or refrain from nursing.

Habit-Forming Potential: None.

Effects of Overdosage: Headache, painful sensations in hands and feet, flushing of the face, gum soreness and bleeding, nausea, abdominal discomfort.

Possible Effects of Long-Term Use: Irreversible kidney damage, severe hypertension.

Suggested Periodic Examinations While Taking This Drug
  (atphysician's discretion)
  Measurement of cyclosporine blood levels.
  Complete blood cell counts.
  Liver and kidney function tests.
  Measurement of magnesium, potassium and uric acid blood levels.
  Serial blood pressure measurements.

▷ **While Taking This Drug, Observe the Following**
  Foods: Avoid excessive intake of high-potassium foods. See Section Six, Table 6.
  Beverages: No restrictions. May be taken with milk.
▷ *Alcohol:* No interactions expected.
  Tobacco Smoking: No interactions expected.
▷ *Other Drugs*
  Cyclosporine *taken concurrently* with
  • aspirin substitutes (anti-inflammatory drugs) may increase kidney toxicity.
  • aminoglycoside antibiotics may increase kidney toxicity.
  • sulfamethoxazole and/or trimethoprim may increase kidney toxicity.
  • methylprednisolone may cause seizures.
  • azathioprine may increase immunosuppression.
  • cyclophosphamide may increase immunosuppression.
  • verapamil may increase immunosuppression.
  • lovastatin may cause muscle destruction and acute kidney failure.
  The following drugs may *increase* the effects of cyclosporine
  • danazol.
  • diltiazem.
  • erythromycin.
  • ketoconazole.
  • methyltestosterone.
  • metoclopramide.
  • oral contraceptives.
  The following drugs may *decrease* the effects of cyclosporine
  • carbamazepine.
  • isoniazid.

- phenobarbital.
- phenytoin.
- rifampin.
- sulfadimidine and/or trimethoprim.

▷ *Driving, Hazardous Activities:* This drug may cause confusion or seizures. Restrict activities as necessary.

Aviation Note: The use of this drug **may be a disqualification** for piloting. Consult a designated Aviation Medical Examiner.

Exposure to Sun: No restrictions.

Discontinuation: Do not discontinue this drug without your physician's guidance.

Special Storage Instructions: Keep the gelatin capsules in the blister packets until ready for use. Store below 77 degrees F (25 degrees C).

Keep the oral solution in a tightly closed container. Store below 86 degrees F (30 degrees C). Do not refrigerate.

Observe the Following Expiration Times: The oral solution must be used within 2 months after opening.

DEMECLOCYCLINE
(dem e kloh SI kleen)

Introduced: 1959

Class: Antibiotic, tetracyclines

Prescription: USA: Yes
Canada: Yes

Controlled Drug: USA: No
Canada: No

Available as Generic: No

Brand Name: Declomycin

BENEFITS versus RISKS	
Possible Benefits	*Possible Risks*
EFFECTIVE TREATMENT OF INFECTIONS due to susceptible microorganisms	Allergic reactions
	Drug-induced colitis
	Drug-induced diabetes insipidus (water diabetes)
	Fungal superinfections

▷ **Principal Uses**

As a Single Drug Product: This member of the tetracycline drug class is used primarily to (1) treat a broad range of infections caused by susceptible bacteria and protozoa and (2) treat the syndrome of inappropriate secretion of antidiuretic hormone, a condition that reduces the normal production of urine.

How This Drug Works: This drug prevents the growth and multiplication of susceptible bacteria by interfering with their formation of essential proteins.

Available Dosage Forms and Strengths
Capsules — 150 mg
Tablets, film-coated — 150 mg, 300 mg

▷ **Usual Adult Dosage Range:** 150 mg/6 hours or 300 mg/12 hours. Total daily dosage should not exceed 2400 mg. **Note: Actual dosage and administration schedule must be determined by the physician for each patient individually.**

▷ **Dosing Instructions:** Preferably taken on an empty stomach, 1 hour before or 2 hours after eating. However, if stomach irritation occurs, it may be taken with crackers or light food (not milk or milk products). Take at same time each day, with a full glass of water. Take the full course prescribed. The tablet may be crushed and the capsule may be opened for administration.

Usual Duration of Use: The time required to control the infection and be free of fever and symptoms for 48 hours. This varies with the nature of the infection.

▷ **This Drug Should Not Be Taken If**
- you are allergic to any tetracycline drug (see Drug Class, Section Four).
- you are pregnant or breast-feeding.

▷ **Inform Your Physician Before Taking This Drug If**
- it is prescribed for a child under 8 years of age.
- you have a history of liver or kidney disease.
- you have systemic lupus erythematosus.
- you are taking any penicillin drug.
- you are taking any anticoagulant drug.
- you plan to have surgery under general anesthesia in the near future.

Possible Side-Effects (natural, expected and unavoidable drug actions)
Superinfections (see Glossary), often due to yeast organisms. These can occur in the mouth, intestinal tract, rectum and/or vagina, resulting in rectal and vaginal itching.

▷ **Possible Adverse Effects** (unusual, unexpected and infrequent reactions)
If any of the following develop, consult your physician promptly for guidance.
Mild Adverse Effects
Allergic Reactions: Skin rash, hives, itching of hands and feet, swelling of face or extremities.
Loss of appetite, nausea, vomiting, diarrhea.
Irritation of mouth or tongue, "black tongue," sore throat, abdominal cramping or pain.

Serious Adverse Effects
Allergic Reactions: Anaphylactic reaction (see Glossary), asthma, fever, swollen joints, abnormal bleeding or bruising, jaundice (see Glossary).
Permanent discoloration and/or malformation of teeth when taken under 8 years of age, including unborn child and infant.
Drug-induced diabetes insipidus (water diabetes).

▷ **Possible Effects on Sexual Function:**   Questionable decrease of libido (1 report only).

Natural Diseases or Disorders That May Be Activated by This Drug
Systemic lupus erythematosus.

Possible Effects on Laboratory Tests
Complete blood cell counts: decreased red cells, hemoglobin, white cells and platelets; increased eosinophils (all rare).
Prothrombin time: increased.
Blood lupus erythematosus (LE) cells: positive (rare).
Kidney function tests: blood creatinine and urea nitrogen (BUN) levels increased.

CAUTION
1. Antacids, dairy products and preparations containing aluminum, bismuth, calcium, iron, magnesium or zinc can prevent adequate absorption of this drug and reduce its effectiveness significantly.
2. Troublesome and persistent diarrhea can develop in sensitive individuals. If diarrhea persists for more than 24 hours, discontinue this drug and consult your physician.
3. If surgery under general anesthesia is required while taking this drug, the choice of anesthetic agent must be considered carefully to prevent serious kidney damage.

Precautions for Use
By Infants and Children: If possible, tetracyclines should not be given to children under 8 years of age because of the risk of permanent discoloration and deformity of the teeth. Rarely, young infants may develop increased intracranial pressure within the first 4 days of receiving this drug. Tetracyclines may inhibit normal bone growth and development.
By Those over 60 Years of Age: Dosage must be carefully individualized and based upon determinations of kidney function. Natural skin changes may predispose to severe and prolonged itching reactions in the genital and anal regions.

▷ **Advisability of Use During Pregnancy**
Pregnancy Category: D (tentative). See Pregnancy Code inside back cover.
Animal studies: Tetracycline causes limb defects in rats, rabbits and chickens.
Human studies: Information from studies of pregnant women indicates

that this drug can cause impaired development and discoloration of teeth and other developmental defects.

It is advisable to avoid this drug completely during entire pregnancy.

Advisability of Use if Breast-Feeding
Presence of this drug in breast milk: Yes.
Avoid drug or refrain from nursing.

Habit-Forming Potential: None.

Effects of Overdosage: Nausea, vomiting, diarrhea, acute liver damage (rare).

Possible Effects of Long-Term Use: Superinfections; rarely, impairment of bone marrow, liver or kidney function.

Suggested Periodic Examinations While Taking This Drug (at physician's discretion)
Complete blood cell counts, liver and kidney function tests.
During extended use, sputum and stool examinations may detect early superinfection due to yeast organisms.

▷ **While Taking This Drug, Observe the Following**
Foods: Avoid cheeses, yogurt, ice cream, iron-fortified cereals and supplements and meats for 2 hours before and after taking this drug.
Beverages: Avoid all forms of milk for 2 hours before and after taking this drug.
▷ *Alcohol:* No interactions expected. However, it is best avoided if you have active liver disease.
Tobacco Smoking: No interactions expected.
▷ *Other Drugs*
Tetracyclines may *increase* the effects of
• oral anticoagulants, and make it necessary to reduce their dosage.
• digoxin (Lanoxin), and cause digitalis toxicity.
• lithium (Eskalith, Lithane, etc.), and increase the risk of lithium toxicity.
Tetracyclines may *decrease* the effects of
• oral contraceptives, and impair their effectiveness in preventing pregnancy.
• penicillins, and impair their effectiveness in treating infections.
Tetracyclines *taken concurrently* with
• methoxyflurane anesthesia may impair kidney function.
The following drugs may *decrease* the effects of tetracyclines
• antacids (aluminum and magnesium preparations, sodium bicarbonate, etc.) may reduce drug absorption.
• iron and mineral preparations may reduce drug absorption.
▷ *Driving, Hazardous Activities:* Usually no restrictions. Be alert to the possible occurrence of nausea or diarrhea.
Aviation Note: The use of this drug *may be a disqualification* for piloting. Consult a designated Aviation Medical Examiner.

Exposure to Sun: Use caution until sensitivity has been determined. Tetracyclines can cause photosensitivity (see Glossary).

DESIPRAMINE
(des IP ra meen)

Introduced: 1964

Class: Antidepressant

Prescription: USA: Yes
Canada: Yes

Controlled Drug: USA: No
Canada: No

Available as Generic: USA: No
Canada: No

Brand Names: Norpramin, Pertofrane

BENEFITS versus RISKS

Possible Benefits	*Possible Risks*
EFFECTIVE RELIEF OF ENDOGENOUS DEPRESSION	ADVERSE BEHAVIORAL EFFECTS: confusion, disorientation, delusions, hallucinations
Possibly beneficial in other depressive disorders	CONVERSION OF DEPRESSION TO MANIA in bipolar affective disorders
	Aggravation of paranoia and schizophrenia
	Drug-induced heart rhythm disorders
	Abnormally low white blood cell and platelet counts

▷ **Principal Uses**

As a Single Drug Product: Used primarily to relieve severe emotional depression and to initiate gradual restoration of normal mood. This drug is more likely to be effective in primary (endogenous) depression than in secondary, reactive (exogenous) depression. It is also being used to treat attention deficit disorder in children over 6 years of age and in adolescents.

How This Drug Works: Not completely established. It is thought that by increasing brain tissue concentrations of certain nerve impulse transmitters (norepinephrine and serotonin), this drug relieves the symptoms associated with depression.

Available Dosage Forms and Strengths
Capsules — 25 mg, 50 mg
Tablets — 10 mg, 25 mg, 50 mg, 75 mg, 100 mg, 150 mg

▷ **Usual Adult Dosage Range:**   Initially 25 mg 2 to 4 times daily. Dose may be increased cautiously as needed and tolerated by 25 mg daily at intervals of 1 week. The usual maintenance dose is 100 mg to 200 mg/24 hours. The total daily dosage should not exceed 300 mg. (When determined, the optimal daily requirement may be given at bedtime as a single dose.) **Note: Actual dosage and administration schedule must be determined by the physician for each patient individually.**

▷ **Dosing Instructions:**   May be taken without regard to meals. The capsule may be opened and the tablet may be crushed for administration.

Usual Duration of Use: Continual use on a regular schedule for 3 to 4 weeks is usually necessary to determine this drug's effectiveness in relieving depression; optimal response may require 3 months of use. Long-term use (months to years) requires periodic evaluation of response and dosage adjustment. Consult your physician on a regular basis.

▷ **This Drug Should Not Be Taken If**
• you have had an allergic reaction to it previously.
• you are taking, or have taken within the past 14 days, any monoamine oxidase (MAO) type A inhibitor drug (see Drug Class, Section Four).
• you have had a recent heart attack (myocardial infarction).
• you have narrow-angle glaucoma.

▷ **Inform Your Physician Before Taking This Drug If**
• you have had an adverse reaction to any other antidepressant drug.
• you have any type of seizure disorder.
• you have increased internal eye pressure.
• you have any type of heart disease, especially a heart rhythm disorder.
• you have any type of thyroid disorder or are taking thyroid medication.
• you have diabetes or sugar intolerance.
• you have prostatism (see Glossary).
• you plan to have surgery under general anesthesia in the near future.

Possible Side-Effects (natural, expected and unavoidable drug actions)
Mild drowsiness, light-headedness (low blood pressure), blurred vision, dry mouth, constipation, impaired urination.

▷ **Possible Adverse Effects** (unusual, unexpected and infrequent reactions)
If any of the following develop, consult your physician promptly for guidance.
Mild Adverse Effects
Allergic Reactions: Skin rash, hives, swelling of face or tongue, drug fever (see Glossary).
Headache, dizziness, weakness, unsteadiness, tremors, fainting.
Irritation of tongue or mouth, altered taste, indigestion, nausea.
Fluctuations of blood sugar.

Serious Adverse Effects
Allergic Reactions: Drug-induced hepatitis, with or without jaundice; anaphylactoid reaction (see terms in Glossary).
Adverse behavioral effects: confusion, disorientation, delusions, hallucinations.
Seizures; reduced control of epilepsy.
Aggravation of paranoid psychoses and schizophrenia.
Heart rhythm disturbances.
Parkinsonlike disorders, peripheral neuritis (see both terms in Glossary).
Abnormally low white blood cell and platelet counts: fever, sore throat, infections, abnormal bleeding or bruising.

▷ **Possible Effects on Sexual Function:** Decreased libido, increased libido (antidepressant effect), impotence, painful male orgasm, male breast enlargement, female breast enlargement with milk production, swelling of testicles.

▷ **Adverse Effects That May Mimic Natural Diseases or Disorders**
Liver toxicity may suggest viral hepatitis.

Natural Diseases or Disorders That May Be Activated by This Drug
Latent diabetes, epilepsy, glaucoma, prostatism.

Possible Effects on Laboratory Tests
Complete blood cell counts: decreased red cells, hemoglobin, white cells and platelets; increased eosinophils (allergic reaction).
Blood glucose levels: unexplained fluctuations.
Liver function tests: increased liver enzymes (ALT/GPT, AST/GOT and alkaline phosphatase), increased bilirubin (all rare).

CAUTION
1. This drug should be used only when a true, primary, endogenous depression has been diagnosed. It should *not* be used to treat the symptoms of reactive depression that may be associated with many life situations in the absence of a true bona fide affective illness.
2. Observe for early indications of toxicity or overdosage: confusion, agitation, rapid heart rate, heart irregularity. Measurement of the blood level of the drug will clarify the situation.
3. It is advisable to withhold this drug if electroconvulsive therapy (ECT) is to be used to treat the depression.

Precautions for Use
By Infants and Children: Safety and effectiveness for use by those under 6 years of age have not been established. This drug is being used experimentally to treat children who have attention deficit syndrome, with or without hyperactivity. Dosage and management must be supervised by a properly trained pediatrician.
By Those over 60 Years of Age: Initiate treatment with 25 mg 1 or 2 times daily to evaluate tolerance. During the first 2 weeks of treatment, observe for confusional reactions—restlessness, agitation, forgetfulness, disorientation, delusions or hallucinations. Also observe for unsteadi-

ness and instability that may predispose to falling. This drug may aggravate prostatism.

▷ **Advisability of Use During Pregnancy**
   Pregnancy Category: C (tentative). See Pregnancy Code inside back cover.
   Animal studies: Birth defects reported in rat and rabbit studies.
   Human studies: Information from adequate studies of pregnant women is not available.
   Use only if clearly needed. Avoid during the first 3 months if possible.

Advisability of Use if Breast-Feeding
   Presence of this drug in breast milk: Yes, in small amounts.
   Monitor nursing infant closely and discontinue drug or nursing if adverse effects develop.

Habit-Forming Potential: Psychological or physical dependence is rare and unexpected. This drug is not liable to abuse.

Effects of Overdosage: Confusion, hallucinations, drowsiness, tremors, heart irregularity, seizures, stupor, hypothermia (see Glossary).

Possible Effects of Long-Term Use: None reported.

Suggested Periodic Examinations While Taking This Drug (at physician's discretion)
   Complete blood cell counts, liver function tests.
   Serial blood pressure readings and electrocardiograms.

▷ **While Taking This Drug, Observe the Following**
   Foods: No specific restrictions. May need to limit food intake to avoid excessive weight gain.
   Beverages: No restrictions. May be taken with milk.
▷ *Alcohol:* Avoid completely. This drug can markedly increase the intoxicating effects of alcohol; the combination can depress brain function significantly.
   Tobacco Smoking: May accelerate the elimination of this drug and require increased dosage.
   Marijuana Smoking
      Occasional (once or twice weekly): Transient increase in drowsiness and mouth dryness. *Daily:* Persistent drowsiness and mouth dryness; possible reduced effectiveness of this drug.
▷ *Other Drugs*
   Desipramine may *increase* the effects of
   • all drugs with sedative effects; observe for excessive sedation.
   • all drugs with atropinelike effects (see Drug Class, Section Four).
   Desipramine may *decrease* the effects of
   • clonidine (Catapres).
   • guanethidine (Ismelin, Esimil).
   Desipramine *taken concurrently* with

- anticonvulsants requires careful monitoring for changes in seizure patterns and need to adjust anticonvulsant dosage.
- ethchlorvynol (Placidyl) may cause delirium; avoid concurrent use.
- monoamine oxidase (MAO) type A inhibitor drugs (see Drug Class, Section Four) may cause high fever, seizures and excessive rise in blood pressure; avoid concurrent use of these drugs and provide periods of 14 days between administration of either.
- stimulant drugs (amphetamine, cocaine, epinephrine, phenylpropanolamine, etc.) may cause severe high blood pressure and/or high fever.
- thyroid preparations may increase the risk of heart rhythm disorders.

The following drugs may *increase* the effects of desipramine
- methylphenidate (Ritalin).
- phenothiazines (see Drug Class, Section Four).

The following drugs may *decrease* the effects of desipramine
- barbiturates (see Drug Class, Section Four).
- chloral hydrate (Noctec, Somnos, etc.).
- estrogen (see Drug Profile for brand names).
- lithium (Lithobid, Lithotab, etc.).
- oral contraceptives (see Drug Profile for brand names).
- reserpine (Serpasil, Ser-Ap-Es, etc.).

▷ *Driving, Hazardous Activities:* This drug may impair mental alertness, judgment, physical coordination and reaction time. Restrict activities as necessary.

Aviation Note: The use of this drug *is a disqualification* for piloting. Consult a designated Aviation Medical Examiner.

Exposure to Sun: Use caution until sensitivity has been determined. This drug may cause photosensitivity (see Glossary).

Exposure to Heat: Use caution. This drug can inhibit sweating and impair the body's adaptation to hot environments, increasing the risk of heat stroke. Avoid saunas.

Exposure to Cold: The elderly should use caution and avoid conditions conducive to hypothermia (see Glossary).

Exposure to Environmental Chemicals: This drug may mask the symptoms of poisoning due to handling certain insecticides (organophosphorus types). Read their labels carefully.

Discontinuation: It is advisable to discontinue this drug gradually. Abrupt withdrawal after prolonged use may cause headache, malaise and nausea. When this drug is stopped, it may be necessary to adjust the dosages of other drugs taken concurrently.

DEXAMETHASONE
(dex a METH a sohn)

Introduced: 1958

Class: Cortisonelike drugs

Prescription: USA: Yes
Canada: Yes

Controlled Drug: USA: No
Canada: No

Available as Generic: USA: Yes
Canada: Yes

Brand Names: ✦Ak-Dex, Decaderm, Decadron, Decadron-LA, Decadron Phosphate Ophthalmic, Decadron Phosphate Respihaler, Decadron Phosphate Turbinaire, Decadron w/Xylocaine [CD], Decaspray, ✦Deronil, Dexasone, Dexone, Hexadrol, Maxidex

---

BENEFITS versus RISKS

Possible Benefits	*Possible Risks*
EFFECTIVE RELIEF OF SYMPTOMS IN A WIDE VARIETY OF INFLAMMATORY AND ALLERGIC DISORDERS	Short-term use (up to 10 days) is usually well tolerated
EFFECTIVE IMMUNOSUPPRESSION in selected benign and malignant disorders	Long-term use (exceeding 2 weeks) is associated with many possible adverse effects:
	ALTERED MOOD AND PERSONALITY
	CATARACTS, GLAUCOMA
	HYPERTENSION
	OSTEOPOROSIS
	ASEPTIC BONE NECROSIS
	INCREASED SUSCEPTIBILITY TO INFECTIONS
	(See Possible Adverse Effects and Possible Effects of Long-Term Use below)

▷ **Principal Uses**

As a Single Drug Product: This potent drug of the cortisone class is used in the treatment of a wide variety of allergic and inflammatory conditions. It is used most commonly in the management of serious skin disorders, asthma, regional enteritis, ulcerative colitis and all types of major rheumatic disorders including bursitis, tendonitis and most forms of arthritis.

How This Drug Works: Not fully established. It is thought that this drug's anti-inflammatory effect is due to its ability to inhibit the normal defensive functions of certain white blood cells. Its immunosuppressant effect is attributed to a reduced production of lymphocytes and antibodies.

Available Dosage Forms and Strengths

Aerosol — 0.01%, 0.04%

Aerosol inhaler — 84 mcg per spray

Cream — 0.1%

Elixir — 0.5 mg per 5-ml teaspoonful

Eye ointment — 0.05%

Gel — 0.1%

Injection — 4 mg per ml, 8 mg per ml, 10 mg per ml, 16 mg per ml, 20 mg per ml, 24 mg per ml

Oral solution — 0.5 mg per 0.5 ml, 0.5 mg per 5 ml

Solution — 0.1%

Suspension — 0.1%

Tablets — 0.25 mg, 0.5 mg, 0.75 mg, 1 mg, 1.5 mg, 2 mg, 4 mg, 6 mg

▷ **Usual Adult Dosage Range:**   0.5 to 9 mg daily as a single dose or in divided doses. **Note: Actual dosage and administration schedule must be determined by the physician for each patient individually.**

▷ **Dosing Instructions:**   Take with or following food to prevent stomach irritation, preferably in the morning. The tablet may be crushed for administration.

Usual Duration of Use: For acute disorders: 4 to 10 days. For chronic disorders: according to individual requirements. The duration of use should not exceed the time necessary to obtain adequate symptomatic relief in acute self-limiting conditions; or the time required to stabilize a chronic condition and permit gradual withdrawal. Because of its long duration of action, this drug is not appropriate for alternate day administration. Consult your physician on a regular basis.

▷ **This Drug Should Not Be Taken If**
• you have had an allergic reaction to any dosage form of it previously.
• you have active peptic ulcer disease.
• you have an active infection of the eye caused by the herpes simplex virus.
• you have active tuberculosis.

▷ **Inform Your Physician Before Taking This Drug If**
• you have had an unfavorable reaction to any cortisonelike drug in the past.
• you have a history of peptic ulcer disease, thrombophlebitis or tuberculosis.
• you have any of the following: diabetes, glaucoma, high blood pressure, deficient thyroid function or myasthenia gravis.
• you plan to have surgery of any kind in the near future.

Possible Side-Effects (natural, expected and unavoidable drug actions)
Increased appetite, weight gain, retention of salt and water, excretion of potassium, increased susceptibility to infection.

▷ **Possible Adverse Effects** (unusual, unexpected and infrequent reactions)
   If any of the following develop, consult your physician promptly for guidance.
   Mild Adverse Effects
   Allergic Reaction: Skin rash.
   Headache, dizziness, insomnia.
   Acid indigestion, abdominal distention.
   Muscle cramping and weakness.
   Acne, excessive growth of facial hair.
   Serious Adverse Effects
   Mental and emotional disturbances of serious magnitude.
   Reactivation of latent tuberculosis.
   Development of peptic ulcer.
   Increased blood pressure.
   Development of inflammation of the pancreas.
   Thrombophlebitis (inflammation of a vein with the formation of blood clot)—pain or tenderness in thigh or leg, with or without swelling of the foot, ankle or leg.
   Pulmonary embolism (movement of a blood clot to the lung)—sudden shortness of breath, pain in the chest, coughing, bloody sputum.

▷ **Possible Effects on Sexual Function:**   Altered timing and pattern of menstruation.

▷ **Adverse Effects That May Mimic Natural Diseases or Disorders**
   Pattern of symptoms and signs resembling Cushing's syndrome.

Natural Diseases or Disorders That May Be Activated by This Drug
   Latent diabetes, glaucoma, peptic ulcer disease, tuberculosis.

Possible Effects on Laboratory Tests
   Blood amylase level: increased (possible pancreatitis).
   Blood glucose level: increased.
   Glucose tolerance test (GTT): decreased.
   Blood potassium level: decreased.

CAUTION
   1. It is advisable to carry a card of personal identification with a notation that you are taking this drug, if your course of treatment is to exceed 1 week.
   2. Do not discontinue this drug abruptly if you are using it for long-term treatment.
   3. If vaccination against measles, rabies, smallpox or yellow fever is required, discontinue this drug 72 hours before vaccination and do not resume it for at least 14 days after vaccination.

Precautions for Use
   By Infants and Children: Avoid prolonged use if possible. During long-term use, observe for suppression of normal growth and the possibility of increased intracranial pressure. Following long-term use, the child

may be at risk for adrenal gland deficiency during stress for as long as 18 months after cessation of this drug.

By Those over 60 Years of Age: Cortisonelike drugs should be used very sparingly after 60 and only when the disorder under treatment is unresponsive to adequate trials of unrelated drugs. Avoid prolonged use of this drug. Continual use (even in small doses) can increase the severity of diabetes, enhance fluid retention, raise blood pressure, weaken resistance to infection, induce stomach ulcer and accelerate the development of cataract and osteoporosis.

▷ **Advisability of Use During Pregnancy**
Pregnancy Category: C (tentative). See Pregnancy Code inside back cover.
Animal studies: Birth defects reported in mice, rats and rabbits.
Human studies: Information from adequate studies of pregnant women is not available.

Avoid completely during the first 3 months. Limit use during the last 6 months as much as possible. If used, examine infant for possible deficiency of adrenal gland function.

Advisability of Use if Breast-Feeding
Presence of this drug in breast milk: Yes.
Avoid drug or refrain from nursing.

Habit-Forming Potential: Use of this drug to suppress symptoms over an extended period of time may produce a state of functional dependence (see Glossary). In the treatment of conditions like asthma and rheumatoid arthritis, it is advisable to keep the dose as small as possible and to attempt drug withdrawal after periods of reasonable improvement. Such procedures may reduce the degree of "steroid rebound"—the return of symptoms as the drug is withdrawn.

Effects of Overdosage: Fatigue, muscle weakness, stomach irritation, acid indigestion, excessive sweating, facial flushing, fluid retention, swelling of extremities, increased blood pressure.

Possible Effects of Long-Term Use: Increased blood sugar (possible diabetes), increased fat deposits on the trunk of the body ("buffalo hump"), rounding of the face ("moon face"), thinning and fragility of skin, loss of texture and strength of bones (osteoporosis, aseptic necrosis), cataracts, glaucoma, retarded growth and development in children.

Suggested Periodic Examinations While Taking This Drug (at physician's discretion)
Measurements of blood pressure, blood sugar and potassium levels.
Complete eye examinations at regular intervals.
Chest X-ray if history of tuberculosis.
Determination of the rate of development of the growing child to detect retardation of normal growth.

▷ **While Taking This Drug, Observe the Following**

Foods: No interactions expected. Ask physician regarding need to restrict salt intake or to eat potassium-rich foods. During long-term use of this drug, it is advisable to eat a high-protein diet.

Nutritional Support: During long-term use, take a vitamin D supplement. During wound repair, take a zinc supplement.

Beverages: No restrictions. Drink all forms of milk liberally.

▷ *Alcohol:* No interactions expected. Use caution if you are prone to peptic ulcer disease.

Tobacco Smoking: Nicotine increases the blood levels of naturally produced cortisone and related hormones. Heavy smoking may add to the expected actions of this drug and requires close observation for excessive effects.

Marijuana Smoking: May cause additional impairment of immunity.

▷ *Other Drugs*

Dexamethasone may *decrease* the effects of
- isoniazid (INH, Niconyl, etc.)
- salicylates (aspirin, sodium salicylate, etc.)

Dexamethasone *taken concurrently* with
- oral anticoagulants may either increase or decrease their effectiveness; consult physician regarding the need for prothrombin time testing and dosage adjustment.

The following drugs may *decrease* the effects of dexamethasone
- antacids may reduce its absorption.
- barbiturates (Amytal, Butisol, phenobarbital, etc.).
- phenytoin (Dilantin, etc.).
- rifampin (Rifadin, Rimactane, etc.).

▷ *Driving, Hazardous Activities:* Usually no restrictions. Be alert to the rare occurrence of dizziness.

Aviation Note: The use of this drug *may be a disqualification* for piloting. Consult a designated Aviation Medical Examiner.

Exposure to Sun: No restrictions.

Occurrence of Unrelated Illness: This drug may decrease natural resistance to infection. Inform your physician if you develop an infection of any kind. It may also reduce your body's ability to respond to the stress of acute illness, injury or surgery. Keep your physician fully informed of any significant changes in your state of health.

Discontinuation: If you have been taking this drug for an extended period of time, do not discontinue it abruptly. Ask physician for guidance regarding gradual withdrawal. For a period of 2 years after discontinuing this drug, it is essential in the event of illness, injury or surgery that you inform attending medical personnel that you have used this drug in the past. The period of impaired response to stress following the use of cortisonelike drugs may last for 1 to 2 years.

DIAZEPAM
(di AZ e pam)

Introduced: 1963

Class: Mild tranquilizer, benzodiazepines

Prescription: USA: Yes
Canada: Yes

Controlled Drug: USA: C-IV*
Canada: No

Available as Generic: Yes

Brand Names: ✦Apo-Diazepam, ✦Diazemuls, Diazepam Intensol, ✦E-Pam, ✦Meval, ✦Novodipam, ✦Rival, Valium, Valrelease, Vazepam, ✦Vivol

---

BENEFITS versus RISKS

Possible Benefits	*Possible Risks*
RELIEF OF ANXIETY AND NERVOUS TENSION in 70% to 80% of users	Habit-forming potential with prolonged use
Wide margin of safety with therapeutic doses	Minor impairment of mental functions
Very few drug interactions	Very rare jaundice
	Very rare blood cell disorders

▷ **Principal Uses**

As a Single Drug Product: Used primarily to (1) provide short-term relief of mild to moderate anxiety; (2) relieve the symptoms of acute alcohol withdrawal: agitation, tremors, hallucinations, incipient delirium tremens; (3) relieve skeletal muscle spasm; (4) provide short-term control of certain types of seizures (epilepsy).

How This Drug Works: It is thought that this drug produces a calming effect by enhancing the action of the nerve transmitter gamma-aminobutyric acid (GABA), which in turn blocks the arousal of higher brain centers.

Available Dosage Forms and Strengths
Capsules, prolonged-action — 15 mg
Concentrate — 5 mg per ml
Injection — 5 mg per ml
Oral solution — 5 mg per ml, 5 mg per 5-ml teaspoonful
Tablets — 2 mg, 5 mg, 10 mg

▷ **Usual Adult Dosage Range:** 2 to 10 mg, 2 to 4 times daily. Dose may be increased cautiously as needed and tolerated. After 1 week of continual use, the total daily dose may be taken at bedtime. Total daily dose should not exceed 60 mg. **Note: Actual dosage and administration schedule must be determined by the physician for each patient individually.**

*See Schedules of Controlled Drugs inside back cover.

▷ **Dosing Instructions:** May be taken on empty stomach or with food or milk. The prolonged-action capsule should not be opened, but the tablet may be crushed for administration. Do not discontinue this drug abruptly if taken for more than 4 weeks.

Usual Duration of Use: Continual use on a regular schedule for 3 to 5 days is usually necessary to determine this drug's effectiveness in relieving moderate anxiety. Limit continual use to 1 to 3 weeks. Avoid uninterrupted and prolonged use.

▷ **This Drug Should Not Be Taken If**
  • you have had an allergic reaction to any dosage form of it previously.
  • you have acute narrow-angle glaucoma.
  • it is prescribed for a child under 6 months of age.

▷ **Inform Your Physician Before Taking This Drug If**
  • you are allergic to any benzodiazepine drug (see Drug Class, Section Four).
  • you have a history of alcoholism or drug abuse.
  • you are pregnant or planning pregnancy.
  • you have impaired liver or kidney function.
  • you have a history of serious depression or mental disorder.
  • you have any of the following: asthma, emphysema, epilepsy, myasthenia gravis.

Possible Side-Effects (natural, expected and unavoidable drug actions)
Drowsiness (5%), lethargy, unsteadiness (0.2%), "hangover" effects on the day following bedtime use.

▷ **Possible Adverse Effects** (unusual, unexpected and infrequent reactions)
If any of the following develop, consult your physician promptly for guidance.
Mild Adverse Effects
Allergic Reactions: Rashes (0.4%), hives.
Dizziness, fainting, blurred vision, double vision, slurred speech, sweating, nausea.
Serious Adverse Effects
Allergic Reactions: Liver damage with jaundice (see Glossary), abnormally low blood platelet count.
Bone marrow depression—impaired production of white blood cells, fever, sore throat.
Paradoxical responses of excitement, agitation, anger, rage.

▷ **Possible Effects on Sexual Function**
Altered timing and pattern of menstruation.
Small doses (2 to 5 mg/day) are used to allay the anxiety that accounts for many cases of impotence in the male and inhibited sexual responsiveness in the female.
Larger doses (10 mg/day or more) can decrease libido, impair potency in the male and inhibit orgasm in the female.

▷ **Adverse Effects That May Mimic Natural Diseases or Disorders**
Liver reaction with jaundice may suggest viral hepatitis.

Possible Effects on Laboratory Tests
White blood cell counts: decreased.
Blood thyroxine (T^4) level: decreased.
Liver function tests: increased liver enzymes (ALT/GPT, AST/GOT and alkaline phosphatase), increased bilirubin (all rare).
Urine sugar tests: no drug effect with TesTape; low test results with Clinistix and Diastix.
Urine screening tests for drug abuse: may be **positive**. (Test results depend upon amount of drug taken and testing method used.)

CAUTION
1. This drug should not be discontinued abruptly if it has been taken continually for more than 4 weeks.
2. The concurrent use of some over-the-counter drug products that contain antihistamines (allergy and cold preparations, sleep aids) can cause excessive sedation in sensitive individuals.

Precautions for Use
By Infants and Children: Safety and effectiveness for use by those under 6 months of age have not been established. This drug should not be used in the hyperactive or psychotic child of any age. Observe for excessive sedation and incoordination.
By Those over 60 Years of Age: It is advisable to use smaller doses at longer intervals to avoid overdosage. Observe for the possible development of lethargy, indifference, fatigue, weakness, unsteadiness, disturbing dreams, nightmares and paradoxical reactions of excitement, agitation, anger, hostility and rage.

▷ **Advisability of Use During Pregnancy**
Pregnancy Category: D (tentative). See Pregnancy Code inside back cover.
Animal studies: Cleft palate reported in mice; skeletal defects reported in rats.
Human studies: Available information is conflicting and inconclusive. Some studies found an increase in serious birth defects associated with the use of this drug. Other studies have found no significant increase in birth defects.
Frequent use in late pregnancy can cause the "floppy infant" syndrome in the newborn: weakness, lethargy, unresponsiveness, depressed breathing, low body temperature.
Avoid use during entire pregnancy.

Advisability of Use if Breast-Feeding
Presence of this drug in breast milk: Yes.
Avoid drug or refrain from nursing.

Habit-Forming Potential: This drug can produce psychological and/or physical dependence (see Glossary) if used in large doses for an extended period of time.

Effects of Overdosage: Marked drowsiness, weakness, feeling of drunkenness, staggering gait, tremor, stupor progressing to deep sleep or coma.

Possible Effects of Long-Term Use: Psychological and/or physical dependence, rare blood cell disorders.

Suggested Periodic Examinations While Taking This Drug (at physician's discretion)
Complete blood cell counts during long-term use.

▷ **While Taking This Drug, Observe the Following**
Foods: No restrictions.
Beverages: Avoid excessive intake of caffeine-containing beverages: coffee, tea, cola. May be taken with milk.
▷ *Alcohol:* Use with extreme caution until the combined effect is determined. Alcohol may increase the absorption of this drug and add to its depressant effects on the brain. It is advisable to avoid alcohol completely—throughout the day and night—if it is necessary to drive or to engage in any hazardous activity.
Tobacco Smoking: Heavy smoking may reduce the calming action of this drug.
Marijuana Smoking: Increased sedation and significant impairment of intellectual and physical performance.
▷ *Other Drugs*
Diazepam may *increase* the effects of
• digoxin (Lanoxin), and cause digoxin toxicity.
• phenytoin (Dilantin), and cause phenytoin toxicity.
Diazepam may *decrease* the effects of
• levodopa (Sinemet, etc.), and reduce its effectiveness in treating Parkinson's disease.
The following drugs may *increase* the effects of diazepam
• cimetidine (Tagamet).
• disulfiram (Antabuse).
• isoniazid (INH, Rifamate, etc.).
• oral contraceptives.
• valproic acid (Depakene).
The following drugs may *decrease* the effects of diazepam
• rifampin (Rimactane, etc.).
• theophylline (aminophylline, Theo-Dur, etc.).
▷ *Driving, Hazardous Activities:* This drug can impair mental alertness, judgment, physical coordination and reaction time. Avoid hazardous activities accordingly.
Aviation Note: The use of this drug *is a disqualification* for piloting. Consult a designated Aviation Medical Examiner.
Exposure to Sun: No restrictions.

Exposure to Heat: Use caution until the effect of excessive perspiration is determined. Because of reduced urine volume, this drug may accumulate in the body and produce effects of overdosage.

Discontinuation: Avoid sudden discontinuation if this drug has been taken for over 4 weeks without interruption. Dosage should be tapered gradually to prevent a withdrawal syndrome that could include depression, confusion, hallucinations, tremor, seizures, muscle cramping, sweating and vomiting.

DICLOFENAC
(di KLOH fen ak)

Introduced: 1976

Class: Mild analgesic, anti-inflammatory

Prescription: USA: Yes
Canada: Yes

Controlled Drug: USA: No
Canada: No

Available as Generic: USA: No
Canada: No

Brand Name: Voltaren

BENEFITS versus RISKS	
Possible Benefits	*Possible Risks*
EFFECTIVE RELIEF OF SYMPTOMS ASSOCIATED WITH MAJOR TYPES OF ARTHRITIS	PEPTIC ULCER DISEASE (less than 2%); associated bleeding and perforation
Effective relief of symptoms associated with bursitis, tendinitis and related conditions	Liver toxicity with jaundice (less than 1%)
Effective relief of menstrual cramps	Rare aplastic anemia (see Glossary)
	Water retention
	Rare kidney toxicity

▷ **Principal Uses**

As a Single Drug Product: Used primarily to relieve the symptoms associated with (1) rheumatoid arthritis, osteoarthritis and ankylosing spondylitis; (2) bursitis, tendinitis, capsulitis and tenosynovitis; (3) painful menstruation.

How This Drug Works: Not completely established. It is thought that this drug reduces the tissue concentrations of prostaglandins (and related compounds), chemicals involved in the production of inflammation and pain.

Available Dosage Forms and Strengths
Suppositories (Canada) — 50 mg, 100 mg
Tablets, enteric-coated — 25 mg, 50 mg, 75 mg
Tablets, prolonged-action (Canada) — 100 mg

▷ **Usual Adult Dosage Range:** Initially 100 to 200 mg/24 hours, in 2 to 5 divided doses. After a satisfactory response has been achieved, dosage should be reduced to the minimum that will sustain adequate relief. The usual maintenance dose is 50 to 100 mg/24 hours. **Note: Actual dosage and administration schedule must be determined by the physician for each patient individually.**

▷ **Dosing Instructions:** Take either on an empty stomach or with food or milk if necessary to prevent stomach irritation. Take with a full glass of water and remain upright (do not lie down) for 15 to 30 minutes to prevent lodging of the tablet in the esophagus (food tube). Take the tablet whole; do not crush for administration.

Usual Duration of Use: Continual use on a regular schedule for 1 to 2 weeks is usually necessary to determine this drug's effectiveness in relieving the symptoms of arthritis, bursitis, etc. Severe arthritis may require continual use for 3 to 4 weeks to obtain maximal relief. Long-term use (months to years) requires periodic evaluation of response and dosage adjustment. Consult your physician on a regular basis.

▷ **This Drug Should Not Be Taken If**
- you have had an allergic reaction to it previously.
- you are subject to asthma or nasal polyps caused by aspirin.
- you have active peptic ulcer disease or any form of gastrointestinal bleeding.
- you have active liver disease.
- you have a bleeding disorder or a blood cell disorder.
- you have severe impairment of kidney function.
- you have porphyria (see Glossary).

▷ **Inform Your Physician Before Taking This Drug If**
- you are allergic to aspirin or to other aspirin substitutes.
- you have a history of peptic ulcer disease or any type of bleeding disorder.
- you have impaired liver or kidney function.
- you have high blood pressure or a history of heart failure.
- you have systemic lupus erythematosus (SLE).
- you are taking any of the following drugs: acetaminophen, aspirin or other aspirin substitutes, anticoagulants, cyclosporine, digoxin, diuretics, insulin, lithium, methotrexate, oral antidiabetic drugs.

Possible Side-Effects (natural, expected and unavoidable drug actions)
Fluid retention (weight gain).

▷ **Possible Adverse Effects** (unusual, unexpected and infrequent reactions)
 If any of the following develop, consult your physician promptly for guidance.

Mild Adverse Effects

Allergic Reactions: Skin rash, hives, itching.

Headache, dizziness, drowsiness, depression, anxiety, insomnia, blurred vision, double vision, reversible hearing loss, ear ringing, altered taste.

Mouth soreness, stomach discomfort, nausea, vomiting, indigestion, constipation, diarrhea.

Serious Adverse Effects

Allergic Reactions: Severe skin reactions, eczema, bruising, erythema multiforme, Stevens-Johnson syndrome, hair loss; swelling of lips, tongue, vocal cords; anaphylactoid reaction (see Glossary).

Drug-induced peptic ulcers, with bleeding and perforation; colitis with bloody diarrhea.

Abnormally low red blood cell, white blood cell and blood platelet counts; rare aplastic anemia (see Glossary).

Liver injury with jaundice.

Kidney injury with significantly impaired function.

▷ **Possible Effects on Sexual Function:**   Impotence reported (less than 1%), but causal relationship not established.

 Possible Delayed Adverse Effects: Mild anemia due to "silent" blood loss from the stomach (less than that caused by aspirin).

▷ **Adverse Effects That May Mimic Natural Diseases or Disorders**

Liver reactions may suggest viral hepatitis.

▷ **Natural Diseases or Disorders That May Be Activated by This Drug**

Peptic ulcer disease, Crohn's disease, ulcerative colitis, porphyria, kidney failure associated with systemic lupus erythematosus.

 Possible Effects on Laboratory Tests

Complete blood cell counts: decreased red cells, hemoglobin, white cells and platelets.

Blood cholesterol level: increased.

Blood lithium level: increased.

Blood urea nitrogen (BUN) level: increased.

Liver function tests: increased liver enzymes (ALT/GPT, AST/GOT and alkaline phosphatase), increased bilirubin.

CAUTION

1. Dosage should always be limited to the smallest amount that produces reasonable improvement.
2. This drug may mask early indications of infection. In- form your physician if you think you are developing an infection of any kind.
3. Observe for a pattern of symptoms that may indicate the development of liver toxicity: fatigue, lethargy, "flu-like" symptoms, nausea,

itching, tenderness under the right rib cage, jaundice (see Glossary). Report such symptoms promptly.

4. Observe for possible drug-induced bleeding in the gastrointestinal tract: bloody (reddish) or tarry (black) stools.

Precautions for Use
By Infants and Children: Safety and effectiveness for use by those under 12 years of age have not been established.

By Those over 60 Years of Age: Small doses are advisable initially until tolerance is determined. Observe for any indications of liver or kidney toxicity, fluid retention, dizziness, confusion, impaired memory, stomach bleeding or constipation.

▷ Advisability of Use During Pregnancy
Pregnancy Category: B (tentative). See Pregnancy Code inside back cover.

Animal studies: Mouse, rat and rabbit studies reveal toxic effects on the embryo but no birth defects due to this drug.

Human studies: Information from adequate studies of pregnant women is not available.

Avoid this drug completely during the last 3 months. Use it during the first 6 months only if clearly needed. Ask your physician for guidance.

Advisability of Use if Breast-Feeding
Presence of this drug in breast milk: Yes.

Avoid drug or refrain from nursing.

Habit-Forming Potential: None.

Effects of Overdosage: Probable drowsiness, dizziness, ear ringing, nausea, vomiting, diarrhea, confusion, unsteadiness, stupor.

Possible Effects of Long-Term Use: Secondary anemia (chronic blood loss from stomach), fluid retention, elevated blood pressure.

Suggested Periodic Examinations While Taking This Drug (at physician's discretion)
Complete blood cell counts; liver function tests within the first 8 weeks of use and periodically thereafter; kidney function tests.

Complete eye examinations if vision is altered in any way.

▷ While Taking This Drug, Observe the Following
Foods: No restrictions.

Nutritional Support: Supplemental iron if anemia develops.

Beverages: No restrictions. May be taken with milk.

▷   *Alcohol:* Use sparingly and with caution. The irritant action of alcohol on the stomach lining, added to the irritant action of this drug in sensitive individuals, can increase the risk of stomach ulceration and/or bleeding.

Tobacco Smoking: No interactions expected.

▷   *Other Drugs*

Diclofenac may ***increase*** the effects of

- acetaminophen (Tylenol, etc.), and increase the risk of liver or kidney damage; avoid prolonged use of this combination.
- anticoagulants (Coumadin, etc.), and increase the risk of bleeding; monitor prothrombin time, adjust dose accordingly.
- aspirin, and increase the risk of stomach ulceration and/or bleeding; avoid this combination.

Diclofenac may *decrease* the effects of

- amiloride (Midamor, Moduretic), and raise blood potassium levels.
- oral antidiabetic drugs (see Drug Class, Section Four), and alter control of blood sugar unpredictably.
- bumetanide (Bumex).
- chlorthalidone (Hygroton, etc.).
- ethacrynic acid (Edecrin).
- furosemide (Lasix).
- indapamide (Lozol).
- metolazone (Diulo, Zaroxolyn).
- spironolactone (Aldactone, Aldactazide), and raise blood potassium levels.
- thiazide diuretics (see Drug Class, Section Four).
- triamterene (Dyazide, Maxzide), and raise blood potassium levels.

Diclofenac *taken concurrently* with the following drugs may increase the risk of bleeding (antiplatelet effect); monitor these combinations closely:

- aspirin.
- colchicine (ColBenemid, etc.).
- dipyridamole (Persantine).
- indomethacin (Indocin).
- sulfinpyrazone (Anturane).
- valproic acid (Depakene).

Diclofenac *taken concurrently* with the following drugs may increase their toxicity; monitor these combinations closely:

- cyclosporine (Sandimmune).
- digoxin (Lanoxin).
- lithium (Lithane, etc.).
- methotrexate (Folex, Mexate).

The following drug may *increase* the effects of diclofenac

- probenecid (Benemid), by slowing its elimination.

▷ *Driving, Hazardous Activities:* This drug may cause dizziness, drowsiness or blurred vision.
Restrict activities as necessary.

Aviation Note: The use of this drug *may be a disqualification* for piloting. Consult a designated Aviation Medical Examiner.

Exposure to Sun: Use caution until sensitivity is determined. Photosensitivity (see Glossary) has been reported.

DICYCLOMINE
(di SI kloh meen)

Introduced: 1952

Class: Antispasmodic, atropinelike drugs

Prescription: USA: Yes
Canada: No

Controlled Drug: USA: No
Canada: No

Available as Generic: Yes

Brand Names: Bentyl, ✦Bentylol, Byclomine, ✦Formulex, ✦Lomine, ✦Protylol, ✦Spasmoban, ✦Viscerol

---

BENEFITS versus RISKS

Possible Benefits	*Possible Risks*
EFFECTIVE RELIEF OF GASTROINTESTINAL SPASM	Increased internal eye pressure (important in glaucoma) Constipation Urinary retention (in predisposed persons)

▷ **Principal Uses**

As a Single Drug Product: Used primarily for its atropinelike antispasmodic effect in the management of functional disorders of the gastrointestinal tract, notably the irritable bowel syndrome (spastic colon). It is also used to relieve cramping and pain in infant colic.

How This Drug Works: Not completely established. It has been suggested that this drug may relax gastrointestinal muscle by means of a local anesthetic action that blocks reflex activity responsible for contraction and motility.

Available Dosage Forms and Strengths
Capsules — 10 mg, 20 mg
Injection — 10 mg per ml
Syrup — 10 mg per 5-ml teaspoonful
Tablets — 20 mg

▷ **Usual Adult Dosage Range:** 10 to 20 mg, 3 or 4 times daily. Total daily dosage should not exceed 160 mg. **Note: Actual dosage and administration schedule must be determined by the physician for each patient individually.**

▷ **Dosing Instructions:** May be taken with or following food to prevent stomach irritation. The syrup may be diluted with an equal amount of water. The capsule may be opened and the tablet may be crushed for administration.

Usual Duration of Use: Continual use on a regular schedule for 2 to 5 days is usually necessary to determine this drug's effectiveness in relieving the symptoms of spastic disorders of the digestive system. Limit use to the relief of symptoms as necessary. Ask physician for guidance regarding long-term use.

▷ **This Drug Should Not Be Taken If**
- you have had an allergic reaction to any dosage form of it previously.
- your stomach cannot empty properly into the intestine (pyloric obstruction).
- you are unable to empty the urinary bladder completely.
- you have ulcerative colitis.

▷ **Inform Your Physician Before Taking This Drug If**
- you have a history of peptic ulcer disease.
- you have impaired liver or kidney function.
- you have glaucoma, myasthenia gravis or prostatism (see Glossary).

Possible Side-Effects (natural, expected and unavoidable drug actions)
Dryness of the mouth, blurred vision, constipation.

▷ **Possible Adverse Effects** (unusual, unexpected and infrequent reactions)
If any of the following develop, consult your physician promptly for guidance.
Mild Adverse Effects
Allergic Reactions: Skin rash, hives.
Headache, dizziness, drowsiness, weakness.
Reduced appetite, nausea, vomiting.
Difficult urination.
Serious Adverse Effects
Allergic Reaction: Anaphylactic reaction (see Glossary).
Idiosyncratic Reactions: Excitement, confusion, disturbed behavior.
Increased internal eye pressure (significant in glaucoma).

▷ **Possible Effects on Sexual Function**
Impotence (6-hour effect following dosage).
Suppression of milk production.

Natural Diseases or Disorders That May Be Activated by This Drug
Glaucoma, prostatism (see Glossary).

Possible Effects on Laboratory Tests
None reported.

CAUTION
Many over-the-counter medications (see OTC drugs in Glossary) for allergies, colds and coughs contain drugs that can interact unfavorably with this drug. Ask your physician or pharmacist for guidance before using any such medications.

Precautions for Use

By Infants and Children: Use extreme care in giving syrup to infants so as to prevent aspiration (inhalation) of the drug. Serious reactions have occurred as a result of this accident during administration.

By Those over 60 Years of Age: Begin treatment with small doses until tolerance is determined. You may be more susceptible to the development of confusion, excitement, constipation and prostatism.

▷ **Advisability of Use During Pregnancy**

Pregnancy Category: B (tentative). See Pregnancy Code inside back cover.

Animal studies: No birth defects reported.

Human studies: Information from adequate studies of pregnant women is not available.

Use only if clearly needed. Ask physician for guidance.

Advisability of Use if Breast-Feeding

Presence of this drug in breast milk: Unknown.

Avoid drug or refrain from nursing.

Habit-Forming Potential: None.

Effects of Overdosage: Headache, dizziness, nausea, dry mouth, difficulty in swallowing, excitement, restlessness, dilated pupils, hot and dry skin.

Possible Effects of Long-Term Use: None reported.

Suggested Periodic Examinations While Taking This Drug (at physician's discretion)

Measurements of internal eye pressure (in presence of glaucoma or suspected glaucoma).

▷ **While Taking This Drug, Observe the Following**

Foods: No interactions. Follow prescribed diet.

Beverages: No interactions. May be taken with milk.

▷ *Alcohol:* Use caution until combined effects have been determined. Observe for increased drowsiness.

Tobacco Smoking: No interactions expected. Follow physician's advice regarding smoking.

Marijuana Smoking: Possible increase in drowsiness and dryness of mouth.

▷ *Other Drugs*

Dicyclomine may *increase* the effects of

• other drugs that have atropinelike actions (see Drug Class, Section Four).

Dicyclomine may *decrease* the effects of

• levodopa (Larodopa, Sinemet, etc.).

▷ *Driving, Hazardous Activities:* This drug may cause drowsiness, dizziness or blurred vision. Restrict activities accordingly.

Aviation Note: The use of this drug *may be a disqualification* for piloting. Consult a designated Aviation Medical Examiner.

Exposure to Sun: No restrictions.

Exposure to Heat: Use caution. The use of this drug in hot environments may impair normal perspiration and interfere with the regulation of body temperature, thus increasing the risk of heat stroke.

DIFLUNISAL
(di FLOO ni sal)

Introduced: 1977

Class: Mild analgesic, anti-inflammatory

Prescription: USA: Yes
Canada: Yes

Controlled Drug: USA: No
Canada: No

Available as Generic: No

Brand Name: Dolobid

BENEFITS versus RISKS	
Possible Benefits	*Possible Risks*
EFFECTIVE RELIEF OF MILD TO MODERATE PAIN AND INFLAMMATION	Gastrointestinal pain, ulceration, bleeding (rare) Rare liver or kidney damage Rare fluid retention

▷ **Principal Uses**

As a Single Drug Product: Used primarily to relieve mild to moderately severe pain associated with (1) musculoskeletal injuries; (2) acute and chronic rheumatoid arthritis and osteoarthritis; and (3) dental, obstetrical and orthopedic surgery.

How This Drug Works: Not completely established. It is thought that this drug reduces the tissue concentrations of prostaglandins (and related compounds), chemicals involved in the production of inflammation and pain.

Available Dosage Forms and Strengths
Tablets — 250 mg, 500 mg

▷ **Usual Adult Dosage Range:** Initially 500 to 1000 mg (loading dose), then 250 to 500 mg/8 to 12 hours. Total daily dosage should not exceed 1500 mg. **Note: Actual dosage and administration schedule must be determined by the physician for each patient individually.**

▷ **Dosing Instructions:** Take either on an empty stomach or with food or milk to prevent stomach irritation. Swallow tablets whole; do not crush or chew. Take with a full glass of water and remain upright (do not lie down) for 30 minutes.

Usual Duration of Use: Continual use on a regular schedule for 1 to 2 weeks is usually necessary to determine this drug's effectiveness in relieving the discomfort of arthritis. Long-term use requires supervision and periodic evaluation by the physician. Consult your physician on a regular basis.

▷ **This Drug Should Not Be Taken If**
- you have had an allergic reaction to it previously.
- you are subject to asthma or nasal polyps caused by aspirin.
- you have active peptic ulcer disease or any form of gastrointestinal bleeding.

▷ **Inform Your Physician Before Taking This Drug If**
- you are allergic to aspirin or to other aspirin substitutes.
- you have a history of peptic ulcer disease or any type of bleeding disorder.
- you have impaired liver or kidney function.
- you have high blood pressure or a history of heart failure.
- you are pregnant.
- you are taking any of the following: acetaminophen, aspirin or other aspirin substitutes, anticoagulants, oral antidiabetic drugs.

Possible Side-Effects (natural, expected and unavoidable drug actions)
Drowsiness, ringing in ears, fluid retention.

▷ **Possible Adverse Effects** (unusual, unexpected and infrequent reactions)
If any of the following develop, consult your physician promptly for guidance.
Mild Adverse Effects
Allergic Reactions: Skin rash, hives, itching.
Headache, dizziness, altered or blurred vision, depression.
Mouth sores, indigestion, nausea, vomiting, constipation, diarrhea.
Serious Adverse Effects
Allergic Reactions: Severe skin reactions, swollen lymph glands, drug fever (see Glossary), asthma, anaphylaxis (see Glossary).
Active peptic ulcer, with or without bleeding.
Liver damage with jaundice (see Glossary).
Kidney damage with painful urination, bloody urine, reduced urine formation.
Reduced blood platelet (see Glossary) count with abnormal bleeding or bruising.

▷ **Possible Effects on Sexual Function:**   None reported.

▷ **Adverse Effects That May Mimic Natural Diseases or Disorders**
Liver reaction may suggest viral hepatitis.

Natural Diseases or Disorders That May Be Activated by This Drug
Peptic ulcer disease, ulcerative colitis.

Possible Effects on Laboratory Tests
Blood uric acid level: decreased (maximal effect within 2 weeks).

CAUTION
1. Inform your physician promptly if flulike symptoms develop in association with a skin rash; this could represent a serious allergic reaction.
2. This drug may mask early indications of infection. Inform your physician if you think you are developing an infection of any kind.

Precautions for Use
By Infants and Children: Safety and effectiveness for use by those under 12 years of age have not been established.
By Those over 60 Years of Age: Small doses are advisable until tolerance is determined. Observe for any indications of liver or kidney toxicity.

▷ ## Advisability of Use During Pregnancy
Pregnancy Category: C (tentative). See Pregnancy Code inside back cover.
Animal studies: Skeletal birth defects reported in rabbits.
Human studies: Information from adequate studies of pregnant women is not available.
Avoid this drug during the first and last 3 months. Use it during the middle 3 months only if clearly needed. Ask physician for guidance.

Advisability of Use if Breast-Feeding
Presence of this drug in breast milk: Yes.
Avoid drug or refrain from nursing.

Habit-Forming Potential: None.

Effects of Overdosage: Drowsiness, confusion, disorientation, nausea, vomiting, stupor.

Possible Effects of Long-Term Use: None reported.

Suggested Periodic Examinations While Taking This Drug (at physician's discretion)
Complete blood cell counts, liver and kidney function tests.
Complete eye examinations if vision is altered in any way.

▷ ## While Taking This Drug, Observe the Following
Foods: No restrictions.
Beverages: No restrictions. May be taken with milk.
▷ *Alcohol:* Use with caution. The irritant action of alcohol on the stomach lining, added to the irritant action of this drug in sensitive individuals, can increase the risk of stomach ulceration and/or bleeding.
Tobacco Smoking: No interactions expected.
▷ *Other Drugs*
Diflunisal may *increase* the effects of
• acetaminophen (Tylenol, etc.), and increase the risk of liver damage; avoid this combination.

- anticoagulants (Coumadin, etc.), and increase the risk of bleeding; monitor prothrombin time, adjust dose accordingly.
- hydrochlorothiazide (Esidrix, HydroDiuril, etc.).

Diflunisal **taken concurrently** with the following drugs may increase the risk of bleeding; avoid these combinations:

- aspirin.
- dipyridamole (Persantine).
- indomethacin (Indocin).
- sulfinpyrazone (Anturane).
- valproic acid (Depakene).

The following drugs may **decrease** the effects of diflunisal

- aluminum antacids may decrease its absorption.

▷ *Driving, Hazardous Activities:* This drug may cause drowsiness, dizziness or altered vision. Restrict activities as necessary.

Aviation Note: The use of this drug **may be a disqualification** for piloting. Consult a designated Aviation Medical Examiner.

Exposure to Sun: Use caution until sensitivity is determined. This drug may cause photosensitivity (see Glossary).

DIGOXIN
(di JOX in)

Introduced: 1934

Class: Digitalis preparations

Prescription: USA: Yes
Canada: No

Controlled Drug: USA: No
Canada: No

Available as Generic: Yes

Brand Names: Lanoxicaps, Lanoxin, ✦Novodigoxin

BENEFITS versus RISKS	
Possible Benefits	*Possible Risks*
EFFECTIVE HEART STIMULANT IN CONGESTIVE HEART FAILURE	NARROW TREATMENT RANGE (treatment dose is 60% of toxic dose)
EFFECTIVE PREVENTION AND TREATMENT OF CERTAIN HEART RHYTHM DISORDERS	Frequent and sometimes serious disturbances of heart rhythm

▷ **Principal Uses**

As a Single Drug Product: This drug has two primary uses: (1) the treatment of congestive heart failure; (2) the restoration and maintenance of normal heart rate and rhythm in such disorders as atrial fibrillation, atrial flutter and atrial/supraventricular tachycardia.

How This Drug Works: By increasing the availability of calcium within the heart muscle, this drug improves the efficiency of the conversion of chemical energy to mechanical energy, thus increasing the force of heart muscle contraction. By slowing the activity of the pacemaker and delaying the transmission of electrical impulses through the conduction system of the heart, this drug assists in restoring normal heart rate and rhythm.

Available Dosage Forms and Strengths
Elixir, pediatric — 0.05 mg per ml
Capsules — 0.05 mg, 0.1 mg, 0.2 mg
Injection — 0.1 mg per ml, 0.25 mg per ml
Tablets — 0.125 mg, 0.25 mg, 0.5 mg

▷ **Usual Adult Dosage Range:**   Rapid digitalization—1 to 1.5 mg divided into 2 or 3 doses given every 6 to 8 hours in 1 day. Slow digitalization—0.125 to 0.5 mg/day for 7 days. Maintenance—0.125 to 0.5 mg/day. Total daily dosage should not exceed 2 mg. **Note: Actual dosage and administration schedule must be determined by the physician for each patient individually.**

▷ **Dosing Instructions:**   Take at the same time each day, or preferably on an empty stomach to ensure uniform absorption. May be taken with or following food if desired (not milk dairy products). The tablet may be crushed for administration; the capsule should be swallowed whole.

Usual Duration of Use: Continual use on a regular schedule for 7 to 10 days is usually necessary to determine this drug's effectiveness in relieving heart failure or controlling heart rhythm disorders. Long-term use requires physician supervision and periodic assessment of continued need. The use of this drug is not necessarily "for life." Consult your physician on a regular basis.

▷ **This Drug Should Not Be Taken If**
• you have had an allergic reaction to any dosage form of it previously.

▷ **Inform Your Physician Before Taking This Drug If**
• you have experienced any unfavorable reaction to a digitalis preparation in the past.
• you have taken any digitalis preparation within the past 2 weeks.
• you are now taking (or have recently taken) any diuretic (urine-producing) drug.
• you have impaired liver or kidney function.
• you have a history of thyroid function disorder.

Possible Side-Effects (natural, expected and unavoidable drug actions)
Slow heart rate, rare enlargement and/or sensitivity of the male breast tissue.

▷ **Possible Adverse Effects** (unusual, unexpected and infrequent reactions)
If any of the following develop, consult your physician promptly for guidance.
Mild Adverse Effects
Allergic Reactions: Skin rash, hives.
Headache, drowsiness, lethargy, confusion, changes in vision: "halo" effect, blurring, spots, double vision, yellow-green vision.
Loss of appetite, nausea, vomiting, diarrhea—early indications of toxicity in adults.
Serious Adverse Effects
Idiosyncratic Reactions: Hallucinations, facial neuralgias, peripheral neuralgias, blindness (very rare).
Disorientation, most common in the elderly.
Heart rhythm disturbances.

▷ **Possible Effects on Sexual Function**
Decreased libido and impotence in 35% of male users.
Enlargement and tenderness of male breasts.
Both effects are attributed to digoxin's estrogenlike action.

▷ **Adverse Effects That May Mimic Natural Diseases or Disorders**
Drug-induced mental disturbances in the elderly may be mistaken for senile dementia or psychosis.

Natural Diseases or Disorders That May Be Activated by This Drug
Digitalis may induce a cutaneous lupus-erythematosuslike syndrome.

Possible Effects on Laboratory Tests
White blood cell counts: decreased.
Blood testosterone level: decreased 30% in men with long-term use.

CAUTION
1. This drug has a narrow margin of safe use. Adhere strictly to prescribed dosage schedules. Do not raise or lower the dose without first consulting your physician.
2. If you are taking calcium supplements, ask your physician for guidance. Avoid large doses.
3. It is advisable to carry a card of personal identification with a notation that you are taking this drug.
4. Avoid taking over-the-counter antacids and cold, cough and allergy remedies without consulting your physician.

Precautions for Use
By Infants and Children: Observe carefully for indications of toxicity: slow heart rate (below 60 beats/minute), irregular heart rhythms.
By Those over 60 Years of Age: You may have a reduced tolerance for this drug; smaller doses are advisable. Observe for indications of early toxicity: headache, dizziness, fatigue, weakness, lethargy, depression, confusion, nervousness, agitation, delusions, difficulty with reading. Report the development of any of these effects promptly to your physician.

▷ **Advisability of Use During Pregnancy**
    Pregnancy Category: C (tentative). See Pregnancy Code inside back cover.
        Animal studies: No birth defects reported.
        Human studies: Information from adequate studies of pregnant women
            is not available. However, no birth defects attributable to the therapeu-
            tic use of this drug have been reported.
        Use this drug only if clearly needed. Overdosage can be harmful to the
            fetus.

Advisability of Use if Breast-Feeding
    Presence of this drug in breast milk: Yes.
    Monitor nursing infant closely and discontinue drug or nursing if ad-
        verse effects develop.

Habit-Forming Potential: None.

Effects of Overdosage: Loss of appetite, excessive saliva, nausea, vomiting,
    diarrhea, serious disturbances of heart rate and rhythm, intestinal
    bleeding, drowsiness, headache, confusion, delirium, hallucinations,
    convulsions.

Possible Effects of Long-Term Use: None reported.

Suggested Periodic Examinations While Taking This Drug (at physician's
    discretion)
        Measurements of blood levels of digoxin, calcium, magnesium and potas-
            sium; electrocardiograms.

▷ **While Taking This Drug, Observe the Following**
    Foods: Avoid all cheeses, yogurt and ice cream for 2 hours before and after
        taking this drug. Consult physician regarding the advisability of eating
        high-potassium foods.
    Beverages: Avoid all forms of milk for 2 hours before and after taking this
        drug. Avoid excessive amounts of caffeine-containing beverages: cof-
        fee, tea, cola.
▷ *Alcohol:* No interactions expected.
    Tobacco Smoking: Nicotine can cause irritability of the heart muscle and
        can predispose to serious rhythm disturbances. It is advisable to ab-
        stain from all forms of tobacco.
    Marijuana Smoking: Possible accentuation of heart failure; reduced di-
        goxin effect; possible changes in electrocardiogram, confusing inter-
        pretation.
▷ *Other Drugs*
    Digoxin *taken concurrently* with
        • diuretics (other than spironolactone and triamterene) may result in
            serious heart rhythm disturbances due to excessive loss of potassium.
        • quinidine may result in decreased digoxin effectiveness and increased
            digoxin toxicity; careful dosage adjustments are necessary.
    The following drugs may *increase* the effects of digoxin
        • amiodarone (Cordarone).
        • benzodiazepines (Librium, Valium, etc.; see Drug Class, Section Four).

- captopril (Capoten, Capazide).
- diltiazem (Cardizem).
- erythromycin (EES, Erythrocin, etc.).
- flecainide (Tambocor).
- hydroxychloroquine.
- ibuprofen (Advil, Medipren, Motrin, Nuprin, etc.).
- indomethacin (Indocin).
- methimazole (Tapazole).
- nifedipine (Adalat, Procardia).
- propylthiouracil (Propacil).
- quinine.
- tetracyclines (see Drug Class, Section Four).
- tolbutamide (Orinase).
- verapamil (Isoptin).

The following drugs may **decrease** the effects of digoxin
- aluminum-containing antacids (Amphojel, Maalox, etc.).
- bleomycin (Blenoxane).
- carmustine (Bicnu).
- cholestyramine (Questran).
- colestipol (Colestid).
- cyclophosphamide (Cytoxan).
- cytarabine (Cytosar).
- doxorubicin (Adriamycin).
- methotrexate (Mexate).
- penicillamine (Cuprimine, Depen).
- procarbazine (Matulane).
- thyroid hormones.
- vincristine (Oncovin).

▷ *Driving, Hazardous Activities:* Usually no restrictions. However, this drug may cause drowsiness, vision changes and nausea. Restrict activities as necessary.

Aviation Note: Heart function disorders **are a disqualification** for piloting. Consult a designated Aviation Medical Examiner.

Exposure to Sun: No restrictions.

Occurrence of Unrelated Illness: Any illness that causes vomiting or diarrhea can seriously alter this drug's effectiveness. Notify your physician promptly.

Discontinuation: This drug must be continued indefinitely. Do not discontinue it without consulting your physician.

DILTIAZEM
(dil TI a zem)

Introduced: 1977

Class: Antianginal, antihypertensive, calcium channel blocker

Prescription: USA: Yes
Canada: Yes

Controlled Drug: USA: No
Canada: No

Available as Generic: No

Brand Names: Cardizem, Cardizem SR

BENEFITS versus RISKS

Possible Benefits	*Possible Risks*
EFFECTIVE PREVENTION OF BOTH MAJOR TYPES OF ANGINA	Depression, confusion
	Low blood pressure
	Heart rhythm disturbance (2%)
EFFECTIVE CONTROL OF MILD TO MODERATE HYPERTENSION	Fluid retention (2.4%)
	Liver damage (very rare)

▷ **Principal Uses**

As a Single Drug Product: Used primarily to treat (1) angina pectoris due to coronary artery spasm (Prinzmetal's variant angina) that occurs spontaneously and is not associated with exertion; (2) classical angina-of-effort (due to atherosclerotic disease of the coronary arteries) in individuals who have not responded to or cannot tolerate the nitrates and beta blocker drugs customarily used to treat this disorder; (3) mild to moderately severe hypertension.

How This Drug Works: Not completely established. It is thought that by blocking the normal passage of calcium through certain cell walls (which is necessary for the function of nerve and muscle tissue), this drug slows the spread of electrical activity through the conduction system of the heart and inhibits the contraction of coronary arteries and peripheral arterioles. As a result of these combined effects, this drug

• prevents spontaneous spasm of the coronary arteries (Prinzmetal's type of angina).
• reduces the rate and contraction force of the heart during exertion, thus lowering the oxygen requirement of the heart muscle; this reduces the occurrence of effort-induced angina (classical angina pectoris).
• reduces the degree of contraction of peripheral arterial walls, resulting in their relaxation and consequent lowering of blood pressure. This further reduces the work load of the heart during exertion and contributes to the prevention of angina.

Available Dosage Forms and Strengths
Tablets — 30 mg, 60 mg, 90 mg, 120 mg
Capsules, prolonged-action — 60 mg, 90 mg, 120 mg

▷ **Usual Adult Dosage Range:**   Initially 30 mg, 3 or 4 times daily. Dose may be increased gradually at 1- to 2-day intervals as needed and tolerated. Total daily dosage should not exceed 360 mg. **Note: Actual dosage and administration schedule must be determined by the physician for each patient individually.**

▷ **Dosing Instructions:**   Preferably taken before meals and at bedtime. Tablet may be crushed for administration.

Usual Duration of Use: Continual use on a regular schedule for 2 to 4 weeks is usually necessary to determine this drug's effectiveness in reducing the frequency and severity of angina and in lowering elevated blood pressure. For long-term use (months to years), determine the smallest effective dose. Consult your physician on a regular basis.

Possible Advantages of This Drug
Often effective as single drug therapy.
Does not reduce blood supply to kidneys.
Does not raise blood cholesterol levels.
Does not induce asthma in susceptible individuals.

▷ **This Drug Should Not Be Taken If**
  • you have had an allergic reaction to it previously.
  • you have a "sick sinus" syndrome (and are not wearing an artificial pacemaker).
  • you have been told that you have a second-degree or third-degree heart block.
  • you have low blood pressure—systolic pressure below 90.

▷ **Inform Your Physician Before Taking This Drug If**
  • you have had an unfavorable response to any calcium blocker drug in the past.
  • you are currently taking any form of digitalis or a beta blocker drug (see Drug Class, Section Four).
  • you have a history of congestive heart failure.
  • you have impaired liver or kidney function.
  • you have a history of drug-induced liver damage.

Possible Side-Effects (natural, expected and unavoidable drug actions)
Fatigue (1.2%), light-headedness, heart rate and rhythm changes in predisposed individuals (1.1%).

▷ **Possible Adverse Effects** (unusual, unexpected and infrequent reactions)
If any of the following develop, consult your physician promptly for guidance.
Mild Adverse Effects
Allergic Reactions: Skin rash (1.3%), hives, itching.

Headache (2.1%), drowsiness, dizziness (1.5%), nervousness, insomnia, depression, confusion, hallucinations.

Flushing, palpitations, fainting, slow heart rate, low blood pressure.

Nausea (1.9%), indigestion, heartburn, vomiting, diarrhea, constipation.

Serious Adverse Effects

Serious disturbances of heart rate and/or rhythm, fluid retention (edema) (2.4%), congestive heart failure.

Drug-induced liver damage (very rare).

▷ **Possible Effects on Sexual Function:**   Impotence is reported in less than 1% of users.

Possible Effects on Laboratory Tests

Blood total cholesterol and triglyceride levels: no effects.

Blood HDL cholesterol level: increased.

Blood LDL and VLDL cholesterol levels: no effects.

CAUTION

1. Be sure to inform all physicians and dentists you consult that you are taking this drug. Note the use of this drug on your card of personal identification.

2. You may use nitroglycerin and other nitrate drugs as needed to relieve acute episodes of angina pain. However, if you detect that your angina attacks are becoming more frequent or intense, notify your physician promptly.

Precautions for Use

By Infants and Children: Safety and effectiveness for use by those under 12 years of age have not been established.

By Those over 60 Years of Age: You may be more susceptible to the development of weakness, dizziness, fainting and falling. Take necessary precautions to prevent injury. Report promptly any changes in your pattern of thirst and urination.

▷ **Advisability of Use During Pregnancy**

Pregnancy Category: C (tentative). See Pregnancy Code inside back cover.

Animal studies: Embryo and fetal deaths and skeletal birth defects reported in mice, rats and rabbits.

Human studies: Information from adequate studies of pregnant women is not available.

Avoid this drug during the first 3 months.

Use during the last 6 months only if clearly needed. Ask physician for guidance.

Advisability of Use if Breast-Feeding

Presence of this drug in breast milk: Yes.

Avoid drug or refrain from nursing.

Habit-Forming Potential: None.

Effects of Overdosage: Weakness, light-headedness, fainting, slow pulse, low blood pressure, shortness of breath, congestive heart failure.

Possible Effects of Long-Term Use: None reported.

Suggested Periodic Examinations While Taking This Drug (at physician's discretion)

Evaluations of heart function, including electrocardiograms; liver and kidney function tests, with long-term use.

▷ **While Taking This Drug, Observe the Following**

Foods: No restrictions. Avoid excessive salt intake.

Beverages: No restrictions. May be taken with milk.

▷ *Alcohol:* Use with caution until combined effects have been determined. Alcohol may exaggerate the drop in blood pressure experienced by some individuals.

Tobacco Smoking: Nicotine may reduce the effectiveness of this drug. Follow your physician's advice regarding smoking.

Marijuana Smoking: Possible reduced effectiveness of this drug; mild to moderate increase in angina; possible changes in electrocardiogram, confusing interpretation.

▷ *Other Drugs*

Diltiazem *taken concurrently* with

• beta blocker drugs or digitalis preparations (see Drug Classes, Section Four) may affect heart rate and rhythm adversely. Careful monitoring by your physician is necessary if these drugs are taken concurrently.

The following drugs may *increase* the effects of diltiazem

• cimetidine (Tagamet).

▷ *Driving, Hazardous Activities:* Usually no restrictions. This drug may cause drowsiness or dizziness. Restrict activities as necessary.

Aviation Note: Coronary artery disease *is a disqualification* for piloting. Consult a designated Aviation Medical Examiner.

Exposure to Sun: Use caution until sensitivity has been determined. This drug may cause photosensitivity (see Glossary).

Exposure to Heat: Caution advised. Hot environments can exaggerate the blood-pressure-lowering effects of this drug. Observe for light-headedness or weakness.

Heavy Exercise or Exertion: This drug may improve your ability to be more active without resulting angina pain. Use caution and avoid excessive exercise that could impair heart function in the absence of warning pain.

Discontinuation: Do not discontinue this drug abruptly. Consult your physician regarding gradual withdrawal.

DIPHENHYDRAMINE
(di fen HI dra meen)

Introduced: 1946

Prescription: USA: Varies
Canada: No

Available as Generic: Yes

Class: Hypnotic, antihistamines

Controlled Drug: USA: No*
Canada: No

Brand Names: ✦Allerdryl, ✦Ambenyl Expectorant [CD], Ambenyl Syrup [CD], Benadryl, Benadryl 25, Benylin, ✦Benylin Decongestant [CD], ✦Benylin Pediatric Syrup, ✦Benylin Syrup w/Codeine [CD], ✦Caladryl [CD], Compoz, Diphenhist, ✦Ergodryl [CD], Excedrin P.M. [CD], Genahist, ✦Insomnal, ✦Mandrax [CD], Nytol, Sleep-Eze 3, Sominex 2, Twilite, Valdrene

---

BENEFITS versus RISKS

Possible Benefits	*Possible Risks*
EFFECTIVE RELIEF OF ALLERGIC RHINITIS AND ALLERGIC SKIN DISORDERS	Marked sedation (50%)
	Atropinelike effects
EFFECTIVE, NONADDICTIVE SEDATIVE AND HYPNOTIC	Accentuation of prostatism (see Glossary)
Prevention and relief of motion sickness	Rare blood cell disorders: abnormally low white blood cell and platelet counts
Partial relief of symptoms of Parkinson's disease	

▷ **Principal Uses**

As a Single Drug Product: This versatile antihistamine is used primarily for (1) the safe and effective induction of sleep (mild to moderate sedation); (2) the prevention and treatment of motion sickness (control of dizziness, nausea and vomiting); (3) the relief of symptoms associated with Parkinson's disease; (4) the treatment of drug-induced parkinsonian reactions, especially in children and the elderly.

As a Combination Drug Product [CD]: This drug may have a mild suppressant effect on coughing, but its actual effectiveness is questionable. It is combined with expectorants and either codeine or dextromethorphan in some cough preparations.

How This Drug Works: This drug reduces the intensity of allergic response by blocking the action of histamine after it has been released from sensitized tissue cells. Its natural side-effects are used to advantage: its sedative action is used to induce drowsiness and sleep; its atropinelike

*Ambenyl Syrup is C-V. See Schedules of Controlled Drugs inside back cover.

action is used in the management of motion sickness and Parkinson-related disorders.

Available Dosage Forms and Strengths
  Capsules — 25 mg, 50 mg
    Cream — 1%
    Elixir — 12.5 mg per 5-ml teaspoonful (14% alcohol)
    Spray — 1%
    Syrup — 12.5 mg, 13.3 mg per 5-ml teaspoonful
  Tablets — 25 mg, 50 mg

▷ **Usual Adult Dosage Range:** 25 to 50 mg/4 to 6 hours. Total daily dosage should not exceed 300 mg. **Note: Actual dosage and administration schedule must be determined by the physician for each patient individually.**

▷ **Dosing Instructions:** Preferably taken with or following food to reduce stomach irritation. Tablet may be crushed and capsule may be opened for administration.

Usual Duration of Use: Continual use on a regular schedule for 2 to 3 days is usually necessary to determine this drug's effectiveness in relieving the symptoms of allergic rhinitis and dermatosis. If not effective after 5 days, this drug should be discontinued. As a bedtime sedative (hypnotic), use only as needed. Avoid long-term use without interruption.

▷ **This Drug Should Not Be Taken If**
  • you have had an allergic reaction to any dosage form of it previously.
  • you are taking, or have taken during the past 2 weeks, any monoamine oxidase (MAO) type A inhibitor drug (see Drug Class, Section Four).

▷ **Inform Your Physician Before Taking This Drug If**
  • you have had an unfavorable response to any antihistamine drug in the past.
  • you have narrow-angle glaucoma.
  • you have peptic ulcer disease, with any degree of pyloric obstruction.
  • you have prostatism (see Glossary).
  • you are subject to bronchial asthma or seizures (epilepsy).

Possible Side-Effects (natural, expected and unavoidable drug actions)
  Drowsiness; sense of weakness; dryness of nose, mouth and throat; constipation.

▷ **Possible Adverse Effects** (unusual, unexpected and infrequent reactions)
  If any of the following develop, consult your physician promptly for guidance.
  Mild Adverse Effects
  Allergic Reactions: Skin rash, hives.
  Headache, dizziness, inability to concentrate, nervousness, blurred or double vision, difficult urination.

Reduced tolerance for contact lenses.

Nausea, vomiting, diarrhea.

Serious Adverse Effects

Allergic Reaction: Anaphylactic reaction (see Glossary).

Idiosyncratic Reactions: Insomnia, excitement, confusion.

Hemolytic anemia (see Glossary).

Reduced white blood cell count—fever, sore throat, infections.

Blood platelet destruction (see Glossary)—abnormal bleeding or bruising.

▷ **Possible Effects on Sexual Function:** Shortened menstrual cycle (early arrival of expected menstrual onset).

Natural Diseases or Disorders That May Be Activated by This Drug

Latent epilepsy, glaucoma, prostatism.

Possible Effects on Laboratory Tests

Red blood cell counts and hemoglobin: decreased.

Urine screening tests for drug abuse: *initial* test result may be falsely **positive**; *confirmatory* test result will be **negative**. (Test results depend upon amount of drug taken and testing method used.)

CAUTION

1. Discontinue this drug 5 days before diagnostic skin testing procedures in order to prevent false negative test results.
2. Do not use this drug if you have active bronchial asthma, bronchitis or pneumonia. It can thicken bronchial mucous and make it more difficult to remove (by absorption or coughing).

Precautions for Use

By Infants and Children: This drug should not be used in premature or full-term newborn infants. Doses for children should be small. The young child is especially sensitive to the effects of antihistamines on the brain and nervous system. Avoid the use of this drug in the child with chicken pox or a flulike infection; although unproven, this drug may adversely affect the course of Reye syndrome should the child develop it during the course of illness.

By Those over 60 Years of Age: You may be more susceptible to the development of drowsiness, dizziness and unsteadiness, and to impairment of thinking, judgment and memory. This drug can increase the degree of impaired urination associated with prostate gland enlargement (prostatism). The sedative effects of antihistamines in the elderly can cause a syndrome of underactivity that may be misinterpreted as senility or emotional depression.

▷ **Advisability of Use During Pregnancy**

Pregnancy Category: B (tentative). See Pregnancy Code inside back cover.

Animal studies: No birth defects reported in rats or rabbits.

Human studies: Information from studies of pregnant women indicates no significant increase in birth defects in 2948 exposures to this drug.

A withdrawal syndrome of tremor and diarrhea has been reported in a 5-day-old infant whose mother used this drug (150 mg daily) during pregnancy.

Avoid drug during the last 3 months. Use sparingly during the first 6 months only if clearly needed.

Advisability of Use if Breast-Feeding
Presence of this drug in breast milk: Yes.
Avoid drug or refrain from nursing.

Habit-Forming Potential: None.

Effects of Overdosage: Marked drowsiness, confusion, incoordination, unsteadiness, muscle tremors, stupor, coma, seizures, fever, flushed face, dilated pupils, weak pulse, shallow breathing.

Possible Effects of Long-Term Use: The development of tolerance (see Glossary) and reduced effectiveness of drug.

Suggested Periodic Examinations While Taking This Drug (at physician's discretion)
Complete blood cell counts.

▷ **While Taking This Drug, Observe the Following**
Foods: No restrictions.
Beverages: No restrictions. May be taken with milk.
▷ *Alcohol:* Use with extreme caution until the combined effect has been determined. The combination of alcohol and antihistamines can cause rapid and marked sedation.
Tobacco Smoking: No interactions expected.
Marijuana Smoking: Increased drowsiness and mouth dryness; possible accentuation of impaired thinking.
▷ *Other Drugs*
Diphenhydramine may *increase* the effects of
• all drugs with a sedative effect, and cause oversedation.
• atropine and atropinelike drugs (see Drug Class, Section Four).
The following drugs may *increase* the effects of diphenhydramine
• monoamine oxidase (MAO) type A inhibitor drugs (see Drug Class, Section Four) may delay its elimination, thus exaggerating and prolonging its action.
▷ *Driving, Hazardous Activities:* This drug may impair mental alertness, judgment, physical coordination and reaction time. Restrict activities as necessary.
Aviation Note: The use of this drug *is a disqualification* for piloting. Consult a designated Aviation Medical Examiner.
Exposure to Sun: Use caution until sensitivity has been determined. This drug may cause photosensitivity (see Glossary).
Exposure to Environmental Chemicals: The insecticides Aldrin, Dieldrin and Chlordane may decrease the effectiveness of this drug. The insecticide Sevin may increase the sedative effects of this drug.

DIPHENOXYLATE
(di fen OX i layt)

Introduced: 1960

Class: Antidiarrheal

Prescription: USA: Yes
Canada: Yes

Controlled Drug: USA: C-V*
Canada: <N>

Available as Generic: USA: Yes
Canada: No

Brand Names: Lomotil [CD], ✦Lomotil

BENEFITS versus RISKS	
Possible Benefits	*Possible Risks*
EFFECTIVE RELIEF OF INTESTINAL CRAMPING AND DIARRHEA	Drowsiness Constipation Low habit-forming potential

▷ **Principal Uses**
As a Single Drug Product: Used primarily for the control of overactivity of the intestinal tract, cramping and diarrhea. Because of its potential for abuse, this drug is not marketed as a single-entity product in the USA.
As a Combination Drug Product [CD]: This drug, in therapeutically effective dosage, is combined with a small amount of atropine to discourage abusive overdosage. The accumulative effects of atropine overdosage would make the combination intolerable.

How This Drug Works: Not completely established. It is thought that this drug acts directly on the nerve supply of the gastrointestinal tract to reduce its motility and propulsive contractions, thus relieving cramping and diarrhea.

Available Dosage Forms and Strengths
Liquid — 2.5 mg (0.025 mg atropine) per 5-ml teaspoonful
Tablets — 2.5 mg (0.025 mg atropine)

▷ **Usual Adult Dosage Range:** Initially 2.5 to 5 mg/4 hours as needed for acute diarrhea; then 2.5 mg/6 to 8 hours as needed for chronic diarrhea. **Note: Actual dosage and administration schedule must be determined by the physician for each patient individually.**

▷ **Dosing Instructions:** May be taken on an empty stomach or with food if stomach irritation occurs. Tablet may be crushed for administration.

*See Schedules of Controlled Drugs inside back cover.

Usual Duration of Use: Continual use on a regular schedule for 24 to 36 hours is usually necessary to determine this drug's effectiveness in controlling acute diarrhea. If diarrhea persists, consult your physician. Avoid prolonged and uninterrupted use.

▷ **This Drug Should Not Be Taken If**
  • you are allergic to either component of this combination drug (single component in Canada).
  • you have active liver disease.
  • it is prescribed for a child under 2 years of age.

▷ **Inform Your Physician Before Taking This Drug If**
  • you have a history of liver disease or impaired liver function.
  • you have regional enteritis or ulcerative colitis.
  • you have chronic lung disease of any kind.

Possible Side-Effects (natural, expected and unavoidable drug actions)
  Drowsiness, constipation.

▷ **Possible Adverse Effects** (unusual, unexpected and infrequent reactions)
  If any of the following develop, consult your physician promptly for guidance.
  Mild Adverse Effects
  Allergic Reactions: Skin rash, hives, localized swellings, itching.
  Headache, dizziness, weakness, euphoria.
  Reduced appetite, nausea, vomiting, bloating.
  Serious Adverse Effects
  "Toxic megacolon" (distended, immobile colon with fluid retention) may develop in acute ulcerative colitis.

▷ **Possible Effects on Sexual Function:**   None reported.

Possible Effects on Laboratory Tests
  Urine screening tests for drug abuse: *initial* test result may be falsely **positive**; *confirmatory* test result will be **negative**. (Test results depend upon amount of drug taken and testing method used.)

CAUTION
  1. Do not exceed recommended doses.
  2. Use with caution in the presence of chronic lung disease (asthma, bronchitis, emphysema). This drug may impair respiration.
  3. If used to treat chronic diarrhea, report promptly any development of bloating, abdominal distension, nausea, vomiting, constipation or abdominal pain.

Precautions for Use
  By Infants and Children: Do not use in those under 2 years of age. Use with caution (especially in children with Down's syndrome); observe closely for any indications of atropine overdosage: excitement, overactivity, hallucinations, fever, flushed face, dilated pupils.

By Those over 60 Years of Age: Start treatment with small doses. You may be more sensitive to the sedative and constipating effects of this drug.

▷ **Advisability of Use During Pregnancy**
Pregnancy Category: C (tentative). See Pregnancy Code inside back cover.
Animal studies: No information available.
Human studies: Information from adequate studies of pregnant women is not available.
Use sparingly and only if clearly needed. Ask physician for guidance.

Advisability of Use if Breast-Feeding
Presence of this drug in breast milk: Yes.
Avoid drug or refrain from nursing.

Habit-Forming Potential: Because of its similarity to meperidine, this drug may cause physical dependence (see Glossary) if used in large doses over an extended period of time.

Effects of Overdosage: Marked drowsiness, lethargy, depression, numbness in arms and legs, dry skin and mouth, flushing, fever, rapid pulse, slow and shallow breathing, stupor progressing to coma.

Possible Effects of Long-Term Use: The development of tolerance with loss of drug effectiveness. Physical dependence is a remote possibility.

Suggested Periodic Examinations While Taking This Drug (at physician's discretion)
None required.

▷ **While Taking This Drug, Observe the Following**
Foods: No restrictions. Follow prescribed diet.
Beverages: No restrictions. May be taken with milk.
▷ *Alcohol:* Use with extreme caution until combined effects have been determined. This drug may increase the depressant action of alcohol on the brain.
Tobacco Smoking: No interactions expected.
▷ *Other Drugs*
Diphenoxylate may *increase* the effects of
• all drugs with a sedative effect, and cause oversedation.
Diphenoxylate *taken concurrently* with
• monoamine oxidase (MAO) type A inhibitor drugs (see Drug Class, Section Four) will require close observation for excessive rise in blood pressure.
▷ *Driving, Hazardous Activities:* This drug may cause drowsiness or dizziness. Restrict activities as necessary.
Aviation Note: The use of this drug *is a disqualification* for piloting. Consult a designated Aviation Medical Examiner.
Exposure to Sun: No restrictions.

DIPYRIDAMOLE
(di peer ID a mohl)

Introduced: 1959

Class: Platelet inhibitor

Prescription: USA: Yes
Canada: No

Controlled Drug: USA: No
Canada: No

Available as Generic: USA: Yes
Canada: No

Brand Names: ✦Apo-Dipyridamole, ✦Asasantine [CD], Persantine, Pyrida-mole

---

BENEFITS versus RISKS

Possible Benefits	*Possible Risks*
EFFECTIVE PREVENTION OF THROMBOEMBOLISM (BLOOD CLOTS) FOLLOWING HEART VALVE SURGERY	Mild low blood pressure with dizziness and fainting (infrequent) Mild indigestion

---

▷ **Principal Uses**

As a Single Drug Product: This drug is used primarily for (1) the prevention of thromboembolism (blood clot formation and migration) following heart valve surgery; (2) the prevention of thromboembolism thought to be responsible for transient ischemic attacks in brain circulation (ministrokes). It may be used together with aspirin or with anticoagulants such as warfarin (Coumadin).

How This Drug Works: Not completely established. It is thought that by inhibiting the actions of certain enzymes, this drug prevents the aggregation of blood platelets (see Glossary) and thereby reduces the tendency to blood clot formation.

Available Dosage Forms and Strengths
Tablets — 25 mg, 50 mg, 75 mg

▷ **Usual Adult Dosage Range:** 50 to 100 mg, 3 or 4 times daily. Total daily dosage should not exceed 400 mg. **Note: Actual dosage and administration schedule must be determined by the physician for each patient individually.**

▷ **Dosing Instructions:** Preferably taken with a full glass of water on an empty stomach, 1 hour before or 2 hours after eating. However, it may be taken with or following food to reduce stomach irritation. The tablet may be crushed for administration.

Usual Duration of Use: Significant reduction in platelet aggregation is thought to occur in 1 week. Long-term use (months to years) requires supervision and periodic evaluation by your physician.

▷ **This Drug Should Not Be Taken If**
- you have had an allergic reaction to it previously.
- you have just experienced an acute heart attack (myocardial infarction).
- you have uncontrolled high blood pressure.

▷ **Inform Your Physician Before Taking This Drug If**
- you have low blood pressure.
- you have impaired liver function.
- you have any type of bleeding disorder.

Possible Side-Effects (natural, expected and unavoidable drug actions)
Flushing, light-headedness, weakness.

▷ **Possible Adverse Effects** (unusual, unexpected and infrequent reactions)
If any of the following develop, consult your physician promptly for guidance.
Mild Adverse Effects
Allergic Reaction: Skin rash.
Headache, dizziness, fainting.
Stomach irritation, nausea, diarrhea.
Serious Adverse Effects
Significant low blood pressure with large doses.
Paradoxical increase in angina on starting treatment (infrequent).
Aggravation of migraine headaches.

▷ **Possible Effects on Sexual Function:**   None reported.

Possible Effects on Laboratory Tests
Blood platelet counts: increased.

CAUTION
1. Occasionally this drug may cause an ***increase*** in the frequency and/or severity of preexisting angina. If this response occurs, inform your physician promptly.
2. Anyone with low blood pressure should avoid large doses of this drug.

Precautions for Use
By Infants and Children: Observe closely for indications of excessively low blood pressure.
By Those over 60 Years of Age: Begin treatment with small doses (25 mg twice daily) to evaluate effect on blood pressure. Avoid doses that cause excessively low blood pressure. Observe for any tendency to develop hypothermia (see Glossary) in cold environments.

▷ **Advisability of Use During Pregnancy**
Pregnancy Category: B (tentative). See Pregnancy Code inside back cover.
Animal studies: Mouse, rat and rabbit studies show no birth defects due to this drug.

Human studies: Information from adequate studies of pregnant women is not available.

Use this drug only if clearly needed. If possible, avoid use during the last month of pregnancy and during labor and delivery because of possible prolongation of bleeding following delivery.

Advisability of Use if Breast-Feeding
Presence of this drug in breast milk: Yes, in small amounts.
Monitor nursing infant closely and discontinue drug or nursing if adverse effects develop.

Habit-Forming Potential: None.

Effects of Overdosage: Flushing, stomach irritation, nausea, vomiting, stomach cramps, diarrhea, rapid heart rate, low blood pressure, weakness, fainting.

Possible Effects of Long-Term Use: None reported.

Suggested Periodic Examinations While Taking This Drug (at physician's discretion)
Measurements of blood pressure in lying, sitting and standing positions.

▷ **While Taking This Drug, Observe the Following**
Foods: No restrictions.
Beverages: No restrictions. May be taken with milk.
▷ *Alcohol:* Use with caution until the combined effect has been determined. Alcohol may enhance the ability of this drug to lower blood pressure.
Tobacco Smoking: Nicotine can reduce the effectiveness of this drug. Follow physician's advice regarding smoking.
Marijuana Smoking: Possible reduced effectiveness of this drug; mild to moderate increase in angina; possible changes in electrocardiogram, confusing interpretation.
▷ *Other Drugs*
Dipyridamole may *increase* the effects of
• oral anticoagulants (warfarin, etc.), when doses of dipyridamole approach or exceed 400 mg/day; observe for abnormal bleeding or bruising.
• other drugs that inhibit platelet activity; observe for abnormal bleeding or bruising.
Dipyridamole *taken concurrently* with
• aspirin makes it possible to reduce the dose of dipyridamole and thus lessen any side-effects that may occur.
▷ *Driving, Hazardous Activities:* This drug may cause light-headedness or dizziness. Restrict activities as necessary.
Aviation Note: The use of this drug *may be a disqualification* for piloting. Consult a designated Aviation Medical Examiner.
Exposure to Sun: No restrictions.
Exposure to Heat: Use caution. Hot environments can cause significant drop in blood pressure.

Exposure to Cold: Use caution. This drug may increase the risk of hypothermia (see Glossary) in the elderly.

Discontinuation: Following long-term use, this drug should not be discontinued abruptly. It should be withdrawn gradually over a period of 2 to 3 weeks. Ask your physician for guidance.

DISOPYRAMIDE
(di so PEER a mide)

Introduced: 1969

Class: Antiarrhythmic

Prescription: USA: Yes
Canada: Yes

Controlled Drug: USA: No
Canada: No

Available as Generic: USA: Yes
Canada: No

Brand Names: Napamide, Norpace, Norpace CR, ✦Rythmodan, ✦Rythmodan-LA

BENEFITS versus RISKS

Possible Benefits	*Possible Risks*
EFFECTIVE TREATMENT OF SELECTED HEART RHYTHM DISORDERS	NARROW TREATMENT RANGE FREQUENT ADVERSE EFFECTS (10–40%) LOW BLOOD PRESSURE CONGESTIVE HEART FAILURE Heart conduction and rhythm abnormalities Frequent atropinelike side-effects

---

▷ **Principal Uses**

As a Single Drug Product: This drug is classified as a Type 1 antiarrhythmic agent, similar to procainamide and quinidine in its actions. It is used primarily to abolish and prevent the recurrence of premature beats arising in the atria (upper chambers) and the ventricles (lower chambers) of the heart. It is also useful in the treatment and prevention of abnormally rapid heart rates (tachycardia) that originate in the atria or the ventricles.

How This Drug Works: By slowing the activity of the pacemaker and delaying the transmission of electrical impulses through the conduction system and muscle of the heart, this drug assists in restoring normal heart rate and rhythm.

Available Dosage Forms and Strengths

Capsules — 100 mg, 150 mg
Capsules, prolonged-action — 100 mg, 150 mg

▷ **Usual Adult Dosage Range:**   100 to 200 mg/6 hours. Dosage should not exceed 200 mg/6 hours or 800 mg/24 hours (1600 mg/24 hours have been used occasionally). **Note: Actual dosage and administration schedule must be determined by the physician for each patient individually.**

▷ **Dosing Instructions:**   Preferably taken on an empty stomach, hour before or 2 hours after eating. However, it may be taken with or following food to reduce stomach irritation. The regular capsules may be opened for administration; however, the prolonged-action capsules should not be opened, chewed or crushed.

Usual Duration of Use: Continual use on a regular schedule for 2 to 4 days is usually necessary to determine this drug's effectiveness in correcting or preventing responsive rhythm disorders. Long-term use requires supervision and periodic evaluation by your physician.

▷ **This Drug Should Not Be Taken If**
  • you have had an allergic reaction to it previously.
  • you have second-degree or third-degree heart block (determined by electrocardiogram).

▷ **Inform Your Physician Before Taking This Drug If**
  • you have had any unfavorable reactions to other antiarrhythmic drugs in the past.
  • you have a history of heart disease of any kind, especially "heart block."
  • you have a history of low blood pressure.
  • you have impaired liver or kidney function.
  • you have glaucoma, or a family history of glaucoma.
  • you have an enlarged prostate gland.
  • you have myasthenia gravis.
  • you are taking any form of digitalis or any diuretic drug that can cause excessive loss of body potassium (ask physician).

Possible Side-Effects (natural, expected and unavoidable drug actions)
Drop in blood pressure in susceptible individuals.
Dry mouth (32%), constipation (11%), blurred vision (3–9%), impaired urination (14%).

▷ **Possible Adverse Effects** (unusual, unexpected and infrequent reactions)
If any of the following develop, consult your physician promptly for guidance.
Mild Adverse Effects
Allergic Reactions: Skin rash (1–3%), itching.
Headache, nervousness, fatigue, muscular weakness, mild aches.

Loss of appetite, indigestion, nausea, vomiting, diarrhea.
Lowered blood sugar level (hypoglycemia).
Serious Adverse Effects
Idiosyncratic Reaction: Acute psychotic behavior (rare).
Severe drop in blood pressure, fainting.
Progressive heart weakness, predisposing to congestive heart failure.
Inability to empty urinary bladder, prostatism (see Glossary).
Jaundice (see Glossary).
Abnormally low white blood cell count (rare).

▷ **Possible Effects on Sexual Function:**   Rare reports of impotence (300 mg/
day); enlargement and tenderness of male breasts.

▷ **Adverse Effects That May Mimic Natural Diseases or Disorders**
Reversible jaundice may suggest viral hepatitis.

Natural Diseases or Disorders That May Be Activated by This Drug
Glaucoma, myasthenia gravis.

Possible Effects on Laboratory Tests
White blood cell counts: decreased.
Liver function tests: increased liver enzymes (ALT/GPT, AST/GOT and
alkaline phosphatase), increased bilirubin.

CAUTION
1. Thorough evaluation of your heart function (including electrocardiograms) is necessary prior to using this drug.
2. Periodic evaluation of your heart function is necessary to determine
   your response to this drug. Some individuals may experience worsening of their heart rhythm disorder and/or deterioration of heart
   function. Close monitoring of heart rate, rhythm and overall performance is essential.
3. Dosage must be adjusted carefully for each individual. Do not change
   your dosage without the knowledge and supervision of your physician.
4. Do not take any other antiarrhythmic drug while taking this drug
   unless directed to do so by your physician.

Precautions for Use
By Infants and Children: Safety and effectiveness for use by those under 12
years of age have not been established. Initial use of this drug requires
hospitalization and supervision by a qualified pediatrician.
By Those over 60 Years of Age: Reduced kidney function may require reduction in dosage. This drug can aggravate existing prostatism (see Glossary) and promote constipation. Observe carefully for light-headedness, dizziness, unsteadiness and tendency to fall.

▷ **Advisability of Use During Pregnancy**
Pregnancy Category: B (tentative). See Pregnancy Code inside back cover.
Animal studies: No birth defects reported in rats and rabbits.

Human studies: Information from adequate studies of pregnant women is not available. It has been reported that this drug can cause contractions of the pregnant uterus.
Use this drug only if clearly needed. Ask your physician for guidance.

Advisability of Use if Breast-Feeding
Presence of this drug in breast milk: Yes.
Avoid drug or refrain from nursing.

Habit-Forming Potential: None.

Effects of Overdosage: Dryness of eyes, nose, mouth and throat; impaired urination; constipation; marked drop in blood pressure; abnormal heart rhythms; congestive heart failure.

Possible Effects of Long-Term Use: None reported.

Suggested Periodic Examinations While Taking This Drug (at physician's discretion)
Electrocardiograms, complete blood cell counts, measurements of potassium blood levels.

▷ **While Taking This Drug, Observe the Following**
Foods: No restrictions. Ask physician regarding need for salt restriction and advisability of eating potassium-rich foods.
Beverages: No restrictions. May be taken with milk.
▷ *Alcohol:* Use caution until the combined effects have been determined. Alcohol can increase the blood-pressure-lowering effects and the blood-sugar-lowering effects of this drug.
Tobacco Smoking: Nicotine can cause irritability of the heart and reduce the effectiveness of this drug. Follow physician's advice regarding smoking.
▷ *Other Drugs*
Disopyramide may *increase* the effects of
• antihypertensive drugs, and cause excessive lowering of blood pressure.
• atropinelike drugs (see Drug Class, Section Four).
• warfarin (Coumadin, etc.); monitor prothrombin times, adjust dosage accordingly.
Disopyramide may *decrease* the effects of
• ambenonium (Mytelase).
• neostigmine (Prostigmin).
• pyridostigmine (Mestinon).
The beneficial effects of these three drugs in the treatment of myasthenia gravis may be reduced.
The following drugs may *decrease* the effects of disopyramide
• all diuretics that promote potassium loss.
• rifampin (Rimactane, Rifadin).
▷ *Driving, Hazardous Activities:* This drug may cause dizziness or blurred vision. Restrict activities as necessary.

Aviation Note: The use of this drug *may be a disqualification* for piloting. Consult a designated Aviation Medical Examiner.

Exposure to Sun: Use caution. This drug is reported to cause photosensitization (see Glossary) in susceptible individuals.

Exposure to Heat: Use caution. The use of this drug in hot environments may increase the risk of heat stroke.

Occurrence of Unrelated Illness: Disorders that cause vomiting, diarrhea or dehydration can affect this drug's action adversely. Report such developments promptly.

Discontinuation: This drug should not be discontinued abruptly following long-term use. Ask your physician for guidance regarding gradual dose reduction.

DISULFIRAM
(di SULF i ram)

Introduced: 1948

Prescription: USA: Yes
Canada: Yes

Available as Generic: USA: Yes
Canada: No

Brand Name: Antabuse

Class: Antialcoholism

Controlled Drug: USA: No
Canada: No

BENEFITS versus RISKS

Possible Benefits	*Possible Risks*
EFFECTIVE ADJUNCT IN THE TREATMENT OF CHRONIC ALCOHOLISM	DANGEROUS REACTIONS WITH ALCOHOL INGESTION Acute psychotic reactions (uncommon) Drug-induced liver damage (rare) Drug-induced optic and/or peripheral neuritis (rare)

▷ **Principal Uses**

As a Single Drug Product: This drug is used for one purpose only—to deter the abusive drinking of alcoholic beverages. It does not abolish the craving or impulse to drink. It is of value in the treatment of alcoholism because of the psychological reinforcement it provides by reminding the patient of the dire consequences of ingesting alcohol.

How This Drug Works: Following the ingestion of alcohol, this drug interrupts normal liver enzyme activity after the conversion of alcohol to acetaldehyde. This causes excessive accumulation of acetaldehyde, a highly toxic substance that produces the disulfiram (Antabuse) reaction (see Glossary).

Available Dosage Forms and Strengths
Tablets — 250 mg, 500 mg

▷ **Usual Adult Dosage Range:**   In the absence of all signs of alcoholic intoxication and no less than 12 hours after the last ingestion of alcohol, treatment is started with a single dose of 500 mg/day for 1 to 2 weeks. This is followed by a maintenance dose of 250 mg/day. The range of the maintenance dose is 125 mg to 500 mg/day and is determined by experience with each patient individually. The total daily dosage should not exceed 1000 mg. **Note: Actual dosage and administration schedule must be determined by the physician for each patient individually.**

▷ **Dosing Instructions:**   May be taken with or following food to reduce stomach irritation. Tablet may be crushed for administration.

Usual Duration of Use: Continual use on a regular schedule for several months is usually necessary to determine this drug's effectiveness in deterring the drinking of alcohol. If tolerated well, use should continue until a basis for permanent self-control and sobriety is established. Consult your physician on a regular basis.

▷ **This Drug Should Not Be Taken If**
- you have experienced a severe allergic reaction to disulfiram in the past. (Note: The interaction of disulfiram and alcohol is *not an allergic* reaction.)
- you have ingested any form of alcohol in any amount within the past 12 hours.
- you are pregnant.
- you are taking (or have taken recently) metronidazole (Flagyl).
- you have coronary heart disease or a serious heart rhythm disorder.

▷ **Inform Your Physician Before Taking This Drug If**
- you have used disulfiram in the past.
- you do not intend to avoid alcohol completely while taking this drug.
- you have not been given a full explanation of the reaction you will experience if you drink alcohol while taking this drug.
- you are planning pregnancy in the near future.
- you have a history of diabetes, epilepsy, kidney or liver disease.
- you are currently taking oral anticoagulants, digitalis, isoniazid, paraldehyde or phenytoin (Dilantin).
- you plan to have surgery under general anesthesia while taking this drug.

Possible Side-Effects (natural, expected and unavoidable drug actions)
Drowsiness, lethargy during early use.
Offensive breath and body odor.

▷ **Possible Adverse Effects** (unusual, unexpected and infrequent reactions)
  If any of the following develop, consult your physician promptly for guidance.
  Mild Adverse Effects
  Allergic Reactions: Skin rash, hives.
  Headache, dizziness, restlessness, tremor.
  Metallic or garliclike taste, indigestion. (These usually subside after 2 weeks of use.)
  Serious Adverse Effects
  Allergic Reactions: Severe skin rashes, drug-induced hepatitis (rare).
  Idiosyncratic Reaction: Acute toxic effect on brain; psychotic behavior.
  Optic or peripheral neuritis (see Glossary).

▷ **Possible Effects on Sexual Function:** Decreased libido and/or impaired erection in 30% of users taking recommended doses of 125 to 500 mg/day.

▷ **Adverse Effects That May Mimic Natural Diseases or Disorders**
  Liver reaction may suggest viral hepatitis.
  Brain toxicity may suggest spontaneous psychosis.

Possible Effects on Laboratory Tests
  Blood cholesterol level: increased.
  Prothrombin time: increased (taken concurrently with warfarin).
  Liver function tests: liver enzymes increased (ALT/GPT, AST/GOT and alkaline phosphatase), increased bilirubin.

CAUTION
  1. This drug should never be taken by anyone who is in a state of alcoholic intoxication.
  2. The patient should be fully informed regarding the purpose and actions of this drug *before* treatment is started.
  3. During long-term use of this drug, examine for any indication of reduced thyroid function.
  4. Carry a card of personal identification with the notation that you are taking this drug.

Precautions for Use
  By Infants and Children: Safety and effectiveness for use by those under 12 years of age have not been established.
  By Those over 60 Years of Age: Observe for excessive sedation during the early use of this drug. *Do not* perform an "alcohol trial" to determine the effects of this drug.

▷ **Advisability of Use During Pregnancy**
  Pregnancy Category: X (tentative). See Pregnancy Code inside back cover.
  Animal studies: No defects reported in rats and hamsters.
  Human studies: Two reports indicate that 4 of 8 fetuses exposed to this drug had serious birth defects. Information from adequate studies of pregnant women is not available.
  Avoid this drug completely if possible.

Advisability of Use if Breast-Feeding
    Presence of this drug in breast milk: Unknown.
    Avoid drug or refrain from nursing.

Habit-Forming Potential: None.

Effects of Overdosage: Marked lethargy, impaired memory, altered behavior, confusion, unsteadiness, weakness, stomach pain, nausea, vomiting, diarrhea.

Possible Effects of Long-Term Use: Decreased function of thyroid gland.

Suggested Periodic Examinations While Taking This Drug (at physician's discretion)
    Visual acuity, liver function tests.

▷ **While Taking This Drug, Observe the Following**
    Foods: Avoid all foods prepared with alcohol, including sauces, marinades, vinegars, desserts, etc. Inquire when dining out regarding the use of alcohol in food preparation.
    Beverages: Avoid all punches, fruit drinks, etc., that may contain alcohol. This drug may be taken with milk.
▷   *Alcohol: **Avoid completely in all forms*** while taking this drug and for 14 days following the last dose. The combination of disulfiram and alcohol—even in small amounts—produces the disulfiram (Antabuse) reaction. This begins within 5 to 10 minutes after ingesting alcohol and consists of intense flushing and warming of the face, a severe throbbing headache, shortness of breath, chest pains, nausea, repeated vomiting, sweating and weakness. If the amount of alcohol ingested is large enough, the reaction may progress to blurred vision, vertigo, confusion, marked drop in blood pressure and loss of consciousness. Severe reactions may lead to convulsions and death. The reaction may last from 30 minutes to several hours, depending upon the amount of alcohol and disulfiram in the body. As the symptoms subside, the individual is exhausted and usually sleeps for several hours.
    Tobacco Smoking: No interactions expected.
    Marijuana Smoking: Possible increase in drowsiness and lethargy.
▷   *Other Drugs*
    Disulfiram may *increase* the effects of
    • oral anticoagulants (warfarin, etc.), and increase the risk of bleeding; dosage adjustments may be necessary.
    • barbiturates, and cause oversedation (see Drug Class, Section Four).
    • chlordiazepoxide (Librium) and diazepam (Valium), and cause oversedation.
    • paraldehyde, and cause excessive depression of brain function.
    • phenytoin (Dilantin), and cause toxic effects on the brain; dosage adjustments may be necessary.
    Disulfiram may *decrease* the effects of
    • perphenazine (Tilafon, etc.).

Disulfiram *taken concurrently* with
- isoniazid (INH, etc.) may cause acute mental disturbance and incoordination, making it necessary to discontinue treatment.
- metronidazole (Flagyl) may cause acute mental and behavioral disturbances, making it necessary to discontinue treatment.
- OTC cough syrups, tonics, etc., containing alcohol may cause a disulfiram (Antabuse) reaction; avoid concurrent use. (See OTC Drugs in Glossary.)

The following drugs may *increase* the effects of disulfiram
- amitriptyline (Elavil) may enhance the disulfiram alcohol interaction; avoid concurrent use of these drugs.

▷ *Driving, Hazardous Activities:* This drug may cause drowsiness or dizziness. Restrict activities as necessary.

Aviation Note: Alcoholism *is a disqualification* for piloting. Consult a designated Aviation Medical Examiner.

Exposure to Sun: No restrictions.

Exposure to Environmental Chemicals: Thiram, a pesticide, and carbon disulfide, a pesticide and industrial solvent, can have additive toxic effects during use of this drug. Observe for toxic effects on the brain and nervous system.

Discontinuation: Treatment with this drug is only part of your total treatment program. Do not discontinue it without the knowledge and guidance of your physician. Abrupt withdrawal does not cause any symptoms. However, no alcohol should be ingested for 14 days following discontinuation.

DOXAZOSIN
(dox AY zoh sin)

Introduced: 1986

Class: Antihypertensive

Prescription: USA: Yes

Controlled Drug: USA: No

Available as Generic: No

Brand Name: Cardura

BENEFITS versus RISKS

Possible Benefits	*Possible Risks*
EFFECTIVE TREATMENT OF MILD TO MODERATE HYPERTENSION when used alone or in combination with other antihypertensive drugs	"First dose" drop in blood pressure, but without fainting (4%) Dizziness (19%) Fluid retention (4.0%) Rapid heart rate (0.3%)

▷ **Principal Uses**
   As a Single Drug Product: Used primarily as a "step 1" antihypertensive drug to initiate treatment of mild to moderate hypertension. Also used in conjunction with other drugs to treat moderate to severe hypertension.

   How This Drug Works: It is thought that by blocking certain actions of the sympathetic nervous system, this drug causes direct relaxation and expansion of blood vessel walls, thus lowering the pressure of the blood within the vessels.

   Available Dosage Forms and Strengths
   Tablets — 1 mg, 2 mg, 4 mg, 8 mg

▷ **Usual Adult Dosage Range:**   Initiate treatment with a "test dose" of 1 mg to determine the patient's response within the first 6 hours. If tolerated satisfactorily, increase dose cautiously (as needed and tolerated) by doubling it every 2 weeks and taking as a single dose at bedtime. Doses in excess of 4 mg may increase the occurrence of light-headedness or dizziness, indicating low blood pressure. Total daily dosage should not exceed 16 mg. **Note: Actual dosage and administration schedule must be determined by the physician for each patient individually.**

▷ **Dosing Instructions:**   Preferably taken at bedtime to avoid orthostatic hypotension (see Glossary). May be taken without regard to food. The tablet may be crushed for administration.

   Usual Duration of Use: Continual use on a regular schedule for 6 to 8 weeks is usually necessary to determine this drug's effectiveness in controlling hypertension. Long-term use (months to years) requires supervision and periodic evaluation by your physician. Consult your physician on a regular basis.

   Possible Advantages of This Drug
   May be used to initiate treatment.
   Effective with once-a-day dosage.
   Causes depression or impotence infrequently.
   Lowers blood cholesterol and sugar levels.
   Does not lose effectiveness with long-term use.

▷ **This Drug Should Not Be Taken If**
   • you have had an allergic reaction to this drug or to prazosin (Minipress) or terazosin (Hytrin) previously.
   • you are experiencing mental depression.
   • you have active liver disease.
   • you have angina (active coronary artery disease) and you are not taking a beta-blocking drug. (Consult your physician.)

▷ **Inform Your Physician Before Taking This Drug If**
   • you have experienced orthostatic hypotension (see Glossary) when using other antihypertensive drugs.
   • you have a history of mental depression.

- you have impaired circulation to the brain, or a history of stroke.
- you have coronary artery disease.
- you have active liver disease or impaired liver function.
- you have impaired kidney function.
- you plan to have surgery under general anesthesia in the near future.

Possible Side-Effects (natural, expected and unavoidable drug actions)
Orthostatic hypotension (0.3%), drowsiness (5%), salt and water retention (4%), dry mouth (2%), nasal congestion (3%), constipation (1%).

▷ **Possible Adverse Effects** (unusual, unexpected and infrequent reactions)
If any of the following develop, consult your physician promptly for guidance.

Mild Adverse Effects
Allergic Reaction: Skin rash (1%), itching (1%).
Headache (14%), dizziness (19%), fatigue (12%), weakness (1%), nervousness (2%), numbness and tingling (1%), blurred vision (2%).
Palpitation (2%), rapid heart rate (0.3%), shortness of breath (1%).
Nausea (3%), diarrhea (2%), indigestion (1%).

Serious Adverse Effects
Mental depression (1%).

▷ **Possible Effects on Sexual Function:** Impotence (2%).

Natural Diseases or Disorders That May Be Activated by This Drug
Latent coronary artery insufficiency.

Possible Effects on Laboratory Tests
White blood cell counts: rare occurrence of mild decrease while taking drug.
Blood lipid tests: decreased total cholesterol, LDL-cholesterol and cholesterol/HDL ratio; decreased triglycerides.
Blood sugar level: small decrease.

CAUTION
1. Observe for the possible "first dose" response of precipitous drop in blood pressue, with or without fainting; this usually occurs within the first 6 hours. Limit initial doses to 1 mg taken at bedtime for the first week; remain supine after taking these trial doses.
2. Impaired liver function may increase your sensitivity to this drug and require smaller than usual doses.
3. Consult your physician if you plan to use over-the-counter remedies for allergic rhinitis or head colds; these preparations contain drugs that may interact with doxazosin.

Precautions for Use
By Infants and Children: Safety and effectiveness for use by those under 12 years of age have not been established.
By Those over 60 Years of Age: Begin treatment with no more than 1 mg/day for the first week. Subsequent increases in dose must be very gradual and carefully supervised by your physician. The occurrence of

orthostatic hypotension can cause unexpected falls and injury; sit or lie down promptly if you feel light-headed or dizzy. Report any indications of dizziness or chest pain promptly.

▷ **Advisability of Use During Pregnancy**
Pregnancy Category: B (tentative). See Pregnancy Code inside back cover.
Animal studies: No birth defects found in rat or rabbit studies.
Human studies: Information from adequate studies of pregnant women is not available.
Use this drug only if clearly needed. Ask your physician for guidance.

Advisability of Use if Breast-Feeding
Presence of this drug in breast milk: Unknown.
Monitor nursing infant closely and discontinue drug or nursing if adverse effects develop.

Habit-Forming Potential: None.

Effects of Overdosage: Orthostatic hypotension, headache, generalized flushing, rapid heart rate, extreme weakness, irregular heart rhythm, circulatory collapse.

Possible Effects of Long-Term Use: None reported.

Suggested Periodic Examinations While Taking This Drug (at physician's discretion)
Measurements of blood pressure in lying, sitting and standing positions.
Measurements of body weight to detect fluid retention.

▷ **While Taking This Drug, Observe the Following**
Foods: No restrictions. Avoid excessive salt intake.
Beverages: No restrictions. May be taken with milk.
▷ *Alcohol:* Use with extreme caution until the combined effects have been determined. Alcohol can exaggerate the blood-pressure-lowering actions of this drug and cause excessive reduction.
Tobacco Smoking: Nicotine can contribute significantly to this drug's ability to intensify coronary insufficiency in susceptible individuals. All forms of tobacco should be avoided.
▷ *Other Drugs*
The following drugs may *increase* the effects of doxazosin
• beta-adrenergic-blocking drugs (see Drug Class, Section Four); the severity and duration of the "first dose" hypotensive response may be increased.
The following drugs may *decrease* the effects of doxazosin
• estrogens.
• indomethacin (Indocin).
▷ *Driving, Hazardous Activities:* This drug may cause dizziness or drowsiness. Restrict activities as necessary.
Aviation Note: The use of this drug *is a disqualification* for piloting. Consult a designated Aviation Medical Examiner.

Exposure to Sun: No restrictions.

Exposure to Cold: Use caution until combined effect has been determined. Cold environments may increase this drug's ability to cause coronary insufficiency (angina) and hypothermia (see Glossary) in susceptible individuals.

Heavy Exercise or Exertion: Excessive exertion can augment this drug's ability to induce angina. See Angina in Section Two.

Discontinuation: If you are taking this drug as part of your treatment program for congestive heart failure, do not discontinue it abruptly. Ask your physician for guidance.

DOXEPIN
(DOX e pin)

Introduced: 1969   **Class:** Antidepressant

Prescription: USA: Yes   **Controlled Drug:** USA: No
Canada: Yes   Canada: No

Available as Generic: USA: Yes
Canada: No

Brand Names: Adapin, Sinequan, ✦Triadapin

BENEFITS versus RISKS	
Possible Benefits	*Possible Risks*
EFFECTIVE RELIEF OF ENDOGENOUS DEPRESSION	ADVERSE BEHAVIORAL EFFECTS: Confusion, disorientation, hallucinations, delusions
EFFECTIVE RELIEF OF ANXIETY AND NERVOUS TENSION	CONVERSION OF DEPRESSION TO MANIA in manic-depressive disorder
Possibly beneficial in other depressive disorders	Aggravation of schizophrenia and paranoia
	Rare blood cell disorders

▷ **Principal Uses**

As a Single Drug Product: To relieve the symptoms associated with spontaneous (endogenous) depression, and to initiate the restoration of normal mood. This drug should be used only when a diagnosis of a true, primary depression of significant degree has been established. It should not be used to treat the symptoms of mild and transient (reactive) depression that may be associated with many life situations in the absence of a bona fide affective illness.

How This Drug Works: Not completely established. It is thought that this drug relieves depression by slowly restoring to normal levels certain constituents of brain tissue (norepinephrine and serotonin) that transmit nerve impulses.

Available Dosage Forms and Strengths
>   Capsules — 10 mg, 25 mg, 50 mg, 75 mg, 100 mg, 150 mg
> Oral concentrate — 10 mg per ml

▷ **Usual Adult Dosage Range:**   Initially 25 mg 2 to 4 times daily. Dose may be increased cautiously as needed and tolerated by 10 to 25 mg daily at intervals of 1 week. Usual maintenance dose is 75 to 150 mg/24 hours. Total dose should not exceed 300 mg/24 hours. When the optimal requirement is determined, it may be taken at bedtime as one dose. **Note: Actual dosage and administration schedule must be determined by the physician for each patient individually.**

▷ **Dosing Instructions:**   May be taken without regard to meals. Capsule may be opened for administration.

Usual Duration of Use: Some benefit may be apparent within to 2 weeks, but adequate response may require continual use for 10 to 12 weeks or longer. Long-term use should not exceed 6 months without evaluation regarding the need for continuation of the drug. Consult your physician on a regular basis.

▷ **This Drug Should Not Be Taken If**
- you have had an allergic reaction to it previously.
- you are taking or have taken within the past 14 days any monoamine oxidase (MAO) type A inhibitor drug (see Drug Class, Section Four).
- you are recovering from a recent heart attack.
- you have narrow-angle glaucoma.

▷ **Inform Your Physician Before Taking This Drug If**
- you are allergic or sensitive to any other tricyclic antidepressant (see Drug Class, Section Four).
- you have a history of any of the following: diabetes, epilepsy, glaucoma, heart diseae, prostate gland enlargement or overactive thyroid function.
- you plan to have surgery under general anesthesia in the near future.

Possible Side-Effects (natural, expected and unavoidable drug actions)
Drowsiness, blurred vision, dry mouth, constipation, impaired urination.

▷ **Possible Adverse Effects** (unusual, unexpected and infrequent reactions)
If any of the following develop, consult your physician promptly for guidance.
Mild Adverse Effects
Allergic Reactions: Skin rash, hives, swelling of face or tongue, drug fever (see Glossary).

Headache, dizziness, weakness, fainting, unsteady gait, tremors.
Peculiar taste, irritation of tongue or mouth, nausea, indigestion.
Fluctuation of blood sugar levels.
Serious Adverse Effects
Allergic Reactions: Hepatitis, with or without jaundice (see Glossary).
Confusion, hallucinations, agitation, restlessness, delusions.
Bone marrow depression (see Glossary)—fatigue, weakness, fever, sore throat, abnormal bleeding or bruising (reported for other drugs of this class).
Peripheral neuritis (see Glossary)—numbness, tingling, pain, loss of strength in arms and legs.
Parkinson-like disorders (see Glossary)—usually mild and infrequent; more likely to occur in the elderly.

▷ **Possible Effects on Sexual Function:** Female breast enlargement with milk production; swelling of testicles.

▷ **Adverse Effects That May Mimic Natural Diseases or Disorders**
Liver toxicity may suggest viral hepatitis.

Natural Diseases or Disorders That May Be Activated by This Drug
Latent diabetes, epilepsy, glaucoma, impaired urination due to prostate gland enlargement (prostatism, see Glossary).

Possible Effects on Laboratory Tests
White blood cell and platelet counts: decreased.

CAUTION
1. Dosage must be adjusted for each person individually. Report for follow-up evaluation and laboratory tests as directed by your physician.
2. It is advisable to withhold this drug if electroconvulsive therapy (ECT, "shock" treatment) is to be used to treat your depression.

Precautions for Use
By Infants and Children: Safety and effectiveness for use by those under 12 years of age have not been established.
By Those over 60 Years of Age: During the first 2 weeks of treatment, observe for the development of confusion, agitation, forgetfulness, disorientation, delusions and hallucinations. Reduction of dosage or discontinuation may be necessary. Unsteadiness may predispose to falling and injury. This drug can increase the degree of impaired urination associated with prostate gland enlargement (prostatism).

▷ **Advisability of Use During Pregnancy**
Pregnancy Category: B (tentative). See Pregnancy Code inside back cover.
Animal studies: No birth defects reported in rats, rabbits, dogs or monkeys.
Human studies: Information from adequate studies of pregnant women is not available.

Use this drug only if clearly needed. If possible, avoid use during the first 3 months and the last month. Ask physician for guidance.

Advisability of Use if Breast-Feeding
Presence of this drug in breast milk: Yes, in small amounts.
Monitor nursing infant closely and discontinue drug or nursing if adverse effects develop.

Habit-Forming Potential: None.

Effects of Overdosage: Confusion, hallucinations, marked drowsiness, heart palpitations, dilated pupils, tremors, stupor, deep sleep, coma, convulsions.

Suggested Periodic Examinations While Taking This Drug (at physician's discretion)
Complete blood cell counts, liver function tests, serial blood pressure readings and electrocardiograms.

▷ **While Taking This Drug, Observe the Following**
Foods: No restrictions. This drug may increase the appetite and cause excessive weight gain.
Beverages: No restrictions. May be taken with milk.
▷ *Alcohol:* Avoid completely. This drug can markedly increase the intoxicating effects of alcohol and accentuate its depressant action on brain function.
Tobacco Smoking: May hasten the elimination of this drug. Higher doses may be necessary.
▷ *Other Drugs*
Doxepin may *increase* the effects of
• atropinelike drugs (see Drug Class, Section Four).
• dicumarol, and increase the risk of bleeding; dosage adjustments may be necessary.
• thyroid hormones.
Doxepin may *decrease* the effects of
• clonidine (Catapres).
• guanethidine (Ismelin).
Doxepin *taken concurrently* with
• monoamine oxidase (MAO) type A inhibitor drugs may cause high fever, delirium and convulsions (see Drug Class, Section Four).
▷ *Driving, Hazardous Activities:* This drug may impair mental alertness, judgment, physical coordination and reaction time. Avoid hazardous activities.
Aviation Note: The use of this drug *is a disqualification* for piloting. Consult a designated Aviation Medical Examiner.
Exposure to Sun: Use caution until sensitivity to sun has been determined. This drug may cause photosensitivity (see Glossary).
Exposure to Heat: This drug can inhibit sweating and impair the body's adaptation to hot environments, increasing the risk of heat stroke. Avoid saunas.

Exposure to Cold: The elderly should use caution and avoid conditions conducive to hypothermia (see Glossary).

Discontinuation: It is advisable to discontinue this drug gradually. Abrupt withdrawal after long-term use can cause headache, malaise and nausea.

DOXYCYCLINE
(dox ee SI kleen)

Introduced: 1967

Class: Antibiotic, tetracyclines

Prescription: USA: Yes
Canada: Yes

Controlled Drug: USA: No
Canada: No

Available as Generic: USA: Yes
Canada: No

Brand Names: Doryx, Doxychel, Vibramycin, Vibra-Tabs, Vivox

BENEFITS versus RISKS

Possible Benefits	*Possible Risks*
EFFECTIVE TREATMENT OF INFECTIONS due to susceptible microorganisms	ALLERGIC REACTIONS, mild to severe
	Liver reaction with jaundice (rare)
	Fungal superinfections
	Drug-induced colitis
	Blood cell disorders

▷ **Principal Uses**

As a Single Drug Product: This member of the tetracycline drug class is used primarily to (1) treat a broad range of infections caused by susceptible bacteria and protozoa; (2) treat and prevent "traveler's diarrhea." It is often used to treat acute and chronic sinusitis and bronchitis.

How This Drug Works: This drug prevents the growth and multiplication of susceptible bacteria by interfering with their formation of essential proteins.

Available Dosage Forms and Strengths
Capsules — 50 mg, 100 mg
Capsules, coated pellets — 100 mg
Injection — 100 mg per vial, 200 mg per vial
Oral suspension — 25 mg per 5-ml teaspoonful
Syrup — 50 mg per 5-ml teaspoonful
Tablets — 50 mg, 100 mg

▷ **Usual Adult Dosage Range:**   100 mg/12 hours the first day; then 100 to 200 mg once daily or 50 to 100 mg/12 hours. Total daily dosage should not exceed 300 mg. **Note: Actual dosage and administration schedule must be determined by the physician for each patient individually.**

▷ **Dosing Instructions:**   Preferably taken on an empty stomach, hour before or 2 hours after eating. However, if stomach irritation occurs, it may be taken with food or milk. Take at same time each day, with a full glass of water. Take the full course prescribed. The tablet may be crushed and the capsule may be opened for administration.

Usual Duration of Use: The time required to control the infection and be free of fever and symptoms for 48 hours. This varies with the nature of the infection.

▷ **This Drug Should Not Be Taken If**
   • you are allergic to any tetracycline drug (see Drug Class, Section Four).
   • you are pregnant or breast-feeding.

▷ **Inform Your Physician Before Taking This Drug If**
   • it is prescribed for a child under 8 years of age.
   • you have a history of liver or kidney disease.
   • you have systemic lupus erythematosus.
   • you are taking any penicillin drug.
   • you are taking any anticoagulant drug.
   • you plan to have surgery under general anesthesia in the near future.

Possible Side-Effects (natural, expected and unavoidable drug actions)
   Superinfections (see Glossary), often due to yeast organisms. These can occur in the mouth, intestinal tract, rectum and/or vagina, resulting in rectal and vaginal itching.

▷ **Possible Adverse Effects** (unusual, unexpected and infrequent reactions)
   If any of the following develop, consult your physician promptly for guidance.
   Mild Adverse Effects
   Allergic Reactions: Skin rash, hives, itching of hands and feet, swelling of face or extremities.
   Loss of appetite, nausea, vomiting, diarrhea.
   Irritation of mouth or tongue, "black tongue," sore throat, abdominal cramping or pain.
   Serious Adverse Effects
   Allergic Reactions: Anaphylactic reaction (see Glossary), asthma, fever, swollen joints, abnormal bleeding or bruising, jaundice (see Glossary).
   Permanent discoloration and/or malformation of teeth when taken by children under 8 years of age, including unborn child and infant.

▷ **Possible Effects on Sexual Function:**   None reported.

Natural Diseases or Disorders That May Be Activated by This Drug
Systemic lupus erythematosus.

Possible Effects on Laboratory Tests
Complete blood cell counts: decreased red cells, hemoglobin, white cells and platelets; increased eosinophils (allergic reaction).
Prothrombin time: increased.
Kidney function tests: increased blood creatinine and urea nitrogen (BUN) levels; increased urine protein (kidney damage).

CAUTION
1. Antacids and preparations containing aluminum, bismuth, iron, magnesium or zinc can prevent adequate absorption of this drug and reduce its effectiveness significantly.
2. Troublesome and persistent diarrhea can develop in sensitive individuals. If diarrhea persists for more than 24 hours, discontinue this drug and consult your physician.

Precautions for Use
By Infants and Children: If possible, tetracyclines should not be given to children under 8 years of age because of the risk of permanent discoloration and deformity of the teeth. Rarely, young infants may develop increased intracranial pressure within the first 4 days of receiving this drug. Tetracyclines may inhibit normal bone growth and development.
By Those over 60 Years of Age: Natural skin changes may predispose to severe and prolonged itching reactions in the genital and anal regions.

▷ **Advisability of Use During Pregnancy**
Pregnancy Category: D (tentative). See Pregnancy Code inside back cover.
Animal studies: Tetracycline causes limb defects in rats, rabbits and chickens.
Human studies: Information from studies of pregnant women indicates that drugs of this class can cause impaired development and discoloration of teeth and other developmental defects.
It is advisable to avoid this drug completely during entire pregnancy.

Advisability of Use if Breast-Feeding
Presence of this drug in breast milk: Yes.
Avoid drug or refrain from nursing.

Habit-Forming Potential: None.

Effects of Overdosage: Nausea, vomiting, diarrhea, acute liver damage (rare).

Possible Effects of Long-Term Use: Superinfections (see Glossary), prolongation of prothrombin time.

Suggested Periodic Examinations While Taking This Drug (at physician's discretion)

Complete blood cell counts, liver and kidney function tests.

During extended use, sputum and stool examinations may detect early superinfection due to yeast organisms.

▷ **While Taking This Drug, Observe the Following**

Foods: Avoid meats and iron-fortified cereals and supplements for 2 hours before and after taking this drug.

Beverages: No restrictions. May be taken with milk.

▷ *Alcohol:* No interactions expected. However, it is best avoided if you have active liver disease.

Tobacco Smoking: No interactions expected.

▷ *Other Drugs*

Doxycycline may *increase* the effects of
- oral anticoagulants, and make it necessary to reduce their dosage.
- digoxin (Lanoxin), and cause digitalis toxicity.
- lithium (Eskalith, Lithane, etc.), and increase the risk of lithium toxicity.

Doxycycline may *decrease* the effects of
- oral contraceptives, and impair their effectiveness in preventing pregnancy.
- penicillins, and impair their effectiveness in treating infections.

The following drugs may *decrease* the effects of doxycycline
- antacids (aluminum and magnesium preparations, sodium bicarbonate, etc.) may reduce drug absorption.
- barbiturates (see Drug Class, Section Four).
- bismuth preparations (Pepto-Bismol, etc.).
- carbamazepine (Tegretol).
- cimetidine (Tagamet).
- phenytoin (Dilantin).
- iron and mineral preparations may reduce drug absorption.

▷ *Driving, Hazardous Activities:* Usually no restrictions. Be alert to the possible occurrence of nausea or diarrhea.

Aviation Note: The use of this drug *may be a disqualification* for piloting. Consult a designated Aviation Medical Examiner.

Exposure to Sun: Use caution until sensitivity has been determined. Tetracyclines can cause photosensitivity (see Glossary).

ENALAPRIL
(e NAL a pril)

Introduced: 1981

Class: Antihypertensive, ACE inhibitor

Prescription: USA: Yes

Controlled Drug: USA: No

Available as Generic: No

Brand Names: Vaseretic [CD], Vasotec

BENEFITS versus RISKS	
Possible Benefits	*Possible Risks*
EFFECTIVE CONTROL OF MILD TO SEVERE HIGH BLOOD PRESSURE	Headache (4.8%), dizziness (4.6%), fatigue (2.8%)
Possibly beneficial as adjunctive treatment in selected cases of congestive heart failure	Low blood pressure (2.3%)
	Bone marrow depression (rare)
	Allergic swelling of face, tongue or vocal cords (0.2%)

▷ **Principal Uses**
As a Single Drug Product
Used primarily to treat all degrees of high blood pressure. Mild to moderate high blood pressure usually responds to low doses; severe high blood pressure may require higher doses, with greater risk of serious adverse effects.
This drug is also used adjunctively to treat heart failure that is not responding adequately to digitalis and diuretics.

How This Drug Works: Not completely known. It is thought that by blocking certain enzyme systems that influence arterial function, this drug contributes to the relaxation of arterial walls throughout the body and thus lowers the resistance to blood flow that causes high blood pressure. This, in turn, reduces the workload of the heart and improves its performance.

Available Dosage Forms and Strengths
Tablets — 5 mg, 10 mg, 20 mg

▷ **Usual Adult Dosage Range:** Initially 5 mg once daily for weeks. Usual maintenance dose is 10 to 40 mg/day in a single dose or in 2 divided doses. Total daily dose should not exceed 40 mg if kidney function is impaired. **Note: Actual dosage and administration schedule must be determined by the physician for each patient individually.**

▷ **Dosing Instructions:** Take on an empty stomach or with food, at same time each day. Tablet may be crushed for administration.

Usual Duration of Use: Continual use on a regular schedule for several weeks is usually necessary to determine this drug's effectiveness in controlling high blood pressure. The proper treatment of high blood pressure usually requires the long-term use of effective medications. Consult your physician on a regular basis.

▷ **This Drug Should Not Be Taken If**
  • you have had an allergic reaction to it previously.
  • you currently have a blood cell or bone marrow disorder.
  • you have active liver disease.
  • you have an abnormally high level of blood potassium.

▷ **Inform Your Physician Before Taking This Drug If**
  • you have a history of kidney disease or impaired kidney function.
  • you have scleroderma or systemic lupus erythematosus.
  • you have any form of heart disease.
  • you have diabetes.
  • you are taking any of the following drugs: other antihypertensives, diuretics, nitrates or potassium supplements.
  • you plan to have surgery under general anesthesia in the near future.

Possible Side-Effects (natural, expected and unavoidable drug actions)
  Dizziness, light-headedness, fainting (excessive drop in blood pressure).

▷ **Possible Adverse Effects** (unusual, unexpected and infrequent reactions)
  If any of the following develop, consult your physician promptly for guidance.
  Mild Adverse Effects
  Allergic Reactions: Skin rash, itching.
  Headache, fatigue, drowsiness, nervousness, numbness and tingling, insomnia.
  Rapid heart rate, palpitation.
  Indigestion, stomach pain, nausea, vomiting, diarrhea.
  Excessive sweating, muscle cramps.
  Serious Adverse Effects
  Allergic Reactions: Swelling (angioedema) of face, tongue and/or vocal cords: can be life threatening.
  Bone marrow depression—fatigue, weakness, fever, sore throat, abnormal bleeding or bruising (very rare).

▷ **Possible Effects on Sexual Function:** Rare report of impotence.

Possible Effects on Laboratory Tests
  Blood eosinophil counts: increased (allergic reaction).
  Blood creatinine level: increased.
  Blood potassium level: increased.
  Blood uric acid level: decreased.

CAUTION
1. Consult your physician regarding the advisability of discontinuing other antihypertensive drugs (especially diuretics) for 1 week before starting this drug.
2. **Report promptly** any indications of infection (fever, sore throat), and any indications of water retention (weight gain, puffiness, swollen feet or ankles).
3. Do not use a salt substitute without your physician's knowledge and approval. (Many salt substitutes contain potassium.)
4. It is advisable to obtain blood cell counts and urine analyses **before** starting this drug.

Precautions for Use
By Infants and Children: Safety and effectiveness for use by those in this age group have not been established.
By Those over 60 Years of Age: Small doses are advisable until tolerance has been determined. Sudden and excessive lowering of blood pressure can predispose to stroke or heart attack in those with impaired brain circulation or coronary artery heart disease.

▷ **Advisability of Use During Pregnancy**
Pregnancy Category: C (tentative). See Pregnancy Code inside back cover.
Animal studies: No birth defects found in rat or rabbit studies.
Human studies: Information from adequate studies of pregnant women is not available.
Avoid during first 3 months if possible.

Advisability of Use if Breast-Feeding
Presence of this drug in breast milk: Not known.
Monitor nursing infant closely and discontinue drug or nursing if adverse effects develop.

Habit-Forming Potential: None.

Effects of Overdosage: Excessive drop in blood pressure—light-headedness, dizziness, fainting.

Possible Effects of Long-Term Use: Gradual increase in blood potassium level.

Suggested Periodic Examinations While Taking This Drug (at physician's discretion)
Before starting drug: Complete blood cell counts; urine analysis with measurement of protein content; blood potassium level.
During use of drug: Blood cell counts; measurements of blood potassium.

▷ **While Taking This Drug, Observe the Following**

Foods: Consult physician regarding salt intake.

Nutritional Support: Do not take potassium supplements unless directed by your physician.

Beverages: No restrictions. May be taken with milk.

▷ *Alcohol:* Use caution until combined effect has been determined. Alcohol may enhance the blood-pressure-lowering effect of this drug.

Tobacco Smoking: No interactions expected.

▷ *Other Drugs*

Enalapril *taken concurrently* with

- potassium preparations (K-Lyte, Slow-K, etc.) may cause increased blood levels of potassium with risk of serious heart rhythm disturbances.

- potassium-sparing diuretics: amiloride (Moduretic), spironolactone (Aldactazide), triamterene (Dyazide) may cause increased blood levels of potassium with risk of serious heart rhythm disturbances.

▷ *Driving, Hazardous Activities:* Usually no restrictions. Be aware of possible drops in blood pressure with resultant dizziness or faintness.

Aviation Note: The use of this drug *may be a disqualification* for piloting. Consult a designated Aviation Medical Examiner.

Exposure to Sun: Caution advised. A similar drug of this class can cause photosensitivity.

Exposure to Heat: Caution advised. Avoid excessive perspiring with resultant loss of body water and drop in blood pressure.

Occurrence of Unrelated Illness: Report promptly any disorder that causes nausea, vomiting or diarrhea. Fluid and chemical imbalances must be corrected as soon as possible.

EPINEPHRINE
(ep i NEF rin)

Other Name: Adrenaline

Introduced: 1900

Class: Antiasthmatic, anti-glaucoma, decongestant

Prescription: USA: Varies
Canada: No

Controlled Drug: USA: No
Canada: No

Available as Generic: USA: Yes
Canada: No

Brand Names: Adrenalin, Bronkaid Mist, ✦Bronkaid Mistometer, ✦Dysne-Inhal, Epifrin, E-Pilo Preparations [CD], EpiPen, Epitrate, Glaucon, Medihaler-Epi Preparations, Primatene Mist, Sus-Phrine, Vaponefrin

---

BENEFITS versus RISKS

Possible Benefits	*Possible Risks*
EFFECTIVE RELIEF OF SEVERE ALLERGIC (ANAPHYLACTIC) REACTIONS	Significant increase in blood pressure (in sensitive individuals)
TEMPORARY RELIEF OF ACUTE BRONCHIAL ASTHMA	Idiosyncratic Reaction: pulmonary edema (fluid formation in lungs)
Reduction of internal eye pressure (treatment of glaucoma)	Heart rhythm disorders (in sensitive individuals)
Relief of allergic congestion of the nose and sinuses	

▷ **Principal Uses**

As a Single Drug Product: This drug is used most commonly by inhalation to relieve acute attacks of bronchial asthma. It is used less frequently as a decongestant for symptomatic relief of allergic nasal congestion and as eye drops in the management of glaucoma.

How This Drug Works: By stimulating certain sympathetic nerve terminals, this drug acts to
- contract blood vessel walls and raise the blood pressure.
- inhibit the release of harmful amounts of histamine into the skin and internal organs.
- dilate those bronchial tubes that are in sustained constriction, thereby increasing the size of the airways and improving the ability to breathe.
- decrease the formation of fluid within the eye, increase its outflow from the eye and thereby reduce internal eye pressure.
- decrease the volume of blood in nasal tissue, thereby shrinking the tissue mass (decongestion) and expanding the nasal airway.

Available Dosage Forms and Strengths

Aerosol — 0.2 mg, 0.27 mg, 0.3 mg per spray
Eye drops — 0.1%, 0.25%, 0.5%, 1%, 2%
Injection — 0.01 mg, 0.1 mg, 1 mg, 5 mg per ml
Nose drops — 0.1%
Solution for nebulizer — 1%, 1.25%, 2.25%

▷ **Usual Adult Dosage Range:** Aerosols: 1 inhalation, repeated in 1 to 2 minutes if needed; wait 4 hours before next inhalation. Eye drops: 1 drop/12 hours. Dosage may vary with product; follow printed instructions and label directions. **Note: Actual dosage and administration schedule must be determined by the physician for each patient individually.**

▷ **Dosing Instructions:** Aerosols and inhalation solutions: After first inhalation, wait 1 to 2 minutes to determine if a second inhalation is necessary. If relief does not occur within 20 minutes of use, and difficult breathing persists, discontinue this drug and seek medical attention promptly. Avoid prolonged and excessive use. Eye drops: During instillation of drops and for 2 minutes following, press finger against the tear sac (inner corner of eye) to prevent rapid absorption of drug into body circulation.

Usual Duration of Use: According to individual needs. Long-term use requires supervision and periodic evaluation by your physician.

▷ **This Drug Should Not Be Taken If**
- you have had an allergic reaction to any dosage form of it previously.
- you have narrow-angle glaucoma.
- you have experienced a recent stroke or heart attack.

▷ **Inform Your Physician Before Taking This Drug If**
- you have any degree of high blood pressure.
- you have any form of heart disease, especially coronary heart disease (with or without angina), or a heart rhythm disorder.
- you have diabetes or overactive thyroid function (hyperthyroidism).
- you have a history of stroke.
- you are taking any of the following drugs: monoamine oxidase (MAO) type A inhibitors, phenothiazines (see Drug Classes, Section Four), digitalis preparations or quinidine.

Possible Side-Effects (natural, expected and unavoidable drug actions)
In sensitive individuals—restlessness, anxiety, headache, tremor, palpitation, coldness of hands and feet, dryness of mouth and throat (with use of aerosol).

▷ **Possible Adverse Effects** (unusual, unexpected and infrequent reactions)
If any of the following develop, consult your physician promptly for guidance.
Mild Adverse Effects
Allergic Reactions: Skin rash; eye drops may cause redness, swelling and itching of the eyelids.
Weakness, dizziness, pallor.
Serious Adverse Effects
Idiosyncratic Reaction: Sudden development of excessive fluid in the lungs (pulmonary edema).
In predisposed individuals—excessive rise in blood pressure with risk of stroke (cerebral hemorrhage).

▷ **Possible Effects on Sexual Function:**   None reported.

Possible Effects on Laboratory Tests
Complete blood cell counts: red cells and white cells increased; eosinophils decreased.
Blood glucose level: increased.
Urine sugar tests: false low or negative results with Clinistix; true positive with Benedict's or Fehling's solution.

CAUTION
1. The frequently repeated use of this drug at short intervals can pro-

duce a condition of unresponsiveness and result in medication failure. If this develops, avoid use completely for 12 hours, at which time a normal response should return.

2. Excessive use of aerosol preparations in the treatment of asthma has been associated with sudden death.

3. This drug can cause significant irritability of the nerve pathways (conduction system) and muscles of the heart, predisposing to serious heart rhythm disorders. If you have any form of heart disorder, consult your physician.

4. This drug can increase the blood sugar level. If you have diabetes, test for urine sugar frequently to detect significant changes.

5. If you become unresponsive to this drug and you intend to substitute isoproterenol (Isuprel), allow an interval of 4 hours between using these two drugs.

6. Promptly discard all preparations of this drug at the first appearance of discoloration (pink to red to brown) or cloudiness (precipitation). Such changes indicate drug deterioration.

Precautions for Use

By Infants and Children: Use cautiously in small doses until tolerance is determined. Observe for any indications of weakness, light-headedness or inclination to faint.

By Those over 60 Years of Age: Use cautiously in small doses until tolerance is determined. Observe for excessive stimulation: nervousness, headache, tremor, rapid heart rate. If you have hardening of the arteries (arteriosclerosis), heart disease, high blood pressure, Parkinson's disease or prostatism (see Glossary), this drug may aggravate your disorder. Ask your physician for guidance.

▷ Advisability of Use During Pregnancy

Pregnancy Category: C (tentative). See Pregnancy Code inside back cover.
Animal studies: Birth defects reported in rats.
Human studies: Information from adequate studies of pregnant women is not available.
This drug can cause significant reduction of oxygen supply to the fetus. Use it only if clearly needed and in small, infrequent doses. Avoid during the first 3 months and during labor and delivery.

Advisability of Use if Breast-Feeding

Presence of this drug in breast milk: Yes.
Avoid drug or refrain from nursing.

Habit-Forming Potential: Tolerance to this drug can develop with frequent use (see Glossary), but dependence does not occur.

Effects of Overdosage: Nervousness, throbbing headache, dizziness, tremor, palpitation, disturbance of heart rhythm, difficult breathing, abdominal pain, vomiting of blood.

Possible Effects of Long-Term Use: "Epinephrine-fastness": loss of ability to respond to this drug's bronchodilator effect. With long-term treatment of glaucoma: pigment deposits on eyeball and eyelids, possible damage to retina, impaired vision, blockage of tear ducts.

Suggested Periodic Examinations While Taking This Drug (at physician's discretion)

Blood pressure measurements; blood or urine sugar measurements in presence of diabetes; vision testing and measurement of internal eye pressure in presence of glaucoma.

▷ **While Taking This Drug, Observe the Following**

Foods: No restrictions, except those that have been shown to cause you to have asthma.

Beverages: No restrictions.

▷ *Alcohol:* Alcoholic beverages can increase the urinary excretion of this drug.

Tobacco Smoking: No interactions expected. Follow physician's advice regarding smoking as it affects the condition under treatment.

▷ *Other Drugs*

Epinephrine *taken concurrently* with

• certain beta blocker drugs (nadolol, propranolol) may cause increased blood pressure and decreased heart rate.

• chlorpromazine (Thorazine) may cause decreased blood pressure and increased heart rate.

• furazolidone (Furoxone) may cause increased blood pressure and high fever.

• guanethidine (Esimil, Ismelin) may cause increased blood pressure.

• tricyclic antidepressants (amitriptyline, etc.) may cause increased blood pressure and heart rhythm disturbances.

▷ *Driving, Hazardous Activities:* This drug may cause dizziness or excessive nervousness. Restrict activities as necessary.

Aviation Note: The use of this drug *may be a disqualification* for piloting. Consult a designated Aviation Medical Examiner.

Exposure to Sun: No restrictions.

Heavy Exercise or Exertion: No interactions expected. However, exercise can induce asthma in sensitive individuals.

Occurrence of Unrelated Illness: Use caution in presence of severe burns. This drug can increase drainage from burned tissue and cause significant loss of tissue fluids and blood proteins.

Discontinuation: If this drug fails to provide relief after an adequate trial, discontinue it and consult your physician. It is dangerous to increase the dosage or frequency of use.

Special Storage Instructions: Protect drug from exposure to air, light and heat. Keep in a cool place, preferably in the refrigerator.

ERGOTAMINE
(er GOT a meen)

Introduced: 1926

Class: Antimigraine, ergot preparations

Prescription: USA: Yes
Canada: Yes

Controlled Drug: USA: No
Canada: No

Available as Generic: No

Brand Names: ✦Bellergal [CD], Bellergal-S [CD], ✦Bellergal Spacetabs [CD], Cafergot [CD], Cafergot P-B [CD], Ercaf [CD], ✦Ergodryl [CD], Ergomar, Ergostat, ✦Gynergen, Medihaler Ergotamine, Wigraine [CD], Wigrettes

---

BENEFITS versus RISKS

Possible Benefits	*Possible Risks*
PREVENTION AND RELIEF OF VASCULAR HEADACHES: MIGRAINE, MIGRAINELIKE AND HISTAMINE HEADACHES	GANGRENE OF THE FINGERS, TOES OR INTESTINE AGGRAVATION OF CORONARY ARTERY DISEASE (ANGINA) ABORTION

▷ **Principal Uses**

As a Single Drug Product: This drug is used primarily in the treatment of vascular headaches, especially migraine and "cluster" headaches. It should not be used on a continual basis to prevent migraine attacks, but it is often effective in terminating the headache if taken within the first hour following the onset of pain. It may be used on a short-term basis in an attempt to prevent or abort "cluster" headaches during the period of their occurrence. The inhalation form provides rapid onset of action.

As a Combination Drug Product [CD]: This drug is combined with caffeine to take advantage of caffeine's ability to enhance its absorption. This permits a smaller dose of ergotamine to be effective and reduces the risk of adverse effects with repeated use. This drug is also combined with belladonna (atropine) and one of the barbiturates to provide preparations that are useful in relieving the symptoms of premenstrual tension and the menopausal syndrome: nervousness, nausea, hot flushes and sweating.

How This Drug Works: Not completely established. It is thought that by constricting the walls of blood vessels in the head, this drug prevents or relieves the excessive expansion (dilation) that is responsible for the pain of migrainelike headaches.

Available Dosage Forms and Strengths
Aerosol — 9 mg per ml (0.36 mg/inhalation)
Suppositories — 2 mg (in combination with caffeine)
Tablets, sublingual — 2 mg

▷ **Usual Adult Dosage Range:** Inhalation: 1 spray (0.36 mg) at the onset of headache; repeat 1 spray every 5 to 10 minutes as needed for relief, up to a maximum of 6 sprays/24 hours. Do not exceed 15 sprays/week. Sublingual tablets: Dissolve 1 mg under tongue at the onset of headache; repeat 1 mg every 30 to 60 minutes as needed, up to a maximum of 5 mg/attack. Do not exceed 5 mg/24 hours or 10 mg/week. Try to determine the optimal dose required (up to 5 mg) that will abort the headache when taken as a single dose at the onset of pain. **Note: Actual dosage and administration schedule must be determined by the physician for each patient individually.**

▷ **Dosing Instructions:** Follow written instructions carefully. Do not exceed prescribed doses. The regular tablets (combination drug) may be crushed for administration; the sustained-release tablets should be taken whole (not crushed). Sublingual tablets should be dissolved under the tongue, not swallowed.

Usual Duration of Use: Continual use on a regular schedule for several episodes of headache is usually necessary to determine this drug's effectiveness in aborting or relieving the pain of vascular headache. Do not exceed recommended dosage schedules. If headaches are not controlled after several trials of maximal doses, consult your physician for alternative treatment.

▷ **This Drug Should Not Be Taken If**
   • you have had an allergic reaction to any dosage form of it previously.
   • you are pregnant.
   • you have a severe infection.
   • you have any of the following conditions:
   angina pectoris (coronary artery disease)
   Buerger's disease
   hardening of the arteries (arteriosclerosis)
   high blood pressure (severe hypertension)
   kidney disease or impaired kidney function
   liver disease or impaired liver function
   Raynaud's phenomenon
   thrombophlebitis
   severe itching

▷ **Inform Your Physician Before Taking This Drug If**
   • you are allergic or overly sensitive to *any* ergot preparation.

Possible Side-Effects (natural, expected and unavoidable drug actions)
   Usually infrequent and mild with recommended doses.
   Susceptible individuals may notice a sensation of cold hands and feet, with mild numbness and tingling.

▷ **Possible Adverse Effects** (unusual, unexpected and infrequent reactions)
   If any of the following develop, consult your physician promptly for guidance.

Mild Adverse Effects
Allergic Reactions: Localized swellings (angioedema), itching.
Headache, drowsiness, dizziness, confusion.
Chest pain, numbness and tingling of fingers and toes, muscle pains in arms or legs.
Nausea, vomiting, diarrhea.

Serious Adverse Effects
Gangrene of the extremities—coldness; numbness; pain; dark discoloration; eventual loss of fingers, toes or feet.
Gangrene of the intestine—severe abdominal pain and swelling; emergency surgery required.

▷ **Possible Effects on Sexual Function:**   None reported.

Natural Diseases or Disorders That May Be Activated by This Drug
Angina pectoris (coronary artery insufficiency), Buerger's disease, Raynaud's syndrome.

Possible Effects on Laboratory Tests
None reported.

CAUTION
1. The excessive use of this drug can actually provoke migraine headache and increase the frequency of its occurrence.
2. Do not exceed a total dose of 5 mg/24 hours or 10 mg/week.
3. Individual sensitivity to the effects of this drug vary greatly. Some may experience early toxic effects even while taking recommended doses. Report promptly any indications of impaired circulation: numbness in fingers or toes, muscle cramping, chest pain.

Precautions for Use
By Infants and Children: Safety and effectiveness for use by those under 12 years of age have not been established.
By Those over 60 Years of Age: Natural changes in blood vessels and circulation may make you more susceptible to the serious adverse effects of this drug. See the preceding list of disorders that are contraindications for the use of this drug.

▷ **Advisability of Use During Pregnancy**
Pregnancy Category: X. See Pregnancy Code inside back cover.
Animal studies: Fetal deaths reported due to this drug.
Human studies: Information from studies of pregnant women indicates that this drug can cause abortion.
This drug should be avoided during the entire pregnancy.

Advisability of Use if Breast-Feeding
Presence of this drug in breast milk: Yes.
Avoid drug or refrain from nursing.

Habit-Forming Potential: None.

Effects of Overdosage: Manifestations of "ergotism": coldness of skin, severe muscle pains, tingling and burning pain in hands and feet, loss of blood supply to extremities resulting in tissue death (gangrene) in fingers and toes. Acute ergot poisoning: nausea, vomiting, diarrhea, cold skin, numbness extremities, confusion, seizures, coma.

Possible Effects of Long-Term Use: A form of functional dependence (see Glossary) may develop, resulting in withdrawal headaches when the drug is discontinued.

Suggested Periodic Examinations While Taking This Drug (at physician's discretion)
Evaluation of circulation (blood flow) to the extremities.

▷ **While Taking This Drug, Observe the Following**
Foods: No interactions expected. Avoid all foods to which you are allergic; some migraine headaches are due to food allergies.
Beverages: No restrictions.
▷ *Alcohol:* Best avoided; alcohol can intensify vascular headache.
Tobacco Smoking: Best avoided; nicotine can further reduce the restricted blood flow produced by this drug.
Marijuana Smoking: Best avoided; additive effects can increase the coldness of hands and feet.
▷ *Other Drugs*
Ergotamine may *decrease* the effects of
• nitroglycerin, and reduce its effectiveness in preventing or relieving angina pain.
The following drugs may *increase* the effects of ergotamine
• erythromycin (E-Mycin, Eryc, etc.).
• troleandomycin (TAO).
▷ *Driving, Hazardous Activities:* This drug may cause drowsiness or dizziness. Restrict activities as necessary.
Aviation Note: Vascular headache *is a disqualification* for piloting. Consult a designated Aviation Medical Examiner.
Exposure to Sun: No restrictions.
Exposure to Cold: Avoid as much as possible. Cold environments and handling cold objects will further reduce the restricted blood flow to the extremities.
Discontinuation: Following long-term use, it may be necessary to withdraw this drug gradually to prevent withdrawal headache. Ask physician for guidance.

ERYTHROMYCIN
(er ith roh MY sin)

Introduced: 1952

Class: Antibiotic, erythromycins

Prescription: USA: Yes
Canada: Yes

Controlled Drug: USA: No
Canada: No

Available as Generic: Yes

Brand Names: ✦Apo-Erythro Base, ✦Apo-Erythro-ES, ✦Apo-Erythro-S, E.E.S., E-Mycin, E-Mycin E, E-Mycin 333, Eryc, Eryderm, Erygel, Erypar, EryPed, Ery-Tab, Erythrocin, ✦Erythromid, Eryzole [CD], Ilosone, Ilotycin, ✦Novorythro, PCE Dispertab, PCE500, Pediamycin, Pediazole [CD], Robimycin, Wyamycin E, Wyamycin S

BENEFITS versus RISKS

Possible Benefits	*Possible Risks*
EFFECTIVE TREATMENT OF INFECTIONS DUE TO SUSCEPTIBLE MICROORGANISMS	Allergic reactions, mild and infrequent Liver reaction (most common with erythromycin estolate) Drug-induced colitis (rare) Superinfections (rare)

▷ **Principal Uses**

As a Single Drug Product: This well-tolerated and versatile antibiotic is used to treat a broad variety of common infections. The more important among these are (1) skin and skin structure infections; (2) upper and lower respiratory tract infections, including "strep" throat, diphtheria and several types of pneumonia; (3) gonorrhea and syphilis; and (4) amebic dysentery. It is also used for the long-term prevention of recurrences of rheumatic fever. Effective use requires the precise identification of the causative organism and determination of its sensitivity to erythromycin.

How This Drug Works: This drug prevents the growth and multiplication of susceptible organisms by interfering with their formation of essential proteins.

Available Dosage Forms and Strengths
Capsules — 125 mg, 250 mg
Capsules, enteric-coated — 125 mg, 250 mg
Drops — 100 mg per ml
Eye ointment — 5 mg per gram
Gel — 2%
Oral suspension — 125 mg, 250 mg per 5-ml teaspoonful
Skin ointment — 2%

Tablets — 500 mg
Tablets, chewable — 125 mg, 200 mg, 250 mg
Tablets, enteric-coated — 250 mg, 333 mg, 500 mg
Tablets, film-coated — 250 mg, 500 mg
Topical solution — 1.5%, 2%

▷ **Usual Adult Dosage Range:**   250 to 1000 mg/6 hours, according to nature and severity of infection. Total daily dosage should not exceed 8 grams. For endocarditis prophylaxis: 1 gram 2 hours before procedure and 500 mg 6 hours later. **Note: Actual dosage and administration schedule must be determined by the physician for each patient individually.**

▷ **Dosing Instructions:**   Nonenteric-coated preparations should be taken 1 hour before or 2 hours after eating. Enteric-coated preparations may be taken without regard to food. Regular uncoated capsules may be opened and tablets may be crushed for administration; coated and prolonged-action preparations should be swallowed whole. Ask pharmacist for guidance.

Usual Duration of Use: Continual use on a regular schedule for 3 to 5 days is usually necessary to determine this drug's effectiveness in controlling responsive infections. For streptococcal infections: not less than 10 consecutive days (without interruption) to reduce the possibility of developing rheumatic fever or glomerulonephritis. The duration of use should not exceed the time required to eliminate the infection.

▷ **This Drug Should Not Be Taken If**
  • you have had an allergic reaction to any form of erythromycin previously.
  • you have active liver disease.

▷ **Inform Your Physician Before Taking This Drug If**
  • you have a history of a previous "reaction" to erythromycin.
  • you are allergic by nature: hay fever, asthma, hives, eczema.
  • you have taken the estolate form of erythromycin previously.

Possible Side-Effects (natural, expected and unavoidable drug actions)
Superinfections (see Glossary).

▷ **Possible Adverse Effects** (unusual, unexpected and infrequent reactions)
If any of the following develop, consult your physician promptly for guidance.
Mild Adverse Effects
Allergic Reactions: Skin rash, hives, itching.
Nausea, vomiting, diarrhea, abdominal cramping.
Serious Adverse Effects
Allergic Reaction: Rare anaphylactic reaction (see Glossary).
Idiosyncratic Reactions: Liver reaction—nausea, vomiting, fever, jaundice (usually but not exclusively associated with erythromycin estolate).
Drug-induced colitis, transient loss of hearing.

▷ **Possible Effects on Sexual Function:** None reported.

▷ **Adverse Effects That May Mimic Natural Diseases or Disorders**
Liver toxicity may resemble acute gallbladder disease or viral hepatitis.

Possible Effects on Laboratory Tests
Complete blood cell counts: white cells may increase or decrease; eosinophils increased (allergic reaction); platelets decreased.
Prothrombin time: increased (drug taken concurrently with warfarin).
Liver function tests: liver enzymes increased (ALT/GPT, AST/GOT and alkaline phosphatase), increased bilirubin.

CAUTION
1. Take the full dosage prescribed to prevent the possible emergence of resistant bacterial strains.
2. If you have a history of liver disease or impaired liver function, avoid any form of erythromycin estolate.
3. If diarrhea develops and continues for more than 24 hours, consult your physician promptly.

Precautions for Use
By Infants and Children: Observe allergic children closely for indications of developing allergy to this drug. Observe also for evidence of gastrointestinal irritation.
By Those over 60 Years of Age: Observe for indications of itching reactions in the genital and anal regions, often due to yeast superinfections. Observe also for evidence of hearing loss. Report such developments promptly.

▷ **Advisability of Use During Pregnancy**
Pregnancy Category: B (tentative). See Pregnancy Code inside back cover.
Animal studies: Studies of rats are inconclusive.
Human studies: No increase in birth defects reported in 230 exposures. Information from adequate studies of pregnant women is not available.
Generally thought to be safe during entire pregnancy, *except for erythromycin estolate*; this form of erythromycin can cause toxic liver reactions during pregnancy and should be avoided.

Advisability of Use if Breast-Feeding
Presence of this drug in breast milk: Yes.
Monitor nursing infant closely and discontinue drug or nursing if adverse effects develop.

Habit-Forming Potential: None.

Effects of Overdosage: Possible nausea, vomiting, diarrhea and abdominal discomfort.

Possible Effects of Long-Term Use: Superinfections (see Glossary).

Suggested Periodic Examinations While Taking This Drug (at physician's discretion)
Liver function tests if the estolate form is used.

▷ **While Taking This Drug, Observe the Following**
Foods: No restrictions.
Beverages: Avoid fruit juices and carbonated beverages for hour after taking any nonenteric-coated preparation. May be taken with milk.
▷ *Alcohol:* Avoid if you have impaired liver function or are taking the estolate form of this drug.
Tobacco Smoking: No interactions expected.
▷ *Other Drugs*
Erythromycin may *increase* the effects of
• carbamazepine (Tegretol), and cause toxicity.
• digoxin (Lanoxin), and cause toxicity.
• ergotamine (Cafergot, Ergostat, etc.), and cause impaired circulation to extremities.
• methylprednisolone (Medrol), and cause excess steroid effects.
• theophylline (aminophylline, Theo-Dur, etc.), and cause toxicity.
• warfarin (Coumadin), and increase the risk of bleeding.
Erythromycin may *decrease* the effects of
• clindamycin.
• lincomycin.
• penicillins.
▷ *Driving, Hazardous Activities:* This drug may cause nausea and/or diarrhea. Restrict activities as necessary.
Aviation Note: The use of this drug *may be a disqualification* for piloting. Consult a designated Aviation Medical Examiner.
Exposure to Sun: No restrictions.
Special Storage Instructions: Keep liquid forms refrigerated.
Observe the Following Expiration Times: Freshly mixed oral suspension— 14 days. Premixed oral suspension—18 months. Ask pharmacist for guidance.

ESTROGENS
(ES troh jenz)

Other Names: Chlorotrianisene, conjugated estrogens, esterified estrogens, estradiol, estriol, estrone, estropipate, quinestrol

Introduced: 1933

Class: Female sex hormones

Prescription: USA: Yes
Canada: Yes

Controlled Drug: USA: No
Canada: No

Available as Generic: USA: Yes
Canada: No

Brand Names: ✦C.E.S., ✦Climestrone, ✦Delestrogen, DV, Estinyl, Estrace, Estraderm, Estraguard, Estratab, Estrovis, Feminone, ✦Femogen, ✦Femogex, Menest, Menrium [CD], Milprem [CD], ✦Oestrilin, Ogen, PMB [CD], Premarin, TACE

BENEFITS versus RISKS

Possible Benefits	*Possible Risks*
EFFECTIVE RELIEF OF MENOPAUSAL HOT FLUSHES AND NIGHT SWEATS	INCREASED RISK OF CANCER OF THE UTERUS with 3 years of continual use
PREVENTION OR RELIEF OF ATROPHIC VAGINITIS, ATROPHY OF THE VULVA AND URETHRA	Increased frequency of gallstones
	Accelerated growth of preexisting fibroid tumors of the uterus
PREVENTION OF OSTEOPOROSIS (62% reduction of fracture risk)	Fluid retention
	Postmenopausal bleeding
Prevention of thinning of the skin	Deep vein thrombophlebitis and thromboembolism (less likely with conjugated estrogens, more likely with synthetic unconjugated hormones)
Mental tonic effect	Increased blood pressure (rare)
	Decreased sugar tolerance (rare)

▷ **Principal Uses**

As a Single Drug Product: This widely used hormone is very effective when administered in proper dosage and carefully supervised. Its primary use is supplemental ("replacement" therapy) when used to treat the following conditions: (1) ovarian failure or removal in the young woman; (2) the menopausal syndrome; (3) postmenopausal atrophy of genital tissues; and (4) postmenopausal osteoporosis. It is also used in selected cases of breast cancer and prostate cancer.

As a Combination Drug Product [CD]: Estrogen is available in combination with chlordiazepoxide (Librium) and with meprobamate (Equanil, Miltown). These mild tranquilizers are added to provide a calming effect that makes the combination more effective in treating selected cases of the menopausal syndrome. See the Drug Profile of the Oral Contraceptives for a discussion of the combination of estrogens and progestins.

How This Drug Works: When used to correct hormonal deficiency states, estrogens restore normal cellular activity by increasing the synthesis of chromatin, RNA and cellular proteins. The frequency and intensity of menopausal symptoms are significantly reduced when normal tissue levels of estrogen are restored.

Available Dosage Forms and Strengths
Capsules — 12 mg, 25 mg, 72 mg (TACE)
Tablets — 0.02 mg, 0.05 mg, 0.1 mg, 0.3 mg, 0.5 mg, 0.625 mg, 0.9 mg, 1.25 mg, 2.5 mg, 5 mg
Transdermal patch — 0.05 mg, 0.1 mg
Vaginal cream — 0.1 mg, 0.625 mg, 1.5 mg per gram

▷ **Usual Adult Dosage Range:**   For conjugated and esterified estrogens: 0.3 to 1.25 mg daily for 21 days. Omit for 7 days. Repeat cyclically as needed. For other forms of estrogen: consult your physician. **Note: Actual dosage and administration schedule must be determined by the physician for each patient individually.**

▷ **Dosing Instructions:**   May be taken without regard to food. The tablets may be crushed for administration. The capsules should be taken whole.

Usual Duration of Use: Continual use on a regular schedule for 10 to 20 days is usually necessary to determine this drug's effectiveness in relieving menopausal symptoms. Long-term use requires supervision and periodic evaluation by your physician every 6 months. Consult your physician on a regular basis.

▷ **This Drug Should Not Be Taken If**
• you have had a significant allergic reaction to any dosage form of it previously.
• you have a history of thrombophlebitis, embolism, heart attack or stroke.
• you have seriously impaired liver function.
• you have abnormal and unexplained vaginal bleeding.
• you have sickle cell disease.
• you are pregnant.

▷ **Inform Your Physician Before Taking This Drug If**
• you have had an unfavorable reaction to estrogen therapy previously.
• you have a history of cancer of the breast or reproductive organs.
• you have any of the following conditions: fibrocystic breast changes, fibroid tumors of the uterus, endometriosis, migrainelike headaches, epilepsy, asthma, heart disease, high blood pressure, gallbladder disease, diabetes or porphyria.

- you smoke tobacco on a regular basis.
- you plan to have surgery in the near future.

Possible Side-Effects (natural, expected and unavoidable drug actions)
Fluid retention, weight gain, "breakthrough" bleeding (spotting in middle of menstrual cycle), altered menstrual pattern, resumption of menstrual flow (bleeding from the uterus) after a period of natural cessation (postmenopausal bleeding), increased susceptibility to yeast infection of the genital tissues.

▷ **Possible Adverse Effects** (unusual, unexpected and infrequent reactions)
If any of the following develop, consult your physician promptly for guidance.
Mild Adverse Effects
Allergic Reactions: Skin rash, hives, itching.
Headache, nervous tension, irritability, accentuation of migraine headaches.
Nausea, vomiting, bloating, diarrhea.
Tannish pigmentation of the face.
Serious Adverse Effects
Idiosyncratic Reaction: Cutaneous porphyria—fragility and scarring of the skin.
Emotional depression, rise in blood pressure (in susceptible individuals).
Gallbladder disease, benign liver tumors, jaundice, rise in blood sugar.
Erosion of uterine cervix, enlargement of uterine fibroid tumors.
Thrombophlebitis (inflammation of a vein with formation of blood clot)—pain or tenderness in thigh or leg, with or without swelling of foot or leg.
Pulmonary embolism (movement of blood clot to lung)—sudden shortness of breath, pain in chest, coughing, bloody sputum.
Stroke (blood clot in brain)—headaches, blackout, sudden weakness or paralysis of any part of the body, severe dizziness, altered vision, slurred speech, inability to speak.
Retinal thrombosis (blood clot in eye vessels)—sudden impairment or loss of vision.
Heart attack (blood clot in coronary artery)—sudden pain in chest, neck, jaw or arm; weakness; sweating; nausea.

▷ **Possible Effects on Sexual Function**
Swelling and tenderness of breasts, milk production.
Increased vaginal secretions.

Possible Delayed Adverse Effects: Estrogens taken during pregnancy can predispose the female child to the later development of cancer of the vagina or cervix following puberty.

▷ **Adverse Effects That May Mimic Natural Diseases or Disorders**
Liver reactions may suggest viral hepatitis.

Natural Diseases or Disorders That May Be Activated by This Drug
Latent hypertension, diabetes mellitus, acute intermittent porphyria.

Possible Effects on Laboratory Tests
Red blood cells, hemoglobin and platelets: decreased.
Blood calcium level: increased.
Blood total cholesterol level: decreased (treatment effect); increased in post-menopausal women.
Blood LDL cholesterol level: decreased in post-menopausal women.
Blood triglyceride level: no drug effect in post-menopausal women.
Blood glucose level: increased.
Glucose tolerance test (GTT): decreased.
Blood thyroid hormone (T^3 and T^4) levels: increased.
Blood uric acid level: decreased.
Liver function tests: increased liver enzymes (ALT/GPT, AST/GOT and alkaline phosphatase), increased bilirubin.

CAUTION
1. To avoid prolonged (uninterrupted) stimulation of breast and uterine tissues, estrogen should be taken in cycles of 3 weeks on and 1 week off of medication.
2. The estrogen in estrogen vaginal creams is absorbed systemically by the woman. It may also be absorbed through the penis during sexual intercourse and can cause enlargement and tenderness of male breast tissue.

Precautions for Use
By Those over 60 Years of Age: This drug has very limited usefulness after 60. Its use should be restricted to those women who are at increased risk for developing osteoporosis. In this age group, it is advisable to attempt relief of hot flushes with nonestrogenic medications. During use, report promptly any indications of impaired circulation: speech disturbances, altered vision, sudden hearing loss, vertigo, sudden weakness or paralysis, angina, leg pains.

▷ Advisability of Use During Pregnancy
Pregnancy Category: X. See Pregnancy Code inside back cover.
Animal studies: Genital defects reported in mice and guinea pigs; cleft palate reported in rodents.
Human studies: Information from studies of pregnant women indicates that estrogens can masculinize the female fetus. In addition, limb defects and heart malformations have been reported.
It is now known that estrogens taken during pregnancy can predispose the female child to the development of cancer of the vagina or cervix following puberty. *Avoid estrogens completely during entire pregnancy.*

Advisability of Use if Breast-Feeding
Presence of this drug in breast milk: Yes, in minute amounts.

Estrogens in large doses can suppress milk formation.
Breast-feeding is considered to be safe during the use of estrogens.

Habit-Forming Potential: None.

Effects of Overdosage: Headache, drowsiness, nausea, vomiting, fluid retention, abnormal vaginal bleeding, breast enlargement and discomfort.

Possible Effects of Long-Term Use: High blood pressure, gallbladder disease with gallstone formation, increased growth of benign fibroid tumors of the uterus. Several reports suggest possible association between the long-term use (3+ years) of estrogens and the development of cancer of the lining of the uterus. Further studies are needed to establish a definite cause-and-effect relationship (see Glossary). Prudence dictates that women with uterus intact should use estrogens only when symptoms justify it and with proper supervision.

Suggested Periodic Examinations While Taking This Drug (at physician's discretion)
Regular (every 6 months) evaluation of the breasts and pelvic organs, including Pap smears. Liver function tests as indicated.

▷ **While Taking This Drug, Observe the Following**
Foods: Avoid excessive use of salt if fluid retention occurs.
Beverages: No restrictions. May be taken with milk.
▷ *Alcohol:* No interactions expected.
Tobacco Smoking: Recent studies indicate that heavy smoking (15 or more cigarettes daily) in association with the use of estrogen-containing oral contraceptives significantly increases the risk of heart attack (coronary thrombosis). Avoid heavy smoking during long-term estrogen therapy.
▷ *Other Drugs*
Estrogens *taken concurrently* with
• antidiabetic drugs may cause unpredictable fluctuations of blood sugar.
• tricyclic antidepressants (Elavil, Sinequan, etc.) may enhance their adverse effects and reduce their antidepressant effectiveness.
• warfarin (Coumadin) may cause unpredictable alterations of prothrombin activity.
The following drugs may *decrease* the effects of estrogens
• carbamazepine (Tegretol).
• phenobarbital.
• phenytoin (Dilantin).
• primidone (Mysoline).
• rifampin (Rifadin, Rimactane).
▷ *Driving, Hazardous Activities:* Usually no restrictions. Consult your physician for assessment of individual risk and for guidance regarding specific restrictions.
Aviation Note: Usually no restrictions. However, it is advisable to observe

for the rare occurrence of disturbed vision and to restrict activities accordingly. Consult a designated Aviation Medical Examiner.

Exposure to Sun: Use caution until full effect is known. These drugs can cause photosensitivity (see Glossary).

Discontinuation: It is advisable to discontinue estrogens periodically to determine if a need for them still exists. Reduce the dose gradually to prevent acute withdrawal hot flushes. Avoid continual, uninterrupted use of large doses. Discontinue altogether when a definite indication for replacement therapy no longer exists. Ask your physician for guidance.

ETHOSUXIMIDE
(eth oh SUX i mide)

Introduced: 1960

Class: Anticonvulsant, succinimides

Prescription: USA: Yes
Canada: Yes

Controlled Drug: USA: No
Canada: No

Available as Generic: No

Brand Name: Zarontin

BENEFITS versus RISKS	
Possible Benefits	*Possible Risks*
EFFECTIVE CONTROL OF ABSENCE SEIZURES (PETIT MAL EPILEPSY) in 70% of cases EFFECTIVE CONTROL OF MYOCLONIC AND AKINETIC EPILEPSY in some individuals	RARE APLASTIC ANEMIA (See Aplastic Anemia and Bone Marrow Depression in Glossary) Rare decrease in white blood cells and blood platelets

▷ **Principal Uses**

As a Single Drug Product: This is the drug of first choice by many physicians for the management of absence seizures. It causes serious adverse effects less frequently than other drugs used for this disorder, and it is quite effective in the presence of structural abnormalities of the brain.

How This Drug Works: Not completely established. It is thought that by altering the transmission of certain nerve impulses, this drug suppresses the abnormal showers of electrical activity responsible for the absence seizures of petit mal epilepsy.

Available Dosage Forms and Strengths
Capsules — 250 mg
Syrup — 250 mg per 5-ml teaspoonful

▷ **Usual Adult Dosage Range:**   20 to 40 mg per kilogram of body weight/24 hours. Initially 500 mg/24 hours. Dosage may be increased cautiously by 250 mg every 4 to 7 days until satisfactory control is achieved. The total daily dosage should not exceed 1500 mg. **Note: Actual dosage and administration schedule must be determined by the physician for each patient individually.**

▷ **Dosing Instructions:**   May be taken with food to reduce stomach irritation. Capsule may be opened for administration.

Usual Duration of Use: Continual use on a regular schedule for 1 to 2 weeks is usually necessary to determine this drug's effectiveness in reducing the frequency of absence seizures. Long-term use requires supervision and periodic evaluation by your physician. Consult your physician on a regular basis.

▷ **This Drug Should Not Be Taken If**
• you are allergic to this or any other succinimide drug (See Drug Class, Section Four).
• you have active liver disease.
• you currently have a blood cell or bone marrow disorder.

▷ **Inform Your Physician Before Taking This Drug If**
• you have a history of liver or kidney disease.
• you have a history of any type of blood cell disorder, especially one induced by drugs.
• you have a history of serious depression or other mental illness.

Possible Side-Effects (natural, expected and unavoidable drug actions)
Drowsiness, lethargy, fatigue.

▷ **Possible Adverse Effects** (unusual, unexpected and infrequent reactions)
If any of the following develop, consult your physician promptly for guidance.
Mild Adverse Effects
Allergic Reactions: Skin rash, hives.
Headache, dizziness, unsteadiness, euphoria, impaired vision, numbness and tingling in extremities.
Loss of appetite, nausea, vomiting, hiccups, stomach pain, diarrhea.
Excessive growth of hair.
Serious Adverse Effects
Allergic Reaction: Swelling of tongue.
Thickening and overgrowth of gums.
Nervousness, hyperactivity, disturbed sleep, night terrors.
Aggravation of emotional depression and paranoid mental disorders.

Severe bone marrow depression—fatigue, weakness, fever, sore throat, abnormal bleeding or bruising.

▷ **Possible Effects on Sexual Function:**   Increased libido (questionable); non-menstrual vaginal bleeding.

Natural Diseases or Disorders That May Be Activated by This Drug
Latent psychosis, systemic lupus erythematosus.

Possible Effects on Laboratory Tests
Complete blood cell counts: decreased red cells, hemoglobin, white cells and platelets; increased eosinophils.
Blood aspartate aminotransferase (AST) level: increased in 33% of users.
Blood bilirubin level: increased (rare liver damage).
Blood lupus erythematosus (LE) cells: positive (rare).
Kidney function tests: increased blood urea nitrogen (BUN) level, increased urine protein content.

CAUTION
1. This drug may increase the frequency of grand mal seizures in individuals with mixed seizure disorders.
2. It is mandatory that you comply with your physician's request for periodic blood counts and other tests that are deemed necessary.

Precautions for Use
By Infants and Children: If a single daily dose causes nausea or vomiting, give in 2 or 3 divided doses 8 to 12 hours apart. Marked individual variation in response occurs; the use of blood levels for monitoring is advised. Observe for a possible lupuslike reaction: fever, rash, arthritis.
By Those over 60 Years of Age: Rarely used in this age group.

▷ **Advisability of Use During Pregnancy**
Pregnancy Category: C (tentative). See Pregnancy Code inside back cover.
Animal studies: Bone defects reported in rodents.
Human studies: Three instances of birth defects have been reported. Information from adequate studies of pregnant women is not available.
Avoid during first 3 months. Use only if clearly needed during the last 6 months.

Advisability of Use if Breast-Feeding
Presence of this drug in breast milk: Yes.
Monitor nursing infant closely and discontinue drug or nursing if adverse effects develop. If mother requires high doses, refrain from nursing. Ask physician for guidance.

Habit-Forming Potential: None.

Effects of Overdosage: Increased drowsiness, lethargy, weakness, dizziness, unsteadiness, nausea, vomiting, stupor progressing to coma.

Possible Effects of Long-Term Use: Systemic lupus erythematosus.

Suggested Periodic Examinations While Taking This Drug (at physician's discretion)
   Complete blood cell counts every 2 weeks during the first months of use, then monthly thereafter; liver and kidney function tests.

▷ **While Taking This Drug, Observe the Following**
   Foods: No restrictions.
   Beverages: No restrictions. May be taken with milk.
▷ *Alcohol:* Use caution until the combined effects have been determined. This drug may increase the sedative effects of alcohol. Excessive alcohol may precipitate seizures.
   Tobacco Smoking: No interactions expected.
▷ *Other Drugs*
   Ethosuximide may *increase* the effects of
   • phenytoin (Dilantin), by slowing its elimination.
   Ethosuximide *taken concurrently* with
   • valproic acid (Depakene) may alter the effects of ethosuximide unpredictably.
   The following drugs may *increase* the effects of ethosuximide
   • isoniazid (INH, Niconyl, etc.).
▷ *Driving, Hazardous Activities:* This drug may cause drowsiness, dizziness, unsteadiness and impaired vision. Restrict activities as necessary.
   Aviation Note: Seizure disorders and the use of this drug *are disqualifications* for piloting. Consult a designated Aviation Medical Examiner.
   Exposure to Sun: No restrictions.
   Discontinuation: Do not stop taking this drug abruptly. Ask your physician for guidance regarding gradual reduction of dosage.

ETRETINATE
(e TRET i nayt)

Introduced: 1976

Class: Antipsoriasis

Prescription: USA: Yes
   Canada: Yes

Controlled Drug: USA: No
   Canada: No

Available as Generic: USA: No
   Canada: No

Brand Name: Tegison

```
┌─────────────────────────────────────────────────────────────────┐
│                      BENEFITS versus RISKS                        │
│                                                                   │
│     Possible Benefits              Possible Risks                 │
│  EFFECTIVE TREATMENT FOR      MAJOR DRUG-INDUCED BIRTH            │
│    SEVERE, RESISTANT            DEFECTS                           │
│  PSORIASIS in the majority of  RARE DRUG-INDUCED                  │
│  all cases treated             HEPATITIS                          │
│                               Adverse effects on eyes and vision │
│                               Adverse effects on musculoskeletal │
│                                 structures                        │
│                               Adverse effects on blood           │
│                                 cholesterol and triglycerides     │
│                               Increased intracranial pressure     │
│                                 (very rare)                       │
└─────────────────────────────────────────────────────────────────┘
```

▷ **Principal Uses**

As a Single Drug Product: Used primarily to treat severe, generalized forms of psoriasis (and related skin disorders) that have failed to respond to conventional, less hazardous treatments.

How This Drug Works: Not completely established. Its principal action is the regulation of cell differentiation in the skin; this results in a more normal pattern of cell growth, with reduction of inflammation and scale formation.

Available Dosage Forms and Strengths

Capsules — 10 mg, 25 mg

▷ **Usual Adult Dosage Range:**   Initially 0.75 to 1 mg/kg/day, in divided doses, until satisfactory response is obtained (usually 8 to 16 weeks). Maintenance: 0.5 to 0.75 mg/kg/day, beginning after initial response. Total daily dosage should not exceed 75 mg. **Note: Actual dosage and administration schedule must be determined by the physician for each patient individually.**

▷ **Dosing Instructions:**   Take with or immediately following meals, preferably with whole milk. Do not suck or chew the capsule; swallow it whole.

Usual Duration of Use: Continual use on a regular schedule for 2 to 4 weeks is usually necessary to determine this drug's effectiveness in reversing the skin changes of psoriasis. The full effect of treatment may not be apparent until after 2 to 3 months of continual use. Long-term use (months to years) requires periodic evaluation of response and dosage adjustment. Due to the potential for drug accumulation and toxicity with long-term use, this drug should be temporarily discontinued after 18 months of treatment; it may be resumed as needed. Consult your physician on a regular basis.

Possible Advantages of This Drug: When used in conjunction with other antipsoriasis drugs and procedures, this drug can enhance the therapeutic response and reduce the total dosage and length of treatment required for satisfactory management.

▷ **This Drug Should Not Be Taken If**
- you have had an allergic reaction to any dosage form of it previously.
- you are pregnant or breast-feeding.
- you plan to donate blood in the near future.

▷ **Inform Your Physician Before Taking This Drug If**
- you are allergic to vitamin A or other vitamin A derivatives: isotretinoin (Accutane), tretinoin (Retin-A).
- you are allergic to parabens (preservatives).
- you have cerebral or coronary artery disease.
- you have high blood cholesterol or triglyceride levels.
- you have diabetes.
- you have impaired liver or kidney function.
- you have alcoholism.
- you have a history of Crohn's disease or ulcerative colitis.

Possible Side-Effects (natural, expected and unavoidable drug actions)
Dry nose, nosebleed, dry lips, sore mouth and tongue, bleeding gums.
Loss of hair, skin peeling of hands and feet, dry skin, itching, bruising, nail deformities.
Thickening of bone (hyperostosis), calcification of tendons and ligaments, bone and joint pain.

▷ **Possible Adverse Effects** (unusual, unexpected and infrequent reactions)
If any of the following develop, consult your physician promptly for guidance.
Mild Adverse Effects
Allergic Reactions: Skin rash, hives, itching.
Headache, dizziness, fatigue, fever, emotional irritability.
Eye irritation, blurred or double vision, sensitivity to bright light, decreased tolerance for contact lenses, earache, impaired hearing.
Altered taste, loss of appetite, nausea, stomach pain, constipation, diarrhea.
Painful urination.
Serious Adverse Effects
Increased intracranial pressure (less than 1%): headache, nausea, vomiting, visual disturbances.
Hepatitis (1.5%); 4 reported deaths worldwide.
Eye reactions: corneal erosion, abrasion, staining; cataract; retinal hemorrhage; visual field defects; reduced night vision.
Inflammatory bowel disease (Crohn's disease), rare.
Altered blood fat levels: increased triglycerides (45%), increased total cholesterol (16%), decreased HDL cholesterol (37%); any of these changes may increase the risk for the development of atherosclerotic heart disease.

▷ **Possible Effects on Sexual Function:**   Altered timing and pattern of menstruation.

Possible Delayed Adverse Effects: This drug has been found in the blood 2.9 years following termination of its use and has the potential for inducing birth defects during this time. It has not been determined how long pregnancy should be avoided after discontinuation of treatment.

▷ **Adverse Effects That May Mimic Natural Diseases or Disorders**
Increased intracranial pressure may suggest brain tumor.
Liver reactions may suggest viral hepatitis.
Joint pains due to calcification of ligaments and tendons may suggest the onset of arthritis.

Natural Diseases or Disorders That May Be Activated by This Drug
Angina may develop in the presence of coronary artery heart disease. Heart attack (myocardial infarction) has been associated with the use of this drug.

Possible Effects on Laboratory Tests
Red blood cell counts: decreased.
Blood eosinophil counts: increased.
Blood total cholesterol, LDL cholesterol and triglyceride levels: increased.
Liver function tests: increased liver enzymes (ALT/GPT, AST/GOT and alkaline phosphatase.

CAUTION
1. *This drug should not be taken during pregnancy.* A pregnancy test should be performed within 2 weeks prior to taking this drug. In the absence of pregnancy, the drug should be started on the second or third day of the next normal menstrual period. An effective form of contraception should be used for 1 month before the drug is started, during the entire period of treatment, and for an indefinite period (minimum of 3 years) after the drug is discontinued. If pregnancy does occur, discontinue this drug immediately and consult your physician.
2. *Do not donate blood to a blood bank if you are taking this drug.* Blood containing this drug could pose a serious risk to the developing fetus of a pregnant patient who received it. Avoid blood donation for a minimum of 3 years if use of the blood is beyond your control.
3. *Comply fully with your physician's recommendations for periodic examinations before, during and following treatment with this drug.* These are mandatory for safe and effective use.
4. Avoid the concurrent use of vitamin A supplements while taking this drug.
5. If you experience significant eye reactions or altered vision, consult your physician promptly.
6. Your psoriasis may appear to worsen during the early period of

treatment with this drug. This is a common response. Consult your physician if symptoms become severe or prolonged.

7. If dry mouth or sore and bleeding gums persist, consult your dentist.

Precautions for Use

By Infants and Children: This drug should be used only after all less hazardous treatments have failed. It is advisable to obtain pretreatment X-rays to determine bone age and to monitor bone growth and development by yearly X-ray studies. This drug can impair normal bone maturation.

By Those over 60 Years of Age: Monitor for the possible development of anemia, impaired kidney function and fluctuation of blood potassium levels.

▷ **Advisability of Use During Pregnancy**

Pregnancy Category: X. See Pregnancy Code inside back cover.

Animal studies: No information available.

Human studies: Major birth defects occur in association with the use of this drug: malformations of the skull, vertebrae, face, extremities, brain and spinal cord.

Avoid this drug completely during entire pregnancy. See *CAUTION.*

Advisability of Use if Breast-Feeding

Presence of this drug in breast milk: Unknown.

Avoid drug or refrain from nursing.

Habit-Forming Potential: None.

Effects of Overdosage: Severe headache, irritability, drowsiness, itching, nausea, vomiting.

Possible Effects of Long-Term Use: Hyperostosis (84%): abnormal thickening of bone (pelvis), calcification of ligaments and tendons (knees and ankles).

Suggested Periodic Examinations While Taking This Drug (at physician's discretion)

Complete blood cell counts; measurements of blood sugar, potassium, sodium and chloride.

Blood cholesterol profiles, before and during treatment.

Liver and kidney function tests.

Complete eye examinations.

Bone X-rays, especially children.

▷ **While Taking This Drug, Observe the Following**

Foods: No restrictions. High-fat foods increase absorption of this drug.

Beverages: No restrictions. Whole milk increases absorption of this drug.

▷ *Alcohol:* No interactions expected. Use moderately; excessive intake can increase blood triglyceride levels.

Tobacco Smoking: No interactions expected.

▷ *Other Drugs*

Etretinate may *increase* the effects of
- vitamin A and its derivatives (isotretinoin and tretinoin) and increase the risk of vitamin A toxicity.

Etretinate *taken concurrently* with
- methotrexate may increase the risk of liver toxicity.
- tetracyclines may increase the risk of elevated intracranial pressure.

▷ *Driving, Hazardous Activities:* This drug may cause dizziness and blurred vision. Restrict activities as necessary.

Aviation Note: The use of this drug *may be a disqualification* for piloting. Consult a designated Aviation Medical Examiner.

Exposure to Sun: Use caution. This drug can cause photosensitivity (see Glossary).

Discontinuation: If this drug is not significantly beneficial after 4 months of continual use, it should be discontinued. If response is adequate to justify its long-term use, it should be discontinued temporarily ("drug holiday") after 18 months of continual treatment. Once the skin has cleared satisfactorily, this drug should be discontinued. The majority of individuals will experience some degree of recurrence by the end of 2 months. Subsequent treatment courses of 4 to 9 months can be instituted as required.

FAMOTIDINE
(fa MOH te deen)

Introduced: 1986

Class: Antiulcer, H-2 receptor blocker

Prescription: USA: Yes

Controlled Drug: USA: No

Available as Generic: USA: No

Brand Name: Pepcid

BENEFITS versus RISKS

Possible Benefits	*Possible Risks*
EFFECTIVE TREATMENT OF PEPTIC ULCER DISEASE: relief of symptoms, acceleration of healing, prevention of recurrence	Headache, dizziness
CONTROL OF HYPERSECRETORY STOMACH DISORDERS	
Beneficial in treatment of reflux esophagitis	

▷ **Principal Uses**

As a Single Drug Product: Used primarily in the treatment of peptic ulcer disease, both benign stomach (gastric) ulcer and duodenal ulcer. It is used specifically to hasten the healing of ulcer and to prevent recurrence. Also used to control the excessive production of stomach acid in the Zollinger-Ellison syndrome. Though its effectiveness has not been fully established, this drug is also used in the management of esophagitis (as with hiatal hernia) and upper gastrointestinal bleeding.

How This Drug Works: By blocking the action of histamine, this drug effectively inhibits the secretion of stomach acid and thus creates a more favorable environment for the healing of peptic ulcers.

Available Dosage Forms and Strengths
Injection — 10 mg per ml
Oral suspension — 40 mg per 5-ml teaspoonful
Tablets — 20 mg, 40 mg

▷ **Usual Adult Dosage Range:** For active peptic ulcer: 20 mg twice daily, or 40 mg at bedtime. For prevention of recurrent ulcer: 20 mg at bedtime. For hypersecretory states: 20 mg/6 hours. **Note: Actual dosage and administration schedule must be determined by the physician for each patient individually.**

▷ **Dosing Instructions:** To obtain the longest period of stomach acid reduction, this drug should be taken with or immediately following food. The tablet may be crushed for administration. If needed, antacids may be taken concurrently with this drug to relieve ulcer pain.

Usual Duration of Use: Continual use on a regular schedule for 4 to 6 weeks is usually necessary to determine this drug's effectiveness in healing active peptic ulcer. Long-term use (months to years) for prevention of ulcer recurrence requires individual consideration by your physician.

▷ **This Drug Should Not Be Taken If**
• you have had an allergic reaction to any dosage form of it previously.

▷ **Inform Your Physician Before Taking This Drug If**
• you are allergic to cimetidine (Tagamet) or ranitidine (Zantac).
• you have impaired liver or kidney function.

Possible Side-Effects (natural, expected and unavoidable drug actions)
None reported.

▷ **Possible Adverse Effects** (unusual, unexpected and infrequent reactions)
If any of the following develop, consult your physician promptly for guidance.
Mild Adverse Effects
Allergic Reactions: Skin rash, swelling of eyelids.
Headache (4.7%), dizziness (1.3%), fatigue.
Nausea, constipation (1.2%), diarrhea (1.7%).

Serious Adverse Effects
   Rare decrease in blood platelet counts: abnormal bleeding or bruising (questionable).

▷ **Possible Effects on Sexual Function:**   Decreased libido.

Possible Effects on Laboratory Tests
   No authoritative reports found.

CAUTION
   1. Do not discontinue this drug abruptly. (Ulcer activation and perforation have occurred following abrupt cessation of cimetidine, a closely related drug.)
   2. After discontinuation of this drug, inform your physician promptly if you experience a return of symptoms indicative of ulcer reactivation.
   3. Inform your allergist that you are taking this drug if allergy skin tests are to be done; this drug may interfere with skin testing and cause false negative results.

Precautions for Use
   By Infants and Children: Safety and effectiveness for use by those under 12 years of age have not been established.
   By Those over 60 Years of Age: This drug may contribute to the formation of stomach phytobezoars (masses of undigested vegetable fibers). Individuals with poor chewing ability (missing teeth) and those who have had partial gastrectomy or vagotomy (stomach surgery) are most susceptible. Observe for loss of appetite, stomach fullness, nausea and vomiting.

▷ **Advisability of Use During Pregnancy**
   Pregnancy Category: B (tentative). See Pregnancy Code inside back cover.
   Animal studies: No birth defects reported.
   Human studies: Information from adequate studies of pregnant women is not available.
   Use this drug only if clearly needed. Ask physician for guidance.

Advisability of Use if Breast-Feeding
   Presence of this drug in breast milk: Probably yes.
   Avoid drug or refrain from nursing.

Habit-Forming Potential: None.

Effects of Overdosage: Related drugs (cimetidine, ranitidine) may cause confusion, delirium, slurred speech, flushing, sweating, drowsiness, muscle twitching, seizures, coma.

Possible Effects of Long-Term Use: Impaired absorption of vitamin B-12.

Suggested Periodic Examinations While Taking This Drug (at physician's discretion)
Complete blood cell counts.

▷ **While Taking This Drug, Observe the Following**
Foods: Protein-rich foods produce maximal stomach acid secretion. Follow the diet prescribed to derive optimal benefit from this drug.
Beverages: No restrictions. May be taken with milk.
▷ *Alcohol:* No interactions with drug. However, alcoholic beverages increase stomach acidity and can reduce the effectiveness of this drug.
Tobacco Smoking: Decreased effectiveness of this drug, especially in its ability to reduce nocturnal stomach acid secretion. Avoid smoking during periods of active peptic ulcer disease.
▷ *Other Drugs:* No significant drug interactions reported to date.
▷ *Driving, Hazardous Activities:* This drug may cause dizziness. Restrict activities as necessary.
Aviation Note: The use of this drug *may be a disqualification* for piloting. Consult a designated Aviation Medical Examiner.
Exposure to Sun: No restrictions.
Discontinuation: Do not discontinue this drug suddenly if taken for peptic ulcer disease. Consult physician for withdrawal instructions. This drug does not provide an extended protective effect. Be alert to the possibility of ulcer recurrence anytime after discontinuation.

FENOPROFEN
(fen oh PROH fen)

Introduced: 1976

Class: Mild analgesic, anti-inflammatory

Prescription: USA: Yes
Canada: Yes

Controlled Drug: USA: No
Canada: No

Available as Generic: Yes

Brand Name: Nalfon

BENEFITS versus RISKS

Possible Benefits	*Possible Risks*
EFFECTIVE RELIEF OF MILD TO MODERATE PAIN AND INFLAMMATION	Gastrointestinal pain, ulceration, bleeding (rare)
	Rare liver or kidney damage
	Rare fluid retention
	Rare bone marrow depression

▷ **Principal Uses**

As a Single Drug Product: Used primarily to relieve mild to moderately severe pain associated with (1) musculoskeletal injuries; (2) acute and chronic gout, rheumatoid arthritis and osteoarthritis; (3) dental, obstetrical and orthopedic surgery; (4) menstrual cramps; and (5) vascular (migrainelike) headaches.

How This Drug Works: Not completely established. It is thought that this drug reduces the tissue concentrations of prostaglandins (and related compounds), chemicals involved in the production of inflammation and pain.

Available Dosage Forms and Strengths
Capsules — 200 mg, 300 mg
Tablets — 600 mg

▷ **Usual Adult Dosage Range:**   300 to 600 mg 3 or 4 times/day. Total daily dosage should not exceed 3200 mg. **Note: Actual dosage and administration schedule must be determined by the physician for each patient individually.**

▷ **Dosing Instructions:**   Take either on an empty stomach or with food or milk to prevent stomach irritation. Take with a full glass of water and remain upright (do not lie down) for 30 minutes. The tablet may be crushed and the capsule may be opened for administration.

Usual Duration of Use: Continual use on a regular schedule for 2 to 3 weeks is usually necessary to determine this drug's effectiveness in relieving the discomfort of arthritis. Long-term use requires supervision and periodic evaluation by the physician. Consult your physician on a regular basis.

▷ **This Drug Should Not Be Taken If**
• you have had an allergic reaction to it previously.
• you are subject to asthma or nasal polyps caused by aspirin.
• you have active peptic ulcer disease or any form of gastrointestinal bleeding.
• you have a bleeding disorder or a blood cell disorder.
• you have severe impairment of kidney function.

▷ **Inform Your Physician Before Taking This Drug If**
• you are allergic to aspirin or to other aspirin substitutes.
• you have a history of peptic ulcer disease or any type of bleeding disorder.
• you have impaired liver or kidney function.
• you have high blood pressure or a history of heart failure.
• you are taking any of the following: acetaminophen, aspirin or other aspirin substitutes, anticoagulants, oral antidiabetic drugs.

Possible Side-Effects (natural, expected and unavoidable drug actions)
Drowsiness (15%), ringing in ears, fluid retention.

▷ **Possible Adverse Effects** (unusual, unexpected and infrequent reactions)
If any of the following develop, consult your physician promptly for guidance.
Mild Adverse Effects
Allergic Reactions: Skin rash, hives, itching (9%).
Headache (15%), dizziness, altered or blurred vision, depression.
Mouth sores, indigestion, nausea, vomiting, constipation, diarrhea.
Serious Adverse Effects
Allergic Reaction: Anaphylaxis (see Glossary).
Blurred vision, impaired hearing.
Active peptic ulcer, with or without bleeding.
Liver damage with jaundice (questionable).
Kidney damage with painful urination, bloody urine, reduced urine formation.
Rare bone marrow depression (see Glossary)—fatigue, weakness, fever, sore throat, abnormal bleeding or bruising.

▷ **Possible Effects on Sexual Function:**   None reported.

Possible Delayed Adverse Effects: Mild anemia due to "silent" blood loss from the stomach (less than that caused by aspirin).

▷ **Adverse Effects That May Mimic Natural Diseases or Disorders**
Liver reaction may suggest viral hepatitis.

Natural Diseases or Disorders That May Be Activated by This Drug
Peptic ulcer disease, ulcerative colitis.

Possible Effects on Laboratory Tests
Complete blood cell counts: decreased red cells, hemoglobin, white cells and platelets.
Kidney function tests: urine analysis—increased protein and white blood cells (kidney damage, rare).

CAUTION
1. Dosage should always be limited to the smallest amount that produces reasonable improvement.
2. This drug may mask early indications of infection. Inform your physician if you think you are developing an infection of any kind.

Precautions for Use
By Infants and Children: Safety and effectiveness for use by those under 12 years of age have not been established.
By Those over 60 Years of Age: Small doses are advisable until tolerance is determined. Observe for any indications of liver or kidney toxicity, fluid retention, dizziness, confusion, impaired memory, stomach bleeding or constipation.

▷ **Advisability of Use During Pregnancy**
Pregnancy Category: B (tentative). See Pregnancy Code inside back cover.
Animal studies: No birth defects reported.

Human studies: Information from adequate studies of pregnant women is not available.

Avoid this drug during the last 3 months. Use it during the first 6 months only if clearly needed. Ask physician for guidance.

The manufacturer does not recommend the use of this drug during pregnancy.

Advisability of Use if Breast-Feeding
Presence of this drug in breast milk: Yes, in minute amounts.
Avoid drug or refrain from nursing.

Habit-Forming Potential: None.

Effects of Overdosage: Drowsiness, nausea, vomiting, diarrhea.

Possible Effects of Long-Term Use: Cataracts have been reported, but a definite cause-and-effect relationship (see Glossary) has not been established.

Suggested Periodic Examinations While Taking This Drug (at physician's discretion)
Complete blood cell counts, liver and kidney function tests, complete eye examinations if vision is altered in any way.

▷ **While Taking This Drug, Observe the Following**
Foods: No restrictions.
Beverages: No restrictions. May be taken with milk.
▷   *Alcohol:* Use with caution. The irritant action of alcohol on the stomach lining, added to the irritant action of this drug in sensitive individuals, can increase the risk of stomach ulceration and/or bleeding.
Tobacco Smoking: No interactions expected.
▷   *Other Drugs*
Fenoprofen may *increase* the effects of
- acetaminophen (Tylenol, etc.), and increase the risk of kidney damage; avoid prolonged use of this combination.
- anticoagulants (Coumadin, etc.), and increase the risk of bleeding; monitor prothrombin time, adjust dose accordingly.

Fenoprofen *taken concurrently* with the following drugs may increase the risk of bleeding; avoid these combinations:
- aspirin.
- dipyridamole (Persantine).
- indomethacin (Indocin).
- sulfinpyrazone (Anturane).
- valproic acid (Depakene).
▷   *Driving, Hazardous Activities:* This drug may cause drowsiness or dizziness. Restrict activities as necessary.
Aviation Note: The use of this drug *may be a disqualification* for piloting. Consult a designated Aviation Medical Examiner.
Exposure to Sun: No restrictions.

FLUOXETINE
(flu OX e teen)

Introduced: 1978

Prescription: USA: Yes

Available as Generic: USA: No

Brand Name: Prozac

Class: Antidepressant

Controlled Drug: USA: No

BENEFITS versus RISKS

Possible Benefits	*Possible Risks*
EFFECTIVE TREATMENT OF MAJOR DEPRESSIVE DISORDERS in 60% to 75% of cases	Serious allergic reactions (4%)
Possibly effective in relieving the symptoms of obsessive-compulsive disorder	Conversion of depression to mania in manic-depressive disorders (1%)
	Seizures (0.2%)

▷ **Principal Uses**

As a Single Drug Product: Used primarily to treat major forms of depression that have not responded well to other therapies. This drug should be used only when a diagnosis of a true, primary depression of significant degree has been established. It should not be used to treat the symptoms of mild and transient (reactive) depression that may be associated with many life situations in the absence of a bona fide affective illness.

How This Drug Works: It is thought that this drug relieves depression by slowly restoring to normal levels a specific constituent of brain tissue (serotonin) that transmits nerve impulses.

Available Dosage Forms and Strengths
Capsules — 20 mg

▷ **Usual Adult Dosage Range:** Initially 20 mg every 1 to 3 days as a single morning dose; if no improvement after 4 weeks of treatment, the dose may be increased by 20 mg/day as needed and tolerated. Doses over 20 mg/day should be taken in 2 divided doses, early morning and noon. Total daily dosage should not exceed 80 mg. **Note: Actual dosage and administration schedule must be determined by the physician for each patient individually.**

▷ **Dosing Instructions:** May be taken without regard to food. The capsule may be opened for administration and the contents mixed with any convenient food. To facilitate smaller doses, the contents may be mixed with orange juice or apple juice and refrigerated; doses of 5 mg to 10 mg may prove effective and better tolerated.

Usual Duration of Use: Continual use on a regular schedule for 4 to 8 weeks is usually necessary to determine (1) this drug's effectiveness in relieving depression; (2) the pattern of both favorable and unfavorable drug effects. Long-term use (months to years) requires periodic evaluation of response and dosage adjustment. Consult your physician on a regular basis.

Possible Advantages of This Drug

Does not cause weight gain, a common side-effect of tricyclic antidepressants.

Less likely to cause dry mouth, constipation, urinary retention, orthostatic hypotension (see Glossary) and heart rhythm disturbances than tricyclic antidepressants.

Does not cause Parkinson-like reactions.

▷ **This Drug Should Not Be Taken If**

• you have had an allergic reaction to any dosage form of it previously.
• you are currently taking or have taken within the past 14 days any monoamine oxidase (MAO) type A inhibitor drug (see Drug Class, Section Four).

▷ **Inform Your Physician Before Taking This Drug If**

• you have experienced any adverse effects from antidepressant drugs used in the past.
• you have impaired liver or kidney function.
• you have Parkinson's disease.
• you have a seizure disorder.
• you are pregnant or plan pregnancy while taking this drug.

Possible Side-Effects (natural, expected and unavoidable drug actions)
Decreased appetite (8.7%), weight loss (13%).

▷ **Possible Adverse Effects** (unusual, unexpected and infrequent reactions)
If any of the following develop, consult your physician promptly for guidance.
Mild Adverse Effects
Allergic Reactions: Skin rash (2.7%), hives (2%), itching (2.4%).
Headache (20%), nervousness (14%), insomnia (13%), drowsiness (11%), tremor (7%), dizziness (5%), fatigue (4%), impaired concentration (1.5%).
Altered taste (1.8%), nausea (21%), vomiting (2.4%), diarrhea (12%).
Serious Adverse Effects
Allergic Reactions: Serum sickness-like syndrome (2% to 3%): fever, weakness, joint pain and swelling, swollen lymph glands, fluid retention, skin rash and/or hives.
Drug-induced seizures (0.2%).
Worsening of Parkinson's disease.
Intense suicidal preoccupation in those with severe depression that does not respond to this drug. (See Current Controversies at the end of this Profile.)

▷ **Possible Effects on Sexual Function:** Impaired erection (1.9%), inhibited orgasm in men and women.

Natural Diseases or Disorders That May Be Activated by This Drug
Latent epilepsy.

Possible Effects on Laboratory Tests
Blood glucose level: decreased.
Blood sodium level: decreased.

CAUTION
1. If any type of skin reaction develops (rash, hives, etc.), discontinue this drug and inform your physician promptly.
2. If dryness of the mouth develops and persists for more than 2 weeks, consult your dentist for guidance.
3. Consult your physician before taking any other prescription or over-the-counter drug while taking this drug.
4. If you are advised to take any monoamine oxidase (MAO) type A inhibitor drug (see Drug Class, Section Four), allow an interval of 5 weeks after discontinuing this drug before starting the MAO inhibitor.
5. It is advisable to withhold this drug if electroconvulsive therapy (ECT, "shock" treatment) is to be used to treat your depression.

Precautions for Use
By Infants and Children: Safety and effectiveness for use by those under 12 years of age have not been established.
By Those over 60 Years of Age: Total daily dosage should not exceed 60 mg.

▷ **Advisability of Use During Pregnancy**
Pregnancy Category: B (tentative). See Pregnancy Code inside back cover.
Animal studies: No birth defects due to this drug found in rat or rabbit studies.
Human studies: Information from adequate studies of pregnant women is not available.
Use this drug only if clearly needed.

Advisability of Use if Breast-Feeding
Presence of this drug in breast milk: Unknown.
Avoid drug or refrain from nursing.

Habit-Forming Potential: None.

Effects of Overdosage: Agitation, restlessness, excitement, nausea, vomiting, seizures.

Possible Effects of Long-Term Use: None reported.

Suggested Periodic Examinations While Taking This Drug (at physician's discretion)
None.

▷ **While Taking This Drug, Observe the Following**
Foods: No restrictions.
Beverages: No restrictions. May be taken with milk.
▷ *Alcohol:* Avoid completely.
Tobacco Smoking: No interactions expected.
▷ *Other Drugs*
Fluoxetine may ***increase*** the effects of
• diazepam (Valium).
• digitalis preparations (digitoxin, digoxin).
• warfarin (Coumadin) and related oral anticoagulants.
Fluoxetine ***taken concurrently*** with
• antidiabetic drugs (insulin, oral hypoglycemics) may increase the risk of hypoglycemic reactions; monitor blood and urine sugar levels carefully.
• monoamine oxidase (MAO) type A inhibitor drugs may cause confusion, agitation, high fever, seizures and dangerous elevations of blood pressure. Avoid the concurrent use of these drugs.
▷ *Driving, Hazardous Activities:* This drug may cause drowsiness, dizziness, impaired judgment and delayed reaction time. Restrict activities as necessary.
Aviation Note: The use of this drug ***is a disqualification*** for piloting. Consult a designated Aviation Medical Examiner.
Exposure to Sun: No restrictions.
Discontinuation: The slow elimination of this drug from the body makes it unlikely that any withdrawal effects will result from abrupt discontinuation. However, consult your physician if you plan to discontinue this drug for any reason.

Current Controversies in Drug Management

In 1990 it was reported that six patients being treated with fluoxetine experienced the onset of intense suicidal preoccupation. All six had severe depression that had not responded to the use of fluoxetine for 2 to 7 weeks. For most of them, suicidal mentality persisted for 2 to 3 months after discontinuation of the drug. The resultant adverse publicity suggested that this experience may be somewhat characteristic of fluoxetine in contrast to other antidepressant drugs. A review of relevant literature on this subject reveals that the development or intensification of suicidal thoughts during treatment (regardless of the severity of depression) has been documented repeatedly for many antidepressant drugs in wide use. It is apparent that suicidal thinking may emerge during treatment with any antidepressant. Recent reports establish that some patients who become suicidal while taking one antidepressant can be switched to fluoxetine and experience cessation of suicidal thinking and satisfactory relief of depression.

This experience is yet another example of the marked variability of individual response to drug therapy. The choice of a drug to treat many serious disorders remains an experiment of trial and error. Successful management requires clinical judgment (based on experience), close monitoring and appropriate dosage adjustments.

FLUPHENAZINE
(flu FEN a zeen)

Introduced: 1959

Class: Strong tranquilizer, phenothiazines

Prescription: USA: Yes
Canada: Yes

Controlled Drug: USA: No
Canada: No

Available as Generic: USA: No
Canada: Yes

Brand Names: ✦Apo-Fluphenazine, ✦Modecate, ✦Moditen, Permitil, Prolixin

---

BENEFITS versus RISKS

Possible Benefits	*Possible Risks*
EFFECTIVE CONTROL OF ACUTE MENTAL DISORDERS in the majority of patients	SERIOUS TOXIC EFFECTS ON BRAIN with long-term use
Beneficial effects on thinking, mood and behavior	Liver damage with jaundice (less than 0.5%)
	Rare blood cell disorders: abnormally low white blood cell counts

---

▷ **Principal Uses**

As a Single Drug Product: This antipsychotic drug is used primarily to treat
acute and chronic psychotic disorders such as schizophrenia, mania
and similar states of mental dysfunction.

How This Drug Works: Not completely established. Present theory is that
by inhibiting the action of dopamine, this drug acts to correct an imbalance of nerve impulse transmissions that is thought to be responsible
for certain mental disorders.

Available Dosage Forms and Strengths
Concentrate — 5 mg per ml (1% alcohol)
Elixir — 2.5 mg per 5-ml teaspoonful (14% alcohol)
Injection — 2.5 mg per ml
Tablets — 1 mg, 2.5 mg, 5 mg, 10 mg

▷ **Usual Adult Dosage Range:**   0.5 to 2.5 mg 1 to 4 times/day; adjust dosage
as needed and tolerated. Total daily dosage should not exceed 20 mg.
**Note: Actual dosage and administration schedule must be deter-
mined by the physician for each patient individually.**

▷ **Dosing Instructions:**   May be taken with or following meals to reduce stomach irritation. Regular tablets may be crushed for administration. Prolonged-action tablets should be swallowed whole (not crushed). The

concentrate must be diluted in 4 to 6 ounces of water, milk, fruit juice or carbonated beverage.

Usual Duration of Use: Continual use on a regular schedule for several weeks is usually necessary to determine this drug's effectiveness in controlling psychotic disorders. If not significantly beneficial within 6 weeks, it should be discontinued. Long-term use (months to years) requires periodic evaluation of response, appropriate dosage adjustment and consideration of continued need. Consult your physician on a regular basis.

▷ **This Drug Should Not Be Taken If**
  • you are allergic to any of the drugs bearing the brand names listed above.
  • you have a history of brain damage.
  • you have active liver disease.
  • you have cancer of the breast.
  • you have a current blood cell or bone marrow disorder.

▷ **Inform Your Physician Before Taking This Drug If**
  • you are allergic or abnormally sensitive to any phenothiazine drug (see Drug Class, Section Four).
  • you have impaired liver or kidney function.
  • you have any type of seizure disorder.
  • you have diabetes, glaucoma, heart disease or chronic lung disease.
  • you have a history of lupus erythematosus.
  • you are taking any drug with sedative effects.
  • you plan to have surgery under general or spinal anesthesia in the near future.

Possible Side-Effects (natural, expected and unavoidable drug actions)
  Drowsiness (usually during the first 2 weeks), orthostatic hypotension (see Glossary), blurred vision, dry mouth, nasal congestion, constipation, impaired urination (all mild).

▷ **Possible Adverse Effects** (unusual, unexpected and infrequent reactions)
  If any of the following develop, consult your physician promptly for guidance.
  Mild Adverse Effects
  Allergic Reactions: Skin rash, hives, itching.
  Lowering of body temperature, especially in the elderly.
  Headache, dizziness, weakness, excitement, restlessness, unusual dreaming.
  Increased appetite and weight gain.
  Serious Adverse Effects
  Allergic Reactions: Hepatitis with jaundice (see Glossary), usually between second and fourth week; anaphylactic reaction (see Glossary).
  Idiosyncratic Reaction: Neuroleptic malignant syndrome (see Glossary).
  Impaired production of white blood cells—fever, sore throat, infections.

Parkinson-like disorders (see Glossary); muscle spasms of face, jaw, neck, back, extremities.

Prolonged drop in blood pressure with weakness, perspiration and fainting.

▷ **Possible Effects on Sexual Function**
Decreased male libido; increased female libido.
Impaired erection (38% to 42%); complete impotence.
Inhibited male orgasm (58%); inhibited female orgasm (22% to 33%).
Inhibited ejaculation (46%).
Altered timing and pattern of menstruation (91%).
Female breast enlargement and milk production.
Male breast enlargement and tenderness.

▷ **Adverse Effects That May Mimic Natural Diseases or Disorders**
Nervous system reactions may suggest Parkinson's disease.
Liver reactions may suggest viral hepatitis.
Reactions resembling systemic lupus erythematosus may occur.

Natural Diseases or Disorders That May Be Activated by This Drug
Latent epilepsy, glaucoma, prostatism (see Glossary).

Possible Effects on Laboratory Tests
Complete blood cell counts: decreased red cells, hemoglobin, white cells and platelets; increased eosinophils (allergic reaction).
Liver function tests: increased liver enzymes (ALT/GPT, AST/GOT and alkaline phosphatase, increased bilirubin.
Urine pregnancy tests: false positive results.
Urine screening test for drug abuse: initial test may be falsely **positive** for barbiturates; the confirmatory test will be **negative**.

CAUTION
1. Many over-the-counter medications (see OTC Drugs in Glossary) for allergies, colds and coughs contain drugs that can interact unfavorably with this drug. Ask your physician or pharmacist for guidance before using any such medications.
2. Antacids that contain aluminum and/or magnesium can prevent the absorption of this drug and reduce its effectiveness.
3. Obtain prompt evaluation of any change or disturbance of vision.

Precautions for Use
By Infants and Children: Do not use this drug in infants under 6 months of age, or in children of any age with symptoms suggestive of Reye syndrome (see Glossary). Monitor carefully for blood cell changes.
By Those over 60 Years of Age: Small doses are advisable until individual response has been determined. You may be more susceptible to the development of drowsiness, lethargy, constipation, lowering of body temperature (hypothermia) and orthostatic hypotension (see Glossary). This drug can enhance existing prostatism (see Glossary). You may also be more susceptible to the development of parkinson-like

reactions and/or tardive dyskinesia (see discussion of these terms in Glossary). These reactions must be recognized early since they may become unresponsive to treatment and irreversible.

▷ **Advisability of Use During Pregnancy**
Pregnancy Category: C (tentative). See Pregnancy Code inside back cover.
Animal studies: Significant birth defects reported in mice.
Human studies: Information from adequate studies of pregnant women is not available.
Avoid drug during the first 3 months and during the last month because of possible effects on the newborn infant.

Advisability of Use if Breast-Feeding
Presence of this drug in breast milk: Unknown.
Avoid drug or refrain from nursing.

Habit-Forming Potential: None.

Effects of Overdosage: Marked drowsiness, weakness, tremor, agitation, unsteadiness, deep sleep, coma, convulsions.

Possible Effects of Long-Term Use: Tardive dyskinesia (see Glossary); eye changes—cataracts and pigmentation of retina; gray to violet pigmentation of skin in exposed areas, more common in women.

Suggested Periodic Examinations While Taking This Drug (at physician's discretion)
Complete blood cell counts, especially between the fourth and tenth weeks of treatment.
Liver function tests, electrocardiograms.
Complete eye examinations—eye structures and vision.
Careful inspection of the tongue for early evidence of fine, involuntary, wavelike movements that could indicate the beginning of tardive dyskinesia.

▷ **While Taking This Drug, Observe the Following**
Foods: No restrictions.
Beverages: No restrictions. May be taken with milk.
▷ *Alcohol:* Avoid completely. Alcohol can increase the sedative action of phenothiazines and accentuate their depressant effects on brain function and blood pressure. Phenothiazines can increase the intoxicating effects of alcohol.
Tobacco Smoking: Possible reduction of drowsiness from drug.
Marijuana Smoking: Moderate increase in drowsiness; accentuation of orthostatic hypotension; increased risk of precipitating latent psychoses, confusing the interpretation of mental status and drug responses.
▷ *Other Drugs*
Fluphenazine may *increase* the effects of

- all sedative drugs, and cause excessive sedation.
- all atropinelike drugs, and cause nervous system toxicity.

Fluphenazine may *decrease* the effects of

- guanethidine (Ismelin, Esimil), and reduce its effectiveness in lowering blood pressure.

Fluphenazine *taken concurrently* with

- beta blocker drugs (see Drug Class, Section Four) may cause increased effects of both drugs; monitor drug effects closely and adjust dosages as necessary.

The following drugs may *decrease* the effects of fluphenazine

- antacids containing aluminum and/or magnesium.
- benztropine (Cogentin).
- trihexyphenidyl (Artane).

▷ *Driving, Hazardous Activities:* This drug can impair mental alertness, judgment and physical coordination. Avoid hazardous activities.

Aviation Note: The use of this drug *is a disqualification* for piloting. Consult a designated Aviation Medical Examiner.

Exposure to Sun: Use caution until sensitivity has been determined. Some phenothiazines can cause photosensitivity (see Glossary).

Exposure to Heat: Use caution and avoid excessive heat as much as possible. This drug may impair the regulation of body temperature and increase the risk of heat stroke.

Exposure to Cold: Use caution and dress warmly. This drug can increase the risk of hypothermia in the elderly.

Discontinuation: After a period of long-term use, do not discontinue this drug suddenly. Gradual withdrawal over 2 to 3 weeks under physician supervision is recommended. Do not discontinue this drug without your physician's knowledge and approval. The relapse rate of schizophrenia after discontinuation is 50% to 60%.

FLURAZEPAM
(floor AZ e pam)

Introduced: 1970

Class: Hypnotic, benzodiazepines

Prescription: USA: Yes
Canada: Yes

Controlled Drug: USA: C-IV*
Canada: No

Available as Generic: USA: Yes
Canada: No

Brand Names: ✦Apo-Flurazepam, Dalmane, Durapam, ✦Novoflupam, ✦Somnol, ✦Som-Pam

*See Schedules of Controlled Drugs inside back cover.

BENEFITS versus RISKS

Possible Benefits	*Possible Risks*
EFFECTIVE HYPNOTIC after 2 weeks of continual use	Habit-forming potential with long-term use
NO SUPPRESSION OF REM (RAPID EYE MOVEMENT) SLEEP	Minor impairment of mental functions ("hangover" effect)
	Very rare jaundice
NO REM SLEEP REBOUND after discontinuation	Very rare blood cell disorder
Wide margin of safety with therapeutic doses	Suppression of stage-4 sleep with reduced "quality" of sleep

---

▷ **Principal Uses**

As a Single Drug Product: This member of the benzodiazepine class of "minor tranquilizers" is used exclusively as a bedtime sedative to induce sleep.

How This Drug Works: It is thought that this drug produces calming effect by enhancing the action of the nerve transmitter gamma-aminobutyric acid (GABA), which in turn blocks the arousal of higher brain centers and helps to induce sleep.

Available Dosage Forms and Strengths

Capsules — 15 mg, 30 mg

▷ **Usual Adult Dosage Range:**   15 to 30 mg at bedtime. Total daily dosage should not exceed 90 mg. **Note: Actual dosage and administration schedule must be determined by the physician for each patient individually.**

▷ **Dosing Instructions:**   May be taken on an empty stomach or with food or milk. The capsule may be opened for administration. Do not discontinue this drug abruptly if taken for more than 4 weeks.

Usual Duration of Use: Periods of 3 to 5 nights intermittently, repeated as needed with appropriate dosage adjustment. Avoid uninterrupted and prolonged use. The duration of use should not exceed 2 weeks without reappraisal of continued need.

▷ **This Drug Should Not Be Taken If**
   • you have had an allergic reaction to it previously.
   • you are pregnant.
   • you have acute narrow-angle glaucoma.

▷ **Inform Your Physician Before Taking This Drug If**
   • you are allergic to any benzodiazepine drug (see Drug Class, Section Four).
   • you have a history of alcoholism or drug abuse.
   • you are planning pregnancy.

- you have impaired liver or kidney function.
- you have a history of serious depression or mental disorder.
- you are taking other drugs with sedative effects.
- you have any of the following: asthma, emphysema, epilepsy, myasthenia gravis.

Possible Side-Effects (natural, expected and unavoidable drug actions)
"Hangover" effects on arising: drowsiness, lethargy and unsteadiness.

▷ **Possible Adverse Effects** (unusual, unexpected and infrequent reactions)
   If any of the following develop, consult your physician promptly for guidance.
   Mild Adverse Effects
   Allergic Reactions: Skin rash, hives, burning eyes, swelling of tongue.
   Dizziness, fainting, blurred vision, double vision, slurred speech, nausea, indigestion.
   Serious Adverse Effects
   Allergic Reactions: Liver damage with jaundice (see Glossary).
   Idiosyncratic Reactions: Nervousness, talkativeness, irritability, apprehension, euphoria, excitement, hallucinations.
   Bone marrow depression—impaired production of white blood cells, fever, sore throat.

▷ **Possible Effects on Sexual Function:**   None reported.

▷ **Adverse Effects That May Mimic Natural Diseases or Disorders**
   Liver reaction with jaundice may suggest viral hepatitis.

Possible Effects on Laboratory Tests
   Liver function tests: increased liver enzymes (ALT/GPT, AST/GOT and alkaline phosphatase, increased bilirubin.
   Urine sugar tests: no drug effect with TesTape; false low results with Clinistix and Diastix; false positive result with Benedict's solution.
   Urine screening tests for drug abuse: may be **positive**. (Test results depend upon amount of drug taken and testing method used.)

CAUTION
   1. This drug should not be discontinued abruptly if it has been taken continually for more than 4 weeks.
   2. The concurrent use of some over-the-counter drug products that contain antihistamines (allergy and cold preparations, sleep aids) can cause excessive sedation in sensitive individuals.
   3. Regular nightly use of any hypnotic drug should be avoided.
   4. This drug is transformed by the liver into long-acting forms that can persist in the body for 24 hours or more. With continual use of this drug daily, these active drug forms accumulate and produce increasing sedation. If you experience a "hangover" effect, avoid hazardous activities (driving, etc.) and the use of alcohol.

Precautions for Use

By Infants and Children: Safety and effectiveness for use by those under 15 years of age have not been established.

By Those over 60 Years of Age: It is advisable to use smaller doses at longer intervals to avoid overdosage. Observe for the possible development of lethargy, indifference, fatigue, weakness, unsteadiness, disturbing dreams, nightmares and paradoxical reactions of excitement, agitation, anger, hostility and rage.

Because this is a long-acting benzodiazepine, it may cause residual sluggishness and unsteadiness with increased risk of falling during the day following bedtime use. This drug may also increase the number of periods of sleep apnea in this age group.

▷ **Advisability of Use During Pregnancy**

Pregnancy Category: X (tentative). See Pregnancy Code inside back cover.

Animal studies: No birth defects reported in rat and rabbit studies.

Human studies: Information from adequate studies of pregnant women is not available.

Several studies indicate an increased risk of birth defects if drugs of this class (benzodiazepines) are used during the first 3 months.

Frequent use in late pregnancy can cause the "floppy infant" syndrome in the newborn: weakness, lethargy, unresponsiveness, depressed breathing, low body temperature.

Avoid use during entire pregnancy.

Advisability of Use if Breast-Feeding

Presence of this drug in breast milk: Probably yes.

Avoid drug or refrain from nursing.

Habit-Forming Potential: This drug can produce psychological and/or physical dependence (see Glossary) if used in large doses for an extended period of time. Avoid continual use.

Effects of Overdosage: Marked drowsiness, weakness, feeling of drunkenness, staggering gait, tremor, stupor progressing to deep sleep or coma.

Possible Effects of Long-Term Use: Psychological and/or physical dependence, impaired liver function.

Suggested Periodic Examinations While Taking This Drug (at physician's discretion)

Complete blood cell counts and liver function tests during long-term use.

▷ **While Taking This Drug, Observe the Following**

Foods: No restrictions.

Beverages: Avoid excessive intake of caffeine-containing beverages (coffee, tea, cola) within 4 hours of taking this drug. May be taken with milk.

▷ *Alcohol:* Use with extreme caution until the combined effect is determined. Alcohol may increase the absorption of this drug and add to its depressant effects on the brain. It is advisable to avoid alcohol completely—throughout the day and night—if it is necessary to drive or to engage in any hazardous activity.

Tobacco Smoking: Heavy smoking may reduce the hypnotic action of this drug.

Marijuana Smoking: Increased sedation and significant impairment of intellectual and physical performance.

▷ *Other Drugs*

Flurazepam may *increase* the effects of
- digoxin (Lanoxin), and cause digoxin toxicity.
- phenytoin (Dilantin), and cause phenytoin toxicity.

Flurazepam may *decrease* the effects of
- levodopa (Sinemet, etc.), and reduce its effectiveness in treating Parkinson's disease.

The following drugs may *increase* the effects of flurazepam
- cimetidine (Tagamet).
- disulfiram (Antabuse).
- isoniazid (INH, Rifamate, etc.).
- oral contraceptives.
- valproic acid (Depakene).

The following drugs may *decrease* the effects of flurazepam
- rifampin (Rimactane, etc.).
- theophylline (aminophylline, Theo-Dur, etc.).

▷ *Driving, Hazardous Activities:* This drug can impair mental alertness, judgment, physical coordination and reaction time. Avoid hazardous activities accordingly.

Aviation Note: The use of this drug *is a disqualification* for piloting. Consult a designated Aviation Medical Examiner.

Exposure to Sun: No restrictions.

Exposure to Heat: Use caution until the effect of excessive perspiration is determined. Because of reduced urine volume, this drug may accumulate in the body and produce effects of overdosage.

Discontinuation: Avoid sudden discontinuation if this drug has been taken for over 4 weeks without interruption. Dosage should be tapered gradually to prevent a withdrawal syndrome that could include depression, confusion, hallucinations, tremor, seizures, muscle cramping, sweating and vomiting.

FLURBIPROFEN
(floor BI pro fen)

Introduced: 1977

Class: Mild analgesic, anti-inflammatory

Prescription: USA: Yes
Canada: Yes

Controlled Drug: USA: No
Canada: No

Available as Generic: USA: No
Canada: No

Brand Names: Ansaid, ✦Froben

```
┌─────────────────────────────────────────────────────────────┐
│                    BENEFITS versus RISKS                      │
│      Possible Benefits              Possible Risks            │
│  EFFECTIVE RELIEF OF          PEPTIC ULCER DISEASE (1% to     │
│   SYMPTOMS ASSOCIATED          4%) with associated bleeding   │
│   WITH MAJOR TYPES OF          and perforation                │
│   ARTHRITIS                   Liver toxicity with jaundice (less│
│  Effective relief of symptoms  than 1%)                       │
│   associated with bursitis,   Water retention                 │
│   tendinitis and related conditions  Rare kidney toxicity     │
│  Effective relief of menstrual  Rare aplastic anemia (see     │
│   cramps                        Glossary)                     │
└─────────────────────────────────────────────────────────────┘
```

▷ **Principal Uses**

As a Single Drug Product: Used primarily to relieve the symptoms associated with (1) rheumatoid arthritis, osteoarthritis and ankylosing spondylitis; (2) bursitis, tendinitis, capsulitis and tenosynovitis; (3) painful menstruation.

How This Drug Works: Not completely established. It is thought that this drug reduces the tissue concentrations of prostaglandins (and related compounds), chemicals involved in the production of inflammation and pain.

Available Dosage Forms and Strengths

Tablets — 50 mg (Canada), 100 mg

▷ **Usual Adult Dosage Range:** Initially 100 to 200 mg/24 hours, in 2 to 4 divided doses. After a satisfactory response has been achieved, dosage should be reduced to the minimum that will sustain adequate relief. Total daily dosage should not exceed 300 mg. **Note: Actual dosage and administration schedule must be determined by the physician for each patient individually.**

▷ **Dosing Instructions:** Take either on an empty stomach or with food or milk if necessary to prevent stomach irritation. Take with a full glass of water and remain upright (do not lie down) for 15 to 30 minutes to prevent lodging of the tablet in the esophagus (food tube). The tablet may be crushed for administration.

Usual Duration of Use: Continual use on a regular schedule for 1 to 2 weeks is usually necessary to determine this drug's effectiveness in relieving the symptoms of arthritis, bursitis, etc. Severe arthritis may require continual use for 3 to 4 weeks to obtain maximal relief. Long-term use (months to years) requires periodic evaluation of response and dosage adjustment. Consult your physician on a regular basis.

▷ **This Drug Should Not Be Taken If**
- you have had an allergic reaction to it previously.
- you are subject to asthma or nasal polyps caused by aspirin.

- you have active peptic ulcer disease or any form of gastrointestinal bleeding.
- you have active liver disease.
- you have a bleeding disorder or a blood cell disorder.
- you have severe impairment of kidney function.

▷ **Inform Your Physician Before Taking This Drug If**
- you are allergic to aspirin or to other aspirin substitutes.
- you have a history of peptic ulcer disease or any type of bleeding disorder.
- you have a history of gout.
- you have impaired liver or kidney function.
- you have high blood pressure or a history of heart failure.
- you have systemic lupus erythematosus (SLE).
- you are taking any of the following drugs: acetaminophen, aspirin or other aspirin substitutes, anticoagulants, diuretics, insulin, lithium, methotrexate, oral antidiabetic drugs.

Possible Side-Effects (natural, expected and unavoidable drug actions)
Fluid retention (1%), increased blood uric acid levels.

▷ **Possible Adverse Effects** (unusual, unexpected and infrequent reactions)
If any of the following develop, consult your physician promptly for guidance.
Mild Adverse Effects
Allergic Reactions: Skin rash (1.4%), hives (0.1%), itching (0.6%).
Headache (1%), dizziness (1%), drowsiness, depression (0.1%), anxiety (0.1%), insomnia (0.3%), blurred vision (1.6%), double vision, reversible hearing loss, ear ringing (1.7%), altered taste (0.2%).
Mouth soreness (0.4%), stomach discomfort (4%), nausea (3.5%), vomiting (0.5%), indigestion (6.9%), constipation (2%), diarrhea (3.8%).
Serious Adverse Effects
Allergic Reactions: Severe skin reactions, eczema, bruising (0.1%), erythema multiforme, Stevens-Johnson syndrome, hair loss; swelling of lips, tongue, vocal cords; anaphylactoid reaction (see Glossary).
Drug-induced gastrointestinal ulceration, with bleeding and perforation (1% after 3 to 6 months of use, up to 4% after 1 year); colitis with bloody diarrhea.
Abnormally low red blood cell (0.3%), white blood cell and blood platelet counts; rare aplastic anemia (see Glossary).
Liver damage with jaundice (0.2%).
Kidney damage with significantly impaired function.

▷ **Possible Effects on Sexual Function:**   None reported to date.

Possible Delayed Adverse Effects: Mild anemia due to "silent" blood loss from the stomach (less than that caused by aspirin).

▷ **Adverse Effects That May Mimic Natural Diseases or Disorders**
Liver reactions may suggest viral hepatitis.

▷ **Natural Diseases or Disorders That May Be Activated by This Drug**
Peptic ulcer disease, Crohn's disease, ulcerative colitis, gout, kidney failure associated with systemic lupus erythematosus.

Possible Effects on Laboratory Tests
Complete blood cell counts: decreased red cells, hemoglobin, white cells and platelets.
Liver function tests: increased liver enzymes (ALT/GPT, AST/GOT and alkaline phosphatase, increased bilirubin.
Kidney function tests: increased blood creatinine and urea nitrogen (BUN) levels.

CAUTION
1. Dosage should always be limited to the smallest amount that produces reasonable improvement.
2. This drug may mask early indications of infection. In- form your physician if you think you are developing an infection of any kind.
3. Observe for a pattern of symptoms that may indicate the development of liver toxicity: fatigue, lethargy, "flu-like" symptoms, nausea, itching, tenderness under the right rib cage, jaundice (see Glossary). Report such symptoms promptly.
4. Observe for possible drug-induced bleeding in the gastrointestinal tract: bloody (reddish) or tarry (black) stools.

Precautions for Use
By Infants and Children: Safety and effectiveness for use by those under 12 years of age have not been established.
By Those over 60 Years of Age: Small doses are advisable initially until tolerance is determined. Observe for any indications of liver or kidney toxicity, fluid retention, dizziness, confusion, impaired memory, stomach bleeding or constipation.

▷ **Advisability of Use During Pregnancy**
Pregnancy Category: B (tentative). See Pregnancy Code inside back cover.
Animal studies: Mouse, rat and rabbit studies reveal no birth defects due to this drug.
Human studies: Information from adequate studies of pregnant women is not available.
The manufacturer does not recommend the use of this drug during pregnancy.

Advisability of Use if Breast-Feeding
Presence of this drug in breast milk: Unknown.
Avoid drug or refrain from nursing.

Habit-Forming Potential: None.

Effects of Overdosage: Probable drowsiness, dizziness, ear ringing, nausea, vomiting, diarrhea, confusion, unsteadiness, stupor.

Possible Effects of Long-Term Use: Secondary anemia (chronic blood loss from stomach), fluid retention, elevated blood pressure.

Suggested Periodic Examinations While Taking This Drug (at physician's discretion)
Complete blood cell counts; liver function tests within the first 8 weeks of use and periodically thereafter; kidney function tests.
Complete eye examinations if vision is altered in any way.

▷ **While Taking This Drug, Observe the Following**
Foods: No restrictions.
Nutritional Support: Supplemental iron if anemia develops.
Beverages: No restrictions. May be taken with milk.
▷ *Alcohol:* Use sparingly and with caution. The irritant action of alcohol on the stomach lining, added to the irritant action of this drug in sensitive individuals, can increase the risk of stomach ulceration and/or bleeding.
Tobacco Smoking: No interactions expected.
▷ *Other Drugs*
Flurbiprofen may *increase* the effects of
- acetaminophen (Tylenol, etc.), and increase the risk of liver or kidney damage; avoid prolonged use of this combination.
- anticoagulants (Coumadin, etc.), and increase the risk of bleeding; monitor prothrombin and bleeding times, adjust dose accordingly.
- oral antidiabetic drugs, and alter control of blood sugar levels unpredictably.
- aspirin, and increase the risk of stomach ulceration and/or bleeding; avoid this combination.

Flurbiprofen may *decrease* the effects of
- amiloride (Midamor, Moduretic).
- bumetanide (Bumex).
- chlorthalidone (Hygroton, etc.).
- ethacrynic acid (Edecrin).
- furosemide (Lasix).
- indapamide (Lozol).
- metolazone (Diulo, Zaroxolyn).
- spironolactone (Aldactone, Aldactazide).
- thiazide diuretics (see Drug Class, Section Four).
- triamterene (Dyazide, Maxzide).

Flurbiprofen *taken concurrently* with the following drugs may increase the risk of bleeding (antiplatelet effect); monitor these combinations closely:
- aspirin.
- colchicine (ColBenemid, etc.).
- dipyridamole (Persantine).
- indomethacin (Indocin).
- sulfinpyrazone (Anturane).
- valproic acid (Depakene).

Flurbiprofen ***taken concurrently*** with the following drugs may increase their toxicity; monitor these combinations closely:
- lithium (Lithane, etc.).
- methotrexate (Folex, Mexate).

The following drug may ***increase*** the effects of flurbiprofen
- probenecid (Benemid), by slowing its elimination.

▷ *Driving, Hazardous Activities:* This drug may cause dizziness, drowsiness or blurred vision.

Restrict activities as necessary.

Aviation Note: The use of this drug ***may be a disqualification*** for piloting. Consult a designated Aviation Medical Examiner.

Exposure to Sun: Use caution until sensitivity is determined. Photosensitivity (see Glossary) has been reported.

FUROSEMIDE
(fur OH se mide)

Introduced: 1964

Class: Antihypertensive, diuretic

Prescription: USA: Yes
Canada: Yes

Controlled Drug: USA: No
Canada: No

Available as Generic: USA: Yes
Canada: Yes

Brand Names: ✦Apo-Furosemide, ✦Furoside, Lasix, ✦Novosemide, ✦Uritol

Warning: The brand names Lasix and Losec are similar and can be mistaken for each other; this can lead to serious medication errors. These names represent very different drugs. Lasix (round white tablets, 3 sizes) is the generic drug furosemide; it is a diuretic. Losec (a purple capsule) is the generic drug omeprazole; it is used to treat several conditions associated with excessive stomach acid production. Verify that you are taking the correct drug.

BENEFITS versus RISKS

Possible Benefits	*Possible Risks*
PROMPT, EFFECTIVE, RELIABLE DIURETIC	WATER AND ELECTROLYTE DEPLETION with excessive use
MODEST ANTIHYPERTENSIVE IN MILD TO MODERATE HYPERTENSION	Excessive potassium loss
	Increased blood sugar level
	Increased blood uric acid level
ENHANCES EFFECTIVENESS OF OTHER ANTIHYPERTENSIVES	Decreased blood calcium level
	Rare liver damage
	Rare blood cell disorder

▷ **Principal Uses**

As a Single Drug Product: This powerful diuretic is used primarily to increase the volume of urine and thereby relieve the body of excessive water retention (edema) that is commonly associated with congestive heart failure and some forms of liver disease and kidney disease. It is also used in the treatment of high blood pressure, but usually in conjunction with other antihypertensive drugs. A less frequent use is to increase the amount of calcium excreted the urine when the blood level of calcium is abnormally high.

How This Drug Works: By increasing the elimination of salt and water from the body (through increased urine production), this drug reduces the volume of fluid in the blood and body tissues and lowers the sodium content throughout the body. These changes contribute to lowering blood pressure.

Available Dosage Forms and Strengths
   Injection — 10 mg per ml
   Solution — 10 mg per ml, 40 mg per 5-ml teaspoonful
   Tablets — 20 mg, 40 mg, 80 mg

▷ **Usual Adult Dosage Range:** As antihypertensive: 40 mg/12 hours initially; increase dose as needed and tolerated. As diuretic: 20 to 80 mg in a single dose initially; if necessary, increase the dose by 20 to 40 mg/6 to 8 hours. The smallest effective dose should be determined. The total daily dose should not exceed 600 mg. **Note: Actual dosage and administration schedule must be determined by the physician for each patient individually.**

▷ **Dosing Instructions:** May be taken with or following meals to reduce stomach irritation. Best taken in the morning to avoid nighttime urination. The tablet may be crushed for administration.

Usual Duration of Use: Continual use on a regular schedule for 2 to 3 weeks is usually necessary to determine this drug's effectiveness in lowering high blood pressure. Long-term use (months to years) requires periodic evaluation of response and possible dosage adjustment. Use as a diuretic should be intermittent with "drug holidays" (no drug taken) to reduce the risk of sodium and potassium imbalance. Consult your physician on a regular basis.

▷ **This Drug Should Not Be Taken If**
   • you have had an allergic reaction to any dosage form of it previously.

▷ **Inform Your Physician Before Taking This Drug If**
   • you are allergic to any form of "sulfa" drug.
   • you are pregnant or planning pregnancy.
   • you have a history of kidney or liver disease.
   • you have diabetes, gout or lupus erythematosus.

- you are taking any form of cortisone, digitalis, oral antidiabetic drug or insulin.
- you plan to have surgery under general anesthesia in the near future.

Possible Side-Effects (natural, expected and unavoidable drug actions)
Light-headedness on arising from sitting or lying position (see Orthostatic Hypotension in Glossary).
Increase in blood sugar level, affecting control of diabetes.
Increase in blood uric acid level, affecting control of gout.
Decrease in blood potassium level, causing muscle weakness and cramping.

▷ **Possible Adverse Effects** (unusual, unexpected and infrequent reactions)
If any of the following develop, consult your physician promptly for guidance.
Mild Adverse Effects
Allergic Reactions: Skin rashes, hives, drug fever.
Headache, dizziness, blurred or yellow vision, ringing in ears, numbness and tingling.
Reduced appetite, indigestion, nausea, vomiting, diarrhea.
Serious Adverse Effects
Allergic Reactions: Hepatitis with jaundice (see Glossary), anaphylactic reaction (see Glossary), severe skin reactions.
Idiosyncratic Reaction: Fluid accumulation in lungs.
Temporary hearing loss.
Inflammation of the pancreas—severe abdominal pain.
Bone marrow depression (see Glossary)—fatigue, weakness, fever, sore throat, abnormal bleeding or bruising.

▷ **Possible Effects on Sexual Function:** Impotence (5%) using recommended dosage of 20 to 80 mg/day.

▷ **Adverse Effects That May Mimic Natural Diseases or Disorders**
Liver reaction may suggest viral hepatitis.

Natural Diseases or Disorders That May Be Activated by This Drug
Diabetes, gout, systemic lupus erythematosus.

Possible Effects on Laboratory Tests
Complete blood cell counts: reduced red cells, hemoglobin, white cells and platelets.
Blood amylase and lipase levels: increased (possible pancreatitis).
Blood sodium and chloride levels: decreased.
Blood levels of total cholesterol, LDL and VLDL cholesterol, and triglycerides: increased.
Blood glucose level: increased.
Glucose tolerance test (GTT): decreased.
Blood potassium level: decreased.
Blood thyroid hormone (T^3 and T^4) levels: decreased.
Blood uric acid level: increased.

Blood urea nitrogen (BUN): increased.

Urine sugar tests: no drug effect with TesTape; false low results with Clinistix and Diastix.

CAUTION

1. Do not exceed recommended doses. Increased dosage can cause excessive loss of sodium and potassium, with resultant loss of appetite, nausea, fatigue, weakness, confusion and tingling in the extremities.
2. If you are also taking a digitalis preparation (digitoxin, digoxin), ensure an adequate intake of high-potassium foods to prevent potassium deficiency—a potential cause of digitalis toxicity. (See Table of High Potassium Foods in Section Six.)

Precautions for Use

By Infants and Children: Avoid overdosage that could cause serious dehydration. Significant potassium loss can occur within the first 2 weeks of drug use.

By Those over 60 Years of Age: Small doses are advisable until your individual response has been determined. You may be more susceptible to the development of impaired thinking, orthostatic hypotension, potassium loss and blood sugar increase. Overdosage and extended use of this drug can cause excessive loss of body water, thickening (increased viscosity) of the blood and an increased tendency for the blood to clot—predisposing to stroke, heart attack or thrombophlebitis (vein inflammation with blood clot).

▷ **Advisability of Use During Pregnancy**

Pregnancy Category: C (tentative). See Pregnancy Code inside back cover.

Animal studies: Significant birth defects have been reported.

Human studies: Information from adequate studies of pregnant women is not available.

It should not be used during pregnancy unless a very serious complication occurs for which this drug is significantly beneficial. Avoid completely during the first 3 months. Ask physician for guidance.

Advisability of Use if Breast-Feeding

Presence of this drug in breast milk: Yes.

Avoid drug or refrain from nursing.

Habit-Forming Potential: None.

Effects of Overdosage: Dry mouth, thirst, lethargy, weakness, muscle cramping, nausea, vomiting, drowsiness progressing to stupor or coma.

Possible Effects of Long-Term Use: Impaired balance of water, salt and potassium in blood and body tissues; dehydration and increased blood coagulability, with predisposition to thromboembolic disorders. Development of diabetes in predisposed individuals.

Suggested Periodic Examinations While Taking This Drug (at physician's discretion)

> Complete blood cell counts, measurements of blood levels of sodium, potassium, chloride, sugar and uric acid.
>
> Kidney and liver function tests.

▷ **While Taking This Drug, Observe the Following**

Foods: Consult your physician regarding the advisability of eating foods rich in potassium. If so advised, see the Table of High Potassium Foods in Section Six. Follow physician's advice regarding the use of salt.

Beverages: No restrictions. This drug may be taken with milk.

▷ *Alcohol:* Use with caution until the combined effects have been determined. Alcohol may exaggerate the blood-pressure-lowering effects of this drug and cause orthostatic hypotension.

Tobacco Smoking: No interactions expected. Follow physician's advice.

▷ *Other Drugs*

Furosemide may *increase* the effects of

- other antihypertensive drugs; dosage adjustments may be necessary to prevent excessive lowering of blood pressure.
- lithium, and cause lithium toxicity.

Furosemide may *decrease* the effects of

- oral antidiabetic drugs (sulfonylureas); dosage adjustments may be necessary for proper control of blood sugar.

Furosemide *taken concurrently* with

- digitalis preparations (digitoxin, digoxin) requires very careful monitoring and dosage adjustments to prevent fluctuations of blood potassium levels and serious disturbances of heart rhythm.

The following drug may *decrease* the effects of furosemide

- indomethacin (Indocin).

▷ *Driving, Hazardous Activities:* Use caution until the possible occurrence of orthostatic hypotension, dizziness or impaired vision has been determined.

Aviation Note: The use of this drug *may be a disqualification* for piloting. Consult a designated Aviation Medical Examiner.

Exposure to Sun: Use caution until sensitivity has been determined. This drug may cause photosensitivity (see Glossary).

Exposure to Heat: Avoid excessive perspiring, which could cause additional loss of salt and water from the body.

Heavy Exercise or Exertion: Avoid exertion that produces light-headedness, excessive fatigue or muscle cramping. Isometric exercises—the "overload" technique for strengthening individual muscles—can raise blood pressure significantly. Ask physician for guidance regarding participation in this form of exercise.

Occurrence of Unrelated Illness: Illnesses that cause vomiting or diarrhea can produce a serious imbalance of important body chemistry. Consult your physician for guidance.

Discontinuation: It may be advisable to discontinue this drug 5 to 7 days before major surgery. Ask your physician, surgeon and/or anesthesiologist for guidance regarding dosage adjustment or drug withdrawal.

GEMFIBROZIL
(jem FI broh zil)

Introduced: 1976

Prescription: USA: Yes
Canada: Yes

Class: Anticholesterol

Controlled Drug: USA: No
Canada: No

Available as Generic: USA: No
Canada: No

Brand Name: Lopid

BENEFITS versus RISKS

Possible Benefits	*Possible Risks*
EFFECTIVE REDUCTION OF TRIGLYCERIDE BLOOD LEVELS AND ELEVATION OF HIGH DENSITY (HDL) CHOLESTEROL BLOOD LEVELS (40% to 50% reduction of triglycerides; 25% to 30% elevation of HDL cholesterol)	May elevate total cholesterol levels in one third of users Gallstone formation with long-term use Increased susceptibility to viral and bacterial infections

---

▷ **Principal Uses**

As a Single Drug Product: Used primarily to reduce abnormally high blood levels of triglycerides in Types IV and V blood lipid (fat) disorders. Its use is recommended as an adjunct to appropriate dietary adjustment in those individuals who are considered to be at high risk for developing coronary artery heart disease.

How This Drug Works: Not completely known. It is thought that this drug reduces blood levels of triglycerides by inhibiting their production in the liver. It addition, it may hasten removal of cholesterol from the liver and increase its excretion in the stool.

Available Dosage Forms and Strengths
Capsules — 300 mg
Tablets — 600 mg

▷ **Usual Adult Dosage Range:**   900 mg to 1500 mg daily in 2 divided doses. The average dose is 1200 mg/24 hours. Dose increases should be made gradually over a period of 2 to 3 months. **Note: Actual dosage and administration schedule must be determined by the physician for each patient individually.**

▷ **Dosing Instructions:**   Take 30 minutes before the morning and evening meals. The capsule may be opened for administration.

Usual Duration of Use: Continual use on a regular schedule for 4 to 8 weeks is usually necessary to determine this drug's effectiveness in reducing blood levels of triglycerides. Long-term use (months to years) requires periodic evaluation of response and dosage adjustment. Consult your physician on a regular basis.

Currently a "Drug of Choice"
for initiating treatment of elevated LDL cholesterol and VLDL triglycerides. See Cholesterol Disorders in Section Two.

▷ **This Drug Should Not Be Taken If**
- you have had an allergic reaction to it previously.
- you have biliary cirrhosis of the liver.

▷ **Inform Your Physician Before Taking This Drug If**
- you have impaired liver or kidney function.
- you have gallbladder disease or gallstones.

Possible Side-Effects (natural, expected and unavoidable drug actions)
Moderate increase in blood sugar levels.

▷ **Possible Adverse Effects** (unusual, unexpected and infrequent reactions)
If any of the following develop, consult your physician promptly for guidance.
Mild Adverse Effects
Allergic Reactions: Skin rash, hives, itching.
Headache, dizziness, blurred vision, fatigue, muscle aches and cramps.
Indigestion, excessive gas, stomach discomfort (6%), nausea (4%), vomiting (1.6%), diarrhea (5%).
Serious Adverse Effects
Abnormally low white blood cell count: fever, chills, sore throat.
Formation of gallstones with long-term use.

▷ **Possible Effects on Sexual Function:**   Decreased libido.

Natural Diseases or Disorders That May Be Activated by This Drug
Latent diabetes, latent urinary tract infections.

Possible Effects on Laboratory Tests
Complete blood cell counts: decreased red cells, hemoglobin, white cells and platelets.
Blood HDL cholesterol levels: increased.
Blood triglyceride levels: decreased.
Liver function tests: increased liver enzymes (ALT/GPT, AST/GOT and alkaline phosphatase, increased bilirubin.

CAUTION
1. This drug should be used only after nondrug methods (primarily diet) have been ineffective in lowering triglyceride levels.
2. If you used the drug clofibrate (Atromid-S) in the past, inform your physician fully regarding your experience.

3. Comply fully with all recommendations for periodic measurements of blood triglyceride and cholesterol levels. These are essential to the proper management of drug therapy for your disorder.

Precautions for Use
By Infants and Children: Safety and effectiveness for use by those under 12 years of age have not been established.
By Those over 60 Years of Age: Observe for any increased tendency to infection; treat all infections promptly.

▷ **Advisability of Use During Pregnancy**
Pregnancy Category: B (tentative). See Pregnancy Code inside back cover.
Animal studies: No significant birth defects found due to this drug.
Human studies: Information from adequate studies of pregnant women is not available.
Use only if clearly needed. Ask your physician for guidance.

Advisability of Use if Breast-Feeding
Presence of this drug in breast milk: Unknown.
Avoid drug or refrain from nursing.

Habit-Forming Potential: None.

Effects of Overdosage: Abdominal pain, nausea, vomiting, diarrhea.

Possible Effects of Long-Term Use: Formation of gallstones.

Suggested Periodic Examinations While Taking This Drug (at physician's discretion)
Complete blood cell counts.
Measurements of blood levels of total cholesterol, HDL and LDL cholesterol fractions, triglycerides and sugar.
Liver function tests.

▷ **While Taking This Drug, Observe the Following**
Foods: Follow the diet prescribed by your physician.
Beverages: No restrictions. May be taken with milk.
▷ *Alcohol:* No interactions expected.
Tobacco Smoking: No interactions expected.
▷ *Other Drugs*
Gemfibrozil may *increase* the effects of
• warfarin (Coumadin), and increase the risk of bleeding; frequent prothrombin time measurements and dosage adjustments are necessary.
Gemfibrozil may *decrease* the effects of
• chenodiol (Chenix), and reduce its effectiveness in the treatment of gallstones.
▷ *Driving, Hazardous Activities:* This drug may cause dizziness and blurred vision. Restrict activities as necessary.
Aviation Note: The use of this drug *is usually not a disqualification* for piloting. Consult a designated Aviation Medical Examiner.

Exposure to Sun: No restrictions.

Discontinuation: If adequate reduction of triglycerides does not occur after 3 months of treatment, this drug should be discontinued. Following withdrawal, blood cholesterol and triglyceride will return to pretreatment levels.

GLIPIZIDE
(GLIP i zide)

Introduced: 1972   **Class:** Antidiabetic, sulfonylureas

Prescription: USA: Yes   **Controlled Drug:** USA: No

Available as Generic: No

Brand Name: Glucotrol

BENEFITS versus RISKS	
Possible Benefits	*Possible Risks*
Assistance in regulating blood sugar in noninsulin-dependent diabetes (adjunctive to appropriate diet and weight control)	HYPOGLYCEMIA, severe and prolonged Allergic skin reactions (some severe) Water retention Rare liver damage Rare blood cell and bone marrow disorders

▷ **Principal Uses**

As a Single Drug Product: To assist in the control of mild to moderately severe type II diabetes mellitus (adult, maturity-onset) that does not require insulin, but that cannot be adequately controlled by diet alone.

How This Drug Works: It is thought that this drug (1) stimulates the secretion of insulin (by a pancreas that is capable of responding to stimulation), and (2) enhances the utilization of insulin by appropriate tissues.

Available Dosage Forms and Strengths
Tablets — 5 mg, 10 mg

▷ **Usual Adult Dosage Range:**   Initially 5 mg daily with breakfast. At 7 day intervals, the dose may be increased by increments of 2.5 to 5 mg daily as needed and tolerated. Total daily dosage should not exceed 40 mg. A "loading" or priming dose is not necessary and should not be given. **Note: Actual dosage and administration schedule must be determined by the physician for each patient individually.**

▷ **Dosing Instructions:**   If the daily maintenance dose is found to be 15 mg or more, the total dose should be divided into 2 equal doses: the first taken with the morning meal, the second with the evening meal. The tablet may be crushed for administration.

Usual Duration of Use: Continual use on a regular schedule for 1 to 2 weeks is usually necessary to determine this drug's effectiveness in controlling diabetes. Failure to respond to maximal doses within 1 month constitutes a primary failure. Up to 10% of those who respond initially may develop secondary failure of the drug later. The duration of effective use can only be determined by periodic measurement of the blood sugar. Consult your physician on a regular basis.

Possible Advantages of This Drug
Effective with once-daily dosing.
Onset of action within 30 minutes.
Near-normal insulin response to eating.
Well tolerated by the elderly diabetic.

Currently a "Drug of Choice"
for initiating treatment in non-insulin-dependent diabetes when diet and weight control fail.

▷ **This Drug Should Not Be Taken If**
- you have had an allergic reaction to it previously.
- you have severe impairment of liver or kidney function.
- you are pregnant.

▷ **Inform Your Physician Before Taking This Drug If**
- you are allergic to other sulfonylurea drugs or to "sulfa" drugs.
- your diabetes has been unstable or "brittle" in the past.
- you do not know how to recognize or treat hypoglycemia (see Glossary).
- you have a history of congestive heart failure, peptic ulcer disease, cirrhosis of the liver, hypothyroidism or porphyria.

Possible Side-Effects (natural, expected and unavoidable drug actions)
If drug dosage is excessive or food intake is delayed or inadequate, abnormally low blood sugar (hypoglycemia) will occur as a predictable drug effect.

▷ **Possible Adverse Effects** (unusual, unexpected and infrequent reactions)
If any of the following develop, consult your physician promptly for guidance.
Mild Adverse Effects
Allergic Reactions: Skin rash, hives, itching.
Headache (1.25%), drowsiness (1.75%), dizziness (2.25%), fatigue (2.13%), sweating (1.25%).
Indigestion, nausea (1.38%), vomiting, diarrhea (1.25%).

Serious Adverse Effects

Allergic Reactions: Hepatitis with jaundice (see Glossary), severe skin reactions.

Idiosyncratic Reaction: Hemolytic anemia (see Glossary).

Disulfiramlike reaction with concurrent use of alcohol (see Glossary), infrequent with this drug.

Water retention (edema), weight gain.

Bone marrow depression (see Glossary)—fatigue, weakness, fever, sore throat, abnormal bleeding or bruising.

▷ **Possible Effects on Sexual Function:**   None reported.

▷ **Adverse Effects That May Mimic Natural Diseases or Disorders**

Liver reactions may suggest viral hepatitis.

Possible Effects on Laboratory Tests

Complete blood cell counts: decreased red cells, hemoglobin, white cells and platelets.

Blood glucose levels: decreased.

Liver function tests: increased liver enzymes (ALT/GPT, AST/GOT and alkaline phosphatase, increased bilirubin.

CAUTION

1. This drug must be regarded as only one part of the total program for the management of your diabetes. It is not a substitute for a properly prescribed diet and regular exercise.

2. Over a period of time (usually several months), this drug may lose its effectiveness in controlling blood sugar levels. Periodic follow-up examinations are necessary to monitor all aspects of response to drug treatment.

Precautions for Use

By Infants and Children: This drug is not effective in type (juvenile, growth-onset) insulin-dependent diabetes.

By Those over 60 Years of Age: This drug should be used with caution in this age group. Start treatment with 2.5 mg/day; increase dosage cautiously and monitor closely to prevent hypoglycemic reactions. Repeated episodes of hypoglycemia in the elderly can cause brain damage.

▷ **Advisability of Use During Pregnancy**

Pregnancy Category: C (tentative). See Pregnancy Code inside back cover.

Animal studies: No birth defects reported in rats and rabbits.

Human studies: Information from adequate studies of pregnant women is not available.

Because uncontrolled blood sugar levels during pregnancy are associated with a higher incidence of birth defects, many experts recommend that insulin (instead of an oral agent) be used as necessary to control diabetes during the entire pregnancy.

Advisability of Use if Breast-Feeding
Presence of this drug in breast milk: Unknown.
Avoid drug or refrain from nursing.

Habit-Forming Potential: None.

Effects of Overdosage: Symptoms of mild to severe hypoglycemia: headache, light-headedness, faintness, nervousness, confusion, tremor, sweating, heart palpitation, weakness, hunger, nausea, vomiting, stupor progressing to coma.

Possible Effects of Long-Term Use: Reduced function of the thyroid gland (hypothyroidism). Reports of increased frequency and severity of heart and blood vessel diseases associated with long-term use of this class of drugs are highly controversial and inconclusive. A direct cause-and-effect relationship (see Glossary) is tenuous. Ask your physician for guidance.

Suggested Periodic Examinations While Taking This Drug (at physician's discretion)
Complete blood cell counts, liver function tests, thyroid function tests, periodic evaluation of heart and circulatory system.

▷ **While Taking This Drug, Observe the Following**
Foods: Follow the diabetic diet prescribed by your physician.
Beverages: As directed in the diabetic diet. May be taken with milk.
▷ *Alcohol:* Use with extreme caution until the combined effect has been determined. Alcohol can exaggerate this drug's hypoglycemic effect. This drug infrequently causes a marked intolerance of alcohol, resulting in a disulfiramlike reaction (see Glossary): facial flushing, sweating, palpitation.
Tobacco Smoking: No interactions expected.
▷ *Other Drugs*
The following drugs may ***increase*** the effects of glipizide
- aspirin, and other salicylates.
- cimetidine (Tagamet).
- clofibrate (Atromid S).
- fenfluramine (Pondimin).
- monoamine oxidase (MAO) type A inhibitor drugs (see Drug Class, Section Four).
- phenylbutazone (Butazolidin).
- ranitidine (Zantac).
The following drugs may ***decrease*** the effects of glipizide
- beta blocker drugs (see Drug Class, Section Four).
- bumetanide (Bumex).
- diazoxide (Proglycem).
- ethacrynic acid (Edecrin).
- furosemide (Lasix).
- phenytoin (Dilantin).
- thiazide diuretics (see Drug Class, Section Four).

▷ *Driving, Hazardous Activities:* Regulate your dosage schedule, eating schedule and physical activities very carefully to prevent hypoglycemia. Be able to recognize the early symptoms of hypoglycemia so you can avoid hazardous activities and take corrective measures.

Aviation Note: Diabetes ***is a disqualification*** for piloting. Consult a designated Aviation Medical Examiner.

Exposure to Sun: Use caution until sensitivity has been determined. Some drugs of this class can cause photosensitivity (see Glossary).

Occurrence of Unrelated Illness: Acute infections, illnesses causing vomiting or diarrhea, serious injuries and surgical procedures can interfere with diabetic control and may require the use of insulin. If any of these conditions occur, consult your physician promptly.

Discontinuation: Because of the possibility of secondary failure, it is advisable to evaluate the continued benefit of this drug every 6 months.

GLYBURIDE
(GLI byoor ide)

Other Name: Glibenclamide

Introduced: 1970

Class: Antidiabetic, sulfonylureas

Prescription: USA: Yes
Canada: Yes

Controlled Drug: USA: No
Canada: No

Available as Generic: No

Brand Names: DiaBeta, ✦Euglucon, Micronase

BENEFITS versus RISKS

Possible Benefits	*Possible Risks*
Assistance in regulating blood sugar in noninsulin-dependent diabetes (adjunctive to appropriate diet and weight control)	HYPOGLYCEMIA, severe and prolonged Allergic skin reactions (some severe) Rare liver damage Rare blood cell and bone marrow disorders

---

▷ **Principal Uses**

As a Single Drug Product: To assist in the control of mild to moderately severe type II diabetes mellitus (adult, maturity-onset) that does not require insulin, but that cannot be adequately controlled by diet alone.

How This Drug Works: It is thought that this drug (1) stimulates the secretion of insulin (by a pancreas that is capable of responding to stimulation), and (2) enhances the utilization of insulin by appropriate tissues.

Available Dosage Forms and Strengths
Tablets — 1.25 mg, 2.5 mg, 5 mg

▷ **Usual Adult Dosage Range:**   Initially 2.5 to 5 mg daily with breakfast. At 7-day intervals the dose may be increased by increments of 2.5 mg daily as needed and tolerated. Total daily dosage should not exceed 20 mg. A "loading" or priming dose is not necessary and should not be given. **Note: Actual dosage and administration schedule must be determined by the physician for each patient individually.**

▷ **Dosing Instructions:**   If the daily maintenance dose is found to be 10 mg or more, the total dose should be divided into 2 equal doses: the first taken with the morning meal, the second with the evening meal. The tablet may be crushed for administration.

Usual Duration of Use: Continual use on a regular schedule for 1 to 2 weeks is usually necessary to determine this drug's effectiveness in controlling diabetes. Failure to respond to maximal doses within 1 month constitutes a primary failure. Up to 10% of those who respond initially may develop secondary failure of the drug later. The duration of effective use can only be determined by periodic measurement of the blood sugar. Consult your physician on a regular basis.

▷ **This Drug Should Not Be Taken If**
  • you have had an allergic reaction to it previously.
  • you have severe impairment of liver and kidney function.
  • you are pregnant.

▷ **Inform Your Physician Before Taking This Drug If**
  • you are allergic to other sulfonylurea drugs or to "sulfa" drugs.
  • your diabetes has been unstable or "brittle" in the past.
  • you do not know how to recognize or treat hypoglycemia (see Glossary).
  • you have a history of congestive heart failure, peptic ulcer disease, cirrhosis of the liver, hypothyroidism or porphyria.

Possible Side-Effects (natural, expected and unavoidable drug actions)
If drug dosage is excessive or food intake is delayed or inadequate, abnormally low blood sugar (hypoglycemia) will occur as a predictable drug effect.

▷ **Possible Adverse Effects** (unusual, unexpected and infrequent reactions)
  If any of the following develop, consult your physician promptly for guidance.
  Mild Adverse Effects
  Allergic Reactions: Skin rash, hives, itching.

Headache, drowsiness, dizziness, fatigue.

Indigestion, heartburn, nausea.

Serious Adverse Effects

Allergic Reactions: Hepatitis with jaundice (see Glossary), severe skin reactions.

Idiosyncratic Reaction: Hemolytic anemia (see Glossary).

Disulfiramlike reaction with concurrent use of alcohol (see Glossary), infrequent with this drug.

Bone marrow depression (see Glossary)—fatigue, weakness, fever, sore throat, abnormal bleeding or bruising.

▷ **Possible Effects on Sexual Function:**   None reported.

▷ **Adverse Effects That May Mimic Natural Diseases or Disorders**

Liver reactions may suggest viral hepatitis.

Possible Effects on Laboratory Tests

Blood platelet counts: decreased.

Blood cholesterol and triglyceride levels: decreased.

Blood glucose levels: decreased.

Liver function tests: increased liver enzymes (ALT/GPT, AST/GOT and alkaline phosphatase), rare and transient.

CAUTION

1. This drug must be regarded as only one part of the total program for the management of your diabetes. It is not a substitute for a properly prescribed diet and regular exercise.

2. Over a period of time (usually several months), this drug may lose its effectiveness in controlling blood sugar levels. Periodic follow-up examinations are necessary to monitor all aspects of response to drug treatment.

Precautions for Use

By Infants and Children: This drug is not effective in type (juvenile, growth-onset) insulin-dependent diabetes.

By Those over 60 Years of Age: This drug should be used with caution in this age group. Start treatment with 1.25 mg/day; increase dosage cautiously and monitor closely to prevent hypoglycemic reactions. Repeated episodes of hypoglycemia in the elderly can cause brain damage.

▷ **Advisability of Use During Pregnancy**

Pregnancy Category: B (tentative). See Pregnancy Code inside back cover.

Animal studies: No birth defects reported in rats and rabbits.

Human studies: Information from adequate studies of pregnant women is not available.

Because uncontrolled blood sugar levels during pregnancy are associated with a higher incidence of birth defects, many experts recommend that insulin (instead of an oral agent) be used as necessary to control diabetes during the entire pregnancy.

Advisability of Use if Breast-Feeding
　Presence of this drug in breast milk: Unknown.
　Avoid drug or refrain from nursing.

Habit-Forming Potential:　None.

Effects of Overdosage:　Symptoms of mild to severe hypoglycemia: head-
　ache, light-headedness, faintness, nervousness, confusion, tremor,
　sweating, heart palpitation, weakness, hunger, nausea, vomiting, stu-
　por progressing to coma.

Possible Effects of Long-Term Use:　Reduced function of the thyroid gland
　(hypothyroidism). Reports of increased frequency and severity of heart
　and blood vessel diseases associated with long-term use of this class of
　drugs are highly controversial and inconclusive. A direct cause-and-
　effect relationship (see Glossary) is tenuous. Ask your physician for
　guidance.

Suggested Periodic Examinations While Taking This Drug (at physician's
　discretion)
　Complete blood cell counts, liver function tests, thyroid function tests,
　periodic evaluation of heart and circulatory system.

▷ **While Taking This Drug, Observe the Following**
　Foods: Follow the diabetic diet prescribed by your physician.
　Beverages: As directed in the diabetic diet. May be taken with milk.
▷　*Alcohol:* Use with extreme caution until the combined effect has been deter-
　　mined. Alcohol can exaggerate this drug's hypoglycemic effect. This
　　drug infrequently causes a marked intolerance of alcohol, resulting in
　　a disulfiramlike reaction (see Glossary): facial flushing, sweating, pal-
　　pitation.
　Tobacco Smoking: No interactions expected.
▷　*Other Drugs*
　　The following drugs may ***increase*** the effects of glyburide
　　• aspirin, and other salicylates.
　　• cimetidine (Tagamet).
　　• clofibrate (Atromid S).
　　• fenfluramine (Pondimin).
　　• monoamine oxidase (MAO) type A inhibitor drugs (see Drug Class,
　　　Section Four).
　　• phenylbutazone (Butazolidin).
　　• ranitidine (Zantac).
　　The following drugs may ***decrease*** the effects of glyburide
　　• beta blocker drugs (see Drug Class, Section Four).
　　• bumetanide (Bumex).
　　• diazoxide (Proglycem).
　　• ethacrynic acid (Edecrin).
　　• furosemide (Lasix).
　　• phenytoin (Dilantin).
　　• thiazide diuretics (see Drug Class, Section Four).

▷ *Driving, Hazardous Activities:* Regulate your dosage schedule, eating schedule and physical activities very carefully to prevent hypoglycemia. Be able to recognize the early symptoms of hypoglycemia so you can avoid hazardous activities and take corrective measures.

Aviation Note: Diabetes **is a disqualification** for piloting. Consult a designated Aviation Medical Examiner.

Exposure to Sun: Use caution until sensitivity has been determined. Some drugs of this class can cause photosensitivity (see Glossary).

Occurrence of Unrelated Illness: Acute infections, illnesses causing vomiting or diarrhea, serious injuries and surgical procedures can interfere with diabetic control and may require the use of insulin. If any of these conditions occur, consult your physician promptly.

Discontinuation: Because of the possibility of secondary failure, it is advisable to evaluate the continued benefit of this drug every 6 months.

GUANFACINE
(GWAHN fa seen)

Introduced: 1980   **Class:** Antihypertensive

Prescription: USA: Yes   **Controlled Drug:** USA: No

Available as Generic: USA: No

Brand Name: Tenex

BENEFITS versus RISKS

Possible Benefits	*Possible Risks*
EFFECTIVE ANTIHYPERTENSIVE in mild to moderate high blood pressure	Amnesia, confusion, mental depression (3% or less)

▷ **Principal Uses**

As a Single Drug Product: This antihypertensive drug is often used as a "step 2" drug in the treatment of mild to moderate high blood pressure. It is generally not used to initiate treatment, but is added when a "step 1" drug proves to be inadequate. It may also be used as a "step 3 or 4" drug in place of drugs that cause marked orthostatic hypotension (see Glossary).

How This Drug Works: By decreasing the activity of the vasomotor center in the brain, this drug reduces the ability of the sympathetic nervous system to maintain the degree of blood vessel constriction responsible for the elevation of blood pressure. This change results in relaxation of blood vessel walls and lowering of blood pressure.

Available Dosage Forms and Strengths
Tablets — 1 mg

▷ **Usual Adult Dosage Range:** Initially 1 mg once daily taken at bedtime. The dose may be increased after 3 to 4 weeks to 2 mg daily, as needed and tolerated. If needed, the dose may be increased again after 3 to 4 weeks to 3 mg daily. The total daily requirement may be taken in 2 divided doses if necessary for stable blood pressure control. **Note: Actual dosage and administration schedule must be determined by the physician for each patient individually.**

▷ **Dosing Instructions:** Tablets may be taken without regard to eating. It is recommended that the daily dose be taken at bedtime to reduce the side-effect of daytime drowsiness. The tablet may be crushed for administration.

Usual Duration of Use: Continual use on a regular schedule for 4 to 6 weeks is usually necessary to determine this drug's effectiveness in controlling high blood pressure. Long-term use (months to years) requires supervision and guidance by the physician. Consult your physician on a regular basis.

▷ **This Drug Should Not Be Taken If**
   • you have had an allergic reaction to it previously.

▷ **Inform Your Physician Before Taking This Drug If**
   • you have a circulatory disorder of the brain.
   • you have angina or coronary artery disease.
   • you have or have had serious emotional depression.
   • you have impaired liver or kidney function.
   • you are taking any sedative or hypnotic drugs or an antidepressant.
   • you plan to have surgery under general anesthesia in the near future.

Possible Side-Effects (natural, expected and unavoidable drug actions)
Drowsiness (21%), dry nose and mouth (30%), constipation (10%), decreased heart rate, mild orthostatic hypotension (see Glossary).

▷ **Possible Adverse Effects** (unusual, unexpected and infrequent reactions)
   If any of the following develop, consult your physician promptly for guidance.
   Mild Adverse Effects
   Allergic Reactions: Skin rash, itching.
   Headache (4%), dizziness (11%), fatigue (9%), insomnia (4%).
   Indigestion, nausea, diarrhea.
   Serious Adverse Effects
   Amnesia, confusion, depression.

▷ **Possible Effects on Sexual Function:** Decreased libido, impotence.

Possible Effects on Laboratory Tests
Blood cholesterol and triglyceride levels: decreased.

CAUTION
1. ***Do not discontinue this drug suddenly.*** Sudden withdrawal can produce anxiety, nervousness, tremors, fast or irregular heart action, nausea, stomach cramps, vomiting and rebound hypertension.
2. Hot weather and the fever associated with infection can reduce blood pressure significantly. Dosage adjustments may be necessary.
3. Report the development of any tendency to emotional depression.

Precautions for Use
By Infants and Children: Safety and effectiveness for use by those under 12 years of age have not been established.

By Those over 60 Years of Age: ***Proceed cautiously*** with the use of any antihypertensive drug. Unacceptably high blood pressure should be reduced without creating the risks associated with excessively low blood pressure. Start treatment with small doses and monitor the blood pressure response frequently. Observe for the development of light-headedness, dizziness, unsteadiness, fainting and falling. Sedation and dry mouth occur commonly in elderly users. Report promptly any changes in mood or behavior: depression, delusions, hallucinations.

▷ Advisability of Use During Pregnancy
Pregnancy Category: B (tentative). See Pregnancy Code inside back cover.
Animal studies: No birth defects due to this drug reported in rat and rabbit studies.
Human studies: Information from adequate studies of pregnant women is not available.
Use this drug only if clearly needed. Ask your physician for guidance.

Advisability of Use if Breast-Feeding
Presence of this drug in breast milk: Probably yes.
Avoid drug or refrain from nursing.

Habit-Forming Potential: None.

Effects of Overdosage: Marked drowsiness, weakness, dry mouth, slow pulse, low blood pressure, vomiting, stupor progressing to coma.

Possible Effects of Long-Term Use: Development of tolerance (see Glossary) with loss of drug effectiveness.

Suggested Periodic Examinations While Taking This Drug (at physician's discretion)
Blood pressure measurements.

▷ While Taking This Drug, Observe the Following
Foods: Avoid excessive salt. Ask physician for guidance regarding degree of salt restriction.
Beverages: No restrictions. May be taken with milk.

▷   *Alcohol:* Use with extreme caution. The combined effects can cause marked drowsiness and exaggerated reduction of blood pressure.

Tobacco Smoking: No interactions expected. Follow your physician's advice regarding use of tobacco.

▷   *Other Drugs:* No significant drug interactions reported to date.

▷   *Driving, Hazardous Activities:* Use caution. This drug can cause drowsiness and can impair mental alertness, judgment and coordination.

Aviation Note: Hypertension (high blood pressure) *is a disqualification* for piloting. Consult a designated Aviation Medical Examiner.

Exposure to Sun: No restrictions.

Exposure to Heat: Use caution. Hot environments may reduce the blood pressure significantly; be alert to the possibility of orthostatic hypotension (see Glossary).

Heavy Exercise or Exertion: Use caution. Isometric exercises—the "overload" technique for strengthening individual muscles—can raise blood pressure significantly. The use of this drug may intensify the hypertensive response to isometric exercise. Ask physician for guidance.

Occurrence of Unrelated Illness: Fever associated with infections may lower the blood pressure significantly. Repeated vomiting may prevent the regular use of this drug and result in an acute withdrawal reaction. Consult your physician.

*Discontinuation: **Do not discontinue this drug suddenly.*** A significant withdrawal reaction can occur within 2 to 7 days after the last dose. The dose should be reduced gradually over 3 to 4 days, with periodic monitoring of the blood pressure.

HALOPERIDOL
(hal oh PER i dohl)

Introduced: 1958

Class: Strong tranquilizer, butyrophenones

Prescription: USA: Yes
Canada: Yes

Controlled Drug: USA: No
Canada: No

Available as Generic: USA: Yes
Canada: No

Brand Names: ✦Apo-Haloperidol, Haldol, ✦Haldol LA, Halperon, ✦Novoperidol, ✦Peridol

```
┌─────────────────────────────────────────────────────────────┐
│                   BENEFITS versus RISKS                       │
│                                                               │
│      Possible Benefits              Possible Risks            │
│   EFFECTIVE CONTROL OF         FREQUENT PARKINSON-LIKE        │
│     ACUTE FREQUENT               SIDE-EFFECTS                 │
│     PSYCHOSES in majority of   SERIOUS TOXIC EFFECTS ON       │
│     patients: beneficial effects on  BRAIN with long-term use │
│     thinking, mood and behavior   Rare blood cell disorders   │
│   EFFECTIVE CONTROL OF SOME    Abnormally low white blood cell│
│     CASES OF TOURETTE'S          count                        │
│     DISORDER                                                  │
│   Beneficial in the management of                            │
│     the hyperactive child                                     │
└─────────────────────────────────────────────────────────────┘
```

▷ **Principal Uses**

As a Single Drug Product: Used primarily to control the psychotic thinking and abnormal behavior associated with acute psychosis of unknown nature, acute schizophrenia, paranoid states and the manic phase of manic-depressive disorders. It is also used to treat the hyperactivity syndrome in children. A less frequent use is to control the tics and offensive language characteristic of Gilles de la Tourette's syndrome.

How This Drug Works: Not completely established. It is thought that by interfering with the action of dopamine as nerve impulse transmitter in certain areas of the brain, this drug reduces anxiety and agitation, improves coherence and organization of thinking and abolishes delusions and hallucinations.

Available Dosage Forms and Strengths

Concentrate — 2 mg per ml

Injection — 5 mg per ml, 50 mg per ml

Tablets — 0.5 mg, 1 mg, 2 mg, 5 mg, 10 mg, 20 mg

▷ **Usual Adult Dosage Range:**   Initially 0.5 to 2 mg 2 or 3 times daily. Dose may be increased by 0.5 mg/day at 3- to 4-day intervals as needed and tolerated. The usual dosage range is 0.5 to 30 mg/24 hours. The total daily dosage should not exceed 100 mg. **Note: Actual dosage and administration schedule must be determined by the physician for each patient individually.**

▷ **Dosing Instructions:**   May be taken with or following food to reduce stomach irritation. The concentrate may be diluted in 2 ounces of water or fruit juice; do not add it to coffee or tea. The tablet may be crushed for administration.

Usual Duration of Use: Continual use on a regular schedule for several weeks is usually necessary to determine this drug's effectiveness in controlling the symptoms of psychotic or psychoneurotic behavior. If not significantly beneficial within 6 weeks, it should be discontinued.

Long-term use requires supervision and periodic evaluation by your physician. Consult your physician on a regular basis.

▷ **This Drug Should Not Be Taken If**
- you have had an allergic reaction to any dosage form of it previously.
- you are experiencing mental depression.
- you have any form of Parkinson's disease.
- you have cancer of the breast.
- you have active liver disease.
- you currently have a bone marrow or blood cell disorder.

▷ **Inform Your Physician Before Taking This Drug If**
- you are allergic or abnormally sensitive to phenothiazine drugs.
- you have a history of mental depression.
- you have any type of heart disease.
- you have impaired liver or kidney function.
- you have low blood pressure, epilepsy or glaucoma.
- you are taking any drugs with a sedative effect.
- you plan to have surgery under general or spinal anesthesia in the near future.

Possible Side-Effects (natural, expected and unavoidable drug actions)
Mild drowsiness, low blood pressure, blurred vision, dry mouth, constipation, marked and frequent Parkinson-like reactions (see Glossary).

▷ **Possible Adverse Effects** (unusual, unexpected and infrequent reactions)
If any of the following develop, consult your physician promptly for guidance.
Mild Adverse Effects
Allergic Reactions: Skin rash, hives.
Dizziness, weakness, agitation, insomnia.
Loss of appetite, indigestion, nausea, vomiting, diarrhea.
Urinary retention.
Serious Adverse Effects
Allergic Reactions: Rare liver reaction with jaundice, asthma, spasm of vocal cords.
Idiosyncratic Reactions: Neuroleptic malignant syndrome (see Glossary).
Depression, disorientation, eye damage (deposits in cornea, lens and retina).
Blood cell disorders: anemia, fluctuation in number of white blood cells.
Nervous system reactions: rigidity of extremities, tremors, restlessness, constant movement, facial grimacing, eye-rolling, spasm of neck muscles, tardive dyskinesia (see Glossary).

▷ **Possible Effects on Sexual Function**
Decreased libido; impotence (10% to 20%); painful ejaculation; priapism (see Glossary).
Male breast enlargement and tenderness; female breast enlargement with milk production.
Altered timing and pattern of menstruation.

▷ **Adverse Effects That May Mimic Natural Diseases or Disorders**
Liver reaction may suggest viral hepatitis.
Nervous system reactions may suggest Parkinson's disease or Reye syndrome.

Natural Diseases or Disorders That May Be Activated by This Drug
Latent epilepsy, glaucoma, diabetes.

Possible Effects on Laboratory Tests
Complete blood cell counts: decreased red cells, hemoglobin and white cells; increased eosinophils.
Prothrombin time: decreased.
Blood cholesterol level: decreased.
Blood glucose level: increased.
Liver function tests: increased liver enzymes (ALT/GPT, AST/GOT and alkaline phosphatase), increased bilirubin.

CAUTION
1. It is advisable to use the smallest dose that is effective for long-term treatment.
2. Use with extreme caution in epilepsy; this drug can alter the pattern of seizures.
3. Individuals with lupus erythematosus and those taking prednisone are more susceptible to nervous system reactions.
4. Do not use levodopa to treat Parkinson-like reactions; it can cause agitation and worsening of the psychotic disorder.
5. Obtain prompt evaluation of any change or disturbance in vision.

Precautions for Use
By Infants and Children: This drug should not be used in children under 3 years of age or 15 kilograms in weight. Avoid this drug in the presence of symptoms suggestive of Reye syndrome. Children are quite susceptible to nervous system reactions induced by this drug.
By Those over 60 Years of Age: Initiate treatment with small doses. This drug can cause significant changes in mood and behavior; observe for confusion, disorientation, agitation, restlessness, aggression and paranoia. You may be more susceptible to the development of drowsiness, lethargy, orthostatic hypotension (see Glossary), hypothermia (see Glossary), Parkinson-like reactions and prostatism (see Glossary).

▷ **Advisability of Use During Pregnancy**
Pregnancy Category: C (tentative). See Pregnancy Code inside back cover.
Animal studies: Cleft palate reported in mouse studies.
Human studies: No increase in birth defects reported in 100 exposures. Information from adequate studies of pregnant women is not available.
Avoid during the first trimester. Use only if clearly needed. Ask physician for guidance.

Advisability of Use if Breast-Feeding
Presence of this drug in breast milk: Yes.
Monitor nursing infant closely and discontinue drug or nursing if adverse effects develop.

Habit-Forming Potential: None.

Effects of Overdosage: Marked drowsiness, weakness, tremor, unsteadiness, agitation, stupor, coma, convulsions.

Possible Effects of Long-Term Use: Eye damage: deposits in cornea, lens or retina; tardive dyskinesia (see Glossary).

Suggested Periodic Examinations While Taking This Drug (at physician's discretion)
Complete blood cell counts, liver function tests, eye examinations, electrocardiograms.
Careful inspection of the tongue for early evidence of fine, involuntary, wavelike movements that could indicate the beginning of tardive dyskinesia.

▷ **While Taking This Drug, Observe the Following**
Foods: No restrictions.
Beverages: No restrictions. May be taken with milk.
▷ *Alcohol:* Avoid completely. Alcohol can increase the sedative action of haloperidol and accentuate its depressant effects on brain function. Haloperidol can increase the intoxicating effects of alcohol.
Tobacco Smoking: No interactions expected.
Marijuana Smoking: Moderate increase in drowsiness; accentuation of orthostatic hypotension; increased risk of precipitating latent psychosis, confusing interpretation of mental status and of drug response.
▷ *Other Drugs*
Haloperidol may *increase* the effects of
• all drugs with sedative actions, and cause excessive sedation.
• some antihypertensive drugs, and cause excessive lowering of blood pressure; monitor the combined effects carefully.
Haloperidol may *decrease* the effects of
• guanethidine (Esimil, Ismelin), and reduce its antihypertensive effect.
Haloperidol *taken concurrently* with
• beta blocker drugs may cause excessive lowering of blood pressure.
• lithium may cause toxic effects on the brain and nervous system.
• methyldopa (Aldomet) may cause serious dementia.
The following drugs may *decrease* the effects of haloperidol
• antacids containing aluminum and/or magnesium may reduce its absorption.
• barbiturates.
• benztropine (Cogentin).
• phenytoin (Dilantin).
• trihexyphenidyl (Artane).

▷ *Driving, Hazardous Activities:* This drug may impair mental alertness, judgment and physical coordination. Restrict activities as necessary.

Aviation Note: The use of this drug *is a disqualification* for piloting. Consult a designated Aviation Medical Examiner.

Exposure to Sun: Use caution until sensitivity has been determined. This drug can cause photosensitivity.

Exposure to Heat: Use caution in hot environments. This drug may impair the regulation of body temperature and increase the risk of heat stroke.

Exposure to Cold: The elderly are advised to use caution; this drug can increase the risk of hypothermia (see Glossary).

Discontinuation: This drug should not be discontinued abruptly following long-term use. Gradual withdrawal over a period of 2 to 3 weeks is advised. Ask physician for guidance.

HYDRALAZINE
(hi DRAL a zeen)

Introduced: 1950

Class: Antihypertensive

Prescription: USA: Yes
Canada: Yes

Controlled Drug: USA: No
Canada: No

Available as Generic: USA: Yes
Canada: No

Brand Names: Alazine, Apresazide [CD], Apresoline, Apresoline-Esidrix [CD], Ser-Ap-Es [CD], Serpasil-Apresoline [CD], Unipres [CD]

BENEFITS versus RISKS

Possible Benefits	*Possible Risks*
EFFECTIVE STEP 2 OR 3 ANTIHYPERTENSIVE FOR MODERATE TO SEVERE HYPERTENSION when used adjunctively with other antihypertensive drugs	DRUG-INDUCED LUPUS ERYTHEMATOSUSLIKE SYNDROME (up to 13%)
Possibly beneficial in the management of severe congestive heart failure	Intensification of angina pectoris Rare blood cell disorders Rare liver damage

---

▷ **Principal Uses**

As a Single Drug Product: Used primarily as a step 2 or antihypertensive drug in conjunction with other antihypertensives in the treatment of moderate to severe high blood pressure.

As a Combination Drug Product [CD]: This drug is available in combination with hydrochlorothiazide (a diuretic) and with reserpine (another type of antihypertensive). When used in combination, several different types of drug action occur concurrently to reduce blood pressure: hydralazine relaxes and expands blood vessel walls; the diuretic reduces the amount of water and sodium in the body; reserpine reduces the rate and contraction force of the heart and enhances the expansion of blood vessels.

How This Drug Works: By causing direct relaxation of arterial walls (mechanism unknown), this drug dilates peripheral blood vessels, with resultant lowering of blood pressure. The dilation of blood vessels can also be beneficial in some cases of heart failure by reducing the workload of the heart and increasing its output.

Available Dosage Forms and Strengths
Tablets — 10 mg, 25 mg, 50 mg, 100 mg

▷ **Usual Adult Dosage Range:**   Initially 10 mg 4 times daily for 2 to 4 days; then increase to 25 mg 4 times daily for the balance of the first week. During the second week the dose may be increased to 50 mg 4 times daily if needed and tolerated. The total daily dosage should not exceed 300 mg for fast acetylators or 200 mg for slow acetylators. Ask your physician for guidance. **Note: Actual dosage and administration schedule must be determined by the physician for each patient individually.**

▷ **Dosing Instructions:**   Preferably taken with or following meals to enhance absorption and reduce stomach irritation. The tablet may be crushed and the capsule [CD] may be opened for administration.

Usual Duration of Use: Continual use on a regular schedule for several weeks is usually necessary to determine this drug's effectiveness in lowering blood pressure. Long-term use requires supervision and periodic evaluation by your physician. Consult your physician on a regular basis.

▷ **This Drug Should Not Be Taken If**
 • you have had an allergic reaction to it previously.
 • you have active angina pectoris.
 • you have mitral valvular heart disease.

▷ **Inform Your Physician Before Taking This Drug If**
 • you have a history of any type of heart disease.
 • you have lupus erythematosus.
 • you have impaired brain circulation.
 • you are subject to migraine headaches.
 • you have impaired kidney function.
 • you have a history of liver sensitivity to other drugs.
 • you plan to have surgery under general anesthesia in the near future.

Possible Side-Effects (natural, expected and unavoidable drug actions)
Orthostatic hypotension (see Glossary), nasal congestion, constipation, delayed or impaired urination, increased heart rate of 10 to 25 beats/minute.

▷ **Possible Adverse Effects** (unusual, unexpected and infrequent reactions)
If any of the following develop, consult your physician promptly for guidance.
Mild Adverse Effects
Allergic Reactions: Skin rash, hives, itching, drug fever.
Headache, dizziness, flushing of face, palpitation.
Loss of appetite, nausea, vomiting, diarrhea.
Tremors, muscle cramps.
Serious Adverse Effects
Allergic Reactions: Liver reaction, with or without jaundice.
Idiosyncratic Reactions: Behavioral changes: nervousness, confusion, emotional depression. Bleeding into lung tissue: densities found on X-ray examination. A syndrome resembling rheumatoid arthritis or lupus erythematosus (see Glossary).
Intensification of coronary artery disease.
Peripheral neuropathy (see Glossary): weakness, numbness and/or pain in extremities.
Rare bone marrow depression (see Glossary): fatigue, weakness, fever, sore throat, abnormal bleeding or bruising.

▷ **Possible Effects on Sexual Function:**   Rare reports of impotence and priapism (see Glossary).

▷ **Adverse Effects That May Mimic Natural Diseases or Disorders**
Drug fever may suggest systemic infection. Liver reaction may suggest viral hepatitis. Skin and joint symptoms may suggest lupus erythematosus.

Natural Diseases or Disorders That May Be Activated by This Drug
Latent coronary artery disease.

Possible Effects on Laboratory Tests
Complete blood cell counts: decreased red cells, hemoglobin, white cells and platelets.
Blood antinuclear antibodies (ANA): positive.
Blood cholesterol level: decreased.
Blood lupus erythematosus (LE) cells: positive.
Blood urea nitrogen (BUN) level: increased (kidney damage).
Liver function tests: increased liver enzymes (ALT/GPT, AST/GOT and alkaline phosphatase), increased bilirubin.

CAUTION
1. Toxic reactions are more likely to occur with large doses. Adhere strictly to prescribed dosage schedules. Keep appointments for periodic follow-up examinations.
2. Report the development of any tendency to emotional depression.

3. This drug can cause salt and water retention if a diuretic is not taken concurrently.
4. This drug can provoke migraine headache.

Precautions for Use
By Infants and Children: Dosage is based upon age, weight and kidney function status. Observe for the possible development of a lupus erythematosuslike reaction.
By Those over 60 Years of Age: Initiate treatment with low doses and proceed cautiously. Unacceptably high blood pressure should be reduced without creating the risks associated with excessively low blood pressure. Sudden, rapid and excessive reduction of blood pressure can predispose to stroke or heart attack. Observe for possible dizziness, unsteadiness, fainting or falling. Headache, palpitation and rapid heart rates are more common in the elderly and can mimic acute anxiety states.

▷ **Advisability of Use During Pregnancy**
Pregnancy Category: C (tentative). See Pregnancy Code inside back cover.
Animal studies: Birth defects of head and facial bones reported in mice.
Human studies: Information from adequate studies of pregnant women is not available.
Avoid use during the first and last 3 months; if taken late in pregnancy, this drug can cause a deficiency of blood platelets (see Glossary) in the newborn infant.

Advisability of Use if Breast-Feeding
Presence of this drug in breast milk: Yes.
Avoid drug or refrain from nursing.

Habit-Forming Potential: None.

Effects of Overdosage: Marked light-headedness, dizziness, headache, flushing of skin, nausea, vomiting, collapse of circulation: loss of consciousness, cold and sweaty skin, weak and rapid pulse, irregular heart rhythm.

Possible Effects of Long-Term Use: An acute or subacute syndrome resembling rheumatoid arthritis or lupus erythematosus, usually seen in slow acetylators taking daily doses of over 200 mg.

Suggested Periodic Examinations While Taking This Drug (at physician's discretion)
Complete blood cell counts, liver function tests, blood tests for evidence of lupus erythematosus.

▷ **While Taking This Drug, Observe the Following**
Foods: No restrictions.
Nutritional Support: Monitor for peripheral neuropathy and take a supplement of pyridoxine (vitamin B-6) as needed. Ask physician for guidance.
Beverages: No restrictions. May be taken with milk.

▷ *Alcohol:* Use with extreme caution until the combined effect has been determined. Alcohol can exaggerate the blood-pressure-lowering effect of
this drug and cause excessive reduction.

Tobacco Smoking: Avoid completely. Nicotine can contribute significantly
to this drug's ability to intensify angina in susceptible individuals.

▷ *Other Drugs*

Hydralazine may *increase* the effects of

- metoprolol (Lopressor).
- oxprenolol (Trasicor).
- propranolol (Inderal).

▷ *Driving, Hazardous Activities:* This drug may cause light-headedness or
dizziness. Restrict activities as necessary.

Aviation Note: Hypertension and the use of this drug *are disqualifications*
for piloting. Consult a designated Aviation Medical Examiner.

Exposure to Sun: No restrictions.

Exposure to Heat: Caution advised. Hot environments may reduce blood
pressure significantly.

Exposure to Cold: Caution advised. Cold environments may increase this
drug's ability to cause angina in susceptible individuals.

Heavy Exercise or Exertion: Caution advised. Excessive exertion can increase this drug's ability to cause angina in susceptible individuals.
Also, isometric exercises can raise blood pressure significantly.

HYDROCHLOROTHIAZIDE
(hi droh klor oh THI a zide)

Introduced: 1959

Class: Antihypertensive, diuretic,
thiazides

Prescription: USA: Yes
Canada: Yes

Controlled Drug: USA: No
Canada: No

Available as Generic: USA: Yes
Canada: Yes

Brand Names: Aldactazide [CD], Aldoril-15/25 [CD], Aldoril D30/D50
[CD], ✦Apo-Hydro, ✦Apo-Methazide [CD], ✦Apo-Triazide [CD], Apresa-
zide [CD], Apresoline-Esidrix [CD], Capozide [CD], ✦Co-Betaloc [CD],
✦Diuchlor H, Dyazide [CD], Esidrix, Hydral [CD], HydroDIURIL, Hy-
dropres [CD], Hydro-Z-50, Inderide [CD], Inderide LA [CD], ✦Ismelin-
Esidrix [CD], Lopressor HCT [CD], Maxzide [CD], Maxzide-25 [CD],
✦Moduret [CD], Moduretic [CD], ✦Natrimax, ✦Neo-Codema, Normo-
zide [CD], ✦Novodoparil [CD], ✦Novohydrazide, ✦Novospirozine [CD],
✦Novotriamzide [CD], Oretic, Oreticyl [CD], ✦PMS Dopazide [CD],
Prinzide [CD], Ser-Ap-Es [CD], Serpasil-Esidrix [CD], Thiuretic, Timo-
lide [CD], Trandate HCT [CD], Unipres [CD], ✦Urozide, Vaseretic [CD],
✦Viskazide [CD], Zestoretic [CD], Zide

```
┌────────────────────────────────────────────────────────────┐
│                    BENEFITS versus RISKS                     │
│                                                              │
│      Possible Benefits              Possible Risks           │
│  EFFECTIVE, WELL-TOLERATED      Loss of body potassium       │
│     DIURETIC                    Increased blood sugar        │
│  POSSIBLY EFFECTIVE IN MILD     Increased blood uric acid    │
│     HYPERTENSION                Increased blood calcium      │
│  ENHANCES EFFECTIVENESS OF      Rare blood cell disorders    │
│     OTHER ANTIHYPERTENSIVES                                  │
│  Beneficial in treatment of diabetes                         │
│    insipidus                                                 │
└────────────────────────────────────────────────────────────┘
```

▷ **Principal Uses**

As a Single Drug Product: Thiazide diuretics are used primarily to (1) increase the volume of urine (diuresis) to correct the excessive fluid retention associated with congestive heart failure and certain types of liver and kidney disease; and (2) initiate treatment for high blood pressure (hypertension). They are often the first drugs tried in treating mild to moderate hypertension. Less frequent uses include the treatment of diabetes insipidus and the prevention of kidney stones that contain calcium.

As a Combination Drug Product [CD]: When this drug is used alone to treat hypertension, it is referred to as a "step 1" antihypertensive. Should it fail to reduce the blood pressure adequately, a "step 2" antihypertensive drug is added to be taken concurrently with the "step 1" drug. These drugs may be combined into one drug product. Thiazides are available in combination with beta blockers, hydralazine, methyldopa, reserpine and other diuretics to increase their effectiveness in treating hypertension.

How This Drug Works: By increasing the elimination of salt and water from the body (through increased urine production), this drug reduces the volume of fluid in the blood and body tissues and lowers the sodium content throughout the body. By relaxing the walls of smaller arteries and allowing them to expand, this drug increases the total capacity of the arterial system. The combined effect of these two actions (reduced blood volume in expanded space) results in lowering of the blood pressure.

Available Dosage Forms and Strengths

Solution — 50 mg per 5-ml teaspoonful

Solution, intensol — 100 mg per ml

Tablets — 25 mg, 50 mg, 100 mg

▷ **Usual Adult Dosage Range:**   As antihypertensive: 50 to 100 mg/day initially; 50 to 200 mg/day for maintenance. As diuretic: 50 to 200 mg/day initially; the smallest effective dose should be determined. The total daily dose should not exceed 200 mg. **Note: Actual dosage and administration schedule must be determined by the physician for each patient individually.**

▷ **Dosing Instructions:**   May be taken with or following meals to reduce stomach irritation. Best taken in the morning to avoid nighttime urination. The tablet may be crushed for administration.

Usual Duration of Use: Continual use on a regular schedule for 2 to 3 weeks is usually necessary to determine this drug's effectiveness in lowering high blood pressure. Long-term use (months to years) requires periodic evaluation of response and possible dosage adjustment. Use as a diuretic should be intermittent with "drug holidays" (no drug taken) to reduce the risk of sodium and potassium imbalance. Consult your physician on a regular basis.

▷ **This Drug Should Not Be Taken If**
- you have had an allergic reaction to any dosage form of it previously.

▷ **Inform Your Physician Before Taking This Drug If**
- you are allergic to any form of "sulfa" drug.
- you are pregnant or planning pregnancy.
- you have a history of kidney or liver disease.
- you have a history of pancreatitis.
- you have diabetes, gout or lupus erythematosus.
- you are taking any form of cortisone, digitalis, oral antidiabetic drug or insulin.
- you plan to have surgery under general anesthesia in the near future.

Possible Side-Effects (natural, expected and unavoidable drug actions)
Light-headedness on arising from sitting or lying position (see Orthostatic Hypotension in Glossary).
Increase in blood sugar level, affecting control of diabetes.
Increase in blood uric acid level, affecting control of gout.
Decrease in blood potassium level, causing muscle weakness and cramping.

▷ **Possible Adverse Effects** (unusual, unexpected and infrequent reactions)
If any of the following develop, consult your physician promptly for guidance.
Mild Adverse Effects
Allergic Reactions: Skin rashes, hives, drug fever.
Headache, dizziness, blurred or yellow vision.
Reduced appetite, indigestion, nausea, vomiting, diarrhea.
Serious Adverse Effects
Allergic Reactions: Hepatitis with jaundice (see Glossary), anaphylactic reaction (see Glossary), severe skin reactions.
Inflammation of the pancreas—severe abdominal pain.
Bone marrow depression (see Glossary)—fatigue, weakness, fever, sore throat, abnormal bleeding or bruising.

▷ **Possible Effects on Sexual Function:**   Decreased libido (12%); impotence (3%).

▷ **Adverse Effects That May Mimic Natural Diseases or Disorders**
Liver reaction may suggest viral hepatitis.

Natural Diseases or Disorders That May Be Activated by This Drug
Diabetes, gout, systemic lupus erythematosus.

Possible Effects on Laboratory Tests
Complete blood cell counts: decreased red cells, hemoglobin, white cells and platelets.
Blood amylase level: increased (possible pancreatitis).
Blood calcium level: increased.
Blood sodium and chloride levels: decreased.
Blood cholesterol and triglyceride levels: increased.
Blood glucose level: increased.
Glucose tolerance test (GTT): decreased.
Blood lithium level: increased.
Blood potassium level: decreased.
Blood urea nitrogen (BUN) level: increased with long-term use.
Blood uric acid level: increased.
Liver function tests: increased liver enzymes (ALT/GPT, AST/GOT and alkaline phosphatase), increased bilirubin.

CAUTION
1. Do not exceed recommended doses. Increased dosage can cause excessive loss of sodium and potassium, with resultant loss of appetite, nausea, fatigue, weakness, confusion and tingling in the extremities.
2. If you are also taking a digitalis preparation (digitoxin, digoxin), ensure an adequate intake of high-potassium foods to prevent potassium deficiency—a potential cause of digitalis toxicity. (See Table of High Potassium Foods in Section Six.)

Precautions for Use
By Infants and Children: Avoid overdosage that could cause serious dehydration. Significant potassium loss can occur within the first 2 weeks of drug use.
By Those over 60 Years of Age: Small doses are advisable until your individual response has been determined. You may be more susceptible to the development of impaired thinking, orthostatic hypotension, potassium loss and blood sugar increase. Overdosage and extended use of this drug can cause excessive loss of body water, thickening (increased viscosity) of the blood and an increased tendency for the blood to clot—predisposing to stroke, heart attack or thrombophlebitis (vein inflammation with blood clot).

▷ **Advisability of Use During Pregnancy**
Pregnancy Category: D (tentative). See Pregnancy Code inside back cover.
Animal studies: No birth defects found in rat studies.
Human studies: Reports are conflicting and inconclusive. This drug does not seem to carry the risk of birth defects that has been found with other related diuretics. However, other types of fetal injury are possible with this drug. It should not be used during pregnancy unless a very serious complication occurs for which this drug is significantly beneficial. Ask physician for guidance.

Advisability of Use if Breast-Feeding
Presence of this drug in breast milk: Yes.
Avoid drug or refrain from nursing.

Habit-Forming Potential: None.

Effects of Overdosage: Dry mouth, thirst, lethargy, weakness, muscle cramping, nausea, vomiting, drowsiness progressing to stupor or coma.

Possible Effects of Long-Term Use: Impaired balance of water, salt and potassium in blood and body tissues. Development of diabetes in predisposed individuals. Pathological changes in parathyroid glands with increased blood calcium levels and decreased blood phosphate levels.

Suggested Periodic Examinations While Taking This Drug (at physician's discretion)
Complete blood cell counts, measurements of blood levels of sodium, potassium, chloride, sugar and uric acid.
Kidney and liver function tests.

▷ **While Taking This Drug, Observe the Following**
Foods: Consult your physician regarding the advisability of eating foods rich in potassium. If so advised, see the Table of High Potassium Foods in Section Six. Follow physician's advice regarding the use of salt.
Beverages: No restrictions. This drug may be taken with milk.
▷ *Alcohol:* Use with caution until the combined effects have been determined. Alcohol may exaggerate the blood-pressure-lowering effects of this drug and cause orthostatic hypotension.
Tobacco Smoking: No interactions expected. Follow physician's advice.
▷ *Other Drugs*
Hydrochlorothiazide may *increase* the effects of
• other antihypertensive drugs; dosage adjustments may be necessary to prevent excessive lowering of blood pressure.
• lithium, and cause lithium toxicity.
Hydrochlorothiazide may *decrease* the effects of
• oral antidiabetic drugs (sulfonylureas); dosage adjustments may be necessary for proper control of blood sugar.
Hydrochlorothiazide *taken concurrently* with
• digitalis preparations (digitoxin, digoxin) requires very careful monitoring and dosage adjustments to prevent fluctuations of blood potassium levels and serious disturbances of heart rhythm.
The following drugs may *decrease* the effects of hydrochlorothiazide
• cholestyramine (Cuemid, Questran) may interfere with its absorption.
• colestipol (Colestid) may interfere with its absorption.
Take cholestyramine and colestipol 1 hour before any oral diuretic.
▷ *Driving, Hazardous Activities:* Use caution until the possible occurrence of orthostatic hypotension, dizziness or impaired vision has been determined.

Aviation Note: The use of this drug *may be a disqualification* for piloting. Consult a designated Aviation Medical Examiner.

Exposure to Sun: Use caution until sensitivity has been determined. This drug can cause photosensitivity (see Glossary).

Exposure to Heat: Avoid excessive perspiring, which could cause additional loss of salt and water from the body.

Heavy Exercise or Exertion: Avoid exertion that produces light-headedness, excessive fatigue or muscle cramping. Isometric exercises—the "overload" technique for strengthening individual muscles—can raise blood pressure significantly. Ask physician for guidance regarding participation in this form of exercise.

Occurrence of Unrelated Illness: Illnesses that cause vomiting or diarrhea can produce a serious imbalance of important body chemistry. Consult your physician for guidance.

Discontinuation: This drug should not be stopped abruptly following long-term use; sudden discontinuation can cause serious thiazide-withdrawal fluid retention (edema). The dose should be reduced gradually. It may be advisable to discontinue this drug 5 to 7 days before major surgery. Ask your physician, surgeon and/or anesthesiologist for guidance regarding dosage adjustment or drug withdrawal.

HYDROCODONE
(hi droh KOH dohn)

Other Name: Dihydrocodeinone

Introduced: 1951

Class: Analgesic, narcotic; cough suppressant

Prescription: USA: Yes
Canada: Yes

Controlled Drug: USA: C-III*
Canada: < N >

Available as Generic: USA: Yes
Canada: No

Brand Names: Anexsia [CD], Anexsia 7.5 [CD], Azdone, ✦Biohisdex DHC [CD], ✦Biohisdine DHC [CD], Dimetane Expectorant-DC [CD], Duocet [CD], ✦Hycodan, Hycodan [CD], ✦Hycomine [CD], Hycomine Compound [CD], Hycomine Pediatric Syrup [CD], ✦Hycomine-S [CD], Hycomine Syrup [CD], Hycotuss Expectorant [CD], Lorcet-HD [CD], Lorcet Plus [CD], Lortab [CD], Lortab ASA [CD], Norcet 7 [CD], ✦Novahistex DH [CD], ✦Novahistine DH [CD], ✦Robidone, T-Gesic [CD], Triaminic Expectorant DH [CD], Tussend [CD], Tussend Expectorant [CD], Tussionex [CD], Tycolet [CD], Vicodin [CD], Vicodin ES [CD], Zydone [CD]

*See Schedules of Controlled Drugs inside back cover.

BENEFITS versus RISKS

Possible Benefits	*Possible Risks*
EFFECTIVE RELIEF OF MILD TO MODERATE PAIN	Low potential for habit formation (dependence)
EFFECTIVE CONTROL OF COUGH	Mild allergic reactions (infrequent)
	Nausea, constipation

▷ **Principal Uses**

As a Single Drug Product: Used primarily to (1) control cough; (2) relieve mild to moderate pain. Its widest use is as an ingredient in cough remedies.

As a Combination Drug Product [CD]: Hydrocodone is frequently added to cough mixtures containing antihistamines, decongestants and expectorants to make these "shotgun" preparations more effective in reducing the frequency and severity of cough. It is also combined with milder analgesics, such as acetaminophen and aspirin, to enhance pain relief.

How This Drug Works: Acting primarily as a depressant of certain brain functions, this drug suppresses the perception of pain, calms the emotional response to pain and reduces the sensitivity of the cough reflex.

Available Dosage Forms and Strengths

Syrup — 5 mg per 5-ml teaspoonful

Tablets — 5 mg

▷ **Usual Adult Dosage Range:** As analgesic—5 to 10 mg/4 to hours as needed. For cough—5 mg/4 to 6 hours as needed. Total daily dosage should not exceed 60 mg. **Note: Actual dosage and administration schedule must be determined by the physician for each patient individually.**

▷ **Dosing Instructions:** May be taken with or following food to reduce stomach irritation or nausea. Tablet may be crushed for administration.

Usual Duration of Use: As required, to control pain or cough. Continual use should not exceed 5 to 7 days without interruption and reassessment of need.

▷ **This Drug Should Not Be Taken If**
- you have had an allergic reaction to any dosage form of it previously.
- you are having an acute attack of asthma.

▷ **Inform Your Physician Before Taking This Drug If**
- you have had an unfavorable reaction to any narcotic drug in the past.
- you have a history of drug abuse or alcoholism.
- you have chronic lung disease with impaired breathing.
- you have impaired liver or kidney function.
- you have gallbladder disease, a seizure disorder or an underactive thyroid gland.
- you have difficulty emptying the urinary bladder.

- you are taking any other drugs that have a sedative effect.
- you plan to have surgery under general anesthesia in the near future.

Possible Side-Effects (natural, expected and unavoidable drug actions)
Drowsiness, light-headedness, dry mouth, urinary retention, constipation.

▷ **Possible Adverse Effects** (unusual, unexpected and infrequent reactions)
If any of the following develop, consult your physician promptly for guidance.
Mild Adverse Effects
Allergic Reactions: Skin rash, hives, itching.
Dizziness, impaired concentration, sensation of drunkenness, confusion, depression, blurred or double vision, facial flushing, sweating.
Nausea, vomiting.
Serious Adverse Effects
Allergic Reactions: Anaphylaxis (rare), severe skin reactions.
Idiosyncratic Reactions: Delirium, hallucinations, excitement, increased sensitivity to pain after the analgesic effect has worn off.
Seizures (rare), impaired breathing.

▷ **Possible Effects on Sexual Function:** None reported.

▷ **Adverse Effects That May Mimic Natural Diseases or Disorders**
Paradoxical behavioral disturbances may suggest psychotic disorder.

Possible Effects on Laboratory Tests
Blood amylase and lipase levels: increased (natural side-effect).
Urine screening tests for drug abuse: *initial* test result may be falsely **positive**; *confirmatory* test result will be **negative**. (Test results depend upon amount of drug taken and testing method used.)

CAUTION
1. If you have asthma, chronic bronchitis or emphysema, the excessive use of this drug may cause significant respiratory difficulty, thickening of bronchial secretions and suppression of coughing.
2. The concurrent use of this drug with atropinelike drugs can increase the risk of urinary retention and reduced intestinal function.
3. Do not take this drug following acute head injury.

Precautions for Use
By Infants and Children: Do not use this drug in children under 2 years of age because of their vulnerability to life-threatening respiratory depression.
By Those over 60 Years of Age: Use small doses initially and increase dosage as needed and tolerated. Limit use to short-term treatment only. There may be increased susceptibility to the development of drowsiness, dizziness, unsteadiness, falling, urinary retention and constipation (often leading to fecal impaction).

▷ **Advisability of Use During Pregnancy**
Pregnancy Category: C (tentative). See Pregnancy Code inside back cover.

Animal studies: Birth defects reported in hamster studies.

Human studies: Information from adequate studies of pregnant women is not available. Hydrocodone taken repeatedly during the last few weeks before delivery may cause withdrawal symptoms in the newborn infant.

Use this drug only if clearly needed and in small, infrequent doses.

Advisability of Use if Breast-Feeding
Presence of this drug in breast milk: Unknown.

Monitor nursing infant closely and discontinue drug or nursing if adverse effects develop. Ask physician for guidance.

Habit-Forming Potential: Psychological and/or physical dependence can develop with use of large doses for an extended period of time. However, true dependence is infrequent and unlikely with prudent use.

Effects of Overdosage: Drowsiness, restlessness, agitation, nausea, vomiting, dry mouth, vertigo, weakness, lethargy, stupor, coma, seizures.

Possible Effects of Long-Term Use: Psychological and physical dependence, chronic constipation.

Suggested Periodic Examinations While Taking This Drug (at physician's discretion)
None.

▷ **While Taking This Drug, Observe the Following**
Foods: No restrictions.
Beverages: No restrictions. May be taken with milk.
▷   *Alcohol:* Use extreme caution until the combined effects have been determined. Hydrocodone can intensify the intoxicating effects of alcohol, and alcohol can intensify the depressant effects of hydrocodone on brain function, breathing and circulation.
Tobacco Smoking: No interactions expected.
Marijuana Smoking: Increase in drowsiness and pain relief; impairment of mental and physical performance.
▷   *Other Drugs*
Hydrocodone may *increase* the effects of
• other drugs with sedative effects.
• atropinelike drugs, and increase the risk of constipation and urinary retention.
▷   *Driving, Hazardous Activities:* This drug can impair mental alertness, judgment, reaction time and physical coordination. Avoid hazardous activities accordingly.
Aviation Note: The use of this drug *is a disqualification* for piloting. Consult a designated Aviation Medical Examiner.
Exposure to Sun: No restrictions.
Discontinuation: It is advisable to limit this drug to short-term use. If it is necessary to use it for extended periods of time, discontinuation should be gradual to minimize possible effects of withdrawal (usually mild with this drug).

HYDROXYCHLOROQUINE
(hi drox ee KLOR oh kwin)

Introduced: 1967

Class: Antimalarial, lupus suppressant, rheumatoid arthritis suppressant

Prescription: USA: Yes
Canada: Yes

Controlled Drug: USA: No
Canada: No

Available as Generic: USA: No
Canada: No

Brand Name: Plaquenil

BENEFITS versus RISKS

Possible Benefits	*Possible Risks*
EFFECTIVE PREVENTION AND TREATMENT OF CERTAIN FORMS OF MALARIA	INFREQUENT BUT SERIOUS DAMAGE OF CORNEAL AND RETINAL EYE TISSUES
Possibly effective in the management of acute and chronic rheumatoid arthritis and juvenile arthritis	RARE BUT SERIOUS BONE MARROW DEPRESSION: aplastic anemia, deficient white blood cells and platelets
Possibly effective in the management of chronic discoid and systemic lupus erythematosus	Rare heart muscle damage
	Rare ear damage: hearing loss, ringing in ears

▷ **Principal Uses**

As a Single Drug Product: Used primarily to (1) suppress the development of and to treat acute attacks of certain types of malarial infection; (2) reduce disease activity in rheumatoid and juvenile arthritis; (3) suppress disease activity in chronic discoid and systemic lupus erythematosus. It is also used in the treatment of sarcoidosis, polymorphous light eruption, porphyria, solar urticaria and chronic vasculitis.

How This Drug Works: Not completely established. As an anti-infective in treating malaria, it is thought that this drug binds to and impairs the function of DNA in the protozoa that cause this disease.

As an antiarthritic and antilupus drug, it is thought to act as a mild immunosuppressant. It accumulates in white blood cells and inhibits many enzymes involved in tissue destruction.

Available Dosage Forms and Strengths

Tablets — 200 mg

▷ **Usual Adult Dosage Range:**   For malaria suppression: 400 mg once every 7 days.

For malaria treatment: (1) 800 mg as a single dose; or (2) initially 800 mg, followed by 400 mg in 6 to 8 hours; then 400 mg once a day on the second and third days.

For rheumatoid arthritis: Up to 6.5 mg per kilogram of lean body weight daily.

For lupus erythematosus: Up to 6.5 mg per kilogram of lean body weight daily. **Note: Actual dosage and administration schedule must be determined by the physician for each patient individually.**

▷ **Dosing Instructions:**   Take with food or milk to reduce stomach irritation. The tablet may be crushed and mixed with jam, jelly or jello for administration. Take full course of treatment as prescribed.

Note: For malaria prevention, begin medication 2 weeks before entering malarious area; continue medication while in the area and for 4 weeks after leaving the area. For treating arthritis and lupus, take medication on a regular schedule daily; continual use for 6 months may be necessary to determine maximal benefit.

Usual Duration of Use:

Continual use on a regular schedule for 2 weeks before exposure, during period of exposure, and 4 weeks after exposure is usually necessary to determine this drug's effectiveness in preventing attacks of malaria. Continual use on a regular schedule for periods up to 6 months may be required to evaluate the potential benefits in reducing the activity of rheumatoid arthritis and lupus erythematosus. If significant improvement is not achieved within this time, this drug should be discontinued. Long-term use (months to years) requires periodic evaluation of response and dosage adjustment. Consult your physician on a regular basis.

Possible Advantages of This Drug

Considered to have less potential for retinal toxicity than chloroquine.

Currently a "Drug of Choice"

for the treatment of chronic discoid and systemic lupus erythematosus.

▷ **This Drug Should Not Be Taken If**
- you have had an allergic reaction to either chloroquine or hydroxychloroquine previously.
- you have an active bone marrow or blood cell disorder.

▷ **Inform Your Physician Before Taking This Drug If**
- you are pregnant or planning pregnancy.
- you have a history of bone marrow depression or a blood cell disorder previously.
- you have a deficiency of glucose-6-phosphate dehydrogenase.
- you have any disorder of the eyes, especially disease of the cornea or retina, or visual field changes.

- you have impaired hearing or ringing in the ears.
- you have a seizure disorder of any kind.
- you have a history of peripheral neuritis.
- you have low blood pressure or a heart rhythm disorder.
- you have a history of peptic ulcer disease, Crohn's disease or ulcerative colitis.
- you have impaired liver or kidney function.
- you have a history of porphyria.
- you have any form of psoriasis.
- you are taking antacids, cimetidine, digoxin or penicillamine.

Possible Side-Effects
(natural, expected and unavoidable drug actions)
Light-headedness (low blood pressure); blue-black discoloration of skin, fingernails, or mouth lining with long-term use.

▷ **Possible Adverse Effects**
(unusual, unexpected and infrequent reactions)
If any of the following develop, consult your physician promptly for guidance.
Mild Adverse Effects
Allergic Reactions: Skin rash, itching (more common in Afro-Americans).
Loss of hair color, loss of hair.
Headache, blurring of near vision (reading), ringing in ears.
Loss of appetite, nausea, vomiting, stomach cramps, diarrhea.
Serious Adverse Effects
Allergic Reactions: Severe skin rash, exfoliative dermatitis.
Idiosyncratic Reactions: Hemolytic anemia in those with glucose-6-phosphate dehydrogenase deficiency in red blood cells.
Emotional or psychotic mental changes; seizures.
Loss of hearing.
Excessive muscle weakness.
Eye tissue damage, specifically cornea and retina, with significant impairment of vision.
Heart rhythm abnormalities.
Aplastic anemia (see Glossary): abnormally low red blood cell counts (fatigue and weakness), abnormally low white blood cell counts (fever, sore throat, infections), abnormally low platelet counts (abnormal bruising or bleeding).

▷ **Possible Effects on Sexual Function:**   None reported.

Possible Delayed Adverse Effects: Irreversible retinal damage has developed 7 years after discontinuation of chloroquine, a closely related drug. Retinal damage is more likely to occur following high-dose and/ or long-term use.

▷ **Adverse Effects That May Mimic Natural Diseases or Disorders**
Central nervous system toxicity may suggest unrelated neuropsychiatric disorder. Seizures may suggest the onset of epilepsy.

Natural Diseases or Disorders That May Be Activated by This Drug
Porphyria, psoriasis.

Possible Effects on Laboratory Tests
Complete blood cell counts: decreased red cells, hemoglobin, white cells and platelets.
Liver function tests: increased liver enzymes (ALT/GPT, AST/GOT and alkaline phosphatase), increased bilirubin.
Electrocardiogram: conduction abnormalities, prolonged QRS interval, T wave changes, heart block have all been reported for chloroquine, a closely related drug.

CAUTION
1. This drug does not prevent relapses in certain types of malaria. Consult your physician regarding this.
2. High-dose and/or long-term use of this drug may cause irreversible retinal damage and significant impairment of vision; such use may also cause hearing loss due to nerve damage. Report promptly any changes in vision or hearing so appropriate evaluation can be made.

Precautions for Use
By Infants and Children: This age group is very sensitive to the effects of this drug. Dosages should be determined and therapy should be monitored by a qualified pediatrician.
By Those over 60 Years of Age: Tolerance for this drug during high-dose and/or long-term use may be reduced. Observe for behavioral changes, low blood pressure, heart rhythm disturbances, muscle weakness and changes in vision or hearing.

▷ **Advisability of Use During Pregnancy**
Pregnancy Category: D (tentative). See Pregnancy Code inside back cover.
Animal studies: No information available.
Human studies: Information from adequate studies of pregnant women is not available. However, closely related drugs of this class are known to cause abnormal retinal pigmentation and hemorrhage and congenital deafness in the fetus.
Avoid use during pregnancy except for the suppression or treatment of malaria.

Advisability of Use if Breast-Feeding
Presence of this drug in breast milk: Yes.
Avoid drug or refrain from nursing.

Habit-Forming Potential: None.

Effects of Overdosage: Drowsiness, headache, blurred vision, excitability, low blood pressure, seizures, coma.

Possible Effects of Long-Term Use: Irreversible eye damage (cornea and retina), hearing loss, muscle weakness, aplastic anemia.

Suggested Periodic Examinations While Taking This Drug
(atphysician's discretion)
Complete blood cell counts; liver and kidney function tests.
Serial blood pressure readings and electrocardiograms.
Neurological examinations for significant muscle weakness.
Complete eye examinations before starting high-dose and/or long-term treatment and every 3 to 6 months during drug use.
Hearing tests as indicated.

▷ **While Taking This Drug, Observe the Following**
Foods: No restrictions.
Beverages: No restrictions. May be taken with milk.
▷ *Alcohol:* Use sparingly to minimize stomach irritation.
Tobacco Smoking: No interactions expected.
▷ *Other Drugs*
Hydroxychloroquine may *increase* the effects of
• digoxin (Lanoxin), and increase its toxic potential.
• penicillamine (Cuprimine, Depen), and increase its toxic potential.
The following drug may *increase* the effects of hydroxychloroquine
• cimetidine (Tagamet).
The following drugs may *decrease* the effects of hydroxychloroquine
• magnesium salts and antacids.
▷ *Driving, Hazardous Activities:* This drug may cause light-headedness, blurred vision or impaired hearing. Restrict activities as necessary.
Aviation Note: The use of this drug **may be a disqualification** for piloting. Consult a designated Aviation Medical Examiner.
Exposure to Sun: Use caution until sensitivity has been determined. Closely related drugs of this class may cause photosensitivity (see Glossary).
Discontinuation: This drug should be discontinued and prompt evaluation should be made if any of the following develop: any changes in vision or hearing, seizures, unusual muscle weakness, indications of infection (fever, sore throat, etc.), abnormal bruising or bleeding.

HYDROXYZINE
(hi DROX i zeen)

Introduced: 1953

Class: Mild tranquilizer, antihistamines

Prescription: USA: Yes
Canada: Yes

Controlled Drug: USA: No
Canada: No

Available as Generic: USA: Yes
Canada: No

Brand Names: ✦Apo-Hydroxyzine, Atarax, Marax [CD], Marax DF [CD], ✦Multipax, Vistaril, Vistrax [CD]

BENEFITS versus RISKS

Possible Benefits	*Possible Risks*
EFFECTIVE RELIEF OF ITCHING DUE TO HIVES	Mild atropinelike effects
Moderately effective relief of itching due to allergic skin disorders	Potentiation of other sedative drugs
Moderately effective relief of mild to moderate anxiety and nervous tension	Impaired control of seizure disorders (epilepsy)

▷ **Principal Uses**

As a Single Drug Product: Used primarily as a mild tranquilizer to relieve anxiety and nervous tension, whether occurring independently or in association with a physical disorder. Also used frequently to relieve itching due to allergic skin conditions.

As a Combination Drug Product [CD]: Combined with antispasmodic drugs, this drug helps to allay the anxiety that is conducive to functional disorders of the gastrointestinal tract. Combined with ephedrine and theophylline (bronchodilator drugs), this drug controls the anxiety that is often associated with bronchial spasm in asthma, bronchitis and emphysema.

How This Drug Works: Not completely established. It is thought that this drug may reduce excessive activity in those brain systems that determine the emotional state.

Available Dosage Forms and Strengths

Capsules — 25 mg, 50 mg, 100 mg
Injection — 25 mg per ml, 50 mg per ml
Oral suspension — 25 mg per 5-ml teaspoonful
Syrup — 10 mg per 5-ml teaspoonful
Tablets — 10 mg, 25 mg, 50 mg, 100 mg

▷ **Usual Adult Dosage Range:**   25 to 100 mg 3 or 4 times daily. The total daily dosage should not exceed 600 mg. **Note: Actual dosage and administration schedule must be determined by the physician for each patient individually.**

▷ **Dosing Instructions:**   May be taken without regard to eating. The tablet may be crushed and the capsule may be opened for administration.

Usual Duration of Use: Continual use on a regular schedule for 1 to 3 weeks is usually necessary to determine this drug's effectiveness in relieving anxiety and tension. Relief of itching is usually apparent in 2 to 3 days. Duration of use as a tranquilizer should not exceed 4 months without reappraisal of continued need. Consult your physician on a regular basis.

▷ **This Drug Should Not Be Taken If**
   • you have had an allergic reaction to any dosage form of it previously.

▷ **Inform Your Physician Before Taking This Drug If**
   • you have a seizure disorder (epilepsy).
   • you have prostatism (see Glossary).
   • you are taking any drugs with sedative effects.
   • you plan to have surgery under general anesthesia in the near future.

Possible Side-Effects (natural, expected and unavoidable drug actions)
   Drowsiness (may subside with continued use); "hangover" effect if taken at bedtime for sleep; dry mouth.

▷ **Possible Adverse Effects** (unusual, unexpected and infrequent reactions)
   If any of the following develop, consult your physician promptly for guidance.
   Mild Adverse Effects
   Allergic Reaction: Itching.
   Headache.
   Serious Adverse Effects
   Idiosyncratic Reactions: Involuntary movements, tremors, seizures (with excessive dosage).

▷ **Possible Effects on Sexual Function:**   None reported.

Natural Diseases or Disorders That May Be Activated by This Drug
   Latent epilepsy.

Possible Effects on Laboratory Tests
   Prothrombin time: increased.

CAUTION
   1. This drug can cause excessive sedation if taken concurrently with other sedative drugs.
   2. Use very cautiously if you have a seizure disorder. This drug may increase the frequency of seizures.

3. If pregnancy occurs, discontinue this drug immediately and inform your physician.

Precautions for Use
By Infants and Children: Observe for evidence of excessive sedation.
By Those over 60 Years of Age: There may be increased susceptibility to the development of drowsiness, dizziness and lethargy, and to impairment of thinking, judgment and memory. A pattern of underactivity may be misinterpreted as senility or emotional depression. Observe also for orthostatic hypotension and prostatism (see Glossary).

▷ Advisability of Use During Pregnancy
Pregnancy Category: C (tentative). See Pregnancy Code inside back cover.
Animal studies: Facial bone defects reported in mice, rats and dogs.
Human studies: Information from adequate studies of pregnant women is not available.
Avoid completely during the first 3 months. During the last 6 months, use only if clearly needed. Ask physician for guidance.

Advisability of Use if Breast-Feeding
Presence of this drug in breast milk: Yes.
Monitor nursing infant closely and discontinue drug or nursing if adverse effects (sedation, poor feeding) develop.

Habit-Forming Potential: None.

Effects of Overdosage: Drowsiness, unsteadiness, dry mouth, delirium, stupor, tremors, seizures.

Possible Effects of Long-Term Use: Loss of drug effectiveness due to development of tolerance (see Glossary).

Suggested Periodic Examinations While Taking This Drug (at physician's discretion)
None required.

▷ While Taking This Drug, Observe the Following
Foods: No restrictions.
Beverages: Avoid large amounts of caffeine-containing beverages: coffee, tea, cola, chocolate. May be taken with milk.
▷ *Alcohol:* Use with extreme caution until the combined effects have been determined. Alcohol can increase the sedative action of hydroxyzine. Hydroxyzine can increase the intoxicating effect of alcohol.
Tobacco Smoking: No interactions expected.
Marijuana Smoking: Increased sedative effects.
▷ *Other Drugs*
Hydroxyzine may *increase* the effects of
• ketamine (intravenous anesthetic), and prolong the recovery time.
• other drugs with sedative effects, and cause excessive sedation.
Hydroxyzine may *decrease* the effects of

- phenothiazines (see Drug Class, Section Four), and reduce their antipsychotic effectiveness.
▷ *Driving, Hazardous Activities:* This drug may impair mental alertness, judgment, coordination and reaction time. Restrict activities as necessary.
  Aviation Note: The use of this drug *is a disqualification* for piloting. Consult a designated Aviation Medical Examiner.
  Exposure to Sun: No restrictions.

IBUPROFEN
(i BYU proh fen)

Introduced: 1969

Class: Mild analgesic, antiinflammatory

Prescription: USA: Varies
Canada: Yes

Controlled Drug: USA: No
Canada: No

Available as Generic: Yes

Brand Names: Advil, ✤Amersol, ✤Apo-Ibuprofen, Children's Advil, CoAdvil [CD], Haltran, Ibuprohm, Ibu-Tab, Medipren, Motrin, Motrin IB, ✤Novoprofen, Nuprin, PediaProfen, Rufen

BENEFITS versus RISKS	
Possible Benefits	*Possible Risks*
EFFECTIVE RELIEF OF MILD TO MODERATE PAIN AND INFLAMMATION	Gastrointestinal pain, ulceration, bleeding (rare)
	Rare kidney damage
	Rare fluid retention
	Rare bone marrow depression (less than 1%)

▷ **Principal Uses**
  As a Single Drug Product: Used primarily to relieve mild to moderately severe pain associated with (1) musculoskeletal injuries; (2) acute and chronic gout, rheumatoid arthritis and osteoarthritis; (3) dental, obstetrical and orthopedic surgery; (4) menstrual cramps; (5) vascular (migrainelike) headaches; and (6) to reduce fever.

How This Drug Works: Not completely established. It is thought that this drug reduces the tissue concentrations of prostaglandins (and related compounds), chemicals involved in the production of inflammation and pain.

Available Dosage Forms and Strengths
Caplets — 200 mg

Oral suspension — 100 mg per 5-ml teaspoonful
Tablets — 200 mg, 300 mg, 400 mg, 600 mg, 800 mg

▷ **Usual Adult Dosage Range:** 200 to 800 mg 3 or 4 times/day. Total daily dosage should not exceed 3200 mg (3600 mg in selected individuals). **Note: Actual dosage and administration schedule must be determined by the physician for each patient individually.**

▷ **Dosing Instructions:** Take either on an empty stomach or with food or milk to prevent stomach irritation. Take with a full glass of water and remain upright (do not lie down) for 30 minutes. The tablet may be crushed for administration.

Usual Duration of Use: Continual use on a regular schedule for 1 to 2 weeks is usually necessary to determine this drug's effectiveness in relieving the discomfort of arthritis. Long-term use requires supervision and periodic evaluation by the physician. Consult your physician on a regular basis.

▷ **This Drug Should Not Be Taken If**
- you have had an allergic reaction to it previously.
- you are subject to asthma or nasal polyps caused by aspirin.
- you have active peptic ulcer disease or any form of gastrointestinal bleeding.
- you have a bleeding disorder or a blood cell disorder.
- you have severe impairment of kidney function.

▷ **Inform Your Physician Before Taking This Drug If**
- you are allergic to aspirin or to other aspirin substitutes.
- you have a history of peptic ulcer disease or any type of bleeding disorder.
- you have impaired liver or kidney function.
- you have high blood pressure or a history of heart failure.
- you are taking any of the following: acetaminophen, aspirin or other aspirin substitutes, anticoagulants, oral antidiabetic drugs.

Possible Side-Effects (natural, expected and unavoidable drug actions)
Fluid retention (weight gain); pink, red, purple or rust coloration of urine (of no significance).

▷ **Possible Adverse Effects** (unusual, unexpected and infrequent reactions)
If any of the following develop, consult your physician promptly for guidance.
Mild Adverse Effects
Allergic Reactions: Skin rash, hives, itching.
Headache, dizziness, altered or blurred vision, ringing in the ears, depression.
Mouth sores, indigestion, nausea, vomiting, constipation, diarrhea.
Serious Adverse Effects
Allergic Reactions: Anaphylaxis (see Glossary), severe skin reactions.

Idiosyncratic Reactions: Drug-induced meningitis with fever and coma.
Active peptic ulcer, with or without bleeding.
Liver damage with jaundice (see Glossary).
Kidney damage with painful urination, bloody urine, reduced urine formation.
Rare bone marrow depression (see Glossary)—fatigue, weakness, fever, sore throat, abnormal bleeding or bruising.

▷ **Possible Effects on Sexual Function**
Altered timing and pattern of menstruation (30%); excessive menstrual bleeding.
Male breast enlargement and tenderness.

Possible Delayed Adverse Effects: Mild anemia due to "silent" blood loss from the stomach (less than that caused by aspirin).

▷ **Adverse Effects That May Mimic Natural Diseases or Disorders**
Liver reaction may suggest viral hepatitis.

Natural Diseases or Disorders That May Be Activated by This Drug
Peptic ulcer disease, ulcerative colitis.

Possible Effects on Laboratory Tests
Complete blood cell counts: decreased red cells, hemoglobin, white cells and platelets.
Blood cholesterol level: increased.
Blood lithium level: increased.
Blood uric acid level: increased.
Liver function tests: increased liver enzymes (ALT/GPT, AST/GOT and alkaline phosphatase), increased bilirubin.
Kidney function tests: increased blood creatinine and urea nitrogen (BUN) levels.
Fecal occult blood test: positive.

CAUTION
1. Dosage should always be limited to the smallest amount that produces reasonable improvement.
2. This drug may mask early indications of infection. Inform your physician if you think you are developing an infection of any kind.

Precautions for Use
By Infants and Children: Safety and effectiveness for use by those under 12 years of age have not been established.
By Those over 60 Years of Age: Small doses are advisable until tolerance is determined. Observe for any indications of liver or kidney toxicity, fluid retention, dizziness, confusion, impaired memory, stomach bleeding or constipation.

▷ **Advisability of Use During Pregnancy**
Pregnancy Category: B (tentative). See Pregnancy Code inside back cover.

Animal studies: No birth defects reported in rats or rabbits.

Human studies: Information from adequate studies of pregnant women is not available.

Avoid this drug during the last 3 months. Use it during the first 6 months only if clearly needed. Ask physician for guidance.

The manufacturer does not recommend the use of this drug during pregnancy.

Advisability of Use if Breast-Feeding

Presence of this drug in breast milk: Yes, in minute amounts.

Avoid drug or refrain from nursing.

Habit-Forming Potential: None.

Effects of Overdosage: Drowsiness, dizziness, ringing in the ears, nausea, vomiting, diarrhea, confusion, unsteadiness, stupor progressing to coma.

Possible Effects of Long-Term Use: Fluid retention.

Suggested Periodic Examinations While Taking This Drug (at physician's discretion)

Complete blood cell counts, liver and kidney function tests, complete eye examinations if vision is altered in any way.

▷ **While Taking This Drug, Observe the Following**

Foods: No restrictions.

Beverages: No restrictions. May be taken with milk.

▷ *Alcohol:* Use with caution. The irritant action of alcohol on the stomach lining, added to the irritant action of this drug in sensitive individuals, can increase the risk of stomach ulceration and/or bleeding.

Tobacco Smoking: No interactions expected.

▷ *Other Drugs*

Ibuprofen may *increase* the effects of

- acetaminophen (Tylenol, etc.), and increase the risk of kidney damage; avoid prolonged use of this combination.
- anticoagulants (Coumadin, etc.), and increase the risk of bleeding; monitor prothrombin time, adjust dose accordingly.

Ibuprofen *taken concurrently* with the following drugs may increase the risk of bleeding; avoid these combinations:

- aspirin.
- dipyridamole (Persantine).
- indomethacin (Indocin).
- sulfinpyrazone (Anturane).
- valproic acid (Depakene).

▷ *Driving, Hazardous Activities:* This drug may cause drowsiness or dizziness. Restrict activities as necessary.

Aviation Note: The use of this drug *may be a disqualification* for piloting. Consult a designated Aviation Medical Examiner.

Exposure to Sun: Use caution until sensitivity is determined. Questionable photosensitivity (see Glossary) has been reported.

IMIPRAMINE
(im IP ra meen)

Introduced: 1955

Class: Antidepressant

Prescription: USA: Yes
Canada: Yes

Controlled Drug: USA: No
Canada: No

Available as Generic: USA: Yes
Canada: Yes

Brand Names: ✦Apo-Imipramine, ✦Impril, Janimine, ✦Novopramine, ✦PMS Imipramine, Tipramine, Tofranil, Tofranil-PM,

---

BENEFITS versus RISKS

Possible Benefits	*Possible Risks*
EFFECTIVE RELIEF OF NEUROTIC AND PSYCHOTIC DEPRESSIVE STATES of various causes and degree	ADVERSE BEHAVIORAL EFFECTS: confusion, delirium, disorientation, hallucinations, delusions
EFFECTIVE TREATMENT FOR CHILDHOOD BEDWETTING (enuresis)	CONVERSION OF DEPRESSION TO MANIA in manic-depressive disorders
Possibly effective in the management of chronic, severe pain; in aiding cocaine withdrawal; in relieving symptoms of attention deficit disorder; in preventing panic attacks; in controlling binge eating and purging in bulimia	Aggravation of schizophrenia and paranoia
	Induction of serious heart rhythm abnormalities
	Abnormally low white blood cell and platelet counts (rare)

▷ **Principal Uses**

As a Single Drug Product: Used primarily to (1) relieve severe emotional depression and to initiate gradual restoration of normal mood; (2) aid in the prevention of childhood bedwetting in children over 6 years of age. It is also being used as indicated above (see Possible Benefits).

How This Drug Works: Not completely established. It is thought that by increasing brain tissue concentrations of certain nerve impulse transmitters (norepinephrine and serotonin), this drug relieves the symptoms associated with depression. Beneficial effects in treating bedwetting are thought to be due partially to this drug's atropinelike action.

Available Dosage Forms and Strengths
Capsules — 75 mg, 100 mg, 125 mg, 150 mg
Injection — 25 mg per 2 ml
Tablets — 10 mg, 25 mg, 50 mg, 75 mg

▷ **Usual Adult Dosage Range:**　Initially 75 mg daily, divided into 3 doses. Dose may be increased cautiously as needed and tolerated by 10 mg to 25 mg daily at intervals of 1 week. The usual maintenance dose is 50 mg to 150 mg/24 hours. The total daily dosage should not exceed 200 mg for outpatient therapy. (When determined, the optimal daily requirement may be given at bedtime as a single dose.) **Note: Actual dosage and administration schedule must be determined by the physician for each patient individually.**

▷ **Dosing Instructions:**　May be taken without regard to meals. If necessary, may be taken with food to reduce stomach irritation. The capsule may be opened and the tablet may be crushed for administration. Note: Tofranil-PM capsules should not be used to treat childhood bedwetting.

Usual Duration of Use:

Continual use on a regular schedule for 3 to 4 weeks is usually necessary to determine this drug's effectiveness in relieving depression; optimal response may require 3 or more months of use. Long-term use (months to years) requires periodic evaluation of response and dosage adjustment. Consult your physician on a regular basis.

Possible Advantages of This Drug

Less likely to increase the heart rate than other tricyclic antidepressants. Less hazardous and more easily managed than monoamine oxidase (MAO) inhibitor antidepressants.

Currently a "Drug of Choice"

for adjunctive use in treating childhood bedwetting when organic causes for this disorder have been eliminated.

▷ **This Drug Should Not Be Taken If**
- you have had an allergic reaction to it previously.
- you are taking, or have taken within the past 14 days, any monoamine oxidase (MAO) type A inhibitor drug (see Drug Class, Section Four).
- you have had a recent heart attack (myocardial infarction).
- you have narrow-angle glaucoma.

▷ **Inform Your Physician Before Taking This Drug If**
- you have had an adverse reaction to any other antidepressant drug.
- you have any type of seizure disorder.
- you have increased internal eye pressure.
- you have any type of heart disease, especially coronary artery disease or a heart rhythm disorder.
- you are subject to bronchial asthma.
- you have impaired liver or kidney function.
- you have any type of thyroid disorder or are taking thyroid medication.
- you have diabetes or sugar intolerance.
- you have prostatism (see Glossary).
- you have a history of alcoholism.
- you plan to have surgery under general anesthesia in the near future.

Possible Side-Effects
(natural, expected and unavoidable drug actions)
Moderate drowsiness, light-headedness (low blood pressure), blurred vision, dry mouth, constipation, impaired urination.

▷ **Possible Adverse Effects**
(unusual, unexpected and infrequent reactions)
If any of the following develop, consult your physician promptly for guidance.
Mild Adverse Effects
Allergic Reactions: Skin rash, hives, swelling of face or tongue, drug fever (see Glossary).
Headache, dizziness, nervousness, weakness, unsteadiness, tremors, fainting.
Increased appetite, weight gain.
Irritation of tongue or mouth, altered taste, indigestion, nausea.
Fluctuations of blood sugar.
Serious Adverse Effects
Allergic Reactions: Drug-induced hepatitis, with or without jaundice; anaphylactoid reaction (see terms in Glossary).
Idiosyncratic Reactions: Neuroleptic malignant syndrome (see Glossary).
Adverse behavioral effects: confusion, delirium, disorientation, delusions, hallucinations.
Seizures; reduced control of epilepsy.
Aggravation of paranoid psychoses and schizophrenia.
Heart rhythm disturbances.
Abnormally low white blood cell and platelet counts: fever, sore throat, infections, abnormal bleeding or bruising.

▷ **Possible Effects on Sexual Function**
Decreased libido, increased libido (antidepressant effect), impaired erection (43%), impaired ejaculation (28%), impotence, inhibited male orgasm (20%), inhibited female orgasm (27%), male breast enlargement and tenderness, female breast enlargement with milk production, swelling of testicles.

▷ **Adverse Effects That May Mimic Natural Diseases or Disorders**
Liver toxicity may suggest viral hepatitis.

Natural Diseases or Disorders That May Be Activated by This Drug
Latent diabetes, epilepsy, glaucoma, prostatism.

Possible Effects on Laboratory Tests
Complete blood cell counts: decreased white cells and platelets; increased eosinophils (allergic reaction).
Blood glucose levels: increased and decreased (fluctuations).
Liver function tests: increased liver enzymes (ALT/GPT, AST/GOT and alkaline phosphatase), increased bilirubin.

CAUTION

1. Observe for early indications of toxicity or overdosage: confusion, agitation, rapid heart rate, heart irregularity. Measurement of the blood level of the drug will clarify the situation.
2. Use with caution in treating depression associated with schizophrenia. Observe closely for any deterioration of thinking or behavior.
3. It is advisable to withhold this drug if electroconvulsive therapy is to be used to treat the depression in the near future.

Precautions for Use

By Infants and Children

: Safety and effectiveness for use by those under 6 years of age have not been established. Recent experience indicates that children (6 to 12 years of age) may be more susceptible than adults to heart toxicity from this and related drugs. Dosage and management should be supervised by a properly trained pediatrician.

By Those over 60 Years of Age: Initiate treatment with 25 mg at bedtime. Dosage may be increased gradually as needed and tolerated to 100 mg daily in divided doses. During the first 2 weeks of treatment, observe for behavioral reactions: restlessness, agitation, forgetfulness, disorientation, delusions or hallucinations. Also observe for unsteadiness and instability that may predispose to falling. This drug may aggravate prostatism.

▷ **Advisability of Use During Pregnancy**

Pregnancy Category: C (tentative). See Pregnancy Code inside back cover.

Animal studies: Skeletal defects reported in rabbit studies. No defects reported in mouse, rat and monkey studies.

Human studies: Information from adequate studies of pregnant women is not available. Use only if clearly needed. Avoid use during the first 3 months.

Advisability of Use if Breast-Feeding

Presence of this drug in breast milk: Yes, in small amounts.

Monitor nursing infant closely and discontinue drug or nursing if adverse effects develop.

Habit-Forming Potential: Psychological or physical dependence is rare and unexpected. This drug is not liable to abuse.

Effects of Overdosage: Confusion, hallucinations, drowsiness, tremors, heart irregularity, seizures, stupor, hypothermia (see Glossary) early, fever later.

Possible Effects of Long-Term Use: Neuroleptic malignant syndrome (see Glossary): fever, fast or irregular heartbeat, fast breathing, sweating, weakness, muscle stiffness, seizures, loss of bladder control.

Suggested Periodic Examinations While Taking This Drug (at physician's discretion)

Monitoring of blood drug levels as appropriate.

Complete blood cell counts; liver and kidney function tests.
Serial blood pressure readings and electrocardiograms.
Measurement of internal eye pressure.

▷ **While Taking This Drug, Observe the Following**

Foods: No specific restrictions. May need to limit food intake to avoid excessive weight gain.

Beverages: No restrictions. May be taken with milk.

▷ *Alcohol:* Avoid completely. This drug can markedly increase the intoxicating effects of alcohol; the combination can depress brain function significantly.

Tobacco Smoking: May accelerate the elimination of this drug and require increased dosage.

Marijuana Smoking: Increased drowsiness and mouth dryness; possible reduced effectiveness of this drug.

▷ *Other Drugs*

Imipramine may *increase* the effects of
- all drugs with sedative effects; observe for excessive sedation.
- all drugs with atropinelike effects (see Drug Class, Section Four).

Imipramine may *decrease* the effects of
- clonidine (Catapres).
- guanadrel (Hylorel).
- guanethidine (Ismelin, Esimil).

Imipramine *taken concurrently* with
- anticonvulsants requires careful monitoring for changes in seizure patterns and need to adjust anticonvulsant dosage.
- ethchlorvynol (Placidyl) may cause delirium; avoid concurrent use.
- monoamine oxidase (MAO) type A inhibitor drugs (see Drug Class, Section Four) may cause high fever, seizures and excessive rise in blood pressure; avoid concurrent use of these drugs and provide periods of 14 days between administration of either.
- stimulant drugs (amphetamine, cocaine, epinephrine, phenylpropanolamine, etc.) may cause severe high blood pressure and/or high fever.
- thyroid preparations may increase the risk of heart rhythm disorders.

The following drugs may *increase* the effects of imipramine
- cimetidine (Tagamet).
- estrogens.
- fluoxetine (Prozac)
- methylphenidate (Ritalin).
- oral contraceptives.
- phenothiazines (see Drug Class, Section Four).
- ranitidine (Zantac).

The following drugs may *decrease* the effects of imipramine
- barbiturates (see Drug Class, Section Four).
- carbamazepine (Tegretol).
- chloral hydrate (Noctec, Somnos, etc.).
- lithium (Lithobid, Lithotab, etc.).
- reserpine (Serpasil, Ser-Ap-Es, etc.).

▷ *Driving, Hazardous Activities:* This drug may impair mental alertness, judgment, physical coordination and reaction time. Restrict activities as necessary.

Aviation Note: The use of this drug **is a disqualification** for piloting. Consult a designated Aviation Medical Examiner.

Exposure to Sun: Use caution until sensitivity has been determined. This drug may cause photosensitivity (see Glossary).

Exposure to Heat: Use caution. This drug can inhibit sweating and impair the body's adaptation to hot environments, increasing the risk of heat stroke. Avoid saunas.

Exposure to Cold: The elderly should use caution and avoid conditions conducive to hypothermia (see Glossary).

Exposure to Environmental Chemicals: This drug may mask the symptoms of poisoning due to handling certain insecticides (organophosphorus types). Read their labels carefully.

Discontinuation: It is advisable to discontinue this drug gradually over a period of 3 to 4 weeks. Abrupt withdrawal after prolonged use may cause nausea, vomiting, diarrhea, headache, malaise, disturbed sleep and vivid dreaming. When this drug is stopped, it may be necessary to adjust the dosages of other drugs taken concurrently.

INDAPAMIDE
(in DAP a mide)

Introduced: 1974

Class: Antihypertensive, diuretic

Prescription: USA: Yes
Canada: Yes

Controlled Drug: USA: No
Canada: No

Available as Generic: No

Brand Names: ✦Lozide, Lozol

BENEFITS versus RISKS	
Possible Benefits	*Possible Risks*
EFFECTIVE ONCE-A-DAY TREATMENT OF MILD TO MODERATE HYPERTENSION	Excessive loss of blood potassium (14%)
EFFECTIVE, MILD DIURETIC	Increased blood sugar level
	Increased blood uric acid level

▷ **Principal Uses**

As a Single Drug Product: Used primarily to (1) increase the volume of urine (diuresis) to correct the excessive fluid retention associated with congestive heart failure; and (2) initiate treatment for high blood pressure (hypertension). It may be the first drug tried in treating mild to moderate hypertension.

How This Drug Works: By increasing the elimination of salt and water from the body (through increased urine production), this drug reduces the volume of fluid in the blood and body tissues and lowers the sodium content throughout the body. By relaxing the walls of smaller arteries and allowing them to expand, this drug increases the total capacity of the arterial system. The combined effect of these two actions (reduced blood volume in expanded space) results in lowering of blood pressure.

Available Dosage Forms and Strengths
Tablets — 2.5 mg

▷ **Usual Adult Dosage Range:** Initially 2.5 mg/day, taken as single dose in the morning. If necessary, the dose may be increased to 5 mg/day after 1 week (for diuresis) or after 4 weeks (for hypertension). The total daily dosage should not exceed 5 mg. (In Canada, the total daily dosage limit is given as 2.5 mg.) **Note: Actual dosage and administration schedule must be determined by the physician for each patient individually.**

▷ **Dosing Instructions:** May be taken with or following food to reduce stomach irritation. Best taken in the morning to avoid nighttime urination. The tablet may be crushed for administration.

Usual Duration of Use: Continual use on a regular schedule for 2 to 4 weeks is usually necessary to determine this drug's effectiveness in lowering high blood pressure. Long-term use (months to years) requires periodic evaluation of response and possible dosage adjustment. Use as a diuretic should be intermittent with "drug holidays" (no drug taken) to reduce the risk of sodium and potassium imbalance. Consult your physician on a regular basis.

Possible Advantages of This Drug
Causes no significant increase in blood cholesterol levels.
Less likely to cause significant loss of potassium.

▷ **This Drug Should Not Be Taken If**
• you have had an allergic reaction to it previously.

▷ **Inform Your Physician Before Taking This Drug If**
• you are allergic to any form of "sulfa" drug.
• you are pregnant or planning pregnancy.
• you have a history of kidney or liver disease.
• you have diabetes, gout or lupus erythematosus.
• you are taking any form of cortisone, digitalis, oral antidiabetic drug or insulin.
• you plan to have surgery under general anesthesia in the near future.

Possible Side-Effects (natural, expected and unavoidable drug actions)
Light-headedness on arising from sitting or lying position (see Orthostatic Hypotension in Glossary).
Increase in blood sugar level, affecting control of diabetes.

Increase in blood uric acid level, affecting control of gout.

Decrease in blood potassium level, causing muscle weakness and cramping.

▷ **Possible Adverse Effects** (unusual, unexpected and infrequent reactions)
If any of the following develop, consult your physician promptly for guidance.
Mild Adverse Effects
Allergic Reactions: Skin rashes, hives, itching.
Headache, dizziness, drowsiness, weakness, lethargy, visual disturbance.
Reduced appetite, indigestion, nausea, vomiting, diarrhea.
Serious Adverse Effects
None reported.

▷ **Possible Effects on Sexual Function:** Decreased libido (4%); impotence (less than 1%).

Natural Diseases or Disorders That May Be Activated by This Drug
Diabetes, gout, systemic lupus erythematosus.

Possible Effects on Laboratory Tests
Blood total cholesterol and LDL cholesterol levels: no effect or slightly increased.
Blood HDL cholesterol level: no effect or slightly decreased.
Blood potassium level: slightly decreased.
Blood uric acid level: increased.

CAUTION

1. Do not exceed recommended doses. Increased dosage can cause excessive loss of sodium and potassium, with resultant loss of appetite, nausea, fatigue, weakness, confusion and tingling in the extremities.
2. If you are also taking a digitalis preparation (digitoxin, digoxin), ensure an adequate intake of high-potassium foods to prevent potassium deficiency—a potential cause of digitalis toxicity. (See Table of High Potassium Foods in Section Six.)

Precautions for Use
By Infants and Children: Safety and effectiveness for use by those under 12 years of age have not been established.
By Those over 60 Years of Age: Small doses are advisable until your individual response has been determined. You may be more susceptible to the development of impaired thinking, orthostatic hypotension, potassium loss and blood sugar increase. Overdosage and extended use of this drug can cause excessive loss of body water, thickening (increased viscosity) of the blood and an increased tendency for the blood to clot—predisposing to stroke, heart attack or thrombophlebitis (vein inflammation with blood clot).

▷ **Advisability of Use During Pregnancy**
Pregnancy Category: B (tentative). See Pregnancy Code inside back cover.

Animal studies: No birth defects reported.

Human studies: Information from adequate studies of pregnant women is not available.

This drug should not be used during pregnancy unless a very serious complication occurs for which this drug is significantly beneficial. Ask physician for guidance.

Advisability of Use if Breast-Feeding
Presence of this drug in breast milk: Unknown.

Avoid drug or refrain from nursing.

Habit-Forming Potential: None.

Effects of Overdosage: Dry mouth, thirst, lethargy, weakness, muscle cramping, nausea, vomiting, drowsiness progressing to stupor or coma.

Possible Effects of Long-Term Use: Impaired balance of water, salt and potassium in blood and body tissues. Development of diabetes in predisposed individuals.

Suggested Periodic Examinations While Taking This Drug (at physician's discretion)
Measurements of blood levels of sodium, potassium, chloride, sugar and uric acid.

▷ **While Taking This Drug, Observe the Following**

Foods: Consult your physician regarding the advisability of eating foods rich in potassium. If so advised, see the Table of High Potassium Foods in Section Six. Follow physician's advice regarding the use of salt.

Beverages: No restrictions. This drug may be taken with milk.

▷ *Alcohol:* Use with caution until the combined effects have been determined. Alcohol may exaggerate the blood-pressure-lowering effects of this drug and cause orthostatic hypotension.

Tobacco Smoking: No interactions expected. Follow physician's advice.

▷ *Other Drugs*

Indapamide may *increase* the effects of

- other antihypertensive drugs; dosage adjustments may be necessary to prevent excessive lowering of blood pressure.
- lithium, and cause lithium toxicity.

Indapamide may *decrease* the effects of

- oral antidiabetic drugs (sulfonylureas); dosage adjustments may be necessary for proper control of blood sugar.

Indapamide *taken concurrently* with

- digitalis preparations (digitoxin, digoxin) requires very careful monitoring and dosage adjustments to prevent fluctuations of blood potassium levels and serious disturbances of heart rhythm.

The following drugs may *decrease* the effects of indapamide

- cholestyramine (Cuemid, Questran) may interfere with its absorption.

• colestipol (Colestid) may interfere with its absorption.
Take cholestyramine and colestipol 1 hour before any oral diuretic.

▷ *Driving, Hazardous Activities:* Use caution until the possible occurrence of orthostatic hypotension, drowsiness, dizziness or impaired vision has been determined.

Aviation Note: The use of this drug **may be a disqualification** for piloting. Consult a designated Aviation Medical Examiner.

Exposure to Sun: No restrictions.

Exposure to Heat: Avoid excessive perspiring, which could cause additional loss of salt and water from the body.

Heavy Exercise or Exertion: Avoid exertion that produces light-headedness, excessive fatigue or muscle cramping. Isometric exercises—the "overload" technique for strengthening individual muscles—can raise blood pressure significantly. Ask physician for guidance regarding participation in this form of exercise.

Occurrence of Unrelated Illness: Illnesses that cause vomiting or diarrhea can produce a serious imbalance of important body chemistry. Consult your physician for guidance.

Discontinuation: It may be advisable to discontinue this drug 5 to 7 days before major surgery. Ask your physician, surgeon and/or anesthesiologist for guidance regarding dosage adjustment or drug withdrawal.

INDOMETHACIN
(in doh METH a sin)

Introduced: 1963

Class: Mild analgesic, anti-inflammatory

Prescription: USA: Yes
Canada: Yes

Controlled Drug: USA: No
Canada: No

Available as Generic: USA: Yes
Canada: No

Brand Names: ✦Apo-Indomethacin, Indameth, ✦Indocid, ✦Indocid PDA, Indocin, Indocin-SR, ✦Novomethacin

BENEFITS versus RISKS	
Possible Benefits	*Possible Risks*
EFFECTIVE RELIEF OF MILD TO MODERATE PAIN AND INFLAMMATION	Gastrointestinal pain, ulceration, bleeding (rare)
	Rare liver or kidney damage
	Rare fluid retention
	Rare bone marrow depression
	Mental depression, confusion

▷ **Principal Uses**

As a Single Drug Product: Used primarily to relieve mild to moderately severe pain associated with (1) musculoskeletal injuries; (2) acute and chronic gout, rheumatoid arthritis and osteoarthritis; (3) dental, obstetrical and orthopedic surgery; (4) menstrual cramps; and (5) vascular (migrainelike) headaches.

How This Drug Works: Not completely established. It is thought that this drug reduces the tissue concentrations of prostaglandins (and related compounds), chemicals involved in the production of inflammation and pain.

Available Dosage Forms and Strengths

Capsules — 25 mg, 50 mg, 75 mg

Capsules, prolonged-action — 75 mg

Oral suspension — 25 mg per 5-ml teaspoonful

Suppositories — 50 mg

▷ **Usual Adult Dosage Range:** For arthritis and related conditions: 25 to 50 mg 2 to 4 times daily. If needed and tolerated, dose may be increased by 25 or 50 mg/day at intervals of 1 week. For acute gout: 100 mg initially; then 50 mg 3 times/day until pain is relieved. Total daily dosage should not exceed 200 mg. **Note: Actual dosage and administration schedule must be determined by the physician for each patient individually.**

▷ **Dosing Instructions:** Take with or following food to prevent stomach irritation. Take with a full glass of water and remain upright (do not lie down) for 30 minutes. The regular capsule may be opened for administration, but not the prolonged-action capsule.

Usual Duration of Use: Continual use on a regular schedule for 1 to 2 weeks is usually necessary to determine this drug's effectiveness in relieving the discomfort of arthritis. The usual length of treatment for bursitis or tendinitis is 7 to 14 days. Long-term use requires supervision and periodic evaluation by the physician. Consult your physician on a regular basis.

▷ **This Drug Should Not Be Taken If**

- you have had an allergic reaction to it previously.
- you are subject to asthma or nasal polyps caused by aspirin.
- you are pregnant or breast-feeding.
- you have active peptic ulcer disease or any form of gastrointestinal ulceration or bleeding.
- you have a bleeding disorder or a blood cell disorder.
- you have severe impairment of kidney function.

▷ **Inform Your Physician Before Taking This Drug If**

- you are allergic to aspirin or to other aspirin substitutes.

- you have a history of peptic ulcer disease, Crohn's disease, ulcerative colitis or any type of bleeding disorder.
- you have a history of epilepsy, Parkinson's disease or mental illness (psychosis).
- you have impaired liver or kidney function.
- you have high blood pressure or a history of heart failure.
- you are taking any of the following: acetaminophen, aspirin or other aspirin substitutes, anticoagulants, oral antidiabetic drugs.

Possible Side-Effects (natural, expected and unavoidable drug actions)
Drowsiness, ringing in ears, fluid retention.

▷ **Possible Adverse Effects** (unusual, unexpected and infrequent reactions)
If any of the following develop, consult your physician promptly for guidance.
Mild Adverse Effects
Allergic Reactions: Skin rash, hives, itching, localized swellings of face and/or extremities.
Headache, dizziness, feelings of detachment.
Mouth sores, indigestion, nausea, vomiting, diarrhea.
Temporary loss of hair.
Serious Adverse Effects
Allergic Reactions: Asthma, difficult breathing, mouth irritation.
Blurred vision, confusion, depression.
Active peptic ulcer, with or without bleeding.
Liver damage with jaundice (see Glossary).
Kidney damage with painful urination, bloody urine, reduced urine formation.
Rare bone marrow depression (see Glossary)—fatigue, weakness, fever, sore throat, abnormal bleeding or bruising.
Peripheral neuritis (see Glossary)—numbness, pain or weakness in extremities.

▷ **Possible Effects on Sexual Function**
Enlargement and tenderness of both male and female breasts.
Nonmenstrual vaginal bleeding.

Possible Delayed Adverse Effects: Mild anemia due to "silent" blood loss from the stomach (less than that caused by aspirin).

▷ **Adverse Effects That May Mimic Natural Diseases or Disorders**
Liver reaction may suggest viral hepatitis.

Natural Diseases or Disorders That May Be Activated by This Drug
Peptic ulcer disease, ulcerative colitis.

Possible Effects on Laboratory Tests
Complete blood cell counts: decreased red cells, hemoglobin, white cells and platelets.

Prothrombin time: increased.

Blood lithium level: increased.

Liver function tests: increased liver enzymes (ALT/GPT, AST/GOT and alkaline phosphatase), increased bilirubin.

Kidney function tests: increased blood creatinine and urea nitrogen (BUN) levels (kidney damage).

Fecal occult blood test: positive.

CAUTION

1. Dosage should always be limited to the smallest amount that produces reasonable improvement.
2. This drug may mask early indications of infection. Inform your physician if you think you are developing an infection of any kind.

Precautions for Use

By Infants and Children: This drug frequently causes impairment of kidney function in infants. Fatal liver reactions have occurred in children between 6 and 12 years of age; avoid the use of this drug in this age group.

By Those over 60 Years of Age: Adverse effects are very common in this age group. Small doses are advisable until tolerance is determined. Observe for any indications of liver or kidney toxicity, fluid retention, dizziness, confusion, impaired memory, depression, peptic ulcer or diarrhea, often with rectal bleeding.

▷ **Advisability of Use During Pregnancy**

Pregnancy Category: D (tentative). See Pregnancy Code inside back cover.

Animal studies: Significant toxicity and birth defects reported in mice and rats.

Human studies: Information from adequate studies of pregnant women is not available. However, birth defects have been attributed to the use of this drug during pregnancy.

The manufacturer recommends that this drug not be taken during pregnancy.

Advisability of Use if Breast-Feeding

Presence of this drug in breast milk: Yes.

Avoid drug or refrain from nursing.

The manufacturer recommends that this drug not be taken while breast-feeding.

Habit-Forming Potential: None.

Effects of Overdosage: Drowsiness, agitation, confusion, nausea, vomiting, diarrhea, disorientation, seizures, coma.

Possible Effects of Long-Term Use: Eye changes: deposits in the cornea, alterations in the retina.

Suggested Periodic Examinations While Taking This Drug (at physician's discretion)

Complete blood cell counts, liver and kidney function tests, complete eye examinations if vision is altered in any way.

▷ **While Taking This Drug, Observe the Following**

Foods: No restrictions.

Nutritional Support: Take 50 mg of vitamin C (ascorbic acid) daily.

Beverages: No restrictions. May be taken with milk.

▷ *Alcohol:* Use with caution. The irritant action of alcohol on the stomach lining, added to the irritant action of this drug in sensitive individuals, can increase the risk of stomach ulceration and/or bleeding.

Tobacco Smoking: No interactions expected.

▷ *Other Drugs*

Indomethacin may *increase* the effects of

- acetaminophen (Tylenol, etc.), and increase the risk of kidney damage; avoid prolonged use of this combination.
- anticoagulants (Coumadin, etc.), and increase the risk of bleeding; monitor prothrombin time, adjust dose accordingly.
- lithium, and cause lithium toxicity.

Indomethacin may *decrease* the effects of

- beta blocker drugs (see Drug Class, Section Four), and reduce their antihypertensive effectiveness.
- bumetanide (Bumex).
- captopril (Capoten).
- ethacrynic acid (Edecrin).
- furosemide (Lasix).

Indomethacin *taken concurrently* with the following drugs may increase the risk of bleeding; avoid these combinations:

- aspirin.
- diflunisal (Dolobid).
- dipyridamole (Persantine).
- sulfinpyrazone (Anturane).
- valproic acid (Depakene).

▷ *Driving, Hazardous Activities:* This drug may cause drowsiness, dizziness or impaired vision. Restrict activities as necessary.

Aviation Note: The use of this drug *may be a disqualification* for piloting. Consult a designated Aviation Medical Examiner.

Exposure to Sun: No restrictions.

INSULIN
(IN suh lin)

Introduced: 1922

Class: Antidiabetic

Prescription: USA: No
Canada: No

Controlled Drug: USA: No
Canada: No

Available as Generic: Yes

Brand Names: Humulin BR, Humulin L, Humulin N, Humulin R, Humulin U, Humulin U Ultralente, Humulin 70/30, Iletin I NPH, ✦Initard, Insulatard NPH, ✦Insulin-Toronto, Lente Iletin I, Lente Iletin II Beef, Lente Iletin II Pork, Lente Insulin, Mixtard, Mixtard Human 70/30, Novolin L, Novolin N, NovolinPen, Novolin R, ✦Novolin-Lente, ✦Novolin-NPH, ✦Novolin-30/70, ✦Novolin-Toronto, ✦Novolin-Ultralente, NPH Iletin I, NPH Iletin II Beef, NPH Iletin II Pork, NPH Insulin, NPH Purified Pork, Protamine, Zinc & Iletin I, Protamine, Zinc & Iletin II Beef, Protamine, Zinc & Iletin II Pork, Regular Iletin I, Regular Iletin II Beef, Regular Iletin II Pork, Regular Iletin II U-500, Regular Insulin, Regular Purified Pork Insulin, Semilente Iletin I, Semilente Insulin, Semilente Purified Pork, Ultralente Iletin I, Ultralente Insulin, Ultralente Purified Beef, Velosulin

---

BENEFITS versus RISKS

Possible Benefits	*Possible Risks*
EFFECTIVE CONTROL OF TYPE I (INSULIN-DEPENDENT) DIABETES MELLITUS	HYPOGLYCEMIA WITH EXCESSIVE DOSAGE Infrequent allergic reactions

---

▷ **Principal Uses**

As a Single Drug Product: Insulin is used to control diabetes mellitus in those individuals whose diabetes has been shown to be insulin-dependent. Proper use involves selection of the most appropriate type of insulin for the individual and determination of the optimal dosage schedule for the continuous regulation of blood sugar levels.

How This Drug Works: Not completely established. By direct action on certain cell membranes, insulin facilitates the transport of sugar through the cell wall to the interior of the cell where it is utilized. This occurs primarily in the brain, the voluntary muscles, the heart muscle and the liver.

Available Dosage Forms and Strengths

Injections — 40 units, 100 units, 500 units per ml
PenFil cartridges — 150 units

▷ **Usual Adult Dosage Range:** According to individual requirements for the optimal regulation of blood sugar on a 24-hour basis. **Note: Actual dosage and administration schedule must be determined by the physician for each patient individually.**

▷ **Dosing Instructions:** Inject insulin subcutaneously according to the schedule prescribed by your physician. The timing and frequency of injections will vary with the type of insulin precribed. The following table of insulin actions (according to type) will help you understand the treatment schedule prescribed for you.

Insulin Type	Action Onset	Peak	Duration
Regular	0.5–1 hr	2–4 hrs	5–7 hrs
Isophane (NPH)	3–4 hrs	6–12 hrs	18–28 hrs
Regular 30%/NPH 70%	0.5 hr	4–8 hrs	24 hrs
Semilente	1–3 hrs	2–8 hrs	12–16 hrs
Lente	1–3 hrs	8–12 hrs	18–28 hrs
Ultralente	4–6 hrs	18–24 hrs	36 hrs
Protamine Zinc	4–6 hrs	14–24 hrs	36 hrs

Usual Duration of Use: Type I insulin-dependent (juvenile-onset) diabetes mellitus usually requires insulin treatment for life. Type II noninsulin-dependent (maturity-onset) diabetes is usually controlled by oral antidiabetic drugs and/or diet but may, on occasion, require insulin for adequate control. Such occasions include serious infections, injuries, burns, surgical procedures and other forms of physical stress. Insulin is used as needed on a temporary basis to regulate and normalize the body's use of sugar until recovery is complete and basic health is restored. Consult your physician on a regular basis.

▷ **This Drug Should Not Be Taken If**
  • the need for it and its correct dosage schedule have not been established by a properly qualified physician.

▷ **Inform Your Physician Before Taking This Drug If**
  • you have a history of allergic reaction to any form of insulin on previous use.
  • you do not know how to recognize and treat abnormally low blood sugar (see Hypoglycemia in Glossary).
  • you are taking any of the following drugs: aspirin, beta blockers, fenfluramine (Pondimin), monoamine oxidase (MAO) type A inhibitors (see respective Drug Classes, Section Four).

Possible Side-Effects (natural, expected and unavoidable drug actions)
  In the management of stable diabetes, no side-effects occur when insulin dose, diet and physical activity are correctly balanced and maintained.
  In the management of unstable ("brittle") diabetes, unexpected drops in blood sugar levels can occur, resulting in periods of hypoglycemia (see Glossary).

▷ **Possible Adverse Effects** (unusual, unexpected and infrequent reactions)
If any of the following develop, consult your physician promptly for guidance.
Mild Adverse Effects
Allergic Reactions: Local redness, swelling and itching at site of injection. Occasional hives.
Thinning of subcutaneous tissue at sites of injection.
Serious Adverse Effects
Allergic Reaction: Anaphylactic reactions (see Glossary).
Severe, prolonged hypoglycemia.

▷ **Possible Effects on Sexual Function:**   None reported.

▷ **Adverse Effects That May Mimic Natural Diseases or Disorders**
The early manifestations of hypoglycemia may be mistaken for alcoholic intoxication.

Possible Effects on Laboratory Tests
Blood cholesterol level: decreased.
Blood glucose level: decreased.
Blood potassium level: decreased.

CAUTION
1. It is most important that you carry with you a card of personal identification with a notation that you have diabetes and are taking insulin.
2. Be sure that you know how to recognize the onset of hypoglycemia and how to treat it. Always carry with you a readily available form of sugar, such as hard candy or sugar cubes. Report all episodes of hypoglycemia to your physician; it may be necessary to adjust your insulin dosage or schedule.
3. Improvement in vision may occur during the first several weeks of insulin treatment. It is advisable to defer examination for glasses for 6 weeks after starting insulin.
4. The rates of insulin absorption vary significantly from one anatomic site to another. Absorption is 80% greater from the abdominal wall than from the leg, and 30% greater than from the arm. Individuals with unstable diabetes may achieve better control of blood sugar levels by rotating the injection site within the same anatomic region rather than by rotating from one anatomic region to another.

Precautions for Use
By Infants and Children: Insulin dosages and schedules are modified according to patient size. Adhere strictly to the physician's prescribed routine.
By Those over 60 Years of Age: Insulin requirements may change with aging. Periodic evaluation of individual status is necessary to determine correct insulin dosage and scheduling. The aging brain adapts well to higher blood sugar levels. Attempts to maintain strictly "normal" blood

sugar levels may result in episodes of unrecognized hypoglycemia that is manifested by confusion and abnormal behavior. Repeated episodes of hypoglycemia (especially if severe) in the elderly may cause brain damage.

▷ **Advisability of Use During Pregnancy**
Pregnancy Category: B (tentative). See Pregnancy Code inside back cover. Animal studies: Inconclusive.

Human studies: Information from adequate studies of pregnant women is not available. It is known that birth defects occur 2 to 4 times more frequently in infants of diabetic mothers than in infants of mothers who do not have diabetes. The exact causes of this are not known.

Insulin is the drug of choice for managing diabetes during pregnancy. To preserve the health of the mother and the welfare of the fetus, every effort must be made to establish the optimal dosage of insulin necessary for "good control" and to prevent episodes of hypoglycemia.

Advisability of Use if Breast-Feeding
Presence of this drug in breast milk: No.

Insulin treatment of the mother has no adverse effect on the nursing infant.

Breast-feeding may decrease insulin requirements; dosage adjustment may be necessary.

Habit-Forming Potential: None.

Effects of Overdosage: Hypoglycemia: fatigue, weakness, headache, nervousness, irritability, sweating, tremors, hunger, confusion, delirium, abnormal behavior (resembling alcoholic intoxication), loss of consciousness, seizures.

Possible Effects of Long-Term Use: Thinning of subcutaneous fat tissue at sites of insulin injection.

Suggested Periodic Examinations While Taking This Drug (at physician's discretion)
Monitoring of urine sugar content as a guide to adjustment of diet and insulin dosage. Measurement of blood sugar levels at intervals recommended by physician.

▷ **While Taking This Drug, Observe the Following**
Foods: Follow your prescribed diabetic diet conscientiously. Do not omit snack foods in midafternoon or at bedtime if they are prescribed to prevent hypoglycemia.

Beverages: According to prescribed diabetic diet.
▷ *Alcohol:* Use with caution until the combined effect has been determined. Used excessively, alcohol can induce severe hypoglycemia, resulting in brain damage.

Tobacco Smoking: Regular smoking can decrease insulin absorption and increase insulin requirements by 30%. It is advisable to refrain from smoking altogether.

Marijuana Smoking: Possible increase in blood sugar levels.

▷ *Other Drugs*

The following drugs may *increase* the effects of insulin

- aspirin, and other salicylates.
- some beta blocker drugs (especially the nonselective ones) may prolong insulin-induced hypoglycemia. (See Drug Class, Section Four.)
- fenfluramine (Pondimin).
- monoamine oxidase (MAO) type A inhibitor drugs (see Drug Class, Section Four).

The following drugs may *decrease* the effects of insulin (by raising blood sugar levels)

- chlorthalidone (Hygroton).
- cortisonelike drugs (see Drug Class, Section Four).
- furosemide (Lasix).
- oral contraceptives.
- phenytoin (Dilantin, etc.).
- thiazide diuretics (see Drug Class, Section Four).
- thyroid preparations.

▷ *Driving, Hazardous Activities:* Usually no restrictions. However, be prepared to stop and take corrective action if indications of impending hypoglycemia develop.

Aviation Note: Diabetes and the use of this drug *are disqualifications* for piloting. Consult a designated Aviation Medical Examiner.

Exposure to Sun: No restrictions.

Exposure to Heat: Use caution. Sauna baths can signficantly increase the rate of insulin absorption and cause hypoglycemia.

Heavy Exercise or Exertion: Use caution. Periods of unusual or unplanned heavy physical activity will hasten the utilization of blood sugar and predispose to hypoglycemia.

Occurrence of Unrelated Illness: Report all illnesses that prevent regular eating. The omission of meals as a result of nausea, vomiting or injury may lead to hypoglycemia. Untreated infections can increase insulin requirements. Consult physician for guidance.

Discontinuation: Do not discontinue this drug without consulting your physician. Diabetes that is insulin-dependent requires continual treatment on a regular basis. Omission of insulin may result in life-threatening coma.

Special Storage Instructions: Keep in a cool place, preferably in the refrigerator. Protect from freezing. Protect from strong light and high temperatures when not refrigerated.

Observe the Following Expiration Times: Do not use this drug if it is older than the expiration date on the vial. Always use fresh, "within date" insulin.

IPRATROPIUM
(i pra TROH pee um)

Introduced: 1975

Class: Bronchodilator

Prescription: USA: Yes
Canada: Yes

Controlled Drug: USA: No
Canada: No

Available as Generic: USA: No
Canada: No

Brand Name: Atrovent

BENEFITS versus RISKS

Possible Benefits	*Possible Risks*
EFFECTIVE BRONCHODILATOR FOR TREATMENT OF CHRONIC BRONCHITIS AND EMPHYSEMA Possibly effective as adjunctive treatment in some cases of bronchial asthma	Mild and infrequent adverse effects (see below)

▷ **Principal Uses**

As a Single Drug Product: Used primarily to prevent or relieve episodes of difficult breathing in the maintenance treatment of chronic bronchitis and emphysema. Because of its relatively slow onset of bronchodilation, it should not be used to treat acute attacks of asthma.

How This Drug Works: This drug is a derivative of atropine. Through its atropinelike (anticholinergic) action, it inhibits the effect of acetylcholine on bronchial tube muscles and thereby blocks their constriction throughout the airways. The net result is bronchodilation.

Available Dosage Forms and Strengths

Inhalation aerosol — 14 gram metered dose inhaler; 18 mcg per inhalation

▷ **Usual Adult Dosage Range:** Initially 2 inhalations (36 mcg) 4 times a day, 4 hours apart. If necessary, the dose may be increased to 4 inhalations (80 mcg) at one time to obtain optimal relief. Maintain 4 hour intervals between doses. Total daily dosage should not exceed 12 inhalations (216 mcg). **Note: Actual dosage and administration schedule must be determined by the physician for each patient individually.**

▷ **Dosing Instructions:** Carefully follow the patient instructions provided with the inhaler. Shake well before using.

Usual Duration of Use:
> Continual use on a regular schedule for 48 to 72 hours is usually necessary to determine this drug's effectiveness in achieving sustained relief of difficult breathing associated with chronic bronchitis and emphysema. Long-term use (months to years) requires periodic evaluation of response and dosage adjustment. Consult your physician on a regular basis.

Possible Advantages of This Drug
> Produces a greater degree of bronchodilation than theophylline in patients with chronic bronchitis and emphysema.
> Causes minimal adverse effects.
> Repeated use does not lead to tolerance and loss of effectiveness.
> Suitable for long-term maintenance therapy.

Currently a "Drug of Choice"
> for the management of difficult breathing associated with chronic bronchitis and emphysema.

▷ **This Drug Should Not Be Taken If**
- you have had an allergic reaction to it previously.
- you are allergic to atropine or to aerosol propellants (fluorocarbons).

▷ **Inform Your Physician Before Taking This Drug If**
- you have had an adverse effect from any belladonna derivative previously.
- you have a history of glaucoma.
- you have any form of urinary retention or prostatism (see Glossary).

Possible Side-Effects
(natural, expected and unavoidable drug actions)
Throat dryness (5%), cough (3%), irritation from aerosol (1.6%), blurred vision (1.2%), dry mouth (2.4%), impaired urination (1%).

▷ **Possible Adverse Effects** (unusual, unexpected and infrequent reactions)
> **If any of the following develop, consult your physician promptly for guidance.**
Mild Adverse Effects
Allergic Reactions: Skin rash (1.2%), hives (rare).
Headache (2%), dizziness (1%), nervousness (3%).
Lip and mouth ulcers, unpleasant taste, indigestion (2.4%), nausea (2.8%).
Serious Adverse Effects
None reported.

▷ **Possible Effects on Sexual Function**
None reported.

Natural Diseases or Disorders That May Be Activated by This Drug
Angle-closure glaucoma, prostatism (see Glossary).

Possible Effects on Laboratory Tests
None reported.

CAUTION
1. This drug's onset of action is within 5 to 15 minutes. It should **not** be used alone to treat acute attacks of asthma which require prompt response to medication.
2. When used as an adjunct to beta-adrenergic antiasthmatic drugs (albuterol, terbutaline, metaproterenol, etc.), the beta-adrenergic aerosol should be used approximately 5 minutes before using ipratropium to prevent fluorocarbon toxicity.
3. When used as an adjunct to steroid or cromolyn aerosols (beclomethasone, Intal), ipratropium should be used approximately 5 minutes before using the steroid or cromolyn aerosol to prevent fluorocarbon toxicity.
4. Avoid the accidental spraying of this aerosol into the eyes; temporary blurring of vision may occur.

Precautions for Use
By Infants and Children
: Safety and effectiveness for use by those under 12 years of age have not been established.
By Those over 60 Years of Age: Observe for the possible development of prostatism and adjust dosage as necessary.

▷ **Advisability of Use During Pregnancy**
Pregnancy Category: B (tentative). See Pregnancy Code inside back cover.
Animal studies: No drug-induced birth defects found in mouse, rat or rabbit studies.
Human studies: Information from adequate studies of pregnant women is not available.
Use this drug only if clearly needed.

Advisability of Use if Breast-Feeding
Presence of this drug in breast milk: Possibly yes, but in very small amounts.
Monitor nursing infant closely and discontinue drug or nursing if adverse effects develop.

Habit-Forming Potential: None.

Effects of Overdosage: This drug is not well absorbed into the systemic circulation when it is taken by aerosol inhalation. No systemic effects of overdosage are expected.

Possible Effects of Long-Term Use: No adverse effects reported.

Suggested Periodic Examinations While Taking This Drug
(at physician's discretion)
Internal eye pressure measurements if appropriate.

▷ **While Taking This Drug, Observe the Following**
Foods: No restrictions.
Beverages: No restrictions.
▷ *Alcohol:* No interactions expected.
Tobacco Smoking: No interactions expected. However, smoking should be
avoided completely if you have chronic bronchitis or emphysema.
▷ *Other Drugs*
Ipratropium may *increase* the effects of
• other atropinelike drugs (see Drug Class, Section Four).
▷ *Driving, Hazardous Activities:* This drug may cause dizziness or blurred
vision. Restrict activities as necessary.
Aviation Note: The use of this drug **may be a disqualification** for piloting.
Consult a designated Aviation Medical Examiner.
Exposure to Sun: No restrictions.
Exposure to Cold: Inhaling cold air may cause bronchospasm and induce
asthmatic breathing and cough; dosage adjustment of this drug may be
necessary.
Heavy Exercise or Exertion: This drug is not considered to be consistently
effective in preventing or treating exercise-induced asthma.
Discontinuation: If you plan to discontinue this drug, consult your physi-
cian for guidance. Substitute medication may be advisable.

ISONIAZID
(i soh NI a zid)

Other Names: Isonicotinic acid hydrazide, INH

Introduced: 1956   **Class:** Antitubercular

Prescription: USA: Yes   **Controlled Drug:** USA: No
Canada: Yes   Canada: No

Available as Generic: USA: Yes
Canada: No

Brand Names: ✦Isotamine, Laniazid, Nydrazid, P-I-N Forte [CD], ✦PMS
Isoniazid, Rifamate [CD], Rimactane/INH Dual Pack [CD], Teebaconin, Teebaconin and Vitamin B-6 [CD]

```
┌─────────────────────────────────────────────────────────────┐
│                    BENEFITS versus RISKS                      │
│                                                               │
│      Possible Benefits              Possible Risks            │
│   EFFECTIVE PREVENTION AND      ALLERGIC LIVER REACTION       │
│     TREATMENT OF ACTIVE           (1% to 2%)                  │
│     TUBERCULOSIS                  Peripheral neuropathy (see  │
│                                     Glossary)                 │
│                                   Bone marrow depression (see │
│                                     Glossary)                 │
│                                   Mental and behavioral       │
│                                     disturbances              │
└─────────────────────────────────────────────────────────────┘
```

▷ **Principal Uses**

As a Single Drug Product: Used alone to prevent the development of active tuberculous infection in individuals who are considered to be at high risk because of known exposure to infection or recent conversion of a negative tuberculin skin test to positive.

As a Combination Drug Product [CD]: This drug is available in combination with rifampin, another antitubercular drug that has a different mechanism of action. This combination is more effective than either drug used alone. Isoniazid can cause deficiency of pyridoxine (vitamin B-6); for this reason, a combination of the two drugs is available in tablet form.

How This Drug Works: Not completely established. It is thought that this drug destroys susceptible tuberculosis organisms by interfering with several of their essential metabolic activities and by disrupting their cell wall.

Available Dosage Forms and Strengths
Injection — 100 mg per ml
Syrup — 50 mg per 5-ml teaspoonful
Tablets — 50 mg, 100 mg, 300 mg

▷ **Usual Adult Dosage Range:**   For prevention: 300 mg once daily. For treatment: 5 mg per kilogram of body weight daily. The total daily dosage should not exceed 600 mg. **Note: Actual dosage and administration schedule must be determined by the physician for each patient individually.**

▷ **Dosing Instructions:**   May be taken with food to prevent stomach irritation. The tablet may be crushed for administration.

Usual Duration of Use: Continual use on a regular schedule for 1 or more years is often necessary, depending upon the nature of the infection. Shorter courses of intermittent high dosage may be adequate in some cases. Consult your physician on a regular basis.

▷ **This Drug Should Not Be Taken If**
- you have had an allergic reaction (especially a liver reaction) to any dosage form of it previously.
- you have active liver disease.

▷ **Inform Your Physician Before Taking This Drug If**
- you have serious impairment of liver or kidney function.
- you drink an alcoholic beverage daily.
- you have a seizure disorder.
- you are taking any other drugs on a long-term basis, especially phenytoin (Dilantin).
- you plan to have surgery under general anesthesia in the near future.

Possible Side-Effects (natural, expected and unavoidable drug actions)
None.

▷ **Possible Adverse Effects** (unusual, unexpected and infrequent reactions)
If any of the following develop, consult your physician promptly for guidance.
Mild Adverse Effects
Allergic Reactions: Skin rash, fever, swollen glands, painful muscles and joints.
Dizziness, indigestion, nausea, vomiting.
Serious Adverse Effects
Allergic Reactions: Drug-induced hepatitis (see Glossary): loss of appetite, nausea, fatigue, fever, itching, dark-colored urine, yellow discoloration of eyes and skin.
Peripheral neuritis (see Glossary): numbness, tingling, pain, weakness in hands and/or feet.
Acute mental and behavioral disturbances, impaired vision, increase in epileptic seizures.
Bone marrow depression (see Glossary): fatigue, weakness, fever, sore throat, abnormal bleeding or bruising.

▷ **Possible Effects on Sexual Function:**   Male breast enlargement and tenderness.

Possible Delayed Adverse Effects: An increase in the frequency of cirrhosis of the liver has been reported.

▷ **Adverse Effects That May Mimic Natural Diseases or Disorders**
Drug-induced hepatitis may suggest viral hepatitis.

Natural Diseases or Disorders That May Be Activated by This Drug
Latent epilepsy, systemic lupus erythematosus (questionable).

Possible Effects on Laboratory Tests
Complete blood cell counts: decreased red cells, hemoglobin, white cells and platelets; increased eosinophils (allergic reaction).
Blood amylase level: increased (possible pancreatitis).

Blood antinuclear antibodies (ANA): positive.

Blood lupus erythematosus (LE) cells: positive.

Blood glucose level: increased (with large doses).

Liver function tests: increased liver enzymes (ALT/GPT, AST/GOT and alkaline phosphatase), increased bilirubin.

Urine sugar tests: increased; false positive results with Benedict's solution and Clinitest.

CAUTION

1. Consult your physician regarding the advisability of determining if you are a "slow" or "rapid" inactivator (acetylator) of isoniazid. This has a bearing on your predisposition to developing adverse effects from this drug.

2. Copper sulfate tests for urine sugar may give a false positive test result. (Diabetics please note.)

Precautions for Use

By Infants and Children: Use with caution in children with seizure disorders. "Slow acetylators" are more prone to adverse drug effects. It is advisable to give supplemental pyridoxine (vitamin B-6).

By Those over 60 Years of Age: There is a greater incidence of liver damage in this age group; the liver status should be monitored carefully. Observe for any indications of an "acute brain syndrome" consisting of confusion, delirium and seizures.

▷ **Advisability of Use During Pregnancy**

Pregnancy Category: C (tentative). See Pregnancy Code inside back cover.

Animal studies: No birth defects reported in mice, rats or rabbits.

Human studies: Information from adequate studies of pregnant women is not available.

Earlier reports of human birth defects due to this drug have not been substantiated by later studies. If clearly needed, this drug is now used at any time during pregnancy. Ask your physician for guidance.

Advisability of Use if Breast-Feeding

Presence of this drug in breast milk: Yes.

Avoid drug or refrain from nursing.

Habit-Forming Potential: None.

Effects of Overdosage: Nausea, vomiting, dizziness, blurred vision, hallucinations, slurred speech, stupor, coma, seizures.

Possible Effects of Long-Term Use: Peripheral neuritis due to a deficiency of pyridoxine (vitamin B-6).

Suggested Periodic Examinations While Taking This Drug (at physician's discretion)

Complete blood cell counts, liver function tests, complete eye examinations.

▷ **While Taking This Drug, Observe the Following**

Foods: Eat the following foods cautiously until your tolerance is determined: Swiss and Cheshire cheeses, tuna fish, skipjack fish and Sardinella species. These may interact with the drug to produce skin rash, itching, sweating, chills, headache, light-headedness or rapid heart rate.

Nutritional Support: It is advisable to take a supplement of pyridoxine (vitamin B-6) to prevent peripheral neuritis. Ask your physician for dosage.

Beverages: No restrictions. May be taken with milk.

▷ *Alcohol:* Avoid completely or use very sparingly. Alcohol may reduce the effectiveness of this drug and increase the risk of liver toxicity.

Tobacco Smoking: No interactions expected.

▷ *Other Drugs*

Isoniazid may *increase* the effects of
- carbamazepine (Tegretol), and cause toxicity.
- phenytoin (Dilantin), and cause toxicity.

The following drugs may *decrease* the effects of isoniazid
- cortisonelike drugs (see Drug Class, Section Four).

▷ *Driving, Hazardous Activities:* Usually no restrictions. This drug may cause dizziness. Restrict activities as necessary.

Aviation Note: The use of this drug *may be a disqualification* for piloting. Consult a designated Aviation Medical Examiner.

Exposure to Sun: No restrictions.

Discontinuation: Long-term treatment is required. Do not discontinue this drug without consulting your physician.

ISOSORBIDE DINITRATE
(i soh SOHR bide di NI trayt)

Other Name: Sorbide nitrate

Introduced: 1959

Class: Antianginal, nitrates

Prescription: USA: Yes
Canada: No

Controlled Drug: USA: No
Canada: No

Available as Generic: USA: Yes
Canada: No

Brand Names: ✦Apo-ISDN, ✦Coronex, Dilatrate-SR, Isonate, Isordil, Isordil Tembids, Isordil Titradose, ✦Novosorbide, Sorbitrate

Warning: The brand names Isordil and Isuprel are similar and can be mistaken for each other; this can lead to serious medication errors. These names represent very different drugs. Isordil (white, yellow, blue, green tablets) is the generic drug isosorbide dinitrate; it is used to treat angina. Isuprel (a glosset tablet for dissolving in the mouth) is the generic drug isoproterenol; it is a bronchodilator used to treat asthma. Verify that you are taking the correct drug.

BENEFITS versus RISKS

Possible Benefits

EFFECTIVE RELIEF AND
PREVENTION OF ANGINA
EFFECTIVE ADJUNCTIVE
TREATMENT IN SELECTED
CASES OF CONGESTIVE
HEART FAILURE

Possible Risks

Orthostatic hypotension (see
Glossary)
Rare skin reactions (severe
peeling)

▷ **Principal Uses**

As a Single Drug Product: The sublingual (under-the-tongue) tablets and the chewable tablets are used to prevent and to relieve acute attacks of anginal pain. The longer-acting tablets and capsules are used to prevent the development of angina, but are not effective in relieving acute episodes of anginal pain. This drug is also used to improve heart function in selected cases of congestive heart failure.

How This Drug Works: By direct action on the muscle in blood vessel walls, this drug relaxes and dilates both arteries and veins. It is thought that its beneficial effects in treating angina and heart failure are due to (1) dilation of coronary arteries, and (2) dilation of systemic veins with consequent reduction of volume and pressure of blood in the heart. The net effects are improved blood flow to the heart muscle and reduced workload of the heart.

Available Dosage Forms and Strengths

Capsules — 40 mg
Capsules, prolonged-action — 40 mg
Tablets — 5 mg, 10 mg, 20 mg, 30 mg, 40 mg
Tablets, chewable — 5 mg, 10 mg
Tablets, prolonged-action — 40 mg
Tablets, sublingual — 2.5 mg, 5 mg, 10 mg

▷ **Usual Adult Dosage Range**

Sublingual tablets: 5 to 10 mg dissolved under tongue every to 3 hours; use for relief of acute attack and for prevention of anticipated attack.

Chewable tablets: Initially, 5 mg chewed to evaluate tolerance; increase dose to 5 or 10 mg every 2 to 3 hours as needed and tolerated; use for relief of acute attack and for prevention of anticipated attack.

Tablets: 5 to 30 mg 4 times daily to prevent acute attack; usual dose is 10 to 20 mg 4 times/day.

Prolonged-action capsules and tablets: 40 mg/6 to 12 hours as needed to prevent acute attacks.

The total daily dosage should not exceed 120 mg.**Note: Actual dosage and administration schedule must be determined by the physician for each patient individually.**

▷ **Dosing Instructions:**   Capsules and tablets to be swallowed are best taken on an empty stomach to achieve maximal blood levels. Regular tablets may be crushed for administration; prolonged-action capsules and tablets should be taken whole and not altered.

Usual Duration of Use: Continual use on a regular schedule for 3 to 7 days is usually necessary to (1) determine this drug's effectiveness in preventing or relieving acute anginal pain, and (2) establish the optimal dosage shedule. Long-term use (months to years) requires supervision and periodic evaluation by your physician. Consult your physician on a regular basis.

▷ **This Drug Should Not Be Taken If**
  • you have had an allergic reaction to any dosage form of it previously.
  • you have had a very recent heart attack (myocardial infarction).

▷ **Inform Your Physician Before Taking This Drug If**
  • you have had an unfavorable response to other nitrate drugs or vasodilators in the past.
  • you have a history of low blood pressure.
  • you have any form of glaucoma.

Possible Side-Effects (natural, expected and unavoidable drug actions)
  Flushing of face, throbbing in head, palpitation, rapid heart rate, orthostatic hypotension (see Glossary).

▷ **Possible Adverse Effects** (unusual, unexpected and infrequent reactions)
  If any of the following develop, consult your physician promptly for guidance.
  Mild Adverse Effects
  Allergic Reaction: Skin rash.
  Headache (may be severe and persistent), dizziness, fainting.
  Nausea, vomiting.
  Serious Adverse Effects
  Allergic Reaction: Severe dermatitis with peeling of skin.
  Transient ischemic attacks (TIAs) in presence of impaired circulation within the brain: dizziness, fainting, impaired vision or speech, localized numbness or weakness.

▷ **Possible Effects on Sexual Function:**   None reported.

▷ **Adverse Effects That May Mimic Natural Diseases or Disorders**
  Spells of low blood pressure (due to this drug) may be mistaken for late-onset epilepsy.

Possible Effects on Laboratory Tests
  None reported.

CAUTION
  1. The development of tolerance (see Glossary) to long-acting forms of nitrates may render the sublingual tablets of nitroglycerin less effec-

tive for the relief of acute anginal attacks. Antianginal effectiveness is restored after 1 week of abstinence from long-acting nitrates.

2. Many over-the-counter (OTC) medications for allergies, colds and coughs contain drugs that may counteract the desired effects of this drug. Ask your physician or pharmacist for guidance before using such medications.

Precautions for Use

By Those over 60 Years of Age: Small doses are advisable until your tolerance has been determined. You may be more susceptible to the development of low blood pressure and associated "blackout" spells, fainting and falling. Throbbing headaches and flushing may be more apparent.

▷ **Advisability of Use During Pregnancy**

Pregnancy Category: C (tentative). See Pregnancy Code inside back cover.
Animal studies: No information available.
Human studies: Information from adequate studies of pregnant women is not available.
Use this drug only if clearly needed.

Advisability of Use if Breast-Feeding

Presence of this drug in breast milk: Unknown.
If drug is thought to be necessary, monitor the nursing infant for low blood pressure and poor feeding.

Habit-Forming Potential: None.

Effects of Overdosage: Headache, dizziness, marked flushing of face and skin, vomiting, weakness, fainting, difficult breathing, coma.

Possible Effects of Long-Term Use: Development of tolerance with temporary loss of effectiveness at recommended doses. Development of abnormal hemoglobin (red blood cell pigment).

Suggested Periodic Examinations While Taking This Drug (at physician's discretion)

Measurement of internal eye pressure. Red blood cell counts and hemoglobin evaluation.

▷ **While Taking This Drug, Observe the Following**

Foods: No restrictions.
Beverages: No restrictions. May be taken with milk.

▷ *Alcohol:* Use extreme caution until the combined effects have been determined. Avoid alcohol completely in the presence of any side-effects or adverse effects of this drug. Alcohol may exaggerate the blood-pressure-lowering effect of this drug.

Tobacco Smoking: Nicotine can reduce the effectiveness of this drug. Avoid all forms of tobacco.

Marijuana Smoking: Possible reduced effectiveness of this drug; mild to moderate increase in angina; possible changes in electrocardiogram, confusing interpretation.

▷ *Other Drugs*
   Isosorbide dinitrate *taken concurrently* with
   • antihypertensive drugs may cause excessive lowering of blood pressure; dosage adjustments may be necessary.
▷ *Driving, Hazardous Activities:* Usually no restrictions. This drug may cause dizziness or spells of low blood pressure. Restrict activities as necessary.
   Aviation Note: Coronary artery disease *is a disqualification* for piloting. Consult a designated Aviation Medical Examiner.
   Exposure to Sun: No restrictions.
   Exposure to Heat: Use caution. Hot environments can cause significant drop in blood pressure.
   Exposure to Cold: Cold environments can increase the need for this drug and limit its effectiveness.
   Heavy Exercise or Exertion: This drug may improve your ability to be more active without anginal pain. Use caution and avoid excessive exertion.
   Discontinuation: It is advisable to withdraw this drug gradually after long-term use. The dosage and frequency of prolonged-action dosage forms should be reduced gradually over period of 4 to 6 weeks.

ISOTRETINOIN
(i soh TRET i noin)

Introduced: 1979

Class: Antiacne

Prescription: USA: Yes
Canada: Yes

Controlled Drug: USA: No
Canada: No

Available as Generic: No

Brand Name: Accutane

BENEFITS versus RISKS	
Possible Benefits	*Possible Risks*
EFFECTIVE TREATMENT OF SEVERE CYSTIC ACNE	MAJOR BIRTH DEFECTS
	Initial worsening of acne (transient)
	Inflammation of lips (90%)
	Dry skin, nose and mouth
	Musculoskeletal discomfort
	Corneal opacities (rare)

▷ **Principal Uses**
   As a Single Drug Product: This drug is reserved to treat severe, disfiguring nodular and cystic acne that has failed to respond to all other forms of standard therapy. *It should not be used to treat mild forms of*

acne. It is also used to treat some less common conditions of the skin that are due to disorders of keratin production.

How This Drug Works: Not completely established. By an unknown action, this drug reduces the size of sebaceous glands and inhibits their production of sebum (skin oil). This helps to correct the major feature of acne and its complications.

Available Dosage Forms and Strengths
Capsules — 10 mg, 20 mg, 40 mg

▷ **Usual Adult Dosage Range:**   Initial dosage is individualized according to the patient's weight and the severity of the acne; the usual dose is 1 to 2 mg per kilogram of body weight daily, taken in 2 divided doses for 15 to 20 weeks. After weeks of treatment, the dose should be adjusted according to the response of the acne and the development of adverse effects. **Note: Actual dosage and administration schedule must be determined by the physician for each patient individually.**

▷ **Dosing Instructions:**   Begin treatment only on the second or third day of your next normal menstrual period. Take with meals (morning and evening) to achieve optimal blood levels. The capsule should not be opened for administration.

Usual Duration of Use: Continual use on a regular schedule for 15 to 20 weeks is usually necessary to determine this drug's effectiveness in clearing or improving severe cystic acne. The drug may be discontinued earlier if the total cyst count is reduced by more than 70%. If a repeat course of treatment is necessary, it should not be started until after a period of 2 months without this drug. Long-term use (months to years) requires supervision and periodic evaluation by your physician. Consult your physician on a regular basis.

▷ **This Drug Should Not Be Taken If**
 • you have had an allergic reaction to it previously.
 • you are allergic to parabens, additives that are used to preserve the drug product.
 • you are pregnant, or planning pregnancy.

▷ **Inform Your Physician Before Taking This Drug If**
 • you have had an allergic reaction to any form of vitamin A in the past.
 • you have diabetes mellitus.
 • you have a cholesterol or triglyceride disorder.
 • you have a history of liver or kidney disease.

Possible Side-Effects (natural, expected and unavoidable drug actions)
Dryness of the nose and mouth (80%), inflammation of the lips (90%), dryness of the skin with itching (80%), peeling of the palms and soles (5%).

▷ **Possible Adverse Effects** (unusual, unexpected and infrequent reactions)
   If any of the following develop, consult your physician promptly for guidance.
   Mild Adverse Effects
   Allergic Reaction: Skin rash (less than 10%).
   Thinning of hair, conjunctivitis, intolerance of contact lenses, decreased night vision, muscular and joint aches, headache, fatigue, indigestion.
   Serious Adverse Effects
   Skin infections, worsening of arthritis, inflammatory bowel disorders.
   Abnormal acceleration of bone development in children.
   Development of opacities in the cornea of the eye.
   Reduced red blood cell and white blood cell counts; increased blood platelet count.
   Increased pressure within the head, with associated headache, visual disturbances, nausea and vomiting.
   Drug-induced hepatitis.

▷ **Possible Effects on Sexual Function**
   Decreased male libido (7%), decreased female libido (13%) beginning after 1 month of drug use.
   Impotence (3%) beginning after 3 months of drug use.
   Decreased vaginal secretions (43%).
   Altered timing and pattern of menstruation (22%).
   Female breast discharge (rare).

Possible Effects on Laboratory Tests
   Complete blood cell counts: infrequently decreased red cells and white cells.
   Blood total cholesterol, LDL cholesterol, VLDL cholesterol and triglyceride levels: increased.
   Blood HDL cholesterol levels: decreased.
   Blood thyroid hormones (T^3, T^4 and free T^4 index): decreased.
   Liver function tests: infrequently increased liver enzymes (ALT/GPT, AST/GOT and alkaline phosphatase), increased bilirubin.

CAUTION
   1. This drug should not be used to treat mild forms of acne.
   2. A transient worsening of your acne may occur during the first few weeks of treatment; this will subside with continued use of the drug.
   3. Do not take any other form of vitamin A while taking this drug. (Observe contents of multiple vitamin preparations.)
   4. Women with potential for pregnancy should have a ***blood*** pregnancy test within 2 weeks before taking this drug and should use 2 effective forms of contraception simultaneously during its use. It is recommended that contraception be continued until normal menstruation resumes after discontinuing this drug.
   5. This drug may cause increased blood levels of cholesterol and triglycerides.

6. If repeated courses of this drug are prescribed, wait a minimum of 2 months between courses before resuming medication.

Precautions for Use

By Infants and Children: Long-term use (6 to 12 months) may cause abnormal acceleration of bone growth and development. Your physician can monitor this possibility by periodic X-ray examination of long bones.

▷ **Advisability of Use During Pregnancy**

Pregnancy Category: X. See Pregnancy Code inside back cover.

Animal studies: Birth defects of skull, brain and vertebral column found in rats; skeletal birth defects found in rabbits.

Human studies: Information from adequate studies of pregnant women is not available. However, many serious birth defects (thought to be due to this drug) have been reported. These include major abnormalities of the head, brain, heart, blood vessels and hormone-producing glands.

Avoid this drug completely during entire pregnancy.

Advisability of Use if Breast-Feeding

Presence of this drug in breast milk: Unknown.

Avoid drug or refrain from nursing.

Habit-Forming Potential: None.

Effects of Overdosage: No experience with overdosage in humans to date.

Suggested Periodic Examinations While Taking This Drug (at physician's discretion)

Complete blood cell counts, including platelet counts.

Measurements of blood cholesterol and triglyceride levels.

Complete eye examinations.

Liver and kidney function tests.

▷ **While Taking This Drug, Observe the Following**

Foods: No restrictions.

Beverages: No restrictions.

▷ *Alcohol:* No interactions expected.

Tobacco Smoking: No interactions expected.

▷ *Other Drugs:* No interactions reported to date.

▷ *Driving, Hazardous Activities:* No restrictions.

Exposure to Sun: This drug can cause photosensitivity (see Glossary). Avoid excessive exposure to sun until your sensitivity is determined.

ISRADIPINE
(is RA di peen)

Introduced: 1984

Class: Antihypertensive, calcium channel blocker

Prescription: USA: Yes

Controlled Drug: USA: No

Available as Generic: USA: No

Brand Name: DynaCirc

BENEFITS versus RISKS

Possible Benefits	*Possible Risks*
EFFECTIVE TREATMENT OF MILD TO MODERATE HYPERTENSION	Headache (13.7%) Dizziness (7.3%) Fluid retention (7.2%) Palpitations (4.0%)

▷ **Principal Uses**

As a Single Drug Product: Used primarily to treat mild to moderately severe hypertension, alone or concurrently with thiazide-type diuretics. It has also been used in the management of chronic, stable angina.

How This Drug Works: Not completely established. It is thought that by blocking the normal passage of calcium through certain cell walls (which is necessary for the function of nerve and muscle tissue), this drug inhibits the contraction of coronary arteries and peripheral arterioles. As a result of these effects, this drug
- promotes dilation of the coronary arteries (antianginal effect).
- reduces the degree of contraction of peripheral arterial walls, resulting in their relaxation and consequent lowering of blood pressure. This further reduces the workload of the heart during exertion and contributes to the prevention of angina.

Available Dosage Forms and Strengths
Capsules — 2.5 mg, 5 mg

▷ **Usual Adult Dosage Range:** Initially 2.5 mg 2 times daily, 12 hours apart, for a trial period of 2 to 4 weeks. If necessary, the dose may be increased by 5 mg per day at intervals of 2 to 4 weeks. The usual maintenance dose is 5 to 10 mg daily. The total daily dosage should not exceed 20 mg. **Note: Actual dosage and administration schedule must be determined by the physician for each patient individually.**

▷ **Dosing Instructions:** May be taken with or following food to reduce stomach irritation. The capsule may be opened for administration; mix the contents with food and swallow promptly.

Usual Duration of Use: Continual use on a regular schedule for 2 to 4 weeks is usually necessary to determine this drug's effectiveness in controlling hypertension or in reducing the frequency and severity of angina. For long-term use (months to years), determine the smallest effective dose. Supervision and periodic evaluation are essential. Consult your physician on a regular basis.

Possible Advantages of This Drug
Does not cause orthostatic hypotension (see Glossary).
No adverse effects on heart or kidney function.
No adverse effects on blood cholesterol levels.

▷ **This Drug Should Not Be Taken If**
  • you have had an allergic reaction to it previously.

▷ **Inform Your Physician Before Taking This Drug If**
  • you have had an unfavorable response to any calcium blocker drug in the past (see Drug Class, Section Four).
  • you are currently taking any beta blocker drug (see Drug Class, Section Four).
  • you are taking any drugs that lower blood pressure.
  • you have a history of congestive heart failure, heart attack or stroke.
  • you are subject to disturbances of heart rhythm.
  • you have impaired liver or kidney function.
  • you plan to have surgery under general anesthesia in the near future.

Possible Side-Effects (natural, expected and unavoidable drug actions)
Rapid heart rate (1.5%), swelling of the feet and ankles (7.2%), flushing and sensation of warmth (2.6%).

▷ **Possible Adverse Effects** (unusual, unexpected and infrequent reactions)
  If any of the following develop, consult your physician promptly for guidance.
  Mild Adverse Effects
  Allergic Reactions: Skin rash (1.5%), hives, itching.
  Headache (13.7%), dizziness (7.3%), weakness (1.2%), nervousness (1%), blurred vision (1%). Palpitation (4%), shortness of breath (1.8%).
  Indigestion (1.7%), nausea (1.8%), vomiting (1.1%), constipation (1%).
  Cramps in legs and feet.
  Serious Adverse Effects
  Allergic Reactions: None reported.
  Rare heart rhythm disturbances.
  Increased frequency or severity of angina on initiation of treatment or following an increase in dose (2.4%).
  Marked drop in blood pressure with fainting (1%).

▷ **Possible Effects on Sexual Function:**   Decreased libido, impotence (less than 1%).

▷ **Adverse Effects That May Mimic Natural Diseases or Disorders**
Flushing and warmth may resemble menopausal "hot flushes."

Possible Effects on Laboratory Tests
White blood cell counts: decreased (less than 1% of users).
Liver function tests: increased enzyme levels (infrequent).
Electrocardiogram: slight increase in QT interval

CAUTION
1. If you are monitoring your own blood pressure, make your measurements just before each dose and 2–3 hours after each dose to obtain an accurate picture of this drug's effect. This will detect excessive fluctuations between high and low readings.
2. Be sure to inform all physicians and dentists you consult that you are taking this drug. Note the use of this drug on your card of personal identification.
3. You may use nitroglycerin and other nitrate drugs as needed to relieve acute episodes of angina pain. However, if you detect that your angina attacks are becoming more frequent or intense, notify your physician promptly.

Precautions for Use
By Infants and Children: Safety and effectiveness for use by those under 18 years of age have not been established.
By Those over 60 Years of Age: Usually well tolerated by this age group. However, observe for the development of weakness, dizziness, fainting and falling. Take necessary precautions to prevent injury.

▷ **Advisability of Use During Pregnancy**
Pregnancy Category: C (tentative). See Pregnancy Code inside back cover.
Animal studies: Embryo and fetal toxicity reported in small animals, but no birth defects due to this drug.
Human studies: Information from adequate studies of pregnant women is not available.
Avoid this drug during the first 3 months. Use during the last 6 months only if clearly needed. Ask physician for guidance.

Advisability of Use if Breast-Feeding
Presence of this drug in breast milk: Unknown.
Avoid drug or refrain from nursing.

Habit-Forming Potential: None.

Effects of Overdosage: Weakness, light-headedness, fainting, fast pulse, low blood pressure, shortness of breath, flushed and warm skin, tremors.

Possible Effects of Long-Term Use: None reported.

Suggested Periodic Examinations While Taking This Drug (at physician's discretion)
Evaluations of heart function, including electrocardiograms; measurements of blood pressure in supine, sitting and standing positions.

▷ **While Taking This Drug, Observe the Following**
  Foods: No restrictions. Avoid excessive salt intake.
  Beverages: No restrictions. May be taken with milk.
▷ *Alcohol:* Use with caution until combined effects have been determined. Alcohol may exaggerate the drop in blood pressure experienced by some individuals.
  Tobacco Smoking: Nicotine may reduce the effectiveness of this drug. Follow your physician's advice regarding smoking.
  Marijuana Smoking: Possible reduced effectiveness of this drug; mild to moderate increase in angina; possible changes in electrocardiogram, confusing interpretation.
▷ *Other Drugs*
  Isradipine *taken concurrently* with
  • beta blocker drugs or digitalis preparations (see Drug Classes, Section Four) may affect heart rate and rhythm adversely. Careful monitoring by your physician is necessary if these drugs are taken concurrently.
▷ *Driving, Hazardous Activities:* Usually no restrictions. This drug may cause drowsiness or dizziness. Restrict activities as necessary.
  Aviation Note: Coronary artery disease and hypertension *are disqualifications* for piloting. Consult a designated Aviation Medical Examiner.
  Exposure to Sun: No restrictions.
  Exposure to Heat: Caution advised. Hot environments can exaggerate the blood-pressure-lowering effects of this drug. Observe for light-headedness or weakness.
  Heavy Exercise or Exertion: This drug may improve your ability to be more active without resulting angina pain. Use caution and avoid excessive exercise that could impair heart function in the absence of warning pain.
  Discontinuation: Do not discontinue this drug abruptly. Consult your physician regarding gradual withdrawal. Observe for the possible development of rebound angina.

KETOPROFEN
(kee toh PROH fen)

Introduced: 1973

Class: Mild analgesic, anti-inflammatory

Prescription: USA: Yes
Canada: Yes

Controlled Drug: USA: No
Canada: No

Available as Generic: No

Brand Names: Orudis, ✦Orudis E-50

```
┌─────────────────────────────────────────────────────────────┐
│                   BENEFITS versus RISKS                       │
│                                                               │
│      Possible Benefits              Possible Risks            │
│  EFFECTIVE RELIEF OF MILD     Gastrointestinal pain, ulceration, │
│  TO MODERATE PAIN AND           bleeding (rare)               │
│  INFLAMMATION                 Rare liver or kidney damage     │
│                               Rare fluid retention            │
│                               Rare bone marrow depression     │
└─────────────────────────────────────────────────────────────┘
```

▷ **Principal Uses**

As a Single Drug Product: Used primarily to relieve mild to moderately severe pain associated with (1) rheumatoid arthritis and osteoarthritis; (2) acute gouty arthritis; (3) acute bursitis, tendinitis and related conditions; and (4) menstrual cramps.

How This Drug Works: Not completely established. It is thought that this drug reduces the tissue concentrations of prostaglandins (and related compounds), chemicals involved in the production of inflammation and pain.

Available Dosage Forms and Strengths
Capsules — 50 mg, 75 mg
Suppositories — 100 mg (in Canada)
Tablets, enteric-coated — 50 mg (in Canada)

▷ **Usual Adult Dosage Range:** Initially, 75 mg 3 times/day or 50 mg 4 times/day. Usual daily dose is 150 to 300 mg divided into 3 or 4 doses. Total daily dosage should not exceed 300 mg. **Note: Actual dosage and administration schedule must be determined by the physician for each patient individually.**

▷ **Dosing Instructions:** Take either on an empty stomach or with food or milk to prevent stomach irritation. Take with a full glass of water and remain upright (do not lie down) for 30 minutes. The capsule may be opened for administration; the tablet should not be crushed or altered.

Usual Duration of Use: Continual use on a regular schedule for 1 to 3 weeks is usually necessary to determine this drug's effectiveness in relieving the discomfort of arthritis. Long-term use (months to years) requires supervision and periodic evaluation by the physician. Consult your physician on a regular basis.

▷ **This Drug Should Not Be Taken If**
• you have had an allergic reaction to it previously.
• you are subject to asthma or nasal polyps caused by aspirin.
• you have active peptic ulcer disease or any form of gastrointestinal ulceration or bleeding.
• you have a bleeding disorder or a blood cell disorder.

- you have severe impairment of kidney function.
- you have active liver disease.

▷ **Inform Your Physician Before Taking This Drug If**
- you are allergic to aspirin or to other aspirin substitutes.
- you have a history of peptic ulcer disease or any type of bleeding disorder.
- you have impaired liver or kidney function.
- you have high blood pressure or a history of heart failure.
- you are taking any of the following: acetaminophen, aspirin or other aspirin substitutes, anticoagulants, oral antidiabetic drugs, or probenecid.

Possible Side-Effects (natural, expected and unavoidable drug actions)
Drowsiness (1% to 3%), ringing in ears (1% to 3%), fluid retention (3%).

▷ **Possible Adverse Effects** (unusual, unexpected and infrequent reactions)
If any of the following develop, consult your physician promptly for guidance.
Mild Adverse Effects
Allergic Reactions: Skin rash (1% to 3%), hives, itching.
Headache (less than 1%), dizziness, altered or blurred vision, depression, confusion, impaired memory.
Mouth sores, indigestion (11%), nausea, vomiting, constipation, diarrhea.
Serious Adverse Effects
Allergic Reaction: Anaphylaxis (see Glossary).
Impaired hearing.
Active peptic ulcer, with or without bleeding (2%).
Rare liver damage with jaundice (see Glossary).
Kidney damage with painful urination, bloody urine, reduced urine formation.
Rare bone marrow depression (see Glossary)—fatigue, weakness, fever, sore throat, abnormal bleeding or bruising.

▷ **Possible Effects on Sexual Function**
Decreased libido, impotence, male breast enlargement.
Altered timing and pattern of menstruation, excessive menstrual bleeding.

Possible Delayed Adverse Effects: Mild anemia due to "silent" blood loss from the stomach (less than that caused by aspirin).

▷ **Adverse Effects That May Mimic Natural Diseases or Disorders**
Liver reaction may suggest viral hepatitis.

Natural Diseases or Disorders That May Be Activated by This Drug
Peptic ulcer disease, ulcerative colitis.

Possible Effects on Laboratory Tests
Fecal occult blood test: positive.

CAUTION
1. Dosage should always be limited to the smallest amount that produces reasonable improvement.
2. This drug may mask early indications of infection. Inform your physician if you think you are developing an infection of any kind.

Precautions for Use
By Infants and Children: Safety and effectiveness for use by those under 12 years of age have not been established.
By Those over 60 Years of Age: Small doses are advisable until tolerance is determined. Observe for any indications of liver or kidney toxicity, fluid retention, dizziness, confusion, impaired memory, stomach bleeding or constipation.

▷ **Advisability of Use During Pregnancy**
Pregnancy Category: B (tentative). See Pregnancy Code inside back cover.
Animal studies: No birth defects reported in mouse, rat or rabbit studies.
Human studies: Information from adequate studies of pregnant women is not available.
Avoid this drug during the last 3 months. Use it during the first 6 months only if clearly needed. Ask physician for guidance.

Advisability of Use if Breast-Feeding
Presence of this drug in breast milk: Unknown.
Avoid drug or refrain from nursing.

Habit-Forming Potential: None.

Effects of Overdosage: Drowsiness, nausea, vomiting, diarrhea.

Possible Effects of Long-Term Use: None reported.

Suggested Periodic Examinations While Taking This Drug (at physician's discretion)
Complete blood cell counts, liver and kidney function tests, complete eye examinations if vision is altered in any way.

▷ **While Taking This Drug, Observe the Following**
Foods: No restrictions.
Beverages: No restrictions. May be taken with milk.
▷ *Alcohol:* Use with caution. The irritant action of alcohol on the stomach lining, added to the irritant action of this drug in sensitive individuals, can increase the risk of stomach ulceration and/or bleeding.
Tobacco Smoking: No interactions expected.
▷ *Other Drugs*
Ketoprofen may *increase* the effects of
• acetaminophen (Tylenol, etc.), and increase the risk of kidney damage; avoid prolonged use of this combination.

- anticoagulants (Coumadin, etc.), and increase the risk of bleeding; monitor prothrombin time, adjust dose accordingly.

Ketoprofen *taken concurrently* with the following drugs may increase the risk of bleeding; avoid these combinations:
- aspirin.
- dipyridamole (Persantine).
- indomethacin (Indocin).
- sulfinpyrazone (Anturane).
- valproic acid (Depakene).

▷ *Driving, Hazardous Activities:* This drug may cause drowsiness or dizziness. Restrict activities as necessary.

Aviation Note: The use of this drug *may be a disqualification* for piloting. Consult a designated Aviation Medical Examiner.

Exposure to Sun: This drug can cause photosensitivity (see Glossary). Avoid excessive exposure to sun until tolerance has been determined.

LABETALOL
(la BET a lohl)

Introduced: 1978

Class: Antihypertensive, alpha- and beta-adrenergic blocker

Prescription: USA: Yes
Canada: Yes

Controlled Drug: USA: No
Canada: No

Available as Generic: No

Brand Names: Normodyne, Normozide [CD], Trandate, Trandate HCT [CD]

BENEFITS versus RISKS

Possible Benefits	*Possible Risks*
EFFECTIVE, WELL-TOLERATED ANTIHYPERTENSIVE in mild to moderate high blood pressure	CONGESTIVE HEART FAILURE in advanced heart disease Worsening of angina in coronary heart disease (if drug is abruptly withdrawn) Masking of low blood sugar (hypoglycemia) in drug-treated diabetes

---

▷ **Principal Uses**

As a Single Drug Product: The treatment of mild to moderately severe high blood pressure. May be used alone or concurrently with other antihypertensive drugs, such as diuretics.

How This Drug Works: By blocking certain actions of the sympathetic nervous system, this drug
- reduces the rate and contraction force of the heart, thus lowering the ejection pressure of blood leaving the heart.
- reduces the degree of contraction of blood vessel walls, resulting in their relaxation and expansion and consequent lowering of blood pressure.

Available Dosage Forms and Strengths
Injection — 5 mg per ml
Tablets — 100 mg, 200 mg, 300 mg

▷ **Usual Adult Dosage Range:** Initially, 100 mg twice daily, 12 hours apart; the dose may be increased by 100 mg twice daily every 2 to 3 days as required to reduce blood pressure. The usual maintenance dose is 200 to 400 mg twice daily. The total dose should not exceed 2400 mg/24 hours, given as 800 mg 3 times daily. **Note: Actual dosage and administration schedule must be determined by the physician for each patient individually.**

▷ **Dosing Instructions:** Take at the same times each day, preferably following the morning and evening meals. The tablet may be crushed for administration. Do not discontinue this drug abruptly.

Usual Duration of Use: Continual use on a regular schedule for 10 to 14 days is usually necessary to determine this drug's effectiveness in lowering blood pressure. The long-term use (months to years) of this drug will be determined by the course of your blood pressure over time and your response to the overall treatment program (weight reduction, salt restriction, smoking cessation, etc.). Consult your physician on a regular basis.

Possible Advantages of This Drug
Decreases blood pressure more promptly than other beta blocker drugs. Can be used to treat hypertensive emergencies.

Currently a "Drug of Choice"
for initiating treatment of hypertension with a single drug.

▷ **This Drug Should Not Be Taken If**
- you have had an allergic reaction to it previously.
- you have active bronchial asthma.
- you have congestive heart failure.
- you have an abnormally slow heart rate or a serious form of heart block.

▷ **Inform Your Physician Before Taking This Drug If**
- you have had an adverse reaction to any beta blocker drug in the past (see Drug Class, Section Four).

- you have a history of serious heart disease, with or without episodes of heart failure.
- you have a history of hay fever (allergic rhinitis), asthma, chronic bronchitis or emphysema.
- you have a history of overactive thyroid function (hyperthyroidism).
- you have a history of low blood sugar (hypoglycemia).
- you have impaired liver or kidney function.
- you have diabetes or myasthenia gravis.
- you are currently taking any form of digitalis, quinidine or reserpine, or any calcium blocker drug (see Drug Class, Section Four).
- you plan to have surgery under general anesthesia in the near future.

Possible Side-Effects (natural, expected and unavoidable drug actions)
Lethargy and fatigability (11%), light-headedness in upright position (see Orthostatic Hypotension in Glossary).

▷ **Possible Adverse Effects** (unusual, unexpected and infrequent reactions)
If any of the following develop, consult your physician promptly for guidance.
Mild Adverse Effects
Allergic Reactions: Skin rash, itching.
Headache, drowsiness, dizziness (20%), scalp tingling (during early treatment).
Indigestion, nausea, diarrhea.
Joint and muscle discomfort, fluid retention (edema).
Serious Adverse Effects
Chest pain, shortness of breath, precipitation of congestive heart failure.
Induction of bronchial asthma (in asthmatic individuals).
Liver damage with jaundice (rare).
Difficult urination (urinary bladder retention).

▷ **Possible Effects on Sexual Function**
Impotence (10%), inhibited ejaculation (10%), prolonged erection following orgasm (related to higher doses), Peyronie's disease (see Glossary).
Decreased vaginal secretions (with low doses), inhibited female orgasm (related to higher doses).

Possible Effects on Laboratory Tests
None reported.

CAUTION
1. ***Do not discontinue this drug suddenly*** without the knowledge and guidance of your physician. Carry a notation on your person that you are taking this drug.
2. Consult your physician or pharmacist before using nasal decongestants usually present in over-the-counter cold preparations and nose drops. These can cause sudden increases in blood pressure when taken concurrently with beta blocker drugs.
3. Report the development of any tendency to emotional depression.

Precautions for Use

By Infants and Children: Safety and effectiveness for use by those under 12 years of age have not been established. However, if this drug is used, observe for the development of low blood sugar (hypoglycemia) during periods of reduced food intake.

By Those over 60 Years of Age: Proceed *cautiously* with all antihypertensive drugs. Unacceptably high blood pressure should be reduced without creating the risks associated with excessively low blood pressure. Start treatment with small doses, and monitor the blood pressure response frequently. Sudden, rapid and excessive reduction of blood pressure can predispose to stroke or heart attack. Observe for dizziness, unsteadiness, tendency to fall, confusion, hallucinations, depression or urinary frequency.

▷ **Advisability of Use During Pregnancy**

Pregnancy Category: C (tentative). See Pregnancy Code inside back cover.

Animal studies: No significant increase in birth defects found in rats or rabbits; some increase in fetal deaths reported.

Human studies: Information from adequate studies of pregnant women is not available.

Use this drug only if clearly needed. Ask physician for guidance.

Advisability of Use if Breast-Feeding

Presence of this drug in breast milk: Yes, in very small amounts.

Avoid drug or refrain from nursing.

Habit-Forming Potential: None.

Effects of Overdosage: Weakness, slow pulse, low blood pressure, fainting, cold and sweaty skin, congestive heart failure, possible coma and convulsions.

Possible Effects of Long-Term Use: Reduced heart reserve and eventual heart failure in susceptible individuals with advanced heart disease.

Suggested Periodic Examinations While Taking This Drug (at physician's discretion)

Measurements of blood pressure, evaluation of heart function.

▷ **While Taking This Drug, Observe the Following**

Foods: No restrictions. Avoid excessive salt intake.

Beverages: No restrictions. May be taken with milk.

▷ *Alcohol:* Use with caution until the combined effect has been determined. Alcohol may exaggerate this drug's ability to lower blood pressure and may increase its mild sedative effect.

Tobacco Smoking: Nicotine may reduce this drug's effectiveness in treating high blood pressure. In addition, high doses of this drug may potentiate the constriction of the bronchial tubes caused by regular smoking.

▷ *Other Drugs*

Labetalol may *increase* the effects of

- other antihypertensive drugs and cause excessive lowering of blood pressure. Dosage adjustments may be necessary.

Labetalol *taken concurrently* with

- clonidine (Catapres) requires close monitoring for rebound high blood pressure if clonidine is withdrawn while labetalol is still being taken.
- insulin requires close monitoring to avoid undetected hypoglycemia (see Glossary).

▷ *Driving, Hazardous Activities:* Use caution until the full extent of fatigue, dizziness and blood pressure change has been determined.

Aviation Note: The use of this drug *is a disqualification* for piloting. Consult a designated Aviation Medical Examiner.

Exposure to Sun: No restrictions.

Exposure to Heat: Caution advised. Hot environments can lower the blood pressure and exaggerate the effects of this drug.

Exposure to Cold: Caution advised. Cold environments can enhance the circulatory deficiency in the extremities that may occur with some beta blocker drugs. The elderly should take precautions to prevent hypothermia (see Glossary).

Heavy Exercise or Exertion: It is advisable to avoid exertion that produces light-headedness, excessive fatigue or muscle cramping. The use of this drug may intensify the hypertensive response to isometric exercise.

Occurrence of Unrelated Illness: The fever that accompanies systemic infections can lower the blood pressure and require adjustment of dosage. Illnesses that cause nausea or vomiting may interrupt the regular dosage schedule. Ask your physician for guidance.

Discontinuation: It is advisable to avoid sudden discontinuation of this drug in all situations. If possible, gradual reduction of dose over a period of 2 to 3 weeks is recommended. Ask your physician for specific guidance.

LEVODOPA
(lee voh DOH pa)

Introduced: 1967

Class: Antiparkinsonism

Prescription: USA: Yes
Canada: Yes

Controlled Drug: USA: No
Canada: No

Available as Generic: USA: Yes
Canada: No

Brand Names: Dopar, Larodopa, ✦Prolopa [CD], Sinemet [CD]

BENEFITS versus RISKS

Possible Benefits	*Possible Risks*
EFFECTIVE RELIEF OF SYMPTOMS IN 80% OF CASES OF IDIOPATHIC PARKINSON'S DISEASE	Emotional depression, confusion, abnormal thinking and behavior
	Abnormal involuntary movements
	Heart rhythm disturbance
	Urinary bladder retention
	Induction of peptic ulcer (rare)
	Blood cell abnormalities: hemolytic anemia, reduced white blood cell count (both rare)

▷ **Principal Uses**

As a Single Drug Product: Used exclusively to treat the major types of Parkinson's disease: paralysis agitans ("shaking palsy" of unknown cause), the type that follows encephalitis, the parkinsonism that develops with aging (associated with hardening of the brain arteries), and the forms of parkinsonism that follow poisoning by carbon monoxide or manganese.

As a Combination Drug Product [CD]: This drug is available in combination with carbidopa, a chemical that prevents the decomposition of levodopa before it reaches its site of action in the brain. The addition of carbidopa reduces the amount of levodopa required by 75%. This combination is more effective in smaller doses and reduces the frequency and severity of adverse effects.

How This Drug Works: Not completely established. Present thinking is that levodopa enters the brain tissue and is converted to dopamine. After sufficient dosage, this corrects the deficiency of dopamine (that is thought to be the cause of parkinsonism) and restores a more normal balance of the chemicals responsible for transmission of nerve impulses in appropriate control centers of the brain.

Available Dosage Forms and Strengths

Capsules — 100 mg, 250 mg, 500 mg
Tablets — 100 mg, 250 mg, 500 mg
Tablets, Sinemet — 10-100 mg, 25-100 mg, 25-250 mg

▷ **Usual Adult Dosage Range:**   Initially, 250 mg 2 to 4 times/day. The dose may be increased cautiously by increments of 100 to 750 mg at 3- to 7-day intervals as needed and tolerated. The total dosage should not exceed 8000 mg/24 hours. If the combination drug Sinemet is used, the total levodopa requirement will be considerably less. **Note: Actual dosage and administration schedule must be determined by the physician for each patient individually.**

▷ **Dosing Instructions:** Preferably taken with or following carbohydrate foods to reduce stomach irritation; when possible, do not take this drug concurrently with high-protein foods. The tablet may be crushed for administration.

Usual Duration of Use: Continual use on a regular schedule for 3 to 6 weeks is usually necessary to determine this drug's effectiveness in relieving the major symptoms of parkinsonism. The determination of maximal effectiveness may require continual use for 6 months. Long-term use (months to years) requires supervision and periodic evaluation by your physician; dosage adjustments will be necessary and unavoidable during the course of the disorder. Consult your physician on a regular basis.

▷ **This Drug Should Not Be Taken If**
  • you are allergic to any of the drugs bearing the brand names listed.
  • you have narrow-angle glaucoma (inadequately controlled).
  • you are taking, or have taken within the past 14 days, any monoamine oxidase (MAO) type A inhibitor drug (see Drug Class, Section Four).

▷ **Inform Your Physician Before Taking This Drug If**
  • you have diabetes, epilepsy, heart disease, high blood pressure or chronic lung disease.
  • you have impaired liver or kidney function.
  • you have a history of peptic ulcer disease or malignant melanoma.
  • you plan to have surgery under general anesthesia in the near future.

Possible Side-Effects (natural, expected and unavoidable drug actions)
Fatigue, lethargy, altered taste, offensive body odor, orthostatic hypotension (see Glossary).
Pink to red coloration of urine, turning black on exposure to air (of no significance).

▷ **Possible Adverse Effects** (unusual, unexpected and infrequent reactions)
  If any of the following develop, consult your physician promptly for guidance.
Mild Adverse Effects
Allergic Reactions: Skin rash, itching.
Headache, dizziness, numbness, unsteadiness, insomnia, nightmares, blurred vision, double vision.
Loss of appetite, nausea, vomiting, dry mouth, difficult swallowing, excessive gas, diarrhea, constipation.
Loss of hair (rare).
Serious Adverse Effects
Idiosyncratic Reactions: Hemolytic anemia (see Glossary). Neuroleptic malignant syndrome (see Glossary).
Confusion, delusions, hallucinations, agitation, paranoia, depression, psychotic episodes, seizures.
Abnormal involuntary movements of the head, face and extremities.

Disturbances of heart rhythm, high blood pressure (rare).
Development of peptic ulcer, gastrointestinal bleeding.
Urinary bladder retention.
Abnormally low white blood cell count—lowered resistance to infection, fever, sore throat.

▷ **Possible Effects on Sexual Function:** Increased libido reported by both males and females (24% to 36%); inhibited ejaculation (rare); priapism (see Glossary).

▷ **Adverse Effects That May Mimic Natural Diseases or Disorders**
Mental reactions may resemble idiopathic psychosis.

Natural Diseases or Disorders That May Be Activated by This Drug
Latent peptic ulcer.

Possible Effects on Laboratory Tests
Complete blood cell counts: occasionally decreased white cells; occasionally increased eosinophils (without symptoms).
Blood thyroxine (T^4) level: increased.
Urine sugar tests: no effect with TesTape; false negative with Clinistix; false positive with Clinitest.
Urine ketone tests: false positive with Ketostix and Phenistix.

CAUTION
1. To reduce the high frequency of serious adverse effects, it is advisable to begin treatment with small doses, and to increase dosage gradually until the desired response is achieved.
2. As improvement occurs, avoid excessive and hurried activity (which often causes falls and injury).

Precautions for Use
By Infants and Children: This drug can cause precocious puberty when taken by the prepubertal boy. Observe closely for hypersexual behavior and for premature growth of the genital organs.
By Those over 60 Years of Age: Treatment should begin with half of the usual adult dose; dosage increases should be made cautiously in small increments as needed and tolerated. Observe for the possible development of significant behavioral changes: depression or inappropriate elation, acute confusion, agitation, paranoia, dementia, nightmares and hallucinations. Abnormal involuntary movements may also occur.

▷ **Advisability of Use During Pregnancy**
Pregnancy Category: C (tentative). See Pregnancy Code inside back cover.
Animal studies: Significant birth defects reported in rodent studies.
Human studies: Information from adequate studies of pregnant women is not available.
Avoid use of drug during the first 3 months. Use only if clearly needed during the last 6 months.

Advisability of Use if Breast-Feeding
   Presence of this drug in breast milk: Yes.
   Avoid drug or refrain from nursing.

Habit-Forming Potential: None.

Effects of Overdosage: Muscle twitching, spastic closure of eyelids, nausea, vomiting, diarrhea, weakness, fainting, confusion, agitation, hallucinations.

Possible Effects of Long-Term Use: Development of abnormal involuntary movements involving the head, face, mouth and extremities. These may be reversible and may gradually subside as the drug is withdrawn.

Suggested Periodic Examinations While Taking This Drug (at physician's discretion)
   Complete blood cell counts; measurements of internal eye pressure; blood pressure measurements in lying, sitting and standing positions.

▷ **While Taking This Drug, Observe the Following**
   Foods: No restrictions. Insofar as possible, do not take concurrently with protein foods; proteins compete for absorption.
   Nutritional Support: If taken alone (without carbidopa), monitor for the development of peripheral neuritis and take small supplements of pyridoxine (vitamin B-6) if needed: 10 mg or less; larger doses can decrease the effectiveness of levodopa. If taken in combination with carbidopa (Sinemet), supplemental pyridoxine is not required.
   Beverages: No restrictions. May be taken with milk.
▷ *Alcohol:* No interactions expected.
   Tobacco Smoking: No interactions expected.
   Marijuana Smoking: Increased fatigue and lethargy; possible accentuation of orthostatic hypotension (see Glossary).
▷ *Other Drugs*
   Levodopa *taken concurrently* with
   • monoamine oxidase (MAO) type A inhibitor drugs (see Drug Class, Section Four) may cause a dangerous rise in blood pressure and body temperature. Do not use these drugs concurrently.
   The following drugs may *decrease* the effects of levodopa
   • papaverine (Cerespan, Pavabid, Vasospan, etc.).
   • phenytoin (Dilantin, etc.).
   • pyridoxine (vitamin B-6).
▷ *Driving, Hazardous Activities:* This drug may cause dizziness, impaired vision and orthostatic hypotension. Restrict activities as necessary.
   Aviation Note: Parkinson's disease *is a disqualification* for piloting. Consult a designated Aviation Medical Examiner.
   Exposure to Sun: No restrictions.
   Exposure to Heat: Use caution. This drug can cause flushing and excessive sweating and predispose to heat exhaustion.
   Occurrence of Unrelated Illness: Suspicious dark-colored skin lesions

should be evaluated carefully to exclude the possibility of malignant melanoma. During the course of any intercurrent infection, monitor the white blood cell count carefully for normal response.

LISINOPRIL
(li SIN oh pril)

Introduced: 1988

Class: Antihypertensive, ACE inhibitor

Prescription: USA: Yes

Controlled Drug: USA: No

Available as Generic: No

Brand Names: Prinivil, Prinzide [CD], Zestoretic [CD], Zestril

---

BENEFITS versus RISKS

Possible Benefits	*Possible Risks*
EFFECTIVE CONTROL OF MILD TO SEVERE HIGH BLOOD PRESSURE	Headache (5.3%), dizziness (6.3%), fatigue (3.3%)
	Low blood pressure (1.8%)
	Allergic swelling of face, tongue, throat, vocal cords (0.1%)

▷ **Principal Uses**
As a Single Drug Product: Used primarily to treat all degrees of high blood pressure. Mild to moderate high blood pressure usually responds to low doses; severe high blood pressure may require higher doses and the concurrent use of a thiazide or other class of antihypertensive drug.

How This Drug Works: Not completely known. It is thought that by blocking certain enzyme systems that influence arterial function, this drug contributes to the relaxation of arterial walls throughout the body and thus lowers the resistance to blood flow that causes high blood pressure. This, in turn, reduces the workload of the heart and improves its performance.

Available Dosage Forms and Strengths
Tablets — 5 mg, 10 mg, 20 mg, 40 mg

▷ **Usual Adult Dosage Range:** Initially 10 mg once daily for those not taking a diuretic; 5 mg once daily for those taking a diuretic. Usual maintenance dose is 20 to 40 mg/day taken in a single dose. Total daily dosage should not exceed 80 mg. **Note: Actual dosage and administration schedule must be determined by the physician for each patient individually.**

▷ **Dosing Instructions:**   Take on an empty stomach or with food, at same time each day. The tablet may be crushed for administration.

 Usual Duration of Use: Continual use on a regular schedule for several weeks is usually necessary to determine this drug's effectiveness in controlling high blood pressure. The proper treatment of high blood pressure usually requires the long-term use of effective medications. Consult your physician on a regular basis.

 Possible Advantages of This Drug
 Controls blood pressure effectively with one daily dose.
 Relatively low incidence of adverse effects.
 No adverse influence on asthma, cholesterol blood levels or diabetes.
 Sudden withdrawal does not result in a rapid increase in blood pressure.

▷ **This Drug Should Not Be Taken If**
 • you have had an allergic reaction to it previously.
 • you currently have a blood cell or bone marrow disorder.
 • you have an abnormally high level of blood potassium.

▷ **Inform Your Physician Before Taking This Drug If**
 • you have a history of kidney disease or impaired kidney function.
 • you have scleroderma or systemic lupus erythematosus.
 • you have cerebral artery disease.
 • you have any form of heart disease.
 • you are taking any of the following drugs: other antihypertensives, diuretics, nitrates or potassium supplements.
 • you plan to have surgery under general anesthesia in the near future.

 Possible Side-Effects (natural, expected and unavoidable drug actions)
 Dizziness (6.3%), orthostatic hypotension (1.4%) (see Glossary), increased blood potassium level (2.2%).

▷ **Possible Adverse Effects** (unusual, unexpected and infrequent reactions)
 If any of the following develop, consult your physician promptly for guidance.
 Mild Adverse Effects
 Allergic Reactions: Skin rash (1.5%), itching (0.3% to 1.0%).
 Headache (5.3%), fatigue (3.3%), numbness and tingling (0.8%), weakness (1.3%).
 Chest pain (1.3%), palpitation (0.3% to 1.0%), cough (2.9%).
 Indigestion (1.0%), nausea (2.3%), vomiting (1.3%), diarrhea (3.2%).
 Serious Adverse Effects
 Allergic Reactions: Swelling (angioedema) of face, tongue and/or vocal cords (less than 0.1%); can be life-threatening.
 Impairment of kidney function (0.3% to 1.0%).

▷ **Possible Effects on Sexual Function:**   Decreased libido (0.2%), impotence (0.7%).

Possible Effects on Laboratory Tests
None reported.

CAUTION
1. Consult your physician regarding the advisability of discontinuing other antihypertensive drugs (especially diuretics) for 1 week before starting this drug.
2. **Report promptly** any indications of infection (fever, sore throat), and any indications of water retention (weight gain, puffiness, swollen feet or ankles).
3. Do not use a salt substitute without your physician's knowledge and approval. (Many salt substitutes contain potassium.)
4. It is advisable to obtain blood cell counts and urine analyses **before** starting this drug.

Precautions for Use
By Infants and Children: Safety and effectiveness for use by those in this age group have not been established.
By Those over 60 Years of Age: Small doses are advisable until tolerance has been determined. Sudden and excessive lowering of blood pressure can predispose to stroke or heart attack in those with impaired brain circulation or coronary artery heart disease.

▷ **Advisability of Use During Pregnancy**
Pregnancy Category: C (tentative). See Pregnancy Code inside back cover.
Animal studies: No birth defects found in mouse or rat studies. Impaired bone formation found in rabbit studies.
Human studies: Information from adequate studies of pregnant women is not available.
Avoid during first 3 months if possible.

Advisability of Use if Breast-Feeding
Presence of this drug in breast milk: Unknown.
Avoid drug or refrain from nursing.

Habit-Forming Potential: None.

Effects of Overdosage: Excessive drop in blood pressure, light-headedness, dizziness, fainting.

Possible Effects of Long-Term Use: Gradual increase in blood potassium level.

Suggested Periodic Examinations While Taking This Drug (at physician's discretion)
Before starting drug: Complete blood cell counts; urine analysis with measurement of protein content; blood potassium level.
During use of drug: Blood cell counts; measurements of blood potassium.

▷ **While Taking This Drug, Observe the Following**

Foods: Consult physician regarding salt intake.

Nutritional Support: Do not take potassium supplements unless directed by your physician.

Beverages: No restrictions. May be taken with milk.

▷ *Alcohol:* Use caution until combined effect has been determined. Alcohol may enhance the blood-pressure-lowering effect of this drug.

Tobacco Smoking: No interactions expected.

▷ *Other Drugs*

Lisinopril *taken concurrently* with

• potassium preparations (K-Lyte, Slow-K, etc.) may cause increased blood levels of potassium with risk of serious heart rhythm disturbances.

• potassium-sparing diuretics: amiloride (Moduretic), spironolactone (Aldactazide), triamterene (Dyazide) may cause increased blood levels of potassium with risk of serious heart rhythm disturbances.

▷ *Driving, Hazardous Activities:* Usually no restrictions. Be aware of possible drops in blood pressure with resultant dizziness or faintness.

Aviation Note: The use of this drug *may be a disqualification* for piloting. Consult a designated Aviation Medical Examiner.

Exposure to Sun: Caution advised. A similar drug of this class can cause photosensitivity.

Exposure to Heat: Caution advised. Avoid excessive perspiring with resultant loss of body water and drop in blood pressure.

Occurrence of Unrelated Illness: Report promptly any disorder that causes nausea, vomiting or diarrhea. Fluid and chemical imbalances must be corrected as soon as possible.

Discontinuation: This drug may be stopped abruptly without causing a sudden increase in blood pressure. However, you should consult your physician regarding withdrawal of this drug for any reason.

LITHIUM
(LITH i um)

Introduced: 1949

Class: Antidepressant, antimanic

Prescription: USA: Yes
Canada: Yes

Controlled Drug: USA: No
Canada: No

Available as Generic: USA: Yes
Canada: No

Brand Names: ✦Carbolith, Cibalith-S, ✦Duralith, Eskalith, Eskaylith CR, Lithane, ✦Lithizine, Lithobid, Lithonate, Lithotabs

```
┌─────────────────────────────────────────────────────────────────┐
│                    BENEFITS versus RISKS                          │
│                                                                   │
│      Possible Benefits                  Possible Risks            │
│  RAPID REVERSAL OF ACUTE          VERY NARROW MARGIN              │
│    MANIA in 80% of users            BETWEEN TREATMENT AND         │
│  STABILIZATION OF MOOD in           TOXIC BLOOD LEVELS            │
│    60% to 70% of users with       POTENTIALLY FATAL TOXICITY      │
│    manic-depressive disorder        with inadequate monitoring    │
│  Prevention of recurrent          Infrequent induction of diabetes│
│    depression in "responders"       mellitus, hypothyroidism      │
│                                   Diabetes insipiduslike syndrome  │
│                                     (excessive dilute urine without│
│                                     sugar)                        │
└─────────────────────────────────────────────────────────────────┘
```

▷ **Principal Uses**

As a Single Drug Product: Used primarily in the management of manic-depressive disorders. While its principal use is the prompt correction of acute mania, it is also used to stabilize these disorders by reducing the frequency and severity of recurrent manic-depressive mood swings. It is also beneficial in treating the depression phase of these disorders in individuals who do not experience the manic phase. Additional uses (experimental) include the prevention of cluster headaches and the stimulation of production of white blood cells.

How This Drug Works: Not completely established. It is thought that lithium may act to correct chemical imbalances in certain nerve impulse transmitters (serotonin and norepinephrine) that influence emotional status and behavior.

Available Dosage Forms and Strengths

Capsules — 150 mg, 300 mg, 600 mg
Syrup — 8 mEq per 5-ml teaspoonful
Tablets — 300 mg
Tablets, prolonged-action — 300 mg, 450 mg

▷ **Usual Adult Dosage Range:** First day: 300 mg taken 3 times, 6 hours apart; second day and thereafter: increase dose to 1200 mg/24 hours and later to 1800 mg/24 hours if needed and tolerated. The usual maintenance dose is 600 to 1200 mg/24 hours taken in 3 divided doses. The total daily dosage should not exceed 3600 mg. **Note: Actual dosage and administration schedule must be determined by the physician for each patient individually.**

▷ **Dosing Instructions:** May be taken with or after meals to reduce stomach irritation. The capsules may be opened and the regular tablets may be crushed for administration; the prolonged-action tablets should be swallowed whole and not altered.

Usual Duration of Use: Continual use on a regular schedule for 1 to 3 weeks is usually necessary to determine this drug's effectiveness in correcting acute mania; several months of continual treatment may be required to correct depression. Long-term use (months to years) requires supervision and periodic evaluation by your physician. Consult your physician on a regular basis.

Currently a "Drug of Choice"
for the treatment of acute mania in bipolar manic-depressive disorders.

▷ **This Drug Should Not Be Taken If**
- you have had an allergic reaction to any dosage form of it previously.
- you have uncontrolled diabetes or uncorrected hypothyroidism.
- you are breast-feeding.
- you will be unable to comply with the need for regular monitoring of lithium blood levels.

▷ **Inform Your Physician Before Taking This Drug If**
- you have a history of a schizophreniclike thought disorder.
- you have any type of organic brain disease, or a history of grand mal epilepsy.
- you have diabetes, heart disease, hypothyroidism or impaired kidney function.
- you are on a salt-restricted diet.
- you are pregnant or planning pregnancy.
- you are taking any diuretic drug or a cortisonelike steroid preparation.
- you plan to have surgery under general anesthesia in the near future.

Possible Side-Effects (natural, expected and unavoidable drug actions)
Increased thirst and urine volume may occur in 60% of initial users and in 20% of long-term maintenance users. Weight gain may occur in first few months of use. Drowsiness and lethargy may occur in sensitive individuals.

▷ **Possible Adverse Effects** (unusual, unexpected and infrequent reactions)
If any of the following develop, consult your physician promptly for guidance.
Mild Adverse Effects
Allergic Reactions: Skin rashes, generalized itching.
Skin dryness, loss of hair.
Headache, dullness, dizziness, weakness, blurred vision, ringing in ears, fine hand tremor, unsteadiness.
Metallic taste, loss of appetite, stomach irritation, nausea, vomiting, diarrhea.
Serious Adverse Effects
"Blackout" spells, confusion, stupor, slurred speech, spasmodic movements of extremities, epilepticlike seizures.
Loss of bladder or rectal control.
Diabetes insipiduslike syndrome: loss of kidney concentrating power, excessive dilute urine.

▷ **Possible Effects on Sexual Function:**   Decreased libido (blood level of 0.7 to 0.9 meq/L); inhibited erection: 30% of users (0.6 to 0.8 meq/L); male infertility; female breast swelling with milk production.

▷ **Adverse Effects That May Mimic Natural Diseases or Disorders**
Painful discoloration and coldness of the hands and feet may resemble Raynaud's syndrome.

Natural Diseases or Disorders That May Be Activated by This Drug
Diabetes mellitus may be worsened. Psoriasis may be intensified. Myasthenia gravis may be induced (1 case).

Possible Effects on Laboratory Tests
White blood cell and platelet counts: increased.
Blood alkaline phosphatase (bone isoenzyme): markedly increased in 66% of users.
Blood cholesterol level: increased.
Blood parathyroid hormone level: increased.
Blood thyroid stimulating hormone (TSH) level: increased.
Blood thyroid hormone (T^3 and T^4) levels: decreased.
Blood uric acid level: decreased.

CAUTION
1. This drug has a very narrow margin of safe use. The blood level of drug required to be effective is quite close to the level that can cause toxic effects. Periodic measurements of blood lithium levels are mandatory for appropriate adjustments of dosage. Follow instructions exactly regarding drug dosage and periodic blood examinations.
2. Lithium should be discontinued at the first signs of toxicity: drowsiness, sluggishness, unsteadiness, tremor, muscle twitching, vomiting or diarrhea.
3. The major causes of lithium toxicity are
   • accidental overdose (sometimes due to inadequate monitoring of blood levels).
   • impaired kidney function.
   • salt restriction.
   • inadequate fluid intake, dehydration.
   • concurrent use of diuretics.
   • intercurrent illness.
   • childbirth (rapid decrease in kidney clearance of lithium).
   • initiation of treatment with a new drug.
4. Over-the-counter preparations that contain iodides (some cough products and vitamin-mineral supplements) should be avoided because of the added antithyroid effect when taken with lithium.

Precautions for Use
By Infants and Children: Safety and effectiveness for use by those under 12 years of age have not been established. Follow physician's instructions exactly.

By Those over 60 Years of Age: Initial and maintenance doses should be smaller than standard doses for younger adults; treatment should start with a "test" dose of 75 to 150 mg daily. Observe closely for early indications of toxic effects, especially if on a low-salt diet and using diuretics. Parkinsonian reactions (abnormal gait and movements) occur with greater frequency; coma can develop without warning symptoms.

▷ **Advisability of Use During Pregnancy**
Pregnancy Category: D (tentative). See Pregnancy Code inside back cover.
Animal studies: Cleft palate reported in mice; eye, ear and palate defects reported in rats.
Human studies: Information from adequate studies of pregnant women is not available. However, cardiovascular defects and goiter in newborn infants (of mothers using lithium) have been reported. If the infant's blood level of lithium approaches the toxic range before delivery, the newborn may suffer the "floppy infant" syndrome: weakness, lethargy, unresponsiveness, low body temperature, weak cry and poor feeding ability.
Avoid use of drug during the first 3 months. Use only if clearly necessary during the last 6 months. Monitor mother's blood lithium levels carefully to avoid possible toxicity.

Advisability of Use if Breast-Feeding
Presence of this drug in breast milk: Yes, in significant amounts.
Avoid drug or refrain from nursing.

Habit-Forming Potential: None.

Effects of Overdosage: Drowsiness, weakness, lack of coordination, nausea, vomiting, diarrhea, muscle spasms, blurred vision, dizziness, staggering gait, slurred speech, confusion, stupor, coma, seizures.

Possible Effects of Long-Term Use: Hypothyroidism (5%), goiter, reduced sugar tolerance, diabetes insipiduslike syndrome, serious kidney damage.

Suggested Periodic Examinations While Taking This Drug (at physician's discretion)
Regular determinations of blood lithium levels are absolutely essential to the safe and effective use of this drug.
Periodic evaluation of thyroid gland size and function.
Complete blood cell counts; kidney function tests.

▷ **While Taking This Drug, Observe the Following**
Foods: Maintain a normal diet; **do not** restrict your use of salt.
Beverages: No restrictions. Drink at least 8 to 12 glasses of liquids/24 hours. This drug may be taken with milk.
▷   *Alcohol:* Use with caution until the combined effects have been determined. Avoid alcohol completely if any symptoms of lithium toxicity develop.
Tobacco Smoking: No interactions expected.

Marijuana Smoking: Possible increase in apathy, lethargy, drowsiness or sluggishness; accentuation of lithium-induced tremor; possible increased risk of precipitating psychotic behavior.

▷ *Other Drugs*

Lithium may *increase* the effects of
• tricyclic antidepressants (see Drug Class, Section Four).

Lithium *taken concurrently* with
• carbamazepine (Tegretol) or with
• chlorpromazine (Thorazine, etc.), and other phenothiazines or with
• fluoxetine (Prozac) or with
• haloperidol (Haldol) or with
• methyldopa (Aldomet, etc.) is usually well tolerated; however, it may cause a severe neurotoxic reaction in susceptible individuals. These combinations should be used very cautiously.
• diazepam (Valium) may cause hypothermia.
• verapamil (Calan, Isoptin) may cause unpredictable effects; both lithium toxicity and decreased lithium blood levels have been reported.

The following drugs may *increase* the effects of lithium
• bumetanide (Bumex).
• ethacrynic acid (Edecrin).
• fluoxetine (Prozac).
• furosemide (Lasix, etc.).
• indomethacin (Indocin).
• piroxicam (Feldene).
• thiazide diuretics (see Drug Class, Section Four).

The following drugs may *decrease* the effects of lithium
• acetazolamide (Diamox, etc.).
• sodium bicarbonate.
• theophylline (Theo-Dur, etc.) and related drugs.

▷ *Driving, Hazardous Activities:* This drug may impair mental alertness, judgment, physical coordination and reaction time. Restrict activities as necessary.

Aviation Note: The use of this drug *is a disqualification* for piloting. Consult a designated Aviation Medical Examiner.

Exposure to Sun: No restrictions.

Exposure to Heat: Excessive sweating can cause significant depletion of salt and water and resultant lithium toxicity. Avoid sauna baths.

Occurrence of Unrelated Illness: Any illness that causes fever, sweating, vomiting or diarrhea can result in significant alterations of blood and tissue lithium concentrations. Close monitoring of your physical condition and blood lithium levels is necessary to prevent serious toxicity.

Discontinuation: Sudden discontinuation does not cause withdrawal symptoms. Avoid premature discontinuation; some individuals may require continual treatment for up to a year to achieve maximal response. Discontinuation by "responders" may result in recurrence of either mania or depression. Lithium should be discontinued if symptoms of brain toxicity appear or if an uncorrectable diabetes insipiduslike syndrome develops.

LOPERAMIDE
(loh PER a mide)

Introduced: 1977

Prescription: USA: Yes
Canada: No

Available as Generic: No

Brand Names: Imodium, Imodium AD

Class: Antidiarrheal

Controlled Drug: USA: No
Canada: No

BENEFITS versus RISKS	
Possible Benefits	*Possible Risks*
EFFECTIVE RELIEF OF INTESTINAL CRAMPING AND DIARRHEA	Drowsiness Constipation Induction of toxic megacolon

▷ **Principal Uses**

As a Single Drug Product: Used primarily for the control of cramping and diarrhea associated with acute gastroenteritis and chronic enteritis and colitis. Also used to reduce the volume of discharge from ileostomies.

How This Drug Works: Not completely established. It is thought that this drug acts directly on the nerve supply of the gastrointestinal tract to reduce its motility and propulsive contractions, thus relieving cramping and diarrhea.

Available Dosage Forms and Strengths
Capsules — 2 mg
Liquid — 1 mg per 5-ml teaspoonful (alcohol 5.25%)
Tablets — 2 mg

▷ **Usual Adult Dosage Range:**   For acute diarrhea: 4 mg initially, then 2 mg after each unformed stool until diarrhea is controlled. For chronic diarrhea: 4 to 8 mg/day in divided doses, taken 8 to 12 hours apart. The total daily dosage should not exceed 16 mg. **Note: Actual dosage and administration schedule must be determined by the physician for each patient individually.**

▷ **Dosing Instructions:**   May be taken on an empty stomach or with food if stomach irritation occurs. The capsule may be opened for administration.

Usual Duration of Use: Continual use on a regular schedule for 48 hours is usually necessary to determine this drug's effectiveness in controlling acute diarrhea; continual use for 10 days may be needed to evaluate its effectiveness in controlling chronic diarrhea. If diarrhea persists, consult your physician.

▷ **This Drug Should Not Be Taken If**
- you have had an allergic reaction to it previously.
- it is prescribed for a child under 2 years of age.

▷ **Inform Your Physician Before Taking This Drug If**
- you have a history of liver disease or impaired liver function.
- you have regional enteritis or ulcerative colitis.

Possible Side-Effects (natural, expected and unavoidable drug actions)
Drowsiness, constipation.

▷ **Possible Adverse Effects** (unusual, unexpected and infrequent reactions)
If any of the following develop, consult your physician promptly for guidance.
Mild Adverse Effects
Allergic Reaction: Skin rash.
Fatigue, dizziness.
Reduced appetite, dry mouth, nausea, vomiting, stomach pain, bloating.
Serious Adverse Effects
"Toxic megacolon" (distended, immobile colon with fluid retention) may develop while treating acute ulcerative colitis.

▷ **Possible Effects on Sexual Function:** None reported.

Possible Effects on Laboratory Tests
None reported.

CAUTION
1. Do not exceed recommended doses.
2. If used to treat chronic diarrhea, report promptly any development of bloating, abdominal distension, nausea, vomiting, constipation or abdominal pain.

Precautions for Use
By Infants and Children: Do not use in those under 2 years of age. Follow physician's instructions exactly regarding dosage. Observe for drowsiness, irritability, personality changes and altered behavior.
By Those over 60 Years of Age: Start treatment with small doses. You may be more sensitive to the sedative and constipating effects of this drug.

▷ **Advisability of Use During Pregnancy**
Pregnancy Category: B (tentative). See Pregnancy Code inside back cover.
Animal studies: No birth defects found in rat and rabbit studies.
Human studies: Information from adequate studies of pregnant women is not available.
Use sparingly and only if clearly needed. Ask physician for guidance.

Advisability of Use if Breast-Feeding
Presence of this drug in breast milk: Unknown.
Avoid drug or refrain from nursing.

Habit-Forming Potential: None.

Effects of Overdosage: Drowsiness, lethargy, depression, dry mouth.

Possible Effects of Long-Term Use: None identified.

Suggested Periodic Examinations While Taking This Drug (at physician's discretion)
None required.

▷ **While Taking This Drug, Observe the Following**
Foods: No restrictions. Follow prescribed diet.
Beverages: No restrictions. May be taken with milk.
▷ *Alcohol:* Use with caution until combined effects have been determined. This drug may increase the depressant action of alcohol on the brain.
Tobacco Smoking: No interactions expected.
▷ *Other Drugs:* No significant drug interactions reported.
▷ *Driving, Hazardous Activities:* This drug may cause drowsiness or dizziness. Restrict activities as necessary.
Aviation Note: The use of this drug *is a disqualification* for piloting. Consult a designated Aviation Medical Examiner.
Exposure to Sun: No restrictions.

LORAZEPAM
(lor AZ e pam)

Introduced: 1971

Class: Mild tranquilizer, benzodiazepines

Prescription: USA: Yes
Canada: Yes

Controlled Drug: USA: C-IV*
Canada: No

Available as Generic: USA: Yes
Canada: No

Brand Names: Alzapam, ✦Apo-Lorazepam, Ativan, Loraz, ✦Novolorazepam

BENEFITS versus RISKS	
Possible Benefits	*Possible Risks*
RELIEF OF ANXIETY AND NERVOUS TENSION in 70% to 80% of users	Habit-forming potential with prolonged use
Wide margin of safety with therapeutic doses	Minor impairment of mental functions
Very few drug interactions	

*See Schedules of Controlled Drugs inside back cover.

▷ **Principal Uses**

As a Single Drug Product: Used primarily to provide short-term relief of mild to moderate anxiety. While it is less sedative than the barbiturates, it is also used at bedtime to produce a calming effect that permits natural sleep.

How This Drug Works: It is thought that this drug produces a calming effect by enhancing the action of the nerve transmitter gamma-aminobutyric acid (GABA), which in turn blocks the arousal of higher brain centers.

Available Dosage Forms and Strengths

Injection — 2 mg per ml, 4 mg per ml

Tablets — 0.5 mg, 1 mg, 2 mg

▷ **Usual Adult Dosage Range:** 1 to 10 mg/24 hours. For anxiety: 2 to 3 mg, 2 or 3 times/day. For insomnia: 2 to 4 mg at bedtime. The total daily dose should not exceed 10 mg. **Note: Actual dosage and administration schedule must be determined by the physician for each patient individually.**

▷ **Dosing Instructions:** May be taken on empty stomach or with food or milk. The tablet may be crushed for administration. Do not discontinue this drug abruptly if taken for more than 4 weeks.

Usual Duration of Use: Continual use on a regular schedule for 3 to 5 days is usually necessary to determine this drug's effectiveness in relieving moderate anxiety. Limit continual use to 1 to 3 weeks. Avoid uninterrupted and prolonged use.

▷ **This Drug Should Not Be Taken If**

• you have had an allergic reaction to any dosage form of it previously.
• you have acute narrow-angle glaucoma.
• it is prescribed for a child under 12 years of age.

▷ **Inform Your Physician Before Taking This Drug If**

• you are allergic to any benzodiazepine drug (see Drug Class, Section Four).
• you have a history of alcoholism or drug abuse.
• you are pregnant or planning pregnancy.
• you have impaired liver or kidney function.
• you have a history of serious depression or mental disorder.
• you have any of the following: asthma, emphysema, epilepsy, myasthenia gravis.

Possible Side-Effects (natural, expected and unavoidable drug actions)

Drowsiness, lethargy, unsteadiness, "hangover" effects on the day following bedtime use.

▷ **Possible Adverse Effects** (unusual, unexpected and infrequent reactions)

If any of the following develop, consult your physician promptly for guidance.

Mild Adverse Effects
Allergic Reaction: Skin rash.
Dizziness (6%), fainting, blurred vision, double vision, slurred speech, headache, sweating, nausea, indigestion.
Serious Adverse Effects
Disorientation, emotional depression, agitation, disturbed sleep, periodic amnesia.

▷ **Possible Effects on Sexual Function:** Antianxiety effect can relieve nervous tension that is often responsible for male impotence and female vaginismus (painful spasm of vagina), thus improving sexual performance. (Impaired sexual functioning relieved in 40%.)

Possible Effects on Laboratory Tests
Urine screening tests for drug abuse: may be **positive.** (Test results depend upon amount of drug taken and testing method used.)

CAUTION
1. This drug should not be discontinued abruptly if it has been taken continually for more than 4 weeks.
2. The concurrent use of some over-the-counter drug products that contain antihistamines (allergy and cold preparations, sleep aids) can cause excessive sedation in sensitive individuals.
3. If this drug is taken at bedtime as a hypnotic, significant impairment of intellectual and motor functions may persist into the following day; avoid hazardous activities and the use of alcohol.

Precautions for Use
By Infants and Children: Safety and effectiveness for use by those under 12 years of age have not been established. This drug should not be used in the hyperactive or psychotic child of any age. Observe for excessive sedation and incoordination.
By Those over 60 Years of Age: It is advisable to use smaller doses at longer intervals to avoid overdosage. Observe for the possible development of lethargy, indifference, fatigue, weakness, unsteadiness, disturbing dreams, nightmares and paradoxical reactions of excitement, agitation, anger, hostility and rage.

▷ **Advisability of Use During Pregnancy**
Pregnancy Category: C (tentative). See Pregnancy Code inside back cover.
Animal studies: Skeletal and eye defects reported in rabbits.
Human studies: Information from adequate studies of pregnant women is not available. No birth defects have been reported with the use of this drug.
Avoid drug completely during the first 3 months; avoid during the last 6 months if possible. Frequent use in late pregnancy may cause the "floppy infant" syndrome in the newborn: weakness, lethargy, unresponsiveness, depressed breathing, low body temperature.

Advisability of Use if Breast-Feeding
  Presence of this drug in breast milk: Yes, in small amounts.
  Monitor nursing infant closely and discontinue drug or nursing if adverse effects develop.

Habit-Forming Potential: This drug can produce psychological and/or physical dependence (see Glossary) if used in large doses for an extended period of time.

Effects of Overdosage: Marked drowsiness, weakness, feeling of drunkenness, staggering gait, tremor, stupor progressing to deep sleep or coma.

Possible Effects of Long-Term Use: Psychological and/or physical dependence.

Suggested Periodic Examinations While Taking This Drug (at physician's discretion)
  Complete blood cell counts and liver function tests during long-term use. (Other drugs of this class are known to cause blood cell and liver function disorders rarely.)

▷ **While Taking This Drug, Observe the Following**
  Foods: No restrictions.
  Beverages: Avoid excessive intake of caffeine-containing beverages: coffee, tea, cola. May be taken with milk.
▷ *Alcohol:* Use with extreme caution until the combined effect is determined. Alcohol may increase the absorption of this drug and add to its depressant effects on the brain. It is advisable to avoid alcohol completely—throughout the day and night—if it is necessary to drive or to engage in any hazardous activity.
  Tobacco Smoking: Heavy smoking may reduce the calming action of this drug.
  Marijuana Smoking: Increased sedation and significant impairment of intellectual and physical performance.
▷ *Other Drugs*
  Lorazepam may ***increase*** the effects of
  • other sedatives, hypnotics, tranquilizers, anticonvulsants and narcotic drugs; excessive sedation may result.
▷ *Driving, Hazardous Activities:* This drug can impair mental alertness, judgment, physical coordination and reaction time. Avoid hazardous activities accordingly.
  Aviation Note: The use of this drug ***is a disqualification*** for piloting. Consult a designated Aviation Medical Examiner.
  Exposure to Sun: No restrictions.
  Exposure to Heat: Use caution until the effect of excessive perspiration is determined. Because of reduced urine volume, this drug may accumulate in the body and produce effects of overdosage.
  Discontinuation: Avoid sudden discontinuation if this drug has been taken for over 4 weeks without interruption. Dosage should be tapered gradu-

ally to prevent a withdrawal syndrome that could include depression, confusion, hallucinations, tremor, seizures, muscle cramping, sweating and vomiting.

LOVASTATIN
(loh vah STA tin)

Introduced: 1987

Prescription: USA: Yes

Available as Generic: USA: No

Brand Name: Mevacor

Class: Anticholesterol

Controlled Drug: USA: No

BENEFITS versus RISKS

Possible Benefits
EFFECTIVE REDUCTION OF
TOTAL BLOOD CHOLESTEROL
in selected individuals

Possible Risks
Drug-induced hepatitis (without
jaundice) 1.9%
Drug-induced myositis (muscle
inflammation) 0.5%
Drug-induced stomach ulceration
(rare)

▷ **Principal Uses**

As a Single Drug Product: Used primarily to reduce abnormally high total blood cholesterol levels in individuals with Types IIa and IIb hypercholesterolemia. It is used in conjunction with a cholesterol-lowering diet. It should not be used until a trial of nondrug methods for lowering cholesterol has proved to be inadequate.

How This Drug Works: This drug is converted in the body to mevolinic acid, which inhibits the liver enzyme that initiates the production of cholesterol. Its principal action is the reduction of low-density lipoproteins (LDL), the fraction of total blood cholesterol that is thought to increase the risk of coronary heart disease. This drug may or may not increase the level of high-density lipoproteins (HDL), the cholesterol fraction that is thought to reduce the risk of heart disease.

Available Dosage Forms and Strengths
Tablets — 20 mg, 40 mg

▷ **Usual Adult Dosage Range:** Initially 20 mg once a day; dose may be increased up to 40 mg twice a day as needed and tolerated. Dosage adjustments should be made at 4-week intervals. The total daily dosage should not exceed 80 mg. **Note: Actual dosage and administration schedule must be determined by the physician for each patient individually.**

▷ **Dosing Instructions:**   Take with food, preferably with the evening meal for maximal effectiveness. (The highest rates of cholesterol production occur between midnight and 5 a.m.) The tablet may be crushed for administration.

Usual Duration of Use: Continual use on a regular schedule for 4 to 6 weeks is usually necessary to determine this drug's effectiveness in reducing blood levels of total and LDL cholesterol. Long-term use (months to years) requires periodic evaluation of response and dosage adjustment. Consult your physician on a regular basis.

Possible Advantages of This Drug: Recent studies indicate that this drug is more effective and better tolerated than other drugs currently available for reducing total and LDL cholesterol. Its long-term effects are yet to be determined. See Cholesterol Disorders in Section Two.

▷ **This Drug Should Not Be Taken If**
- you have had an allergic reaction to it previously.
- you have active liver disease.
- you have active peptic ulcer disease.
- you are pregnant or breast-feeding.

▷ **Inform Your Physician Before Taking This Drug If**
- you have a history of liver disease or impaired liver function.
- you have a history of peptic ulcer disease or upper gastrointestinal bleeding.
- you are not using any method of birth control, or you are planning pregnancy.
- you regularly consume substantial amounts of alcohol.
- you have cataracts or impaired vision.
- you have any type of chronic muscular disorder.

Possible Side-Effects (natural, expected and unavoidable drug actions)
Development of abnormal liver function tests without associated symptoms.

▷ **Possible Adverse Effects** (unusual, unexpected and infrequent reactions)
If any of the following develop, consult your physician promptly for guidance.
Mild Adverse Effects
Allergic Reactions: Skin rash, itching (5.2%).
Headache (9.3%), dizziness (2.0%), blurred vision (1.5%), altered taste (0.8%).
Indigestion (3.9%), stomach pain (5.7%), nausea (4.7%), excessive gas (6.4%), constipation (4.9%), diarrhea (5.5%).
Muscle cramps and/or pain (2.4%).
Serious Adverse Effects
Marked and persistent abnormal liver function tests with focal hepatitis (without jaundice) occurred in 1.9% after 1 year of use.

Acute myositis (muscle pain and tenderness) occurred in 0.5% during long-term use.

Cataracts occurred in 8% after 5 to 15 months of continual use; a cause-and-effect relationship (see Glossary) has not been established.

Stomach and duodenal ulceration with bleeding have been reported in a few cases.

▷ **Possible Effects on Sexual Function:** None reported.

Possible Delayed Adverse Effects: None reported to date.

Natural Diseases or Disorders That May Be Activated by This Drug
Latent liver disease; latent peptic ulcer disease; latent cataracts (possibly).

Possible Effects on Laboratory Tests
Blood alanine aminotransferase (ALT) enzyme level: increased (with higher doses of drug).
Blood total cholesterol, LDL cholesterol and triglyceride levels: decreased.
Blood HDL cholesterol level: increased.

CAUTION
1. If pregnancy occurs while taking this drug, discontinue it immediately and consult your physician.
2. Report promptly any development of muscle pain or tenderness, especially if accompanied by fever or malaise.
3. Report promptly the development of altered or impaired vision so that appropriate evaluation can be made.

Precautions for Use
By Infants and Children: Safety and effectiveness for use by those under 20 years of age have not been established.
By Those over 60 Years of Age: Inform your physician regarding any personal or family history of cataracts. Comply with all recommendations regarding periodic eye examinations. Report promptly any alterations in vision.

▷ **Advisability of Use During Pregnancy**
Pregnancy Category: X. See Pregnancy Code inside back cover.
Animal studies: Mouse and rat studies reveal skeletal birth defects due to this drug.
Human studies: Information from adequate studies of pregnant women is not available.
This drug should be avoided during entire pregnancy.

Advisability of Use if Breast-Feeding
Presence of this drug in breast milk: Probably yes.
Avoid drug or refrain from nursing.

Habit-Forming Potential: None.

Effects of Overdosage: Increased indigestion, stomach distress, nausea, diarrhea.

Possible Effects of Long-Term Use: Abnormal liver function with focal hepatitis.

Suggested Periodic Examinations While Taking This Drug (at physician's discretion)
Blood cholesterol studies: total cholesterol, HDL and LDL fractions.
Liver function tests every 4 to 6 weeks during the first 15 months of use and periodically thereafter.
Complete eye examination at beginning of treatment and periodically thereafter. Ask your physician for guidance.

▷ **While Taking This Drug, Observe the Following**
Foods: Follow a standard low-cholesterol diet.
Beverages: No restrictions. May be taken with milk.
▷ *Alcohol:* No interactions expected. Use sparingly.
Tobacco Smoking: No interactions expected.
▷ *Driving, Hazardous Activities:* This drug may cause dizziness or impaired vision. Restrict activities as necessary.
Aviation Note: The use of this drug *may be a disqualification* for piloting. Consult a designated Aviation Medical Examiner.
Exposure to Sun: No restrictions.
Discontinuation: Do not discontinue this drug without your physician's knowledge and guidance.

MAPROTILINE
(ma PROH ti leen)

Introduced: 1974   **Class:** Antidepressant

Prescription: USA: Yes   **Controlled Drug:** USA: No
    Canada: Yes   Canada: No

Available as Generic: No

Brand Name: Ludiomil

```
┌─────────────────────────────────────────────────────────┐
│                 BENEFITS versus RISKS                     │
│                                                           │
│    Possible Benefits              Possible Risks          │
│  EFFECTIVE RELIEF OF ALL     ADVERSE BEHAVIORAL           │
│    TYPES OF DEPRESSION          EFFECTS: confusion,       │
│                                 disorientation, hallucinations │
│                              CONVERSION OF DEPRESSION     │
│                                 TO MANIA in manic-depressive │
│                                 disorders                 │
│                              Irregular heart rhythms      │
│                              Rare liver toxicity with jaundice │
└─────────────────────────────────────────────────────────┘
```

▷ **Principal Uses**

As a Single Drug Product: To relieve the symptoms associated with spontaneous (endogenous) depression and with reactive depressions, and to initiate the restoration of normal mood. This drug should be used only when a diagnosis of true depression of significant degree has been established. It should not be used to treat mild and transient despondency that may be associated with many life situations in the absence of a bona fide affective illness.

How This Drug Works: It is thought that this drug relieves depression by slowly restoring the nerve impulse transmitter norepinephrine to normal levels within brain tissue.

Available Dosage Forms and Strengths

Tablets — 10 mg (in Canada), 25 mg, 50 mg, 75 mg

▷ **Usual Adult Dosage Range:** Initially 25 mg 3 times daily. Dose may be increased cautiously as needed and tolerated by 10 to 25 mg daily at intervals of 1 week. Usual maintenance dose is 50 to 100 mg/24 hours. The total daily dose should not exceed 150 mg. When the optimal requirement is determined, it may be taken at bedtime as one dose. **Note: Actual dosage and administration schedule must be determined by the physician for each patient individually.**

▷ **Dosing Instructions:** May be taken without regard to meals. Tablet may be crushed for administration.

Usual Duration of Use: Some benefit may be apparent within to 2 weeks, but adequate response may require continual use for 4 to 6 weeks or longer. Long-term use should not exceed 6 months without evaluation regarding the need for continuation of the drug. Consult your physician on a regular basis.

▷ **This Drug Should Not Be Taken If**
- you have had an allergic reaction to it previously.
- you are taking or have taken within the past 14 days any monoamine oxidase (MAO) type A inhibitor drug (see Drug Class, Section Four).
- you are recovering from a recent heart attack.

▷ **Inform Your Physician Before Taking This Drug If**
- you are allergic or overly sensitive to any tricyclic antidepressant (see Drug Class, Section Four).
- you have a history of any of the following: alcoholism, asthma, epilepsy, glaucoma, heart disease, paranoia, prostate gland enlargement, schizophrenia or overactive thyroid function.
- you have impaired liver function.
- you plan to have surgery under general anesthesia in the near future.

Possible Side-Effects (natural, expected and unavoidable drug actions)
Drowsiness, blurred vision, dry mouth, constipation, impaired urination.

▷ **Possible Adverse Effects** (unusual, unexpected and infrequent reactions)
If any of the following develop, consult your physician promptly for guidance.
Mild Adverse Effects
Allergic Reactions: Skin rash, itching.
Insomnia, nervousness, palpitations, dizziness, unsteadiness, tremors, fainting, weakness.
Nausea, vomiting, acid indigestion, diarrhea.
Increased sweating.
Serious Adverse Effects
Behavioral effects: anxiety, confusion, hallucinations.
Aggravation of paranoid psychosis and schizophrenia.
Aggravation of seizure disorders (epilepsy).
Liver toxicity with jaundice (see Glossary).

▷ **Possible Effects on Sexual Function:** Decreased libido, increased libido (antidepressant effect), impotence, male breast enlargement and tenderness, female breast enlargement with milk production, swelling of testicles.

▷ **Adverse Effects That May Mimic Natural Diseases or Disorders**
The development of jaundice may suggest viral hepatitis.

Natural Diseases or Disorders That May Be Activated by This Drug
Latent epilepsy, glaucoma, prostatism (see Glossary).

Possible Effects on Laboratory Tests
Liver function tests: rarely increased liver enzymes (ALT/GPT and AST/ GOT).

CAUTION
1. Dosage must be adjusted for each person individually. Report for follow-up evaluation and laboratory tests as directed by your physician.
2. Observe for early indications of toxicity: confusion, agitation, rapid heartbeat.
3. It is advisable to withhold this drug if electroconvulsive therapy (ECT, "shock" treatment) is to be used to treat your depression.

Precautions for Use

By Infants and Children: Safety and effectiveness for use by those under 18 years of age have not been established.

By Those over 60 Years of Age: During the first 2 weeks of treatment, observe for the development of confusion, agitation, forgetfulness, disorientation, delusions and hallucinations. Reduction of dosage or discontinuation may be necessary. Unsteadiness may predispose to falling and injury. This drug can increase the degree of impaired urination associated with prostate gland enlargement (prostatism).

▷ **Advisability of Use During Pregnancy**

Pregnancy Category: B (tentative). See Pregnancy Code inside back cover.

Animal studies: No birth defects found in mouse, rat or rabbit studies.

Human studies: Information from adequate studies of pregnant women is not available.

Avoid use of drug during first 3 months. Use during the last 6 months only if clearly needed.

Advisability of Use if Breast-Feeding

Presence of this drug in breast milk: Yes.

Monitor nursing infant closely for drowsiness or failure to feed properly; discontinue drug or nursing if adverse effects develop.

Habit-Forming Potential: None.

Effects of Overdosage: Confusion, hallucinations, marked drowsiness, heart palpitations, dilated pupils, tremors, stupor, deep sleep, coma, convulsions.

Suggested Periodic Examinations While Taking This Drug (at physician's discretion)

Complete blood cell counts, liver function tests, serial blood pressure readings and electrocardiograms.

▷ **While Taking This Drug, Observe the Following**

Foods: No restrictions.

Beverages: No restrictions. May be taken with milk.

▷   *Alcohol:* Avoid completely. This drug can markedly increase the intoxicating effects of alcohol and accentuate its depressant action on brain function.

Tobacco Smoking: No interactions expected.

Marijuana Smoking: Increased drowsiness and dryness of mouth; possible reduced effectiveness of this drug.

▷   *Other Drugs*

Maprotiline may *increase* the effects of

• atropinelike drugs (see Drug Class, Section Four).

• all drugs with sedative effects, and cause excessive sedation.

Maprotiline may *decrease* the effects of

• clonidine (Catapres).

• guanethidine (Ismelin).

- methyldopa (Aldomet).
- reserpine (Serpasil, Ser-Ap-Es, etc.).

Maprotiline *taken concurrently* with

- amphetaminelike drugs may cause severe high blood pressure and/or high fever (see Drug Class, Section Four).
- antiseizure drugs requires careful monitoring for change in seizure patterns; dosage adjustments may be necessary.
- ethchlorvynol (Placidyl) may cause delirium; avoid concurrent use.
- monoamine oxidase (MAO) type A inhibitor drugs may cause high fever, delirium and convulsions (see Drug Class, Section Four).
- thyroid preparations may impair heart rhythm and function.

Ask physician for guidance regarding adjustment of thyroid dose.

The following drugs may *decrease* the effects of maprotiline

- estrogens.
- oral contraceptives.

▷ *Driving, Hazardous Activities:* This drug may impair mental alertness, judgment, physical coordination and reaction time. Avoid hazardous activities.

Aviation Note: The use of this drug *is a disqualification* for piloting. Consult a designated Aviation Medical Examiner.

Exposure to Sun: Use caution until sensitivity to sun has been determined. This drug may cause photosensitivity (see Glossary).

Exposure to Heat: This drug can inhibit sweating and impair the body's adaptation to hot environments, increasing the risk of heat stroke. Avoid saunas.

Exposure to Cold: The elderly should use caution and avoid conditions conducive to hypothermia (see Glossary).

Discontinuation: It is advisable to discontinue this drug gradually. Abrupt withdrawal after long-term use may cause headache, malaise and nausea.

MECLIZINE
(MEK li zeen)

Other Name: Meclozine

Introduced: 1951

Class: Antinausea, antivertigo, antihistamines

Prescription: USA: Varies
Canada: Yes

Controlled Drug: USA: No
Canada: No

Available as Generic: USA: Yes
Canada: No

Brand Names: Antivert, ✦Bonamine, Bonine, Ru-Vert-M

BENEFITS versus RISKS

Possible Benefits	*Possible Risks*
EFFECTIVE PREVENTION OF MOTION SICKNESS	Mild sedation
Moderately effective relief of nausea and vertigo	Mild atropinelike effects

---

▷ **Principal Uses**

As a Single Drug Product: Used primarily to control dizziness and vertigo associated with disorders of the inner ear. Also used to prevent or relieve the nausea, vomiting and dizziness characteristic of motion sickness.

As a Combination Drug Product [CD]: This drug is available in Canada in combination with niacin (nicotinic acid), which is added because of its ability to dilate blood vessels and (theoretically) improve circulation.

How This Drug Works: Not completely established. It is thought that this drug reduces the sensitivity of the nerve pathways connecting the organ of equilibrium in the inner ear with the vomiting center in the brain; this prevents or reduces the occurrence of nausea, vomiting and vertigo.

Available Dosage Forms and Strengths
　　　　Tablets — 12.5 mg, 25 mg, 50 mg
　Tablets, chewable — 25 mg

▷ **Usual Adult Dosage Range:**   12.5 to 25 mg, once or twice daily as needed for vertigo. For motion sickness: 25 to 50 mg taken 1 hour before travel; repeat once daily if needed. Total daily dosage should not exceed 100 mg. **Note: Actual dosage and administration schedule must be determined by the physician for each patient individually.**

▷ **Dosing Instructions:**   May be taken without regard to food. The regular tablet may be crushed for administration.

Usual Duration of Use: Continual use on a regular schedule for 2 to 4 days is usually necessary to determine this drug's effectiveness in relieving vertigo or preventing motion sickness. Duration of use should not exceed 5 days if this drug is not effective.

▷ **This Drug Should Not Be Taken If**
  • you have had an allergic reaction to it previously.
  • you are taking, or have taken within the past 14 days, any monoamine oxidase (MAO) type A inhibitor drug (see Drug Class, Section Four).
  • you are, or think you may be, pregnant.

▷ **Inform Your Physician Before Taking This Drug If**
  • you have had an unfavorable response to any antihistamine drug in the past.

- you have any of the following: asthma, epilepsy, glaucoma, peptic ulcer disease, prostate gland enlargement.

Possible Side-Effects (natural, expected and unavoidable drug actions)
Mild drowsiness, lethargy, impaired concentration, dry mouth, constipation.

▷ **Possible Adverse Effects** (unusual, unexpected and infrequent reactions)
If any of the following develop, consult your physician promptly for guidance.
Mild Adverse Effects
Allergic Reactions: No significant reactions identified.
Blurred vision.
Serious Adverse Effects
Possible increase in prostatism (see Glossary).

▷ **Possible Effects on Sexual Function:** None reported.

Natural Diseases or Disorders That May Be Activated by This Drug
Latent epilepsy, glaucoma, prostatism.

Possible Effects on Laboratory Tests
None reported.

CAUTION
1. Discontinue this drug 5 days before diagnostic skin testing for allergies.
2. Avoid this drug completely in children with flulike infections or chicken pox. Although a cause-and-effect relationship has not been established, this drug may contribute to the development of Reye syndrome (see Glossary) in susceptible children.

Precautions for Use
By Infants and Children: Safety and effectiveness for use by those under 12 years of age have not been established. See *CAUTION.*
By Those over 60 Years of Age: Observe for increased susceptibility to drowsiness, dizziness and impaired thinking, judgment and memory; the antihistamine-sedative effect can cause a hypoactive syndrome that may be mistaken for emotional depression or senility.

▷ **Advisability of Use During Pregnancy**
Pregnancy Category: C (tentative). See Pregnancy Code inside back cover.
Animal studies: Significant birth defects reported in mouse, rat and ferret studies.
Human studies: Information from studies of pregnant women is inconclusive. No increase in birth defects was reported in 2076 exposures in 2 studies; 12 cleft lips or palates were reported in 3333 exposures in another study.
Avoid this drug completely during the first 3 months. Use it during the

last 6 months only if clearly needed. **Note:** This drug is *contraindicated* during pregnancy by one manufacturer.

Advisability of Use if Breast-Feeding
Presence of this drug in breast milk: Unknown.
Avoid drug or refrain from nursing.

Habit-Forming Potential: None.

Effects of Overdosage: Marked drowsiness, confusion, unsteadiness, tremors, stupor progressing to coma; in children: excitement, hallucinations, overactivity, seizures.

Possible Effects of Long-Term Use: Development of tolerance and loss of effectiveness.

Suggested Periodic Examinations While Taking This Drug (at physician's discretion)
None required.

▷ **While Taking This Drug, Observe the Following**
Foods: No restrictions.
Beverages: No restrictions. May be taken with milk.
▷ *Alcohol:* Use with extreme caution until the combined effects have been determined. The combination of alcohol and antihistamines can cause rapid and marked sedation.
Tobacco Smoking: No interactions expected.
▷ *Other Drugs*
Meclizine may *increase* the effects of
• all other drugs with atropinelike effects.
• all other drugs with sedative effects.
The following drugs may *increase* the effects of meclizine:
• monoamine oxidase (MAO) type A inhibitor drugs may prolong its atropinelike effects (see Drug Class, Section Four).
▷ *Driving, Hazardous Activities:* This drug may impair mental alertness, judgment, physical coordination and reaction time. Restrict activities as necessary.
Aviation Note: The use of this drug *is a disqualification* for piloting. Consult a designated Aviation Medical Examiner.
Exposure to Sun: No restrictions.

MECLOFENAMATE
(me kloh fen AM ayt)

Introduced: 1977

Class: Mild analgesic, anti-inflammatory

Prescription: USA: Yes

Controlled Drug: USA: No

Available as Generic: Yes

Brand Names: Meclodium, Meclomen

BENEFITS versus RISKS

Possible Benefits	*Possible Risks*
EFFECTIVE RELIEF OF MILD TO MODERATE PAIN AND INFLAMMATION	Gastrointestinal pain, ulceration, bleeding (rare) Rare kidney damage Rare fluid retention Rare bone marrow depression

---

▷ **Principal Uses**

As a Single Drug Product: Used primarily to relieve mild to moderately severe pain and inflammation associated with acute and chronic rheumatoid arthritis and osteoarthritis. Also used to relieve mild to moderate pain of any cause.

How This Drug Works: Not completely established. It is thought that this drug reduces the tissue concentrations of prostaglandins (and related compounds), chemicals involved in the production of inflammation and pain.

Available Dosage Forms and Strengths

Capsules — 50 mg, 100 mg

▷ **Usual Adult Dosage Range:** 200 to 400 mg daily, in 3 or 4 divided doses. Total daily dosage should not exceed 400 mg. **Note: Actual dosage and administration schedule must be determined by the physician for each patient individually.**

▷ **Dosing Instructions:** Take with food or milk to prevent stomach irritation. Take with a full glass of water and remain upright (do not lie down) for 30 minutes. The capsule may be opened for administration.

Usual Duration of Use: Continual use on a regular schedule for 2 to 3 weeks is usually necessary to determine this drug's effectiveness in relieving the discomfort of arthritis. Long-term use (months to years) requires supervision and periodic evaluation by your physician. Consult your physician on a regular basis.

▷ **This Drug Should Not Be Taken If**
- you have had an allergic reaction to it previously.
- you are subject to asthma or nasal polyps caused by aspirin.
- you have active peptic ulcer disease, regional enteritis, ulcerative colitis or any form of gastrointestinal bleeding.
- you have a bleeding disorder or a blood cell disorder.
- you have severe impairment of kidney function.

▷ **Inform Your Physician Before Taking This Drug If**
- you are allergic to aspirin or to other aspirin substitutes.
- you have a history of peptic ulcer disease, regional enteritis or ulcerative colitis.
- you have a history of any type of bleeding disorder.
- you have impaired liver or kidney function.
- you have high blood pressure or a history of heart failure.
- you are taking any of the following: acetaminophen, aspirin or other aspirin substitutes, anticoagulants, oral antidiabetic drugs or cortisonelike drugs.

Possible Side-Effects (natural, expected and unavoidable drug actions)
Ringing in ears, fluid retention.

▷ **Possible Adverse Effects** (unusual, unexpected and infrequent reactions)
If any of the following develop, consult your physician promptly for guidance.
Mild Adverse Effects
Allergic Reactions: Skin rash, hives, itching.
Headache, dizziness, altered or blurred vision, depression.
Mouth sores, indigestion, nausea, vomiting (11%), diarrhea (10% to 33%, sometimes severe).
Serious Adverse Effects
Allergic Reactions: Severe skin reactions, drug fever (see Glossary).
Active peptic ulcer, with or without bleeding.
Kidney damage with painful urination, bloody urine, reduced urine formation.
Rare bone marrow depression (see Glossary)—fatigue, weakness, fever, sore throat, abnormal bleeding or bruising.

▷ **Possible Effects on Sexual Function**
None reported.

Possible Delayed Adverse Effects: Mild anemia due to "silent" blood loss from the stomach (less than that caused by aspirin).

Natural Diseases or Disorders That May Be Activated by This Drug
Peptic ulcer disease, ulcerative colitis.

Possible Effects on Laboratory Tests
Complete blood cell counts: decreased red cells, hemoglobin, white cells and platelets (all rare).

CAUTION
1. Dosage should always be limited to the smallest amount that produces reasonable improvement.
2. This drug may mask early indications of infection. Inform your physician if you think you are developing an infection of any kind.

Precautions for Use

By Infants and Children: Safety and effectiveness for use by those under 14 years of age have not been established.

By Those over 60 Years of Age: Small doses are advisable until tolerance is determined. Observe for any indications of liver or kidney toxicity, fluid retention, dizziness, confusion, impaired memory, stomach bleeding or diarrhea.

▷ **Advisability of Use During Pregnancy**

Pregnancy Category: B (tentative). See Pregnancy Code inside back cover.
Animal studies: Some minor birth defects reported in rodents.
Human studies: Information from adequate studies of pregnant women is not available.
Avoid this drug during the first and last 3 months. Use it during the second 3 months only if clearly needed. Ask physician for guidance.
The manufacturer does not recommend the use of this drug during pregnancy.

Advisability of Use if Breast-Feeding

Presence of this drug in breast milk: Unknown.
Avoid drug or refrain from nursing.

Habit-Forming Potential: None.

Effects of Overdosage: Drowsiness, nausea, vomiting, diarrhea, marked agitation, irrational behavior, seizures.

Possible Effects of Long-Term Use: None identified.

Suggested Periodic Examinations While Taking This Drug (at physician's discretion)
Complete blood cell counts, kidney function tests, complete eye examinations if vision is altered in any way.

▷ **While Taking This Drug, Observe the Following**

Foods: No restrictions.
Beverages: No restrictions. May be taken with milk.
▷ *Alcohol:* Use with caution. The irritant action of alcohol on the stomach lining, added to the irritant action of this drug in sensitive individuals, can increase the risk of stomach ulceration and/or bleeding.
Tobacco Smoking: No interactions expected.
▷ *Other Drugs*
Meclofenamate may ***increase*** the effects of
- acetaminophen (Tylenol, etc.), and increase the risk of kidney damage; avoid prolonged use of this combination.

- anticoagulants (Coumadin, etc.), and increase the risk of bleeding; monitor prothrombin time, adjust dose accordingly.

Meclofenamate *taken concurrently* with the following drugs may increase the risk of bleeding; avoid these combinations:

- aspirin.
- dipyridamole (Persantine).
- sulfinpyrazone (Anturane).
- valproic acid (Depakene).

▷   *Driving, Hazardous Activities:* This drug may cause dizziness or altered vision. Restrict activities as necessary.

Aviation Note: The use of this drug *may be a disqualification* for piloting. Consult a designated Aviation Medical Examiner.

Exposure to Sun: No restrictions.

MEDROXYPROGESTERONE
(me DROX ee proh JESS te rohn)

Introduced: 1959

Class: Female sex hormones, progestins

Prescription: USA: Yes
Canada: Yes

Controlled Drug: USA: No
Canada: No

Available as Generic: Yes

Brand Names: Amen, Curretab, Provera

BENEFITS versus RISKS	
Possible Benefits	*Possible Risks*
EFFECTIVE TREATMENT OF ABSENT OR ABNORMAL MENSTRUATION due to hormone imbalance	Thrombophlebitis (rare) Pulmonary embolism (rare) Liver reaction with jaundice (rare)
EFFECTIVE CONTRACEPTION when given by injection	Drug-induced birth defects
Useful adjunctive therapy in selected cases of uterine and kidney cancer	

▷ **Principal Uses**

As a Single Drug Product: Used primarily to initiate and regulate menstruation and to correct abnormal patterns of menstrual bleeding caused by hormonal imbalance (and not by organic disease). The injectable form of this drug is a very effective contraceptive (but is not approved for this use in the USA).

How This Drug Works: By inducing and maintaining a lining in the uterus that resembles pregnancy, this drug can prevent uterine bleeding until it is withdrawn. By suppressing the release of the pituitary gland hormone that induces ovulation, and by stimulating the secretion of mucus by the uterine cervix (to resist the passage of sperm), this drug can prevent pregnancy.

Available Dosage Forms and Strengths
Tablets — 2.5 mg, 5 mg, 10 mg

▷ **Usual Adult Dosage Range:** To initiate menstruation: 5 to 10 mg/day for 5 to 10 days, started at any time; to correct abnormal bleeding: 5 to 10 mg/day for 5 to 10 days, started on the sixteenth or twenty-first day of the menstrual cycle. Withdrawal bleeding usually begins within 3 to 7 days after stopping the drug. **Note: Actual dosage and administration schedule must be determined by the physician for each patient individually.**

▷ **Dosing Instructions:** Take on an empty stomach or with food to prevent nausea. The tablet may be crushed for administration.

Usual Duration of Use: Continual use on a regular schedule for 2 or 3 menstrual cycles is usually necessary to determine this drug's effectiveness in correcting abnormal patterns of menstrual bleeding. Consult your physician on a regular basis.

▷ **This Drug Should Not Be Taken If**
  • you have had an allergic reaction to it previously.
  • you are pregnant.
  • you have seriously impaired liver function.
  • you have a history of cancer of the breast or reproductive organs.
  • you have a history of thrombophlebitis, embolism or stroke.
  • you have abnormal and unexplained vaginal bleeding.

▷ **Inform Your Physician Before Taking This Drug If**
  • you have impaired kidney function.
  • you have any of the following disorders: asthma, diabetes, emotional depression, epilepsy, heart disease, migraine headaches.

Possible Side-Effects (natural, expected and unavoidable drug actions)
  Fluid retention, weight gain, changes in menstrual timing and flow, spotting between periods.

▷ **Possible Adverse Effects** (unusual, unexpected and infrequent reactions)
  If any of the following develop, consult your physician promptly for guidance.
  Mild Adverse Effects
  Allergic Reactions: Skin rash, hives, itching.
  Fatigue, weakness, nausea.
  Acne, excessive hair growth.

Serious Adverse Effects

Liver toxicity with jaundice (see Glossary): yellow eyes and skin, dark-colored urine, light-colored stools.

Thrombophlebitis (inflammation of a vein with blood clot formation): pain or tenderness in thigh or leg, with or without swelling of the foot, ankle or leg.

Pulmonary embolism (movement of blood clot to lung): sudden shortness of breath, chest pain, cough, bloody sputum.

Stroke (blood clot in the brain): sudden headache, blackouts, sudden weakness or paralysis of any part of the body, severe dizziness, double vision, slurred speech, inability to speak.

Retinal thrombosis (blood clot in principal blood vessel to the eye): sudden impairment or loss of vision.

▷ **Possible Effects on Sexual Function**

Altered timing and pattern of menstruation.
Female breast tenderness and secretion.
Decreased vaginal secretions.

▷ **Adverse Effects That May Mimic Natural Diseases or Disorders**

Liver toxicity may suggest viral hepatitis.

Possible Effects on Laboratory Tests

Blood total cholesterol, HDL cholesterol, LDL cholesterol and triglyceride levels: decreased.
Glucose tolerance test (GTT): decreased.

CAUTION

1. There is an increased risk of birth defects in children whose mothers take this drug during the first 4 months of pregnancy.
2. Inform your physician promptly if you think you may be pregnant.
3. This drug should not be used as a test for pregnancy.

Precautions for Use

By Infants and Children: Not used in this age group.
By Those over 60 Years of Age: Used selectively as adjunctive therapy in treating cancer of the breast, uterus and kidney. Observe for excessive fluid retention.

▷ **Advisability of Use During Pregnancy**

Pregnancy Category: X. See Pregnancy Code inside back cover.

Animal studies: Genital defects reported in rat and rabbit studies; masculinization of the female rodent fetus; various defects in chick embryo and rabbit.

Human studies: Masculinization of the female genitals: enlargement of the clitoris, fusion of the labia. Increased risk of heart, nervous system and limb defects also reported.

Avoid this drug completely during entire pregnancy.

Advisability of Use if Breast-Feeding
   Presence of this drug in breast milk: Yes.
   Avoid drug or refrain from nursing.

Habit-Forming Potential: None.

Effects of Overdosage: Nausea, vomiting, fluid retention, breast enlargement and discomfort, abnormal vaginal bleeding.

Possible Effects of Long-Term Use: None reported in humans.

Suggested Periodic Examinations While Taking This Drug (at physician's
   discretion)
   Regular examinations (every 6 to 12 months) of the breasts and reproductive organs (pelvic examination of the uterus and ovaries, including
   Pap smear).

▷ **While Taking This Drug, Observe the Following**
   Foods: No restrictions.
   Beverages: No restrictions.
▷ *Alcohol:* No interactions expected.
   Tobacco Smoking: It is advisable to smoke lightly or not at all.
▷ *Other Drugs*
   The following drugs may *decrease* the effects of medroxyprogesterone
   • rifampin (Rifadin, Rimactane, etc.) may hasten its elimination.
▷ *Driving, Hazardous Activities:* Usually no restrictions. Consult your physi-
   cian for assessment of individual risk and for guidance regarding spe-
   cific restrictions.
   Aviation Note: The use of this drug *may be a disqualification* for piloting.
   Consult a designated Aviation Medical Examiner.
   Exposure to Sun: No restrictions.

MEPERIDINE
(me PER i deen)

Other Name: Pethidine

Introduced: 1939   **Class:**   Strong analgesic, opioids

Prescription: USA: Yes   **Controlled Drug:**   USA: C-II*
   Canada: Yes   Canada: < N >

Available as Generic: Yes

Brand Names: Demerol, Demerol APAP [CD], Pethadol

*See Schedules of Controlled Drugs inside back cover.

```
┌─────────────────────────────────────────────────────────────────┐
│                      BENEFITS versus RISKS                        │
│                                                                   │
│       Possible Benefits              Possible Risks               │
│    EFFECTIVE RELIEF OF            POTENTIAL FOR HABIT             │
│      MODERATE TO SEVERE PAIN        FORMATION (DEPENDENCE)        │
│                                   Weakness, fainting              │
│                                   Disorientation, hallucinations  │
│                                   Interference with urination     │
└─────────────────────────────────────────────────────────────────┘
```

▷ **Principal Uses**

As a Single Drug Product: This potent analgesic is used by mouth or injection to relieve moderate to severe pain of any cause.

As a Combination Drug Product [CD]: This drug is available in combination with acetaminophen (APAP) to create a dosage form that utilizes two pain relievers, one of which also reduces fever.

How This Drug Works: Acting primarily as a depressant of certain brain functions, this drug suppresses the perception of pain and calms the emotional response to pain.

Available Dosage Forms and Strengths

Injection — 10 mg per ml, 25 mg per ml, 50 mg per ml, 75 mg per ml, 100 mg per ml

Syrup — 50 mg per 5-ml teaspoonful

Tablets — 50 mg, 100 mg

▷ **Usual Adult Dosage Range:**   Taken by mouth: 50 to 150 mg/3 to 4 hours as needed to relieve pain; the usual dose is 100 mg. The total daily dosage should not exceed 900 mg. **Note: Actual dosage and administration schedule must be determined by the physician for each patient individually.**

▷ **Dosing Instructions:**   May be taken with or following food to reduce stomach irritation or nausea. The tablet may be crushed for administration. The syrup may be diluted in 4 ounces of water to reduce the numbing effect on the tongue and mouth tissues.

Usual Duration of Use: As required to control pain. Continual use should not exceed 5 to 7 days without interruption and reassessment of need.

▷ **This Drug Should Not Be Taken If**
• you have had an allergic reaction to any dosage form of it previously.
• you are having an acute attack of asthma.
• you are taking, or have taken within the past 14 days, any monoamine oxidase (MAO) type A inhibitor drug (see Drug Class, Section Four).

▷ **Inform Your Physician Before Taking This Drug If**
• you have a history of drug abuse or alcoholism.
• you have impaired liver or kidney function.
• you have a history of asthma, epilepsy or glaucoma.

- you are taking any other drugs that have a sedative effect.
- you plan to have surgery under general anesthesia in the near future.

Possible Side-Effects (natural, expected and unavoidable drug actions)
Drowsiness, light-headedness, weakness, euphoria, dry mouth, urinary retention, constipation.

▷ **Possible Adverse Effects** (unusual, unexpected and infrequent reactions)
If any of the following develop, consult your physician promptly for guidance.
Mild Adverse Effects
Allergic Reactions: Skin rash, hives, itching.
Headache, dizziness, impaired concentration, sensation of drunkenness, confusion, depression, blurred or double vision.
Facial flushing, sweating, heart palpitation.
Nausea, vomiting.
Serious Adverse Effects
Drop in blood pressure, causing severe weakness and fainting.
Disorientation, hallucinations, unstable gait, tremor, muscle twitching.

▷ **Possible Effects on Sexual Function:** None reported.

▷ **Adverse Effects That May Mimic Natural Diseases or Disorders**
Paradoxical behavioral disturbances may suggest psychotic disorder.

Possible Effects on Laboratory Tests
Blood alanine aminotransferase (ALT) and aspartate aminotransferase (AST) levels: increased (natural side-effects).
Blood amylase and lipase levels: increased (natural side-effects).

CAUTION
1. If you have asthma, chronic bronchitis or emphysema, the excessive use of this drug may cause significant respiratory difficulty, thickening of bronchial secretions and suppression of coughing.
2. The concurrent use of this drug with atropinelike drugs can increase the risk of urinary retention and reduced intestinal function.
3. Do not take this drug following acute head injury.

Precautions for Use
By Infants and Children: Do not use this drug in infants under 1 year of age because of their vulnerability to life-threatening respiratory depression.
By Those over 60 Years of Age: Use small doses initially and increase dosage as needed and tolerated. Limit use to short-term treatment only if possible. There may be increased susceptibility to the development of drowsiness, dizziness, unsteadiness, falling, urinary retention and constipation (often leading to fecal impaction).

▷ **Advisability of Use During Pregnancy**
Pregnancy Category: C (tentative). See Pregnancy Code inside back cover.
Animal studies: Significant birth defects reported in hamster studies.

Human studies: Information from adequate studies of pregnant women is not available. However, no significant increase in birth defects was found in 1100 exposures to this drug.
Avoid during the first 3 months. Use sparingly and in small doses during the last 6 months only if clearly needed.

Advisability of Use if Breast-Feeding
Presence of this drug in breast milk: Yes.
Avoid drug or refrain from nursing.

Habit-Forming Potential: This drug can cause psychological and physical dependence (see Glossary).

Effects of Overdosage: Marked drowsiness, confusion, tremors, convulsions, stupor progressing to coma.

Possible Effects of Long-Term Use: Psychological and physical dependence, chronic constipation.

Suggested Periodic Examinations While Taking This Drug (at physician's discretion)
None.

▷ **While Taking This Drug, Observe the Following**
Foods: No restrictions.
Beverages: No restrictions. May be taken with milk.
▷   *Alcohol:* Use extreme caution until the combined effects have been determined. Opioid analgesics can intensify the intoxicating effects of alcohol, and alcohol can intensify the depressant effects of opioids on brain function, breathing and circulation. Alcohol is best avoided.
Tobacco Smoking: No interactions expected.
Marijuana Smoking: Increase in drowsiness and pain relief; impairment of mental and physical performance.
▷   *Other Drugs*
Meperidine may ***increase*** the effects of
• other drugs with sedative effects.
• atropinelike drugs, and increase the risk of constipation and urinary retention.
Meperidine ***taken concurrently*** with
• monoamine oxidase (MAO) type A inhibitor drugs (see Drug Class, Section Four) can cause the equivalent of an acute narcotic overdose: unconsciousness; severe depression of breathing, heart action and circulation. A variation of this reaction can be excitability, convulsions, high fever and rapid heart action.
• phenothiazines (see Drug Class, Section Four) can cause excessive and prolonged depression of brain functions, breathing and circulation.
▷   *Driving, Hazardous Activities:* This drug can impair mental alertness, judgment, reaction time and physical coordination. Avoid hazardous activities.

Aviation Note: The use of this drug *is a disqualification* for piloting. Consult a designated Aviation Medical Examiner.

Exposure to Sun: No restrictions.

Discontinuation: It is advisable to limit this drug to short-term use. If it is necessary to use it for extended periods of time, discontinuation should be gradual to minimize possible effects of withdrawal.

METAPROTERENOL
(met a proh TER e nohl)

Other Name: Orciprenaline

Introduced: 1964

Class: Antiasthmatic, broncho-dilator

Prescription: USA: Yes
Canada: Yes

Controlled Drug: USA: No
Canada: No

Available as Generic: Yes

Brand Names: Alupent, Arm-a-Med, Metaprel, Prometa

BENEFITS versus RISKS

Possible Benefits	*Possible Risks*
VERY EFFECTIVE RELIEF OF BRONCHOSPASM	Increased blood pressure
	Fine hand tremor
	Irregular heart rhythm (with excessive use)

▷ **Principal Uses**

As a Single Drug Product: To relieve acute bronchial asthma and to reduce the frequency and severity of chronic, recurrent asthmatic attacks; also used to relieve reversible bronchospasm associated with chronic bronchitis and emphysema.

How This Drug Works: By stimulating certain sympathetic nerve terminals, this drug acts to dilate those bronchial tubes that are in sustained constriction, thereby increasing the size of the airway and improving the ability to breathe.

Available Dosage Forms and Strengths
Powder for inhalation — 0.65 mg/inhalation
Solution for nebulizer — 0.4%, 0.6%, 5%
Syrup — 10 mg per 5-ml teaspoonful
Tablets — 10 mg, 20 mg

▷ **Usual Adult Dosage Range:**   Inhaler: 2 or 3 inhalations/3 to 4 hours; do not exceed 12 inhalations/day. Hand nebulizer: 5 to 15 inhalations/4 hours; do not exceed 40 inhalations/day. Syrup and tablets: 20 mg/6 to 8 hours. **Note: Actual dosage and administration schedule must be determined by the physician for each patient individually.**

▷ **Dosing Instructions:**   May be taken on empty stomach or with food or milk. Tablets should not be crushed for administration. For aerosol and nebulizer, follow the written instructions carefully. Do not overuse.

Usual Duration of Use: According to individual requirements. Do not use beyond the time necessary to terminate episodes of asthma.

▷ **This Drug Should Not Be Taken If**
  • you have had an allergic reaction to any dosage form of it previously.
  • you currently have an irregular heart rhythm.
  • you are taking, or have taken within the past 2 weeks, any monoamine oxidase (MAO) type A inhibitor drug (see Drug Class, Section Four).

▷ **Inform Your Physician Before Taking This Drug If**
  • you are overly sensitive to other drugs that stimulate the sympathetic nervous system.
  • you are currently using epinephrine (Adrenalin, Primatene Mist, etc.) to relieve asthmatic breathing.
  • you have any type of heart or circulatory disorder, especially high blood pressure or coronary heart disease.
  • you have diabetes or an overactive thyroid gland (hyperthyroidism).
  • you are taking any form of digitalis or any stimulant drug.

Possible Side-Effects (natural, expected and unavoidable drug actions)
Aerosol—dryness or irritation of mouth or throat, altered taste.
Tablet—nervousness, palpitation.

▷ **Possible Adverse Effects** (unusual, unexpected and infrequent reactions)
If any of the following develop, consult your physician promptly for guidance.
Mild Adverse Effects
Headache, dizziness, restlessness, insomnia, fine tremor of hands.
Rapid, pounding heartbeat; increased sweating; muscle cramps in arms and legs.
Nausea, heartburn, vomiting.
Serious Adverse Effects
Rapid or irregular heart rhythm, intensification of angina, increased blood pressure.

▷ **Possible Effects on Sexual Function:**   None reported.

Natural Diseases or Disorders That May Be Activated By This Drug
Latent coronary artery disease, diabetes or high blood pressure.

Possible Effects on Laboratory Tests
Urine sugar tests: positive (unreliable results with Benedict's solution).

CAUTION
1. Concurrent use of this drug by aerosol inhalation with beclomethasone aerosol (Beclovent, Vanceril) may increase the risk of toxicity due to fluorocarbon propellants. It is advisable to use this aerosol 20 to 30 minutes *before* beclomethasone aerosol. This will reduce the risk of toxicity and will enhance the penetration of beclomethasone.
2. *Avoid excessive use of aerosol inhalation.* The excessive or prolonged use of this drug by inhalation can reduce its effectiveness and cause serious heart rhythm disturbances, including cardiac arrest.
3. Do not use this drug concurrently with epinephrine. These two drugs may be used alternately if an interval of 4 hours is allowed between doses.
4. If you do not respond to your usually effective dose, ask your physician for guidance. Do not increase the size or frequency of the dose without your physician's approval.

Precautions for Use
By Infants and Children: Safety and effectiveness of use of the aerosol and nebulized solution have not been established for children under 12 years of age. Safety and effectiveness of use of the syrup and tablet have not been established for children under 6 years of age.
By Those over 60 Years of Age: Avoid excessive and continual use. If acute asthma is not relieved promptly, other drugs will have to be tried. Observe for the development of nervousness, palpitations, irregular heart rhythm and muscle tremors. Use with extreme caution if you have hardening of the arteries, heart disease or high blood pressure.

▷ **Advisability of Use During Pregnancy**
Pregnancy Category: C (tentative). See Pregnancy Code inside back cover.
Animal studies: Significant birth defects reported in rabbit studies.
Human studies: Information from adequate studies of pregnant women is not available.
Avoid use during first 3 months. Use during the last 6 months only if clearly needed.

Advisability of Use if Breast-Feeding
Presence of this drug in breast milk: Unknown.
Avoid drug or refrain from nursing.

Habit-Forming Potential: None.

Effects of Overdosage: Nervousness, palpitation, rapid heart rate, sweating, headache, tremor, vomiting, chest pain.

Possible Effects of Long-Term Use: Loss of effectiveness. See *CAUTION* category.

Suggested Periodic Examinations While Taking This Drug (at physician's discretion)
Blood pressure measurements, evaluation of heart status.

▷ **While Taking This Drug, Observe the Following**
Foods: No restrictions.
Beverages: Avoid excessive use of caffeine-containing beverages: coffee, tea, cola, chocolate.
▷ *Alcohol:* No interactions expected.
Tobacco Smoking: No interactions expected.
▷ *Other Drugs*
Metaproterenol *taken concurrently* with
• monoamine oxidase (MAO) type A inhibitor drugs may cause excessive increase in blood pressure and undesirable heart stimulation.
▷ *Driving, Hazardous Activities:* Usually no restrictions. Use caution if excessive nervousness or dizziness occurs.
Aviation Note: The use of this drug *is a disqualification* for piloting. Consult a designated Aviation Medical Examiner.
Exposure to Sun: No restrictions.
Heavy Exercise or Exertion: Use caution. Excessive exercise can induce asthma in sensitive individuals.

METHADONE
(METH a dohn)

Introduced: 1948

Prescription: USA: Yes

Available as Generic: Yes

Brand Name: Dolophine

Class: Strong analgesic, opioids

Controlled Drug: USA: C-II*

BENEFITS versus RISKS

Possible Benefits
EFFECTIVE RELIEF OF
MODERATE TO SEVERE PAIN

Possible Risks
POTENTIAL FOR HABIT
FORMATION (DEPENDENCE)
Weakness, fainting
Disorientation, hallucinations
Interference with urination

▷ **Principal Uses**
As a Single Drug Product: This potent analgesic is used by mouth or injection to relieve moderate to severe pain of any cause. Its primary use

*See Schedules of Controlled Drugs inside back cover.

today is to provide an appropriate substitute for heroin in treatment programs for drug addiction.

How This Drug Works: Acting primarily as a depressant of certain brain functions, this drug suppresses the perception of pain and calms the emotional response to pain.

Available Dosage Forms and Strengths
Concentrate — 10 mg per ml
Injection — 10 mg per ml
Oral solution — 5 mg, 10 mg per 5-ml teaspoonful (8% alcohol)
Tablets — 5 mg, 10 mg
Tablets, dispersible — 40 mg

▷ **Usual Adult Dosage Range:** Taken by mouth: 2.5 to 10 mg/3 to 4 hours as needed to relieve pain. The total daily dosage should not exceed 80 mg. (Dosage schedules for maintenance treatment during heroin withdrawal must be individualized.) **Note: Actual dosage and administration schedule must be determined by the physician for each patient individually.**

▷ **Dosing Instructions:** May be taken with or following food to reduce stomach irritation or nausea. The tablet may be crushed for administration. The concentrate must be diluted in 3 ounces (or more) of water before swallowing.

Usual Duration of Use: As required to control pain. Continual use should not exceed 5 to 7 days without interruption and reassessment of need.

▷ **This Drug Should Not Be Taken If**
• you have had an allergic reaction to any dosage form of it previously.
• you are having an acute attack of asthma.

▷ **Inform Your Physician Before Taking This Drug If**
• you have a history of drug abuse or alcoholism.
• you have impaired liver or kidney function.
• you have a history of asthma or other chronic lung disease.
• you are taking any other drugs that have a sedative effect.
• you are taking, or have taken within the past 14 days, any monoamine oxidase (MAO) type A inhibitor drug (see Drug Class, Section Four).
• you plan to have surgery under general anesthesia in the near future.

Possible Side-Effects (natural, expected and unavoidable drug actions)
Drowsiness, light-headedness, weakness, euphoria, dry mouth, urinary retention, constipation.

▷ **Possible Adverse Effects** (unusual, unexpected and infrequent reactions)
If any of the following develop, consult your physician promptly for guidance.
Mild Adverse Effects
Allergic Reactions: Skin rash, hives, itching.

Headache, dizziness, impaired concentration, sensation of drunkenness, confusion, depression, blurred or double vision.
Facial flushing, sweating, heart palpitation.
Nausea, vomiting.
Serious Adverse Effects
Drop in blood pressure, causing severe weakness and fainting.
Disorientation, hallucinations, unstable gait, tremor, muscle twitching.

▷ **Possible Effects on Sexual Function:**   Decreased libido, impotence, delayed ejaculation, inhibited female orgasm, male infertility, loss of menstruation. (These effects do not occur with short-term use for pain relief; however, they are very common with long-term use and addiction.)

▷ **Adverse Effects That May Mimic Natural Diseases or Disorders**
Paradoxical behavioral disturbances may suggest psychotic disorder.

Possible Effects on Laboratory Tests
Blood thyroid hormone levels: T^3 and T^4 levels increased; free T^4 level decreased.
Urine pregnancy tests: false positive results with Gravindex.
Urine screening tests for drug abuse: may be **positive.** (Test results depend upon amount of drug taken and testing method used.)

CAUTION
1. If you have asthma, chronic bronchitis or emphysema, the excessive use of this drug may cause significant respiratory difficulty, thickening of bronchial secretions and suppression of coughing.
2. The concurrent use of this drug with atropinelike drugs can increase the risk of urinary retention and reduced intestinal function.
3. Do not take this drug following acute head injury.

Precautions for Use
By Infants and Children: Do not use this drug in infants under 1 year of age because of their vulnerability to life-threatening respiratory depression.
By Those over 60 Years of Age: Use small doses initially and increase dosage as needed and tolerated. Limit use to short-term treatment only if possible. There may be increased susceptibility to the development of drowsiness, dizziness, unsteadiness, falling, urinary retention and constipation (often leading to fecal impaction).

▷ **Advisability of Use During Pregnancy**
Pregnancy Category: C (tentative). See Pregnancy Code inside back cover.
Animal studies: Significant birth defects reported in mice and hamster studies.
Human studies: Information from adequate studies of pregnant women is not available.
Avoid during the first 3 months. Use sparingly and in small doses during the last 6 months only if clearly needed.

Advisability of Use if Breast-Feeding
Presence of this drug in breast milk: Yes.
Avoid drug or refrain from nursing.

Habit-Forming Potential: This drug can cause psychological and physical dependence (see Glossary).

Effects of Overdosage: Marked drowsiness, confusion, tremors, convulsions, stupor progressing to coma.

Possible Effects of Long-Term Use: Psychological and physical dependence, chronic constipation.

Suggested Periodic Examinations While Taking This Drug (at physician's discretion)
None.

▷ **While Taking This Drug, Observe the Following**
Foods: No restrictions.
Beverages: No restrictions. May be taken with milk.
▷   *Alcohol:* Use extreme caution until the combined effects have been determined. Opioid analgesics can intensify the intoxicating effects of alcohol, and alcohol can intensify the depressant effects of opioids on brain function, breathing and circulation. Alcohol is best avoided.
Tobacco Smoking: No interactions expected.
Marijuana Smoking: Increase in drowsiness and pain relief; impairment of mental and physical performance.
▷   *Other Drugs*
Methadone may *increase* the effects of
• other drugs with sedative effects, and cause excessive sedation.
Methadone *taken concurrently* with
• monoamine oxidase (MAO) type A inhibitor drugs (see Drug Class, Section Four) requires cautious observation for indications of nervous system toxicity.
The following drugs may *decrease* the effects of methadone
• phenytoin (Dilantin, etc.).
• rifampin (Rifadin, Rimactane, etc.).
▷   *Driving, Hazardous Activities:* This drug can impair mental alertness, judgment, reaction time and physical coordination. Avoid hazardous activities.
Aviation Note: The use of this drug *is a disqualification* for piloting. Consult a designated Aviation Medical Examiner.
Exposure to Sun: No restrictions.
Discontinuation: It is advisable to limit this drug to short-term use. If it is necessary to use it for extended periods of time, discontinuation should be gradual to minimize possible effects of withdrawal (stomach cramps, tearing eyes, nasal discharge, chills and tremors.

METHOTREXATE
(meth oh TREX ayt)

Other Names: Amethopterin, MTX

Introduced: 1948

Class: Anticancer drugs, antipsoriasis

Prescription: USA: Yes
Canada: Yes

Controlled Drug: USA: No
Canada: No

Available as Generic: Yes

Brand Names: Folex, Mexate, Rheumatrex Dose Pack

BENEFITS versus RISKS

Possible Benefits	*Possible Risks*
EFFECTIVE TREATMENT OF SOME CASES OF SEVERE DISABLING PSORIASIS	GASTROINTESTINAL ULCERATION AND BLEEDING
EFFECTIVE TREATMENT OF CERTAIN ADULT AND CHILDHOOD CANCERS	MOUTH AND THROAT ULCERATON
PREVENTION OF REJECTION OF BONE MARROW TRANSPLANTS	SEVERE BONE MARROW DEPRESSION
Helpful adjunctive therapy in severe, refractory rheumatoid arthritis and related disorders	DAMAGE TO LUNGS, LIVER AND KIDNEYS
	Loss of hair

▷ **Principal Uses**

As a Single Drug Product: This very potent drug is used to treat (1) severe and widespread forms of disabling psoriasis that have failed to respond to all standard treatment procedures; (2) various types of both adult and childhood cancer. In addition, it is used to prevent rejection of transplanted bone marrow. More recently, it is being used in the treatment of connective tissue disorders such as rheumatoid arthritis, scleroderma and related conditions. Its use in rheumatoid arthritis is restricted to the treatment of selected adults with severe active disease that has failed to respond to conventional therapy.

How This Drug Works: By interfering with the normal utilization of folic acid in tissue cell reproduction, this drug retards abnormally rapid tissue growth (as in psoriasis and cancer).

Available Dosage Forms and Strengths
Injections — 2.5 mg per ml, 25 mg per ml
Injections (preservative-free) — 25 mg per ml
Tablets — 2.5 mg

▷ **Usual Adult Dosage Range**

For psoriasis (alternate schedules): (1) 10 to 50 mg once/week; (2) 2.5 to 5 mg/12 hours for 3 doses, or every 8 hours for 4 doses, once a week up to a maximum of 30 mg/week; (3) 2.5 mg/day for 5 days, followed by 2 days without drug, with gradual increase in dosage to a maximum of 6.25 mg/day.

For rheumatoid arthritis (alternate schedules): (1) single oral dose of 7.5 mg once weekly; (2) divided doses of 2.5 mg every 12 hours for 3 doses per week. Dosage may be increased gradually as needed and tolerated. Do not exceed a weekly dose of 20 mg.**Note: Actual dosage and administration schedule must be determined by the physician for each patient individually.**

▷ **Dosing Instructions:** May be taken with food to reduce stomach irritation. Drink at least 2 to 3 quarts of liquids daily. The tablet may be crushed for administration.

Usual Duration of Use: Continual use on a regular schedule for several weeks is usually necessary to determine this drug's effectiveness in reducing the severity and extent of psoriasis. Response in rheumatoid arthritis usually begins after 3 to 6 weeks of treatment. When a favorable response has been achieved, the dosage should be reduced to the smallest amount that will maintain acceptable improvement. Long-term use (months to years) requires supervision and periodic evaluation by your physician. Consult your physician on a regular basis.

▷ **This Drug Should Not Be Taken If**
- you have had an allergic reaction to it previously.
- you currently have, or have had a recent exposure to, either chicken pox or shingles (herpes zoster).
- you are pregnant or planning pregnancy in the near future, and you are taking this drug to treat psoriasis or rheumatoid arthritis.
- you have active liver disease, peptic ulcer, regional enteritis or ulcerative colitis.
- you currently have a blood cell or bone marrow disorder.

▷ **Inform Your Physician Before Taking This Drug If**
- you have a chronic infection of any kind.
- you have impaired liver or kidney function.
- you have a history of bone marrow impairment of any kind, especially drug-induced bone marrow depression.
- you have a history of gout, peptic ulcer disease, regional enteritis or ulcerative colitis.

Possible Side-Effects (natural, expected and unavoidable drug actions)
The following are due to the pharmacological actions of this drug. **Report such developments to your physician promptly.**
Sores on the lips, in the mouth or throat; vomiting; intestinal cramping; diarrhea (may be bloody); painful urination; bloody urine.

Reduced resistance to infection, fatigue, weakness, fever, abnormal bleeding or bruising (bone marrow depression).

▷ **Possible Adverse Effects** (unusual, unexpected and infrequent reactions)
If any of the following develop, consult your physician promptly for guidance.
Mild Adverse Effects
Allergic Reactions: Skin rash, hives, itching.
Headache, drowsiness, blurred vision.
Loss of appetite, nausea, vomiting.
Loss of hair, loss of skin pigmentation, acne.
Serious Adverse Effects
Allergic Reactions: Drug-induced pneumonia: cough, chest pain, shortness of breath.
Nervous system toxicity: speech disturbances, paralysis, seizures.
Liver toxicity with jaundice (see Glossary).
Kidney toxicity: reduced urine volume, kidney failure.

▷ **Possible Effects on Sexual Function:**   Altered timing and pattern of menstruation.

Possible Delayed Adverse Effects: Some reports suggest that methotrexate therapy may contribute to the later development of secondary cancers. Other studies have not confirmed this.

Possible Effects on Laboratory Tests
Complete blood cell counts: decreased red cells, hemoglobin, white cells and platelets.
Blood uric acid level: increased.
Liver function tests: increased liver enzymes (ALT/GPT, AST/GOT and alkaline phosphatase), increased bilirubin.
Kidney function tests: increased blood urea nitrogen (BUN) level; increased urine creatinine content (kidney damage).
Fecal occult blood test: positive.
Sperm count: decreased.

CAUTION
1. This drug has a high potential for serious toxicity. Its use must be monitored carefully and continually by a physician who is skilled in its proper administration. Request the Patient Package Insert that is available with this drug (Rheumatrex Dose Pack) and read it thoroughly.
2. Appropriate laboratory examinations, performed before and during the use of this drug, are mandatory. Comply fully with your physician's instructions regarding periodic studies.
3. Women with potential for pregnancy should have a pregnancy test before taking this drug and should use an effective form of contraception during its use and for 8 weeks following its discontinuation.
4. Administration of live virus vaccines should be avoided during use

of this drug. Because immune functions are suppressed by this drug, live virus vaccines could actually produce infection rather than stimulate an immune response.

Precautions for Use
By Those over 60 Years of Age: Careful evaluation of kidney function should be made before starting treatment and during the entire course of therapy.

▷ Advisability of Use During Pregnancy
Pregnancy Category: D (tentative). See Pregnancy Code inside back cover.
Animal studies: Skull and facial defects reported in mice.
Human studies: This drug is known to cause fetal deaths and birth defects.
Its use during pregnancy to treat psoriasis or rheumatoid arthritis cannot be justified. If its use during pregnancy is deemed necessary to treat a responsive type of cancer, it should be avoided during the first 3 months if possible.

Advisability of Use if Breast-Feeding
Presence of this drug in breast milk: Yes.
Avoid drug or refrain from nursing.

Habit-Forming Potential: None.

Effects of Overdosage: The side-effects and adverse effects listed previously develop earlier and with greater severity.

Possible Effects of Long-Term Use: Liver fibrosis and cirrhosis occur in 3% to 5% of long-term users (35 to 49 months).

Suggested Periodic Examinations While Taking This Drug (at physician's discretion)
Complete blood cell counts, liver and kidney function tests, blood uric acid levels, chest X-ray examinations.

▷ While Taking This Drug, Observe the Following
Foods: Avoid highly seasoned foods that could be irritating. Between courses of treatment, eat liberally of the following foods: beef, chicken, lamb and pork liver, asparagus, navy beans, kale and spinach.
Beverages: No restrictions. This drug may be taken with milk.
▷ *Alcohol:* Avoid completely.
Tobacco Smoking: No interactions expected.
▷ *Other Drugs*
Methotrexate may *decrease* the effects of
- digoxin (Lanoxin).
- phenytoin (Dilantin).

The following drugs may *increase* the effects of methotrexate and enhance its toxicity
- aspirin and other salicylates.
- probenecid (Benemid).

▷ *Driving, Hazardous Activities:* This drug may cause drowsiness, dizziness or blurred vision. Restrict activities as necessary.

Aviation Note: The use of this drug *is a disqualification* for piloting. Consult a designated Aviation Medical Examiner.

Exposure to Sun: Use caution until skin sensitivity has been determined. This drug can cause photosensitivity. Avoid ultraviolet lamps.

METHYCLOTHIAZIDE
(METH ee kloh THI a zide)

Introduced: 1960

Class: Antihypertensive, diuretic, thiazides

Prescription: USA: Yes
Canada: Yes

Controlled Drug: USA: No
Canada: No

Available as Generic: USA: Yes
Canada: No

Brand Names: Aquatensen, Diutensen [CD], Diutensen-R [CD], ✦Duretic, ✦Dureticyl [CD], Enduron, Enduronyl [CD], Enduronyl Forte [CD]

BENEFITS versus RISKS

Possible Benefits	*Possible Risks*
EFFECTIVE, WELL-TOLERATED DIURETIC	Loss of body potassium
POSSIBLY EFFECTIVE IN MILD HYPERTENSION	Increased blood sugar
ENHANCES EFFECTIVENESS OF OTHER ANTIHYPERTENSIVES	Increased blood uric acid
Beneficial in treatment of diabetes insipidus	Increased blood calcium
	Rare blood cell disorders

▷ **Principal Uses**

As a Single Drug Product: Thiazide diuretics are used primarily to (1) increase the volume of urine (diuresis) to correct the excessive fluid retention associated with congestive heart failure and certain types of liver and kidney disease; and (2) initiate treatment for high blood pressure (hypertension). They are often the first drugs tried in treating mild to moderate hypertension. Less frequent uses include the treatment of diabetes insipidus and the prevention of kidney stones that contain calcium.

As a Combination Drug Product [CD]: When this drug is used alone to treat hypertension, it is referred to as a "step 1" antihypertensive. Should it fail to reduce the blood pressure adequately, a "step 2" antihypertensive drug is added to be taken concurrently with the step 1 drug. These drugs may be combined into one drug product. Thiazides are available in combination with beta blockers, hydralazine, methyldopa, reserpine and other diuretics to increase their effectiveness in treating hypertension.

How This Drug Works: By increasing the elimination of salt and water from the body (through increased urine production), this drug reduces the volume of fluid in the blood and body tissues and lowers the sodium content throughout the body. By relaxing the walls of smaller arteries and allowing them to expand, this drug increases the total capacity of the arterial system. The combined effect of these two actions (reduced blood volume in expanded space) results in lowering of blood pressure.

Available Dosage Forms and Strengths
Tablets — 2.5 mg, 5 mg

▷ **Usual Adult Dosage Range:** As antihypertensive: 2.5 to 5 mg/day initially; 2.5 to 10 mg/day for maintenance. As diuretic: 2.5 to 10 mg/day initially; the smallest effective dose should be determined. The total daily dose should not exceed 10 mg. **Note: Actual dosage and administration schedule must be determined by the physician for each patient individually.**

▷ **Dosing Instructions:** May be taken with or following meals to reduce stomach irritation. Best taken in the morning to avoid nighttime urination. The tablet may be crushed for administration.

Usual Duration of Use: Continual use on a regular schedule for 2 to 3 weeks is usually necessary to determine this drug's effectiveness in lowering high blood pressure. Long-term use (months to years) requires periodic evaluation of response and possible dosage adjustment. Use as a diuretic should be intermittent with "drug holidays" (no drug taken) to reduce the risk of sodium and potassium imbalance. Consult your physician on a regular basis.

▷ **This Drug Should Not Be Taken If**
• you have had an allergic reaction to any dosage form of it previously.

▷ **Inform Your Physician Before Taking This Drug If**
• you are allergic to any form of "sulfa" drug.
• you are pregnant or planning pregnancy.
• you have a history of kidney or liver disease.
• you have diabetes, gout or lupus erythematosus.
• you are taking any form of cortisone, digitalis, oral antidiabetic drug or insulin.
• you plan to have surgery under general anesthesia in the near future.

Possible Side-Effects (natural, expected and unavoidable drug actions)
Light-headedness on arising from sitting or lying position (see Orthostatic Hypotension in Glossary).

Increase in blood sugar level, affecting control of diabetes.
Increase in blood uric acid level, affecting control of gout.
Decrease in blood potassium level, causing muscle weakness and cramp-
ing.

▷ **Possible Adverse Effects** (unusual, unexpected and infrequent reactions)
   **If any of the following develop, consult your physician promptly for
   guidance.**
   Mild Adverse Effects
   Allergic Reactions: Skin rashes, hives, drug fever.
   Headache, dizziness, blurred or yellow vision.
   Reduced appetite, indigestion, nausea, vomiting, diarrhea.
   Serious Adverse Effects
   Allergic Reactions: Hepatitis with jaundice (see Glossary), anaphylactic
   reaction (see Glossary), severe skin reactions.
   Inflammation of the pancreas—severe abdominal pain.
   Bone marrow depression (see Glossary)—fatigue, weakness, fever, sore
   throat, abnormal bleeding or bruising.

▷ **Possible Effects on Sexual Function:**   Impotence (rare) with recommended
   dosage.

▷ **Adverse Effects That May Mimic Natural Diseases or Disorders**
   Liver reaction may suggest viral hepatitis.

Natural Diseases or Disorders That May Be Activated by This Drug
   Diabetes, gout, systemic lupus erythematosus.

Possible Effects on Laboratory Tests
   Complete blood cell counts: decreased red cells, hemoglobin, white cells
   and platelets.
   Blood amylase level: increased (possible pancreatitis).
   Blood calcium level: increased.
   Blood sodium and chloride levels: decreased.
   Blood cholesterol and triglyceride levels: increased.
   Blood glucose level: increased.
   Glucose tolerance test (GTT): decreased.
   Blood lithium level: increased.
   Blood potassium level: decreased.
   Blood urea nitrogen (BUN) level: increased with long-term use.
   Blood uric acid level: increased.
   Liver function tests: increased liver enzymes (ALT/GPT, AST/GOT and
   alkaline phosphatase), increased bilirubin.

CAUTION
   1. Do not exceed recommended doses. Increased dosage can cause ex-
      cessive loss of sodium and potassium, with resultant loss of appetite,
      nausea, fatigue, weakness, confusion and tingling in the extremities.
   2. If you are also taking a digitalis preparation (digitoxin, digoxin),

ensure an adequate intake of high-potassium foods to prevent potassium deficiency—a potential cause of digitalis toxicity. (See Table of High Potassium Foods in Section Six.)

Precautions for Use

By Infants and Children: Avoid overdosage that could cause serious dehydration. Significant potassium loss can occur within the first 2 weeks of drug use.

By Those over 60 Years of Age: Small doses are advisable until your individual response has been determined. You may be more susceptible to the development of impaired thinking, orthostatic hypotension, potassium loss and blood sugar increase. Overdosage and extended use of this drug can cause excessive loss of body water, thickening (increased viscosity) of the blood and an increased tendency for the blood to clot—predisposing to stroke, heart attack or thrombophlebitis (vein inflammation with blood clot).

▷ **Advisability of Use During Pregnancy**

Pregnancy Category: D (tentative). See Pregnancy Code inside back cover.

Animal studies: No information available.

Human studies: Information from adequate studies of pregnant women is not available.

This drug should not be used during pregnancy unless a very serious complication occurs for which this drug is significantly beneficial. Ask physician for guidance.

Advisability of Use if Breast-Feeding

Presence of this drug in breast milk: Yes, in small amounts.

Avoid drug or refrain from nursing.

Habit-Forming Potential: None.

Effects of Overdosage: Dry mouth, thirst, lethargy, weakness, muscle cramping, nausea, vomiting, drowsiness progressing to stupor or coma.

Possible Effects of Long-Term Use: Impaired balance of water, salt and potassium in blood and body tissues. Development of diabetes in predisposed individuals. Pathological changes in parathyroid glands with increased blood calcium levels and decreased blood phosphate levels.

Suggested Periodic Examinations While Taking This Drug (at physician's discretion)

Complete blood cell counts, measurements of blood levels of sodium, potassium, chloride, sugar and uric acid.

Kidney and liver function tests.

▷ **While Taking This Drug, Observe the Following**

Foods: Consult your physician regarding the advisability of eating foods rich in potassium. If so advised, see the Table of High Potassium Foods in Section Six. Follow physician's advice regarding the use of salt.

Beverages: No restrictions. This drug may be taken with milk.

▷   *Alcohol:* Use with caution until the combined effects have been determined. Alcohol may exaggerate the blood-pressure-lowering effects of this drug and cause orthostatic hypotension.

Tobacco Smoking: No interactions expected. Follow physician's advice.

▷   *Other Drugs*

Methyclothiazide may ***increase*** the effects of

- other antihypertensive drugs; dosage adjustments may be necessary to prevent excessive lowering of blood pressure.
- lithium, and cause lithium toxicity.

Methyclothiazide may ***decrease*** the effects of

- oral antidiabetic drugs (sulfonylureas); dosage adjustments may be necessary for proper control of blood sugar.

Methyclothiazide ***taken concurrently*** with

- digitalis preparations (digitoxin, digoxin) requires very careful monitoring and dosage adjustments to prevent fluctuations of blood potassium levels and serious disturbances of heart rhythm.

The following drugs may ***decrease*** the effects of methyclothiazide

- cholestyramine (Cuemid, Questran) may interfere with its absorption.
- colestipol (Colestid) may interfere with its absorption.

Take cholestyramine and colestipol 1 hour before any oral diuretic.

▷   *Driving, Hazardous Activities:* Use caution until the possible occurrence of orthostatic hypotension, dizziness or impaired vision has been determined.

Aviation Note: The use of this drug ***may be a disqualification*** for piloting. Consult a designated Aviation Medical Examiner.

Exposure to Sun: Use caution until sensitivity has been determined. This drug can cause photosensitivity (see Glossary).

Exposure to Heat: Avoid excessive perspiring, which could cause additional loss of salt and water from the body.

Heavy Exercise or Exertion: Avoid exertion that produces light-headedness, excessive fatigue or muscle cramping. Isometric exercises—the "overload" technique for strengthening individual muscles—can raise blood pressure significantly. Ask physician for guidance regarding participation in this form of exercise.

Occurrence of Unrelated Illness: Illnesses that cause vomiting or diarrhea can produce a serious imbalance of important body chemistry. Consult your physician for guidance.

Discontinuation: This drug should not be stopped abruptly following long-term use; serious thiazide-withdrawal fluid retention (edema) can develop after sudden withdrawal. The dose should be reduced gradually. It may be advisable to discontinue this drug 5 to 7 days before major surgery. Ask your physician, surgeon and/or anesthesiologist for guidance regarding dosage adjustment or drug withdrawal.

METHYLDOPA
(meth il DOH pa)

Other Name: Alpha-methyldopa

Introduced: 1963

Class: Antihypertensive

Prescription: USA: Yes
Canada: Yes

Controlled Drug: USA: No
Canada: No

Available as Generic: Yes

Brand Names: Aldochlor-150/250 [CD], Aldomet, Aldoril-15/25 [CD], Aldoril D30/D50 [CD], ✦Apo-Methazide [CD], ✦Apo-Methyldopa, ✦Dopa-
met, ✦Medimet-250, ✦Novodoparil [CD], ✦Novomedopa, ✦PMS Dopazide [CD]

BENEFITS versus RISKS

Possible Benefits	*Possible Risks*
EFFECTIVE STEP-2 OR -3 ANTIHYPERTENSIVE IN 66% OF CASES OF MILD TO SEVERE HYPERTENSION when used adjunctively with other drugs	LIVER TOXICITY (may be severe)
	Mental depression
	Water retention
	Hemolytic anemia (less than 1%)
Symptomatic relief in cases of Raynaud's disease	Drug fever
	Blood cell disorders (rare)

▷ **Principal Uses**

As a Single Drug Product: Used as a "step 2" or "step 3" medication in
conjunction with other antihypertensive drugs in the treatment of moderate to severe high blood pressure.

As a Combination Drug Product [CD]: This drug is available in combination
with chlorothiazide and with hydrochlorothiazide, mild diuretics that
represent "step 1" antihypertensive drugs. Combinations of "step 1" and
"step 2" drugs are more effective and more convenient for long-term
use.

How This Drug Works: By decreasing the activity of the vasomotor center
in the brain, this drug reduces the ability of the sympathetic nervous
system to maintain the degree of blood vessel constriction that is responsible for blood pressure elevation. This change results in relaxation of blood vessel walls and lowering of blood pressure.

Available Dosage Forms and Strengths
Injection — 250 mg per 5 ml
Oral suspension — 250 mg per 5-ml teaspoonful (1% alcohol)
Tablets — 125 mg, 250 mg, 500 mg

▷ **Usual Adult Dosage Range:**   Initially, 250 mg 2 or 3 times/day for 2 days; increase dose as needed and tolerated. For maintenance, 500 to 2000 mg/day in 2 to 4 divided doses. The total daily dose should not exceed 3000 mg. **Note: Actual dosage and administration schedule must be determined by the physician for each patient individually.**

▷ **Dosing Instructions:**   May be taken without regard to meals. The tablet may be crushed for administration.

Usual Duration of Use: Continual use on a regular schedule for 2 to 4 weeks is usually necessary to determine this drug's effectiveness in controlling high blood pressure. Long-term use (months to years) requires supervision and periodic evaluation by your physician. Consult your physician on a regular basis.

▷ **This Drug Should Not Be Taken If**
  • you have had an allergic reaction to it previously.
  • you have active liver disease.
  • you have a mild and uncomplicated case of hypertension.

▷ **Inform Your Physician Before Taking This Drug If**
  • you have a history of liver disease or impaired liver function.
  • you have a history of mental depression or porphyria.
  • you are taking any monoamine oxidase (MAO) type A inhibitor drugs, phenothiazines or tricyclic antidepressant drugs (see Drug Classes, Section Four).
  • you plan to have surgery under general anesthesia in the near future.

Possible Side-Effects (natural, expected and unavoidable drug actions)
  Drowsiness, lethargy and weakness; these may occur during the first few weeks and then subside.
  Light-headedness in upright position (see Orthostatic Hypotension in Glossary).
  Nasal stuffiness, dry mouth.

▷ **Possible Adverse Effects** (unusual, unexpected and infrequent reactions)
  If any of the following develop, consult your physician promptly for guidance.
  Mild Adverse Effects
  Allergic Reactions: Skin rash, joint and muscle discomfort, fever.
  Headache, dizziness.
  Irritation of tongue, nausea, vomiting, diarrhea.
  Water retention, weight gain.
  Serious Adverse Effects
  Allergic Reactions: Hepatitis with jaundice (see Glossary).
  Idiosyncratic Reaction: Episodes of high fever (not due to infection), 1% of users.
  Bone marrow depression (see Glossary): fatigue, weakness, fever, sore throat, abnormal bleeding or bruising.
  Inflammation of the pancreas: abdominal pain, fever, nausea, vomiting.

Parkinson-like disorders (see Glossary).
Behavioral changes: depression, confusion, nightmares.

▷ **Possible Effects on Sexual Function:** Decreased male and female libido (14%), impotence (24% to 80%), inhibited ejaculation (rare), inhibited female orgasm (related to higher doses), male breast enlargement and tenderness, female breast enlargement with milk production (26%), loss of menstruation.

▷ **Adverse Effects That May Mimic Natural Diseases or Disorders**
Liver toxicity may suggest viral hepatitis.
Idiosyncratic fever may suggest a viral flulike infection.
Abnormal involuntary movements of extremities may suggest Huntington's disease.

Natural Diseases or Disorders That May Be Activated by This Drug
Porphyria, latent coronary artery insufficiency, lupus erythematosuslike syndrome.

Possible Effects on Laboratory Tests
Complete blood cell counts: decreased red cells, hemoglobin, white cells and platelets; increased eosinophils (allergic reaction).
Blood antinuclear antibodies (ANA): positive.
Blood lupus erythematosus (LE) cells: positive.
Prothrombin time: increased.
Blood total cholesterol, HDL cholesterol, LDL cholesterol, VLDL cholesterol levels: decreased.
Blood triglyceride levels: increased.
Blood sodium level: increased (salt and water retention).
Liver function tests: increased liver enzymes (ALT/GPT, AST/GOT and alkaline phosphatase), increased bilirubin.
Urine sugar tests: false positive result with Clinitest.

CAUTION
1. If this drug is used as the sole agent, the blood pressure may be very erratic. Observe for the development of tolerance and loss of effectiveness.
2. This drug is most effective when combined with a diuretic.
3. Avoid concurrent use with other drugs known to depress bone marrow function.
4. Report the development of any tendency to emotional depression.

Precautions for Use
By Infants and Children: Observe for the development of hemolytic anemia, abnormal liver function, excessive sedation and nightmares.
By Those over 60 Years of Age: The basic rule in treating hypertension after 60 is to proceed cautiously. Unacceptably high blood pressure should be reduced without creating risks associated with excessively low blood pressure. Sudden, rapid and excessive reduction of blood pressure can predispose to stroke or heart attack. Adverse effects are com-

mon: drowsiness (50%), depression (10%), forgetfulness, reduced mental acuity, nasal congestion, dry mouth, hallucinations. This drug can cause parkinsonism or intensify existing parkinsonism.

▷ **Advisability of Use During Pregnancy**
Pregnancy Category: B (tentative). See Pregnancy Code inside back cover.
Animal studies: No birth defects reported in mice, rats or rabbits.
Human studies: Information from adequate studies of pregnant women is not available.
Use this drug only if clearly needed. Use the minimal effective dose.

Advisability of Use if Breast-Feeding
Presence of this drug in breast milk: Yes.
If drug is necessary, monitor infant for drowsiness and inadequate feeding.

Habit-Forming Potential: None.

Effects of Overdosage: Marked drowsiness, weakness, confusion, nausea, vomiting, stupor progressing to coma.

Possible Effects of Long-Term Use: Water retention (if not taken with a diuretic). Development of hemolytic anemia (see Glossary).

Suggested Periodic Examinations While Taking This Drug (at physician's discretion)
Complete blood cell counts, liver function tests.

▷ **While Taking This Drug, Observe the Following**
Foods: Avoid excessive salt. When possible, avoid high-protein foods at the time this drug is taken; this drug competes with proteins for absorption.
Beverages: No restrictions. May be taken with milk.
▷ *Alcohol:* Use with extreme caution until the combined effects have been determined. This combination can cause marked sedation and exaggerated drop in blood pressure.
Tobacco Smoking: No interactions expected.
▷ *Other Drugs*
Methyldopa may *increase* the effects of
• tolbutamide (Orinase), and cause excessive hypoglycemia.
• other drugs with sedative effects, and cause excessive sedation.
Methyldopa *taken concurrently* with
• beta blocker drugs may rarely cause hypertensive reactions (see Drug Class, Section Four).
• haloperidol (Haldol) may cause dementia, disorientation and abnormal behavior.
• monoamine oxidase (MAO) type A inhibitor drugs may cause hallucinations and hypertension (see Drug Class, Section Four).
• phenothiazines may cause hypertension (see Drug Class, Section Four).

The following drugs may *decrease* the effects of methyldopa
  • tricyclic antidepressants (see Drug Class, Section Four).

▷ *Driving, Hazardous Activities:* This drug may cause drowsiness and fatigue. Restrict activities as necessary.

Aviation Note: The use of this drug *may be a disqualification* for piloting. Consult a designated Aviation Medical Examiner.

Exposure to Sun: No restrictions.

Heavy Exercise or Exertion: Use caution. Excessive physical activity may increase the possibility of orthostatic hypotension. Isometric exercises—the "overload" technique for strengthening individual muscles—can raise blood pressure significantly. Ask your physician for guidance.

Discontinuation: It may be advisable to discontinue this drug 5 to 7 days before surgery under general anesthesia. Consult your surgeon and/or anesthesiologist regarding dosage adjustment or withdrawal of this drug prior to surgery.

METHYLPHENIDATE
(meth il FEN i dayt)

Introduced: 1956

Class: Stimulant, amphetamine-like drugs

Prescription: USA: Yes
  Canada: Yes

Controlled Drug: USA: C-II*
  Canada: <C>

Available as Generic: USA: Yes
  Canada: No

Brand Names: Ritalin, Ritalin-SR

BENEFITS versus RISKS	
Possible Benefits	*Possible Risks*
EFFECTIVE CONTROL OF NARCOLEPSY	POTENTIAL FOR SERIOUS PSYCHOLOGICAL DEPENDENCE
USEFUL AS ADJUNCTIVE TREATMENT IN THE ATTENTION DEFICIT DISORDERS OF CHILDHOOD	SUPPRESSION OF GROWTH IN CHILDHOOD
Useful in treatment of mild to moderate depression	Abnormal behavior
Useful in some cases of emotional withdrawal in the elderly	Rare blood cell disorders

*See Schedules of Controlled Drugs inside back cover.

▷ **Principal Uses**

As a Single Drug Product: Used primarily to treat (1) narcolepsy, recurrent spells of uncontrollable drowsiness and sleep; and (2) attention-deficit disorders of childhood, formerly known as the hyperactive child syndrome, minimal brain damage and minimal brain dysfunction. Additional uses include the treatment of mild to moderate depression, and the management of apathetic and withdrawal states in the elderly.

How This Drug Works: Not completely established. It is thought that this drug may increase the release of the nerve impulse transmitter norepinephrine. The resulting stimulation of brain function improves alertness and concentration, and increases learning ability and attention span. The primary action that calms the overactive child is not known.

Available Dosage Forms and Strengths
Tablets — 5 mg, 10 mg, 20 mg
Tablets, prolonged-action — 20 mg

▷ **Usual Adult Dosage Range:**   5 to 20 mg 2 or 3 times/day. **Note: Actual dosage and administration schedule must be determined by the physician for each patient individually.**

▷ **Dosing Instructions:**   Take tablet 30 to 45 minutes before meals. The regular tablet may be crushed for administration; the prolonged-action tablet should be taken whole, not crushed.

Usual Duration of Use: Continual use on a regular schedule for 3 to 4 weeks is usually necessary to determine this drug's effectiveness in controlling the symptoms of narcolepsy or improving the behavior of attention-deficit children. Long-term use (months to years) requires supervision and periodic evaluation by your physician. Consult your physician on a regular basis.

▷ **This Drug Should Not Be Taken If**
• you have had an allergic reaction to it previously.
• you have glaucoma (inadequately treated).
• you are experiencing a period of severe anxiety, nervous tension or emotional depression.

▷ **Inform Your Physician Before Taking This Drug If**
• you have high blood pressure, angina or epilepsy.
• you are taking, or have taken within the past 14 days, any monoamine oxidase (MAO) type A inhibitor drug (see Drug Class, Section Four).

Possible Side-Effects (natural, expected and unavoidable drug actions)
Nervousness, insomnia.

▷ **Possible Adverse Effects** (unusual, unexpected and infrequent reactions)
If any of the following develop, consult your physician promptly for guidance.
Mild Adverse Effects
Allergic Reactions: Skin rash, hives, drug fever, joint pains.

Headache, dizziness, rapid and forceful heart palpitation.
Reduced appetite, nausea, abdominal discomfort.
Serious Adverse Effects
Allergic Reactions: Severe skin reactions, extensive bruising due to allergic destruction of blood platelets (see Glossary).
Idiosyncratic Reaction: Abnormal patterns of behavior.
Abnormally low red blood cell and white blood cell counts.

▷ **Possible Effects on Sexual Function:** None reported.

Natural Diseases or Disorders That May Be Activated by This Drug
Latent epilepsy.

Possible Effects on Laboratory Tests
Blood platelet counts: occasionally decreased.
Prothrombin time: increased.

CAUTION
1. Careful dosage adjustments on an individual basis are mandatory.
2. Paradoxical reactions (see Glossary) can occur, causing aggravation of initial symptoms for which this drug was prescribed.

Precautions for Use
By Infants and Children: Safety and effectiveness for use by those under 6 years of age have not been established. If this drug is not benefical in managing an attention deficit disorder after a trial of one month, it should be discontinued. During long-term use, monitor the child for normal growth and development.
By Those over 60 Years of Age: Start with small doses to determine your tolerance for this drug. You may be more susceptible to the development of nervousness, agitation, insomnia, high blood pressure, angina or disturbance of heart rhythm.

▷ **Advisability of Use During Pregnancy**
Pregnancy Category: B (tentative). See Pregnancy Code inside back cover.
Animal studies: No birth defects found in mouse studies.
Human studies: Information from adequate studies of pregnant women is not available.
Use this drug only if clearly needed. Ask physician for guidance.

Advisability of Use if Breast-Feeding
Presence of this drug in breast milk: Unknown.
Avoid drug or refrain from nursing.

Habit-Forming Potential: This drug can produce tolerance and cause serious psychological dependence (see Glossary), a potentially dangerous characteristic of amphetaminelike drugs (see Drug Class, Section Four).

Effects of Overdosage: Headache, vomiting, agitation, tremors, muscle twitching, dry mouth, sweating, fever, confusion, hallucinations, seizures, coma.

Possible Effects of Long-Term Use: Suppression of growth (in weight and/ or height) has been reported in children during long-term use of this drug.

Suggested Periodic Examinations While Taking This Drug (at physician's discretion)
Complete blood cell counts, blood pressure measurements.

▷ **While Taking This Drug, Observe the Following**
Foods: Avoid foods rich in tyramine (see Glossary); this drug in combination with tyramine may cause an excessive rise in blood pressure.
Beverages: Avoid beverages prepared from meat or meat extracts. This drug may be taken with milk.
▷ *Alcohol:* Avoid beer, Chianti wines and vermouth.
Tobacco Smoking: No interactions expected.
▷ *Other Drugs*
Methylphenidate may *increase* the effects of
• tricyclic antidepressants, and enhance their toxic effects (see Drug Class, Section Four).
Methylphenidate may *decrease* the effects of
• guanethidine (Ismelin), and impair its ability to lower blood pressure.
Methylphenidate *taken concurrently* with
• anticonvulsants may cause a significant change in the pattern of epileptic seizures; dosage adjustments may be necessary for proper control.
• monoamine oxidase (MAO) type A inhibitor drugs (see Drug Class, Section Four) may cause a significant rise in blood pressure. Avoid the concurrent use of these drugs.
▷ *Driving, Hazardous Activities:* This drug may cause dizziness or drowsiness. Restrict activities as necessary.
Aviation Note: The use of this drug *is a disqualification* for piloting. Consult a designated Aviation Medical Examiner.
Exposure to Sun: No restrictions.
Discontinuation: If it has been necessary to use this drug for an extended period of time, do not discontinue it abruptly. Careful supervision is necessary during withdrawal to prevent severe depression and erratic behavior.

METHYLPREDNISOLONE
(meth il pred NIS oh lohn)

Introduced: 1957

Class: Cortisonelike drugs

Prescription: USA: Yes
Canada: Yes

Controlled Drug: USA: No
Canada: No

Available as Generic: USA: Yes
Canada: No

Brand Names: Medrol, Medrol Enpak

BENEFITS versus RISKS

Possible Benefits
EFFECTIVE RELIEF OF
 SYMPTOMS IN A WIDE
 VARIETY OF INFLAMMATORY
 AND ALLERGIC DISORDERS
EFFECTIVE
 IMMUNO-SUPPRESSION in
 selected benign and malignant
 disorders

Possible Risks
Short-term use (up to 10 days) is
 usually well tolerated
Long-term use (exceeding 2
 weeks) is associated with many
 possible adverse effects:
ALTERED MOOD AND
 PERSONALITY
CATARACTS, GLAUCOMA
HYPERTENSION
OSTEOPOROSIS
ASEPTIC BONE NECROSIS
INCREASED SUSCEPTIBILITY
 TO INFECTIONS
(See Possible Adverse Effects and
 Possible Effects of Long-Term
 Use)

▷ **Principal Uses**

As a Single Drug Product: This potent drug of the cortisone class is used in the treatment of a wide variety of allergic and inflammatory conditions. It is used most commonly in the management of serious skin disorders, asthma, regional enteritis, ulcerative colitis and all types of major rheumatic disorders including bursitis, tendinitis and most forms of arthritis.

How This Drug Works: Not fully established. It is thought that this drug's anti-inflammatory effect is due to its ability to inhibit the normal defensive functions of certain white blood cells. Its immunosuppressant effect is attributed to a reduced production of lymphocytes and antibodies.

Available Dosage Forms and Strengths
Ointment — 0.25%, 1%
Retention enema — 40 mg/bottle
Tablets — 2 mg, 4 mg, 8 mg, 16 mg, 24 mg, 32 mg

▷ **Usual Adult Dosage Range:**   4 to 48 mg daily as a single dose or in divided doses. **Note: Actual dosage and administration schedule must be determined by the physician for each patient individually.**

▷ **Dosing Instructions:**   Take with or following food to prevent stomach irritation, preferably in the morning. The tablet may be crushed for administration.

Usual Duration of Use: For acute disorders: 4 to 10 days. For chronic disorders: according to individual requirements. The duration of use should not exceed the time necessary to obtain adequate symptomatic relief in acute self-limiting conditions, or the time required to stabilize a chronic condition and permit gradual withdrawal. Because of its intermediate duration of action, this drug is appropriate for alternate-day administration. Consult your physician on a regular basis.

▷ **This Drug Should Not Be Taken If**
• you have had an allergic reaction to any dosage form of it previously.
• you have active peptic ulcer disease.
• you have an active infection of the eye caused by the herpes simplex virus.
• you have active tuberculosis.

▷ **Inform Your Physician Before Taking This Drug If**
• you have had an unfavorable reaction to any cortisonelike drug in the past.
• you have a history of peptic ulcer disease, thrombophlebitis or tuberculosis.
• you have any of the following: diabetes, glaucoma, high blood pressure, deficient thyroid function or myasthenia gravis.
• you plan to have surgery of any kind in the near future.

Possible Side-Effects (natural, expected and unavoidable drug actions)
Increased appetite, weight gain, retention of salt and water, excretion of potassium, increased susceptibility to infection.

▷ **Possible Adverse Effects** (unusual, unexpected and infrequent reactions)
If any of the following develop, consult your physician promptly for guidance.
Mild Adverse Effects
Allergic Reaction: Skin rash.
Headache, dizziness, insomnia.
Acid indigestion, abdominal distension.
Muscle cramping and weakness.
Acne, excessive growth of facial hair.
Serious Adverse Effects
Mental and emotional disturbances of serious magnitude.
Reactivation of latent tuberculosis.
Development of peptic ulcer.
Increased blood pressure.
Development of inflammation of the pancreas.
Thrombophlebitis (inflammation of a vein with the formation of blood clot)—pain or tenderness in thigh or leg, with or without swelling of the foot, ankle or leg.
Pulmonary embolism (movement of a blood clot to the lung)—sudden shortness of breath, pain in the chest, coughing, bloody sputum.

▷ **Possible Effects on Sexual Function:**   Altered timing and pattern of menstruation.

▷ **Adverse Effects That May Mimic Natural Diseases or Disorders**
Pattern of symptoms and signs resembling Cushing's syndrome.

Natural Diseases or Disorders That May Be Activated by This Drug
Latent diabetes, glaucoma, peptic ulcer disease, tuberculosis.

Possible Effects on Laboratory Tests
Blood amylase and lipase levels: increased (possible pancreatitis).
Glucose tolerance test (GTT): decreased.
Blood potassium level: decreased.
Blood testosterone level: decreased.

CAUTION
1. It is advisable to carry a card of personal identification with a notation that you are taking this drug, if your course of treatment is to exceed 1 week.
2. Do not discontinue this drug abruptly if you are using it for long-term treatment.
3. If vaccination against measles, rabies, smallpox or yellow fever is required, discontinue this drug 72 hours before vaccination and do not resume it for at least 14 days after vaccination.

Precautions for Use
By Infants and Children: Avoid prolonged use if possible. During long-term use, observe for suppression of normal growth and the possibility of increased intracranial pressure. Following long-term use, the child may be at risk for adrenal gland deficiency during stress for as long as 18 months after cessation of this drug.
By Those over 60 Years of Age: Cortisonelike drugs should be used very sparingly after 60 and only when the disorder under treatment is unresponsive to adequate trials of unrelated drugs. Avoid prolonged use of this drug. Continual use (even in small doses) can increase the severity of diabetes, enhance fluid retention, raise blood pressure, weaken resistance to infection, induce stomach ulcer and accelerate the development of cataract and osteoporosis.

▷ **Advisability of Use During Pregnancy**
Pregnancy Category: C (tentative). See Pregnancy Code inside back cover.
Animal studies: Birth defects reported in mice, rats and rabbits.
Human studies: Information from adequate studies of pregnant women is not available.
Avoid completely during the first 3 months. Limit use during the last 6 months as much as possible. If used, examine infant for possible deficiency of adrenal gland function.

Advisability of Use if Breast-Feeding
Presence of this drug in breast milk: Yes.
Avoid drug or refrain from nursing.

Habit-Forming Potential: Use of this drug to suppress symptoms over an extended period of time may produce a state of functional dependence (see Glossary). In the treatment of conditions like asthma and rheumatoid arthritis, it is advisable to keep the dose as small as possible and to attempt drug withdrawal after periods of reasonable improvement. Such procedures may reduce the degree of "steroid rebound"—the return of symptoms as the drug is withdrawn.

Effects of Overdosage: Fatigue, muscle weakness, stomach irritation, acid indigestion, excessive sweating, facial flushing, fluid retention, swelling of extremities, increased blood pressure.

Possible Effects of Long-Term Use: Increased blood sugar (possible diabetes), increased fat deposits on the trunk of the body ("buffalo hump"), rounding of the face ("moon face"), thinning and fragility of skin, loss of texture and strength of bones (osteoporosis, aseptic necrosis), cataracts, glaucoma, retarded growth and development in children.

Suggested Periodic Examinations While Taking This Drug (at physician's discretion)
Measurements of blood pressure, blood sugar and potassium levels.
Complete eye examinations at regular intervals.
Chest X-ray if history of tuberculosis.
Determination of the rate of development of the growing child to detect retardation of normal growth.

▷ **While Taking This Drug, Observe the Following**
Foods: No interactions expected. Ask physician regarding need to restrict salt intake or to eat potassium-rich foods. During long-term use of this drug, it is advisable to eat high-protein diet.
Nutritional Support: During long-term use, take a vitamin supplement. During wound repair, take a zinc supplement.
Beverages: No restrictions. Drink all forms of milk liberally.
▷ *Alcohol:* No interactions expected. Use caution if you are prone to peptic ulcer disease.
Tobacco Smoking: Nicotine increases the blood levels of naturally produced cortisone and related hormones. Heavy smoking may add to the expected actions of this drug and requires close observation for excessive effects.
Marijuana Smoking: May cause additional impairment of immunity.
▷ *Other Drugs*
Methylprednisolone may *decrease* the effects of
• isoniazid (INH, Niconyl, etc.).
• salicylates (aspirin, sodium salicylate, etc.).
Methylprednisolone *taken concurrently* with
• oral anticoagulants may either increase or decrease their effectiveness; consult physician regarding the need for prothrombin time testing and dosage adjustment.
The following drugs may *decrease* the effects of methylprednisolone
• antacids may reduce its absorption.

- barbiturates (Amytal, Butisol, phenobarbital, etc.).
- phenytoin (Dilantin, etc.).
- rifampin (Rifadin, Rimactane, etc.).

▷ *Driving, Hazardous Activities:* Usually no restrictions. Be alert to the rare occurrence of dizziness.

Aviation Note: The use of this drug *may be a disqualification* for piloting. Consult a designated Aviation Medical Examiner.

Exposure to Sun: No restrictions.

Occurrence of Unrelated Illness: This drug may decrease natural resistance to infection. Inform your physician if you develop an infection of any kind. It may also reduce your body's ability to respond to the stress of acute illness, injury or surgery. Keep your physician fully informed of any significant changes in your state of health.

Discontinuation: If you have been taking this drug for an extended period of time, do not discontinue it abruptly. Ask physician for guidance regarding gradual withdrawal. For a period of 2 years after discontinuing this drug, it is essential in the event of illness, injury or surgery that you inform attending medical personnel that you have used this drug in the past. The period of impaired response to stress following the use of cortisonelike drugs may last for 1 to 2 years.

METOCLOPRAMIDE
(met oh kloh PRA mide)

Introduced: 1973

Class: Gastrointestinal stimulant, antivomiting agent

Prescription: USA: Yes
Canada: Yes

Controlled Drug: USA: No
Canada: No

Available as Generic: Yes

Brand Names: ✦Emex, ✦Maxeran, Maxolon, Reglan

BENEFITS versus RISKS

Possible Benefits	*Possible Risks*
EFFECTIVE STOMACH STIMULANT FOR CORRECTING DELAYED EMPTYING	Sedation and fatigue (10%)
	Parkinson-like reactions (see Glossary), 1 in 500
Symptomatic relief in reflux esophagitis	Tardive dyskinesia (see Glossary), rare
Relief of nausea and vomiting associated with migraine headache	

▷ **Principal Uses**

As a Single Drug Product: Used primarily to stimulate contractions of the stomach and thereby facilitate timely emptying of the stomach in disorders such as (1) the stomach retention (gastroparesis) associated with diabetes; (2) acid reflux from the stomach into the esophagus (esophagitis); (3) the nausea and vomiting associated with migraine headaches; and (4) the nausea and vomiting induced by anticancer drugs.

How This Drug Works: Not completely established. It is thought that this drug inhibits relaxation of the stomach muscles and enhances the stimulation of the parasympathetic nervous system that is responsible for stomach muscle contractions. This action accelerates emptying of the stomach into the intestine.

Available Dosage Forms and Strengths
>   Injection — 5 mg per ml, 10 mg per ml
>   Syrup — 5 mg per 5-ml teaspoonful
>   Tablets — 5 mg, 10 mg

▷ **Usual Adult Dosage Range:**   10 to 15 mg 4 times/day. The total daily dose should not exceed 0.5 mg per kilogram of body weight. **Note: Actual dosage and administration schedule must be determined by the physician for each patient individually.**

▷ **Dosing Instructions:**   Take tablet or syrup 30 minutes before each meal and at bedtime. The tablet may be crushed for administration.

Usual Duration of Use: Continual use on a regular schedule for 5 to 7 days is usually necessary to determine this drug's effectiveness in accelerating stomach emptying and relieving symptoms of heartburn, fullness and belching. Long-term use (months to years) requires supervision and periodic evaluation by your physician. Consult your physician on a regular basis.

▷ **This Drug Should Not Be Taken If**
- you have had an allergic reaction to it previously.
- you have a seizure disorder of any kind.
- you have active gastrointestinal bleeding.
- you have a pheochromocytoma (adrenalin-producing tumor).

▷ **Inform Your Physician Before Taking This Drug If**
- you are allergic or overly sensitive to procaine or procainamide.
- you have impaired liver or kidney function.
- you have Parkinson's disease.
- you are taking any atropinelike drugs, antipsychotic drugs or opioid analgesics (see Drug Classes, Section Four).

Possible Side-Effects (natural, expected and unavoidable drug actions)
Drowsiness and lethargy (10%), breast tenderness and swelling, milk production.

▷ **Possible Adverse Effects** (unusual, unexpected and infrequent reactions)
If any of the following develop, consult your physician promptly for guidance.
Mild Adverse Effects
Allergic Reaction: Skin rash.
Headache, dizziness, restlessness, depression, insomnia.
Dry mouth, nausea, diarrhea, constipation.
Serious Adverse Effects
Idiosyncratic Reactions: Neuroleptic malignant syndrome (see Glossary).
Parkinson-like reactions (see Glossary).
Tardive dyskinesia (see Glossary).

▷ **Possible Effects on Sexual Function**
Decreased libido (80%), impaired erection (60%), decreased sperm count.
Altered timing and pattern of menstruation.

Possible Effects on Laboratory Tests
Blood lithium level: increased.
Blood thyroid stimulating hormone (TSH) level: increased.

Precautions for Use
By Infants and Children: Observe for the early development of Parkinson-like reactions soon after starting treatment. Use the smallest effective dose to minimize such reactions.
By Those over 60 Years of Age: Parkinson-like reactions and tardive dyskinesias are more likely to occur with the use of high doses over an extended period of time. Determine the smallest effective dose and use this only when clearly needed.

▷ **Advisability of Use During Pregnancy**
Pregnancy Category: B (tentative). See Pregnancy Code inside back cover.
Animal studies: No birth defects found due to this drug.
Human studies: Information from adequate studies of pregnant women is not available.
Use this drug only if clearly needed.

Advisability of Use if Breast-Feeding
Presence of this drug in breast milk: Yes.
Avoid drug or refrain from nursing.

Habit-Forming Potential: None.

Effects of Overdosage: Marked drowsiness, confusion, muscle spasms, jerking movements of head and face, tremors, shuffling gait.

Possible Effects of Long-Term Use: Parkinson-like reactions may appear within several months of use. Tardive dyskinesias usually occur after a year of continual use; they may persist after this drug is discontinued.

Suggested Periodic Examinations While Taking This Drug (at physician's discretion)
During long-term use, observe for the development of fine, wormlike movements on the surface of the tongue; these may be the first indications of an emerging tardive dyskinesia.

▷ **While Taking This Drug, Observe the Following**
Foods: No restrictions.
Beverages: No restrictions. May be taken with milk.
▷ *Alcohol:* Use with extreme caution. Combined effects can result in excessive sedation and marked intoxication. Alcohol is best avoided.
Tobacco Smoking: No interactions expected.
▷ *Other Drugs*
Metoclopramide may *decrease* the effects of
• cimetidine (Tagamet).
• digoxin (slow-dissolving dosage forms), and reduce its effectiveness.
Metoclopramide *taken concurrently* with
• major antipsychotic drugs (phenothiazines, thiothixenes, haloperidol, etc.) may increase the risk of developing Parkinson-like reactions.
The following drugs may *decrease* the effects of metoclopramide
• atropinelike drugs.
• opioid analgesics (see Drug Class, Section Four).
▷ *Driving, Hazardous Activities:* This drug may cause drowsiness and dizziness. Restrict activities as necessary.
Aviation Note: The use of this drug *may be a disqualification* for piloting. Consult a designated Aviation Medical Examiner.
Exposure to Sun: No restrictions.

METOLAZONE
(me TOHL a zohn)

Introduced: 1974

Class: Antihypertensive, diuretic, sulfonamides

Prescription: USA: Yes
Canada: Yes

Controlled Drug: USA: No
Canada: No

Available as Generic: USA: No
Canada: No

Brand Names: Diulo, Microx, Zaroxolyn

BENEFITS versus RISKS

Possible Benefits	*Possible Risks*
EFFECTIVE, WELL-TOLERATED DIURETIC	Loss of body potassium
	Increased blood sugar
POSSIBLY EFFECTIVE IN MILD HYPERTENSION	Increased blood uric acid
	Rare liver damage, jaundice
ENHANCES EFFECTIVENESS OF OTHER ANTIHYPERTENSIVES	Rare blood cell disorder: abnormally low white blood cell count

---

▷ **Principal Uses**

As a Single Drug Product: Diuretics of this class are used to primarily to (1) increase the volume of urine (diuresis) to correct the excessive fluid retention associated with congestive heart failure and certain types of liver and kidney disease; and (2) initiate treatment for high blood pressure (hypertension). They are often the first drugs tried ("step 1") in treating mild to moderate hypertension.

How This Drug Works: By increasing the elimination of salt and water from the body (through increased urine production), this drug reduces the volume of fluid in the blood and body tissues and lowers the sodium content throughout the body. By relaxing the walls of smaller arteries and allowing them to expand, this drug increases the total capacity of the arterial system. The combined effect of these two actions (reduced blood volume in expanded space) results in lowering of blood pressure.

Available Dosage Forms and Strengths
    Tablets — 0.5 mg, 2.5 mg, 5 mg, 10 mg

▷ **Usual Adult Dosage Range:** As antihypertensive: 2.5 to 5 mg/day initially; 2.5 to 10 mg/day for maintenance. As diuretic: 2.5 to 10 mg/day initially; the smallest effective dose should be determined. The total daily dose should not exceed 20 mg. **Note: Actual dosage and administration schedule must be determined by the physician for each patient individually.**

▷ **Dosing Instructions:** May be taken with or following food to reduce stomach irritation. Best taken as one dose in the morning to avoid nighttime urination. The tablet may be crushed for administration.

Usual Duration of Use: Continual use on a regular schedule for 2 to 3 weeks is usually necessary to determine this drug's effectiveness in lowering high blood pressure. Long-term use (months to years) requires periodic evaluation of response and possible dosage adjustment. Use as a diuretic should be intermittent with "drug holidays" (no drug taken) to reduce the risk of sodium and potassium imbalance. Consult your physician on a regular basis.

▷ **This Drug Should Not Be Taken If**
  • you have had an allergic reaction to it previously.

▷ **Inform Your Physician Before Taking This Drug If**
  • you are allergic to any form of "sulfa" drug.
  • you are pregnant or planning pregnancy.
  • you have a history of kidney or liver disease.
  • you have diabetes, gout or lupus erythematosus.
  • you are taking any form of cortisone, digitalis, oral antidiabetic drug or insulin.
  • you plan to have surgery under general anesthesia in the near future.

Possible Side-Effects (natural, expected and unavoidable drug actions)
  Light-headedness on arising from sitting or lying position (see Ortho-static Hypotension in Glossary).
  Increase in blood sugar level, affecting control of diabetes.
  Increase in blood uric acid level, affecting control of gout.
  Decrease in blood potassium level, causing muscle weakness and cramping.

▷ **Possible Adverse Effects** (unusual, unexpected and infrequent reactions)
  If any of the following develop, consult your physician promptly for guidance.
  Mild Adverse Effects
  Allergic Reactions: Skin rashes, hives.
  Headache, dizziness, blurred vision.
  Reduced appetite, indigestion, nausea, vomiting, diarrhea.
  Serious Adverse Effects
  Allergic Reactions: Hepatitis with jaundice (see Glossary).
  Idiosyncratic Reactions: Muscle pains and cramping, seizures, collapse.
  Acute gout attacks (in susceptible individuals).
  Acute to chronic muscle disorders (due to potassium loss).
  Abnormally low white blood cell count: fever, sore throat, infections.

▷ **Possible Effects on Sexual Function:**   None reported.

▷ **Adverse Effects That May Mimic Natural Diseases or Disorders**
  Liver reaction may suggest viral hepatitis.

Natural Diseases or Disorders That May Be Activated by This Drug
  Diabetes, gout, systemic lupus erythematosus (questionable).

Possible Effects on Laboratory Tests
  Blood sodium and chloride levels: decreased (diuretic effect).
  Blood glucose level: increased.
  Blood potassium level: decreased.
  Blood uric acid level: increased.

CAUTION
  1. Do not exceed recommended doses. Increased dosage can cause ex-

cessive loss of sodium and potassium, with resultant loss of appetite, nausea, fatigue, weakness, confusion and tingling in the extremities.

2. If you are also taking a digitalis preparation (digitoxin, digoxin), ensure an adequate intake of high-potassium foods to prevent potassium deficiency—a potential cause of digitalis toxicity. (See Table of High Potassium Foods in Section Six).

Precautions for Use

By Infants and Children: Safety and effectiveness for use by those under 12 years of age have not been established. Avoid overdosage that could cause serious dehydration. Significant potassium loss can occur within the first 2 weeks of drug use.

By Those over 60 Years of Age: Small doses are advisable until your individual response has been determined. You may be more susceptible to the development of impaired thinking, orthostatic hypotension, potassium loss and blood sugar increase. Overdosage and extended use of this drug can cause excessive loss of body water, thickening (increased viscosity) of the blood and an increased tendency for the blood to clot—predisposing to stroke, heart attack or thrombophlebitis (vein inflammation with blood clot).

▷ **Advisability of Use During Pregnancy**

Pregnancy Category: B (tentative). See Pregnancy Code inside back cover.
Animal studies: No birth defects reported in mouse, rat or rabbit studies.
Human studies: Information from adequate studies of pregnant women is not available.

This drug should not be used during pregnancy unless a very serious complication occurs for which this drug is significantly beneficial. Ask physician for guidance.

Advisability of Use if Breast-Feeding

Presence of this drug in breast milk: Yes.
Avoid drug if possible. If use is necessary, monitor nursing infant closely and discontinue drug or nursing if adverse effects develop.

Habit-Forming Potential: None.

Effects of Overdosage: Dry mouth, thirst, lethargy, weakness, muscle cramping, nausea, vomiting, drowsiness progressing to stupor or coma.

Possible Effects of Long-Term Use: Impaired balance of water, salt and potassium in blood and body tissues. Development of diabetes in predisposed individuals. Pathological changes in the parathyroid glands (with increased blood calcium levels and decreased blood phosphate levels) have been reported with long-term use of thiazide diuretics, a class chemically related to this diuretic.

Suggested Periodic Examinations While Taking This Drug (at physician's discretion)

Complete blood cell counts, measurements of blood levels of sodium, potassium, chloride, sugar and uric acid.

Kidney and liver function tests.

▷ **While Taking This Drug, Observe the Following**

Foods: Consult your physician regarding the advisability of eating foods rich in potassium. If so advised, see the Table of High Potassium Foods in Section Six. Follow physician's advice regarding the use of salt.

Beverages: No restrictions. This drug may be taken with milk.

▷ *Alcohol:* Use with caution until the combined effects have been determined. Alcohol may exaggerate the blood-pressure-lowering effects of this drug and cause orthostatic hypotension.

Tobacco Smoking: No interactions expected. Follow physician's advice.

▷ *Other Drugs*

Metolazone may *increase* the effects of

• other antihypertensive drugs; dosage adjustments may be necessary to prevent excessive lowering of blood pressure.

• lithium, and cause lithium toxicity.

Metolazone may *decrease* the effects of

• oral antidiabetic drugs (sulfonylureas); dosage adjustments may be necessary for proper control of blood sugar.

Metolazone *taken concurrently* with

• digitalis preparations (digitoxin, digoxin) requires very careful monitoring and dosage adjustments to prevent fluctuations of blood potassium levels and serious disturbances of heart rhythm.

The following drugs may *decrease* the effects of metolazone

• cholestyramine (Cuemid, Questran) may interfere with its absorption.

• colestipol (Colestid) may interfere with its absorption.

Take cholestyramine and colestipol 1 hour before any oral diuretic.

▷ *Driving, Hazardous Activities:* Use caution until the possible occurrence of orthostatic hypotension, dizziness or impaired vision has been determined.

Aviation Note: The use of this drug *may be a disqualification* for piloting. Consult a designated Aviation Medical Examiner.

Exposure to Sun: Use caution until sensitivity has been determined. This drug may cause photosensitivity (see Glossary).

Exposure to Heat: Avoid excessive perspiring, which could cause additional loss of salt and water from the body.

Heavy Exercise or Exertion: Avoid exertion that produces light-headedness, excessive fatigue or muscle cramping. Isometric exercises—the "overload" technique for strengthening individual muscles—can raise blood pressure significantly. Ask physician for guidance regarding participation in this form of exercise.

Occurrence of Unrelated Illness: Illnesses that cause vomiting or diarrhea can produce a serious imbalance of important body chemistry. Consult your physician for guidance.

Discontinuation: This drug should not be stopped abruptly following long-term use; serious diuretic-withdrawal fluid retention (edema) can develop after sudden discontinuation. The dose should be reduced gradually. It may be advisable to discontinue this drug 5 to 7 days before major surgery. Ask your physician, surgeon and/or anesthesiologist for guidance regarding dosage adjustment or drug withdrawal.

METOPROLOL
(me TOH proh lohl)

Introduced: 1974

Class: Antihypertensive, beta-adrenergic blocker

Prescription: USA: Yes
Canada: Yes

Controlled Drug: USA: No
Canada: No

Available as Generic: No

Brand Names: ✦Apo-Metoprolol, ✦Betaloc, ✦Co-Betaloc [CD], Lopressor, Lopressor HCT [CD], Lopressor OROS, ✦Novometoprol

---

BENEFITS versus RISKS

Possible Benefits	*Possible Risks*
EFFECTIVE, WELL-TOLERATED ANTIHYPERTENSIVE in mild to moderate high blood pressure	CONGESTIVE HEART FAILURE in advanced heart disease Worsening of angina in coronary heart disease (abrupt withdrawal) Masking of low blood sugar (hypoglycemia) in drug-treated diabetes Provocation of asthma (with high doses)

▷ **Principal Uses**

As a Single Drug Product: The treatment of mild to moderately severe high blood pressure. May be used alone or concurrently with other antihypertensive drugs, such as diuretics. Also used to reduce the risk of recurrent heart attack.

How This Drug Works: By blocking certain actions of the sympathetic nervous system, this drug
- reduces the rate the contraction force of the heart, thus lowering the ejection pressure of the blood leaving the heart.
- reduces the degree of contraction of blood vessel walls, resulting in their relaxation and expansion and consequent lowering of blood pressure.

- prolongs the conduction time of nerve impulses through the heart, of benefit in the management of certain heart rhythm disorders.

Available Dosage Forms and Strengths
                    Injection — 1 mg per ml
                    Tablets — 50 mg, 100 mg
        Tablets, prolonged-action — 100 mg, 200 mg, 300 mg, 400 mg

▷ **Usual Adult Dosage Range:**   Initially, 50 mg twice daily (12 hours apart). The dose may be increased gradually at intervals of 7 to 10 days as needed and tolerated, up to 300 mg/day. For maintenance, 100 mg twice/day. The total daily dose should not exceed 450 mg. **Note: Actual dosage and administration schedule must be determined by the physician for each patient individually.**

▷ **Dosing Instructions:**   May be taken without regard to eating. The regular tablet may be crushed for administration. The prolonged-action tablet should be swallowed whole (not altered). Do not discontinue this drug abruptly.

Usual Duration of Use: Continual use on a regular schedule for 10 to 14 days is usually necessary to determine this drug's effectiveness in lowering blood pressure. The long-term use of this drug (months to years) will be determined by the course of your blood pressure over time and your response to the overall treatment program (weight reduction, salt restriction, smoking cessation, etc.). Consult your physician on a regular basis.

Currently a "Drug of Choice"
    for initiating treatment of hypertension with a single drug, especially for those subject to bronchial asthma or diabetes.

▷ **This Drug Should Not Be Taken If**
- you have had an allergic reaction to it previously.
- you have congestive heart failure.
- you have an abnormally slow heart rate or a serious form of heart block.
- you are taking, or have taken within the past 14 days, any monoamine oxidase (MAO) type A inhibitor drug (see Drug Class, Section Four).

▷ **Inform Your Physician Before Taking This Drug If**
- you have had an adverse reaction to any beta blocker drug in the past (see Drug Class, Section Four).
- you have a history of serious heart disease, with or without episodes of heart failure.
- you have a history of hay fever (allergic rhinitis), asthma, chronic bronchitis or emphysema.
- you have a history of overactive thyroid function (hyperthyroidism).
- you have a history of low blood sugar (hypoglycemia).
- you have impaired liver or kidney function.

- you have diabetes or myasthenia gravis.
- you are currently taking any form of digitalis, quinidine or reserpine, or any calcium blocker drug (see Drug Class, Section Four).
- you plan to have surgery under general anesthesia in the near future.

Possible Side-Effects (natural, expected and unavoidable drug actions)
Lethargy and fatigability (10%), cold extremities, slow heart rate (15%), light-headedness in upright position (see Orthostatic Hypotension in Glossary).

▷ **Possible Adverse Effects** (unusual, unexpected and infrequent reactions)
If any of the following develop, consult your physician promptly for guidance.
Mild Adverse Effects
Allergic Reactions: Skin rash, itching.
Headache, dizziness (10%), insomnia, abnormal dreams.
Indigestion, nausea, vomiting, constipation, diarrhea.
Joint and muscle discomfort, fluid retention (edema).
Serious Adverse Effects
Mental depression (5%), anxiety.
Chest pain, shortness of breath, precipitation of congestive heart failure.
Induction of bronchial asthma (in asthmatic individuals).

▷ **Possible Effects on Sexual Function:** Decreased libido (4 times more common in men); impaired erection (less common with this drug than with most other beta blockers); Peyronie's disease (see Glossary).

Possible Effects on Laboratory Tests
Blood HDL cholesterol level: decreased.
Blood LDL cholesterol level: decreased.
Blood VLDL cholesterol level: increased.
Blood glucose level: increased.
Blood triglyceride levels: increased.

CAUTION
1. *Do not discontinue this drug suddenly* without the knowledge and guidance of your physician. Carry a notation on your person that you are taking this drug.
2. Consult your physician or pharmacist before using nasal decongestants usually present in over-the-counter cold preparations and nose drops. These can cause sudden increases in blood pressure when taken concurrently with beta blocker drugs.
3. Report the development of any tendency to emotional depression.

Precautions for Use
By Infants and Children: Safety and effectiveness for use by those under 12 years of age have not been established. However, if this drug is used, observe for the development of low blood sugar (hypoglycemia) during periods of reduced food intake.
By Those over 60 Years of Age: Proceed *cautiously* with all antihypertensive

drugs. Unacceptably high blood pressure should be reduced without creating the risks associated with excessively low blood pressure. Start treatment with small doses, and monitor the blood pressure response frequently. Sudden, rapid and excessive reduction of blood pressure can predispose to stroke or heart attack. Observe for dizziness, unsteadiness, tendency to fall, confusion, hallucinations, depression or urinary frequency.

▷ **Advisability of Use During Pregnancy**
   Pregnancy Category: B (tentative). See Pregnancy Code inside back cover.
   Animal studies: No significant increase in birth defects due to this drug.
   Human studies: Information from adequate studies of pregnant women is not available.
   Use this drug only if clearly needed. Ask physician for guidance.

Advisability of Use if Breast-Feeding
   Presence of this drug in breast milk: Yes, in large amounts.
   Avoid drug or refrain from nursing.

Habit-Forming Potential: None.

Effects of Overdosage: Weakness, slow pulse, low blood pressure, fainting, cold and sweaty skin, congestive heart failure, possible coma and convulsions.

Possible Effects of Long-Term Use: Reduced heart reserve and eventual heart failure in susceptible individuals with advanced heart disease.

Suggested Periodic Examinations While Taking This Drug (at physician's discretion)
   Measurements of blood pressure, evaluation of heart function.

▷ **While Taking This Drug, Observe the Following**
   Foods: No restrictions. Avoid excessive salt intake.
   Beverages: No restrictions. May be taken with milk.
▷ *Alcohol:* Use with caution until the combined effect has been determined. Alcohol may exaggerate this drug's ability to lower the blood pressure and may increase its mild sedative effect.
   Tobacco Smoking: Nicotine may reduce this drug's effectiveness in treating high blood pressure. In addition, high doses of this drug may potentiate the constriction of the bronchial tubes caused by regular smoking.
▷ *Other Drugs*
   Metoprolol may *increase* the effects of
   • other antihypertensive drugs, and cause excessive lowering of the blood pressure. Dosage adjustments may be necessary.
   • reserpine (Ser-Ap-Es, etc.), and cause sedation, depression, slowing of the heart rate and lowering of the blood pressure.
   • verapamil (Calan, Isoptin), and cause excessive depression of heart function; monitor this combination closely.
   Metoprolol *taken concurrently* with

- clonidine (Catapres) requires close monitoring for rebound high blood pressure if clonidine is withdrawn while metoprolol is still being taken.
- insulin requires close monitoring to avoid undetected hypoglycemia (see Glossary).

The following drugs may *increase* the effects of metoprolol
- cimetidine (Tagamet).
- methimazole (Tapazole).
- oral contraceptives.
- propylthiouracil (Propacil).

The following drugs may *decrease* the effects of metoprolol
- barbiturates (phenobarbital, etc.).
- indomethacin (Indocin), and possibly other "aspirin substitutes," may impair metoprolol's antihypertensive effect.
- rifampin (Rifadin, Rimactane).

▷ *Driving, Hazardous Activities:* Use caution until the full extent of drowsiness, lethargy and blood pressure change has been determined.

Aviation Note: The use of this drug *is a disqualification* for piloting. Consult a designated Aviation Medical Examiner.

Exposure to Sun: No restrictions.

Exposure to Heat: Caution advised. Hot environments can lower the blood pressure and exaggerate the effects of this drug.

Exposure to Cold: Caution advised. Cold environments can enhance the circulatory deficiency in the extremities that may occur with this drug. The elderly should take precautions to prevent hypothermia (see Glossary).

Heavy Exercise or Exertion: It is advisable to avoid exertion that produces light-headedness, excessive fatigue or muscle cramping. The use of this drug may intensify the hypertensive response to isometric exercise.

Occurrence of Unrelated Illness: The fever that accompanies systemic infections can lower the blood pressure and require adjustment of dosage. Illnesses that cause nausea or vomiting may interrupt the regular dosage schedule. Ask your physician for guidance.

Discontinuation: It is advisable to avoid sudden discontinuation of this drug in all situations. If possible, gradual reduction of dose over a period of 2 to 3 weeks is recommended. Ask your physician for specific guidance.

METRONIDAZOLE
(me troh NI da zohl)

Introduced: 1960   **Class:** Anti-infective

Prescription: USA: Yes   **Controlled Drug:** USA: No
    Canada: Yes   Canada: No

Available as Generic: Yes

Brand Names: ✦Apo-Metronidazole, Flagyl, Metizol, MetroGel, Metryl, ✦Neo-Tric, ✦Novonidazole, ✦PMS-Metronidazole, Protostat

```
┌─────────────────────────────────────────────────────────────┐
│                    BENEFITS versus RISKS                      │
│                                                               │
│        Possible Benefits              Possible Risks          │
│   EFFECTIVE TREATMENT FOR        Superinfection with yeast    │
│     TRICHOMONAS INFECTIONS,        organisms                  │
│     AMEBIC DYSENTERY AND         Peripheral neuropathy (see   │
│     GIARDIASIS                     Glossary)                  │
│   Effective treatment for some   Abnormally low white blood cell │
│     anaerobic bacterial infections  count (transient)         │
│   Effective local treatment for  Aggravation of epilepsy      │
│     rosacea.                                                  │
└─────────────────────────────────────────────────────────────┘
```

▷ **Principal Uses**

As a Single Drug Product: Used primarily to treat trichomonas infections of the vaginal canal and cervix and of the male urethra. It is also used to treat amebic dysentery, giardia infections of the intestine and serious infections caused by certain strains of anaerobic bacteria. A more recent use is the treatment of rosacea with local application of a gel dosage form.

How This Drug Works: By interacting with DNA, this drug destroys essential components of the nucleus that are necessary for the cell life and growth of infecting organisms.

Available Dosage Forms and Strengths
    Gel — 0.75%
  Injection — 500 mg per 100 ml
  Tablets — 250 mg, 500 mg

▷ **Usual Adult Dosage Range:** Varies with infection to be treated.
    For trichomoniasis: One-day course—2 grams as a single dose; or 1 gram for 2 doses 12 hours apart. Seven-day course—250 mg 3 times/day for 7 consecutive days. (The 7-day course is preferred.)
    For amebiasis: 500 to 750 mg 3 times/day for 5 to 10 consecutive days.
    For giardiasis: 2 grams once/day for 3 days; or 250 to 500 mg 3 times/day for 5 to 7 days.
    The total daily dosage should not exceed 4 grams (4000 mg).**Note: Actual dosage and administration schedule must be determined by the physician for each patient individually.**

▷ **Dosing Instructions:** May be taken with or following food to reduce stomach irritation. The tablet may be crushed for administration.

Usual Duration of Use: Continual use on a regular schedule as outlined is necessary to ensure this drug's effectiveness. Do not repeat the course of treatment without your physician's approval.

▷ **This Drug Should Not Be Taken If**
  • you have had an allergic reaction to it previously.

- you currently have a bone marrow or blood cell disorder.
- you have any type of central nervous system disorder, including epilepsy.

▷ **Inform Your Physician Before Taking This Drug If**
- you have a history of any type of blood cell disorder, especially one induced by drugs.
- you have impaired liver or kidney function.
- you are pregnant or breast-feeding.

Possible Side-Effects (natural, expected and unavoidable drug actions)
A sharp, metallic, unpleasant taste.
Dark discoloration of the urine (of no significance).
Superinfection (see Glossary) by yeast organisms in the mouth or vagina.

▷ **Possible Adverse Effects** (unusual, unexpected and infrequent reactions)
If any of the following develop, consult your physician promptly for guidance.
Mild Adverse Effects
Allergic Reactions: Skin rash, hives, flushing, itching.
Headache, dizziness, incoordination, unsteadiness.
Loss of appetite, nausea, vomiting, abdominal cramps, diarrhea.
Irritation of mouth and tongue, possibly due to yeast infection.
Serious Adverse Effects
Idiosyncratic Reactions: Abnormal behavior, confusion, depression.
Peripheral neuropathy (see Glossary).
Abnormally low white blood cell count (transient): fever, sore throat, infections.

▷ **Possible Effects on Sexual Function:**   Decreased libido; decreased vaginal secretions (difficult or painful intercourse).

Possible Delayed Adverse Effects: Studies have shown that this drug can cause cancer in mice and possibly in rats. There is no evidence to date that this drug causes cancer in man when used in the dosages specified earlier. Follow your physician's instructions exactly. Avoid unnecessary or prolonged use.

▷ **Adverse Effects That May Mimic Natural Diseases or Disorders**
Behavioral changes may suggest spontaneous psychosis.

Natural Diseases or Disorders That May Be Activated by This Drug
Latent yeast infections.

Possible Effects on Laboratory Tests
White blood cell counts: decreased.
Prothrombin time: increased.

CAUTION
1. Troublesome and persistent diarrhea can develop in sensitive in-

704   Metronidazole

dividuals. If diarrhea persists for more than 24 hours, discontinue this drug and consult with your physician.

2. Discontinue this drug immediately if you develop any indications of toxic effects on the brain or nervous system: confusion, irritability, dizziness, incoordination, unsteady stance or gait, muscle jerking or twitching, numbness or weakness in the extremities.

Precautions for Use

By Infants and Children: Avoid use in those with a history of bone marrow or blood cell disorders.

By Those over 60 Years of Age: Natural changes in the skin may predispose to yeast infections in the genital and anal regions. Report the development of rashes and itching promptly.

▷ Advisability of Use During Pregnancy

Pregnancy Category: B (tentative). See Pregnancy Code inside back cover.

Animal studies: No birth defects reported in rat studies. However, this drug is known to cause cancer in mice and possibly in rats.

Human studies: No increase in birth defects reported in 206 exposures to this drug during the first 3 months. However, information from adequate studies of pregnant women is not available.

The manufacturer advises against the use of this drug during the first 3 months. Use during the last 6 months is not advised unless it is absolutely essential to the mother's health.

Advisability of Use if Breast-Feeding

Presence of this drug in breast milk: Yes.

Avoid drug or refrain from nursing.

Habit-Forming Potential: None.

Effects of Overdosage: Weakness, stomach irritation, nausea, vomiting, confusion, disorientation.

Possible Effects of Long-Term Use: None reported. Avoid long-term use.

Suggested Periodic Examinations While Taking This Drug (at physician's discretion)

Complete blood cell counts.

▷ While Taking This Drug, Observe the Following

Foods: No restrictions.

Beverages: No restrictions. May be taken with milk.

▷ *Alcohol:* Use caution until combined effects have been determined. A disulfiramlike reaction has been reported (see Glossary).

Tobacco Smoking: No interactions expected.

▷ *Other Drugs*

Metronidazole may *increase* the effects of

- warfarin (Coumadin, etc.), and cause abnormal bleeding. The prothrombin time should be monitored closely, especially during the first 10 days of concurrent use.

Metronidazole *taken concurrently* with
  • disulfiram (Antabuse) may cause severe emotional and behavioral disturbances.
▷ *Driving, Hazardous Activities:* This drug may cause dizziness or incoordination. Restrict activities as necessary.
Aviation Note: The use of this drug *may be a disqualification* for piloting. Consult a designated Aviation Medical Examiner.
Exposure to Sun: No restrictions.

MEXILETINE
(mex IL e teen)

Introduced: 1973

Class: Antiarrhythmic

Prescription: USA: Yes
    Canada: Yes

Controlled Drug: USA: No
    Canada: No

Available as Generic: No

Brand Name: Mexitil

BENEFITS versus RISKS

Possible Benefits	*Possible Risks*
EFFECTIVE TREATMENT IN 30% OF SELECTED HEART RHYTHM DISORDERS	NARROW TREATMENT RANGE FREQUENT ADVERSE EFFECTS (up to 40% of users) WORSENING OF SOME ARRHYTHMIAS Rare seizures, liver injury and reduced white blood cell count

---

▷ **Principal Uses**
  As a Single Drug Product: This drug is classified as a Class 1B agent, similar to lidocaine in its actions. It is used primarily to correct and prevent the recurrence of (1) abnormally rapid heart rates (tachycardia) that arise in the ventricles (lower heart chambers); and (2) premature beats arising in the ventricles.

How This Drug Works: By slowing the transmission of electrical impulses throughout the conduction system of the heart, this drug assists in restoring normal heart rate and rhythm in selected types of arrhythmia.

Available Dosage Forms and Strengths
  Capsules — 150 mg, 200 mg, 250 mg

▷ **Usual Adult Dosage Range:** Initiate treatment with 200 mg/8 hours. At intervals of 2 to 3 days, increase dose by 50 to 100 mg as needed and tolerated. The total daily dosage should not exceed 1200 mg. Measurement of drug blood levels is advised (when available) to determine the optimal dose and schedule. **Note: Actual dosage and administration schedule must be determined by the physician for each patient individually.**

▷ **Dosing Instructions:** Take with food or antacid to reduce stomach irritation. Take at same times each day to obtain uniform results. The capsule may be opened for administration.

Usual Duration of Use: Continual use on a regular schedule for 1 to 2 weeks is usually necessary to determine this drug's effectiveness in correcting or preventing responsive rhythm disorders. Long-term use requires supervision and periodic evaluation by your physician. Consult your physician on a regular basis.

▷ **This Drug Should Not Be Taken If**
- you have had an allergic reaction to it previously.
- you have second-degree or third-degree heart block (determined by electrocardiogram), uncorrected by a pacemaker.

▷ **Inform Your Physician Before Taking This Drug If**
- you have had any unfavorable reactions to other antiarrhythmic drugs in the past.
- you have a history of heart disease of any kind, especially "heart block" or heart failure.
- you have impaired liver function.
- you have a seizure disorder of any kind.
- you are taking any form of digitalis, a potassium supplement or any diuretic drug that can cause excessive loss of body potassium (ask physician).

Possible Side-Effects (natural, expected and unavoidable drug actions)
Nervousness (11%), light-headedness (10%).

▷ **Possible Adverse Effects** (unusual, unexpected and infrequent reactions)
If any of the following develop, consult your physician promptly for guidance.
Mild Adverse Effects
Allergic Reaction: Skin rash (4%).
Headache (7%), dizziness (26%), visual disturbance (7%), fatigue (3%), weakness (5%), tremor (13%).
Loss of appetite, indigestion, nausea (39%), vomiting, constipation (4%), diarrhea (5%), abdominal pain (1%).
Serious Adverse Effects
Idiosyncratic Reactions: Depression, confusion, amnesia, hallucinations, seizures (all rare).

Drug-induced heart rhythm disorders (1%), shortness of breath (5%), palpitations (7%), chest pain (7%), swelling of feet.
Urinary retention.
Liver damage with jaundice (see Glossary).
Abnormally low white blood cell and blood platelet counts (rare): fever, sore throat, abnormal bleeding or bruising.

▷ **Possible Effects on Sexual Function:**   Decreased libido, impotence (rare).

▷ **Adverse Effects That May Mimic Natural Diseases or Disorders**
Liver toxicity may suggest viral hepatitis.

Natural Diseases or Disorders That May Be Activated by This Drug
Latent epilepsy.

Possible Effects on Laboratory Tests
Blood white cell and platelet counts: decreased.
Liver function tests: increased liver enzymes (ALT/GPT, AST/GOT) increased in less than 1% of users.

CAUTION
1. Thorough evaluation of your heart function (including electrocardiograms) is necessary prior to using this drug.
2. Periodic evaluation of your heart function is necessary to determine your response to this drug. Some individuals may experience worsening of their heart rhythm disorder and/or deterioration of heart function. Close monitoring of heart rate, rhythm and overall performance is essential.
3. Dosage must be adjusted carefully for each individual. Do not change your dosage without the knowledge and supervision of your physician.
4. Do not take any other antiarrhythmic drug while taking this drug unless you are directed to do so by your physician.
5. Carry a card of personal identification with the notation that you are taking this drug. Inform all attending medical personnel that you are taking this drug, especially if you require surgery of any kind.

Precautions for Use
By Infants and Children: Safety and effectiveness for use by those under 12 years of age have not been established. Initial use of this drug requires hospitalization and supervision by a qualified cardiologist.
By Those over 60 Years of Age: Reduced liver function may require reduction in dosage. Observe carefully for light-headedness, dizziness, unsteadiness and tendency to fall.

▷ **Advisability of Use During Pregnancy**
Pregnancy Category: C (tentative). See Pregnancy Code inside back cover.
Animal studies: No birth defects reported in mice, rats or rabbits. However, an increased rate of fetal resorption was found.

Human studies: Information from adequate studies of pregnant women is not available.
Avoid during first 3 months. Use this drug only if clearly needed. Ask physician for guidance.

Advisability of Use if Breast-Feeding
Presence of this drug in breast milk: Yes.
Avoid drug or refrain from nursing.

Habit-Forming Potential: None.

Effects of Overdosage: Impaired urination, constipation, marked drop in blood pressure, abnormal heart rhythms, congestive heart failure, dizziness, incoordination, seizures.

Possible Effects of Long-Term Use: None reported.

Suggested Periodic Examinations While Taking This Drug (at physician's discretion)
Electrocardiograms, complete blood cell counts, liver function tests.

▷ **While Taking This Drug, Observe the Following**
Foods: No restrictions. Ask physician regarding need for salt restriction.
Beverages: No restrictions. May be taken with milk.
▷ *Alcohol:* Use caution until the combined effects have been determined. Alcohol can increase the blood-pressure-lowering effects of this drug.
Tobacco Smoking: Nicotine can cause irritability of the heart and reduce the effectiveness of this drug. Follow physician's advice regarding smoking.
▷ *Other Drugs*
Mexiletine may *increase* the effects of
• antihypertensive drugs, and cause excessive lowering of blood pressure.
• beta blocker drugs (see Drug Class, Section Four).
The following drugs may *decrease* the effects of mexiletine
• phenytoin (Dilantin, etc.).
• rifampin (Rifadin, Rimactane).
▷ *Driving, Hazardous Activities:* This drug may cause weakness, dizziness or blurred vision. Restrict activities as necessary.
Aviation Note: The use of this drug *may be a disqualification* for piloting. Consult a designated Aviation Medical Examiner.
Exposure to Sun: No restrictions.
Occurrence of Unrelated Illness: Disorders that cause vomiting, diarrhea or dehydration can affect this drug's action adversely. Report such developments promptly.
Discontinuation: This drug should not be discontinued abruptly following long-term use. Ask your physician for guidance regarding gradual dose reduction.

MINOCYCLINE
(min oh SI kleen)

Introduced: 1970

Prescription: USA: Yes
Canada: Yes

Available as Generic: Yes

Brand Name: Minocin

Class: Antibiotic, tetracyclines

Controlled Drug: USA: No
Canada: No

BENEFITS versus RISKS

Possible Benefits	*Possible Risks*
EFFECTIVE TREATMENT OF INFECTIONS due to susceptible microorganisms	Allergic reactions
	Drug-induced colitis
	Drug-induced dizziness and unsteadiness
	Fungal superinfections

▷ **Principal Uses**

As a Single Drug Product: This member of the tetracycline drug class is used primarily to treat (1) a broad range of infections caused by susceptible bacteria and protozoa, and (2) severe, resistant pustular acne.

How This Drug Works: This drug prevents the growth and multiplication of susceptible bacteria by interfering with their formation of essential proteins.

Available Dosage Forms and Strengths

Capsules — 50 mg, 100 mg
Capsules, prolonged-action (Minocin) — 50 mg, 100 mg
Oral suspension — 50 mg per 5-ml teaspoonful (5% alcohol)
Tablets, film-coated — 50 mg, 100 mg

▷ **Usual Adult Dosage Range:** Initially, 200 mg; then 100 mg/12 hours or 50 mg/6 hours. The total daily dosage should not exceed 350 mg the first day or 200 mg thereafter. **Note: Actual dosage and administration schedule must be determined by the physician for each patient individually.**

▷ **Dosing Instructions:** May be taken without regard to food. Take at same time each day, with a full glass of water or milk. Take the full course prescribed. The tablet may be crushed and the capsule may be opened for administration. However, the pellets in Minocin capsules should not be chewed or crushed; mix with soft food and swallow unaltered.

Usual Duration of Use: The time required to control the infection and be free of fever and symptoms for 48 hours. This varies with the nature of the infection.

▷ **This Drug Should Not Be Taken If**
- you are allergic to any tetracycline drug (see Drug Class, Section Four).
- you are pregnant or breast-feeding.

▷ **Inform Your Physician Before Taking This Drug If**
- it is prescribed for a child under 8 years of age.
- you have a history of liver or kidney disease.
- you have systemic lupus erythematosus.
- you are taking any penicillin drug.
- you are taking any anticoagulant drug.
- you plan to have surgery under general anesthesia in the near future.

Possible Side-Effects (natural, expected and unavoidable drug actions)
Superinfections (see Glossary), often due to yeast organisms. These can occur in the mouth, intestinal tract, rectum and/or vagina, resulting in rectal and vaginal itching.

▷ **Possible Adverse Effects** (unusual, unexpected and infrequent reactions)
If any of the following develop, consult your physician promptly for guidance.
Mild Adverse Effects
Allergic Reactions: Skin rash, hives, itching of hands and feet, swelling of face or extremities.
Marked dizziness, unsteadiness, incoordination (usually occurs during the first 3 days).
Pigmentation of skin.
Loss of appetite, stomach irritation, nausea, vomiting, diarrhea.
Irritation of mouth or tongue, "black tongue," sore throat, abdominal cramping or pain.
Serious Adverse Effects
Allergic Reactions: Anaphylactic reaction (see Glossary), asthma, fever, swollen joints, abnormal bleeding or bruising.
Permanent discoloration and/or malformation of teeth when taken under 8 years of age, including unborn child and infant.

▷ **Possible Effects on Sexual Function:**   None reported.

Natural Diseases or Disorders That May Be Activated by This Drug
Systemic lupus erythematosus.

Possible Effects on Laboratory Tests
Complete blood cell counts: decreased red cells, hemoglobin, white cells and platelets; increased eosinophils (allergic reaction).
Blood lupus erythematosus (LE) cells: positive.
Prothrombin time: increased.

Liver function tests: increased liver enzymes (AST/GOT and alkaline phosphatase).

CAUTION

1. Antacids, dairy products and preparations containing aluminum, bismuth, calcium, iron, magnesium or zinc can prevent adequate absorption of this drug and reduce its effectiveness significantly.
2. Troublesome and persistent diarrhea can develop in sensitive individuals. If diarrhea persists for more than 24 hours, discontinue this drug and consult your physician.
3. If surgery under general anesthesia is required while taking this drug, the choice of anesthetic agent must be considered carefully to prevent serious kidney damage.

Precautions for Use

By Infants and Children: If possible, tetracyclines should not be given to children under 8 years of age because of the risk of permanent discoloration and deformity of the teeth. Rarely, young infants may develop increased intracranial pressure within the first 4 days of receiving this drug. Tetracyclines may inhibit normal bone growth and development.

By Those over 60 Years of Age: Dosage must be carefully individualized and based upon determinations of kidney function. Natural skin changes may predispose to severe and prolonged itching reactions in the genital and anal regions.

▷ **Advisability of Use During Pregnancy**

Pregnancy Category: D (tentative). See Pregnancy Code inside back cover.
Animal studies: Tetracycline causes limb defects in rats, rabbits and chickens.
Human studies: Information from studies of pregnant women indicates that this drug can cause impaired development and discoloration of teeth and other developmental defects.
It is advisable to avoid this drug completely during entire pregnancy.

Advisability of Use if Breast-Feeding

Presence of this drug in breast milk: Yes.
Avoid drug or refrain from nursing.

Habit-Forming Potential: None.

Effects of Overdosage: Dizziness, nausea, vomiting, diarrhea.

Possible Effects of Long-Term Use: Superinfections; rarely, impairment of bone marrow, liver or kidney function.

Suggested Periodic Examinations While Taking This Drug (at physician's discretion)
Complete blood cell counts, liver and kidney function tests.

During extended use, sputum and stool examinations may detect early superinfection due to yeast organisms.

▷ **While Taking This Drug, Observe the Following**
Foods: No restrictions.
Beverages: No restrictions.
▷ *Alcohol:* No interactions expected. However, it is best avoided if you have active liver disease.
Tobacco Smoking: No interactions expected.
▷ *Other Drugs*
Tetracyclines may *increase* the effects of
- oral anticoagulants, and make it necessary to reduce their dosage.
- digoxin (Lanoxin), and cause digitalis toxicity.
- lithium (Eskalith, Lithane, etc.), and increase the risk of lithium toxicity.

Tetracyclines may *decrease* the effects of
- oral contraceptives, and impair their effectiveness in preventing pregnancy.
- penicillins, and impair their effectiveness in treating infections.

Tetracyclines *taken concurrently* with
- methoxyflurane anesthesia may impair kidney function.

The following drugs may *decrease* the effects of tetracyclines
- antacids (aluminum and magnesium preparations, sodium bicarbonate, etc.) may reduce drug absorption.
- iron and mineral preparations may reduce drug absorption.

▷ *Driving, Hazardous Activities:* This drug may cause marked dizziness or incoordination. Restrict activities as necessary.
Aviation Note: The use of this drug *may be a disqualification* for piloting. Consult a designated Aviation Medical Examiner.
Exposure to Sun: Use caution until sensitivity has been determined. Some tetracyclines can cause photosensitivity (see Glossary).

MINOXIDIL
(min OX i dil)

Introduced: 1972

Class: Antihypertensive, hair growth stimulant

Prescription: USA: Yes
Canada: Yes

Controlled Drug: USA: No
Canada: No

Available as Generic: Yes

Brand Names: Loniten, Minodyl, Rogaine

```
                    BENEFITS versus RISKS

        Possible Benefits              Possible Risks
A POTENT, LONG-ACTING          EXCESSIVE BODY HAIR
   ANTIHYPERTENSIVE               GROWTH (in 80% of users)
EFFECTIVE IN 75% OF CASES      SALT AND WATER RETENTION
   OF SEVERE HYPERTENSION      Excessively rapid heart rate
EFFECTIVE IN ACCELERATED       Aggravation of angina
   AND MALIGNANT               Local scalp irritation (topical use)
   HYPERTENSION
Moderately effective in treating
   male-pattern baldness in 39% of
   users
```

▷ **Principal Uses**
   As a Single Drug Product: Principal uses include (1) the treatment of severe high blood pressure that cannot be controlled by conventional therapy; (2) the treatment of male-pattern baldness, using a topical solution applied to the scalp.

How This Drug Works: (1) By causing direct relaxation of the constricted muscles within the walls of small arteries throughout the body, this drug permits expansion of the arteries with resultant lowering of blood pressure. (2) The exact mechanism by which this drug stimulates hair growth is not completely known. It is thought that it may increase the size of previously closed small blood vessels in the scalp (improve blood flow) and restore small hair follicles to normal size and activity.

Available Dosage Forms and Strengths
         Tablets — 2.5 mg, 10 mg
   Topical solution — 2%

▷ **Usual Adult Dosage Range:**   For hypertension: Initially, 5 mg/24 hours in one dose. Gradually increase dose to 10 mg, 20 mg, then 40 mg/24 hours, taken in 1 or 2 divided doses daily, as needed and tolerated. The usual maintenance dose is 10 to 40 mg/24 hours. The total daily dosage should not exceed 50 mg. For male-pattern baldness: Apply thinly 1 ml of topical solution to the balding area of the scalp twice daily. The total daily dosage should not exceed 2 ml. **Note: Actual dosage and administration schedule must be determined by the physician for each patient individually.**

▷ **Dosing Instructions:**   For hypertension: Tablets may be taken with or following food to prevent nausea. Take at the same time each day. The tablet may be crushed for administration. For baldness: *The topical solution is for external, local use only; it is not to be swallowed.* Begin application at the center of the bald area; apply thinly to cover the entire area. The scalp and hair must be dry at the time of application. Follow carefully the instructions that accompany the applicator you have purchased.

Usual Duration of Use: Continual use on a regular schedule for 3 to 7 days is usually necessary to determine this drug's effectiveness in controlling severe hypertension. Continual use of the topical solution for at least 4 months is necessary to determine its ability to promote hair growth. Long-term use (months to years) of both dosage forms requires supervision and periodic evaluation by your physician. Consult your physician on a regular basis.

▷ **This Drug Should Not Be Taken If**
  • you have had an allergic reaction to it previously.
  • you are known to have a pheochromocytoma (an adrenalin-producing tumor).
  • you have pulmonary hypertension due to mitral valve stenosis.

▷ **Inform Your Physician Before Taking This Drug If**
  • you are pregnant or planning pregnancy.
  • you have a history of coronary artery disease or impaired heart function.
  • you have a history of stroke or impaired brain circulation.
  • you have impaired liver or kidney function.

Possible Side-Effects (natural, expected and unavoidable drug actions)
  Increased heart rate, fluid retention with weight gain (7%), excessive hair growth on face, arms, legs and back (80%).

▷ **Possible Adverse Effects** (unusual, unexpected and infrequent reactions)
  If any of the following develop, consult your physician promptly for guidance.
  Mild Adverse Effects
  Allergic Reactions: Skin rash (less than 1%). Localized dermatitis at site of application of topical solution.
  Headache, dizziness, fainting (1% to 2%).
  Nausea, increased thirst.
  Serious Adverse Effects
  Idiosyncratic Reaction: Fluid formation around the heart (pericardial effusion) (3%).
  Development of angina pectoris; development of high blood pressure in the lung circulation (pulmonary hypertension).

▷ **Possible Effects on Sexual Function:**   Breast tenderness (less than 1%).

Natural Diseases or Disorders That May Be Activated by This Drug
  Latent coronary artery disease with symptomatic angina.

Possible Effects on Laboratory Tests
  Blood HDL cholesterol level: increased.
  Blood LDL cholesterol level: decreased.

CAUTION
1. The long-term use of this drug for hypertension usually requires the concurrent use of an effective diuretic to counteract salt and water retention.
2. The long-term use of this drug for hypertension often requires the concurrent use of a beta blocker drug to control excessive acceleration of the heart rate.
3. It is best to avoid the concurrent use of this drug and guanethidine; the combination can cause severe orthostatic hypotension (see Glossary).
4. Consult your physician regarding the advisability of using a "no salt added" diet.
5. Only very small amounts of this drug are absorbed into the general circulation when the topical solution is applied to the scalp. However, some systemic effects have been reported. Inform your physician promptly if you experience any unusual symptoms while using the topical solution.

Precautions for Use
By Infants and Children: Dosage schedules should be determined by a qualified pediatrician. Monitor closely for salt and water retention.
By Those over 60 Years of Age: This drug must be used very cautiously by this age group. Start treatment with small doses and limit the total daily dose to 75 mg. Headache, palpitation and rapid heart rate due to this drug are more common in this age group and can mimic acute anxiety states. Observe for dizziness, unsteadiness, fainting and falling.

▷ Advisability of Use During Pregnancy
Pregnancy Category: C (tentative). See Pregnancy Code inside back cover.
Animal studies: No birth defects reported in rats or rabbits. However, studies did reveal decreased fertility and increased fetal deaths.
Human studies: Information from adequate studies of pregnant women is not available.
Avoid during the first 3 months. Use only if clearly needed during the last 6 months.

Advisability of Use if Breast-Feeding
Presence of this drug in breast milk: Yes.
Avoid drug or refrain from nursing.

Habit-Forming Potential: None.

Effects of Overdosage: Headache, dizziness, weakness, nausea, marked low blood pressure, weak and rapid pulse, loss of consciousness.

Possible Effects of Long-Term Use: Excessive growth of body hair occurs in 80% of users after 1 to 2 months of continual treatment for hypertension. Close to 100% of users will experience this effect after 1 year of continual treatment. This may be accompanied by darkening of the skin and coarsening of facial features.

Suggested Periodic Examinations While Taking This Drug (at physician's discretion)

Body weight measurement for insidious gain due to water retention. Electrocardiographic and echocardiographic heart examinations.

▷ **While Taking This Drug, Observe the Following**

Foods: Avoid excessive salt and heavily salted foods.

Beverages: No restrictions. May be taken with milk.

▷ *Alcohol:* Use with extreme caution until combined effects have been determined. Alcohol can exaggerate the blood-pressure-lowering effects of this drug.

Tobacco Smoking: Best avoided. Nicotine can contribute significantly to the development of angina in susceptible individuals.

▷ *Other Drugs*

Minoxidil may *increase* the effects of

• all other antihypertensive drugs; careful dosage adjustments are mandatory.

Minoxidil *taken concurrently* with

• guanethidine (Ismelin, Esimil) may cause severe orthostatic hypotension; avoid this combination.

▷ *Driving, Hazardous Activities:* This drug may cause dizziness and fatigue. Restrict activities as necessary.

Aviation Note: The use of this drug *is a disqualification* for piloting. Consult a designated Aviation Medical Examiner.

Exposure to Sun: No restrictions.

Discontinuation: This drug should not be stopped abruptly. If it is to be discontinued, consult your physician regarding gradual reduction in dosage and appropriate replacement with other drugs for the management of hypertension. Following discontinuation of the topical solution, the pretreatment pattern of baldness may return within 3 to 4 months.

MISOPROSTOL
(mi soh PROH stohl)

Introduced: 1987

Class: Stomach ulcer preventive, antiulcer

Prescription: USA: Yes
Canada: Yes

Controlled Drug: USA: No
Canada: No

Available as Generic: USA: No
Canada: No

Brand Name: Cytotec

```
┌─────────────────────────────────────────────────────────────────────┐
│                      BENEFITS versus RISKS                            │
│                                                                       │
│      Possible Benefits                    Possible Risks              │
│  EFFECTIVE PREVENTION OF          ABORTION (11%)                      │
│     STOMACH ULCERATION            Diarrhea (14% to 40%), transient    │
│     WHILE TAKING                                                      │
│     ANTI-INFLAMMATORY DRUGS                                           │
│     (93% reduction of ulcer                                           │
│     development)                                                      │
│  Effective treatment of duodenal                                     │
│     ulcer                                                             │
└─────────────────────────────────────────────────────────────────────┘
```

▷ **Principal Uses**

As a Single Drug Product: Used primarily to prevent development of stomach ulcers during long-term use of anti-inflammatory drugs as therapy for arthritis and related conditions. Also used (in Canada and other countries) for treatment of active duodenal ulcer unrelated to use of anti-inflammatory drugs.

How This Drug Works: This drug protects the lining tissues of the stomach and duodenum and prevents ulceration due to anti-inflammatory drugs by using several mechanisms: (1) replacing tissue prostaglandins that are depleted by anti-inflammatory drugs; (2) inhibiting the secretion of stomach acid; (3) increasing the local production of bicarbonate (to neutralize acids) and of mucus (to protect stomach and duodenal tissues). The combined effects prevent new ulcer formation and promote healing of existing ulcer(s).

Available Dosage Forms and Strengths

Tablets — 100 mcg, 200 mcg

▷ **Usual Adult Dosage Range**

For prevention of stomach ulcer—100 to 200 mcg 4 times daily, taken concurrently during the use of any anti-inflammatory drug (see Antiarthritic/Anti-inflammatory Drug Class, Section Four).

For treatment of duodenal ulcer—200 mcg 4 times daily for 4 to 8 weeks.-**Note: Actual dosage and administration schedule must be determined by the physician for each patient individually.**

▷ **Dosing Instructions:** Take the prescribed dose with each of 3 daily meals; take the last (fourth) dose of the day with food at bedtime. The tablet may be crushed for administration.

Usual Duration of Use: For prevention of stomach ulcer, continual use on a regular schedule is recommended for the entire period of anti-inflammatory drug use. For treatment of duodenal ulcer, continual use on a regular schedule for 4 weeks is recommended; if ulcer healing is not complete, a second course of 4 weeks is advised. Long-term use (months to years) requires periodic evaluation of response and dosage adjustment. Consult your physician on a regular basis.

Possible Advantages of This Drug: Significantly more effective than histamine (H-2)-blocking drugs (cimetidine, famotidine, nizatidine, ranitidine) or sucralfate in preventing the development of stomach ulcers.

Currently a "Drug of Choice"
for the routine prevention of stomach ulcers induced by long-term use of antiarthritic/anti-inflammatory drugs.

▷ **This Drug Should Not Be Taken If**
  • you have had an allergic reaction to it previously.
  • you are allergic to any type of prostaglandin.
  • you are pregnant or breast-feeding.
  • you are not able or willing to use effective contraception (oral contraceptives or intrauterine device) while taking this drug.

▷ **Inform Your Physician Before Taking This Drug If**
  • you have a history of peptic ulcer disease or Crohn's disease.
  • you have impaired kidney function.
  • you have a seizure disorder.

Possible Side-Effects (natural, expected and unavoidable drug actions)
  Diarrhea (14% to 40% of users), usually beginning after 13 days of use and subsiding spontaneously after 8 days.
  Abortion (miscarriage) of pregnancy (11% of users); this is often incomplete and accompanied by serious uterine bleeding that may require hospitalization and urgent treatment.

▷ **Possible Adverse Effects** (unusual, unexpected and infrequent reactions)
  If any of the following develop, consult your physician promptly for guidance.
  Mild Adverse Effects
  Allergic Reaction: Skin rash.
  Headache (2.4%), dizziness.
  Abdominal pain (12.8%), indigestion (2%), nausea (3.2%), vomiting (1.3%), flatulence (2.9%), constipation (1.1%).
  Menstrual irregularity (0.3%), menstrual cramps (0.6%), heavy menstrual flow (0.5%), spotting between periods (0.7%).
  Serious Adverse Effects
  Allergic Reactions: None reported.
  Post-menopausal vaginal bleeding; this may require further evaluation.

▷ **Possible Effects on Sexual Function:** Reduced libido and impotence reported rarely, but causal relationship not established.

▷ **Natural Diseases or Disorders That May Be Activated by This Drug**
  Latent epilepsy.

Possible Effects on Laboratory Tests
  None reported.

▷ *CAUTION*
1. Do not take this drug if you are pregnant. It can cause abortion.
2. Do not make this drug available to others who may be pregnant or who may become pregnant.
3. If your physician prescribes this drug for you, it is advisable that you have a negative serum pregnancy test within 2 weeks before starting treatment.
4. Start taking this drug only on the second or third day of your next normal menstrual period.
5. Also initiate effective contraceptive measures when you begin to take this drug. Discuss the use of oral contraceptives or intrauterine devices with your physician.
6. Should pregnancy occur while you are taking this drug, discontinue it immediately and inform your physician.

Precautions for Use
By Infants and Children: Safety and effectiveness for use by those under 18 years of age have not been established.
By Those over 60 Years of Age: This drug is usually well tolerated by this age group. However, some forms of prostaglandins can cause drops in blood pressure; observe for periods of light-headedness or faintness that may indicate low blood pressure. Report any such development to your physician.

▷ **Advisability of Use During Pregnancy**
Pregnancy Category: X. See Pregnancy Code inside back cover.
Animal studies: No birth defects due to this drug found in rat or rabbit studies.
Human studies: Information from studies of pregnant women confirms that this drug can cause abortion, sometimes incomplete; unpassed products of conception can cause life-threatening complications.
Avoid this drug completely.

Advisability of Use if Breast-Feeding
Presence of this drug in breast milk: Unknown.
Avoid drug or refrain from nursing.

Habit-Forming Potential: None.

Effects of Overdosage: Abdominal pain, diarrhea, fever, drowsiness, weakness, tremor, convulsions, difficult breathing.

Possible Effects of Long-Term Use: Unknown at this time.

Suggested Periodic Examinations While Taking This Drug (at physician's discretion)
Monitoring for accidental pregnancy.

▷ **While Taking This Drug, Observe the Following**
Foods: No restrictions.
Beverages: No restrictions. May be taken with milk.

▷ *Alcohol:* No interactions expected. However, use sparingly if at all; alcohol can promote the development of stomach ulcer and reduce the effectiveness of this drug.

Tobacco Smoking: No interactions expected. However, nicotine is conducive to the development of stomach ulcer. Smoking should be avoided.

▷ *Other Drugs*

Misoprostol *taken concurrently* with

• antacids that contain magnesium may increase the risk of diarrhea; avoid this combination.

▷ *Driving, Hazardous Activities:* This drug may cause dizziness, light-headedness, stomach pain or diarrhea. Restrict activities as necessary.

Aviation Note: The use of this drug *may be a disqualification* for piloting. Consult a designated Aviation Medical Examiner.

Exposure to Sun: No restrictions.

Discontinuation: This drug should be taken concurrently while you are taking antiarthritic/anti-inflammatory drugs that can induce stomach ulceration. Consult your physician if you have reason to discontinue it prematurely.

MOLINDONE
(moh LIN dohn)

Introduced: 1971

Class: Strong tranquilizer, antipsychotic

Prescription: USA: Yes

Controlled Drug: USA: No

Available as Generic: No

Brand Name: Moban

BENEFITS versus RISKS

Possible Benefits	*Possible Risks*
EFFECTIVE TREATMENT OF SOME CASES OF ACUTE AND CHRONIC SCHIZOPHRENIA	NARROW TREATMENT MARGIN SERIOUS TOXIC EFFECTS ON BRAIN:
May be effective in schizophrenia that has not responded to other drugs	PARKINSON-LIKE REACTIONS SEVERE RESTLESSNESS ABNORMAL INVOLUNTARY MOVEMENTS TARDIVE DYSKINESIAS (see Glossary) Liver toxicity, jaundice Atropinelike side-effects

---

▷ **Principal Uses**

As a Single Drug Product: Used primarily in the management of acute and chronic schizophrenia to control thought disorder, disorientation, hallucinations, perceptual distortions and hostility. It is sometimes effective in chronic schizophrenic individuals who have not responded to other antipsychotic drugs.

How This Drug Works: Not completely established. It is thought that by decreasing dopamine activity in the reticular activating system of the brain, this drug improves distorted patterns of thinking and behavior.

Available Dosage Forms and Strengths
  Concentrate — 20 mg per ml
    Tablets — 5 mg, 10 mg, 25 mg, 50 mg, 100 mg

▷ **Usual Adult Dosage Range:** Initially, 50 to 75 mg/day in 3 or 4 divided doses; dose may be increased gradually in 3 to days to 100 mg/day as needed and tolerated. For maintenance: mild psychosis—5 to 15 mg, 3 or 4 times/day; moderate psychosis—10 to 25 mg, 3 or 4 times/day; severe psychosis—up to 225 mg/day, in 3 or 4 divided doses. The total daily dosage should not exceed 225 mg. **Note: Actual dosage and administration schedule must be determined by the physician for each patient individually.**

▷ **Dosing Instructions:** Take with food or milk to reduce stomach irritation. The liquid concentrate may be diluted with water, milk, fruit juice or carbonated beverages. The tablet may be crushed for administration.

Usual Duration of Use: Continual use on a regular schedule for 3 to 6 weeks is usually necessary to determine this drug's effectiveness in controlling the features of schizophrenia. Long-term use (months to years) requires supervision and periodic evaluation by your physician. Consult your physician on a regular basis.

▷ **This Drug Should Not Be Taken If**
  • you have had an allergic reaction to it previously.
  • you have acute alcoholic intoxication.

▷ **Inform Your Physician Before Taking This Drug If**
  • you are taking any drugs that have sedative effects.
  • you use alcohol excessively.
  • you have any type of seizure disorder.
  • you have any type of glaucoma.
  • you have Parkinson's disease or an enlarged prostate gland.
  • you have impaired liver or kidney function.
  • you have a history of breast cancer.

Possible Side-Effects (natural, expected and unavoidable drug actions)
  Drowsiness, dry mouth, nasal congestion, constipation, impaired urination.
  Parkinson-like reactions (see Glossary).

▷ **Possible Adverse Effects** (unusual, unexpected and infrequent reactions)
    **If any of the following develop, consult your physician promptly for
    guidance.**
    Mild Adverse Effects
    Allergic Reaction: Skin rash.
    Headache, dizziness, blurred vision, lethargy, unsteadiness, insomnia,
    depression, euphoria, ringing in ears.
    Rapid heartbeat, low blood pressure, fainting.
    Loss of appetite, indigestion, nausea.
    Serious Adverse Effects
    Allergic Reactions: Liver reaction with jaundice (rare, questionable).
    Idiosyncratic Reactions: Neuroleptic malignant syndrome (see Glos-
    sary).
    Spasms of face and neck muscles, abnormal involuntary movements of
    extremities, severe restlessness.
    Development of tardive dyskinesias (see Glossary).

▷ **Possible Effects on Sexual Function**
    Increased libido; male breast enlargement and tenderness; female breast
    enlargement with milk formation.
    Altered timing and pattern of menstruation.

▷ **Adverse Effects That May Mimic Natural Diseases or Disorders**
    Parkinson-like reactions may be mistaken for naturally occurring Par-
    kinson's disease.
    Rare liver reaction may suggest viral hepatitis.

Possible Effects on Laboratory Tests
    None reported.

CAUTION
    1. This drug may alter the pattern of epileptic seizures and require
       dosage adjustments of anticonvulsant drugs.
    2. Obtain prompt evaluation of any change or disturbance of vision.
    3. There is a very narrow margin between the effective therapeutic dose
       and the dose that can cause Parkinson-like reactions. Inform your
       physician promptly if suggestive symptoms develop.

Precautions for Use
    By Infants and Children: Safety and effectiveness for use by those under 12
    years of age have not been established.
    By Those over 60 Years of Age: Start treatment with small doses. This drug
    can aggravate an existing prostatism (see Glossary). You may be more
    susceptible to the development of Parkinson-like reactions or tardive
    dyskinesia. Report any suggestive symptoms promptly.

▷ **Advisability of Use During Pregnancy**
    Pregnancy Category: B (tentative). See Pregnancy Code inside back cover.
    Animal studies: No birth defects reported in mice, rats or rabbits.

Human studies: Information from adequate studies of pregnant women is not available.

Because of its inherent toxicity for brain tissue, avoid use during pregnancy if possible.

Advisability of Use if Breast-Feeding
Presence of this drug in breast milk: Unknown.
Avoid drug or refrain from nursing.

Habit-Forming Potential: None.

Effects of Overdosage: Marked drowsiness, weakness, tremor, agitation, impaired stance and gait, stupor progressing to coma, possible seizures.

Possible Effects of Long-Term Use: Development of tardive dyskinesias.

Suggested Periodic Examinations While Taking This Drug (at physician's discretion)
Complete blood cell counts, liver function tests.

▷ **While Taking This Drug, Observe the Following**
Foods: No restrictions.
Beverages: No restrictions. May be taken with milk.
▷ *Alcohol:* Avoid completely. Alcohol can increase the sedative action of this drug and enhance its depressant effects on brain function. Also, this drug can increase the intoxicating effects of alcohol.
Tobacco Smoking: No interactions expected.
▷ *Other Drugs*
Molindone may *increase* the effects of
• all drugs containing atropine or having atropinelike effects (see Drug Class, Section Four).
• all drugs with sedative effects, and cause excessive sedation.
Molindone *taken concurrently* with
• antiepileptic drugs (anticonvulsants) may require close monitoring for changes in seizure patterns and need for dosage adjustments.
▷ *Driving, Hazardous Activities:* This drug may cause dizziness and drowsiness. Restrict activities as necessary.
Aviation Note: The use of this drug *is a disqualification* for piloting. Consult a designated Aviation Medical Examiner.
Exposure to Sun: No restrictions.
Exposure to Heat: Use caution and avoid excessive heat as much as possible. This drug may impair the regulation of body temperature and increase the risk of heat stroke.
Discontinuation: Do not stop taking this drug suddenly after long-term use. Ask your physician for guidance regarding gradual dosage reduction and withdrawal.

NADOLOL
(nay DOH lohl)

Introduced: 1976

Class: Antianginal, antihypertensive, beta-adrenergic blocker

Prescription: USA: Yes
Canada: Yes

Controlled Drug: USA: No
Canada: No

Available as Generic: No

Brand Names: Corgard, Corzide [CD]

BENEFITS versus RISKS

Possible Benefits	*Possible Risks*
EFFECTIVE, WELL-TOLERATED ANTIHYPERTENSIVE in mild to moderate high blood pressure EFFECTIVE ANTIANGINAL DRUG IN CLASSICAL CORONARY ARTERY DISEASE with moderate to severe angina	CONGESTIVE HEART FAILURE in advanced heart disease Provocation of asthma (in predisposed individuals) Masking of hypoglycemia in drug-dependent diabetes Worsening of angina following abrupt withdrawal

---

▷ **Principal Uses**

As a Single Drug Product: This beta blocker drug is used primarily to (1) treat moderately high blood pressure, and (2) contribute to the management of coronary artery disease by preventing attacks of effort-induced angina. (This drug is contraindicated in Prinzmetal's vasospastic angina.)

As a Combination Drug Product [CD]: This drug is available in combination with bendroflumethiazide, a mild diuretic "step 1" antihypertensive drug. This combination product is more effective and more convenient for long-term use.

How This Drug Works: By blocking certain actions of the sympathetic nervous system, this drug

- reduces the rate and contraction force of the heart, thus lowering the oxygen requirement of the heart muscle and reducing the ejection pressure of the blood leaving the heart; these actions reduce the frequency of angina and lower blood pressure.
- reduces the degree of contraction of blood vessel walls, resulting in their relaxation and expansion and consequent lowering of blood pressure.
- prolongs the conduction time of nerve impulses through the heart, of benefit in the management of certain heart rhythm disorders.

Available Dosage Forms and Strengths
    Tablets — 20 mg, 40 mg, 80 mg, 120 mg, 160 mg

▷ **Usual Adult Dosage Range:**   For hypertension: Initially, 40 mg daily in one dose; this may be increased gradually as needed and tolerated, up to 640 mg/24 hours. The usual maintenance dose is 80 to 320 mg/24 hours. The total daily dosage should not exceed 640 mg. For angina: Initially, 40 mg daily in one dose; increase gradually at intervals of 3 to 7 days up to 240 mg/24 hours. The usual maintenance dose is 80 to 240 mg/24 hours. The total daily dose should not exceed 240 mg. **Note: Actual dosage and administration schedule must be determined by the physician for each patient individually.**

▷ **Dosing Instructions:**   May be taken without regard to eating. The tablet may be crushed for administration. Do not discontinue this drug abruptly.

Usual Duration of Use: Continual use on a regular schedule for 10 to 14 days is usually necessary to determine this drug's effectiveness in lowering blood pressure and preventing effort-induced angina. The long-term use of this drug (months to years) will be determined by the course of your blood pressure and angina over time and your response to the overall treatment program (weight reduction, salt restriction, smoking cessation, etc.). Consult your physician on a regular basis.

Possible Advantages of This Drug
    Does not reduce blood flow to the kidney.
    Can be used concurrently with other drugs that may reduce blood flow to the kidney (such as most anti-inflammatory aspirin substitutes).

Currently a "Drug of Choice"
    for initiating treatment of hypertension with a single drug.

▷ **This Drug Should Not Be Taken If**
    • you have had an allergic reaction to it previously.
    • you have congestive heart failure.
    • you have an abnormally slow heart rate or a serious form of heart block.
    • you are subject to bronchial asthma.
    • you are presently experiencing seasonal hay fever.
    • you are taking, or have taken within the past 14 days, any monoamine oxidase (MAO) type A inhibitor drug (see Drug Class, Section Four).

▷ **Inform Your Physician Before Taking This Drug If**
    • you have had an adverse reaction to any beta blocker drug in the past (see Drug Class, Section Four).
    • you have a history of serious heart disease, with or without episodes of heart failure.
    • you have a history of hay fever (allergic rhinitis), asthma, chronic bronchitis or emphysema.
    • you have a history of overactive thyroid function (hyperthyroidism).

- you have a history of low blood sugar (hypoglycemia).
- you have impaired liver or kidney function.
- you have diabetes or myasthenia gravis.
- you are currently taking any form of digitalis, quinidine or reserpine, or any calcium blocker drug (see Drug Class, Section Four).
- you plan to have surgery under general anesthesia in the near future.

Possible Side-Effects (natural, expected and unavoidable drug actions)
Lethargy and fatigability, cold extremities, slow heart rate, light-headedness in upright position (see Orthostatic Hypotension in Glossary).

▷ **Possible Adverse Effects** (unusual, unexpected and infrequent reactions)
If any of the following develop, consult your physician promptly for guidance.
Mild Adverse Effects
Allergic Reactions: Skin rash, itching, drug fever.
Headache, dizziness, insomnia, vivid dreaming, visual disturbances, ringing in ears, slurred speech.
Indigestion, nausea, vomiting, diarrhea, abdominal pain.
Numbness and tingling of extremities.
Serious Adverse Effects
Allergic Reaction: Facial swelling.
Chest pain, shortness of breath, precipitation of congestive heart failure.
Intensification of heart block.
Induction of bronchial asthma (in asthmatic individuals).
Masking of warning indications of acute hypoglycemia in drug-treated diabetes.

▷ **Possible Effects on Sexual Function:**   Decreased libido, impotence (4%), impaired erection (36%).

▷ **Adverse Effects That May Mimic Natural Diseases or Disorders**
Impaired circulation to the extremities may resemble Raynaud's phenomenon.

Natural Diseases or Disorders That May Be Activated by This Drug
Bronchial asthma, Prinzmetal's variant (vasospastic) angina, latent Raynaud's disease, myasthenia gravis (questionable).

Possible Effects on Laboratory Tests
Blood HDL cholesterol level: decreased.
Blood VLDL cholesterol level: increased.
Blood triglyceride levels: increased.

CAUTION
   1. ***Do not discontinue this drug suddenly*** without the knowledge and guidance of your physician. Carry a notation on your person that you are taking this drug.
   2. Consult your physician or pharmacist before using nasal decongestants usually present in over-the-counter cold preparations and nose

drops. These can cause sudden increases in blood pressure when taken concurrently with beta blocker drugs.

3. Report the development of any tendency to emotional depression.

Precautions for Use

By Infants and Children: Safety and effectiveness for use by those under 12 years of age have not been established. However, if this drug is used, observe for the development of low blood sugar (hypoglycemia) during periods of reduced food intake.

By Those over 60 Years of Age: Proceed **cautiously** with all antihypertensive drugs. Unacceptably high blood pressure should be reduced without creating the risks associated with excessively low blood pressure. Start treatment with small doses, and monitor the blood pressure response frequently. Sudden, rapid and excessive reduction of blood pressure can predispose to stroke or heart attack. Observe for dizziness, unsteadiness, tendency to fall, confusion, hallucinations, depression or urinary frequency.

▷ **Advisability of Use During Pregnancy**

Pregnancy Category: C (tentative). See Pregnancy Code inside back cover.

Animal studies: No significant increase in birth defects due to this drug, but embryotoxicity reported in rabbits.

Human studies: Information from adequate studies of pregnant women is not available.

Avoid use during the first 3 months if possible. Use this drug only if clearly needed. Ask physician for guidance.

Advisability of Use if Breast-Feeding

Presence of this drug in breast milk: Yes, in large amounts.

Avoid drug or refrain from nursing.

Habit-Forming Potential: None.

Effects of Overdosage: Weakness, slow pulse, low blood pressure, fainting, cold and sweaty skin, congestive heart failure, possible coma and convulsions.

Possible Effects of Long-Term Use: Reduced heart reserve and eventual heart failure in susceptible individuals with advanced heart disease.

Suggested Periodic Examinations While Taking This Drug (at physician's discretion)

Measurements of blood pressure, evaluation of heart function.

▷ **While Taking This Drug, Observe the Following**

Foods: No restrictions. Avoid excessive salt intake.

Beverages: No restrictions. May be taken with milk.

▷   *Alcohol:* Use with caution until the combined effect has been determined. Alcohol may exaggerate this drug's ability to lower blood pressure and may increase its mild sedative effect.

Tobacco Smoking: Nicotine may reduce this drug's effectiveness in treating high blood pressure and angina. In addition, high doses of this drug may potentiate the constriction of the bronchial tubes caused by regular smoking.

▷ *Other Drugs*

Nadolol may *increase* the effects of
- other antihypertensive drugs, and cause excessive lowering of blood pressure. Dosage adjustments may be necessary.
- reserpine (Ser-Ap-Es, etc.), and cause sedation, depression, slowing of the heart rate and lowering of blood pressure.
- verapamil (Calan, Isoptin), and cause excessive depression of heart function; monitor this combination closely.

Nadolol may *decrease* the effects of
- theophyllines (Aminophyllin, Theo-Dur, etc.), and reduce their effectiveness in treating asthma.

Nadolol *taken concurrently* with
- clonidine (Catapres) requires close monitoring for rebound high blood pressure if clonidine is withdrawn while nadolol is still being taken.
- insulin requires close monitoring to avoid undetected hypoglycemia (see Glossary).

The following drugs may *decrease* the effects of nadolol
- indomethacin (Indocin), and possibly other "aspirin substitutes," may impair nadolol's antihypertensive effect.

▷ *Driving, Hazardous Activities:* Use caution until the full extent of drowsiness, lethargy and blood pressure change has been determined.

Aviation Note: The use of this drug *is a disqualification* for piloting. Consult a designated Aviation Medical Examiner.

Exposure to Sun: No restrictions.

Exposure to Heat: Caution advised. Hot environments can lower the blood pressure and exaggerate the effects of this drug.

Exposure to Cold: Caution advised. Cold environments can enhance the circulatory deficiency in the extremities that may occur with this drug. The elderly should take precautions to prevent hypothermia (see Glossary).

Heavy Exercise or Exertion: It is advisable to avoid exertion that produces light-headedness, excessive fatigue or muscle cramping. The use of this drug may intensify the hypertensive response to isometric exercise.

Occurrence of Unrelated Illness: The fever that accompanies systemic infections can lower the blood pressure and require adjustment of dosage. Illnesses that cause nausea or vomiting may interrupt the regular dosage schedule. Ask your physician for guidance.

Discontinuation: It is advisable to avoid sudden discontinuation of this drug in all situations. If possible, gradual reduction of dose over a period of 2 to 3 weeks is recommended. Ask your physician for specific guidance.

NAFARELIN
(NAF a re lin)

Introduced: 1984

Class: Gonadotropin-releasing hormone

Prescription: USA: Yes

Controlled Drug: USA: No

Available as Generic: USA: No

Brand Name: Synarel

BENEFITS versus RISKS

Possible Benefits	*Possible Risks*
VERY EFFECTIVE TREATMENT OF ENDOMETRIOSIS: Relief of symptoms (94%); reduction of lesions (86%)	Symptoms of estrogen deficiency (during treatment) Masculinizing effects (during treatment) Minor loss of vertebral bone density (at 6 months after treatment)

▷ **Principal Uses**

As a Single Drug Product: Used primarily to treat the manifestations of endometriosis: reduction in the size and activity of endometrial implants within the pelvis; relief of pelvic pain associated with menstruation.

This drug is also used to treat precocious puberty due to excessive production of gonadotropic hormones.

How This Drug Works: This drug is a potent analog of the naturally occurring gonadotropin-releasing hormone (made in the hypothalamus of the brain) that stimulates the pituitary gland to secrete two additional hormones that regulate production of estrogen by the ovaries. Initially this drug causes an increase in the production of estrogen, but with continued use the high levels of estrogen suppress (via a feed-back mechanism) the production of hormones that stimulate the ovary and thus estrogen production is significantly reduced. The implants of endometrium (from the lining of the uterus) that are attached to the pelvic wall are stimulated by the cyclic rise and fall of estrogen that accompanies menstruation. As a result of suppressing estrogen production, the displaced endometrial tissue (endometriosis) becomes dormant; the conditions responsible for premenstrual and menstrual pain are no longer active.

Available Dosage Forms and Strengths

Nasal solution — 2 mg per ml (10 ml bottle)

▷ **Usual Adult Dosage Range:**   400 mcg daily. Spray 1 dose of 200 mcg into one nostril in the morning and 1 dose of 200 mcg into the other nostril in the evening, 12 hours apart. Begin treatment between days 2 and 4 of the menstrual cycle.

If regular menstruation persists after 2 months of treatment, the dose may be increased to 800 mcg daily: 1 spray into each nostril (a total of 2 sprays, 400 mcg) in the morning and again in the evening. **Note: Actual dosage and administration schedule must be determined by the physician for each patient individually.**

▷ **Dosing Instructions:**   Carefully read and follow the patient instructions provided with this drug. The solution is to be sprayed directly into the nostrils where it is absorbed into the blood stream; it is not to be swallowed. Time the beginning of treatment and your daily dosage exactly as directed.

If the use of a nasal decongestant (spray or drops, as for a headcold) is necessary, the decongestant should not be used for at least 30 minutes after administration of the nafarelin spray; earlier use could impair absorption of nafarelin.

Usual Duration of Use:

Continual use on a regular schedule for 2 to 3 months is usually necessary to determine this drug's effectiveness in relieving the symptoms associated with endometriosis. The standard course of treatment is limited to 6 months. On completion of 6 months of treatment, 60% of users are free of symptoms, 32% have mild symptoms, 7% have moderate symptoms and 1% will have severe symptoms. Six months after discontinuing this drug, of the 60% who obtain complete relief 50% will remain free of symptoms, 33% will have mild symptoms and 17% will have moderate symptoms.

If symptoms of endometriosis recur following a 6 month course of treatment and a repeat course is considered, it is advisable to measure bone density before retreatment is started.

Possible Advantages of This Drug

Causes fewer masculinizing effects than danazol.

Less tendency than danazol to increase blood cholesterol levels.

Unlike danazol, this drug does not cause abnormally low HDL cholesterol levels or abnormally high LDL cholesterol levels.

Currently a "Drug of Choice"

for the management of symptoms associated with endometriosis.

▷ **This Drug Should Not Be Taken If**
  • you have had an allergic reaction to it previously.
  • you are pregnant or breast-feeding.
  • you have abnormal vaginal bleeding of unknown cause.

▷ **Inform Your Physician Before Taking This Drug If**
  • you have used this drug, danazol or similar drugs previously.
  • you are taking any type of estrogen, progesterone or oral contraceptive.

- you are planning pregnancy in the near future.
- you have a family history of osteoporosis.
- you use alcohol or tobacco regularly.
- you are using anticonvulsants or cortisonelike drugs.
- you are subject to allergic or infectious rhinitis and use nasal decongestants frequently.

Possible Side-Effects
(natural, expected and unavoidable drug actions)
Effects due to reduced estrogen production: hot flashes (90%), headaches (19%), emotional lability (15%), insomnia (8%).
Masculinizing effects: acne (13%), muscle aches (10%), fluid retention (8%), increased skin oil (8%), weight gain (8%), excessive hair growth (2%).

▷ **Possible Adverse Effects**
(unusual, unexpected and infrequent reactions)
If any of the following develop, consult your physician promptly for guidance.
Mild Adverse Effects
Allergic Reactions: Skin rash, hives (less than 1%).
Nasal irritation (10%).
Depression (2%).
Serious Adverse Effects
Loss of vertebral bone density: at completion of 6 months of treatment, bone density decreases an average of 8.7% and bone mass decreases an average of 4.3%; partial recovery during the post-treatment period restores bone density loss to 4.9% and bone mass loss to 3.3%.

▷ **Possible Effects on Sexual Function**
Decreased libido (22%), vaginal dryness (19%), reduced breast size (10%).

Natural Diseases or Disorders That May Be Activated by This Drug
Latent osteoporosis could be worsened.

Possible Effects on Laboratory Tests
Blood testosterone level: decreased in men with benign enlargement of prostate gland.

CAUTION
1. With continual use of this drug in proper dosage, menstruation will cease. If regular menstruation persists, inform your physician. Dosage adjustment may be necessary.
2. Use this drug consistently on a regular basis. Missed doses can result in breakthrough bleeding and ovulation.
3. It is advisable to avoid pregnancy during the course of treatment. Use a nonhormonal method of birth control; do not use oral contraceptives. Inform your physician promptly if you think you may be pregnant.

4. If you find it necessary to use nasal decongestant sprays or drops, delay their use for at least 30 minutes following the intranasal spray of nafarelin.

Precautions for Use
By Infants and Children
: Safety and effectiveness for use by those under 18 years of age have not been established.
By Those over 60 Years of Age: No indications for use of this drug by this age group.

▷ **Advisability of Use During Pregnancy**
Pregnancy Category: X. See Pregnancy Code inside back cover.
Animal studies: Major fetal abnormalities and increased fetal deaths due to this drug have been demonstrated in rat studies.
Human studies: Information from adequate studies of pregnant women is not available.
Avoid this drug during entire pregnancy.

Advisability of Use if Breast-Feeding
Presence of this drug in breast milk: Unknown.
Avoid drug or refrain from nursing.

Habit-Forming Potential: None.

Effects of Overdosage: No significant effects expected.

Possible Effects of Long-Term Use: Continual use should be limited to 6 months. If repeated courses of treatment are considered, careful determination of bone density and mass should be made to assess the risk of possible bone loss and predisposition to osteoporosis.

Suggested Periodic Examinations While Taking This Drug
(at physician's discretion)
Blood cholesterol and triglyceride profiles.
Bone density and mass measurements.

▷ **While Taking This Drug, Observe the Following**
Foods: No restrictions.
Beverages: No restrictions.
▷ *Alcohol:* No interactions expected.
Tobacco Smoking: No interactions expected.
▷ *Other Drugs*
The following drugs will *decrease* the effects of nafarelin
• estrogens
• oral contraceptives
▷ *Driving, Hazardous Activities:* No restrictions.
Aviation Note: The use of this drug **is not a disqualification** for piloting. Consult a designated Aviation Medical Examiner for confirmation.
Exposure to Sun: No restrictions.

Discontinuation: Normal ovarian function (ovulation, menstruation, etc.) is usually restored within 4 to 8 weeks after discontinuation of this drug.

Special Storage Instructions: Store in an upright position at room temperature. Protect from light.

NAPROXEN
(na PROX en)

Introduced: 1974

Class: Mild analgesic, anti-inflammatory

Prescription: USA: Yes
Canada: Yes

Controlled Drug: USA: No
Canada: No

Available as Generic: No

Brand Names: Anaprox, Anaprox DS, ✦Apo-Naproxen, Naprosyn, ✦Naxen, ✦Novoanaprox

---

BENEFITS versus RISKS

Possible Benefits	*Possible Risks*
EFFECTIVE RELIEF OF MILD TO MODERATE PAIN AND INFLAMMATION	Gastrointestinal pain, ulceration, bleeding (rare) Drug-induced hepatitis with jaundice (rare) Rare kidney damage Mild fluid retention Reduced white blood cell and platelet counts

---

▷ **Principal Uses**

As a Single Drug Product: Used primarily to relieve mild to moderately severe pain associated with (1) musculoskeletal injuries; (2) acute and chronic gout, rheumatoid arthritis and osteoarthritis; (3) dental, obstetrical and orthopedic surgery; and (4) menstrual cramps. It is also used to prevent and relieve migrainelike headaches.

How This Drug Works: Not completely established. It is thought that this drug reduces the tissue concentrations of prostaglandins (and related compounds), chemicals involved in the production of inflammation and pain.

Available Dosage Forms and Strengths

Oral suspension — 125 mg per 5-ml teaspoonful
Tablets — 250 mg, 275 mg, 375 mg, 500 mg, 550 mg

▷ **Usual Adult Dosage Range**
As analgesic: initially, 500 mg; then 250 mg every 6 to 8 hours as needed.
As antiarthritic: 250, 375 or 500 mg twice/day, 12 hours apart.
As antigout: initially, 750 mg; then 250 mg/8 hours until acute attack is relieved.
For menstrual pain: initially, 500 mg; then 250 mg every 6 to 8 hours as needed.
The total daily dosage should not exceed 1650 mg.**Note: Actual dosage and administration schedule must be determined by the physician for each patient individually.**

▷ **Dosing Instructions:**   Take either on an empty stomach or with food or milk to prevent stomach irritation. Take with a full glass of water and remain upright (do not lie down) for 30 minutes. The tablet may be crushed for administration.

Usual Duration of Use: Continual use on a regular schedule for 1 to 2 weeks is usually necessary to determine this drug's effectiveness in relieving the discomfort of arthritis. Long-term use requires supervision and periodic evaluation by the physician. Consult your physician on a regular basis.

Possible Advantages of This Drug
Concentrates in the diseased joint tissues.
Lower incidence of adverse effects on the stomach, liver and kidney.
Well tolerated by the elderly.

▷ **This Drug Should Not Be Taken If**
• you have had an allergic reaction to it previously.
• you are subject to asthma or nasal polyps caused by aspirin.
• you have active peptic ulcer disease or any form of gastrointestinal bleeding.
• you have a bleeding disorder or a blood cell disorder.
• you have active liver disease.
• you have severe impairment of kidney function.

▷ **Inform Your Physician Before Taking This Drug If**
• you are allergic to aspirin or to other aspirin substitutes.
• you have a history of peptic ulcer disease or any type of bleeding disorder.
• you have impaired liver or kidney function.
• you have high blood pressure or a history of heart failure.
• you are taking any of the following: acetaminophen, aspirin or other aspirin substitutes, anticoagulants, oral antidiabetic drugs.

Possible Side-Effects (natural, expected and unavoidable drug actions)
Fluid retention (weight gain), prolongation of bleeding time.

▷ **Possible Adverse Effects** (unusual, unexpected and infrequent reactions)
If any of the following develop, consult your physician promptly for guidance.

Mild Adverse Effects
  Allergic Reactions: Skin rash, hives, itching, localized swellings, spontaneous bruising.
  Headache, dizziness, altered or blurred vision, ringing in the ears, drowsiness, fatigue, inability to concentrate.
  Mouth sores, indigestion, nausea, vomiting, abdominal pain, diarrhea.
Serious Adverse Effects
  Active peptic ulcer, stomach or intestinal bleeding, diverticulitis.
  Liver damage with jaundice (see Glossary).
  Kidney damage with painful urination, bloody urine, reduced urine formation.
  Visual disturbances due to corneal changes, lens opacities, retinal changes.
  Impaired hearing.
  Reduction of white blood cell and/or platelet counts.

▷ **Possible Effects on Sexual Function**
  Inhibited ejaculation (1 report).
  Altered timing and pattern of menstruation.

Possible Delayed Adverse Effects: Mild anemia due to "silent" blood loss from the stomach (less than that caused by aspirin).

▷ **Adverse Effects That May Mimic Natural Diseases or Disorders**
  Liver reaction may suggest viral hepatitis.

Natural Diseases or Disorders That May Be Activated by This Drug
  Peptic ulcer disease, ulcerative colitis.

Possible Effects on Laboratory Tests
  Blood eosinophil count: increased (allergic reaction).
  Liver function tests: increased liver enzymes (ALT/GPT and AST/GOT), increased bilirubin.
  Fecal occult blood test: positive.

CAUTION
  1. Dosage should always be limited to the smallest amount that produces reasonable improvement.
  2. This drug may mask early indications of infection. Inform your physician if you think you are developing an infection of any kind.

Precautions for Use
  By Infants and Children: Indications and dosage recommendations for use by those under 12 years of age have not been established.
  By Those over 60 Years of Age: Small doses are advisable until tolerance is determined. Observe for any indications of liver or kidney toxicity, fluid retention, dizziness, confusion, impaired memory, stomach bleeding or constipation.

▷ **Advisability of Use During Pregnancy**
  Pregnancy Category: B (tentative). See Pregnancy Code inside back cover.
  Animal studies: No birth defects reported in mice, rats or rabbits.

Human studies: Information from adequate studies of pregnant women is not available.

Avoid this drug during the last 3 months. Use it during the first 6 months only if clearly needed. Ask physician for guidance.

Advisability of Use if Breast-Feeding
Presence of this drug in breast milk: Yes, in minute amounts.
Avoid drug or refrain from nursing.

Habit-Forming Potential: None.

Effects of Overdosage: Possible drowsiness, dizziness, ringing in the ears, nausea, vomiting, indigestion.

Possible Effects of Long-Term Use: Eye changes such as opacities in the cornea or lens, retinal changes in the macular area. Kidney damage.

Suggested Periodic Examinations While Taking This Drug (at physician's discretion)
Complete blood cell counts, liver and kidney function tests.
Complete eye examinations if vision is altered in any way.
Hearing examinations if ringing in the ears or hearing loss develops.

▷ **While Taking This Drug, Observe the Following**
Foods: No restrictions.
Beverages: No restrictions. May be taken with milk.
▷   *Alcohol:* Use with caution. The irritant action of alcohol on the stomach lining, added to the irritant action of this drug in sensitive individuals, can increase the risk of stomach ulceration and/or bleeding.
Tobacco Smoking: No interactions expected.
▷   *Other Drugs*
Naproxen may ***increase*** the effects of
- acetaminophen (Tylenol, etc.), and increase the risk of kidney damage; avoid prolonged use of this combination.
- anticoagulants (Coumadin, etc.), and increase the risk of bleeding; monitor prothrombin time and adjust dose accordingly.

Naproxen ***taken concurrently*** with the following drugs may increase the risk of bleeding; avoid these combinations:
- aspirin.
- dipyridamole (Persantine).
- indomethacin (Indocin).
- sulfinpyrazone (Anturane).
- valproic acid (Depakene).
▷   *Driving, Hazardous Activities:* This drug may cause drowsiness or dizziness. Restrict activities as necessary.
Aviation Note: The use of this drug ***may be a disqualification*** for piloting. Consult a designated Aviation Medical Examiner.
Exposure to Sun: No restrictions.

NEOSTIGMINE
(nee oh STIG meen)

Introduced: 1931

Prescription: USA: Yes
  Canada: No

Available as Generic: USA: Yes
  Canada: No

Brand Name: Prostigmin

Class: Antimyasthenic

Controlled Drug: USA: No
  Canada: No

BENEFITS versus RISKS

Possible Benefits	*Possible Risks*
MODERATELY EFFECTIVE TREATMENT OF OCULAR AND MILD FORMS OF MYASTHENIA GRAVIS (symptomatic relief of muscle weakness)	Cholinergic crisis (overdose): excessive salivation, nausea, vomiting, stomach cramps, diarrhea, shortness of breath (asthmalike wheezing), excessive weakness

---

▷ **Principal Uses**

As a Single Drug Product: Used primarily to treat the ocular and milder forms of myasthenia gravis by providing temporary relief of muscle weakness and fatigability. It is most useful in long-term treatment when there is little or no difficulty in swallowing.

How This Drug Works: This drug inhibits cholinesterase, the enzyme that destroys acetylcholine. This results in higher levels of acetylcholine, the nerve transmitter that facilitates the stimulation of muscular activity. The net effects are increased muscle strength and endurance.

Available Dosage Forms and Strengths
  Injection — 0.25, 0.5, 1.0 mg per ml
  Tablets — 15 mg

▷ **Usual Adult Dosage Range:** Initially: 15 mg/3 to 4 hours; adjust dosage as needed and tolerated. Maintenance: up to 300 mg/24 hours; the average dose is 75 to 150 mg/24 hours. **Note: Actual dosage and administration schedule must be determined by the physician for each patient individually.**

▷ **Dosing Instructions:** Take with food or milk to reduce the intensity of side-effects. Larger portions of the daily maintenance dosage should be timed according to the pattern of fatigue and weakness. The tablet may be crushed for administration.

Usual Duration of Use: Continual use on a regular schedule (with dosage adjustment) for 10 to 14 days is usually necessary to determine this drug's effectiveness in relieving the symptoms of myasthenia gravis. Long-term use (months to years) requires periodic evaluation of response and dosage adjustment. Consult your physician on a regular basis.

▷ **This Drug Should Not Be Taken If**
  • you have had an allergic reaction to it previously.
  • you are known to be allergic to bromide compounds.

▷ **Inform Your Physician Before Taking This Drug If**
  • you have any type of seizure disorder.
  • you are subject to heart rhythm disorders or bronchial asthma.
  • you have recurrent urinary tract infections.
  • you have prostatism (see Glossary).
  • you plan to have surgery under general anesthesia in the near future.

Possible Side-Effects (natural, expected and unavoidable drug actions)
  Small pupils, watering of eyes, slow pulse, excessive salivation, nausea, vomiting, stomach cramps, diarrhea, urge to urinate, increased sweating.

▷ **Possible Adverse Effects** (unusual, unexpected and infrequent reactions)
  If any of the following develop, consult your physician promptly for guidance.
  Mild Adverse Effects
  Allergic Reaction: Skin rash.
  Nervousness, anxiety, unsteadiness, muscle cramps or twitching.
  Serious Adverse Effects
  Confusion, slurred speech, seizures, difficult breathing (asthmatic wheezing).
  Increased muscle weakness or paralysis.
  Excessive vomiting or diarrhea may induce abnormally low blood potassium levels (hypokalemia). This will accentuate muscle weakness.

▷ **Possible Effects on Sexual Function:**   None reported.

▷ **Adverse Effects That May Mimic Natural Diseases or Disorders**
  Seizures may suggest the possibility of epilepsy.

Natural Diseases or Disorders That May Be Activated by This Drug
  Latent bronchial asthma.

Possible Effects on Laboratory Tests
  None reported.

CAUTION
  1. Certain drugs can block the action of this drug and reduce its effectiveness in treating myasthenia gravis. (See *Other Drugs* below.) Con-

sult your physician before starting any new drug, prescription or over-the-counter.
2. The dosage schedule of this drug must be carefully individualized for each patient. Variations in response may occur from time to time. Because generalized muscle weakness is a major symptom of both myasthenia crisis (underdosage) and cholinergic crisis (overdosage), it may be difficult to recognize the correct cause. As a rule, weakness that begins within 1 hour after taking this drug probably represents overdosage; weakness that begins 3 or more hours after taking this drug is probably due to underdosage. Observe these time relationships and inform your physician.
3. During long-term use of this drug, observe for the possible development of resistance to the drug's therapeutic action (loss of effectiveness). Consult your physician regarding the advisability of discontinuing this drug for a few days to see if responsiveness can be restored.

Precautions for Use
By Infants and Children: Dosage and administration schedule must be modified if kidney function is severely impaired.
By Those over 60 Years of Age: The natural decline of kidney function with aging may require smaller doses to prevent accumulation of this drug to toxic levels.

▷ Advisability of Use During Pregnancy
Pregnancy Category: C (tentative). See Pregnancy Code inside back cover.
Animal studies: No information available.
Human studies: Information from adequate studies of pregnant women is not available.
There are no reports of birth defects due to the use of this drug during pregnancy. However, there are reports of significant muscular weakness in 20% of newborn infants whose mothers had taken this drug during pregnancy. Ask your physician for guidance.

Advisability of Use if Breast-Feeding
Presence of this drug in breast milk: Probably not.
Monitor nursing infant closely and discontinue drug or nursing if adverse effects develop.

Habit-Forming Potential: None.

Effects of Overdosage: Generalized muscular weakness, blurred vision, very small pupils, slow heart rate, difficult breathing (wheezing), excessive salivation, nausea, vomiting, stomach cramps, diarrhea, muscle cramps or twitching. This syndrome constitutes the cholinergic crisis.

Possible Effects of Long-Term Use: Development of tolerance (see Glossary) with loss of therapeutic effectiveness.

Suggested Periodic Examinations While Taking This Drug (at physician's discretion)
   Assessment of drug effectiveness and dosage schedule for optimal therapeutic results.

▷ **While Taking This Drug, Observe the Following**
   Foods: No restrictions.
   Beverages: No restrictions. May be taken with milk.
▷ *Alcohol:* Use caution until the combined effects are determined. Weakness and unsteadiness may be accentuated.
   Tobacco Smoking: No interactions expected.
▷ *Other Drugs*
   The following drugs may *decrease* the effects of neostigmine
   • atropine (belladonna).
   • clindamycin (Cleocin).
   • guanadrel (Hylorel).
   • guanethidine (Esimil, Ismelin).
   • procainamide (Procan SR, Pronestyl).
   • quinidine (Cardioquin, Duraquin, etc.).
   • quinine (Quinamm).
▷ *Driving, Hazardous Activities:* This drug may cause blurred vision, confusion or generalized weakness. Restrict activities as necessary.
   Aviation Note: The use of this drug *is a disqualification* for piloting. Consult a designated Aviation Medical Examiner.
   Exposure to Sun: No restrictions.
   Exposure to Heat: Use caution. This may cause excessive sweating and increased weakness.
   Exposure to Environmental Chemicals: Avoid excessive exposure (inhalation, skin contamination) to the insecticides Baygon, Diazinon and Sevin. These can accentuate the potential toxicity of this drug.
   Discontinuation: Do not discontinue this drug abruptly without your physician's knowledge and guidance.

NIACIN
(NI a sin)

Other Names: Nicotinic acid, vitamin B-3

Introduced: 1937

Class: Anticholesterol, vasodilator, vitamins

Prescription: USA: Tablets and liquid—no; capsules—yes
Canada: No

Controlled Drug: USA: No
Canada: No

Available as Generic: USA: Yes
Canada: Yes

Brand Names: ✦Antivert [CD], Niac, Nicobid, Nico-400, Nicolar, Nicotinex, ✦Novoniacin, Slo-Niacin, Span-Niacin-150

BENEFITS versus RISKS

Possible Benefits	*Possible Risks*
EFFECTIVE REDUCTION OF TOTAL CHOLESTEROL, LOW DENSITY CHOLESTEROL AND TRIGLYCERIDES IN TYPES II, III, IV AND V CHOLESTEROL DISORDERS (25% reduction of total cholesterol, 35% reduction of LDL cholesterol, and 20% elevation of HDL cholesterol, a beneficial effect)	Activation of peptic ulcer Drug-induced hepatitis Aggravation of diabetes or gout
Specific prevention and treatment of pellagra (niacin-deficiency disease)	

▷ **Principal Uses**

As a Single Drug Product: This drug is used to treat three unrelated disorders: (1) certain patterns of abnormally high blood levels of cholesterol and triglycerides in individuals considered to be at high risk for the development of coronary artery heart disease; (2) pellagra, a niacin (vitamin B-3) deficiency disorder characterized by dementia, dermatitis and diarrhea; and (3) certain types of vertigo and tinnitus (ringing in the ears).

As a Combination Drug Product [CD]: In Canada this drug is combined with meclizine to enhance its effectiveness in the treatment of motion sickness and vertigo.

How This Drug Works

The mechanism by which this drug reduces cholesterol and triglyceride blood levels is not completely known. It is thought that it may inhibit the initial production of triglycerides and impair the conversion of fatty tissue to cholesterol and triglycerides.

This drug corrects the specific deficiency of vitamin B-3 that is responsible for the symptoms of pellagra.

This drug causes direct dilation of peripheral blood vessels in the skin of the face and neck; for this reason it has been used to increase the blood flow to the inner ear in an attempt to relieve some types of vertigo and ringing in the ears. The effectiveness of this application is questionable.

Available Dosage Forms and Strengths

Capsules, prolonged-action — 125 mg, 250 mg, 300 mg, 400 mg, 500 mg

Oral solution — 50 mg per 5-ml teaspoonful

Tablets — 20 mg, 25 mg, 50 mg, 100 mg, 500 mg

Tablets, prolonged-action — 150 mg, 250 mg, 500 mg, 750 mg

▷ **Usual Adult Dosage Range**

For cholesterol disorders: Initially 100 mg 3 times daily. Dose may be increased in increments of 300 mg daily at intervals of 4 to 7 days as needed and tolerated. The usual maintenance dose is 1 to 2 grams 3 times daily. The total daily dosage should not exceed 6 grams.

For prevention of pellagra: 10 to 20 mg daily.

For treatment of pellagra: 50 mg 3 to 10 times daily.**Note: Actual dosage and administration schedule must be determined by the physician for each patient individually.**

▷ **Dosing Instructions:**   Take with or immediately following meals to prevent stomach irritation. Also take one-half of an adult's aspirin tablet or 1 children's aspirin tablet with each dose of niacin to prevent facial flushing and itching. Dosage should be increased very slowly over 2 to 3 months as needed. The prolonged-action form of niacin is preferable to improve tolerance. The regular tablet may be crushed for administration, but the prolonged-action capsules and tablets should not be altered.

Usual Duration of Use: Continual use on a regular schedule for 3 to 5 weeks is usually necessary to determine this drug's effectiveness in reducing elevated levels of cholesterol and triglycerides. Long-term use (months to years) requires periodic evaluation of response and dosage adjustment. Consult your physician on a regular basis.

Currently a "Drug of Choice"
for initiating treatment of elevated LDL cholesterol and VLDL triglycerides. See Cholesterol Disorders in Section Two.

▷ **This Drug Should Not Be Taken If**
- you have had an allergic reaction to it previously.
- you have active peptic ulcer disease or inflammatory bowel disease.
- you have active liver disease.

▷ **Inform Your Physician Before Taking This Drug If**
- you are prone to low blood pressure.
- you have a heart rhythm disorder of any kind.
- you have a history of peptic ulcer disease, inflammatory bowel disease, liver disease, jaundice or gallbladder disease (with or without gallstones).
- you have diabetes or gout.

Possible Side-Effects (natural, expected and unavoidable drug actions)
Flushing, itching, tingling and feeling of warmth usually in the face and neck. Sensitive individuals may experience orthostatic hypotension (see Glossary).

▷ **Possible Adverse Effects** (unusual, unexpected and infrequent reactions)
If any of the following develop, consult your physician promptly for guidance.
Mild Adverse Effects
Allergic Reactions: Skin rash, itching, hives.

Headache, dizziness, faintness, impaired vision.

Indigestion, nausea, vomiting, diarrhea.

Dryness of skin, grayish-black pigmentation of skin folds.

Serious Adverse Effects

Drug-induced hepatitis with jaundice (see Glossary): yellow eyes and skin, dark-colored urine, light-colored stools.

Worsening of diabetes and gout.

Development of heart rhythm disorders.

▷ **Possible Effects on Sexual Function:**   None reported.

▷ **Adverse Effects That May Mimic Natural Diseases or Disorders**

Liver reactions may suggest viral hepatitis.

Natural Diseases or Disorders That May Be Activated by This Drug

Latent diabetes, gout, inflammatory bowel disease or peptic ulcer.

Possible Effects on Laboratory Tests

Complete blood cell counts: decreased eosinophils and lymphoctes.

Blood total cholesterol, LDL cholesterol and triglyceride levels: decreased.

Blood HDL cholesterol level: increased.

Blood glucose level: increased.

Glucose tolerance test (GGT): decreased.

Blood uric acid level: increased.

Liver function tests: increased liver enzymes (ALT/GPT, AST/GOT and alkaline phosphatase), increased bilirubin.

Urine sugar tests: inaccurate test results with Benedict's solution.

CAUTION

1. Large doses may cause significant increases in blood levels of sugar and uric acid. Those who have diabetes or gout should monitor their status regularly.
2. Comply fully with all recommendations for periodic measurements of blood cholesterol and triglyceride levels. These are essential to monitoring your response to treatment and determining the need for changes in dosage or medication.
3. Recent reports indicate that the prolonged-action dosage forms of niacin may be more likely to cause liver damage than the rapidly absorbed (crystalline) forms. Consult your physician regarding the most appropriate dosage form and schedule for you.

Precautions for Use

By Infants and Children: Safety and effectiveness for use of large doses by those under 12 years of age have not been established.

By Those over 60 Years of Age: Observe for the possible development of low blood pressure (light-headedness, dizziness, faintness) and heart rhythm disorders.

▷ **Advisability of Use During Pregnancy**
Pregnancy Category: C (tentative). See Pregnancy Code inside back cover.
Animal studies: Significant birth defects due to this drug were found in chicks.
Human studies: Information from adequate studies of pregnant women is not available.
Use this drug only if clearly needed. Avoid completely during the first 3 months.

Advisability of Use if Breast-Feeding
Presence of this drug in breast milk: Unknown.
Avoid drug or refrain from nursing.

Habit-Forming Potential: None.

Effects of Overdosage: Generalized flushing, nausea, vomiting, stomach cramps, diarrhea, weakness, fainting.

Possible Effects of Long-Term Use: Increased blood levels of sugar and uric acid; liver damage.

Suggested Periodic Examinations While Taking This Drug (at physician's discretion)
Measurements of blood levels of total cholesterol, HDL and LDL cholesterol fractions, triglycerides, sugar and uric acid.
Liver function tests.

▷ **While Taking This Drug, Observe the Following**
Foods: Follow the low-cholesterol diet prescribed by your physician.
Beverages: No restrictions. May be taken with milk.
▷ *Alcohol:* Use with caution until the combined effects have been determined. Alcohol used with large doses of this drug may cause excessive lowering of blood pressure.
Tobacco Smoking: No interactions expected.
▷ *Other Drugs*
Niacin may *increase* the effects of
• some antihypertensive drugs, and cause excessive lowering of blood pressure.
Niacin may *decrease* the effects of
• antidiabetic drugs (insulin and sulfonylureas), by raising the level of blood sugar.
• probenecid (Benemid) and sulfinpyrazone (Anturane), by raising the level of blood uric acid.
▷ *Driving, Hazardous Activities:* This drug may cause dizziness and faintness. Restrict activities as necessary.
Aviation Note: The use of this drug *may be a disqualification* for piloting. Consult a designated Aviation Medical Examiner.
Exposure to Sun: No restrictions.
Discontinuation: Do not discontinue this drug without your physician's knowledge and guidance. Abrupt withdrawal may be followed by excessive increase in blood cholesterol and triglyceride levels.

NICARDIPINE
(ni KAR de peen)

Introduced: 1984

Class: Antianginal, antihypertensive, calcium channel blocker

Prescription: USA: Yes

Controlled Drug: USA: No

Available as Generic: USA: No

Brand Name: Cardene

BENEFITS versus RISKS	
Possible Benefits	*Possible Risks*
EFFECTIVE PREVENTION OF CLASSICAL ANGINA-OF-EFFORT EFFECTIVE TREATMENT OF HYPERTENSION	Increase in angina upon starting treatment (7%) Water retention, ankle swelling (8%)

▷ **Principal Uses**

As a Single Drug Product: Used primarily to treat (1) classical angina-of-effort (due to atherosclerotic disease of the coronary arteries) in individuals who have not responded to or cannot tolerate the nitrates and beta blocker drugs customarily used to treat this disorder; (2) mild to moderately severe hypertension.

How This Drug Works: Not completely established. It is thought that by blocking the normal passage of calcium through certain cell walls (which is necessary for the function of nerve and muscle tissue), this drug inhibits the contraction of coronary arteries and peripheral arterioles. As a result of these effects, this drug
- promotes dilation of the coronary arteries (antianginal effect).
- reduces the degree of contraction of peripheral arterial walls, resulting in their relaxation and consequent lowering of blood pressure. This further reduces the workload of the heart during exertion and contributes to the prevention of angina.

Available Dosage Forms and Strengths
Capsules — 20 mg, 30 mg

▷ **Usual Adult Dosage Range:** Initially 20 mg 3 times daily, 6 to 8 hours apart. Dose may be increased gradually at 3-day intervals (as needed and tolerated) up to 40 mg 3 times daily. The total daily dosage should not exceed 120 mg. **Note: Actual dosage and administration schedule must be determined by the physician for each patient individually.**

▷ **Dosing Instructions:** May be taken with or following food to reduce stomach irritation. However, if taken after a high-fat meal, total absorption of this drug may be reduced by 20% to 30%. The capsule should be swallowed whole (not altered).

Usual Duration of Use: Continual use on a regular schedule for 2 to 4 weeks is usually necessary to determine this drug's effectiveness in reducing the frequency and severity of angina or controlling hypertension. For long-term use (months to years), determine the smallest effective dose. Supervision and periodic evaluation are essential. Consult your physician on a regular basis.

Possible Advantages of This Drug
Does not impair heart function or cause heart rhythm abnormalities. Can be used safely with beta blocker drugs, digoxin, diuretics and nitrate drugs.

▷ **This Drug Should Not Be Taken If**
- you have had an allergic reaction to it previously.
- you have advanced aortic stenosis.

▷ **Inform Your Physician Before Taking This Drug If**
- you have had an unfavorable response to any calcium blocker drug in the past (see Drug Class, Section Four).
- you are currently taking any form of digitalis or a beta blocker drug (see Drug Class, Section Four).
- you are taking any drugs that lower blood pressure.
- you are taking cimetidine (Tagamet) or cyclosporine (Sandimmune).
- you have a history of congestive heart failure, heart attack or stroke.
- you are subject to disturbances of heart rhythm.
- you have impaired liver or kidney function.

Possible Side-Effects (natural, expected and unavoidable drug actions)
Rapid heart rate (3.4%), swelling of the feet and ankles (8%), flushing and sensation of warmth (9.7%).

▷ **Possible Adverse Effects** (unusual, unexpected and infrequent reactions)
If any of the following develop, consult your physician promptly for guidance.
Mild Adverse Effects
Allergic Reaction: Skin rash (0.4% to 1.2%).
Headache (6.4% to 8.2%), dizziness (4% to 6.9%), weakness (4.2% to 5.8%), nervousness (0.6%), blurred vision, confusion.
Palpitation (3.3% to 4.1%), shortness of breath (0.6%).
Indigestion (0.8% to 1.5%), nausea (1.9% to 2.2%), vomiting (0.4%), constipation (0.6%).
Serious Adverse Effects
Allergic Reactions: None reported.
Increased frequency or severity of angina on initiation of treatment or following an increase in dose (7%).
Marked drop in blood pressure with fainting (0.8%).

▷ **Possible Effects on Sexual Function:** Rare impotence (less than 1%).

▷ **Adverse Effects That May Mimic Natural Diseases or Disorders**
Flushing and warmth may resemble menopausal "hot flushes."

Possible Effects on Laboratory Tests
None reported.

CAUTION
1. If you are monitoring your own blood pressure, make your measurements just before each dose and 1–2 hours after each dose to obtain an accurate picture of this drug's effect. This will detect excessive fluctuations between high and low readings.
2. Be sure to inform all physicians and dentists you consult that you are taking this drug. Note the use of this drug on your card of personal identification.
3. You may use nitroglycerin and other nitrate drugs as needed to relieve acute episodes of angina pain. However, if you detect that your angina attacks are becoming more frequent or intense, notify your physician promptly.

Precautions for Use
By Infants and Children: Safety and effectiveness for use by those under 18 years of age have not been established.
By Those over 60 Years of Age: Usually well tolerated by this age group. However, observe for the development of weakness, dizziness, fainting and falling. Take necessary precautions to prevent injury. Report promptly any changes in your pattern of thirst and urination.

▷ **Advisability of Use During Pregnancy**
Pregnancy Category: C (tentative). See Pregnancy Code inside back cover.
Animal studies: Embryo and fetal toxicity reported in small animals, but no birth defects due to this drug.
Human studies: Information from adequate studies of pregnant women is not available.
Avoid this drug during the first 3 months. Use during the last 6 months only if clearly needed. Ask physician for guidance.

Advisability of Use if Breast-Feeding
Presence of this drug in breast milk: Probably yes.
Avoid drug or refrain from nursing.

Habit-Forming Potential: None.

Effects of Overdosage: Weakness, light-headedness, fainting, fast pulse, low blood pressure, shortness of breath, flushed and warm skin, tremors.

Possible Effects of Long-Term Use: None reported.

Suggested Periodic Examinations While Taking This Drug (at physician's discretion)
Evaluations of heart function, including electrocardiograms; measurements of blood pressure in supine, sitting and standing positions.

▷ **While Taking This Drug, Observe the Following**

Foods: No restrictions. Avoid excessive salt intake.

Beverages: No restrictions. May be taken with milk.

▷ *Alcohol:* Use with caution until combined effects have been determined. Alcohol may exaggerate the drop in blood pressure experienced by some individuals.

Tobacco Smoking: Nicotine may reduce the effectiveness of this drug. Follow your physician's advice regarding smoking.

Marijuana Smoking: Possible reduced effectiveness of this drug; mild to moderate increase in angina; possible changes in electrocardiogram, confusing interpretation.

▷ *Other Drugs*

Nicardipine may *increase* the effects of
- cyclosporine (Sandimmune), and cause kidney toxicity.

Nicardipine *taken concurrently* with
- beta blocker drugs or digitalis preparations (see Drug Classes, Section Four) may affect heart rate and rhythm adversely. Careful monitoring by your physician is necessary if these drugs are taken concurrently.

The following drugs may *increase* the effects of nicardipine
- cimetidine (Tagamet).

▷ *Driving, Hazardous Activities:* Usually no restrictions. This drug may cause drowsiness or dizziness. Restrict activities as necessary.

Aviation Note: Coronary artery disease and hypertension *are disqualifications* for piloting. Consult a designated Aviation Medical Examiner.

Exposure to Sun: No restrictions.

Exposure to Heat: Caution advised. Hot environments can exaggerate the blood-pressure-lowering effects of this drug. Observe for light-headedness or weakness.

Heavy Exercise or Exertion: This drug may improve your ability to be more active without resulting angina pain. Use caution and avoid excessive exercise that could impair heart function in the absence of warning pain.

Discontinuation: Do not discontinue this drug abruptly. Consult your physician regarding gradual withdrawal. Observe for the possible development of rebound angina.

NIFEDIPINE
(ni FED i peen)

Introduced: 1972

Class: Antianginal, antihypertensive, calcium channel blocker

Prescription: USA: Yes
Canada: Yes

Controlled Drug: USA: No
Canada: No

Available as Generic: Yes

Brand Names: Adalat, Procardia, Procardia XL

BENEFITS versus RISKS	
Possible Benefits	*Possible Risks*
EFFECTIVE PREVENTION OF BOTH MAJOR TYPES OF ANGINA	Rare increase in angina upon starting treatment
EFFECTIVE TREATMENT OF HYPERTENSION	Rare precipitation of congestive heart failure
	Very rare drug-induced hepatitis

▷ **Principal Uses**

As a Single Drug Product: Used primarily to treat (1) angina pectoris due to coronary artery spasm (Prinzmetal's variant angina) that occurs spontaneously and is not associated with exertion; and (2) classical angina-of-effort (due to atherosclerotic disease of the coronary arteries) in individuals who have not responded to or cannot tolerate the nitrates and beta blocker drugs customarily used to treat this disorder. The sustained release tablets are used to treat mild to moderate hypertension.

How This Drug Works: Not completely established. It is thought that by blocking the normal passage of calcium through certain cell walls (which is necessary for the function of nerve and muscle tissue), this drug slows the spread of electrical activity through the conduction system of the heart and inhibits the contraction of coronary arteries and peripheral arterioles. As a result of these combined effects, this drug

- prevents spontaneous spasm of the coronary arteries (Prinzmetal's type of angina).
- reduces the rate and contraction force of the heart during exertion, thus lowering the oxygen requirement of the heart muscle; this reduces the occurrence of effort-induced angina (classical angina pectoris).
- reduces the degree of contraction of peripheral arterial walls, resulting in their relaxation and consequent lowering of blood pressure. This further reduces the workload of the heart during exertion and contributes to the prevention of angina.

Available Dosage Forms and Strengths

Capsules — 10 mg, 20 mg

Tablets, sustained release — 30 mg, 60 mg, 90 mg

▷ **Usual Adult Dosage Range:** Initially, 10 mg 3 times daily. Dose may be increased gradually at 7- to 14-day intervals (as needed and tolerated) up to 30 mg 3 or 4 times/day. The usual maintenance dose is 10 to 20 mg 3 times/day. The total daily dosage should not exceed 180 mg.

For hypertension: Initially a single 30-mg or 60-mg sustained release tablet taken once daily. Gradually increase the single daily dose as needed and tolerated.**Note: Actual dosage and administration schedule must be determined by the physician for each patient individually.**

▷ **Dosing Instructions:**   May be taken with or following food to reduce stomach irritation. The capsule should be swallowed whole (not altered). The sustained release tablet should be taken whole (not altered).

Usual Duration of Use: Continual use on a regular schedule for 2 to 4 weeks is usually necessary to determine this drug's effectiveness in reducing the frequency and severity of angina and in controlling hypertension. For long-term use (months to years), determine the smallest effective dose. Supervision and periodic evaluation by your physician are essential. Consult your physician on a regular basis.

Possible Advantages of This Drug
The sustained release form of this drug permits effective once-a-day treatment for both angina and hypertension.

▷ **This Drug Should Not Be Taken If**
   • you have had an allergic reaction to it previously.
   • you have active liver disease.
   • you have low blood pressure—systolic pressure below 90.

▷ **Inform Your Physician Before Taking This Drug If**
   • you have had an unfavorable response to any calcium blocker drug in the past.
   • you are currently taking any form of digitalis or a beta blocker drug (see Drug Class, Section Four).
   • you are taking any drugs that lower blood pressure.
   • you have a history of congestive heart failure, heart attack or stroke.
   • you are subject to disturbances of heart rhythm.
   • you have impaired liver or kidney function.
   • you have diabetes.
   • you have a history of drug-induced liver damage.

Possible Side-Effects (natural, expected and unavoidable drug actions)
Low blood pressure, rapid heart rate, swelling of the feet and ankles (7%), flushing and sensation of warmth (25%), sweating.

▷ **Possible Adverse Effects** (unusual, unexpected and infrequent reactions)
   If any of the following develop, consult your physician promptly for guidance.
   Mild Adverse Effects
   Allergic Reactions: Skin rash, hives, itching, fever.
   Headache (23%), dizziness (27%), weakness (12%), nervousness (7%), blurred vision.
   Palpitation (7%), shortness of breath, wheezing (6%), cough.
   Heartburn (11%), nausea, cramps, diarrhea (2%).
   Tremors, muscle cramps (8%).
   Serious Adverse Effects
   Allergic Reaction: Drug-induced hepatitis (very rare).
   Idiosyncratic Reactions: Joint stiffness and inflammation.

Increased frequency or severity of angina on initiation of treatment or following an increase in dose.
Marked drop in blood pressure with fainting.

▷ **Possible Effects on Sexual Function:** Altered timing and pattern of menstruation; excessive menstrual bleeding.

▷ **Adverse Effects That May Mimic Natural Diseases or Disorders**
An allergic rash and swelling of the legs may resemble erysipelas.
Drug-induced hepatitis may suggest viral hepatitis.

Possible Effects on Laboratory Tests
Bleeding time: increased.
Blood total cholesterol level: no effect in age group under 60 years old; decreased in those over 60 years old.
Blood HDL cholesterol level: no effect or increased.
Blood LDL and VLDL cholesterol levels: no effect.
Blood triglyceride levels: no effect or decreased.

CAUTION
1. Be sure to inform all physicians and dentists you consult that you are taking this drug. Note the use of this drug on your card of personal identification.
2. You may use nitroglycerin and other nitrate drugs as needed to relieve acute episodes of angina pain. However, if you detect that your angina attacks are becoming more frequent or intense, notify your physician promptly.

Precautions for Use
By Infants and Children: Safety and effectiveness for use by those under 12 years of age have not been established.
By Those over 60 Years of Age: You may be more susceptible to the development of weakness, dizziness, fainting and falling. Take necessary precautions to prevent injury. Report promptly any changes in your pattern of thirst and urination.

▷ **Advisability of Use During Pregnancy**
Pregnancy Category: C (tentative). See Pregnancy Code inside back cover.
Animal studies: Embryo and fetal deaths reported in mice, rats and rabbits; birth defects reported in rats.
Human studies: Information from adequate studies of pregnant women is not available.
Avoid this drug during the first 3 months. Use during the last 6 months only if clearly needed. Ask physician for guidance.

Advisability of Use if Breast-Feeding
Presence of this drug in breast milk: Unknown.
Avoid drug or refrain from nursing.

Habit-Forming Potential: None.

Effects of Overdosage: Weakness, light-headedness, fainting, fast pulse, low blood pressure, shortness of breath, flushed and warm skin, tremors.

Possible Effects of Long-Term Use: None reported.

Suggested Periodic Examinations While Taking This Drug (at physician's discretion)
Evaluations of heart function, including electrocardiograms; measurements of blood pressure in supine, sitting and standing positions.

▷ **While Taking This Drug, Observe the Following**
Foods: No restrictions. Avoid excessive salt intake.
Beverages: No restrictions. May be taken with milk.
▷ *Alcohol:* Use with caution until combined effects have been determined. Alcohol may exaggerate the drop in blood pressure experienced by some individuals.
Tobacco Smoking: Nicotine may reduce the effectiveness of this drug. Follow your physician's advice regarding smoking.
Marijuana Smoking: Possible reduced effectiveness of this drug; mild to moderate increase in angina; possible changes in electrocardiogram, confusing interpretation.
▷ *Other Drugs*
Nifedipine *taken concurrently* with
• beta blocker drugs or digitalis preparations (see Drug Classes, Section Four) may affect heart rate and rhythm adversely. Careful monitoring by your physician is necessary if these drugs are taken concurrently.
The following drugs may *increase* the effects of nifedipine
• cimetidine (Tagamet).
▷ *Driving, Hazardous Activities:* Usually no restrictions. This drug may cause drowsiness or dizziness. Restrict activities as necessary.
Aviation Note: Coronary artery disease *is a disqualification* for piloting. Consult a designated Aviation Medical Examiner.
Exposure to Sun: No restrictions.
Exposure to Heat: Caution advised. Hot environments can exaggerate the blood-pressure-lowering effects of this drug. Observe for light-headedness or weakness.
Heavy Exercise or Exertion: This drug may improve your ability to be more active without resulting angina pain. Use caution and avoid excessive exercise that could impair heart function in the absence of warning pain.
Discontinuation: Do not discontinue this drug abruptly. Consult your physician regarding gradual withdrawal. Observe for the possible development of rebound angina.

NITROFURANTOIN
(ni troh fyur AN toin)

Introduced: 1953

Class: Urinary anti-infective

Prescription: USA: Yes
Canada: Yes

Controlled Drug: USA: No
Canada: No

Available as Generic: Yes

Brand Names: ✦Apo-Nitrofurantoin, Furadantin, Furalan, Macrodantin, Macrodantin MACPAC, ✦Nephronex, ✦Novofuran

```
┌─────────────────────────────────────────────────────────────┐
│                   BENEFITS versus RISKS                        │
│                                                                 │
│      Possible Benefits            Possible Risks               │
│   EFFECTIVE TREATMENT OF       ALLERGIC REACTIONS:             │
│     SOME URINARY TRACT           Anaphylaxis                   │
│     INFECTIONS                   Rashes, hives                 │
│                                  Repetitive asthma             │
│                                  Lung inflammation             │
│                                  Drug-induced hepatitis        │
│                                  Peripheral neuropathy (see    │
│                                    Glossary)                   │
│                                  Blood cell disorders: hemolytic│
│                                    anemia (see Glossary)       │
│                                  Reduced white blood cell count│
│                                  Superinfections               │
└─────────────────────────────────────────────────────────────┘
```

▷ **Principal Uses**

As a Single Drug Product: Because this drug is concentrated in the urine and attains only low levels in the blood, its use is limited to the prevention or treatment of infections in the urinary tract.

How This Drug Works: Not completely established. It is thought that by interfering with some bacterial enzyme systems, this drug is bacteriostatic (growth retarding) in low to moderate concentrations and bactericidal (killing) in high concentrations.

Available Dosage Forms and Strengths
Capsules — 25 mg, 50 mg, 100 mg
Oral suspension — 25 mg per 5-ml teaspoonful
Tablets — 50 mg, 100 mg

▷ **Usual Adult Dosage Range:** For treatment of active infections: 50 to 100 mg/6 hours. For prevention: 50 to 100 mg once/day at bedtime. The total daily dosage should not exceed 600 mg. **Note: Actual dosage and administration schedule must be determined by the physician for each patient individually.**

▷ **Dosing Instructions:**   Preferably taken with or following food to facilitate absorption and reduce stomach irritation. The tablet may be crushed and the capsule opened for administration, but this drug can stain the teeth yellow on contact.

Usual Duration of Use: Continual use on a regular schedule for 7 to 10 days is usually necessary to determine this drug's effectiveness in curing urinary tract infections. Long-term use for prevention (months to years) requires supervision and periodic evaluation by your physician. Consult your physician on a regular basis.

▷ **This Drug Should Not Be Taken If**
   • you have had an allergic reaction to it previously.
   • you have severely impaired kidney function.
   • you have active liver disease.
   • you are in the last month of pregnancy.

▷ **Inform Your Physician Before Taking This Drug If**
   • you are allergic to any nitrofuran drug.
   • you have impaired liver or kidney function.
   • you have a deficiency of glucose-6-phosphate dehydrogenase in your red blood cells.
   • you have chronic anemia or diabetes.

Possible Side-Effects (natural, expected and unavoidable drug actions)
   Superinfections (see Glossary) in the urinary tract.
   Brown discoloration of the urine, of no significance.

▷ **Possible Adverse Effects** (unusual, unexpected and infrequent reactions)
   If any of the following develop, consult your physician promptly for guidance.
   Mild Adverse Effects
   Allergic Reactions: Skin rashes, hives, localized swellings, itching, fever.
   Headache, dizziness, drowsiness, burning and tearing of eyes, impaired color vision, muscle aching, loss of hair.
   Loss of appetite, nausea, vomiting, diarrhea, abdominal cramping.
   Serious Adverse Effects
   Allergic Reactions: Anaphylaxis (see Glossary), interstitial pneumonitis (lung inflammation), asthma, hepatitis.
   Idiosyncratic Reaction: Hemolytic anemia (see Glossary).
   Peripheral neuropathy (see Glossary).
   Blood cell disorders: reduced red and white blood cell counts.

▷ **Possible Effects on Sexual Function:**   None reported.

▷ **Adverse Effects That May Mimic Natural Diseases or Disorders**
   Allergic pneumonitis may suggest an infectious pneumonia.
   Allergic hepatitis may suggest viral hepatitis.

Natural Diseases or Disorders That May Be Activated by This Drug
Latent asthma.

Possible Effects on Laboratory Tests
Complete blood cell counts: decreased red cells, hemoglobin, white cells and platelets; increased white cells and eosinophils (allergic reactions and drug-induced lung inflammation).
Blood amylase level: increased (pancreatic reaction).
Liver function tests: increased liver enzymes (ALT/GPT, AST/GOT and alkaline phosphatase), increased bilirubin.
Kidney function tests: increased blood creatinine and urea nitrogen (BUN) levels (kidney damage).
Urine sugar tests: false positive result with Benedict's solution.

CAUTION
Troublesome and persistent diarrhea can develop in sensitive individuals. If diarrhea persists for more than 24 hours, discontinue this drug and consult your physician.

Precautions for Use
By Infants and Children: This drug should not be used in infants under 1 month of age. Observe closely for the possible development of increased intracranial pressure.
By Those over 60 Years of Age: Dosage must be carefully individualized on the basis of kidney function. This age group is more susceptible to skin rashes, nausea, vomiting and constipation.

▷ **Advisability of Use During Pregnancy**
Pregnancy Category: C (tentative). See Pregnancy Code inside back cover.
Animal studies: No information available.
Human studies: No significant increase in birth defects reported in 590 exposures. Information from adequate studies of pregnant women is not available.
Avoid use of drug during the last few weeks of pregnancy. Use otherwise only if clearly needed. Ask your physician for guidance.

Advisability of Use if Breast-Feeding
Presence of this drug in breast milk: Yes, in small amounts.
Avoid drug or refrain from nursing.

Habit-Forming Potential: None.

Effects of Overdosage: Nausea, vomiting, diarrhea.

Possible Effects of Long-Term Use: Allergic reactions in lungs or liver, peripheral neuropathy, superinfections within the urinary tract.

Suggested Periodic Examinations While Taking This Drug (at physician's discretion)
Complete blood cell counts, liver function tests, X-ray examinations of lungs during long-term use.

▷ **While Taking This Drug, Observe the Following**

Foods: No restrictions. Eat liberally of the following foods: beef, chicken, lamb and pork liver, asparagus, navy beans (good sources of folic acid).

Beverages: No restrictions. May be taken with milk.

▷ *Alcohol:* Use with extreme caution until the combined effects have been determined. This drug, in combination with alcohol, may cause a disulfiramlike reaction (see Glossary) in sensitive individuals.

Tobacco Smoking: No interactions expected.

▷ *Other Drugs*

The following drugs may *decrease* the effects of nitrofurantoin

• antacids that contain magnesium can prevent the absorption of nitrofurantoin and reduce its effectiveness.

▷ *Driving, Hazardous Activities:* This drug may cause dizziness. Restrict activities as necessary.

Aviation Note: The use of this drug *may be a disqualification* for piloting. Consult a designated Aviation Medical Examiner.

Exposure to Sun: No restrictions.

NITROGLYCERIN
(ni troh GLIS er in)

Introduced: 1847   **Class:** Antianginal, nitrates

Prescription: USA: Yes   **Controlled Drug:** USA: No
Canada: No   Canada: No

Available as Generic: Yes

Brand Names: Deponit, Minitran Transdermal Delivery System, Nitro-Bid, Nitrodisc, Nitro-Dur, Nitro-Dur II, Nitrogard, ✦Nitrogard-SR, Nitroglyn, Nitrol, Nitrolingual Spray, Nitrong, ✦Nitrong SR, Nitrospan, ✦Nitrostabilin, Nitrostat, Transderm-Nitro, ✦Tridil

---

BENEFITS versus RISKS

Possible Benefits	*Possible Risks*
EFFECTIVE RELIEF AND PREVENTION OF ANGINA EFFECTIVE ADJUNCTIVE TREATMENT IN SELECTED CASES OF CONGESTIVE HEART FAILURE	Orthostatic hypotension (see Glossary) with and without fainting Skin rash (rare) Altered hemoglobin with large doses (very rare)

▷ **Principal Uses**

As a Single Drug Product: Used primarily in the treatment of symptomatic coronary artery disease. The rapid-action forms are used to relieve acute attacks of anginal pain at their onset. The sustained-action forms are used to prevent the development of angina.

How This Drug Works:　By direct action on the muscles in blood vessel walls, this drug relaxes and dilates both arteries and veins. Its beneficial effects in the management of angina are due to two mechanisms of action: (1) dilation of narrowed coronary arteries; (2) dilation of veins in the general circulation, with consequent reduction of the volume and pressure of blood entering the heart. The net effects are improved blood supply to the heart muscle and reduced workload for the heart. Both actions reduce the frequency and severity of angina.

Available Dosage Forms and Strengths
　　Canisters, translingual spray — 13.8 grams (200 doses), 0.4 mg per metered dose
　　Capsules, prolonged-action — 2.5 mg, 2.6 mg, 6.5 mg, 9 mg
　　Ointment — 2%
　　Tablets, buccal — 1 mg, 2 mg, 3 mg
　　Tablets, prolonged-action — 2.6 mg, 6.5 mg, 9 mg
　　Tablets, sublingual — 0.15 mg, 0.3 mg, 0.4 mg, 0.6 mg
　　Transdermal systems — 2.5 mg, 5 mg, 7.5 mg, 10 mg, 15 mg (all per 24 hours)

▷ **Usual Adult Dosage Range:**　According to dosage form:
　　Sublingual spray—1 metered spray (0.4 mg) under tongue/3 to 5 minutes, up to 3 doses within 15 minutes, to relieve acute angina. To prevent angina, 1 spray taken 5 to 10 minutes before exertion.
　　Sublingual tablets—0.15 to 0.6 mg dissolved under tongue at 5-minute intervals to relieve acute angina.
　　Prolonged-action tablets—1.3 to 6.5 mg at 8- to 12-hour intervals to prevent angina.
　　Prolonged-action capsules—2.5 to 9 mg at 8- to 12-hour intervals to prevent angina.
　　Ointment—2.5 to 5 cm (1 to 2 inches, 15 to 30 mg) applied in a thin, even layer of uniform size to hairless skin at 3- to 4-hour intervals to prevent angina.
　　Buccal tablets—1 to 2 mg/4 to 5 hours placed between cheek and gum.
　　Transdermal patches—5-sq.-cm to 30-sq.-cm patch applied to hairless skin once/24 hours to prevent angina.**Note: Actual dosage and administration schedule must be determined by the physician for each patient individually.**

▷ **Dosing Instructions:**　Dosage forms to be swallowed are best taken when stomach is empty (1 hour before or 2 hours after eating) to obtain maximal blood levels. Tablets should not be crushed for administration. Capsules may be opened, but the contents should not be crushed or chewed before swallowing.

Usual Duration of Use: Continual use on a regular schedule for 3 to 5 days is usually necessary to determine this drug's effectiveness in preventing and relieving acute anginal attacks. Individual dosage adjustments will be necessary for optimal results. Long-term use (months to years) requires supervision and periodic evaluation by your physician. Consult your physician on a regular basis.

▷ **This Drug Should Not Be Taken If**
   • you have had an allergic reaction to it previously.
   • you are severely anemic.
   • you have closed-angle glaucoma (inadequately treated).

▷ **Inform Your Physician Before Taking This Drug If**
   • you have had an unfavorable response to other nitrate drugs in the past.
   • you have low blood pressure.
   • you have any form of glaucoma.

Possible Side-Effects (natural, expected and unavoidable drug actions)
   Flushing of face, headaches (50%), orthostatic hypotension (see Glossary), rapid heart rate, palpitation.

▷ **Possible Adverse Effects** (unusual, unexpected and infrequent reactions)
   If any of the following develop, consult your physician promptly for guidance.
   Mild Adverse Effects
   Allergic Reaction: Skin rash.
   Throbbing headaches (may be severe and persistent), dizziness, fainting.
   Nausea, vomiting.
   Serious Adverse Effects
   Allergic Reactions: Severe skin reactions with peeling.
   Idiosyncratic Reaction: Methemoglobinemia (very rare).

▷ **Possible Effects on Sexual Function**
   Correction of impotence (1 report following sublingual use).
   The preventive use of nitroglycerin prior to sexual activity has been recommended to eliminate or reduce the risk of angina. Consult your physician for guidance.

▷ **Adverse Effects That May Mimic Natural Diseases or Disorders**
   Hypotensive spells (sudden drops in blood pressure) due to this drug may be mistaken for late-onset epilepsy.

Possible Effects on Laboratory Tests
   Blood platelet count: decreased.

CAUTION
   1. This drug can provoke migraine headaches in susceptible individuals.
   2. In the presence of impaired brain circulation (cerebral arteriosclero-

sis), this drug can cause transient ischemic attacks—periods of temporary speech impairment, paralysis, numbness, etc.

3. The development of tolerance to long-acting forms of nitrates will render the sublingual tablets ineffective for the relief of acute angina. Sensitivity to the drug's antianginal effect is restored after one week of abstinence from the long-acting forms.

4. Many over-the-counter (OTC) drug products for allergies, colds and coughs contain drugs that may counteract the desired effects of this drug. Ask your physician or pharmacist for guidance before using any such medications.

Precautions for Use

By Infants and Children: Limited usefulness and experience in this age group. Dosage schedules not established.

By Those over 60 Years of Age: Begin treatment with small doses and increase dose cautiously as needed and tolerated. You may be more susceptible to the development of flushing, throbbing headache, dizziness, "blackout" spells, fainting and falling.

▷ **Advisability of Use During Pregnancy**

Pregnancy Category: C (tentative). See Pregnancy Code inside back cover.
Animal studies: No information available.
Human studies: Information from adequate studies of pregnant women is not available.
Use this drug only if clearly needed. Ask physician for guidance.

Advisability of Use if Breast-Feeding

Presence of this drug in breast milk: Unknown.
Monitor nursing infant closely and discontinue drug or nursing if adverse effects develop.

Habit-Forming Potential: None.

Effects of Overdosage: Throbbing headache, dizziness, marked flushing, nausea, vomiting, abdominal cramps, confusion, delirium, paralysis, seizures, circulatory collapse.

Possible Effects of Long-Term Use: The development of tolerance (see Glossary) and the temporary loss of effectiveness.

Suggested Periodic Examinations While Taking This Drug (at physician's discretion)
Measurements of blood pressure and internal eye pressures.
Evaluation of hemoglobin.

▷ **While Taking This Drug, Observe the Following**

Foods: No restrictions.
Beverages: No restrictions. May be taken with milk.

▷ *Alcohol:* Use extreme caution until the combined effects have been determined. Avoid alcohol completely in the presence of any side-effects or adverse effects from nitroglycerin. Never use alcohol in the presence of a nitroglycerin headache.

Tobacco Smoking: Nicotine can reduce the effectiveness of this drug. Follow your physician's advice regarding smoking.

Marijuana Smoking: Possible reduced effectiveness of this drug; mild to moderate increase in angina; possible changes in the electrocardiogram, confusing interpretation.

▷ *Other Drugs*

Nitroglycerin *taken concurrently* with

- antihypertensive drugs may cause excessive lowering of blood pressure. Careful dosage adjustments may be necessary.

The following drugs may *increase* the effects of nitroglycerin

- aspirin, in analgesic doses (500 mg or more).

▷ *Driving, Hazardous Activities:* Usually no restrictions. This drug may cause dizziness or faintness. Restrict activities as necessary.

Aviation Note: Coronary artery disease *is a disqualification* for piloting. Consult a designated Aviation Medical Examiner.

Exposure to Sun: No restrictions.

Exposure to Heat: Use caution. Hot environments can cause significant lowering of blood pressure.

Exposure to Cold: Cold environments can increase the need for this drug and limit its effectiveness.

Heavy Exercise or Exertion: This drug can increase your tolerance for exercise. Use good judgment regarding excessive exertion in the absence of anginal pain.

Discontinuation: Do not stop this drug abruptly after long-term use. It is advisable to reduce the dose (of the prolonged-action dosage forms) gradually over a period of to 6 weeks. Observe for rebound angina.

Special Storage Instructions: For sublingual tablets, to prevent loss of strength

- keep tablets in the original glass container.
- do not transfer tablets to a plastic or metallic container (such as a pillbox).
- do not place absorbent cotton, paper (such as the prescription label), or other material inside the container.
- do not store other drugs in the same container.
- close the container tightly immediately after each use.
- store at room temperature.

NIZATIDINE
(ni ZA te deen)

Introduced: 1986

Class: Antiulcer, H-2 receptor blocker

Prescription: USA: Yes

Controlled Drug: USA: No

Available as Generic: No

Brand Name: Axid

BENEFITS versus RISKS

Possible Benefits
EFFECTIVE TREATMENT OF
  PEPTIC ULCER DISEASE: relief
  of symptoms, acceleration of
  healing (in 80% to 90% of
  cases), prevention of recurrence
  (in 65% to 80% of cases)
CONTROL OF
  HYPERSECRETORY STOMACH
  DISORDERS
Beneficial in treatment of reflux
  esophagitis

Possible Risks
Drug-induced liver damage (rare)
Abnormally low blood platelet
  count (rare)

▷ **Principal Uses**
  As a Single Drug Product: Used primarily in the treatment of peptic ulcer
    disease, both benign stomach (gastric) ulcer and duodenal ulcer. It is
    used specifically to hasten the healing of ulcer and to prevent recur-
    rence. Also used to control the excessive production of stomach acid in
    the Zollinger-Ellison syndrome. Though its effectiveness has not been
    fully established, this drug is also used in the management of esophagi-
    tis (as with hiatal hernia) and upper gastrointestinal bleeding.

How This Drug Works: By blocking the action of histamine, this drug
  effectively inhibits the secretion of stomach acid and thus creates a
  more favorable environment for the healing of peptic ulcers.

Available Dosage Forms and Strengths
  Capsules — 150 mg, 300 mg

▷ **Usual Adult Dosage Range:** For active peptic ulcer: 150 mg 2 times daily,
    12 hours apart; or 300 mg once daily at bedtime. For prevention of
    recurrent ulcer: 150 mg at bedtime. **Note: Actual dosage and adminis-
    tration schedule must be determined by the physician for each pa-
    tient individually.**

▷ **Dosing Instructions:**   To obtain the longest period of stomach acid reduction, this drug should be taken with or immediately following food. The capsule may be opened for administration.

Usual Duration of Use: Continual use on a regular schedule for 4 to 6 weeks is usually necessary to determine this drug's effectiveness in healing active peptic ulcer. Long-term use (months to years) for prevention of ulcer recurrence requires individual consideration by your physician.

Possible Advantages of This Drug
Effective ulcer treatment with once-a-day dosage.
Minimal adverse effects.
Does not cause confusion; does not reduce sperm count or sexual potency.
No significant drug interactions.

▷ **This Drug Should Not Be Taken If**
• you have had an allergic reaction to any dosage form of it previously.

▷ **Inform Your Physician Before Taking This Drug If**
• you are allergic to other H-2 receptor blockers: cimetidine (Tagamet), famotidine (Pepcid), ranitidine (Zantac).
• you have impaired liver or kidney function.
• you are taking large doses of aspirin.

Possible Side-Effects (natural, expected and unavoidable drug actions)
None reported.

▷ **Possible Adverse Effects** (unusual, unexpected and infrequent reactions)
If any of the following develop, consult your physician promptly for guidance.
Mild Adverse Effects
Allergic Reaction: Skin rash, hives (0.5%).
Drowsiness (2.4%), sweating (1.0%).
Serious Adverse Effects
Allergic Reaction: Exfoliative dermatitis.
Drug-induced liver injury (without jaundice), reversible.
Reduced blood platelet count: abnormal bleeding or bruising (rare).

▷ **Possible Effects on Sexual Function:**   Male breast enlargement (rare).

Possible Effects on Laboratory Tests
Blood platelet count: decreased.
Liver function tests: increased liver enzymes (ALT/GPT, AST/GOT).

CAUTION
1. Do not discontinue this drug abruptly. (Ulcer activation and perforation have occurred following abrupt cessation of cimetidine, a closely related drug.)
2. After discontinuation of this drug, inform your physician promptly

if you experience a return of symptoms indicative of ulcer reactivation.

Precautions for Use
By Infants and Children: Safety and effectiveness for use by those under 12 years of age have not been established.

By Those over 60 Years of Age: This drug may contribute to the formation of stomach phytobezoars (masses of undigested vegetable fibers). Individuals with poor chewing ability (missing teeth) and those who have had partial gastrectomy or vagotomy (stomach surgery) are most susceptible. Observe for loss of appetite, stomach fullness, nausea and vomiting.

▷ **Advisability of Use During Pregnancy**
Pregnancy Category: C (tentative). See Pregnancy Code inside back cover.
Animal studies: Rabbit studies revealed significant birth defects of the heart, brain and spinal cord.
Human studies: Information from adequate studies of pregnant women is not available.
Avoid drug during the first 3 months if possible. Use this drug only if clearly needed. Ask physician for guidance.

Advisability of Use if Breast-Feeding
Presence of this drug in breast milk: Probably yes.
Avoid drug or refrain from nursing.

Habit-Forming Potential: None.

Effects of Overdosage: Based on animal studies: excessive tearing, salivation, vomiting, diarrhea.

Possible Effects of Long-Term Use: None reported.

Suggested Periodic Examinations While Taking This Drug (at physician's discretion)
Complete blood cell counts, liver function tests.

▷ **While Taking This Drug, Observe the Following**
Foods: Protein-rich foods produce maximal stomach acid secretion. Follow the diet prescribed to derive optimal benefit from this drug.
Beverages: No restrictions. May be taken with milk.
▷ *Alcohol:* No interactions with drug. However, alcoholic beverages increase stomach acidity and can reduce the effectiveness of this drug.
▷ *Other Drugs*
Nizatidine may *increase* the effects of
• aspirin (when aspirin is taken in large doses—3900 mg/day).
The following drugs may *decrease* the effects of nizatidine
• antacids containing aluminum and magnesium hydroxide can reduce

absorption of nizatidine by 10%. Avoid antacids for 2 hours before and after taking nizatidine.

▷ *Driving, Hazardous Activities:* This drug may cause drowsiness. Restrict activities as necessary.

Aviation Note: The use of this drug *may be a disqualification* for piloting. Consult a designated Aviation Medical Examiner.

Exposure to Sun: No restrictions.

Discontinuation: Do not discontinue this drug suddenly if taken for peptic ulcer disease. Consult physician for withdrawal instructions. This drug does not provide an extended protective effect. Be alert to the possibility of ulcer recurrence anytime after discontinuation.

NORFLOXACIN
(nor FLOX a sin)

Introduced: 1986

Class: Anti-infectives

Prescription: USA: Yes
Canada: Yes

Controlled Drug: USA: No
Canada: No

Available as Generic: USA: No
Canada: No

Brand Name: Noroxin

BENEFITS versus RISKS

Possible Benefits	*Possible Risks*
HIGH CURE RATE (95%) IN TREATMENT OF URINARY TRACT INFECTIONS	Infrequent nausea, indigestion
	Rare impairment of vision
	Rare seizure
Effective treatment of bacterial gastroenteritis and gonorrhea	

▷ **Principal Uses**

As a Single Drug Product: Used primarily to treat urinary tract infections (in adults) caused by a wide variety of bacteria sensitive to the action of this drug. It is also used to treat acute gastroenteritis caused by certain bacteria, to prevent traveler's diarrhea and to treat gonorrhea.

How This Drug Works: By inhibiting essential enzyme systems of bacterial nucleic acids (DNA), this drug prevents bacterial reproduction (with low doses) and destroys bacteria (with higher doses).

Available Dosage Forms and Strengths
Tablets — 400 mg

▷ **Usual Adult Dosage Range:** Uncomplicated urinary tract infections—400 mg/12 hours for 3 days. Complicated urinary tract infections—400 mg/12 hours for 10 to 21 days. Total daily dosage should not exceed 800 mg. **Note: Actual dosage and administration schedule must be determined by the physician for each patient individually.**

▷ **Dosing Instructions:** Preferably taken with a full glass of water 1 hour before or 2 hours after eating. Avoid antacids for 2 hours after taking this drug. The tablet may be crushed for administration. Take the full course prescribed.

Usual Duration of Use: Continual use on a regular schedule for 3 to 21 days (depending upon the nature of the infection) is usually necessary to determine this drug's effectiveness in eradicating the infection.

Possible Advantages of This Drug: Highly effective in treating adults with urinary tract infections due to virtually all varieties of causative bacteria. This drug kills bacteria rapidly, preventing the development of bacterial resistance to the action of the drug.

Currently a "Drug of Choice"
for starting anti-infective treatment prior to obtaining the results of urine bacterial culture and sensitivity tests.

▷ **This Drug Should Not Be Taken If**
• you have had an allergic reaction to any dosage form of it previously.
• you are pregnant or breast-feeding.
• it is prescribed for a child under 18 years of age.

▷ **Inform Your Physician Before Taking This Drug If**
• you are allergic to cinoxacin (Cinobac) or nalidixic acid (NegGram).
• you have a seizure disorder.
• you have impaired liver or kidney function.

Possible Side-Effects (natural, expected and unavoidable drug actions)
None reported.

▷ **Possible Adverse Effects** (unusual, unexpected and infrequent reactions)
If any of the following develop, consult your physician promptly for guidance.
Mild Adverse Effects
Allergic Reactions: Skin rash (0.4%), hives (0.1%), localized swelling, itching (0.1%).
Headache (1.6%), dizziness (1.2%), mental depression (4 reports), seizures (3 reports).
Drowsiness, mood alterations, nervousness, insomnia, hallucinations (all less than 1%).
Visual disturbances: blurred or double vision, altered color vision, increased sensitivity to light (all less than 0.1%).

Dry mouth, decreased appetite (0.1%), nausea (2%), indigestion (0.3%), vomiting, (0.2%), diarrhea (0.2%).
Swollen or painful tendons and joints (0.1%).
Serious Adverse Effects
Allergic Reactions: Exfoliative dermatitis (1 report), anaphylactic reaction (see Glossary; 1 report).

▷ **Possible Effects on Sexual Function:**   None reported.

Natural Diseases or Disorders That May Be Activated by This Drug
Latent epilepsy.

Possible Effects on Laboratory Tests
Red and white blood cell counts: rarely decreased.
Liver function tests: rarely increased liver enzymes (ALT/GPT, AST/GOT).
Kidney function tests: rarely increased blood creatinine and urea nitrogen (BUN) levels.

CAUTION
1. With high doses or prolonged use, crystal formation in the kidney can occur. This can be prevented by drinking copious amounts of water, up to 2 quarts/24 hours.
2. This drug may decrease the formation of saliva and predispose to the formation of dental cavities or gum disease. Consult your dentist if mouth dryness persists.

Precautions for Use
By Infants and Children: Safety for use by those who have not attained complete bone growth has not been established. This drug can impair normal bone growth and development in test animals. Avoid its use in children until complete bone development is assured.
By Those over 60 Years of Age: Impaired kidney function may require dosage reduction. Consult your physician.

▷ **Advisability of Use During Pregnancy**
Pregnancy Category: C (tentative). See Pregnancy Code inside back cover.
Animal studies: Mouse, rat, rabbit and monkey studies reveal no birth defects due to this drug. However, this drug can cause impaired bone development in immature dogs.
Human studies: Information from adequate studies of pregnant women is not available.
This drug should be avoided during entire pregnancy.

Advisability of Use if Breast-Feeding
Presence of this drug in breast milk: Unknown.
Avoid drug or refrain from nursing.

Habit-Forming Potential: None.

Effects of Overdosage: No information available.

Possible Effects of Long-Term Use: Crystal formation in kidneys with high doses and inadequate fluid intake.

Suggested Periodic Examinations While Taking This Drug (at physician's discretion)
Liver function tests, urine analysis.

▷ **While Taking This Drug, Observe the Following**
Foods: No restrictions.
Beverages: No restrictions.
▷ *Alcohol:* No interactions expected.
Tobacco Smoking: No interactions expected.
▷ *Other Drugs*
Nitrofurantoin (Macrodantin, etc.) *taken concurrently* with norfloxacin may antagonize the antibacterial action of norfloxacin in the urinary tract. Avoid this combination.
The following drug may *increase* the effects of norfloxacin
• probenecid (Benemid).
The following drugs may *decrease* the effects of norfloxacin
• antacids may reduce its absorption.
▷ *Driving, Hazardous Activities:* This drug may cause dizziness or impaired vision. Restrict activities as necessary.
Aviation Note: The use of this drug *may be a disqualification* for piloting. Consult a designated Aviation Medical Examiner.
Exposure to Sun: Sunglasses advised if eyes are overly sensitive to bright light.
Discontinuation: If you experience no adverse effects from this drug, take the full course prescribed for maximal results. Consult your physician regarding termination of treatment.

NORTRIPTYLINE
(nor TRIP ti leen)

Introduced: 1963

Class: Antidepressant

Prescription: USA: Yes
Canada: Yes

Controlled Drug: USA: No
Canada: No

Available as Generic: USA: No
Canada: No

Brand Names: Aventyl, Pamelor

BENEFITS versus RISKS

Possible Benefits	*Possible Risks*
EFFECTIVE RELIEF OF ENDOGENOUS DEPRESSION	ADVERSE BEHAVIORAL EFFECTS: confusion, disorientation, hallucinations, delusions
Possibly beneficial in other depressive disorders	CONVERSION OF DEPRESSION TO MANIA in manic-depressive disorders
Possibly beneficial in the management of some types of chronic, severe pain	Aggravation of schizophrenia
	Irregular heart rhythms
	Rare blood cell abnormalities

▷ **Principal Uses**

As a Single Drug Product

Used primarily to relieve the symptoms associated with spontaneous (endogenous) depression, and to initiate the restoration of normal mood. This drug should be used only when a diagnosis of a true, primary depression of significant degree has been established. It should not be used to treat the symptoms of mild and transient (reactive) depression that may be associated with many life situations in the absence of a bona fide affective illness.

It is also used in conjunction with other drugs to manage chronic, severe pain associated with such conditions as cancer, migraine headache, severe arthritis, peripheral neuropathy, AIDS, etc.

How This Drug Works: It is thought that this drug relieves depression by slowly restoring to normal levels certain constituents of brain tissue (norepinephrine and serotonin) that transmit nerve impulses.

Available Dosage Forms and Strengths

Capsules — 10 mg, 25 mg, 50 mg, 75 mg
Oral solution — 10 mg per 5-ml teaspoonful (alcohol 4%)

▷ **Usual Adult Dosage Range:** Initially 25 mg 3 or 4 times daily. Dose may be increased cautiously as needed and tolerated by 10 to 25 mg daily at intervals of 1 week. Usual maintenance dose is 50 to 100 mg/24 hours. Total dose should not exceed 150 mg/24 hours. When the optimal requirement is determined, it may be taken at bedtime as one dose. **Note: Actual dosage and administration schedule must be determined by the physician for each patient individually.**

▷ **Dosing Instructions:** May be taken without regard to meals. The capsule may be opened for administration.

Usual Duration of Use: Some benefit may be apparent within 1 to 2 weeks, but adequate response may require continual use for 3 months or longer. Long-term use should not exceed 6 months without evaluation regarding the need for continuation of the drug. Consult your physician on a regular basis.

Possible Advantages of This Drug
Causes less daytime sedation.
Causes fewer atropinelike side-effects.
Causes orthostatic hypotension infrequently (see Glossary).

▷ **This Drug Should Not Be Taken If**
• you have had an allergic reaction to it previously.
• you are taking or have taken within the past 14 days any monoamine oxidase (MAO) type A inhibitor drug (see Drug Class, Section Four).
• you are recovering from a recent heart attack.
• you have narrow-angle glaucoma.

▷ **Inform Your Physician Before Taking This Drug If**
• you are allergic or sensitive to any other tricyclic antidepressant (see Drug Class, Section Four).
• you have a history of any of the following: diabetes, epilepsy, glaucoma, heart disease, prostate gland enlargement or overactive thyroid function.
• you plan to have surgery under general anesthesia in the near future.

Possible Side-Effects (natural, expected and unavoidable drug actions)
Light-headedness, drowsiness, blurred vision, dry mouth, constipation, impaired urination (see Prostatism in Glossary).

▷ **Possible Adverse Effects** (unusual, unexpected and infrequent reactions)
If any of the following develop, consult your physician promptly for guidance.
Mild Adverse Effects
Allergic Reactions: Skin rash, hives, swelling of face or tongue, drug fever (see Glossary).
Headache, dizziness, weakness, fainting, unsteady gait, tremors.
Peculiar taste, irritation of tongue or mouth, nausea, indigestion.
Fluctuation of blood sugar levels.
Serious Adverse Effects
Allergic Reactions: Hepatitis, with or without jaundice (see Glossary).
Confusion, disorientation, hallucinations, delusions.
Aggravation of paranoid psychoses and schizophrenia; seizures.
Heart palpitation and irregular rhythm.
Bone marrow depression (see Glossary)—fatigue, weakness, fever, sore throat, abnormal bleeding or bruising.
Peripheral neuritis (see Glossary)—numbness, tingling, pain, loss of strength in arms and legs.
Parkinson-like disorders (see Glossary)—usually mild and infrequent; more likely to occur in the elderly.

▷ **Possible Effects on Sexual Function:** Decreased libido, increased libido (antidepressant effect), male impotence, inhibited female orgasm, male and female breast enlargement, milk production, swelling of testicles.

▷ **Adverse Effects That May Mimic Natural Diseases or Disorders**
Liver toxicity may suggest viral hepatitis.

Natural Diseases or Disorders That May Be Activated by This Drug
Latent diabetes, epilepsy, glaucoma, prostatism.

Possible Effects on Laboratory Tests
White blood cell and platelet counts: decreased.
Blood glucose levels: increased and decreased (fluctuations).
Liver function tests: increased liver enzymes (ALT/GPT, AST/GOT and alkaline phosphatase), increased bilirubin.

CAUTION
1. Dosage must be adjusted for each person individually. Report for follow-up evaluation and laboratory tests as directed by your physician.
2. It is advisable to withhold this drug if electroconvulsive therapy (ECT, "shock" treatment) is to be used to treat your depression.

Precautions for Use
By Infants and Children: Safety and effectiveness for use by those under 6 years of age have not been established.
By Those over 60 Years of Age: Usual dosage is 30 to 50 mg daily in divided doses. During the first 2 weeks of treatment, observe for the development of confusion, agitation, forgetfulness, disorientation, delusions and hallucinations. Reduction of dosage or discontinuation may be necessary. Unsteadiness may predispose to falling and injury. This drug can increase the degree of impaired urination associated with prostate gland enlargement (prostatism).

▷ **Advisability of Use During Pregnancy**
Pregnancy Category: C (tentative). See Pregnancy Code inside back cover.
Animal studies: Results are inconclusive.
Human studies: No defects reported in 21 exposures to amitriptyline, a closely related drug. Information from adequate studies of pregnant women is not available for this drug.
Avoid use of drug during first 3 months. Use during last 6 months only if clearly needed. Ask your physician for guidance.

Advisability of Use if Breast-Feeding
Presence of this drug in breast milk: Yes, in small amounts.
Monitor nursing infant closely and discontinue drug or nursing if adverse effects develop: excessive drowsiness and failure to feed.

Habit-Forming Potential: Psychological or physical dependence is rare and unexpected.

Effects of Overdosage: Confusion, hallucinations, marked drowsiness, heart palpitations, dilated pupils, tremors, stupor, deep sleep, coma, convulsions.

Suggested Periodic Examinations While Taking This Drug (at physician's discretion)
Complete blood cell counts, liver function tests, serial blood pressure readings and electrocardiograms.

▷ **While Taking This Drug, Observe the Following**
Foods: No restrictions. This drug may increase the appetite and cause excessive weight gain.
Beverages: No restrictions. May be taken with milk.
▷ *Alcohol:* Avoid completely. This drug can markedly increase the intoxicating effects of alcohol and accentuate its depressant action on brain function.
Tobacco Smoking: May hasten the elimination of this drug. Higher doses may be necessary.
▷ *Other Drugs*
Nortriptyline may *increase* the effects of
• atropinelike drugs (see Drug Class, Section Four).
• dicoumarol, and increase the risk of bleeding.
• epinephrine (Adrenalin).
Nortriptyline may *decrease* the effects of
• clonidine (Catapres).
• ephedrine (Primatene tablets).
• guanethidine (Ismelin).
Nortriptyline *taken concurrently* with
• disulfiram (Antabuse) may cause acute dementia: confusion, disorientation, hallucinations.
• monoamine oxidase (MAO) inhibitor drugs may cause high fever, delirium and convulsions (see Drug Class, Section Four).
• thyroid preparations may impair heart rhythm and function. Ask physician for guidance regarding adjustment of thyroid dose.
The following drugs may *increase* the effects of nortriptyline
• cimetidine (Tagamet), and cause nortriptyline toxicity.
• quinidine (Quinaglute, etc,), and cause nortriptyline toxicity.
The following drugs may *decrease* the effects of nortriptyline
• barbiturates (see Drug Class, Section Four), and reduce its effectiveness.
▷ *Driving, Hazardous Activities:* This drug may impair mental alertness, judgment, physical coordination and reaction time. Avoid hazardous activities.
Aviation Note: The use of this drug *is a disqualification* for piloting. Consult a designated Aviation Medical Examiner.
Exposure to Sun: Use caution until sensitivity to sun has been determined. This drug may cause photosensitivity (see Glossary).
Exposure to Heat: This drug can inhibit sweating and impair the body's

adaptation to hot environments, increasing the risk of heat stroke. Avoid saunas.

Exposure to Cold: The elderly should use caution and avoid conditions conducive to hypothermia (see Glossary).

Discontinuation: It is advisable to discontinue this drug gradually. Abrupt withdrawal after long-term use can cause headache, malaise and nausea.

OFLOXACIN
(oh FLOX a sin)

Introduced: 1984

Class: Anti-infective

Prescription: USA: Yes

Controlled Drug: USA: No

Available as Generic: USA: No

Brand Name: Floxin

BENEFITS versus RISKS

Possible Benefits	*Possible Risks*
HIGHLY EFFECTIVE TREATMENT FOR INFECTIONS OF THE LOWER RESPIRATORY TRACT, URINARY TRACT, SKIN AND SKIN STRUCTURES, due to susceptible organisms	Rare but serious allergic reactions
	Rare seizures and hallucinations
	Headache (1–9%), dizziness (1–5%)
	Nausea (3–10%), diarrhea (1–4%)
EFFECTIVE TREATMENT FOR SOME SEXUALLY TRANSMITTED DISEASES	
Effective treatment for some infections of the prostate gland	

▷ **Principal Uses**

As a Single Drug Product: Used primarily to treat responsive infections (in adults) of: (1) the lower respiratory tract (lungs and bronchial tubes); (2) the urinary tract (kidneys, bladder, urethra and prostate gland); (3) skin and related tissues; (4) certain sexually transmitted diseases: gonorrheal and chlamydial infections of the urethra and cervix.

How This Drug Works: By interfering with the bacterial enzyme DNA gyrase (which is required for DNA synthesis and cell reproduction), this drug arrests bacterial growth (in low concentrations) and destroys bacteria (in high concentrations).

Available Dosage Forms and Strengths
   Tablets — 200 mg, 300 mg, 400 mg

▷ **Usual Adult Dosage Range:**   200 mg to 400 mg/12 hours, depending upon
   the nature and severity of the infection. The total daily dosage should
   not exceed 800 mg. **Note: Actual dosage and administration schedule
   must be determined by the physician for each patient individually.**

▷ **Dosing Instructions:**   Do not take with food. Preferably it should be taken
   1 hour before or 2 hours after eating. Drink fluids liberally during the
   entire course of treatment. Avoid antacids containing aluminum or
   magnesium and supplements containing iron or zinc for 2 hours before
   and after dosing. The tablet may be crushed for administration.

   Usual Duration of Use: Continual use on a regular schedule for up to 10
   days is usually necessary to determine this drug's effectiveness in eradicating the infection. The drug should be continued for at least 2 days
   after all indications of infection have disappeared. Prostate gland infections may require continual treatment for 6 weeks. Long-term use
   requires periodic evaluation of response and dosage adjustment. Consult your physician on a regular basis.

Possible Advantages of This Drug
   Very broad spectrum of antibacterial activity. Capable of establishing
   effective drug levels throughout the prostate gland. Effective one-dose
   treatment for uncomplicated gonorrheal infection of the urethra.
   No significant effect on kidney function.
   No reports of serious drug-induced colitis.

Currently a "Drug of Choice"
   for (1) starting treatment of urinary tract infections prior to obtaining the
   results of urine bacterial culture and sensitivity tests; (2) treating infections due to *Pseudomonas* bacterial strains often resistant to other
   anti-infective drugs.

▷ **This Drug Should Not Be Taken If**
   • you have had an allergic reaction to it previously.
   • you are pregnant or breast-feeding.
   • you have a seizure disorder that is not adequately controlled.
   • it is prescribed for a person under 18 years of age.

▷ **Inform Your Physician Before Taking This Drug If**
   • you are allergic to cinoxacin (Cinobac), nalidixic acid (NegGram), cip-
     rofloxacin (Cipro) or norfloxacin (Noroxin).
   • you have a history of a seizure disorder or a circulatory disorder of the
     brain.
   • you have impaired liver or kidney function.
   • you are taking any form of probenecid or theophylline.

Possible Side-Effects (natural, expected and unavoidable drug actions)
Superinfections: vaginitis (1–3%). (See Superinfection in the Glossary.)

▷ **Possible Adverse Effects** (unusual, unexpected and infrequent reactions)
If any of the following develop, consult your physician promptly for guidance.
Mild Adverse Effects
Allergic Reactions: Rash (1–3%), itching (1–3%), fever (1–3%).
Headache (1–9%), dizziness (1–5%), weakness (1–3%), drowsiness (1–3%), nervousness (1–3%), insomnia (3–7%), visual disturbances (1–3%).
Decreased appetite (1–3%), altered taste (1–3%), dry mouth (1–3%), nausea (3–10%), vomiting (1–3%), indigestion (1%), diarrhea (1–4%).
Serious Adverse Effects
Allergic Reactions: Anaphylactoid reactions (see Glossary).
Idiosyncratic Reactions: None reported.
Central nervous system stimulation: restlessness, tremor, confusion, hallucinations, seizures (all very rare).

▷ **Possible Effects on Sexual Function:**   Painful menstruation, excessive menstrual bleeding.

▷ **Natural Diseases or Disorders That May Be Activated by This Drug**
Latent epilepsy.

Possible Effects on Laboratory Tests
Complete blood cell counts: rarely decreased lymphocytes; rarely increased eosinophils.
Liver function tests: rarely increased liver enzymes (ALT/GPT, AST/GOT).
Blood creatinine level: rarely increased.
Blood glucose levels: rare fluctuations.

CAUTION
1. With high doses or prolonged use of other drugs of this class, crystal formation in the kidney may occur. This can be prevented by drinking copious amounts of water, up to 2 quarts/24 hours.
2. Drugs of this class may decrease the formation of saliva and predispose to the development of dental cavities or gum disease. Consult your dentist if dry mouth persists.

Precautions for Use
By Infants and Children: Safety and effectiveness for use by those under 18 years of age have not been established. Avoid the use of this drug completely. It can impair normal bone growth and development in immature animals.
By Those over 60 Years of Age: Impaired kidney function may require dosage reduction.
If you are taking theophylline concurrently with this drug, observe closely for possible theophylline accumulation and toxicity.

▷ **Advisability of Use During Pregnancy**
Pregnancy Category: C (tentative). See Pregnancy Code inside back cover.
    Animal studies: Mild skeletal defects due to this drug were found in rat
    studies; toxic effects on the fetus were shown in rat and rabbit studies.
    This drug can impair normal bone development in immature dogs.
    Human studies: Information from adequate studies of pregnant women
    is not available. However, the potential for adverse effects on fetal bone
    development contraindicates the use of this drug during entire preg-
    nancy.

Advisability of Use if Breast-Feeding
    Presence of this drug in breast milk: Yes.
    Avoid drug or refrain from nursing.

Habit-Forming Potential: None.

Effects of Overdosage: No information available.

Possible Effects of Long-Term Use: Superinfections (see Glossary).

Suggested Periodic Examinations While Taking This Drug (at physician's
    discretion)
    Liver function tests, urine analysis.

▷ **While Taking This Drug, Observe the Following**
    Foods: No restrictions.
    Beverages: No restrictions. May be taken with milk.
▷   *Alcohol:* No interactions expected.
    Tobacco Smoking: No interactions expected.
▷   *Other Drugs*
        Ofloxacin may *increase* the effects of
        • theophylline, and cause theophylline toxicity.
        The following drug may *increase* the effects of ofloxacin
        • probenecid (Benemid).
        The following drugs may *decrease* the effects of ofloxacin
        • antacids containing aluminum or magnesium can reduce the absorp-
         tion of ofloxacin and lessen its effectiveness.
▷   *Driving, Hazardous Activities:* This drug may cause drowsiness, dizziness
        and impaired vision. Restrict activities as necessary.
    Aviation Note: The use of this drug *may be a disqualification* for piloting.
        Consult a designated Aviation Medical Examiner.
    Exposure to Sun: This drug may rarely cause photosensitivity (see Glos-
        sary). Sunglasses are advised if eyes are overly sensitive to bright light.
    Discontinuation: If you experience no adverse effects from this drug, take
        the full course prescribed for maximal results. Consult your physician
        regarding termination of treatment.

OMEPRAZOLE
(oh ME pra zohl)

Introduced: 1986

Class: Antiulcer, gastric acid inhibitor

Prescription: USA: Yes
Canada: Yes

Controlled Drug: USA: No
Canada: No

Available as Generic: USA: No
Canada: No

Brand Name: Prilosec (formerly Losec)

BENEFITS versus RISKS

Possible Benefits	*Possible Risks*
VERY EFFECTIVE TREATMENT OF CONDITIONS ASSOCIATED WITH EXCESSIVE PRODUCTION OF GASTRIC ACID: Zollinger-Ellison syndrome, mastocytosis, endocrine adenoma	RARE APLASTIC ANEMIA (see Glossary) Urinary tract infection
VERY EFFECTIVE TREATMENT OF REFLUX ESOPHAGITIS	
VERY EFFECTIVE TREATMENT OF GASTRIC AND DUODENAL ULCERS	

▷ **Principal Uses**

As a Single Drug Product: Used primarily to inhibit the secretion of stomach acid, an important first step in the treatment of several conditions associated with excessive stomach acid production: acute and chronic gastritis, reflux esophagitis, Zollinger-Ellison syndrome, mastocytosis, endocrine adenomas, active gastric and duodenal ulcer.

How This Drug Works: By inhibiting the action of a specific enzyme system in the acid-secreting cells of the stomach lining, this drug arrests the production of stomach acid and thereby (1) eliminates a principal cause of the condition under treatment, and (2) creates an environment conducive to healing.

Available Dosage Forms and Strengths

Capsules, delayed-release — 20 mg

▷ **Usual Adult Dosage Range:** Reflux esophagitis: 20 mg to 40 mg once daily for 4 to 8 weeks.

Excessive stomach acid conditions: 60 mg once daily for as long as necessary.

Gastric and duodenal ulcer: 20 mg to 40 mg once daily for 4 to 8 weeks. In extreme conditions, doses of 120 mg daily, in divided doses, have been used.**Note: Actual dosage and administration schedule must be determined by the physician for each patient individually.**

▷ **Dosing Instructions:**   Take immediately before eating, preferably the morning meal. The capsule should be swallowed whole without opening; the contents should not be crushed or chewed. This drug may be taken concurrently with antacids if they are needed to relieve stomach pain.

Usual Duration of Use:
Continual use on a regular schedule for 2 to 3 weeks is usually necessary to determine this drug's effectiveness in suppressing stomach acid production. Long-term use (months to years) requires periodic evaluation of response and dosage adjustment. Consult your physician on a regular basis.

Possible Advantages of This Drug
Effectively inhibits acid secretion at all times: basal conditions (stomach empty and at rest) and following food, alcohol, smoking or other stimulants.
Is more effective than H-2 receptor blocking drugs in treating severe reflux esophagitis and refractory duodenal ulcer.

Currently a "Drug of Choice"
for the short-term treatment of severe reflux esophagitis and for the long-term treatment of Zollinger-Ellison syndrome.

▷ **This Drug Should Not Be Taken If**
  • you have had an allergic reaction to it previously.
  • you have a currently active bone marrow or blood cell disorder.

▷ **Inform Your Physician Before Taking This Drug If**
  • you have a history of liver disease or impaired liver function.
  • you have a history of any type of bone marrow or blood cell disorder, especially one that is drug-induced.
  • you are currently taking any anticoagulant medication, diazepam (Valium) or phenytoin (Dilantin, etc.).

Possible Side-Effects
(natural, expected and unavoidable drug actions)
None reported.

▷ **Possible Adverse Effects**
(unusual, unexpected and infrequent reactions)
If any of the following develop, consult your physician promptly for guidance.
Mild Adverse Effects
Allergic Reactions: Skin rash (1.5%), itching.
Headache (6.9%), dizziness (1.5%), drowsiness, weakness (1.1%).

Indigestion (2.4%), nausea (2.2%), vomiting (1.5%), diarrhea (3%), constipation (1.1%).

Serious Adverse Effects

Rare bone marrow depression (see Glossary): fatigue, weakness, fever, sore throat, infections, abnormal bleeding or bruising.

Rare liver damage with jaundice (see Glossary).

Urinary tract infection: painful urination, cloudy or bloody urine.

▷ **Possible Effects on Sexual Function**

One case of drug-induced male breast enlargement and tenderness (gynecomastia) has been reported; this occurred on two separate occasions in association with the use of this drug.

▷ **Adverse Effects That May Mimic Natural Diseases or Disorders**

Persistent infection or bruising may reflect bone marrow depression; blood counts advisable.

Liver reactions may suggest viral hepatitis.

Possible Effects on Laboratory Tests

Complete blood cell counts: decreased red cells, hemoglobin, white cells and platelets.

Blood glucose level: decreased.

Liver function tests: increased liver enzymes (ALT/GPT, AST/GOT and alkaline phosphatase), increased bilirubin.

CAUTION

1. Follow your physician's instructions exactly regarding the length of time you take this drug. Do not extend its use without his guidance.
2. Report promptly any indications of infection.
3. Inform your physician if you plan to take any other medications (prescription or over-the-counter) while taking omeprazole.

Precautions for Use

By Infants and Children

: Safety and effectiveness for use by those under 12 years of age have not been established.

By Those over 60 Years of Age: Slower elimination of this drug makes it possible to achieve satisfactory response with smaller doses; this reduces the risk of adverse effects. Limit the daily dose to 20 mg if possible.

▷ **Advisability of Use During Pregnancy**

Pregnancy Category: C (tentative). See Pregnancy Code inside back cover.

Animal studies: No drug-induced birth defects found in rats; drug-induced embryo and fetal toxicity were demonstrated in rats and rabbits.

Human studies: Information from adequate studies of pregnant women is not available.

Avoid use if possible. Use only if clearly necessary and for the shortest possible time.

Advisability of Use if Breast-Feeding
Presence of this drug in breast milk: Unknown.
Avoid drug or refrain from nursing.

Habit-Forming Potential: None.

Effects of Overdosage: Possible drowsiness, dizziness, lethargy, abdominal pain, nausea.

Possible Effects of Long-Term Use: Some long-term (2 year) studies in rats revealed the development of drug-induced carcinoid tumors in the stomach. To date, long-term use of this drug (more than 5 years) in humans has not revealed any drug-induced tumor potential. Pending more studies of long-term human use, it is advisable to limit the use of this drug to the shortest duration possible to obtain optimal results.

Suggested Periodic Examinations While Taking This Drug
(at physician's discretion)
Complete blood cell counts.

▷ **While Taking This Drug, Observe the Following**
Foods: No restrictions.
Beverages: No restrictions. May be taken with milk.
▷ *Alcohol:* No interactions expected. However, alcohol is best avoided; it stimulates the secretion of stomach acid.
Tobacco Smoking: No interactions expected. However, smoking is best avoided; it may stimulate the secretion of stomach acid.
▷ *Other Drugs*
Omeprazole may *increase* the effects of
• anticoagulants (warfarin, etc.) and increase the risk of bleeding.
• diazepam (Valium) and cause excessive sedation.
• phenytoin (Dilantin, etc.) and cause phenytoin toxicity.
Omeprazole may *decrease* the effects of
• ampicillin.
• iron preparations.
• ketoconazole (Nizoral).
▷ *Driving, Hazardous Activities:* This drug may cause drowsiness and dizziness. Restrict activities as necessary.
Aviation Note: The use of this drug **may be a disqualification** for piloting. Consult a designated Aviation Medical Examiner.
Exposure to Sun: No restrictions.
Discontinuation: Follow your physician's instructions. The duration of use will vary according to the condition under treatment and individual patient response. Premature discontinuation could result in incomplete healing or prompt recurrence of symptoms.

ORAL CONTRACEPTIVES
(or al kon tra SEP tivs)

Other Names: Estrogens/progestins

Introduced: 1956

Class: Female sex hormones

Prescription: USA: Yes
Canada: Yes

Controlled Drug: USA: No
Canada: No

Available as Generic: USA: No
Canada: No

Brand Names: Brevicon, Demulen, Enovid, Levlen, Loestrin, Lo/Ovral, Mi-cronor*, ✦Minestrin 1/20, Modicon, Nelova, Nelova 1/50 M, Nelova 10/11, Norcept-E 1/35, Nordette, Norethin 1/35E, Norethin 1/50M, Norinyl, Norlestrin, Nor-Q.D.*, Ortho Cyclen, Ortho-Novum, Ovcon, Ovral, Ovrette*, ✦Synphasic, Tri-Levlen, Tri-Norinyl, Triphasil

BENEFITS versus RISKS	
Possible Benefits	*Possible Risks*
HIGHLY EFFECTIVE FOR CONTRACEPTIVE PROTECTION Moderately effective as adjunctive treatment in management of excessive menses and endometriosis	SERIOUS, LIFE-THREATENING THROMBOEMBOLIC DISORDERS in susceptible individuals Hypertension Fluid retention Intensification of migrainelike headaches Intensification of fibrocystic breast changes Accelerated growth of uterine fibroid tumors Drug-induced hepatitis with jaundice Benign liver tumors (rare)

▷ **Principal Uses**

As a Single Drug Product: The "Mini-Pill" contains only one component—a progestin. This has been shown to be slightly less effective than the combination of estrogen and progestin in preventing pregnancy.

As a Combination Drug Product [CD]: Most oral contraceptives consist of a combination of a type of estrogen and a type of progestin. These products are the most effective form of contraception available. While used primarily to prevent pregnancy, they are sometimes used to treat menstrual irregularity, excessively heavy menstrual flow and endometriosis.

*"Mini-Pill" type, contains progestin only.

How This Drug Works: When the combination of an estrogen and a progestin is taken in sufficient dosage and on a regular basis, the blood and tissue levels of these hormones increase to resemble those that occur during pregnancy. This results in suppression of the two pituitary gland hormones that normally produce ovulation (the formation and release of an egg by the ovary). In addition, these drugs may (1) alter the cervical mucus so that it resists the passage of sperm, and (2) alter the lining of the uterus so that it resists implantation of the egg (if ovulation occurs).

Available Dosage Forms and Strengths

Tablets — several combinations of synthetic estrogens and progestins in varying strengths; see the package label of the brand prescribed.

▷ **Usual Adult Dosage Range:**   Initiate treatment with the first tablet on the fifth day after the onset of menstruation. Follow with 1 tablet daily (taken at the same time each day) for 21 consecutive days. Resume treatment on the eighth day following the last tablet taken during the preceding cycle. The schedule is to take the drug daily for 3 weeks and to omit it for 1 week. For the Mini-Pill (progestin only), initiate treatment on the first day of menstruation and take 1 tablet daily, every day, throughout the year (no interruption). **Note: Actual dosage and administration schedule must be determined by the physician for each patient individually.**

▷ **Dosing Instructions:**   May be taken with or after food to reduce stomach irritation. To ensure regular (every day) use and uniform blood levels, it is advisable to take the tablet at the same time daily. The tablets may be crushed for administration.

Usual Duration of Use: According to individual needs and circumstances. Long-term use (months to years) requires supervision and periodic evaluation by your physician every 6 months.

▷ **This Drug Should Not Be Taken If**
- you have had a significant allergic reaction to any dosage form of it previously.
- you have a history of thrombophlebitis, embolism, heart attack or stroke.
- you have breast cancer.
- you have active liver disease, seriously impaired liver function or a history of liver tumor.
- you have abnormal and unexplained vaginal bleeding.
- you have sickle cell disease.
- you are pregnant.

▷ **Inform Your Physician Before Taking This Drug If**
- you have had an unfavorable reaction to any oral contraceptive previously.
- you have a history of cancer of the breast or reproductive organs.

- you have any of the following conditions: fibrocystic breast changes, fibroid tumors of the uterus, endometriosis, migrainelike headaches, epilepsy, asthma, heart disease, high blood pressure, gallbladder disease, diabetes or porphyria.
- you smoke tobacco on a regular basis.
- you plan to have surgery in the near future.

Possible Side-Effects (natural, expected and unavoidable drug actions)
Fluid retention, weight gain, "breakthrough" bleeding (spotting in middle of menstrual cycle), altered menstrual pattern, lack of menstruation (during and following cessation of drug), increased susceptibility to yeast infection of the genital tissues.

▷ **Possible Adverse Effects** (unusual, unexpected and infrequent reactions)
If any of the following develop, consult your physician promptly for guidance.
Mild Adverse Effects
Allergic Reactions: Skin rash, hives, itching.
Headache, nervous tension, irritability, accentuation of migraine headaches.
Nausea, vomiting, bloating, diarrhea.
Tannish pigmentation of the face.
Reduced tolerance to contact lenses.
Impaired color vision: blue tinge to objects, blue halo around lights.
Serious Adverse Effects
Allergic Reactions: Erythema multiforme and nodosum (skin reactions), loss of scalp hair.
Idiosyncratic Reactions: Joint and muscle pains.
Emotional depression, rise in blood pressure (in susceptible individuals).
Eye changes: optic neuritis, retinal thrombosis, altered curvature of the cornea, cataracts.
Gallbladder disease, benign liver tumors, jaundice, rise in blood sugar.
Erosion of uterine cervix, enlargement of uterine fibroid tumors, cystitis-like syndrome.
Thrombophlebitis (inflammation of a vein with formation of blood clot)—pain or tenderness in thigh or leg, with or without swelling of foot or leg.
Pulmonary embolism (movement of blood clot to lung)—sudden shortness of breath, pain in chest, coughing, bloody sputum.
Stroke (blood clot in brain)—headaches, blackout, sudden weakness or paralysis of any part of the body, severe dizziness, altered vision, slurred speech, inability to speak.
Heart attack (blood clot in coronary artery)—sudden pain in chest, neck, jaw or arm; weakness; sweating; nausea.
Mesenteric thrombosis—blood clot in abdominal artery.

▷ **Possible Effects on Sexual Function**
Decreased libido (14% to 50%).
Altered character of menstruation; midcycle spotting.

Breast enlargement and tenderness with milk production.
Absent menstruation and infertility (temporary) after discontinuation of drug.

Possible Delayed Adverse Effects: Estrogens taken during pregnancy can predispose the female child to the later development of cancer of the vagina or cervix following puberty.

▷ **Adverse Effects That May Mimic Natural Diseases or Disorders**
Liver reactions may suggest viral hepatitis.

Natural Diseases or Disorders That May Be Activated by This Drug
Latent hypertension, diabetes mellitus, acute intermittent porphyria, lupus erythematosuslike syndrome.

Possible Effects on Laboratory Tests
Blood lupus erythematosus (LE) cells: positive.
Blood clotting time: decreased.
Blood prothrombin time: decreased.
Blood amylase and lipase levels: increased (very rare pancreatitis).
Blood total cholesterol, HDL cholesterol, LDL and VLDL cholesterol levels: usually no effects; some variability depending upon estrogen and progestin content of preparation used.
Blood triglyceride levels: no effect to increased, depending upon estrogen and progestin content of preparation used.
Blood glucose level: increased.
Blood thyroid stimulating hormone (TSH) level: no effect.
Blood thyroid hormone levels: T^3 and T^4 increased; free T^4 either no effect or decreased.
Liver function tests: increased liver enzymes (ALT/GPT, AST/GOT and alkaline phosphatase), increased bilirubin.

CAUTION
1. The incidence of serious adverse effects due to the use of these drugs is very low. However, any unusual development should be reported and evaluated promptly.
2. Studies indicate that women over 30 years of age who smoke and use oral contraceptives are at significantly greater risk of having a serious cardiovascular event than are nonusers.
3. The risk of thromboembolism increases with the amount of estrogen in the product and with the age of the user. Low-estrogen combinations are advised.
4. It is advisable to discontinue these drugs 1 month prior to elective surgery to reduce the risk of postsurgical thromboembolism.
5. Investigate promptly any alteration or disturbance of vision that occurs during the use of these drugs.
6. Investigate promptly the nature of recurrent, persistent or severe headaches that develop while taking these drugs.

7. Observe for significant change of mood. Discontinue this drug if depression develops.
8. Certain commonly used drugs may reduce the effectiveness of oral contraceptives. Some of these are listed in the category of *Other Drugs.*
9. Diarrhea lasting more than a few hours (and occurring during the days the drug is taken) can prevent adequate absorption of these drugs and impair their effectiveness as contraceptives.
10. If 2 consecutive menstrual periods are missed, consult your physician regarding the advisability of performing a pregnancy test. Do not continue to use these drugs until your pregnancy status is determined.

▷ **Advisability of Use During Pregnancy**
Pregnancy Category: X. See Pregnancy Code inside back cover.
Animal studies: Genital defects reported in mice and guinea pigs; cleft palate reported in rodents.
Human studies: Information from studies of pregnant women indicates that estrogens can masculinize the female fetus. In addition, limb defects and heart malformations have been reported.
It is now known that estrogens taken during pregnancy can predispose the female child to the development of cancer of the vagina or cervix following puberty. *Avoid these drugs completely during entire pregnancy.*

Advisability of Use if Breast-Feeding
Presence of these drugs in breast milk: Yes, in minute amounts.
These drugs may suppress milk formation if started early following delivery.
Breast-feeding is considered to be safe during the use of oral contraceptives.

Habit-Forming Potential: None.

Effects of Overdosage: Headache, drowsiness, nausea, vomiting, fluid retention, abnormal vaginal bleeding, breast enlargement and discomfort.

Possible Effects of Long-Term Use: High blood pressure, gallbladder disease with stones, accelerated growth of uterine fibroid tumors, absent menstruation and impaired fertility after discontinuation of drug.

Suggested Periodic Examinations While Taking This Drug (at physician's discretion)
Regular (every 6 months) evaluation of the breasts and pelvic organs, including Pap smears. Liver function tests as indicated.

▷ **While Taking This Drug, Observe the Following**
Foods: Avoid excessive use of salt if fluid retention occurs.
Beverages: No restrictions. May be taken with milk.

▷   *Alcohol:* No interactions expected.

   Tobacco Smoking: Recent studies indicate that heavy smoking (15 or more cigarettes daily) in association with the use of oral contraceptives significantly increases the risk of heart attack (coronary thrombosis). Heavy smoking should be considered a contraindication to the use of oral contraceptives.

▷   *Other Drugs*

   Oral contraceptives may *increase* the effects of

   • some benzodiazepines, and cause excessive sedation.
   • metoprolol (Lopressor), and cause excessive beta blocker effects.
   • prednisolone and prednisone, and cause excessive cortisonelike effects.
   • theophyllines, and increase the risk of toxic effects.

   Oral contraceptives *taken concurrently* with

   • antidiabetic drugs may cause unpredictable fluctuations of blood sugar.
   • tricyclic antidepressants (Elavil, Sinequan, etc.) may enhance their adverse effects and reduce their antidepressant effectiveness.
   • troleandomycin (TAO) may increase the incidence of liver toxicity and jaundice.
   • warfarin (Coumadin) may cause unpredictable alterations of prothrombin activity.

   The following drugs may *decrease* the effects of oral contraceptives (and impair their effectiveness)

   • barbiturates (phenobarbital, etc.; see Drug Class, Section Four).
   • carbamazepine (Tegretol).
   • griseofulvin (Fulvicin, etc.).
   • penicillins (ampicillin, penicillin V).
   • phenytoin (Dilantin).
   • primidone (Mysoline).
   • rifampin (Rifadin, Rimactane).
   • tetracyclines (see Drug Class, Section Four).

▷   *Driving, Hazardous Activities:* Usually no restrictions. Consult your physician for assessment of individual risk and for guidance regarding specific restrictions.

   Aviation Note: Usually no restrictions. However, it is advisable to observe for the rare occurrence of disturbed vision and to restrict activities accordingly. Consult a designated Aviation Medical Examiner.

   Exposure to Sun: Use caution until full effect is known. These drugs can cause photosensitivity (see Glossary).

   Discontinuation: Do not discontinue this drug if "breakthrough" bleeding occurs. If spotting or bleeding continues, consult your physician. A preparation with a higher estrogen content may be required. Remember: Omitting this drug for only 1 day may allow pregnancy to occur. It is advisable to avoid pregnancy for 3 to 6 months after discontinuing these drugs; aborted fetuses from women who became pregnant within 6 months after discontinuation reveal significantly increased chromosome abnormalities.

OXAZEPAM
(ox AZ e pam)

Introduced: 1965

Class: Mild tranquilizer, benzodiazepines

Prescription: USA: Yes
Canada: Yes

Controlled Drug: USA: C-IV*
Canada: No

Available as Generic: USA: Yes
Canada: Yes

Brand Names: ✦Apo-Oxazepam, ✦Novoxapam, ✦Oxpam, Serax, ✦Zapex,
Zaxopam

BENEFITS versus RISKS

Possible Benefits	*Possible Risks*
RELIEF OF ANXIETY AND NERVOUS TENSION in 70% to 80% of users	Habit-forming potential with prolonged use
Wide margin of safety with therapeutic doses	Minor impairment of mental functions
Very few drug interactions	Very rare jaundice
	Very rare blood cell disorders

▷ **Principal Uses**

As a Single Drug Product: Used primarily to (1) provide short-term relief of
mild to moderate anxiety; (2) relieve the symptoms of acute alcohol
withdrawal: agitation, tremors, hallucinations, incipient delirium tremens.

How This Drug Works: It is thought that this drug produces a calming effect
by enhancing the action of the nerve transmitter gamma-aminobutyric
acid (GABA), which in turn blocks the arousal of higher brain centers.

Available Dosage Forms and Strengths
Capsules — 10 mg, 15 mg, 30 mg
Tablets — 15 mg

▷ **Usual Adult Dosage Range:**   30 to 120 mg/24 hours, in 3 or 4 divided doses.
The total daily dosage should not exceed 180 mg. **Note: Actual dosage
and administration schedule must be determined by the physician
for each patient individually.**

▷ **Dosing Instructions:**   May be taken on empty stomach or with food or milk
as needed to prevent stomach irritation. The tablet may be crushed and
the capsule may be opened for administration. Do not discontinue this
drug abruptly if taken for more than 4 weeks.

*See Schedules of Controlled Drugs inside back cover.

Usual Duration of Use: Continual use on a regular schedule for 3 to 5 days is usually necessary to determine this drug's effectiveness in relieving moderate anxiety. Limit continual use to 1 to 3 weeks. Avoid uninterrupted and prolonged use.

▷ **This Drug Should Not Be Taken If**
  • you have had an allergic reaction to any dosage form of it previously.
  • you have acute narrow-angle glaucoma.
  • it is prescribed for a child under 6 years of age.

▷ **Inform Your Physician Before Taking This Drug If**
  • you are allergic to any benzodiazepine drug (see Drug Class, Section Four).
  • you have a history of alcoholism or drug abuse.
  • you are pregnant or planning pregnancy.
  • you have impaired liver or kidney function.
  • you have a history of serious depression or mental disorder.
  • you have any of the following: asthma, emphysema, epilepsy, myasthenia gravis.
  • you are taking any drugs with sedative effects.

Possible Side-Effects (natural, expected and unavoidable drug actions)
  Drowsiness, lethargy, unsteadiness, "hangover" effects on the day following bedtime use.

▷ **Possible Adverse Effects** (unusual, unexpected and infrequent reactions)
  If any of the following develop, consult your physician promptly for guidance.
  Mild Adverse Effects
  Allergic Reactions: Skin rashes, hives.
  Dizziness, fainting, blurred vision, double vision, slurred speech, sweating, nausea.
  Serious Adverse Effects
  Allergic Reactions: Liver reaction with jaundice (see Glossary).
  Abnormally low white blood cell count: fever, sore throat, infections.
  Paradoxical responses of excitement, agitation, anger, rage.

▷ **Possible Effects on Sexual Function:**   Altered timing and pattern of menstruation.

▷ **Adverse Effects That May Mimic Natural Diseases or Disorders**
  Liver reaction with jaundice may suggest viral hepatitis.

Possible Effects on Laboratory Tests
  Complete blood cell counts: decreased white cells; increased eosinophils (allergic reaction).
  Liver function tests: increased liver enzymes (ALT/GPT, AST/GOT and alkaline phosphatase), increased bilirubin.
  Urine screening tests for drug abuse: may be **positive.** (Test results depend upon amount of drug taken and testing method used.)

CAUTION
1. This drug should not be discontinued abruptly if it has been taken continually for more than 4 weeks.
2. The concurrent use of some over-the-counter drug products that contain antihistamines (allergy and cold preparations, sleep aids) can cause excessive sedation in sensitive individuals.

Precautions for Use
By Infants and Children: Safety and effectiveness for use by those under 6 years of age have not been established. This drug should not be used in the hyperactive or psychotic child of any age. Observe for excessive sedation and incoordination.

By Those over 60 Years of Age: It is advisable to use smaller doses at longer intervals to avoid overdosage. Observe for the possible development of lethargy, indifference, fatigue, weakness, unsteadiness, disturbing dreams, nightmares and paradoxical reactions of excitement, agitation, anger, hostility and rage.

▷ **Advisability of Use During Pregnancy**
Pregnancy Category: C (tentative). See Pregnancy Code inside back cover.
Animal studies: No birth defects found in mice, rats or rabbits.

Human studies: Information from adequate studies of pregnant women is not available. No birth defects have been reported with the use of this drug. However, available information regarding the use of other drugs of this class (benzodiazepines) is conflicting and inconclusive. Some studies found an increase in serious birth defects associated with the use of 2 benzodiazepines. Other studies have found no significant increase in birth defects.

Frequent use in late pregnancy can cause the "floppy infant" syndrome in the newborn: weakness, lethargy, unresponsiveness, depressed breathing, low body temperature. Avoid use during entire pregnancy if possible.

Advisability of Use if Breast-Feeding
Presence of this drug in breast milk: Yes.
Avoid drug or refrain from nursing.

Habit-Forming Potential: This drug can produce psychological and/or physical dependence (see Glossary) if used in large doses for an extended period of time.

Effects of Overdosage: Marked drowsiness, weakness, feeling of drunkenness, staggering gait, tremor, stupor progressing to deep sleep or coma.

Possible Effects of Long-Term Use: Psychological and/or physical dependence, rare blood cell disorders.

Suggested Periodic Examinations While Taking This Drug (at physician's discretion)

Complete blood cell counts during long-term use.

Liver function tests.

▷ **While Taking This Drug, Observe the Following**

Foods: No restrictions.

Beverages: Avoid excessive intake of caffeine-containing beverages: coffee, tea, cola. May be taken with milk.

▷ *Alcohol:* Use with extreme caution until the combined effect is determined. Alcohol may increase the depressant effects of this drug on the brain. It is advisable to avoid alcohol completely—throughout the day and night—if it is necessary to drive or to engage in any hazardous activity.

Tobacco Smoking: Heavy smoking may reduce the calming action of this drug.

Marijuana Smoking: Increased sedation and significant impairment of intellectual and physical performance.

▷ *Other Drugs*

Oxazepam may *increase* the effects of

• digoxin (Lanoxin), and cause digoxin toxicity.

• phenytoin (Dilantin), and cause phenytoin toxicity.

Oxazepam may *decrease* the effects of

• levodopa (Sinemet, etc.), and reduce its effectiveness in treating Parkinson's disease.

The following drugs may *decrease* the effects of oxazepam

• oral contraceptives.

• theophylline (Aminophylline, Theo-Dur, etc.).

▷ *Driving, Hazardous Activities:* This drug can impair mental alertness, judgment, physical coordination and reaction time. Avoid hazardous activities accordingly.

Aviation Note: The use of this drug *is a disqualification* for piloting. Consult a designated Aviation Medical Examiner.

Exposure to Sun: No restrictions.

Exposure to Heat: Use caution until the effect of excessive perspiration is determined. Because of reduced urine volume, this drug may accumulate in the body and produce effects of overdosage.

Discontinuation: Avoid sudden discontinuation if this drug has been taken for over 4 weeks without interruption. Dosage should be tapered gradually to prevent a withdrawal syndrome that could include depression, confusion, hallucinations, tremor, seizures, muscle cramping, sweating and vomiting.

OXYCODONE
(ox ee KOH dohn)

Introduced: 1950

Prescription: USA: Yes
Canada: Yes

Available as Generic: USA: Yes
Canada: No

Class: Analgesic, narcotic

Controlled Drug: USA: C-II*
Canada: <N>

Brand Names: ✦Oxycocet [CD], ✦Oxycodan [CD], Percocet [CD], ✦Percocet-Demi [CD], Percodan [CD], Percodan-Demi [CD], Roxicodone, Roxiprin [CD], ✦Supeudol, Tylox [CD]

BENEFITS versus RISKS

Possible Benefits	*Possible Risks*
EFFECTIVE RELIEF OF MODERATE TO SEVERE PAIN	POTENTIAL FOR HABIT FORMATION (DEPENDENCE)
	Sedative effects
	Mild allergic reactions (infrequent)
	Nausea, constipation

▷ **Principal Uses**

As a Single Drug Product: Used primarily in tablet and suppository form (Canada) to relieve moderate to severe pain.

As a Combination Drug Product [CD]: Oxycodone is available in combinations with acetaminophen and with aspirin. These milder pain relievers are added to enhance the analgesic effect and to reduce fever when present.

How This Drug Works: Acting primarily as a depressant of certain brain functions, this drug suppresses the perception of pain and calms the emotional response to pain.

Available Dosage Forms and Strengths

Solution — 5 mg per 5-ml teaspoonful
Suppositories — 10 mg, 20 mg (Canada)
Tablets — 5 mg, 10 mg (Canada)
Tablets — 2.44 mg, 4.88 mg (in combination drugs)

▷ **Usual Adult Dosage Range:** 5 mg/3 to 6 hours as needed. May be increased to 10 mg/4 hours if needed for severe pain. The total daily dosage should not exceed 60 mg. **Note: Actual dosage and administration**

---

*See Schedules of Controlled Drugs inside back cover.

schedule must be determined by the physician for each patient individually.

▷ **Dosing Instructions:**   May be taken with or following food to reduce stomach irritation or nausea. The tablet may be crushed for administration.

Usual Duration of Use: As required to control pain. Continual use should
not exceed 5 to 7 days without interruption and reassessment of need.

▷ **This Drug Should Not Be Taken If**
• you have had an allergic reaction to any dosage form of it previously.
• you are having an acute attack of asthma.

▷ **Inform Your Physician Before Taking This Drug If**
• you have had an unfavorable reaction to any narcotic drug in the past.
• you have a history of drug abuse or alcoholism.
• you have chronic lung disease with impaired breathing.
• you have impaired liver or kidney function.
• you have gallbladder disease, a seizure disorder or an underactive
thyroid gland.
• you have difficulty emptying the urinary bladder.
• you are taking any other drugs that have a sedative effect.
• you plan to have surgery under general anesthesia in the near future.

Possible Side-Effects (natural, expected and unavoidable drug actions)
Drowsiness, light-headedness, dry mouth, urinary retention, constipation.

▷ **Possible Adverse Effects** (unusual, unexpected and infrequent reactions)
**If any of the following develop, consult your physician promptly for
guidance.**
Mild Adverse Effects
Allergic Reactions: Skin rash, hives, itching.
Idiosyncratic Reactions: Skin rash and itching when combined with
dairy products (milk or cheese).
Dizziness, impaired concentration, sensation of drunkenness, confusion,
depression, blurred or double vision.
Nausea, vomiting.
Serious Adverse Effects
Impaired breathing: use with caution in chronic lung disease.

▷ **Possible Effects on Sexual Function:**   None reported.

Possible Effects on Laboratory Tests
Urine screening tests for drug abuse: *initial* test result may be falsely
positive; *confirmatory* test result will be **negative**. (Test results depend
upon amount of drug taken and testing method used.)

CAUTION
1. If you have asthma, chronic bronchitis or emphysema, the excessive

use of this drug may cause significant respiratory difficulty, thickening of bronchial secretions and suppression of coughing.
2. The concurrent use of this drug with atropinelike drugs can increase the risk of urinary retention and reduced intestinal function.
3. Do not take this drug following acute head injury.

Precautions for Use

By Infants and Children: Do not use this drug in children under 2 years of age because of their vulnerability to life-threatening respiratory depression.

By Those over 60 Years of Age: Use small doses initially and increase dosage as needed and tolerated. Limit use to short-term treatment only. There may be increased susceptibility to the development of drowsiness, dizziness, unsteadiness, falling, urinary retention and constipation (often leading to fecal impaction).

▷ **Advisability of Use During Pregnancy**

Pregnancy Category: C (tentative). See Pregnancy Code inside back cover.
Animal studies: No information available.
Human studies: Information from adequate studies of pregnant women is not available. Oxycodone taken repeatedly during the last few weeks before delivery may cause withdrawal symptoms in the newborn infant.
Use this drug only if clearly needed and in small, infrequent doses.

Advisability of Use if Breast-Feeding

Presence of this drug in breast milk: Unknown.
Avoid drug or refrain from nursing.

Habit-Forming Potential: Psychological and/or physical dependence can develop with use of large doses for an extended period of time.

Effects of Overdosage: Drowsiness, restlessness, agitation, nausea, vomiting, dry mouth, vertigo, weakness, lethargy, stupor, coma, seizures.

Possible Effects of Long-Term Use: Psychological and physical dependence, chronic constipation.

Suggested Periodic Examinations While Taking This Drug (at physician's discretion)
None.

▷ **While Taking This Drug, Observe the Following**

Foods: No restrictions.
Beverages: No restrictions. May be taken with milk.
▷ *Alcohol:* Use extreme caution until the combined effects have been determined. Oxycodone can intensify the intoxicating effects of alcohol, and alcohol can intensify the depressant effects of oxycodone on brain function, breathing and circulation.
Tobacco Smoking: No interactions expected.

Marijuana Smoking: Increase in drowsiness and pain relief; impairment of mental and physical performance.

▷ *Other Drugs*

Oxycodone may *increase* the effects of
- other drugs with sedative effects.
- atropinelike drugs, and increase the risk of constipation and urinary retention.

▷ *Driving, Hazardous Activities:* This drug can impair mental alertness, judgment, reaction time and physical coordination. Avoid hazardous activities accordingly.

Aviation Note: The use of this drug *is a disqualification* for piloting. Consult a designated Aviation Medical Examiner.

Exposure to Sun: No restrictions.

Discontinuation: It is advisable to limit this drug to short-term use. If it is necessary to use it for extended periods of time, discontinuation should be gradual to minimize possible effects of withdrawal.

PENBUTOLOL
(pen BYU toh lohl)

Introduced: 1976

Class: Antihypertensive, beta-adrenergic blocker

Prescription: USA: Yes

Controlled Drug: USA: No

Available as Generic: No

Brand Name: Levatol

BENEFITS versus RISKS

Possible Benefits	*Possible Risks*
EFFECTIVE, WELL-TOLERATED ANTIHYPERTENSIVE in mild to moderate high blood pressure	CONGESTIVE HEART FAILURE in advanced heart disease Worsening of angina in coronary heart disease (abrupt withdrawal) Masking of low blood sugar (hypoglycemia) in drug-treated diabetes Provocation of asthma

---

▷ **Principal Uses**

As a Single Drug Product: The treatment of mild to moderately severe high blood pressure. May be used alone or concurrently with other antihypertensive drugs, such as diuretics.

How This Drug Works: By blocking certain actions of the sympathetic nervous system, this drug
- reduces the rate and contraction force of the heart, thus lowering the ejection pressure of the blood leaving the heart.
- reduces the degree of contraction of blood vessel walls, resulting in their relaxation and expansion and consequent lowering of blood pressure.

Available Dosage Forms and Strengths
Tablets — 20 mg

▷ **Usual Adult Dosage Range:**   Initially 20 mg once daily. The dose may be increased gradually by 10 mg/day at intervals of 2 weeks as needed and tolerated up to 80 mg/day. For maintenance, 20 to 40 mg once daily is usually adequate. The total daily dose should not exceed 80 mg. **Note: Actual dosage and administration schedule must be determined by the physician for each patient individually.**

▷ **Dosing Instructions:**   May be taken without regard to eating. The tablet may be crushed for administration. Do not discontinue this drug abruptly.

Usual Duration of Use: Continual use on a regular schedule for 2 to 3 weeks is usually necessary to determine this drug's effectiveness in lowering blood pressure. The long-term use of this drug (months to years) will be determined by the course of your blood pressure over time and your response to the overall treatment program (weight reduction, salt restriction, smoking cessation, etc.). Consult your physician on a regular basis.

Possible Advantages of This Drug
Adequate control of blood pressure with a single daily dose.
Causes less slowing of the heart rate than most other beta blocker drugs.

Currently a "Drug of Choice"
for initiating treatment of hypertension with a single drug.

▷ **This Drug Should Not Be Taken If**
- you have had an allergic reaction to it previously.
- you have congestive heart failure.
- you have an abnormally slow heart rate or a serious form of heart block.
- you are subject to bronchial asthma.

▷ **Inform Your Physician Before Taking This Drug If**
- you have had an adverse reaction to any beta blocker drug in the past (see Drug Class, Section Four).
- you have a history of serious heart disease, with or without episodes of heart failure.
- you have a history of hay fever (allergic rhinitis), asthma, chronic bronchitis or emphysema.

- you have a history of overactive thyroid function (hyperthyroidism).
- you have a history of low blood sugar (hypoglycemia).
- you have impaired liver or kidney function.
- you have diabetes or myasthenia gravis.
- you have impaired circulation in the extremities (Raynaud's disorder, claudication pains in legs).
- you are currently taking any form of digitalis, quinidine or reserpine, or any calcium blocker drug (see Drug Class, Section Four).
- you plan to have surgery under general anesthesia in the near future.

Possible Side-Effects (natural, expected and unavoidable drug actions)
Lethargy and fatigability, cold extremities, slow heart rate, light-headedness in upright position (see Orthostatic Hypotension in Glossary).

▷ **Possible Adverse Effects** (unusual, unexpected and infrequent reactions)
If any of the following develop, consult your physician promptly for guidance.
Mild Adverse Effects
Allergic Reactions: Skin rash, itching, reversible hair loss.
Headache, dizziness, blurred vision, insomnia, abnormal dreams.
Indigestion, nausea, vomiting, constipation, diarrhea.
Joint and muscle discomfort.
Serious Adverse Effects
Allergic Reactions: Anaphylactoid reaction (see Glossary).
Mental depression, anxiety, disorientation, short-term memory loss, hallucinations.
Chest pain, shortness of breath, precipitation of congestive heart failure.
Induction of bronchial asthma (in asthmatic individuals).
Aggravation of myasthenia gravis.
Abnormally low white blood cell and platelet counts: fever, sore throat, abnormal bleeding or bruising.

▷ **Possible Effects on Sexual Function:**   Decreased libido and impotence, rare but more common with higher doses; Peyronie's disease (see Glossary).

▷ **Adverse Effects That May Mimic Natural Diseases or Disorders**
Reduced blood flow to extremities may resemble Raynaud's phenomenon (see Glossary).

Natural Diseases or Disorders That May Be Activated by This Drug
Raynaud's disease, intermittent claudication, myasthenia gravis.

Possible Effects on Laboratory Tests
White blood cell and platelet counts: decreased.

CAUTION
1. *Do not discontinue this drug suddenly* without the knowledge and guidance of your physician. Carry a notation on your person that you are taking this drug.
2. Consult your physician or pharmacist before using nasal deconges-

tants usually present in over-the-counter cold preparations and nose drops. These can cause sudden increases in blood pressure when taken concurrently with beta blocker drugs.
3. Report the development of any tendency to emotional depression.

Precautions for Use
By Infants and Children: Safety and effectiveness for use by those under 12 years of age have not been established. However, if this drug is used, observe for the development of low blood sugar (hypoglycemia) during periods of reduced food intake.
By Those over 60 Years of Age: Proceed *cautiously* with all antihypertensive drugs. Unacceptably high blood pressure should be reduced without creating the risks associated with excessively low blood pressure. Start treatment with small doses, and monitor the blood pressure response frequently. Sudden, rapid and excessive reduction of blood pressure can predispose to stroke or heart attack. Observe for dizziness, unsteadiness, tendency to fall, confusion, hallucinations, depression or urinary frequency.

▷ **Advisability of Use During Pregnancy**
Pregnancy Category: C (tentative). See Pregnancy Code inside back cover.
  Animal studies: No birth defects due to this drug found in rat or rabbit studies.
  Human studies: Information from adequate studies of pregnant women is not available.
  Use this drug only if clearly needed. Ask physician for guidance.

Advisability of Use if Breast-Feeding
Presence of this drug in breast milk: Unknown.
Avoid drug or refrain from nursing.

Habit-Forming Potential: None.

Effects of Overdosage: Weakness, slow pulse, low blood pressure, fainting, cold and sweaty skin, congestive heart failure, possible coma and convulsions.

Possible Effects of Long-Term Use: Reduced heart reserve and eventual heart failure in susceptible individuals with advanced heart disease.

Suggested Periodic Examinations While Taking This Drug (at physician's discretion)
Measurements of blood pressure, evaluation of heart function.
Complete blood cell counts.

▷ **While Taking This Drug, Observe the Following**
Foods: No restrictions. Avoid excessive salt intake.
Beverages: No restrictions. May be taken with milk.
▷ *Alcohol:* Use with caution until the combined effect has been determined. Alcohol may exaggerate this drug's ability to lower the blood pressure and may increase its mild sedative effect.

Tobacco Smoking: Nicotine may reduce this drug's effectiveness in treating high blood pressure. In addition, high doses of this drug may potentiate the constriction of the bronchial tubes caused by regular smoking.

▷ *Other Drugs*

Penbutolol may *increase* the effects of

- other antihypertensive drugs, and cause excessive lowering of the blood pressure. Dosage adjustments may be necessary.
- reserpine (Ser-Ap-Es, etc.), and cause sedation, depression, slowing of the heart rate and lowering of the blood pressure. This combination is best avoided.
- verapamil (Calan, Isoptin), and cause excessive depression of heart function; monitor this combination closely.

Penbutolol *taken concurrently* with

- clonidine (Catapres) requires close monitoring for rebound high blood pressure if clonidine is withdrawn while penbutolol is still being taken.
- insulin requires close monitoring to avoid undetected hypoglycemia (see Glossary).

The following drugs may *increase* the effects of penbutolol

- methimazole (Tapazole).
- oral contraceptives.
- propylthiouracil (Propacil).

The following drugs may *decrease* the effects of penbutolol

- barbiturates (phenobarbital, etc.).
- indomethacin (Indocin), and possibly other "aspirin substitutes," may impair penbutolol's antihypertensive effect.
- rifampin (Rifadin, Rimactane).

▷ *Driving, Hazardous Activities:* Use caution until the full extent of fatigue, dizziness and blood pressure change have been determined.

Aviation Note: The use of this drug *is a disqualification* for piloting. Consult a designated Aviation Medical Examiner.

Exposure to Sun: No restrictions.

Exposure to Heat: Caution advised. Hot environments can lower the blood pressure and exaggerate the effects of this drug.

Exposure to Cold: Caution advised. Cold environments can enhance the circulatory deficiency in the extremities that may occur with this drug. The elderly should take precautions to prevent hypothermia (see Glossary).

Heavy Exercise or Exertion: It is advisable to avoid exertion that produces light-headedness, excessive fatigue or muscle cramping. The use of this drug may intensify the hypertensive response to isometric exercise.

Occurrence of Unrelated Illness: The fever that accompanies systemic infections can lower the blood pressure and require adjustment of dosage. Illnesses that cause nausea or vomiting may interrupt the regular dosage schedule. Ask your physician for guidance.

Discontinuation: It is advisable to avoid sudden discontinuation of this drug in all situations. If possible, gradual reduction of dose over a period of 2 to 3 weeks is recommended. Ask your physician for specific guidance.

PENICILLIN V
(pen i SIL in VEE)

Introduced: 1953

Class: Antibiotic, penicillins

Prescription: USA: Yes
Canada: Yes

Controlled Drug: USA: No
Canada: No

Available as Generic: USA: Yes
Canada: Yes

Brand Names: ✦Apo-Penicillin VK, Beepen VK, Betapen-VK, Ledercillin VK, ✦Nadopen-V, ✦Novopen-VK, Penapar VK, ✦Pen-Vee, Pen-Vee K, ✦PVF, ✦PVF K, Robicillin VK, Uticillin VK, V-Cillin K, ✦VC-K 500, Veetids

---

BENEFITS versus RISKS

Possible Benefits	*Possible Risks*
EFFECTIVE TREATMENT OF INFECTIONS due to susceptible microorganisms	ALLERGIC REACTIONS, mild to severe, in 3% of the general population and 15% of allergic individuals Superinfections (yeast) Drug-induced colitis

---

▷ **Principal Uses**

As a Single Drug Product: This type of penicillin is used primarily to treat responsive infections of the upper and lower respiratory tract, the middle ear and the skin. Equally important uses are the prevention of rheumatic fever and the prevention of bacterial endocarditis in individuals with valvular heart disease.

How This Drug Works: This drug destroys susceptible infecting bacteria by interfering with their ability to produce new protective cell walls as they multiply and grow.

Available Dosage Forms and Strengths
Oral solution — 125 mg, 250 mg per 5-ml teaspoonful
Tablets — 125 mg, 250 mg, 500 mg

▷ **Usual Adult Dosage Range:** Dosage is based upon the results of sensitivity testing of the causative organism, the severity of the infection and the response of the patient. Depending upon the specific infection, the dosage range is 125 to 500 mg/6 to 8 hours. For the prevention of bacterial endocarditis: 2 grams (2000 mg) taken 1 hour before the procedure, followed by 1 gram 6 hours later. The total daily dosage should not exceed 7 grams (7000 mg). **Note: Actual dosage and administration schedule must be determined by the physician for each patient individually.**

▷ **Dosing Instructions:**   May be taken on an empty stomach or with food or milk. Absorption may be slightly faster if taken when stomach is empty. The tablet may be crushed for administration.

Usual Duration of Use: For all streptococcal infections—not less than 10 consecutive days (without interruption) to reduce the possibility of developing rheumatic fever or glomerulonephritis. For all other infections—as long as necessary to eradicate the infection.

▷ **This Drug Should Not Be Taken If**
  • you have had an allergic reaction to any dosage form of it previously.
  • you are certain you are allergic to *any* form of penicillin.

▷ **Inform Your Physician Before Taking This Drug If**
  • you suspect you may be allergic to penicillin or you have a history of a previous "reaction" of any type to penicillin.
  • you are allergic to any cephalosporin antibiotic (Ancef, Anspor, Ceclor, Ceporan, Ceporex, Kafocin, Keflex, Keflin, Kefzol, Loridine, Ultracef, Velosef; see Drug Class, Section Four).
  • you are allergic by nature (hay fever, asthma, hives, eczema).

Possible Side-Effects (natural, expected and unavoidable drug actions)
  Superinfections (see Glossary), often due to yeast organisms.

▷ **Possible Adverse Effects** (unusual, unexpected and infrequent reactions)
  If any of the following develop, consult your physician promptly for guidance.
  Mild Adverse Effects
  Allergic Reactions: Skin rashes, hives, itching.
  Irritations of mouth and tongue, "black tongue," nausea, vomiting, mild diarrhea, dizziness (rare).
  Serious Adverse Effects
  Allergic Reactions: Anaphylactic reaction (see Glossary), severe skin reactions, drug fever, swollen painful joints, sore throat, abnormal bleeding or bruising.
  Drug-induced colitis.

▷ **Possible Effects on Sexual Function:**   None reported.

Possible Effects on Laboratory Tests
  Complete blood cell counts: decreased red cells, hemoglobin, white cells and platelets; increased eosinophils (allergic reaction).
  Prothrombin time: occasionally increased.
  Liver function tests: increased aspartate aminotransferase (AST/GOT) and bilirubin.

CAUTION
  1. Take the exact dose and the full course prescribed.
  2. This drug should not be used concurrently with antibiotics like erythromycin or tetracycline.

Precautions for Use

By Infants and Children: Observe the allergic child closely for evidence of a developing allergy to penicillin. This drug may cause diarrhea, which sometimes necessitates discontinuation.

By Those over 60 Years of Age: Natural changes in the skin may predispose to prolonged itching reactions in the genital and anal regions. Report such reactions promptly.

▷ **Advisability of Use During Pregnancy**

Pregnancy Category: B (tentative). See Pregnancy Code inside back cover.

Animal studies: Birth defects of the limbs reported in mice. (Not confirmed in other studies.)

Human studies: Information from adequate studies of pregnant women indicates no increased risk of birth defects in 3546 pregnancies exposed to penicillin derivatives.

This drug is considered safe for use during any period of pregnancy.

Advisability of Use if Breast-Feeding

Presence of this drug in breast milk: Yes.

The nursing infant may be sensitized to penicillin and be at risk for developing diarrhea or yeast infections.

Avoid drug if possible or refrain from nursing.

Habit-Forming Potential: None.

Effects of Overdosage: Possible nausea, vomiting and/or diarrhea.

Possible Effects of Long-Term Use: Superinfections, often due to yeast organisms.

Suggested Periodic Examinations While Taking This Drug (at physician's discretion)

Complete blood cell counts, kidney function tests.

▷ **While Taking This Drug, Observe the Following**

Foods: No restrictions.

Beverages: No restrictions. May be taken with milk.

▷ *Alcohol:* No interactions expected.

Tobacco Smoking: No interactions expected.

▷ *Other Drugs*

Penicillin V may *decrease* the effects of

• oral contraceptives in some women, and impair their effectiveness in preventing pregnancy.

The following drugs may *decrease* the effects of penicillin V

• antacids may reduce the absorption of penicillin V.
• chloramphenicol (Chloromycetin).
• erythromycin (Erythrocin, E-Mycin, etc.).
• tetracyclines (Achromycin, Declomycin, Minocin, etc.). (See Drug Class, Section Four.)

▷ *Driving, Hazardous Activities:* Usually no restrictions. Be alert to the rare occurrence of dizziness and/or nausea, and restrict activities accordingly.

Aviation Note: The use of this drug *may be a disqualification* for piloting. Consult a designated Aviation Medical Examiner.

Exposure to Sun: No restrictions.

Special Storage Instructions: Oral solutions should be refrigerated.

Observe the Following Expiration Times: Do not take the oral solution of this drug if older than 7 days when kept at room temperature or 14 days when kept refrigerated.

PENTAZOCINE
(pen TAZ oh seen)

Introduced: 1967

Prescription: USA: Yes
Canada: Yes

Available as Generic: USA: No
Canada: No

Class: Analgesic, narcotic

Controlled Drug: USA: C-IV*
Canada: < N >

Brand Names: Talacen [CD], Talwin, Talwin Compound [CD], ✦Talwin Compound-50 [CD], Talwin Nx [CD]

BENEFITS versus RISKS

Possible Benefits	*Possible Risks*
EFFECTIVE RELIEF OF MODERATE TO SEVERE PAIN	POTENTIAL FOR HABIT FORMATION (DEPENDENCE)
	Sedative effects
	Mental and behavioral disturbances
	Low blood pressure, fainting
	Nausea, constipation

▷ **Principal Uses**

As a Single Drug Product: Used exclusively to relieve acute or chronic pain of moderate to severe degree from any cause.

As a Combination Drug Product [CD]: Pentazocine is available in combinations with acetaminophen and with aspirin. These milder pain relievers are added to enhance the analgesic effect and to reduce fever when present. In the USA the tablet form of pentazocine also contains naloxone (Talwin Nx), a narcotic antagonist that renders the drug ineffective if abused.

*See Schedules of Controlled Drugs inside back cover.

How This Drug Works: Acting primarily as a depressant of certain brain functions, this drug suppresses the perception of pain and calms the emotional response to pain.

Available Dosage Forms and Strengths
   Injection — 30 mg per ml
   Tablets — 50 mg (Canada)
   Tablets — 50 mg with 0.5 mg of naloxone (USA)

▷ **Usual Adult Dosage Range:**   50 mg/3 to 4 hours as needed. May be increased to 100 mg/4 hours if needed for severe pain. The total daily dosage should not exceed 600 mg. **Note: Actual dosage and administration schedule must be determined by the physician for each patient individually.**

▷ **Dosing Instructions:**   May be taken with or following food to reduce stomach irritation or nausea. The tablet may be crushed for administration.

Usual Duration of Use: As required to control pain. Continual use should not exceed 5 to 7 days without interruption and reassessment of need.

▷ **This Drug Should Not Be Taken If**
   • you have had an allergic reaction to any dosage form of it previously.
   • you are having an acute attack of asthma.

▷ **Inform Your Physician Before Taking This Drug If**
   • you have had an unfavorable reaction to any narcotic drug in the past.
   • you have a history of drug abuse or alcoholism.
   • you have chronic lung disease with impaired breathing.
   • you have impaired liver or kidney function.
   • you have gallbladder disease, a seizure disorder or an underactive thyroid gland.
   • you have difficulty emptying the urinary bladder.
   • you are taking any other drugs that have a sedative effect.
   • you plan to have surgery under general anesthesia in the near future.

Possible Side-Effects (natural, expected and unavoidable drug actions)
   Drowsiness, light-headedness, weakness, urinary retention, constipation.

▷ **Possible Adverse Effects** (unusual, unexpected and infrequent reactions)
   If any of the following develop, consult your physician promptly for guidance.
   Mild Adverse Effects
   Allergic Reactions: Skin rash, hives, itching, swelling of face.
   Headache, dizziness, impaired concentration, sensation of drunkenness, blurred or double vision, flushing, sweating.
   Nausea, vomiting, indigestion, diarrhea.
   Serious Adverse Effects
   Marked drop in blood pressure, possible fainting.

Impaired breathing: use with caution in chronic lung disease.
Mental and behavioral disturbances, hallucinations, tremor.
Bone marrow depression (see Glossary) of a mild and reversible nature
(rare).
Aggravation of prostatism (see Glossary).

▷ **Possible Effects on Sexual Function:**   None reported.

Natural Diseases or Disorders That May Be Activated by This Drug
Porphyria (see Glossary).

Possible Effects on Laboratory Tests
White blood cell count: rarely decreased.
Blood amylase and lipase levels: increased (natural side-effects).

CAUTION
  1. The use of this drug with atropinelike drugs may increase the risk of
     urinary retention and reduced intestinal function.
  2. Do not take this drug following acute head injury.

Precautions for Use
By Infants and Children: Safety and effectiveness for use by those under 12
  years of age have not been established.
By Those over 60 Years of Age: Use small doses initially and increase dosage
  as needed and tolerated. Limit use to short-term treatment only. There
  may be increased susceptibility to the development of drowsiness, dizziness, unsteadiness, falling, urinary retention and constipation.

▷ **Advisability of Use During Pregnancy**
Pregnancy Category: C (tentative). See Pregnancy Code inside back cover.
  Animal studies: Significant birth defects reported in hamsters.
  Human studies: Information from adequate studies of pregnant women
    is not available. Pentazocine taken repeatedly during the last few weeks
    before delivery may cause withdrawal symptoms in the newborn in-
    fant.
  Avoid this drug during the first 3 months. Use only if clearly needed and
    in small, infrequent doses during the last 6 months.

Advisability of Use if Breast-Feeding
Presence of this drug in breast milk: Unknown.
Avoid drug or refrain from nursing.

Habit-Forming Potential: Psychological and/or physical dependence can
  develop with use of large doses for an extended period of time.

Effects of Overdosage: Anxiety, disturbed thoughts, hallucinations, progressive drowsiness, stupor, depressed breathing.

Possible Effects of Long-Term Use: Psychological and physical dependence, chronic constipation.

Suggested Periodic Examinations While Taking This Drug (at physician's discretion)

Complete blood cell counts, if used for an extended period of time.

▷ **While Taking This Drug, Observe the Following**

Foods: No restrictions.

Beverages: No restrictions. May be taken with milk.

▷ *Alcohol:* Use extreme caution until the combined effects have been determined. Pentazocine can intensify the intoxicating effects of alcohol, and alcohol can intensify the depressant effects of pentazocine on brain function, breathing and circulation.

Tobacco Smoking: Heavy smoking may reduce the effectiveness of pentazocine and make larger doses necessary.

Marijuana Smoking: Increase in drowsiness and pain relief; impairment of mental and physical performance.

▷ *Other Drugs*

Pentazocine may *increase* the effects of
- other drugs with sedative effects.
- atropinelike drugs, and increase the risk of constipation and urinary retention.

▷ *Driving, Hazardous Activities:* This drug can impair mental alertness, judgment, reaction time and physical coordination. Avoid hazardous activities accordingly.

Aviation Note: The use of this drug *is a disqualification* for piloting. Consult a designated Aviation Medical Examiner.

Exposure to Sun: No restrictions.

Discontinuation: It is advisable to limit this drug to short-term use. If it is necessary to use it for extended periods of time, discontinuation should be gradual to minimize possible effects of withdrawal.

PENTOXIFYLLINE
(pen tox I fi leen)

Other Name: Oxpentifylline

Introduced: 1972   **Class:** Blood flow agent, xanthines

Prescription: USA: Yes   **Controlled Drug:** USA: No
  Canada: Yes   Canada: No

Available as Generic: No

Brand Name: Trental

```
┌─────────────────────────────────────────────────────────────┐
│                   BENEFITS versus RISKS                       │
│                                                               │
│      Possible Benefits              Possible Risks            │
│   IMPROVED BLOOD FLOW IN        Reduced blood pressure, angina,│
│     PERIPHERAL ARTERIAL           abnormal heart rhythms (in  │
│     DISEASE                       susceptible individuals)    │
│   REDUCTION OF INTERMITTENT     Indigestion, nausea, vomiting │
│     CLAUDICATION PAIN           Dizziness, flushing           │
└─────────────────────────────────────────────────────────────┘
```

▷ **Principal Uses**

As a Single Drug Product: Used primarily (as adjunctive treatment) in the management of peripheral obstructive arterial disease to improve arterial blood flow and reduce the frequency and severity of muscle pain due to intermittent claudication.

How This Drug Works: This drug is thought to improve blood flow through the microcirculation and to increase the oxygen supply to working muscles by way of three mechanisms: (1) reduction of blood viscosity due to decreased levels of fibrinogen in the blood; (2) increased flexibility of the red blood cells (carrying oxygen) due to an increase in cyclic AMP (enzyme) within red blood cells; this permits easier passage through the minute blood vessels of the microcirculation; and (3) prevention of red blood cell and platelet aggregation.

Available Dosage Forms and Strengths

Tablets, prolonged-action — 400 mg

▷ **Usual Adult Dosage Range:** 400 mg 3 times/day. If adverse nervous system or gastrointestinal effects occur, reduce the dose to 400 mg twice/day. **Note: Actual dosage and administration schedule must be determined by the physician for each patient individually.**

▷ **Dosing Instructions:** Take with or following food to reduce stomach irritation. Swallow the tablet whole without breaking, crushing or chewing.

Usual Duration of Use: Continual use on a regular schedule for 2 to 4 weeks is usually necessary to determine this drug's effectiveness in preventing or delaying the pains of intermittent claudication associated with walking. Treatment for a minimum of 3 months is recommended to determine full effectiveness. Long-term use (months to years) requires supervision and periodic evaluation by your physician. Consult your physician on a regular basis.

Possible Advantages of This Drug

Reduces blood viscosity and thereby improves blood flow through small vessels.

Increases supply of oxygen to working muscles.

Currently a "Drug of Choice"
for treating peripheral arterial disease and reducing the frequency and severity of intermittent claudication pain.

▷ **This Drug Should Not Be Taken If**
• you have had an allergic reaction to it previously.

▷ **Inform Your Physician Before Taking This Drug If**
• you are allergic to other xanthine drugs: caffeine, theophylline, theobromine.
• you have impaired kidney function.
• you have low blood pressure, impaired brain circulation or coronary artery disease.
• you smoke tobacco.
• you are taking any antihypertensive drugs.

Possible Side-Effects (natural, expected and unavoidable drug actions)
Usually none with recommended doses.

▷ **Possible Adverse Effects** (unusual, unexpected and infrequent reactions)
If any of the following develop, consult your physician promptly for guidance.
Mild Adverse Effects
Allergic Reaction: Skin rash.
Headache (1.2%), dizziness (1.9%), tremor.
Indigestion (2.8%), nausea (2.2%), vomiting (1.2%).
Serious Adverse Effects
Development of angina or heart rhythm disorders in the presence of coronary artery disease.

▷ **Possible Effects on Sexual Function**
None reported.

Possible Effects on Laboratory Tests
Complete blood cell counts: rarely decreased red cells, hemoglobin, white cells and platelets.

CAUTION
Use this drug with caution in the presence of impaired circulation within the brain (cerebral arteriosclerosis) or coronary artery disease. If any related symptoms develop, consult your physician for prompt evaluation.

Precautions for Use
By Infants and Children: Safety and effectiveness for use by those under 18 years of age have not been established. Use by this age group is not anticipated.
By Those over 60 Years of Age: You may be more susceptible to the adverse effects listed. Observe closely for any indications of dizziness or chest pain and report these promptly.

▷ **Advisability of Use During Pregnancy**
  Pregnancy Category: C (tentative). See Pregnancy Code inside back cover.
    Animal studies: Increased fetal resorptions reported in rats, but no birth
    defects found in rats or rabbits.
    Human studies: Information from adequate studies of pregnant women
    is not available.
    Avoid use during the first 3 months. Use otherwise only if clearly needed.

Advisability of Use if Breast-Feeding
  Presence of this drug in breast milk: Yes.
  Avoid drug or refrain from nursing.

Habit-Forming Potential: None.

Effects of Overdosage: Drowsiness, flushing, faintness, excitement, seizures.

Possible Effects of Long-Term Use: None reported.

Suggested Periodic Examinations While Taking This Drug (at physician's
  discretion)
  Blood pressure measurements, evaluation of heart status.

▷ **While Taking This Drug, Observe the Following**
  Foods: No restrictions.
  Beverages: No restrictions. May be taken with milk.
▷ *Alcohol:* Use caution until the combined effects have been determined.
    Alcohol may increase the blood-pressure-lowering effect of this drug.
  Tobacco Smoking: Nicotine constricts arteries and will impair the effec-
    tiveness of this drug significantly. Avoid all use of tobacco.
▷ *Other Drugs*
    Pentoxifylline may *increase* the effects of
    • antihypertensive drugs, and cause excessive lowering of blood pres-
      sure.
    • warfarin (Coumadin, etc.), and increase the possibility of unwanted
      bleeding; monitor prothrombin times as appropriate.
▷ *Driving, Hazardous Activities:* This drug may cause drowsiness or dizziness.
    Restrict activities as necessary.
  Aviation Note: The use of this drug *may be a disqualification* for piloting.
    Consult a designated Aviation Medical Examiner.
  Exposure to Sun: No restrictions.

PERGOLIDE
(PER go lide)

Introduced: 1980

Class: Antiparkinsonism, dopamine agonist, ergot derivative

Prescription: USA: Yes

Controlled Drug: USA: No

Available as Generic: USA: No

Brand Name: Permax

BENEFITS versus RISKS

Possible Benefits	*Possible Risks*
ADDITIVE RELIEF OF SYMPTOMS OF PARKINSON'S DISEASE when used concurrently with levodopa/carbidopa (Sinemet) PERMITS A 5% TO 30% REDUCTION IN SINEMET DOSAGE	ABNORMAL INVOLUNTARY MOVEMENTS (62%) HALLUCINATIONS (14%) INITIAL FALL IN BLOOD PRESSURE/ORTHOSTATIC HYPOTENSION (10%)

▷ **Principal Uses**

As a Single Drug Product: Used solely as an adjunct to levodopa/carbidopa treatment of Parkinson's disease for those individuals who experience intolerable abnormal movements (dyskinesia) and/or increasing "on-off" episodes due to levodopa. The addition of pergolide (1) permits reduction of the daily dose of levodopa with consequent lessening of dyskinesia and erratic drug response, and (2) provides additional relief of parkinsonian symptoms.

How This Drug Works: By directly stimulating the dopamine receptor sites in the corpus striatum of the brain, this drug helps to compensate for the deficiency of dopamine that is responsible for the rigidity, tremor and sluggish movement characteristic of Parkinson's disease.

Available Dosage Forms and Strengths

Tablets — 0.05 mg, 0.25 mg, 1 mg

▷ **Usual Adult Dosage Range**

Initially 0.05 mg daily for the first 2 days; gradually increase the daily dose by 0.1 mg or 0.15 mg every third day over the next 12 days. If needed and tolerated, the daily dose may be increased further by 0.25 mg every third day until an optimal respose is achieved. The total daily dosage should be divided into 3 equal portions and given at 6 to 8 hour intervals. The usual maintenance dose is 3 mg/24 hours; do not exceed 5 mg/24 hours.

During the gradual introduction of pergolide, the concurrent dose of levodopa/carbidopa (Sinemet) may be cautiously decreased in accord with your physician's instructions.**Note: Actual dosage and administration schedule must be determined by the physician for each patient individually.**

▷ **Dosing Instructions:** Take with food or milk to reduce stomach irritation. The tablet may be crushed for administration.

Usual Duration of Use: Continual use on a regular schedule for 4 to 6 weeks is usually necessary to determine this drug's effectiveness in controlling the symptoms of Parkinson's disease and permitting reduction of levodopa/carbidopa dosage. Long-term use (months to years) requires periodic evaluation of response and dosage adjustment. Consult your physician on a regular basis.

Possible Advantages of This Drug: It may provide a more effective and uniform control of parkinsonian symptoms and a significant reduction of some adverse effects of long-term levodopa therapy.

▷ **This Drug Should Not Be Taken If**
- you have had an allergic reaction to it previously.
- you have had a serious adverse effect from any ergot preparation in the past.
- you have severe coronary artery disease or peripheral vascular disease.

▷ **Inform Your Physician Before Taking This Drug If**
- you have constitutionally low blood pressure.
- you are pregnant or breast-feeding.
- you are taking any antihypertensive drugs or antipsychotic drugs (see Drug Classes, Section Four).
- you have any degree of coronary artery disease, especially angina or a history of heart attack.
- you have any type of heart rhythm disorder.
- you have impaired liver or kidney function.
- you have a seizure disorder.

Possible Side-Effects (natural, expected and unavoidable drug actions)
Weakness (4.2%), chest pain—possibly anginal (3.7%), peripheral edema (7.4%), orthostatic hypotension (see Glossary) (10%).

▷ **Possible Adverse Effects** (unusual, unexpected and infrequent reactions)
If any of the following develop, consult your physician promptly for guidance.
Mild Adverse Effects
Allergic Reactions: Skin rash (3.2%), facial swelling (1.1%).
Headache (5.3%), dizziness (19%), hallucinations (14%), confusion (11%), drowsiness (10%), insomnia (8%), anxiety (6%), double vision (2%).

Nasal congestion (12%), shortness of breath (5%), palpitation (2%), fainting (2%).

Altered taste (1.6%), loss of appetite (4.8%), dry mouth (3.7%), indigestion (6.4%), nausea (24%), vomiting (2.7%), constipation (10%), diarrhea (6.4%).

Serious Adverse Effects

Allergic Reactions: None reported.

Idiosyncratic Reactions: "Flu-like" symptoms (3%).

Abnormal involuntary movements (dyskinesia) (62%), psychotic behavior (2%).

▷ **Possible Effects on Sexual Function:** Infrequent reports of altered libido (both increased and decreased), impotence, breast pain, priapism (see Glossary).

▷ **Adverse Effects That May Mimic Natural Diseases or Disorders**

Effects on mental function and behavior may resemble psychotic disorders.

▷ **Natural Diseases or Disorders That May Be Activated by This Drug**

Coronary artery disease with anginal syndrome, heart rhythm disorders, Raynaud's syndrome (see Glossary), seizure disorders.

Possible Effects on Laboratory Tests

Blood prolactin level: decreased (marked reduction).

CAUTION

1. This drug can initiate dyskinesias and can intensify existing dyskinesias. Observe carefully for the development of tremors, twitching or abnormal, involuntary movements of any kind. Report these promptly.
2. Begin treatment with low doses to prevent the possibility of excessive drop in blood pressure. See dosage routine outlined above.
3. Inform your physician promptly if you become pregnant or plan pregnancy. This drug has been reported (rarely) to cause abortion and birth defects.

Precautions for Use

By Infants and Children: This drug is not utilized by this age group.

By Those over 60 Years of Age: Small initial doses are mandatory. Observe closely for any tendency to light-headedness or faintness, especially on arising from a lying or sitting position. You may be more susceptible to the development of impaired thinking, confusion, agitation, nightmares or hallucinations.

▷ **Advisability of Use During Pregnancy**

Pregnancy Category: B (tentative). See Pregnancy Code inside back cover.

Animal studies: No birth defects due to this drug were found in mouse or rabbit studies.

Human studies: Information from adequate studies of pregnant women is not available. However, there are four reports of birth defects associated with the use of this drug and infrequent reports of abortion. Causal relationships have not been established, but prudence advises against the use of this drug during pregnancy. Consult your physician for guidance.

Advisability of Use if Breast-Feeding
Presence of this drug in breast milk: Unknown.
Avoid drug or refrain from nursing.

Habit-Forming Potential: None.

Effects of Overdosage: Nausea, vomiting, palpitations, low blood pressure, agitation, severe involuntary movements, hallucinations, seizures.

Possible Effects of Long-Term Use: Increased risk of developing dyskinesias.

Suggested Periodic Examinations While Taking This Drug (at physician's discretion)
Regular evaluation of drug response, heart function and blood pressure status.

▷ **While Taking This Drug, Observe the Following**
Foods: No restrictions.
Beverages: No restrictions. May be taken with milk.
▷   *Alcohol:* Use caution until the combined effects have been determined. Alcohol can exaggerate the blood-pressure-lowering and sedative effects of this drug.
Tobacco Smoking: No interactions expected.
▷   *Other Drugs*
Pergolide *taken concurrently* with
- antihypertensive drugs (and other drugs that can lower blood pressure) requires careful monitoring for excessive drops in pressure. Dosage adjustments may be necessary.
The following drugs may *decrease* the effects of pergolide and diminish its effectiveness
- chlorprothixene (Taractan).
- haloperidol (Haldol).
- metoclopramide (Reglan).
- phenothiazines (see Drug Class, Section Four).
- thiothixene (Navane).
▷   *Driving, Hazardous Activities:* This drug may cause dizziness, drowsiness, impaired coordination or fainting. Restrict activities as necessary.
Aviation Note: The use of this drug *is a disqualification* for piloting. Consult a designated Aviation Medical Examiner.
Exposure to Sun: No restrictions.
Exposure to Heat: Use caution until the combined effects have been determined. Hot environments can cause lowering of blood pressure.
Discontinuation: Do not discontinue this drug abruptly. Sudden withdrawal can cause confusion, paranoid thinking and severe hallucinations. Consult your physician regarding a schedule for gradual withdrawal.

PERPHENAZINE
(per FEN a zeen)

Introduced: 1957

Class: Strong tranquilizer, phenothiazines

Prescription: USA: Yes
Canada: Yes

Controlled Drug: USA: No
Canada: No

Available as Generic: USA: No
Canada: Yes

Brand Names: ✦Apo-Perphenazine, ✦Elavil Plus [CD], Etrafon [CD], Etrafon-A [CD], Etrafon Forte [CD], ✦Phenazine, ✦PMS Levazine, Triavil
[CD], Trilafon

BENEFITS versus RISKS

Possible Benefits	*Possible Risks*
EFFECTIVE CONTROL OF ACUTE MENTAL DISORDERS in the majority of patients	SERIOUS TOXIC EFFECTS ON BRAIN with long-term use
Beneficial effects on thinking, mood and behavior	Liver damage with jaundice (infrequent)
Relief of anxiety and tension	Rare blood cell disorders: hemolytic anemia, abnormally low white blood cell and platelet counts
Moderately effective control of nausea and vomiting	

▷ **Principal Uses**

As a Single Drug Product: This antipsychotic drug is used primarily to treat
acute and chronic psychotic disorders such as agitated depression,
schizophrenia and similar states of mental dysfunction. It may be used
as a tranquilizer in the management of agitated and disruptive behavior in the absence of true psychosis. Less frequently, it may be used to
relieve severe nausea or vomiting.

As a Combination Drug Product [CD]: This drug is available in combination
with amitriptyline, an effective antidepressant. In some cases of severe
agitated depression, the combination of a specific antipsychotic drug
and a specific antidepressant drug will be more effective than either
drug used alone.

How This Drug Works: Not completely established. Present theory is that
by inhibiting the action of dopamine, this drug acts to correct an imbalance of nerve impulse transmissions that is thought to be responsible
for certain mental disorders.

Available Dosage Forms and Strengths

Concentrate — 16 mg per 5-ml teaspoonful
Injection — 5 mg per ml
Tablets — 2 mg, 4 mg, 8 mg, 16 mg
Tablets, prolonged-action — 8 mg

▷ **Usual Adult Dosage Range:**   Initially 2 to 16 mg 2 to 4 times daily. Dose may be increased by 4 mg at 3- to 4-day intervals as needed and tolerated. Usual dosage range is 8 to 24 mg daily. The total daily dosage should not exceed 64 mg. **Note: Actual dosage and administration schedule must be determined by the physician for each patient individually.**

▷ **Dosing Instructions:**   May be taken with or following meals to reduce stomach irritation. The regular tablets may be crushed for administration; the prolonged-action tablets should be taken whole, not broken, crushed or chewed.

Usual Duration of Use: Continual use on a regular schedule for several weeks is usually necessary to determine this drug's effectiveness in controlling psychotic disorders. If it is not significantly beneficial within 6 weeks, it should be discontinued. Long-term use (months to years) requires periodic evaluation of response, appropriate dosage adjustment and consideration of continued need. Consult your physician on a regular basis.

▷ **This Drug Should Not Be Taken If**
  • you are allergic to any of the drugs bearing the brand names listed.
  • you have active liver disease.
  • you have cancer of the breast.
  • you have a current blood cell or bone marrow disorder.

▷ **Inform Your Physician Before Taking This Drug If**
  • you are allergic or abnormally sensitive to any phenothiazine drug (see Drug Class, Section Four).
  • you have impaired liver or kidney function.
  • you have any type of seizure disorder.
  • you have diabetes, glaucoma or heart disease.
  • you have a history of lupus erythematosus.
  • you are taking any drug with sedative effects.
  • you plan to have surgery under general or spinal anesthesia in the near future.

Possible Side-Effects (natural, expected and unavoidable drug actions)
  Drowsiness (usually during the first 2 weeks), orthostatic hypotension (see Glossary), blurred vision, dry mouth, nasal congestion, constipation, impaired urination.
  Pink or purple coloration of urine, of no significance.

▷ **Possible Adverse Effects** (unusual, unexpected and infrequent reactions)
  If any of the following develop, consult your physician promptly for guidance.
  Mild Adverse Effects
  Allergic Reactions: Skin rash, hives, low-grade fever.
  Lowering of body temperature, especially in the elderly. (See Hypothermia in Glossary).
  Increased appetite and weight gain.

Dizziness, weakness, agitation, insomnia, impaired day and night vision. Chronic constipation, fecal impaction.

Serious Adverse Effects

Allergic Reactions: Hepatitis with jaundice (see Glossary), severe skin reactions, anaphylactic reaction (see Glossary).

Idiosyncratic Reactions: Neuroleptic malignant syndrome (see Glossary).

Depression, disorientation, seizures, deposits in cornea, lens and retina.

Rapid heart rate, heart rhythm disorders.

Blood cell disorders: hemolytic anemia, reduced white blood cell and blood platelet counts.

Nervous system reactions: Parkinson-like disorders (see Glossary), severe restlessness, muscle spasms involving the face and neck, tardive dyskinesia (see Glossary).

▷ **Possible Effects on Sexual Function**

Altered timing and pattern of menstruation.
Female breast enlargement with milk production.
Male breast enlargement and tenderness.
Inhibited ejaculation.
False positive pregnancy test results.

▷ **Adverse Effects That May Mimic Natural Diseases or Disorders**

Nervous system reactions may suggest true Parkinson's disease.
Liver reactions may suggest viral hepatitis.
Reactions resembling systemic lupus erythematosus can occur.

Natural Diseases or Disorders That May Be Activated by This Drug

Latent epilepsy, glaucoma, diabetes mellitus, prostatism (see Glossary).

Possible Effects on Laboratory Tests

White blood cell counts: decreased.
Blood bilirubin level: increased (jaundice—see Glossary).
Blood glucose level: increased.
Glucose tolerance test (GTT): decreased in 35% of those taking this drug.

CAUTION

1. Many over-the-counter medications (see OTC Drugs in Glossary) for allergies, colds and coughs contain drugs that can interact unfavorably with this drug. Ask your physician or pharmacist for guidance before using any such medications.
2. Antacids that contain aluminum and/or magnesium can prevent the absorption of this drug and reduce its effectiveness.
3. Obtain prompt evaluation of any change or disturbance of vision.

Precautions for Use

By Infants and Children: Use of this drug is not recommended in children under 12 years of age. Do not use this drug in the presence of symptoms suggestive of Reye syndrome (see Glossary). Children with acute infectious diseases (flulike infections, chicken pox, measles, etc.) are more prone to develop muscular spasms of the face, back and extremities when this drug is given to control nausea or vomiting.

By Those over 60 Years of Age: Small doses are advisable until individual response has been determined. You may be more susceptible to the development of drowsiness, lethargy, constipation, lowering of body temperature (hypothermia) and orthostatic hypotension (see Glossary). This drug can enhance existing prostatism (see Glossary). You may also be more susceptible to the development of Parkinson-like reactions and/or tardive dyskinesia (see discussion of these terms in Glossary). These reactions must be recognized early since they may become unresponsive to treatment and irreversible.

▷ **Advisability of Use During Pregnancy**
Pregnancy Category: C (tentative). See Pregnancy Code inside back cover.
Animal studies: Cleft palate reported in mouse and rat studies.
Human studies: No increase in birth defects reported in 166 exposures. Information from adequate studies of pregnant women is not available.
Avoid drug during the first 3 months; avoid during the last month because of possible effects on the newborn infant.

Advisability of Use if Breast-Feeding
Presence of this drug in breast milk: Yes, in minute amounts.
Monitor nursing infant closely and discontinue drug or nursing if adverse effects develop.

Habit-Forming Potential: None.

Effects of Overdosage: Marked drowsiness, weakness, tremor, agitation, unsteadiness, deep sleep, coma, convulsions.

Possible Effects of Long-Term Use: Opacities in the cornea or lens of the eye, pigmentation of the retina.
Tardive dyskinesia (see Glossary).

Suggested Periodic Examinations While Taking This Drug (at physician's discretion)
Complete blood cell counts, especially between the fourth and tenth weeks of treatment.
Liver function tests, electrocardiograms.
Complete eye examinations—eye structures and vision.
Careful inspection of the tongue for early evidence of fine, involuntary, wavelike movements that could indicate the beginning of tardive dyskinesia.

▷ **While Taking This Drug, Observe the Following**
Foods: No restrictions.
Nutritional Support: A riboflavin (vitamin B-2) supplement should be taken with long-term use.
Beverages: No restrictions. May be taken with milk.
▷ *Alcohol:* Avoid completely. Alcohol can increase the sedative action of

phenothiazines and accentuate their depressant effects on brain function and blood pressure. Phenothiazines can increase the intoxicating effects of alcohol.

Tobacco Smoking: Possible reduction of drowsiness from drug.

Marijuana Smoking: Moderate increase in drowsiness; accentuation of orthostatic hypotension; increased risk of precipitating latent psychoses, confusing the interpretation of mental status and drug responses.

▷ *Other Drugs*

Perphenazine may *increase* the effects of
• all sedative drugs, especially meperidine (Demerol), and cause excessive sedation.
• all atropinelike drugs, and cause nervous system toxicity.

Perphenazine may *decrease* the effects of
• guanethidine (Ismelin, Esimil), and reduce its effectiveness in lowering blood pressure.

Perphenazine *taken concurrently* with
• lithium (Lithobid, Lithotabs) may impair the effectiveness of lithium and cause nervous system toxicity.

The following drugs may *decrease* the effects of perphenazine
• antacids containing aluminum and/or magnesium.
• barbiturates (see Drug Class, Section Four).
• benztropine (Cogentin).
• disulfiram (Antabuse).
• trihexyphenidyl (Artane).

▷ *Driving, Hazardous Activities:* This drug can impair mental alertness, judgment and physical coordination. Avoid hazardous activities.

Aviation Note: The use of this drug *is a disqualification* for piloting. Consult a designated Aviation Medical Examiner.

Exposure to Sun: Use caution until sensitivity has been determined. Some phenothiazines can cause photosensitivity (see Glossary).

Exposure to Heat: Use caution and avoid excessive heat as much as possible. This drug may impair the regulation of body temperature and increase the risk of heat stroke.

Exposure to Cold: Use caution and dress warmly. This drug can increase the risk of hypothermia in the elderly.

Discontinuation: After a period of long-term use, do not discontinue this drug suddenly. Gradual withdrawal over 2 to 3 weeks under physician supervision is recommended. Do not discontinue this drug without your physician's knowledge and approval. The relapse rate of schizophrenia after discontinuation is 50% to 60%.

PHENAZOPYRIDINE
(fen az oh PEER i deen)

Introduced: 1927

Class: Urinary analgesic

Prescription: USA: Varies
Canada: No

Controlled Drug: USA: No
Canada: No

Available as Generic: USA: Yes
Canada: No

Brand Names: Azo Gantanol [CD], Azo Gantrisin [CD], Azo-Standard, Baridium, Di-Azo, ✦Phenazo, Pyridium, Pyridium Plus [CD], ✦Pyronium, Thiosulfil-A [CD], Urobiotic-250 [CD], ✦Uro Gantanol [CD]

BENEFITS versus RISKS

Possible Benefits	*Possible Risks*
EFFECTIVE RELIEF OF URINARY URGENCY AND DISCOMFORT	DRUG-INDUCED HEPATITIS (rare) Hemolytic anemia (rare)

▷ **Principal Uses**

As a Single Drug Product: Used exclusively in the treatment of lower urinary tract infections and irritations to relieve the urgency to urinate and the discomfort that accompanies the passage of urine (as in cystitis, urethritis and prostatitis).

As a Combination Drug Product [CD]: This drug is available in combinations with several anti-infective drugs that are commonly used to treat urinary tract infections. Each combination product provides a drug to eradicate the infection and a drug to relieve the discomfort during the early period of treatment.

How This Drug Works: Not completely established. By its direct local anesthetic effect on the tissues lining the lower urinary tract, this drug provides symptomatic relief of pain, burning, pressure and the sense of urgency to void.

Available Dosage Forms and Strengths
Tablets — 100 mg, 200 mg

▷ **Usual Adult Dosage Range:**   100 to 200 mg 3 or 4 times/day, as needed and tolerated. **Note: Actual dosage and administration schedule must be determined by the physician for each patient individually.**

▷ **Dosing Instructions:**   Take with or after food to reduce stomach irritation. The tablet should be taken whole, not broken or crushed for administration.

Usual Duration of Use: Continual use on a regular schedule for 12 to 24 hours is usually necessary to determine this drug's effectiveness in relieving urinary urgency and discomfort. This drug is intended for short-term use; do not continue to take it after the bladder disorder has been corrected.

▷ **This Drug Should Not Be Taken If**
   • you have had an allergic reaction to it previously.
   • you have active liver disease.

▷ **Inform Your Physician Before Taking This Drug If**
   • you have a history of liver or kidney disease.
   • you have had a drug-induced blood cell disorder in the past.

Possible Side-Effects (natural, expected and unavoidable drug actions)
Reddish-orange discoloration of urine and feces (of no significance).

▷ **Possible Adverse Effects** (unusual, unexpected and infrequent reactions)
   If any of the following develop, consult your physician promptly for guidance.
   Mild Adverse Effects
   Allergic Reaction: Skin rash.
   Headache, dizziness, indigestion, abdominal cramping.
   Serious Adverse Effects
   Allergic Reactions: Drug-induced hepatitis, with or without jaundice (see Glossary).
   Idiosyncratic Reaction: Hemolytic anemia (see Glossary) in sensitive individuals; this is more likely to occur in the presence of impaired kidney function.

▷ **Possible Effects on Sexual Function:**   None reported.

▷ **Adverse Effects That May Mimic Natural Diseases or Disorders**
   Liver reaction may suggest viral hepatitis.

Possible Effects on Laboratory Tests
   Red blood cell count and hemoglobin: decreased.
   Liver function tests: increased liver enzymes (ALT/GPT, AST/GOT and alkaline phosphatase), increased bilirubin.
   Urine sugar tests: false positive result with TesTape; false negative result with Clinistix.
   Urine ketone tests: false positive result with Ketostix.
   Urine protein tests: false positive result with Labstix.

CAUTION
   It is important to understand that this drug is only an analgesic, and that its action is limited to the relief of symptoms. It has no curative effect on the underlying condition that is responsible for the symptoms. Consult your physician regarding the need for specific anti-infective therapy.

Precautions for Use
By Infants and Children: Consult your physician regarding appropriate dosage. Limit use to the time required for adequate relief of symptoms.

By Those over 60 Years of Age: The natural decline in kidney function that occurs after 60 may require that you use smaller doses. Observe for the development of a yellowish coloration of the eyes or skin—an indication of excessive drug accumulation. If this occurs, consult your physician.

▷ **Advisability of Use During Pregnancy**
Pregnancy Category: B (tentative). See Pregnancy Code inside back cover.
Animal studies: No birth defects found.
Human studies: Information from studies of pregnant women indicates no increase in birth defects in 1109 exposures to this drug.
Limit use to small doses for short periods of time. Ask your physician for guidance.

Advisability of Use if Breast-Feeding
Presence of this drug in breast milk: Unknown.
Avoid drug or refrain from nursing.

Habit-Forming Potential: None.

Effects of Overdosage: Nausea, vomiting, abdominal discomfort, skin discoloration, hemolytic anemia (in susceptible individuals), altered hemoglobin resulting in weakness and shortness of breath.

Possible Effects of Long-Term Use: Orange-yellow discoloration of the skin; hemolytic anemia.

Suggested Periodic Examinations While Taking This Drug (at physician's discretion)
None for short-term use; red blood cell counts and liver-function tests during long-term use.

▷ **While Taking This Drug, Observe the Following**
Foods: No restrictions.
Beverages: No restrictions.
▷ *Alcohol:* No interactions expected.
Tobacco Smoking: No interactions expected.
▷ *Other Drugs:* No significant interactions with other drugs have been reported.
▷ *Driving, Hazardous Activities:* Usually no restrictions. This drug may cause dizziness. Restrict activities as necessary.
Aviation Note: The use of this drug **may be a disqualification** for piloting. Consult a designated Aviation Medical Examiner.
Exposure to Sun: No restrictions.

PHENELZINE
(FEN el zeen)

Introduced: 1961

Class: Antidepressant, MAO type A inhibitor

Prescription: USA: Yes
Canada: Yes

Controlled Drug: USA: No
Canada: No

Available as Generic: No

Brand Name: Nardil

BENEFITS versus RISKS

Possible Benefits	*Possible Risks*
EFFECTIVE RELIEF OF REACTIVE, NEUROTIC, ATYPICAL DEPRESSIONS with associated anxiety or phobia Beneficial in some depressions that are not responsive to other treatments	DANGEROUS INTERACTIONS WITH MANY DRUGS AND FOODS CONDUCIVE TO HYPERTENSIVE CRISIS DISORDERED HEART RATE AND RHYTHM Drug-induced hepatitis (rare) Mental changes: agitation, confusion, impaired memory, hypomania

---

▷ **Principal Uses**

As a Single Drug Product: This potent MAO type A inhibitor drug is used exclusively to treat severe situational (reactive or neurotic) depression, atypical depression, and (though less effective) severe endogenous depression. Because of the supervision required during its use and its potential for serious adverse effects, this drug is usually reserved to treat depressions that have not responded satisfactorily to other antidepressant therapy.

How This Drug Works: Not completely established. It is thought that by inhibiting the action of a certain enzyme (monoamine oxidase type A) in brain tissue, this drug produces an increase of those nerve impulse transmitters that maintain normal mood and emotional stability.

Available Dosage Forms and Strengths
Tablets — 15 mg

▷ **Usual Adult Dosage Range:** Initially, 15 mg 3 times/day; increase rapidly up to 60 mg/day, as needed and tolerated, until improvement is apparent. For maintenance, reduce dose gradually over several weeks to the smallest dose that will maintain optimal improvement; this may be as low as 15 mg daily or every other day. The total daily dosage should not exceed 90 mg. **Note: Actual dosage and administration schedule must be determined by the physician for each patient individually.**

▷ **Dosing Instructions:**   May be taken on an empty stomach or with food. Do not take this drug in the late evening; it can interfere with sleep. The tablet may be crushed for administration.

Usual Duration of Use: Continual use on a regular schedule for 3 to 4 weeks is usually necessary to determine this drug's effectiveness in relieving depression. Once the optimal maintenance dose has been determined, it may be continued indefinitely. Long-term use (months to years) requires supervision and periodic evaluation by your physician. Consult your physician on a regular basis.

▷ **This Drug Should Not Be Taken If**
   • you have had an allergic reaction to it previously.
   • you have advanced heart disease.
   • you have active liver disease or impaired liver function.
   • you have an adrenalin-producing tumor (pheochromocytoma).
   • you are taking any of the following drugs: another MAO type A inhibitor, a tricyclic antidepressant, carbamazepine (see Drug Classes, Section Four).

▷ **Inform Your Physician Before Taking This Drug If**
   • you have high blood pressure.
   • you have had a stroke, or you have impaired circulation to the brain.
   • you have coronary heart disease.
   • you have frequent or severe headaches.
   • you have diabetes, epilepsy, schizophrenia or an overactive thyroid gland (hyperthyroidism).
   • you have impaired kidney function.
   • you plan to have surgery under general or spinal anesthesia in the near future.

Possible Side-Effects (natural, expected and unavoidable drug actions)
   Insomnia if taken in the evening.
   Orthostatic hypotension (see Glossary).
   Fluid retention (swelling of feet and ankles).

▷ **Possible Adverse Effects** (unusual, unexpected and infrequent reactions)
   If any of the following develop, consult your physician promptly for guidance.
   Mild Adverse Effects
   Allergic Reaction: Skin rash.
   Headache, dizziness, drowsiness, weakness, agitation, confusion, impaired memory, tremors, muscle twitching, blurred vision, impaired red-green color vision.
   Dry mouth, increased appetite, indigestion, constipation.

Serious Adverse Effects

Drug-induced hepatitis with jaundice (see Glossary).

Hypertensive crisis: rapid and extreme rise in blood pressure, severe throbbing headache, palpitation, nausea, vomiting, sweating, risk of brain hemorrhage.

Unusual excitement or nervousness.

Disturbances of heart rate and rhythm.

▷ **Possible Effects on Sexual Function**

Decreased libido (30% of males, 28% of females).

Impaired erection (50%); inhibited ejaculation (60%).

Inhibited orgasm (30% of males, 35% of females).

▷ **Adverse Effects That May Mimic Natural Diseases or Disorders**

Drug-induced hepatitis may suggest viral hepatitis.

Natural Diseases or Disorders That May Be Activated by This Drug

Latent epilepsy, schizophrenia.

This drug may convert a depression into the manic phase of a manic-depressive disorder.

Possible Effects on Laboratory Tests

White blood cell counts: decreased.

Blood glucose level: increased.

Liver function tests: increased liver enzymes (ALT/GPT and AST/GOT), increased bilirubin.

CAUTION

1. Careful dosage adjustment is mandatory. Determine the lowest effective dose and do not exceed it.

2. The development of a severe headache or palpitation may indicate a dangerous elevation of blood pressure. Discontinue this drug immediately and consult your physician.

3. This drug may suppress anginal pain that would normally serve as a warning of excessive demand on the heart.

4. This drug may increase the possibility of hypoglycemic reactions if used concurrently with insulin or oral antidiabetic drugs (sulfonylureas; see Drug Class, Section Four). It may also delay recovery from hypoglycemia.

5. This drug can alter the threshold for convulsions in anyone with epilepsy or a seizure disorder. Dosages of anticonvulsant drugs may require adjustment.

6. This drug should be discontinued 2 weeks before elective surgery under general or spinal anesthesia. Consult your surgeon or anesthesiologist.

7. Many over-the-counter drug products contain ingredients that can cause serious interactions if taken concurrently with this drug. Avoid use of the following: cold and sinus medications, nasal decongestants, hay fever preparations, asthma inhalants, appetite and weight

control products, "pep" pills. Consult your physician or pharmacist regarding their safe use with this drug.

8. It is advisable to carry a card of personal identification with the notation that you are taking this drug. Notify all medical personnel that may attend you that you are taking this drug.

Precautions for Use

By Infants and Children: Safety and effectiveness for use by those under 16 years of age have not been established.

By Those over 60 Years of Age: This drug is not recommended for use by anyone over 60. However, if poor response to other treatment justifies consideration of a trial of this drug, it is inadvisable to use it in the presence of high blood pressure, hardening of the arteries, impaired circulation within the brain or coronary artery disease. This drug will intensify existing prostatism (see Glossary). Fluid retention is more prominent in this age group.

▷ Advisability of Use During Pregnancy

Pregnancy Category: C (tentative). See Pregnancy Code inside back cover.

Animal studies: No information available.

Human studies: Information from adequate studies of pregnant women is not available. Birth defects have been reported with the use of this drug.

Avoid this drug completely if possible. Ask your physician for guidance.

Advisability of Use if Breast-Feeding

Presence of this drug in breast milk: Probably yes.

Avoid drug or refrain from nursing.

Habit-Forming Potential: None.

Effects of Overdosage: Overstimulation, agitation, anxiety, restlessness, insomnia, confusion, delirium, hallucinations, seizures, high fever, circulatory collapse, coma.

Possible Effects of Long-Term Use: The conversion of mental depression into a state of hypomania: excessive mental and physical activity, excitement, agitation, loud and rapid talking, delusional thinking.

Suggested Periodic Examinations While Taking This Drug (at physician's discretion)

Blood pressure measurements in lying, sitting and standing positions.

Complete blood cell counts, liver function tests.

▷ While Taking This Drug, Observe the Following

*Foods: **All tyramine-rich foods should be avoided completely.*** See Tyramine in the Glossary for a compete list of foods and beverages to avoid while taking this drug.

Beverages: Limit coffee, tea and cola beverages to one serving daily. See Tyramine in the Glossary.

▷   *Alcohol:* Use extreme caution until the combined effects have been determined. Alcohol can increase the depressant effects of this drug on brain
function.

Tobacco Smoking: No interactions expected.

▷   *Other Drugs*

Phenelzine may *increase* the effects of

• amphetamine and related drugs.
• appetite suppressants.
• all drugs with stimulant effects on the nervous system, and cause excessive rise in blood pressure.
• all drugs with sedative effects, and cause excessive sedation.
• insulin.
• sulfonylureas (see Drug Class, Section Four).

Phenelzine *taken concurrently* with

• carbamazepine (Tegretol) may cause severe toxic reactions.
• levodopa (Dopar, Sinemet) may cause a dangerous rise in blood pressure.
• meperidine (Demerol) may cause high fever, seizures and coma.
• methyldopa (Aldomet) may cause a dangerous rise in blood pressure.
• methylphenidate (Ritalin) may cause severe headache, weakness and
numbness in the extremities.
• tricyclic antidepressants may cause severe toxic reactions including
high fever, delirium, tremor, seizures and coma.

Note: Consult your physician before taking *any other drugs* while taking
phenelzine.

▷   *Driving, Hazardous Activities:* This drug may cause dizziness, drowsiness
and blurred vision. Restrict activities as necessary.

Aviation Note: The use of this drug *is a disqualification* for piloting.
Consult a designated Aviation Medical Examiner.

Exposure to Sun: No restrictions.

Occurrence of Unrelated Illness: Because of the very serious and life-threatening interactions that can occur between this drug and many others,
it is mandatory that you inform each physician and dentist you consult
that you are taking this drug.

Discontinuation: If this drug is not effective after 4 weeks of continual use,
it should be discontinued. If it is effective, continue to take it in proper
dosage until advised to stop. Do not discontinue it abruptly. If another
antidepressant is to be tried, a drug-free waiting period of 14 days must
elapse between the discontinuation of this drug and initiation of the
new one. All precautions regarding the avoidance of tyramine-rich
foods and other drugs must be observed during this 14-day period.

PHENOBARBITAL
(fee noh BAR bi tawl)

Other Name: Phenobarbitone

Introduced: 1912

Class: Sedative, anticonvulsant, barbiturates

Prescription: USA: Yes
Canada: Yes

Controlled Drug: USA: C-IV*
Canada: < C >

Available as Generic: Yes

Brand Names: Barbidonna [CD], Barbidonna Elixir [CD], Barbita, Belladenal [CD], Belladenal-S [CD], ◆Belladenal Spacetabs [CD], ◆Bellergal [CD], Bellergal-S [CD], ◆Bellergal Spacetabs [CD], Bronchotabs [CD], Bronkolixir [CD], Chardonna-2 [CD], ◆Diclophen [CD], Dilantin w/Phenobarbital [CD], Donnatal [CD], Donnazyme [CD], ◆Gardenal, Kinesed [CD], Luminal, Mudrane GG Elixir & Tablets [CD], Mudrane Tablets [CD], ◆Neuro-Spasex [CD], ◆Neuro-Trasentin [CD], ◆Neuro-Trasentin Forte [CD], ◆Phenaphen Capsules [CD], ◆Phenaphen No. 2, 3, 4 [CD], Quadrinal [CD], Solfoton, Tedral Preparations [CD]

BENEFITS versus RISKS

Possible Benefits	*Possible Risks*
EFFECTIVE CONTROL OF TONIC-CLONIC SEIZURES AND ALL TYPES OF PARTIAL SEIZURES	POTENTIAL FOR DEPENDENCE LIFE-THREATENING TOXICITY WITH OVERDOSAGE
EFFECTIVE CONTROL OF FEBRILE SEIZURES OF CHILDHOOD	Drug-induced hepatitis
Effective relief of anxiety and nervous tension	Rare blood cell disorders: abnormally low red cell, white cell and platelet counts

---

▷ **Principal Uses**

As a Single Drug Product: This barbiturate drug has two primary uses: (1) as a mild sedative to relieve anxiety, nervous tension and insomnia; and (2) as an anticonvulsant to control grand mal epilepsy and all types of partial seizures. It is also used to control febrile seizures of childhood.

As a Combination Drug Product [CD]: This drug is available in many combinations with derivatives of belladonna, an antispasmodic commonly used to treat functional disorders of the gastrointestinal tract. It is also available in combination with bronchodilators for the treatment of asthma, and with ergotamine for the treatment of headaches.

*See Schedules of Controlled Drugs inside back cover.

How This Drug Works: Not completely established. It is thought that by impeding the transfer of sodium and potassium across cell membranes, this drug selectively blocks the transmission of nerve impulses. This could serve to produce a sedative effect and to suppress the spread of nerve impulses that are responsible for epileptic seizures.

Available Dosage Forms and Strengths
Capsules — 16 mg
  Elixir — 15 mg, 20 mg per 5-ml teaspoonful
  Tablets — 8 mg, 16 mg, 32 mg, 65 mg, 100 mg

▷ **Usual Adult Dosage Range:** As sedative: 15 to 30 mg 2 to 4 times/day. As hypnotic: 100 to 200 mg at bedtime. As anticonvulsant: 100 to 200 mg given as a single dose at bedtime. The total daily dosage should not exceed 600 mg. **Note: Actual dosage and administration schedule must be determined by the physician for each patient individually.**

▷ **Dosing Instructions:** May be taken with or after food to reduce stomach irritation. Regular tablets may be crushed and capsules opened for administration. Prolonged-action dosage forms should be swallowed whole without alteration.

Usual Duration of Use: Continual use on a regular schedule for 3 to 5 days is usually necessary to determine this drug's effectiveness in relieving anxiety and tension, and for 4 to 6 weeks to determine its ability to control seizures. If used to treat anxiety-tension states, its use should not exceed 4 weeks without reappraisal of continued need. Long-term use for seizure control (months to years) requires supervision and periodic evaluation by your physician. Consult your physician on a regular basis.

▷ **This Drug Should Not Be Taken If**
• you have had an allergic reaction to it previously.
• you are subject to acute intermittent porphyria (see Glossary).

▷ **Inform Your Physician Before Taking This Drug If**
• you are allergic or overly sensitive to any barbiturate drug (see Drug Class, Section Four).
• you are pregnant or planning pregnancy.
• you have a history of alcohol or drug abuse.
• you are taking any drugs with sedative effects.
• you have any type of seizure disorder.
• you have myasthenia gravis.
• you have impaired liver, kidney or thyroid gland function.
• you plan to have surgery under general anesthesia in the near future.

Possible Side-Effects (natural, expected and unavoidable drug actions)
Drowsiness, impaired concentration, mental and physical sluggishness.

▷ **Possible Adverse Effects** (unusual, unexpected and infrequent reactions)
If any of the following develop, consult your physician promptly for guidance.

Mild Adverse Effects

Allergic Reactions: Skin rashes, hives, localized swellings of face, drug fever (see Glossary).

Dizziness, unsteadiness, impaired vision, double vision.

Nausea, vomiting, diarrhea.

Shoulder-hand syndrome: pain and stiffness in the shoulder, pain and swelling in the hand.

Serious Adverse Effects

Allergic Reactions: Drug-induced hepatitis with jaundice (see Glossary).

Idiosyncratic Reactions: Paradoxical excitement and delirium (instead of sedation).

Mental depression, abnormal involuntary movements.

Blood cell disorders: deficiencies of all blood cell types causing fatigue, weakness, fever, sore throat, abnormal bleeding or bruising.

▷ **Possible Effects on Sexual Function**

Decreased libido and/or impotence (16%).

Decreased effectiveness of oral contraceptives taken concurrently (71%).

▷ **Adverse Effects That May Mimic Natural Diseases or Disorders**

Liver reactions may suggest viral hepatitis.

Natural Diseases or Disorders That May Be Activated by This Drug

Acute intermittent and/or cutaneous porphyria, systemic lupus erythematosus.

Possible Effects on Laboratory Tests

Complete blood cell counts: decreased red cells, hemoglobin, white cells and platelets.

Blood lupus erythematosus (LE) cells: positive.

Prothrombin time: decreased (when taken concurrently with warfarin).

Blood calcium level: decreased (with long-term use).

Blood thyroxine (T^4) level: decreased.

Liver function tests: increased liver enzymes (ALT/GPT, AST/GOT and alkaline phosphatase), increased bilirubin.

Urine sugar tests: no effect with TesTape; false low results with Clinistix and Diastix.

Urine screening tests for drug abuse: may be **positive**. (Test results depend upon amount of drug taken and testing method used.)

CAUTION

1. Anticonvulsant drug therapy must be carefully individualized. Accurate diagnosis and classification of the seizure pattern are essential to the correct selection of the most appropriate drug for seizure control.

2. Emotional stress or physical trauma (including surgery) may require increased anticonvulsant dosage to control seizures.

3. Prolonged-action dosage forms of this drug are not appropriate for the treatment of seizures and should not be used.

Precautions for Use

By Infants and Children: This drug should not be given to the hyperkinetic child. Observe for possible paradoxical stimulation and hyperactivity; this can occur in 10% to 40% of children. Changes associated with puberty characteristically slow the metabolism of this drug and permit its gradual accumulation. Blood levels of this drug in young adolescents should be monitored every 3 months to detect rising concentrations and early toxicity. Adjust dosage as necessary.

By Those over 60 Years of Age: It is advisable to avoid all barbiturates in the elderly. If use of this drug is attempted, start with small doses until tolerance has been determined. Observe for confusion, delirium, agitation and excitement. Do not use this drug concurrently with other drugs for mental disorders. This drug is conducive to the development of hypothermia (see Glossary).

▷ **Advisability of Use During Pregnancy**

Pregnancy Category: D (tentative). See Pregnancy Code inside back cover.

Animal studies: Conflicting reports of cleft palate and skeletal defects in mouse, rat and rabbit studies.

Human studies: Information from studies of pregnant women indicates no increase in birth defects in 8037 exposures to this drug. However, it is reported that barbiturates can cause fetal damage when taken during pregnancy.

Avoid use of drug during entire pregnancy if possible. If it is clearly needed to control seizures, the mother should receive vitamin K prior to delivery and the infant should receive it at birth.

Advisability of Use if Breast-Feeding

Presence of this drug in breast milk: Yes, in small amounts.

Monitor nursing infant closely and discontinue drug or nursing if adverse effects develop.

Habit-Forming Potential: Psychological and physical dependence can occur with prolonged use of excessive doses—300 to 700 mg/day for 1 to 2 months. Dependence is not likely to occur with usual sedative or anticonvulsant doses.

Effects of Overdosage: Behavior similar to alcoholic intoxication: confusion, slurred speech, physical incoordination, staggering gait, drowsiness, stupor progressing to coma.

Possible Effects of Long-Term Use: Psychological and/or physical dependence; syndrome of chronic intoxication: headache, depression, impaired vision, dizziness, slurred speech, incoordination. Megaloblastic anemia due to folic acid deficiency. Rickets or osteomalacia due to deficiencies of vitamin D and calcium.

Suggested Periodic Examinations While Taking This Drug (at physician's discretion)

Complete blood cell counts, liver function tests.

During long-term use: blood levels of folic acid, vitamin B-12, calcium and phosphorus; skeletal X-ray studies for demineralization of bone.

▷ **While Taking This Drug, Observe the Following**

Foods: No restrictions. Eat liberally of foods rich in folic acid: fortified breakfast cereals, liver, legumes, green leafy vegetables.

Beverages: No restrictions. May be taken with milk or fruit juices.

▷ *Alcohol:* Avoid completely. Alcohol can increase greatly the sedative and depressant actions of this drug on brain functions.

Tobacco Smoking: May enhance the sedative effects of this drug and increase drowsiness.

Marijuana Smoking: Increased drowsiness, unsteadiness; significantly impaired mental and physical performance.

▷ *Other Drugs*

Phenobarbital may *increase* the effects of
• all other drugs with sedative effects, and cause excessive sedation.

Phenobarbital may *decrease* the effects of
• anticoagulants (Coumadin, etc.), and require dosage adjustments.
• certain beta blockers (Inderal, Lopressor), and reduce their effectiveness.
• cortisonelike drugs.
• doxycycline (Vibramycin), and reduce its effectiveness.
• griseofulvin (Fulvicin, etc.), and reduce its effectiveness.
• oral contraceptives, and reduce their effectiveness in preventing pregnancy.
• quinidine (Quinaglute, etc.), and reduce its effectiveness.
• theophyllines (Aminophyllin, Theo-Dur, etc.), and reduce their antiasthmatic effectiveness.

Phenobarbital *taken concurrently* with
• phenytoin (Dilantin) may alter phenytoin blood levels: a high phenobarbital level will increase the phenytoin level; a low phenobarbital level will decrease the phenytoin level. Periodic determination of blood levels of both drugs is advised.

The following drugs may *increase* the effects of phenobarbital
• valproic acid (Depakene).

▷ *Driving, Hazardous Activities:* This drug may cause drowsiness and may impair mental alertness, judgment, physical coordination and reaction time. Restrict activities as necessary.

Aviation Note: The use of this drug *is a disqualification* for piloting. Consult a designated Aviation Medical Examiner.

Exposure to Sun: Use caution until sensitivity has been determined. This drug may cause photosensitivity.

Exposure to Cold: Observe the elderly for possible hypothermia (see Glossary) while taking this drug.

Discontinuation: If used as an anticonvulsant, this drug must not be discontinued abruptly. Sudden withdrawal can precipitate status epilepticus (repetitive seizures). Gradual reduction in dosage should be made over a period of 3 months. Total drug withdrawal may be attempted after a period of 3 to 5 years without a seizure. However, seizures are likely to recur in 40% of adults and in 20% to 30% of children.

PHENYLBUTAZONE
(fen il BYU ta zohn)

Introduced: 1949

Class: Mild analgesic, anti-inflammatory

Prescription: USA: Yes
Canada: Yes

Controlled Drug: USA: No
Canada: No

Available as Generic: Yes

Brand Names: ✦Apo-Phenylbutazone, Azolid, Butazolidin, ✦Butone [CD], ✦Intrabutazone, ✦Neo-Zoline-M [CD], ✦Novobutazone, ✦Phenbuff

---

BENEFITS versus RISKS

Possible Benefits	*Possible Risks*
PROMPT, EFFECTIVE RELIEF OF INFLAMMATION AND PAIN IN MODERATELY SEVERE ARTHRITIS, GOUT, BURSITIS AND SUPERFICIAL PHLEBITIS (FOR SHORT-TERM USE)	BONE MARROW DEPRESSION MAY BE SEVERE DRUG-INDUCED HEPATITIS KIDNEY DAMAGE, IMPAIRED FUNCTION GASTROINTESTINAL ULCER FORMATION AND BLEEDING HYPERTENSION HEART MUSCLE DAMAGE EYE DAMAGE: OPTIC NEURITIS EAR DAMAGE: HEARING LOSS

▷ **Principal Uses**

As a Single Drug Product: This potent anti-inflammatory drug is used primarily for the short-term relief of pain and inflammation associated with moderately severe arthritis, gout, bursitis, tendinitis and superficial phlebitis. Because of its potential for severe toxicity, it is not considered to be an "aspirin substitute." Its use should be limited to those conditions that do not respond to less toxic drugs.

How This Drug Works: Not completely established. It is thought that this drug acts somewhat like aspirin, by suppressing the formation of prostaglandins and related substances that are involved in the production of inflammation.

Available Dosage Forms and Strengths
Capsules — 100 mg
Tablets — 100 mg

▷ **Usual Adult Dosage Range:** For arthritis: Initially, 100 to 200 mg 3 times/day; for maintenance, 100 mg 1 to 4 times/day. For acute gout: Initially, 400 mg as a single dose; then 100 mg/4 hours for 4 days or until the acute attack is relieved; continual use should not exceed 1 week. Alternate course for gout: 200 mg/4 hours for 4 days or until acute attack is relieved; continual use should not exceed 2 weeks. **Note: Actual dosage and administration schedule must be determined by the physician for each patient individually.**

▷ **Dosing Instructions:** Take with or following food to reduce stomach irritation. The tablet may be crushed and the capsule may be opened for administration.

Usual Duration of Use: Continual use on a regular schedule for 2 to 5 days is usually necessary to determine this drug's effectiveness in relieving acute pain in arthritis, gout and related conditions. This drug should be limited to short-term use only. If significant improvement does not occur within 1 week, this drug should be discontinued. The maximal period of continual use should not exceed 10 to 14 days.

▷ **This Drug Should Not Be Taken If**
- you have had an allergic reaction to it previously, or to oxyphenbutazone (Tandearil), a closely related drug.
- you have a history of serious adverse effects from drugs.
- you have a history of a blood cell or bone marrow disorder.
- you have a history of stomach or intestinal ulceration or bleeding.
- you have a history of disease or impaired function of the thyroid, heart, liver or kidneys.
- you have high blood pressure.

▷ **Inform Your Physician Before Taking This Drug If**
- you are allergic to aspirin or aspirin substitutes (anti-inflammatory analgesics).
- you are taking any other drugs at this time, either prescription or over-the-counter drugs.
- you are taking anticoagulants.
- you have glaucoma.

Possible Side-Effects (natural, expected and unavoidable drug actions)
Salt and water retention, reduced urine output.

▷ **Possible Adverse Effects** (unusual, unexpected and infrequent reactions)
If any of the following develop, consult your physician promptly for guidance.
  Mild Adverse Effects
  Allergic Reactions: Skin rashes, hives, itching, drug fever (see Glossary).
  Headache, drowsiness, lethargy, nervousness, confusion, tremors.
  Indigestion, stomach pain, nausea, vomiting, diarrhea.
  Progressive gain in weight and rise in blood pressure; these are indications to discontinue this drug.
  Serious Adverse Effects
  Allergic Reactions: Severe skin reactions, high fever, swollen and painful joints, salivary gland enlargement, anaphylactic reaction (see Glossary).
  Bone marrow depression (see Glossary): fatigue, weakness, fever, sore throat, abnormal bleeding or bruising.
  Drug-induced hepatitis, with or without jaundice (see Glossary).
  Kidney damage, impaired kidney function, kidney failure.
  Stomach and intestinal ulceration and/or bleeding.
  Damage to heart muscle (myocarditis) and heart covering (pericarditis).
  Eye damage: injuries to optic nerve and retina, impaired vision.
  Ear damage: loss of hearing.

▷ **Possible Effects on Sexual Function:**   None reported.

Possible Delayed Adverse Effects: The development of leukemia following the use of this drug has been reported. A cause-and-effect relationship (see Glossary) has not been established.

▷ **Adverse Effects That May Mimic Natural Diseases or Disorders**
  Liver reactions may suggest viral hepatitis.

Natural Diseases or Disorders That May Be Activated by This Drug
  Latent hypertension, peptic ulcer disease, ulcerative colitis.

Possible Effects on Laboratory Tests
  Complete blood cell counts: decreased red cells, hemoglobin, white cells and platelets; increased white cells (drug-induced leukemia); increased eosinophils (allergic reaction).
  Blood lupus erythematosus (LE) cells: positive.
  Prothrombin time: increased (when taken concurrently with warfarin).
  Blood amylase level: increased (salivary gland inflammation).
  Blood glucose level: increased.
  Blood sodium level: increased (salt retention).
  Blood thyroid hormone levels: T^4, free T^4 and free T^4 index decreased.
  Blood uric acid levels: increased with low doses of drug; decreased with high doses of drug. Liver function tests: increased liver enzymes (ALT/GPT, AST/GOT and alkaline phosphatase), increased bilirubin. Kidney function tests: blood creatinine and urea nitrogen (BUN) levels increased (kidney damage).
  Fecal occult blood test: positive.

CAUTION
1. This drug should never be used for mild and trivial conditions. It has high potential for serious and life-threatening adverse effects.
2. Follow your physician's instructions fully regarding periodic examinations while taking this drug. These are essential for the early detection of possible adverse effects.

Precautions for Use
By Infants and Children: Safety and effectiveness for use by those under 15 years of age have not been established.

By Those over 60 Years of Age: Many authorities advise that this drug should not be used by this age group. More than 60% of users over 61 years of age experience adverse effects from this drug. The elderly and the debilitated are clearly more vulnerable to the toxic effects of this drug. Its use is not recommended.

▷ **Advisability of Use During Pregnancy**
Pregnancy Category: D (tentative). See Pregnancy Code inside back cover.
Animal studies: Evidence of embryo toxicity reported.
Human studies: Information from adequate studies of pregnant women is not available. Two cases of birth defects following use of this drug have been reported. A causal relationship has not been established.
One manufacturer of this drug recommends that it not be used during pregnancy.

Advisability of Use if Breast-Feeding
Presence of this drug in breast milk: Yes.
Avoid drug or refrain from nursing.

Habit-Forming Potential: None.

Effects of Overdosage: Headache, dizziness, insomnia, mental and behavioral disturbances, hallucinations, seizures, coma.

Possible Effects of Long-Term Use: Bone marrow depression. Development of thyroid gland enlargement (goiter), with or without altered function.

Suggested Periodic Examinations While Taking This Drug (at physician's discretion)
Complete blood cell counts and urine analysis should be made before the drug is taken and during the course of treatment at intervals of 1 to 2 weeks.
Liver function tests.

▷ **While Taking This Drug, Observe the Following**
Foods: No restrictions. Avoid excessive salt.
Beverages: No restrictions. May be taken with milk.
▷ *Alcohol:* Avoid completely because of its irritant effect on the stomach, increasing the risk of ulceration and bleeding.
Tobacco Smoking: No interactions expected.

▷ *Other Drugs*

Phenylbutazone may *increase* the effects of
- anticoagulants (Coumadin, etc.), and cause bleeding.
- lithium (Lithane, Lithotabs, etc.), and increase the risk of lithium toxicity.
- phenytoin (Dilantin), and cause phenytoin toxicity.
- sulfonylureas (see Drug Class, Section Four), and increase the risk of hypoglycemia.

▷ *Driving, Hazardous Activities:* This drug may cause dizziness, confusion and impaired vision or hearing. Restrict activities as necessary.

Aviation Note: The use of this drug *may be a disqualification* for piloting. Consult a designated Aviation Medical Examiner.

Exposure to Sun: Use caution until sensitivity has been determined. This drug may cause photosensitivity (see Glossary).

PHENYTOIN
(FEN i toh in)

Other Name: Diphenylhydantoin

Introduced: 1938

Class: Anticonvulsant, hydantoins

Prescription: USA: Yes
Canada: Yes

Controlled Drug: USA: No
Canada: No

Available as Generic: USA: Yes
Canada: No

Brand Names: Dilantin, Dilantin w/Phenobarbital [CD], Diphenylan, ✦Mebroin [CD]

BENEFITS versus RISKS	
Possible Benefits	*Possible Risks*
EFFECTIVE CONTROL OF TONIC-CLONIC (GRAND MAL), PSYCHOMOTOR (TEMPORAL LOBE), MYOCLONIC AND FOCAL SEIZURES IN 80% OF USERS	VERY NARROW TREATMENT MARGIN POSSIBLE BIRTH DEFECTS Overgrowth of gums Excessive hair growth Rare blood cell disorders: impaired production of all blood cells Drug-induced hepatitis Drug-induced nephritis

▷ **Principal Uses**

As a Single Drug Product: Used primarily as an antiepileptic drug to control grand mal, psychomotor, myoclonic and focal seizures. Though not officially approved, this drug is also used to initiate treatment of trigeminal neuralgia; it is sometimes effective in relieving the severe facial pain of this disorder. Recent studies show that it is also effective in preventing motion sickness.

As a Combination Drug Product [CD]: This drug is available in combination with phenobarbital, another effective anticonvulsant. Some seizure disorders require the combined actions of these two drugs for effective control.

How This Drug Works: Not completely established. It is thought that by promoting the loss of sodium from nerve fibers, this drug lowers and stabilizes their excitability and thereby inhibits the repetitious spread of electrical impulses along nerve pathways. This action may prevent seizures altogether, or it may reduce their frequency and severity.

Available Dosage Forms and Strengths

Capsules (extended) — 30 mg, 100 mg
Capsules (prompt) — 30 mg, 100 mg
Injection — 50 mg per ml
Oral suspension — 30 mg, 125 mg per 5-ml teaspoonful
Tablets, chewable — 50 mg

▷ **Usual Adult Dosage Range:**   Initially, 100 mg 3 times/day. Dose may be increased cautiously by 100 mg/week as needed and tolerated. After the optimal maintenance dose has been determined, the total daily dose may be taken as a single dose every 24 hours if Dilantin capsules are used. No other formulation is approved for once-a-day use. The total daily dosage should not exceed 600 mg. **Note: Actual dosage and administration schedule must be determined by the physician for each patient individually.**

▷ **Dosing Instructions:**   May be taken with or after food to reduce stomach irritation. The capsule may be opened and the tablet may be crushed for administration.

Usual Duration of Use: Continual use on a regular schedule for 2 to 3 weeks is usually necessary to determine this drug's effectiveness in reducing the frequency and severity of seizures. Optimal control will require careful dosage adjustments over a period of several months. Long-term use (months to years) requires ongoing supervision and periodic evaluation by your physician. Consult your physician on a regular basis.

▷ **This Drug Should Not Be Taken If**

• you have had an allergic reaction to this drug or to other hydantoin drugs previously.

▷ **Inform Your Physician Before Taking This Drug If**
- you are taking any other drugs at this time.
- you have a history of liver disease or impaired liver function.
- you have low blood pressure, diabetes or any type of heart disease.
- you plan to have surgery under general anesthesia in the near future.

Possible Side-Effects (natural, expected and unavoidable drug actions)
Mild fatigue, sluggishness and drowsiness (in sensitive individuals).
Pink to red to brown coloration of urine (of no significance).

▷ **Possible Adverse Effects** (unusual, unexpected and infrequent reactions)
If any of the following develop, consult your physician promptly for guidance.
Mild Adverse Effects
Allergic Reactions: Skin rashes (5% to 10%), hives, drug fever (see Glossary).
Headache, dizziness, nervousness, insomnia, muscle twitching.
Nausea, vomiting, constipation.
Overgrowth of gum tissues (most common in children).
Excessive growth of body hair (most common in young girls).
Serious Adverse Effects
Allergic Reactions: Drug-induced hepatitis, with or without jaundice (see Glossary). Drug-induced nephritis, with acute kidney failure. Severe skin reactions. Generalized enlargement of lymph glands (pseudolymphoma).
Idiosyncratic Reaction: Hemolytic anemia (see Glossary).
Acute psychotic episodes (rare).
Bone marrow depression (see Glossary): fatigue, weakness, fever, sore throat, abnormal bleeding or bruising.
Mental confusion, unsteadiness, double vision, jerky eye movements, slurred speech.
Joint pain and swelling.
Elevated blood sugar, due to inhibition of insulin release.

▷ **Possible Effects on Sexual Function**
Decreased libido and/or impotence (11%).
Peyronie's disease (see Glossary).
Decreased effectiveness of oral contraceptives taken concurrently (24%).

▷ **Adverse Effects That May Mimic Natural Diseases or Disorders**
Drug-induced hepatitis may suggest viral hepatitis.
Skin reactions may resemble lupus erythematosus.

Natural Diseases or Disorders That May Be Activated by This Drug
Latent diabetes, porphyria, systemic lupus erythematosus.

Possible Effects on Laboratory Tests
Complete blood cell counts: decreased red cells, hemoglobin, white cells and platelets; increased eosinophils (allergic reaction).
Blood lupus erythematosus (LE) cells: positive.

Prothrombin time: increased (when taken concurrently with warfarin).
Blood calcium level: decreased.
Blood total cholesterol, LDL and VLDL cholesterol levels: no effects.
Blood HDL cholesterol level: increased.
Blood triglyceride levels: no effect.
Blood glucose level: increased.
Blood thyroid hormone levels: T^3, T^4 and free T^4 increased.
Liver function tests: increased liver enzymes (ALT/GPT, AST/GOT and alkaline phosphatase), increased bilirubin.

CAUTION

1. Some brand name capsules of this drug have a significantly longer duration of action than generic name capsules of the same strength. To assure a correct dosing schedule, it is necessary to distinguish between "prompt" action and "extended" action capsules. Do not substitute one for the other without your physician's knowledge and guidance.
2. When used for the treatment of epilepsy, *this drug must not be stopped abruptly.*
3. The wide variation of this drug's action from person to person requires careful individualization of dosage schedules. Periodic measurements of blood levels of this drug can be very helpful in determining appropriate dosage. (See Therapeutic Drug Monitoring in Section One.)
4. Regularity of drug use is essential for successful management of seizure disorders. Take this drug at the same time each day.
5. Shake the suspension form of this drug thoroughly before measuring the dose. Use a standard measuring device to assure that the dose is based upon a 5-ml teaspoon.
6. Side-effects and mild adverse effects are usually most apparent during the first several days of treatment, and often subside with continued use.
7. It may be necessary to take folic acid to prevent anemia while taking this drug. Consult your physician regarding this.
8. It is advisable to carry a card of personal identification with a notation that you are taking this drug.

Precautions for Use

By Infants and Children: Elimination of this drug varies widely with age. Careful monitoring by periodic measurement of blood levels is essential for all ages. Some children will require more than one dose daily for good control. Observe for early indications of drug toxicity: jerky eye movements, unsteadiness in stance and gait, slurred speech, abnormal involuntary movements of the extremities and odd behavior.

By Those over 60 Years of Age: You may be more sensitive to all of the actions of this drug and require smaller doses. Observe closely for any indications of early toxicity: drowsiness, fatigue, confusion, unsteadiness, disturbances of vision, slurred speech, muscle twitching.

▷ **Advisability of Use During Pregnancy**

Pregnancy Category: D (tentative). See Pregnancy Code inside back cover.

Animal studies: Cleft lip and palate, skeletal and visceral defects in mice; skeletal and visceral defects in rats.

Human studies: Available information is conflicting. Some studies suggest a small but significant increase in the occurrence of birth defects associated with the use of phenytoin during pregnancy. The incidence of birth defects in children of epileptics not taking anticonvulsant drugs is 3.2%; the incidence with the use of anticonvulsant drugs during pregnancy increases to 6.4%. The "fetal hydantoin syndrome" in the newborn infant exposed to phenytoin during pregnancy consists of birth defects of the skull, face and limbs, deficient growth and development, and subnormal intelligence and performance. Other effects on the infant include reduction in blood clotting factors that predispose it to severe bruising and hemorrhage.

Discuss with your physician the advantages and possible disadvantages of using this drug during pregnancy. It is advisable to use the smallest maintenance dose that will control seizures. In addition, you should be given vitamin K during the last month of pregnancy to prevent a deficiency of blood clotting factors in the fetus.

Advisability of Use if Breast-Feeding

Presence of this drug in breast milk: Yes, in trace amounts.

Monitor nursing infant closely and discontinue drug or nursing if adverse effects develop.

Habit-Forming Potential: None.

Effects of Overdosage: Drowsiness, jerky eye movements, hand tremor, unsteadiness, slurred speech, hallucinations, delusions, nausea, vomiting, stupor progressing to coma.

Possible Effects of Long-Term Use: Low blood calcium resulting in rickets or osteomalacia; megaloblastic anemia; peripheral neuropathy (see Glossary); schizophreniclike psychosis. Lymphosarcoma, malignant lymphoma and leukemia have been associated with long-term use; a cause-and-effect relationship (see Glossary) has not been established.

Suggested Periodic Examinations While Taking This Drug (at physician's discretion)

Monitoring of blood phenytoin levels to guide dosage.

Complete blood cell counts, liver function tests.

Measurements of the following blood levels: glucose, calcium, phosphorus, folic acid, vitamin B-12.

Skeletal X-ray studies for demineralization of bone.

▷ **While Taking This Drug, Observe the Following**

Foods: No restrictions.

Nutritional Support: Supplements of folic acid, calcium, vitamin D and vitamin K may be necessary.

Beverages: No restrictions. May be taken with milk.

▷   *Alcohol:* Use extreme caution until the combined effects have been determined. Alcohol (in large quantities or with continual use) may reduce this drug's effectiveness in preventing seizures.

Tobacco Smoking: No interactions expected.

▷ *Other Drugs*

Phenytoin may ***decrease*** the effects of

- cortisonelike drugs (see Drug Class, Section Four).
- cyclosporine.
- doxycycline (Vibramycin, etc.).
- levodopa (Larodopa, Sinemet).
- methadone (Dolophine).
- mexiletine (Mexitil).
- oral contraceptives.
- quinidine (Quinaglute, etc.).

Phenytoin ***taken concurrently*** with

- oral anticoagulants (Coumadin, etc.) can either increase or decrease the anticoagulant effect; monitor this combination very closely with serial prothrombin testing.
- primidone (Mysoline) may alter primidone actions and enhance its toxicity.
- theophyllines (Aminophyllin, Theo-Dur, etc.) may cause a decrease in the effectiveness of both drugs.

The following drugs may ***increase*** the effects of phenytoin

- chloramphenicol (Chloromycetin).
- cimetidine (Tagamet).
- disulfiram (Antabuse).
- isoniazid (INH, Niconyl, etc.).
- phenacemide (Phenurone).
- phenylbutazone (Butazolidin).
- sulfonamides (see Drug Class, Section Four).
- trimethoprim (Proloprim, Trimpex).
- valproic acid (Depakene).

The following drugs may ***decrease*** the effects of phenytoin

- bleomycin.
- carmustine.
- cisplatin.
- diazoxide.
- folic acid.
- methotrexate.
- rifampin.
- vinblastine.

▷ *Driving, Hazardous Activities:* This drug may impair mental alertness, vision and coordination. Restrict activities as necessary.

Aviation Note: The use of this drug ***is a disqualification*** for piloting. Consult a designated Aviation Medical Examiner.

Exposure to Sun: Use caution. This drug may cause photosensitivity (see Glossary).

Occurrence of Unrelated Illness: Intercurrent infections may slow the elimination of this drug and increase the risk of toxicity due to higher blood levels.

*Discontinuation: **This drug must not be discontinued abruptly.*** Sudden withdrawal can precipitate severe and repeated seizures. If this drug is to be discontinued, gradual reduction in dosage should be made over a period of 3 months. Total drug withdrawal may be attempted after a period of 3 to 4 years without a seizure. However, seizures are likely to recur in 40% of adults and in 20% to 30% of children.

PILOCARPINE
(pi loh KAR peen)

Introduced: 1875

Class: Antiglaucoma

Prescription: USA: Yes
Canada: No

Controlled Drug: USA: No
Canada: No

Available as Generic: Yes

Brand Names: Almocarpine, E-Pilo Preparations [CD], Isopto Carpine, ✦Minims, ✦Miocarpine, Ocusert Pilo-20,-40, PE Preparations [CD], Pilagan, Pilocar, ✦Pilopine HS

BENEFITS versus RISKS

Possible Benefits	*Possible Risks*
EFFECTIVE REDUCTION OF INTERNAL EYE PRESSURE FOR CONTROL OF ACUTE AND CHRONIC GLAUCOMA	Mild side-effects with systemic absorption Minor eye discomfort Altered vision

---

▷ **Principal Uses**

As a Single Drug Product: This drug is used exclusively for the management of all types of glaucoma. Selection of the appropriate dosage form and strength must be carefully individualized.

As a Combination Drug Product [CD]: This drug is combined with epinephrine (in eye drop solutions) to utilize the actions of both drugs in lowering internal eye pressure. The opposite effects of these two drugs on the size of the pupil (pilocarpine constricts, epinephrine dilates) provides a balance that prevents excessive constriction or dilation.

How This Drug Works: By directly stimulating constriction of the pupil, this drug enlarges the outflow canal in the anterior chamber of the eye and promotes the drainage of excess fluid (aqueous humor), thus lowering the internal eye pressure.

Available Dosage Forms and Strengths
Eye drop solutions — 0.25%, 0.5%, 1%, 2%, 3%, 4%, 5%, 6%, 8%, 10%
Gel — 4%
Ocuserts — 20 mcg, 40 mcg

▷ **Usual Adult Dosage Range:**   For chronic glaucoma: Eye drop solutions—1 drop of a 0.5% to 4% solution 4 times/day. Eye gel—apply 0.5 inch strip of gel into the eye once daily at bedtime. Ocusert—insert one into affected eye and replace every 7 days with a new one. **Note: Actual dosage and administration schedule must be determined by the physician for each patient individually.**

▷ **Dosing Instructions:**   To avoid excessive absorption into the body, press finger against inner corner of the eye (to close off the tear duct) during and for 2 minutes following instillation of the eye drop. Place the gel and the Ocusert in the eye at bedtime.

Usual Duration of Use: Continual use on a regular schedule for 1 to 2 weeks is usually necessary to determine this drug's effectiveness in controlling internal eye pressure. Long-term use (months to years) requires supervision and periodic evaluation by your physician. Consult your physician on a regular basis.

▷ **This Drug Should Not Be Taken If**
  • you have had an allergic reaction to it previously.
  • you have active bronchial asthma.

▷ **Inform Your Physician Before Taking This Drug If**
  • you have a history of bronchial asthma.
  • you have a history acute iritis.

Possible Side-Effects (natural, expected and unavoidable drug actions)
  Temporary impairment of vision, usually lasting 2 to 3 hours following instillation of drops.

▷ **Possible Adverse Effects** (unusual, unexpected and infrequent reactions)
  If any of the following develop, consult your physician promptly for guidance.
  Mild Adverse Effects
  Allergic Reactions: Itching of the eyes, itching and/or swelling of the eyelids.
  Headache, heart palpitation, tremors.
  Serious Adverse Effects
  Provocation of acute asthma in susceptible individuals.

▷ **Possible Effects on Sexual Function:**   None reported.

Possible Effects on Laboratory Tests
  Red blood cell and white blood cell counts: increased.

Precautions for Use
  By Those over 60 Years of Age: Maintain personal cleanliness to prevent eye infections. Report promptly any indication of possible infection involving the eyes.

▷ **Advisability of Use During Pregnancy**
   Pregnancy Category: C (tentative). See Pregnancy Code inside back cover.
   Animal studies: Significant birth defects due to this drug reported in rats.
   Human studies: Information from adequate studies of pregnant women
   is not available.
   Limit use to the smallest effective dose. Minimize systemic absorption
   (see Dosing Instructions).

Advisability of Use if Breast-Feeding
   Presence of this drug in breast milk: May be present in small amounts.
   Monitor nursing infant closely and discontinue drug or nursing if ad-
   verse effects develop.

Habit-Forming Potential: None.

Effects of Overdosage: Flushing of face, increased flow of saliva, sweating.
   If solution is swallowed: nausea, vomiting, diarrhea, profuse sweating,
   rapid pulse, difficult breathing, loss of consciousness.

Possible Effects of Long-Term Use: Development of tolerance (see Glossary), temporary loss of effectiveness.

Suggested Periodic Examinations While Taking This Drug (at physician's
   discretion)
   Measurement of internal eye pressure on a regular basis.
   Examination of eyes for development of cataracts.

▷ **While Taking This Drug, Observe the Following**
   Foods: No restrictions.
   Beverages: No restrictions.
▷ *Alcohol:* Use caution until the combined effect has been determined. If this
      drug is absorbed, it may prolong the effect of alcohol on the brain.
   Tobacco Smoking: No interactions expected.
   Marijuana Smoking: Sustained additional decrease in internal eye pres-
      sure.
▷ *Other Drugs*
      The following drugs may **decrease** the effects of pilocarpine
      • atropine and drugs with atropinelike actions (see Drug Class, Section
         Four).
▷ *Driving, Hazardous Activities:* This drug may impair your ability to focus
      your vision properly. Restrict activities as necessary.
   Aviation Note: The use of this drug **may be a disqualification** for piloting.
      Consult a designated Aviation Medical Examiner.
   Exposure to Sun: No restrictions.
   Discontinuation: Do not discontinue the regular use of this drug without
      consulting your physician. Periodic discontinuation and temporary
      substitution of another drug may be necessary to preserve its effec-
      tiveness in treating glaucoma.

PINDOLOL
(PIN doh lohl)

Introduced: 1972

Class: Antihypertensive, beta-
adrenergic blocker

Prescription: USA: Yes
Canada: Yes

Controlled Drug: USA: No
Canada: No

Available as Generic: No

Brand Names: ✦Viskazide [CD], Visken

BENEFITS versus RISKS

Possible Benefits	*Possible Risks*
EFFECTIVE, WELL-TOLERATED ANTIHYPERTENSIVE in mild to moderate high blood pressure	CONGESTIVE HEART FAILURE in advanced heart disease
	Worsening of angina in coronary heart disease (abrupt withdrawal)
	Masking of low blood sugar (hypoglycemia) in drug-treated diabetes
	Provocation of asthma (with high doses)

▷ **Principal Uses**

As a Single Drug Product: The treatment of mild to moderately severe high
blood pressure. May be used alone or concurrently with other antihypertensive drugs, such as diuretics.

As a Combination Drug Product [CD]: This drug is available in combination
with hydrochlorothiazide (in Canada). The addition of a thiazide diuretic to this beta blocker drug enhances its effectiveness as an antihypertensive.

How This Drug Works: By blocking certain actions of the sympathetic
nervous system, this drug

• reduces the rate and contraction force of the heart, thus lowering the
ejection pressure of the blood leaving the heart.

• reduces the degree of contraction of blood vessel walls, resulting in
their relaxation and expansion and consequent lowering of blood pressure.

Available Dosage Forms and Strengths

Tablets — 5 mg, 10 mg

▷ **Usual Adult Dosage Range:** Initially, 5 mg twice daily (12 hours apart). The
dose may be increased gradually by 10 mg/day at intervals of 2 to 3

weeks as needed and tolerated up to 60 mg/day. For maintenance, 5 to 10 mg 2 or 3 times/day. The total daily dose should not exceed 60 mg. **Note: Actual dosage and administration schedule must be determined by the physician for each patient individually.**

▷ **Dosing Instructions:**   May be taken without regard to eating. The tablet may be crushed for administration. Do not discontinue this drug abruptly.

Usual Duration of Use: Continual use on a regular schedule for 2 to 3 weeks is usually necessary to determine this drug's effectiveness in lowering blood pressure. The long-term use of this drug (months to years) will be determined by the course of your blood pressure over time and your response to the overall treatment program (weight reduction, salt restriction, smoking cessation, etc.). Consult your physician on a regular basis.

Possible Advantages of This Drug: Causes less slowing of the heart rate than most other beta blocker drugs.

Currently a "Drug of Choice"
for initiating treatment of hypertension with a single drug.

▷ **This Drug Should Not Be Taken If**
- you have had an allergic reaction to it previously.
- you have congestive heart failure.
- you have an abnormally slow heart rate or a serious form of heart block.
- you are taking, or have taken within the past 14 days, any monoamine oxidase (MAO) type A inhibitor drug (see Drug Class, Section Four).

▷ **Inform Your Physician Before Taking This Drug If**
- you have had an adverse reaction to any beta blocker drug in the past (see Drug Class, Section Four).
- you have a history of serious heart disease, with or without episodes of heart failure.
- you have a history of hay fever (allergic rhinitis), asthma, chronic bronchitis or emphysema.
- you have a history of overactive thyroid function (hyperthyroidism).
- you have a history of low blood sugar (hypoglycemia).
- you have impaired liver or kidney function.
- you have diabetes or myasthenia gravis.
- you are currently taking any form of digitalis, quinidine or reserpine, or any calcium blocker drug (see Drug Class, Section Four).
- you plan to have surgery under general anesthesia in the near future.

Possible Side-Effects (natural, expected and unavoidable drug actions)
Lethargy and fatigability (15%), cold extremities, slow heart rate, lightheadedness in upright position (see Orthostatic Hypotension in Glossary).

▷ **Possible Adverse Effects** (unusual, unexpected and infrequent reactions)
 **If any of the following develop, consult your physician promptly for
  guidance.**
 Mild Adverse Effects
  Allergic Reactions: Skin rash, itching.
  Headache (5%), dizziness (17%), insomnia (19%), abnormal dreams.
  Indigestion, nausea (7%), vomiting, constipation, diarrhea.
  Joint and muscle discomfort (11%), fluid retention (edema) (11%).
 Serious Adverse Effects
  Mental depression, anxiety.
  Chest pain, shortness of breath, precipitation of congestive heart failure.
  Induction of bronchial asthma (in asthmatic individuals).

▷ **Possible Effects on Sexual Function:**   Decreased libido, impaired erection
  (rare).

 Possible Effects on Laboratory Tests
  Blood lupus erythematosus (LE) cells: positive (one case of drug-induced
  LE).
  Blood total cholesterol level: decreased (with long-term use).
  Blood HDL cholesterol level: increased.
  Blood LDL and VLDL cholesterol levels: no effects.
  Blood triglyceride levels: no effects.
  Glucose tolerance test (GTT): decreased.
  Liver function tests: slightly increased liver enzymes (ALT/GPT and
  AST/GOT) in 7% of drug users.

 CAUTION
  1. *Do not discontinue this drug suddenly* without the knowledge and
   guidance of your physician. Carry a notation on your person that you
   are taking this drug.
  2. Consult your physician or pharmacist before using nasal decongestants usually present in over-the-counter cold preparations and nose
   drops. These can cause sudden increases in blood pressure when
   taken concurrently with beta blocker drugs.
  3. Report the development of any tendency to emotional depression.

 Precautions for Use
  By Infants and Children: Safety and effectiveness for use by those under 12
   years of age have not been established. However, if this drug is used,
   observe for the development of low blood sugar (hypoglycemia) during
   periods of reduced food intake.
  By Those over 60 Years of Age: Proceed *cautiously* with all antihypertensive
   drugs. Unacceptably high blood pressure should be reduced without
   creating the risks associated with excessively low blood pressure. Start
   treatment with small doses, and monitor the blood pressure response
   frequently. Sudden, rapid and excessive reduction of blood pressure

can predispose to stroke or heart attack. Observe for dizziness, unsteadiness, tendency to fall, confusion, hallucinations, depression or urinary frequency.

▷ **Advisability of Use During Pregnancy**
Pregnancy Category: B (tentative). See Pregnancy Code inside back cover.
Animal studies: No significant increase in birth defects due to this drug.
Human studies: Information from adequate studies of pregnant women is not available.
Use this drug only if clearly needed. Ask physician for guidance.

Advisability of Use if Breast-Feeding
Presence of this drug in breast milk: Yes.
Avoid drug or refrain from nursing.

Habit-Forming Potential: None.

Effects of Overdosage: Weakness, slow pulse, low blood pressure, fainting, cold and sweaty skin, congestive heart failure, possible coma and convulsions.

Possible Effects of Long-Term Use: Reduced heart reserve and eventual heart failure in susceptible individuals with advanced heart disease.

Suggested Periodic Examinations While Taking This Drug (at physician's discretion)
Measurements of blood pressure, evaluation of heart function.

▷ **While Taking This Drug, Observe the Following**
Foods: No restrictions. Avoid excessive salt intake.
Beverages: No restrictions. May be taken with milk.
▷   *Alcohol:* Use with caution until the combined effect has been determined. Alcohol may exaggerate this drug's ability to lower the blood pressure and may increase its mild sedative effect.
Tobacco Smoking: Nicotine may reduce this drug's effectiveness in treating high blood pressure. In addition, high doses of this drug may potentiate the constriction of the bronchial tubes caused by regular smoking.
▷   *Other Drugs*
Pindolol may ***increase*** the effects of
• other antihypertensive drugs, and cause excessive lowering of the blood pressure. Dosage adjustments may be necessary.
• reserpine (Ser-Ap-Es, etc.), and cause sedation, depression, slowing of the heart rate and lowering of the blood pressure.
• verapamil (Calan, Isoptin), and cause excessive depression of heart function; monitor this combination closely.
Pindolol ***taken concurrently*** with
• clonidine (Catapres) requires close monitoring for rebound high blood pressure if clonidine is withdrawn while pindolol is still being taken.
• insulin requires close monitoring to avoid undetected hypoglycemia (see Glossary).

The following drugs may *increase* the effects of pindolol
- cimetidine (Tagamet).
- methimazole (Tapazole).
- oral contraceptives.
- propylthiouracil (Propacil).

The following drugs may *decrease* the effects of pindolol
- barbiturates (phenobarbital, etc.).
- indomethacin (Indocin), and possibly other "aspirin substitutes," may impair pindolol's antihypertensive effect.
- rifampin (Rifadin, Rimactane).

▷ *Driving, Hazardous Activities:* Use caution until the full extent of fatigue, dizziness and blood pressure change have been determined.

Aviation Note: The use of this drug *is a disqualification* for piloting. Consult a designated Aviation Medical Examiner.

Exposure to Sun: No restrictions.

Exposure to Heat: Caution advised. Hot environments can lower the blood pressure and exaggerate the effects of this drug.

Exposure to Cold: Caution advised. Cold environments can enhance the circulatory deficiency in the extremities that may occur with this drug. The elderly should take precautions to prevent hypothermia (see Glossary).

Heavy Exercise or Exertion: It is advisable to avoid exertion that produces light-headedness, excessive fatigue or muscle cramping. The use of this drug may intensify the hypertensive response to isometric exercise.

Occurrence of Unrelated Illness: The fever that accompanies systemic infections can lower the blood pressure and require adjustment of dosage. Illnesses that cause nausea or vomiting may interrupt the regular dosage schedule. Ask your physician for guidance.

Discontinuation: It is advisable to avoid sudden discontinuation of this drug in all situations. If possible, gradual reduction of dose over a period of 2 to 3 weeks is recommended. Ask your physician for specific guidance.

PIRBUTEROL
(peer BYU ter ohl)

Introduced: 1983

Class: Antiasthmatic, bronchodilator

Prescription: USA: Yes

Controlled Drug: USA: No

Available as Generic: No

Brand Name: Maxair

BENEFITS versus RISKS

Possible Benefits	*Possible Risks*
VERY EFFECTIVE RELIEF OF BRONCHOSPASM	Increased blood pressure
	Nervousness
	Fine hand tremor
	Irregular heart rhythm (with excessive use)

▷ **Principal Uses**

As a Single Drug Product: Used primarily to (1) relieve acute attacks of bronchial asthma; (2) reduce the frequency and severity of chronic, recurrent asthmatic attacks (prevention); (3) relieve reversible bronchospasm associated with chronic bronchitis, bronchiectasis and emphysema.

How This Drug Works: It is thought that by increasing the production of cyclic AMP, this drug relaxes constricted bronchial muscles to relieve asthmatic wheezing.

Available Dosage Forms and Strengths

Aerosol — 200 mcg per actuation (in canisters of 300 inhalations)

▷ **Usual Adult Dosage Range:** Inhaler—1 to 2 inhalations (200 to 400 mcg) every 4 to 6 hours. **Do not exceed** 12 inhalations (2400 mcg)/24 hours. **Note: Actual dosage and administration schedule must be determined by the physician for each patient individually.**

▷ **Dosing Instructions:** Carefully follow the "Patient's Instructions for Use"-provided with the inhaler. Do not overuse.

Usual Duration of Use: According to individual requirements. Do not use beyond the time necessary to terminate episodes of asthma.

Possible Advantages of This Drug

Has a more rapid onset of action and a longer duration of effect than most other drugs of this class.

▷ **This Drug Should Not Be Taken If**
- you have had an allergic reaction to it previously.
- you currently have an irregular heart rhythm.
- you are taking, or have taken within the past 2 weeks, any monoamine oxidase (MAO) type A inhibitor drug (see Drug Class, Section Four).

▷ **Inform Your Physician Before Taking This Drug If**
- you have any type of heart or circulatory disorder, especially high blood pressure, coronary heart disease or heart rhythm abnormality.
- you have diabetes or hyperthyroidism.
- you have any type of seizure disorder.
- you are taking any form of digitalis or any stimulant drug.

Possible Side-Effects (natural, expected and unavoidable drug actions)
Aerosol—dryness or irritation of mouth or throat, altered taste.

▷ **Possible Adverse Effects** (unusual, unexpected and infrequent reactions)
**If any of the following develop, consult your physician promptly for
guidance.**
Mild Adverse Effects
Allergic Reactions: Skin rash, itching (less than 1%).
Headache (2%), dizziness (1.2%), nervousness (6.9%), fine tremor of
hands (6%).
Palpitations (1.7%), rapid heart rate (1.2%), chest pain (1.3%), cough
(1.2%).
Nausea (1.7%), diarrhea (1.3%).
Serious Adverse Effects
Irregular heart rhythm, increased blood pressure.

▷ **Possible Effects on Sexual Function:** None reported.

Natural Diseases or Disorders That May Be Activated By This Drug
Latent coronary artery disease, diabetes, epilepsy or high blood pressure.

Possible Effects on Laboratory Tests
None reported.

CAUTION
1. Concurrent use of this drug by inhalation with beclomethasone aerosol (Beclovent, Vanceril) may increase the risk of toxicity due to
fluorocarbon propellants. It is advisable to use pirbuterol aerosol 20
to 30 minutes *before* beclomethasone aerosol. This will reduce the
risk of toxicity and will enhance the penetration of beclomethasone.
2. The excessive or prolonged use of this drug by inhalation can reduce
its effectiveness and cause serious heart rhythm disturbances, including cardiac arrest.

Precautions for Use
By Infants and Children: Safety and effectiveness of use in children under
12 years of age have not been established.
By Those over 60 Years of Age: Avoid excessive and continual use. If acute
asthma is not relieved promptly, other drugs will have to be tried.
Observe for the development of nervousness, palpitations, irregular
heart rhythm and muscle tremors.

▷ **Advisability of Use During Pregnancy**
Pregnancy Category: C (tentative). See Pregnancy Code inside back cover.
Animal studies: High-dose studies in rabbits revealed abortion and in-
creased fetal deaths. Studies in rats and rabbits found no drug as-
sociated birth defects.
Human studies: Information from adequate studies of pregnant women
is not available.
Avoid use during first 3 months if possible.

Advisability of Use if Breast-Feeding
Presence of this drug in breast milk: Unknown.
Avoid drug or refrain from nursing.

Habit-Forming Potential: None.

Effects of Overdosage: Nervousness, palpitation, rapid heart rate, sweating, headache, tremor, vomiting, chest pain.

Possible Effects of Long-Term Use: Loss of effectiveness.

Suggested Periodic Examinations While Taking This Drug (at physician's discretion)
Blood pressure measurements, evaluation of heart status.

▷ **While Taking This Drug, Observe the Following**
Foods: No restrictions.
Beverages: Avoid excessive use of caffeine-containing beverages—coffee, tea, cola, chocolate.
▷   *Alcohol:* No interactions expected.
Tobacco Smoking: No interactions expected.
▷   *Other Drugs*
Pirbuterol *taken concurrently* with
  • monoamine oxidase (MAO) type A inhibitor drugs may cause excessive increase in blood pressure and undesirable heart stimulation.
▷   *Driving, Hazardous Activities:* Use caution if excessive nervousness or dizziness occurs.
Aviation Note: The use of this drug *is a disqualification* for piloting. Consult a designated Aviation Medical Examiner.
Exposure to Sun: No restrictions.
Heavy Exercise or Exertion: Use caution. Excessive exercise can induce asthma in sensitive individuals.

PIROXICAM
(peer OX i kam)

Introduced: 1978

Class: Mild analgesic, anti-inflammatory

Prescription: USA: Yes
Canada: Yes

Controlled Drug: USA: No
Canada: No

Available as Generic: No

Brand Names: ✦Apo-Piroxicam, Feldene, ✦Novopirocam

```
┌─────────────────────────────────────────────────────────────┐
│                   BENEFITS versus RISKS                       │
│                                                               │
│     Possible Benefits              Possible Risks             │
│  EFFECTIVE RELIEF OF MILD      Gastrointestinal pain, ulceration,│
│  TO MODERATE PAIN AND            bleeding.                    │
│  INFLAMMATION                  Drug-induced hepatitis (rare)  │
│                                Rare kidney damage             │
│                                Mild fluid retention           │
│                                Reduced white blood cell and   │
│                                  platelet counts              │
└─────────────────────────────────────────────────────────────┘
```

▷ **Principal Uses**
  As a Single Drug Product: Used primarily to relieve mild to moderately severe pain and inflammation associated with (1) rheumatoid arthritis, (2) osteoarthritis and (3) acute and chronic gout.

  How This Drug Works: Not completely established. It is thought that this drug suppresses the formation of prostaglandins (and related compounds), chemicals involved in the production of inflammation and pain.

  Available Dosage Forms and Strengths
    Capsules — 10 mg, 20 mg

▷ **Usual Adult Dosage Range:**   As antiarthritic: 10 mg twice daily, 12 hours apart; or 20 mg once daily. The total daily dosage should not exceed 40 mg, and then for no more than 5 days. **Note: Actual dosage and administration schedule must be determined by the physician for each patient individually.**

▷ **Dosing Instructions:**   Take with or following food to prevent stomach irritation. Take with a full glass of water and remain upright (do not lie down) for 30 minutes. The capsule may be opened for administration.

  Usual Duration of Use: Continual use on a regular schedule for 2 weeks is usually necessary to determine this drug's effectiveness in relieving the discomfort of arthritis. Long-term use (months to years) requires supervision and periodic evaluation by your physician. Consult your physician on a regular basis.

▷ **This Drug Should Not Be Taken If**
  • you have had an allergic reaction to it previously.
  • you are subject to asthma or nasal polyps caused by aspirin.
  • you have active peptic ulcer disease or any form of gastrointestinal bleeding.
  • you have a bleeding disorder or a blood cell disorder.
  • you have active liver disease.
  • you have severe impairment of kidney function.

▷ **Inform Your Physician Before Taking This Drug If**
- you are allergic to aspirin or to other aspirin substitutes.
- you have a history of peptic ulcer disease, regional enteritis or ulcerative colitis.
- you have a history of any type of bleeding disorder.
- you have impaired liver or kidney function.
- you have high blood pressure or a history of heart failure.
- you are taking any of the following: acetaminophen, aspirin or other aspirin substitutes, anticoagulants, oral antidiabetic drugs.
- you plan to have surgery of any type in the near future.

Possible Side-Effects (natural, expected and unavoidable drug actions)
Fluid retention (weight gain), prolongation of bleeding time.

▷ **Possible Adverse Effects** (unusual, unexpected and infrequent reactions)
If any of the following develop, consult your physician promptly for guidance.
Mild Adverse Effects
Allergic Reactions: Skin rash, itching, spontaneous bruising.
Headache, dizziness, altered or blurred vision, ringing in the ears, drowsiness, fatigue, inability to concentrate.
Indigestion, nausea, vomiting, abdominal pain, diarrhea.
Serious Adverse Effects
Active peptic ulcer, stomach or intestinal bleeding.
Drug-induced liver damage.
Kidney damage with painful urination, bloody urine, reduced urine formation.
Rare bone marrow depression (see Glossary): fatigue, weakness, fever, sore throat, abnormal bleeding or bruising.

▷ **Possible Effects on Sexual Function:**   None reported.

Possible Delayed Adverse Effects: Mild anemia due to "silent" blood loss from the stomach (less than that caused by aspirin).

▷ **Adverse Effects That May Mimic Natural Diseases or Disorders**
Liver reaction may suggest viral hepatitis.

Natural Diseases or Disorders That May Be Activated by This Drug
Peptic ulcer disease, ulcerative colitis.

Possible Effects on Laboratory Tests
Red blood cell count and hemoglobin level: decreased.
Bleeding time: increased.
Blood uric acid level: increased.
Liver function tests: increased liver enzymes (ALT/GPT, AST/GOT and alkaline phosphatase), increased bilirubin.
Kidney function tests: blood creatinine and urea nitrogen (BUN) levels increased; urine analysis positive for red blood cells, casts and increased protein content (kidney damage).
Fecal occult blood test: positive.

CAUTION
1. Dosage should always be limited to the smallest amount that produces reasonable improvement.
2. This drug may mask early indications of infection. Inform your physician if you think you are developing an infection of any kind.

Precautions for Use
By Infants and Children: Indications and dosage recommendations for use by those under 12 years of age have not been established.

By Those over 60 Years of Age: Small doses are advisable until tolerance is determined. Observe for any indications of liver or kidney toxicity, fluid retention, dizziness, confusion, impaired memory, stomach bleeding or constipation.

▷ **Advisability of Use During Pregnancy**
Pregnancy Category: B (tentative). See Pregnancy Code inside back cover.
Animal studies: No birth defects reported due to this drug.
Human studies: Information from adequate studies of pregnant women is not available.
The manufacturer does not recommend the use of this drug during pregnancy.

Advisability of Use if Breast-Feeding
Presence of this drug in breast milk: Unknown.
Avoid drug or refrain from nursing.

Habit-Forming Potential: None.

Effects of Overdosage: Possible drowsiness, dizziness, ringing in the ears, nausea, vomiting, indigestion.

Possible Effects of Long-Term Use: Development of anemia due to "silent" bleeding from the gastrointestinal tract.

Suggested Periodic Examinations While Taking This Drug (at physician's discretion)
Complete blood cell counts, liver and kidney function tests.
Complete eye examinations if vision is altered in any way.
Hearing examinations if ringing in the ears or hearing loss develops.

▷ **While Taking This Drug, Observe the Following**
Foods: No restrictions.
Beverages: No restrictions. May be taken with milk.
▷   *Alcohol:* Use with caution. The irritant action of alcohol on the stomach lining, added to the irritant action of this drug in sensitive individuals, can increase the risk of stomach ulceration and/or bleeding.
Tobacco Smoking: No interactions expected.
▷   *Other Drugs*
Piroxicam may *increase* the effects of
• acetaminophen (Tylenol, etc.), and increase the risk of kidney damage; avoid prolonged use of this combination.

- anticoagulants (Coumadin, etc.), and increase the risk of bleeding; monitor prothrombin time, adjust dose accordingly.

Piroxicam *taken concurrently* with the following drugs may increase the risk of bleeding; avoid these combinations:

- aspirin.
- dipyridamole (Persantine).
- indomethacin (Indocin).
- sulfinpyrazone (Anturane).
- valproic acid (Depakene).

▷ *Driving, Hazardous Activities:* This drug may cause drowsiness or dizziness. Restrict activities as necessary.

Aviation Note: The use of this drug *may be a disqualification* for piloting. Consult a designated Aviation Medical Examiner.

Exposure to Sun: No restrictions.

POTASSIUM
(poh TAS ee um)

Introduced: 1939

Class: Potassium preparations

Prescription: USA: Yes
Canada: No

Controlled Drug: USA: No
Canada: No

Available as Generic: Yes

Brand Names: ✦Apo-K, Kaochlor, Kaochlor-Eff, Kaon, Kaon-Cl, Kay Ciel, K-Dur, K-Lor, Klorvess, Klotrix, K-Lyte, K-Lyte/Cl, K-Lyte DS, K+Care, K+10, K-Tab, Micro-K, Micro-K Extencaps, Micro-K LS, ✦Neo-K, Slow-K, Ten-K, Trikates

---

BENEFITS versus RISKS

Possible Benefits	*Possible Risks*
EFFECTIVE PREVENTION AND TREATMENT OF POTASSIUM DEFICIENCY (HYPOKALEMIA)	DEVELOPMENT OF EXCESSIVELY HIGH BLOOD POTASSIUM LEVEL (HYPERKALEMIA)
	Ulceration and perforation of stomach or intestine with use of slow-release or enteric-coated tablets (these forms no longer recommended)

▷ **Principal Uses**

As a Single Drug Product: This drug is used primarily in conjunction with those diuretics that cause excessive loss of potassium from the body. Potassium preparations are usually given to stabilize the blood level within the normal range. Dosage adjustments may be necessary from time to time.

How This Drug Works: By maintaining or replenishing the normal potassium content of cells, this drug preserves or restores such normal cellular functions as the transmission of nerve impulses, the contraction of muscle fibers, the regulation of kidney function and the secretion of stomach juices.

Available Dosage Forms and Strengths

Capsules, prolonged-action — 8 mEq, 10 mEq

Liquids — 10 mEq, 15 mEq, 20 mEq, 25 mEq, 30 mEq, 40 mEq, 45 mEq per 15-ml tablespoonful

Powders — 15 mEq, 20 mEq, 25 mEq per packet

Suspension, prolonged-action — 20 mEq per packet

Tablets — 2 mEq, 2.5 mEq, 5 mEq

Tablets, chewable — 1 mEq, 2.5 mEq

Tablets, effervescent — 20 mEq, 25 mEq, 50 mEq

Tablets, enteric-coated — 4 mEq

Tablets, prolonged-action — 6.7 mEq, 8 mEq, 10 mEq

Tablets, wax matrix — 6.7 mEq, 8 mEq, 10 mEq

▷ **Usual Adult Dosage Range:** Depends upon the dosage form prescribed. Follow your physician's prescribed dose exactly. **Note: Actual dosage and administration schedule must be determined by the physician for each patient individually.**

▷ **Dosing Instructions:** Take each dose with food or immediately following a meal to reduce stomach irritation. Regular tablets should be swallowed whole. Soluble tablets and powders should be dissolved completely in 4 ounces of cold water or juice and sipped slowly over a period of 5 to 10 minutes. Liquid forms should be diluted in 4 ounces of water or juice. The prolonged-action capsules should be swallowed whole and not opened for administration. Wax matrix and enteric-coated tablets are not recommended because of their potential for causing localized erosion and ulceration of gastrointestinal tissues.

Usual Duration of Use: This must be determined by your physician. Periods of use will depend upon your concurrent use of diuretics, the potassium content of your diet and periodic measurement of your blood potassium level. Consult your physician on a regular basis.

▷ **This Drug Should Not Be Taken If**
- you have had an allergic reaction to it previously.
- you have severe impairment of kidney function.
- you are taking any drug that contains amiloride, spironolactone or triamterene.

▷ **Inform Your Physician Before Taking This Drug If**
- you are taking any of the following: a cortisonelike drug, a digitalis preparation, a diuretic (see Drug Classes, Section Four).
- you have Addison's disease (adrenal gland deficiency).
- you have diabetes or any form of heart disease.
- you have a history of kidney disease or impaired kidney function.
- you have a history of familial periodic paralysis.

Possible Side-Effects (natural, expected and unavoidable drug actions)
A mild laxative effect for some individuals.

▷ **Possible Adverse Effects** (unusual, unexpected and infrequent reactions)
If any of the following develop, consult your physician promptly for guidance.
Mild Adverse Effects
Nausea, vomiting, abdominal discomfort, diarrhea. (These usually occur if potassium is taken undiluted or on an empty stomach.)
Serious Adverse Effects
Potassium accumulation, resulting in abnormally high blood levels. Immediate treatment is mandatory.
Potassium in enteric-coated tablets or slow-release (wax matrix) tablets can cause ulceration of the stomach or intestine with risk of bleeding and/or perforation.

▷ **Possible Effects on Sexual Function:**   None reported.

Possible Effects on Laboratory Tests
Blood glucose level: decreased.
Blood potassium level: increased. **Note:** If you are taking supplemental potassium, monitor the dose and blood levels carefully; an excessively high blood level of potassium is a major cause of fatal drug reactions.

CAUTION
1. Dosage must be carefully individualized. Periodic evaluation of overall condition and blood potassium levels is essential to safe and effective management. Excessively high blood levels of potassium can occur without warning. Do not exceed the prescribed dose.
2. Inform your physician promptly if you are taking a tablet form of this drug and you become aware of any difficulty in swallowing.
3. If you have chronic constipation, it is advisable that you avoid potassium in tablet form.
4. Some salt substitutes contain a large amount of potassium. If you are using a salt substitute, consult your physician regarding its continued use or any necessary adjustment in the dosage of your potassium preparation.

Precautions for Use
By Those over 60 Years of Age: Your potassium balance must be maintained within strict limitations. Serious adverse effects can occur when the potassium level is either above or below the normal range. Adhere to your dosage schedule exactly.

▷ **Advisability of Use During Pregnancy**
Pregnancy Category: A (tentative). See Pregnancy Code inside back cover.
Animal studies: No information available.
Human studies: Information from adequate studies of pregnant women is not available.
Potassium is a normal and essential constituent of body tissues. Potassium preparations can be used safely during pregnancy. Adhere strictly to prescribed dosage schedules.

Advisability of Use if Breast-Feeding
Presence of this drug in breast milk: Yes.
Monitor nursing infant closely and discontinue drug or nursing if adverse effects develop.

Habit-Forming Potential: None.

Effects of Overdosage: Lethargy, weakness and heaviness of legs, numbness and tingling in the extremities, confusion, irregular heart rhythm, drop in blood pressure, seizures, coma, heart arrest.

Possible Effects of Long-Term Use: Reduced absorption of vitamin B-12, resulting in anemia in some individuals.

Suggested Periodic Examinations While Taking This Drug (at physician's discretion)
Measurement of blood potassium levels.

▷ **While Taking This Drug, Observe the Following**
Foods: No restrictions. Consult your physician regarding any special modifications of your diet.
Beverages: No restrictions.
▷ *Alcohol:* No interactions expected.
Tobacco Smoking: No interactions expected.
▷ *Other Drugs*
Potassium ***taken concurrently*** with
• amiloride, spironolactone or triamterene may cause an excessive rise in blood potassium levels. This can be extremely dangerous; avoid the concurrent use of these diuretics and any form of potassium.
• digitalis preparations requires very careful monitoring of dosage and heart status.
▷ *Driving, Hazardous Activities:* No restrictions.
Aviation Note: The use of this drug ***may be a disqualification*** for piloting. Consult a designated Aviation Medical Examiner.
Exposure to Sun: No restrictions.
Discontinuation: Do not discontinue this drug suddenly if you are taking digitalis. Ask your physician for guidance if you find it necessary to discontinue potassium medication for any reason.

PRAZEPAM
(PRA ze pam)

Introduced: 1969

Class: Mild tranquilizer, benzodiazepines

Prescription: USA: Yes

Controlled Drug: USA: C-IV*

Available as Generic: USA: No

Brand Name: Centrax

BENEFITS versus RISKS

Possible Benefits	*Possible Risks*
RELIEF OF ANXIETY AND NERVOUS TENSION in 70% to 80% of users	Habit-forming potential with prolonged use
Wide margin of safety with therapeutic doses	Minor impairment of mental functions
Very few drug interactions	

▷ **Principal Uses**

As a Single Drug Product: Used primarily to (1) provide short-term relief of mild to moderate anxiety; (2) relieve the symptoms of acute alcohol withdrawal: agitation, tremors, hallucinations, incipient delirium tremens.

How This Drug Works: It is thought that this drug produces a calming effect by enhancing the action of the nerve transmitter gamma-aminobutyric acid (GABA), which in turn blocks the arousal of higher brain centers.

Available Dosage Forms and Strengths

Capsules — 5 mg, 10 mg, 20 mg

Tablets — 10 mg

▷ **Usual Adult Dosage Range:**   20 to 60 mg/24 hours, in 3 or 4 divided doses. The total daily dosage should not exceed 60 mg. **Note: Actual dosage and administration schedule must be determined by the physician for each patient individually.**

▷ **Dosing Instructions:**   May be taken on empty stomach or with food or milk as needed to prevent stomach irritation. The tablet may be crushed and the capsule may be opened for administration. Do not discontinue this drug abruptly if taken for more than 4 weeks.

Usual Duration of Use: Continual use on a regular schedule for 3 to 5 days is usually necessary to determine this drug's effectiveness in relieving

*See Schedules of Controlled Drugs inside back cover.

moderate anxiety. Limit continual use to 1 to 3 weeks. Avoid uninterrupted and prolonged use.

▷ **This Drug Should Not Be Taken If**
- you have had an allergic reaction to any dosage form of it previously.
- you have acute narrow-angle glaucoma.
- it is prescribed for a child under 18 years of age.

▷ **Inform Your Physician Before Taking This Drug If**
- you are allergic to any benzodiazepine drug (see Drug Class, Section Four).
- you have a history of alcoholism or drug abuse.
- you are pregnant or planning pregnancy.
- you have impaired liver or kidney function.
- you have a history of serious depression or mental disorder.
- you have any of the following: asthma, emphysema, epilepsy, myasthenia gravis.
- you are taking any drugs with sedative effects.

Possible Side-Effects (natural, expected and unavoidable drug actions)
Drowsiness (6%), lethargy (11%), unsteadiness (5%), "hangover" effects on the day following bedtime use.

▷ **Possible Adverse Effects** (unusual, unexpected and infrequent reactions)
If any of the following develop, consult your physician promptly for guidance.
Mild Adverse Effects
Allergic Reactions: Skin rashes, hives, itching.
Dizziness (8%), fainting, weakness (7%), confusion, blurred vision, double vision, slurred speech, sweating, nausea.
Serious Adverse Effects
Paradoxical responses of excitement, agitation, anger, rage.

▷ **Possible Effects on Sexual Function:** None reported.

Possible Effects on Laboratory Tests
Urine screening tests for drug abuse: may be **positive.** (Test results depend upon amount of drug taken and testing method used.)

CAUTION
1. This drug should not be discontinued abruptly if it has been taken continually for more than 4 weeks.
2. The concurrent use of some over-the-counter drug products that contain antihistamines (allergy and cold preparations, sleep aids) can cause excessive sedation in sensitive individuals.

Precautions for Use
By Infants and Children: Safety and effectiveness for use by those under 18 years of age have not been established. This drug should not be used

in the hyperactive or psychotic child of any age. Observe for excessive sedation and incoordination.

By Those over 60 Years of Age: It is advisable to use smaller doses at longer intervals to avoid overdosage. Observe for the possible development of lethargy, indifference, fatigue, weakness, unsteadiness, disturbing dreams, nightmares and paradoxical reactions of excitement, agitation, anger, hostility and rage.

▷ **Advisability of Use During Pregnancy**

Pregnancy Category: D (tentative). See Pregnancy Code inside back cover. Animal studies: No information available.

Human studies: Information from adequate studies of pregnant women is not available. No birth defects have been reported with the use of this drug. However, available information regarding the use of other drugs of this class (benzodiazepines) is conflicting and inconclusive. Some studies found an increase in serious birth defects associated with the use of 2 benzodiazepines. Other studies have found no significant increase in birth defects.

Frequent use in late pregnancy can cause the "floppy infant" syndrome in the newborn: weakness, lethargy, unresponsiveness, depressed breathing, low body temperature.

Avoid use during entire pregnancy if possible.

Advisability of Use if Breast-Feeding

Presence of this drug in breast milk: Probably yes.

Avoid drug or refrain from nursing.

Habit-Forming Potential: This drug can produce psychological and/or physical dependence (see Glossary) if used in large doses for an extended period of time.

Effects of Overdosage: Marked drowsiness, weakness, feeling of drunkenness, staggering gait, tremor, stupor progressing to deep sleep or coma.

Possible Effects of Long-Term Use: Psychological and/or physical dependence.

Suggested Periodic Examinations While Taking This Drug (at physician's discretion)

Complete blood cell counts during long-term use.

▷ **While Taking This Drug, Observe the Following**

Foods: No restrictions.

Beverages: Avoid excessive intake of caffeine-containing beverages: coffee, tea, cola. May be taken with milk.

▷ *Alcohol:* Use with extreme caution until the combined effect has been determined. Alcohol may increase the depressant effects of this drug on the brain. It is advisable to avoid alcohol completely—throughout the day

and night—if it is necessary to drive or to engage in any hazardous
activity.

Tobacco Smoking: Heavy smoking may reduce the calming action of this
drug.

Marijuana Smoking: Increased sedation and significant impairment of intellectual and physical performance.

▷ *Other Drugs*

The following drugs may ***increase*** the effects of prazepam

- cimetidine (Tagamet).
- disulfiram (Antabuse).
- oral contraceptives.

▷ *Driving, Hazardous Activities:* This drug can impair mental alertness, judgment, physical coordination and reaction time. Avoid hazardous activities accordingly.

Aviation Note: The use of this drug ***is a disqualification*** for piloting.
Consult a designated Aviation Medical Examiner.

Exposure to Sun: No restrictions.

Exposure to Heat: Use caution until the effect of excessive perspiration is
determined. Because of reduced urine volume, this drug may accumulate in the body and produce effects of overdosage.

Exposure to Cold: The elderly should dress warmly and avoid situations and
environments conducive to hypothermia (see Glossary).

Discontinuation: Avoid sudden discontinuation if this drug has been taken
for over 4 weeks without interruption. Dosage should be tapered gradually to prevent a withdrawal syndrome that could include depression,
confusion, hallucinations, tremor, seizures, muscle cramping, sweating and vomiting.

PRAZOSIN
(PRA zoh sin)

Introduced: 1970

Class: Antihypertensive

Prescription: USA: Yes
Canada: Yes

Controlled Drug: USA: No
Canada: No

Available as Generic: Yes

Brand Names: Minipress, Minizide [CD]

BENEFITS versus RISKS

Possible Benefits	*Possible Risks*

EFFECTIVE INITIAL THERAPY FOR MILD TO MODERATE HYPERTENSION

"First dose" drop in blood pressure with fainting (0.15%)

EFFECTIVE "STEP 2 OR 3" ANTIHYPERTENSIVE IN 60% TO 70% OF CASES OF MODERATE TO SEVERE HYPERTENSION when used adjunctively with other antihypertensive drugs

Induction of paroxysmal tachycardia (rare)

EFFECTIVE CONTROL OF HYPERTENSION IN PHEOCHROMOCYTOMA

Effective in presence of impaired kidney function

▷ **Principal Uses**

As a Single Drug Product: Used primarily to initiate treatment in mild to moderate hypertension. Also used as a "step 2" or "step 3" antihypertensive drug, in conjunction with other drugs, to treat moderate to severe hypertension.

As a Combination Drug Product [CD]: This drug is available in combination with polythiazide, a diuretic of the thiazide class of drugs that are usually used as "step 1" medications to initiate treatment for hypertension. By utilizing two different methods of drug action, this combination product is more effective and more convenient for long-term use.

How This Drug Works: It is thought that by blocking certain actions of the sympathetic nervous system, this drug causes direct relaxation and expansion of blood vessel walls, thus lowering the pressure of the blood within the vessels.

Available Dosage Forms and Strengths
Capsules — 1 mg, 2 mg, 5 mg

▷ **Usual Adult Dosage Range:**   Initiate treatment with a "test dose" of 1 mg to determine the patient's response within the first 2 hours. If tolerated satisfactorily, increase dose cautiously up to 15 mg/24 hours in 2 or 3 divided doses. The total daily dosage should not exceed 20 mg. **Note: Actual dosage and administration schedule must be determined by the physician for each patient individually.**

▷ **Dosing Instructions:**   May be taken without regard to food. The capsule may be opened for administration.

Usual Duration of Use: Continual use on a regular schedule for 4 to 6 weeks is usually necessary to determine this drug's effectiveness in controlling hypertension. Long-term use (months to years) requires supervision and periodic evaluation by your physician. Consult your physician on a regular basis.

Possible Advantages of This Drug
Effective initial treatment of hypertension.
Does not alter blood cholesterol, potassium or sugar levels.

▷ **This Drug Should Not Be Taken If**
- you have had an allergic reaction to it previously.
- you are experiencing mental depression.
- you have angina (active coronary artery disease) and you are not taking a beta-blocking drug. (Consult your physician.)

▷ **Inform Your Physician Before Taking This Drug If**
- you have experienced orthostatic hypotension (see Glossary) when using other antihypertensive drugs.
- you have a history of mental depression.
- you have impaired circulation to the brain, or a history of stroke.
- you have coronary artery disease.
- you have active liver disease or impaired liver function.
- you plan to have surgery under general anesthesia in the near future.

Possible Side-Effects (natural, expected and unavoidable drug actions)
Orthostatic hypotension, drowsiness (7%), salt and water retention, dry mouth, nasal congestion, constipation.

▷ **Possible Adverse Effects** (unusual, unexpected and infrequent reactions)
If any of the following develop, consult your physician promptly for guidance.
Mild Adverse Effects
Allergic Reactions: Skin rash, itching.
Headache (7.8%), dizziness (10.3%), fatigue (6.9%), weakness (6.5%), nervousness, sweating, numbness and tingling, blurred vision, reddened eyes, ringing in the ears.
Palpitation (5.3%), rapid heart rate, shortness of breath.
Nausea (4.9%), vomiting, diarrhea, abdominal pain.
Urinary frequency and incontinence.
Serious Adverse Effects
Mental depression, sleep disturbance.
Paroxysmal tachycardia (heart rates of 120 to 160).

▷ **Possible Effects on Sexual Function**
Decreased libido (14%); impotence (less than 1%).
Priapism (see Glossary).

Natural Diseases or Disorders That May Be Activated by This Drug
Latent coronary artery insufficiency.

Possible Effects on Laboratory Tests
Blood total cholesterol level: no effect in some; decrease in others.

Blood HDL cholesterol level: no effect in some; increased in others.
Blood LDL cholesterol level: no effect.
Blood VLDL cholesterol level: no effect in some; decreased in others.
Blood triglyceride levels: no effect in some; decreased in others.
Blood glucose level: increased.
Glucose tolerance test (GTT): decreased.
Blood thyroid stimulating hormone (TSH) level: increased.
Blood thyroxine (T^4) level: increased.

CAUTION

1. Observe for the possible "first dose" response of precipitous drop in blood pressue, with or without fainting; this usually occurs within 30 to 90 minutes. Limit initial doses to 1 mg taken at bedtime for the first 3 days; remain supine after taking these trial doses.
2. Impaired kidney function may increase your sensitivity to this drug and require smaller than usual doses.

Precautions for Use

By Infants and Children: Safety and effectiveness for use by those under 12 years of age have not been established.

By Those over 60 Years of Age: Begin treatment with no more than 1 mg/ day for the first 3 days. Subsequent increases in dose must be very gradual and carefully supervised by your physician. The occurrence of orthostatic hypotension can cause unexpected falls and injury; sit or lie down promptly if you feel light-headed or dizzy. Report any indications of dizziness or chest pain promptly.

▷ ### Advisability of Use During Pregnancy

Pregnancy Category: C (tentative). See Pregnancy Code inside back cover.
Animal studies: No birth defects found.
Human studies: Information from adequate studies of pregnant women is not available.
Use this drug only if clearly needed. Ask your physician for guidance.

Advisability of Use if Breast-Feeding

Presence of this drug in breast milk: Yes, in small amounts.
Monitor nursing infant closely and discontinue drug or nursing if adverse effects develop.

Habit-Forming Potential: None.

Effects of Overdosage: Orthostatic hypotension, headache, generalized flushing, rapid heart rate, extreme weakness, irregular heart rhythm, circulatory collapse.

Possible Effects of Long-Term Use: None reported.

Suggested Periodic Examinations While Taking This Drug (at physician's discretion)

Measurements of blood pressure in lying, sitting and standing positions.
Measurements of body weight to detect fluid retention.

▷ **While Taking This Drug, Observe the Following**

Foods: No restrictions. Avoid excessive salt intake.

Beverages: No restrictions. May be taken with milk.

▷ *Alcohol:* Use with extreme caution until the combined effects have been determined. Alcohol can exaggerate the blood-pressure-lowering actions of this drug and cause excessive reduction.

Tobacco Smoking: Nicotine can contribute significantly to this drug's ability to intensify coronary insufficiency in susceptible individuals. All forms of tobacco should be avoided.

▷ *Other Drugs*

The following drugs may *increase* the effects of prazosin

- beta-adrenergic-blocking drugs (see Drug Class, Section Four); the severity and duration of the "first dose" hypotensive response may be increased.

▷ *Driving, Hazardous Activities:* This drug may cause dizziness or drowsiness. Restrict activities as necessary.

Aviation Note: The use of this drug *is a disqualification* for piloting. Consult a designated Aviation Medical Examiner.

Exposure to Sun: No restrictions.

Exposure to Cold: Use caution until combined effect has been determined. Cold environments may increase this drug's ability to cause coronary insufficiency (angina) in susceptible individuals.

Heavy Exercise or Exertion: Excessive exertion can augment this drug's ability to induce angina. See Profile of Angina in Section Two.

Discontinuation: If you are taking this drug as part of your treatment program for congestive heart failure, do not discontinue it abruptly. Ask your physician for guidance.

PREDNISOLONE
(pred NIS oh lohn)

Introduced: 1955

Class: Cortisonelike drugs

Prescription: USA: Yes
Canada: Yes

Controlled Drug: USA: No
Canada: No

Available as Generic: USA: Yes
Canada: Yes

Brand Names: ✦Ak-Cide [CD], ✦Ak-Tate, Delta-Cortef, ✦Inflamase, ✦Inflamase Forte, ✦Nova-Pred, ✦Novoprednisolone, ✦Pred Forte, Pred-G [CD], ✦Pred Mild, Prelone

```
┌─────────────────────────────────────────────────────────────┐
│                    BENEFITS versus RISKS                      │
│                                                               │
│    Possible Benefits              Possible Risks              │
│  EFFECTIVE RELIEF OF          Short-term use (up to 10 days) is│
│    SYMPTOMS IN A WIDE           usually well tolerated         │
│    VARIETY OF INFLAMMATORY    Long-term use (exceeding 2       │
│    AND ALLERGIC DISORDERS       weeks) is associated with many │
│  EFFECTIVE                      possible adverse effects:      │
│    IMMUNO-SUPPRESSION in        ALTERED MOOD AND               │
│    selected benign and malignant   PERSONALITY                │
│    disorders                    CATARACTS, GLAUCOMA            │
│  Prevention of rejection in organ  HYPERTENSION               │
│    transplantation              OSTEOPOROSIS                   │
│                                 ASEPTIC BONE NECROSIS          │
│                                 INCREASED SUSCEPTIBILITY       │
│                                   TO INFECTIONS                │
│                               (See Possible Adverse Effects and│
│                                 Possible Effects of Long-Term  │
│                                 Use below)                     │
└─────────────────────────────────────────────────────────────┘
```

▷ **Principal Uses**

As a Single Drug Product: This potent drug of the cortisone class is used in the treatment of a wide variety of allergic and inflammatory conditions. It is used most commonly in the management of serious skin disorders, asthma, regional enteritis, ulcerative colitis and all types of major rheumatic disorders including bursitis, tendinitis and most forms of arthritis.

How This Drug Works: Not fully established. It is thought that this drug's anti-inflammatory effect is due to its ability to inhibit the normal defensive functions of certain white blood cells. Its immunosuppressant effect is attributed to a reduced production of lymphocytes and antibodies.

Available Dosage Forms and Strengths

Eye ointment — 0.6%
Eye suspension — 1%
Syrup — 15 mg per 5-ml teaspoonful
Tablets — 5 mg

▷ **Usual Adult Dosage Range:**   5 to 60 mg daily as a single dose or in divided doses. The total daily dosage should not exceed 250 mg. **Note: Actual dosage and administration schedule must be determined by the physician for each patient individually.**

▷ **Dosing Instructions:**   Take with or following food to prevent stomach irritation, preferably in the morning. The tablet may be crushed for administration.

Usual Duration of Use: For acute disorders: 4 to 10 days. For chronic disorders: according to individual requirements. The duration of use should not exceed the time necessary to obtain adequate symptomatic relief in acute self-limiting conditions; or the time required to stabilize a chronic condition and permit gradual withdrawal. Because of its intermediate duration of action, this drug is appropriate for alternate day administration. Consult your physician on a regular basis.

▷ **While Taking This Drug, Observe the Following**
▷ *Other Drugs*
Prednisolone may *decrease* the effects of
• isoniazid (INH, Niconyl, etc.).
• salicylates (aspirin, sodium salicylate, etc.).
Prednisolone *taken concurrently* with
• oral anticoagulants may either increase or decrease their effectiveness; consult physician regarding the need for prothrombin time testing and dosage adjustment.
The following drugs may *decrease* the effects of prednisolone
• antacids may reduce its absorption.
• barbiturates (Amytal, Butisol, phenobarbital, etc.).
• phenytoin (Dilantin, etc.).
• rifampin (Rifadin, Rimactane, etc.).

Note: The information categories provided in this Profile are appropriate for prednisolone. For specific information that is normally found in those categories that have been omitted from this Profile, the reader is referred to the Drug Profile of Prednisone which follows. Prednisolone is a derivative of Prednisone; all significant actions and effects are shared by both drugs.

PREDNISONE
(PRED ni sohn)

Introduced: 1955

Class: Cortisonelike drugs

Prescription: USA: Yes
   Canada: Yes

Controlled Drug: USA: No
   Canada: No

Available as Generic: USA: Yes
   Canada: Yes

Brand Names: ✦Apo-Prednisone, Deltasone, Meticorten, ✦Novoprednisone, Orasone, ✦Winpred

---

BENEFITS versus RISKS

Possible Benefits	*Possible Risks*

Possible Benefits
EFFECTIVE RELIEF OF
SYMPTOMS IN A WIDE
VARIETY OF INFLAMMATORY
AND ALLERGIC DISORDERS
EFFECTIVE
IMMUNOSUPPRESSION in
selected benign and malignant
disorders
Prevention of rejection in organ
transplantation

Possible Risks
Short-term use (up to 10 days) is
usually well tolerated
Long-term use (exceeding 2
weeks) is associated with many
possible adverse effects:
ALTERED MOOD AND
PERSONALITY
CATARACTS, GLAUCOMA
HYPERTENSION
OSTEOPOROSIS
ASEPTIC BONE NECROSIS
INCREASED SUSCEPTIBILITY
TO INFECTIONS
(See Possible Adverse Effects and
Possible Effects of Long-Term
Use below)

▷ **Principal Uses**

As a Single Drug Product: This potent drug of the cortisone class is used in
the treatment of a wide variety of allergic and inflammatory conditions. It is used most commonly in the management of serious skin
disorders, asthma, regional enteritis, ulcerative colitis and all types of
major rheumatic disorders including bursitis, tendinitis and most
forms of arthritis.

How This Drug Works: Not fully established. It is thought that this drug's
anti-inflammatory effect is due to its ability to inhibit the normal defensive functions of certain white blood cells. Its immunosuppressant
effect is attributed to a reduced production of lymphocytes and antibodies.

Available Dosage Forms and Strengths
　　Oral solution — 5 mg per 5-ml teaspoonful
　　　　Syrup — 5 mg per 5-ml teaspoonful (alcohol 5%)
　　　　Tablets — 1 mg, 2.5 mg, 5 mg, 10 mg, 20 mg, 25 mg, 50 mg

▷ **Usual Adult Dosage Range:**   5 to 60 mg daily as a single dose or in divided
doses. The total daily dosage should not exceed 250 mg. **Note: Actual
dosage and administration schedule must be determined by the physician for each patient individually.**

▷ **Dosing Instructions:**   Take with or following food to prevent stomach irritation, preferably in the morning. The tablet may be crushed for administration.

Usual Duration of Use: For acute disorders: 4 to 10 days. For chronic disorders: according to individual requirements. The duration of use should not exceed the time necessary to obtain adequate symptomatic relief in acute self-limiting conditions; or the time required to stabilize a chronic condition and permit gradual withdrawal. Because of its intermediate duration of action, this drug is appropriate for alternate day administration. Consult your physician on a regular basis.

▷ **This Drug Should Not Be Taken If**
- you have had an allergic reaction to any dosage form of it previously.
- you have active peptic ulcer disease.
- you have an active infection of the eye caused by the herpes simplex virus.
- you have active tuberculosis.

▷ **Inform Your Physician Before Taking This Drug If**
- you have had an unfavorable reaction to any cortisonelike drug in the past.
- you have a history of peptic ulcer disease, thrombophlebitis or tuberculosis.
- you have any of the following: diabetes, glaucoma, high blood pressure, deficient thyroid function or myasthenia gravis.
- you plan to have surgery of any kind in the near future.

Possible Side-Effects (natural, expected and unavoidable drug actions)
Increased appetite, weight gain, retention of salt and water, excretion of potassium, increased susceptibility to infection.

▷ **Possible Adverse Effects** (unusual, unexpected and infrequent reactions)
If any of the following develop, consult your physician promptly for guidance.
Mild Adverse Effects
Allergic Reaction: Skin rash.
Headache, dizziness, insomnia.
Acid indigestion, abdominal distention.
Muscle cramping and weakness.
Acne, excessive growth of facial hair.
Serious Adverse Effects
Mental and emotional disturbances of serious magnitude.
Reactivation of latent tuberculosis.
Development of peptic ulcer.
Increased blood pressure.
Development of inflammation of the pancreas.
Thrombophlebitis (inflammation of a vein with the formation of blood clot)—pain or tenderness in thigh or leg, with or without swelling of the foot, ankle or leg.
Pulmonary embolism (movement of a blood clot to the lung)—sudden shortness of breath, pain in the chest, coughing, bloody sputum.

▷ **Possible Effects on Sexual Function**
Altered timing and pattern of menstruation.
Correction of male infertility when due to autoantibodies that suppress sperm activity.

▷ **Adverse Effects That May Mimic Natural Diseases or Disorders**
Pattern of symptoms and signs resembling Cushing's syndrome.

Natural Diseases or Disorders That May Be Activated by This Drug
Latent diabetes, glaucoma, peptic ulcer disease, tuberculosis.

Possible Effects on Laboratory Tests
Complete blood cell counts: decreased eosinophils, lymphocytes and platelets.
Blood amylase level: increased (possible pancreatitis).
Blood total cholesterol and HDL cholesterol levels: increased.
Blood LDL cholesterol level: no effect.
Blood triglyceride levels: no significant effect.
Blood glucose level: increased.
Glucose tolerance test (GTT): decreased.
Blood potassium level: decreased.
Blood testosterone level: decreased.
Blood thyroid hormone (T^3): decreased.
Blood uric acid level: increased.
Urine sugar tests: no effect with TesTape; false low result with Clinistix and Diastix.
Fecal occult blood test: positive (if gastrointestinal bleeding).

CAUTION
1. It is advisable to carry a card of personal identification with a notation that you are taking this drug, if your course of treatment is to exceed 1 week.
2. Do not discontinue this drug abruptly if you are using it for long-term treatment.
3. If vaccination against measles, rabies, smallpox or yellow fever is required, discontinue this drug 72 hours before vaccination and do not resume it for at least 14 days after vaccination.

Precautions for Use
By Infants and Children: Avoid prolonged use if possible. During long-term use, observe for suppression of normal growth and the possibility of increased intracranial pressure. Following long-term use, the child may be at risk for adrenal gland deficiency during stress for as long as 18 months after cessation of this drug.
By Those over 60 Years of Age: Cortisonelike drugs should be used very sparingly after 60 and only when the disorder under treatment is unresponsive to adequate trials of unrelated drugs. Avoid the prolonged use of this drug. Continual use (even in small doses) can increasethe severity of diabetes, enhance fluid retention, raise blood pressure, weaken

resistance to infection, induce stomach ulcer and accelerate development of cataract and osteoporosis.

▷ **Advisability of Use During Pregnancy**
Pregnancy Category: C (tentative). See Pregnancy Code inside back cover.
Animal studies: Birth defects reported in mice, rats and rabbits.
Human studies: Information from adequate studies of pregnant women is not available.
Avoid completely during the first 3 months. Limit use during the last 6 months as much as possible. If used, examine infant for possible deficiency of adrenal gland function.

Advisability of Use if Breast-Feeding
Presence of this drug in breast milk: Yes.
Avoid drug or refrain from nursing.

Habit-Forming Potential: Use of this drug to suppress symptoms over an extended period of time may produce a state of functional dependence (see Glossary). In the treatment of conditions like asthma and rheumatoid arthritis, it is advisable to keep the dose as small as possible and to attempt drug withdrawal after periods of reasonable improvement. Such procedures may reduce the degree of "steroid rebound"—the return of symptoms as the drug is withdrawn.

Effects of Overdosage: Fatigue, muscle weakness, stomach irritation, acid indigestion, excessive sweating, facial flushing, fluid retention, swelling of extremities, increased blood pressure.

Possible Effects of Long-Term Use: Increased blood sugar (possible diabetes), increased fat deposits on the trunk of the body ("buffalo hump"), rounding of the face ("moon face"), thinning and fragility of skin, loss of texture and strength of bones (osteoporosis, aseptic necrosis), cataracts, glaucoma, retarded growth and development in children.

Suggested Periodic Examinations While Taking This Drug (at physician's discretion)
Measurements of blood pressure, blood sugar and potassium levels.
Complete eye examinations at regular intervals.
Chest X-ray if history of tuberculosis.
Determination of the rate of development of the growing child to detect retardation of normal growth.

▷ **While Taking This Drug, Observe the Following**
Foods: No interactions expected. Ask physician regarding need to restrict salt intake or to eat potassium-rich foods. During long-term use of this drug, it is advisable to eat a high-protein diet.
Nutritional Support: During long-term use, take a vitamin D supplement. During wound repair, take a zinc supplement.
Beverages: No restrictions. Drink all forms of milk liberally.
▷ *Alcohol:* No interactions expected. Use caution if you are prone to peptic ulcer disease.

Tobacco Smoking: Nicotine increases the blood levels of naturally produced cortisone and related hormones. Heavy smoking may add to the expected actions of this drug and requires close observation for excessive effects.

Marijuana Smoking: May cause additional impairment of immunity.

▷ *Other Drugs*

Prednisone may *decrease* the effects of
- isoniazid (INH, Niconyl, etc.).
- salicylates (aspirin, sodium salicylate, etc.).

Prednisone *taken concurrently* with
- oral anticoagulants may either increase or decrease their effectiveness; consult physician regarding the need for prothrombin time testing and dosage adjustment.

The following drugs may *decrease* the effects of prednisone
- antacids may reduce its absorption.
- barbiturates (Amytal, Butisol, phenobarbital, etc.).
- phenytoin (Dilantin, etc.).
- rifampin (Rifadin, Rimactane, etc.).

▷ *Driving, Hazardous Activities:* Usually no restrictions. Be alert to the rare occurrence of dizziness.

Aviation Note: The use of this drug *may be a disqualification* for piloting. Consult a designated Aviation Medical Examiner.

Exposure to Sun: No restrictions.

Occurrence of Unrelated Illness: This drug may decrease natural resistance to infection. Inform your physician if you develop an infection of any kind. It may also reduce your body's ability to respond to the stress of acute illness, injury or surgery. Keep your physician fully informed of any significant changes in your state of health.

Discontinuation: If you have been taking this drug for an extended period of time, do not discontinue it abruptly. Ask physician for guidance regarding gradual withdrawal. For a period of 2 years after discontinuing this drug, it is essential in the event of illness, injury or surgery that you inform attending medical personnel that you have used this drug in the past. The period of impaired response to stress following the use of cortisonelike drugs may last for 1 to 2 years.

PRIMIDONE
(PRI mi dohn)

Introduced: 1953   **Class:** Anticonvulsant

Prescription: USA: Yes   **Controlled Drug:** USA: No
Canada: Yes   Canada: No

Available as Generic: USA: Yes
Canada: Yes

Brand Names: ✦Apo-Primidone, Myidone, Mysoline, ✦Sertan

BENEFITS versus RISKS	
Possible Benefits	*Possible Risks*
EFFECTIVE CONTROL OF TONIC-CLONIC (GRAND MAL) AND ALL TYPES OF PARTIAL SEIZURES	Allergic skin reactions Rare blood cell disorders: megaloblastic anemia, deficient white blood cells and platelets

▷ **Principal Uses**

As a Single Drug Product: This drug is used exclusively to control generalized grand mal seizures and all types of partial seizures. It can be used to supplement the anticonvulsant action of phenytoin.

How This Drug Works: Not completely established. This drug reduces and stabilizes the excitability of nerve fibers and inhibits the repetitious spread of electrical impulses along nerve pathways. This action may prevent seizures altogether, or it may reduce their frequency and severity. (Part of this drug's action is attributable to phenobarbital, one of its conversion products in the body.)

Available Dosage Forms and Strengths

Oral suspensions — 250 mg per 5-ml teaspoonful
Tablets — 50 mg, 250 mg

▷ **Usual Adult Dosage Range:** Initially, 250 mg/24 hours as a single dose at bedtime for 1 week; 2nd week, 250 mg/12 hours; 3rd week, 250 mg 3 times/day, 6 to 8 hours apart; 4th week, 250 mg 4 times/day, 4 to 6 hours apart. The total daily dosage should not exceed 2000 mg. **Note: Actual dosage and administration schedule must be determined by the physician for each patient individually.**

▷ **Dosing Instructions:** May be taken with or following food to reduce stomach irritation. The tablet may be crushed for administration. Shake the suspension well before measuring the dose.

Usual Duration of Use: Continual use on a regular schedule for 2 to 4 weeks is usually necessary to determine this drug's effectiveness in reducing the frequency and severity of seizures. Long-term use (months to years) requires supervision and periodic evaluation by your physician. Consult your physician on a regular basis.

▷ **This Drug Should Not Be Taken If**
  • you have had an allergic reaction to it previously.
  • you are allergic to phenobarbital.
  • you have a history of porphyria.

▷ **Inform Your Physician Before Taking This Drug If**
  • you have had an allergic or idiosyncratic reaction to any barbiturate drug in the past.
  • you have a family history of intermittent porphyria.
  • you have impaired liver, kidney or thyroid gland function.

- you have asthma, emphysema or myasthenia gravis.
- you are pregnant or planning pregnancy.
- you plan to have surgery under general anesthesia in the near future.

Possible Side-Effects (natural, expected and unavoidable drug actions)
Drowsiness, impaired concentration, mental and physical sluggishness.

▷ **Possible Adverse Effects** (unusual, unexpected and infrequent reactions)
If any of the following develop, consult your physician promptly for guidance.
Mild Adverse Effects
Allergic Reactions: Skin rashes, hives, localized swellings.
"Hangover" effect, dizziness, unsteadiness, impaired vision, double vision, fatigue, emotional disturbances.
Low blood pressure, faintness.
Nausea, vomiting, thirst, increased urine volume.
Serious Adverse Effects
Allergic Reaction: Swelling of lymph glands.
Idiosyncratic Reactions: Paradoxical anxiety, agitation, restlessness, rage.
Visual hallucinations.
Blood cell disorders: megaloblastic anemia due to folic acid depletion; deficient production of white blood cells and blood platelets.

▷ **Possible Effects on Sexual Function**
Decreased libido and/or impotence (22%).
Decreased effectiveness of oral contraceptives taken concurrently.

▷ **Adverse Effects That May Mimic Natural Diseases or Disorders**
Allergic swelling of lymph glands may suggest a naturally occurring lymphoma.

Natural Diseases or Disorders That May Be Activated by This Drug
Acute intermittent and/or cutaneous porphyria (see Glossary).
Systemic lupus erythematosus.

Possible Effects on Laboratory Tests
Complete blood cell counts: decreased red cells, hemoglobin, white cells and platelets; increased eosinophils.
Blood lupus erythematosus (LE) cells: positive.
Prothrombin time: decreased (when taken concurrently with warfarin).
Urine screening tests for drug abuse: may be **positive** for phenobarbital (a normal derivative of this drug). (Test results depend upon amount of drug taken and testing method used.)

CAUTION
1. This drug must not be stopped abruptly.
2. The wide variation of this drug's action from person to person requires careful individualization of dosage schedules.

3. Regularity of drug use is essential for the successful management of seizure disorders. Take your medication at the same time each day.
4. Side-effects and mild adverse effects are usually most apparent during the first several weeks of treatment and often subside with continued use.
5. It may be necessary to take folic acid to prevent anemia while taking this drug. Consult your physician.
6. It is advisable to carry a card of personal identification with a notation that you are taking this drug.

Precautions for Use

By Infants and Children: This drug should be used with caution in the hyperkinetic (overactive) child. Observe for possible paradoxical hyperactivity. Changes associated with puberty characteristically slow the metabolism of phenobarbital and permit its gradual accumulation. Measurements of blood levels in young adolescents can detect rising concentrations of this drug that could lead to toxicity. (See Therapeutic Drug Monitoring in Section One.)

By Those over 60 Years of Age: It is advisable to avoid all barbiturates in the elderly. If use of this drug is attempted, start with small doses until tolerance has been determined. Observe for confusion, delirium, agitation or paradoxical excitement. This drug may be conducive to hypothermia (see Glossary).

▷ **Advisability of Use During Pregnancy**

Pregnancy Category: D (tentative). See Pregnancy Code inside back cover.

Animal studies: Birth defects due to this drug reported in mice.

Human studies: Information from adequate studies of pregnant women is not available. However, recent reports suggest a possible association between the use of this drug during the first 3 months of pregnancy and the development of birth defects in the fetus. Discuss with your physician the advantages and possible disadvantages of using this drug during pregnancy. If it is used, determine the smallest maintenance dose that will prevent seizures.

The newborn infants of mothers who take this drug during pregnancy may develop abnormal bleeding or bruising due to the deficiency of certain blood clotting factors in the blood. Consult your physician regarding the need to take vitamin K during the last month of pregnancy.

Advisability of Use if Breast-Feeding

Presence of this drug in breast milk: Yes.

Monitor nursing infant closely and discontinue drug or nursing if adverse effects develop.

Habit-Forming Potential: None.

Effects of Overdosage: Drowsiness, jerky eye movements, blurred vision, staggering gait, incoordination, slurred speech, stupor progressing to coma.

Possible Effects of Long-Term Use: Enlargement of lymph glands; enlargement of thyroid gland. Megaloblastic anemia due to folic acid deficiency. Reduced blood levels of calcium and phosphorus, leading to rickets in children and loss of bone texture (osteomalacia) in adults.

Suggested Periodic Examinations While Taking This Drug (at physician's discretion)
Complete blood cell counts. Measurements of blood levels of calcium and phosphorus. Evaluation of lymph and thyroid glands. Skeletal X-ray examinations for bone demineralization during long-term use.

▷ **While Taking This Drug, Observe the Following**
Foods: No restrictions.
Nutritional Support: Consult your physician regarding the need for supplements of calcium, vitamin D, folic acid and vitamin K.
Beverages: No restrictions. May be taken with milk or fruit juice.
▷ *Alcohol:* Avoid completely. Alcohol can increase greatly the sedative and depressant effects of this drug on brain function.
Tobacco Smoking: May enhance the sedative effects of this drug and increase drowsiness.
▷ *Other Drugs*
Note: 15% of primidone is converted to phenobarbital in the body. See the Drug Profile of Phenobarbital for possible interactions with other drugs.
▷ *Driving, Hazardous Activities:* This drug may cause drowsiness and dizziness; it can also impair mental alertness, vision and physical coordination. Restrict activities as necessary.
Aviation Note: The use of this drug *is a disqualification* for piloting. Consult a designated Aviation Medical Examiner.
Exposure to Sun: No restrictions.
Occurrence of Unrelated Illness: Notify your physician of any illness or injury that prevents the use of this drug according to your regular dosage schedule.
Discontinuation: Do not discontinue this drug without your physician's knowledge and approval. Sudden withdrawal of any anticonvulsant drug can cause severe and repeated seizures.

PROBENECID
(proh BEN e sid)

Introduced: 1951

Class: Antigout

Prescription: USA: Yes
Canada: No

Controlled Drug: USA: No
Canada: No

Available as Generic: USA: Yes
Canada: No

Brand Names: ✦Ampicin PRB [CD], Benemid, ✦Benuryl, ColBenemid [CD], Polycillin-PRB [CD], Probalan, ✦Pro-Biosan 500 Kit [CD]

BENEFITS versus RISKS

Possible Benefits	*Possible Risks*
EFFECTIVE LONG-TERM PREVENTION OF ACUTE ATTACKS OF GOUT	Formation of uric acid kidney stones
Useful adjunct to penicillin therapy (to achieve high blood and tissue levels of penicillin)	Bone marrow depression (aplastic anemia) (rare)
	Drug-induced liver and kidney damage (both rare)

▷ **Principal Uses**

As a Single Drug Product: Used primarily in the long-term management of gout to prevent acute attacks. While effective for prevention, it has no beneficial effects in relieving the joint inflammation and pain of the acute episode. In fact, it may aggravate and prolong the symptoms of acute gout.

As a Combination Drug Product [CD]: This drug is available in combination with colchicine, a drug often used for the treatment of acute gout. Each drug has a different mechanism of action; when used in combination they provide both relief of the acute manifestations of gout and some measure of protection from recurrence of acute attacks.

How This Drug Works: By acting on the tubular systems of the kidney to increase the amount of uric acid excreted in the urine, this drug reduces the levels of uric acid in the blood and body tissues. By acting on the tubular systems of the kidney to decrease the amount of penicillin excreted in the urine, this drug prolongs the presence of penicillin in the blood and helps achieve higher concentrations in body tissues.

Available Dosage Forms and Strengths

Tablets — 500 mg

▷ **Usual Adult Dosage Range:** Antigout: Initially, 250 mg twice/day for 1 week; then 500 mg twice/day. Adjunct to penicillin therapy: 500 mg 4 times/day. **Note: Actual dosage and administration schedule must be determined by the physician for each patient individually.**

▷ **Dosing Instructions:** Take with or following food to reduce stomach irritation. Drink 2.5 to 3 quarts of liquids daily. The tablet may be crushed for administration.

Usual Duration of Use: Continual use on a regular schedule for several months is usually necessary to determine this drug's effectiveness in preventing acute attacks of gout. Long-term use (months to years) requires supervision and periodic evaluation by your physician. Consult your physician on a regular basis.

▷ **This Drug Should Not Be Taken If**
- you have had an allergic reaction to it previously.
- you have active liver disease.
- you have an active blood cell or bone marrow disorder.
- you are experiencing an attack of acute gout at the present time.

▷ **Inform Your Physician Before Taking This Drug If**
- you have a history of kidney disease or kidney stones.
- you have a history of liver disease or impaired liver function.
- you have a history of peptic ulcer disease.
- you have a history of a blood cell or bone marrow disorder.
- you are taking any drug product that contains aspirin or aspirinlike drugs.

Possible Side-Effects (natural, expected and unavoidable drug actions)
Development of kidney stones (composed of uric acid); this is preventable. Consult your physician regarding the use of sodium bicarbonate (or other urine alkalizer) to prevent stone formation.

▷ **Possible Adverse Effects** (unusual, unexpected and infrequent reactions)
If any of the following develop, consult your physician promptly for guidance.
Mild Adverse Effects
Allergic Reactions: Skin rash, itching, drug fever (see Glossary).
Headache, dizziness, flushing of face.
Reduced appetite, sore gums, nausea, vomiting.
Serious Adverse Effects
Allergic Reaction: Anaphylactic reaction (see Glossary).
Idiosyncratic Reaction: Hemolytic anemia (see Glossary).
Bone marrow depression (see Glossary): fatigue, weakness, fever, sore throat, abnormal bleeding or bruising.
Drug-induced liver damage with jaundice (see Glossary).
Drug-induced kidney damage: marked fluid retention, reduced urine formation.

▷ **Possible Effects on Sexual Function:** None reported.

▷ **Adverse Effects That May Mimic Natural Diseases or Disorders**
Liver reactions may suggest viral hepatitis.
Kidney reactions may suggest nephrosis.

Possible Effects on Laboratory Tests
> Complete blood cell counts: decreased red cells, hemoglobin, white cells and platelets.
> Prothrombin time: increased (when taken concurrently with warfarin).
> Blood glucose level: decreased.
> Blood urea nitrogen (BUN) level: increased (kidney damage).
> Blood uric acid level: decreased.
> Liver function tests: increased liver enzymes (ALT/GPT, AST/GOT and alkaline phosphatase), increased bilirubin.
> Urine sugar tests: false positive with Benedict's solution and Clinitest.

CAUTION
> 1. This drug should not be started until 2 to 3 weeks after an acute attack of gout has subsided.
> 2. This drug may increase the frequency of acute attacks of gout during the first few months of treatment. Concurrent use of colchicine is advised to prevent acute attacks. See the Profile of Gout in Section Two.
> 3. Aspirin (and aspirin-containing drug products) can reduce the effectiveness of this drug. Use acetaminophen or a nonaspirin analgesic for pain relief as needed.

Precautions for Use
> *By Infants and Children:* Safety and effectiveness for use by those under 2 years of age have not been established.
> *By Those over 60 Years of Age:* The natural decline in kidney function that occurs after 60 may require adjustment of your dosage. You may be more susceptible to the serious adverse effects of this drug. Report any unusual symptoms promptly for evaluation.

▷ **Advisability of Use During Pregnancy**
> *Pregnancy Category:* C (tentative). See Pregnancy Code inside back cover.
> Animal studies: No information available.
> Human studies: Information from adequate studies of pregnant women is not available.
> This drug has been used during pregnancy with no reports of birth defects or adverse effects on the fetus. Ask your physician for guidance.

Advisability of Use if Breast-Feeding
> Presence of this drug in breast milk: Unknown.
> Avoid drug or refrain from nursing.

Habit-Forming Potential: None.

Effects of Overdosage: Stomach irritation, nausea, vomiting, nervous agitation, delirium, seizures, coma.

Possible Effects of Long-Term Use: Formation of kidney stones. Kidney damage in sensitive individuals.

Suggested Periodic Examinations While Taking This Drug (at physician's discretion)

Complete blood cell counts, measurements of blood uric acid, liver and kidney function tests.

▷ **While Taking This Drug, Observe the Following**

Foods: Follow physician's advice regarding the need for a low-purine diet.

Beverages: A large intake of coffee, tea or cola beverages may reduce the effectiveness of treatment.

▷ *Alcohol:* No interactions expected. However, large amounts of alcohol can raise the blood uric acid level and reduce the effectiveness of treatment.

Tobacco Smoking: No interactions expected.

▷ *Other Drugs*

Probenecid may *increase* the effects of
- clofibrate (Atromid S).
- dyphylline (Neothylline).
- methotrexate (Mexate), and increase its toxicity.
- thiopental (Pentothal), and prolong its anesthetic effect.

Probenecid *taken concurrently* with
- penicillins may cause a threefold to fivefold increase in penicillin blood levels, greatly increasing the effectiveness of each penicillin dose.

The following drugs may *decrease* the effects of probenecid
- aspirin and other salicylates may reduce its effectiveness in promoting the excretion of uric acid.

▷ *Driving, Hazardous Activities:* This drug may cause dizziness. Restrict activities as necessary.

Aviation Note: The use of this drug *may be a disqualification* for piloting. Consult a designated Aviation Medical Examiner.

Exposure to Sun: No restrictions.

Discontinuation: Do not discontinue this drug without consulting your physician.

PROBUCOL
(PROH byu kohl)

Introduced: 1971

Class: Anticholesterol

Prescription: USA: Yes
Canada: Yes

Controlled Drug: USA: No
Canada: No

Available as Generic: USA: No
Canada: No

Brand Name: Lorelco

```
┌─────────────────────────────────────────────────────────────┐
│                   BENEFITS versus RISKS                        │
│                                                                │
│      Possible Benefits              Possible Risks            │
│  EFFECTIVE REDUCTION OF        CONCURRENT REDUCTION            │
│  TOTAL CHOLESTEROL AND         (22% to 25%) OF HIGH           │
│  LOW DENSITY CHOLESTEROL       DENSITY (HDL)                   │
│  IN TYPE IIa CHOLESTEROL       CHOLESTEROL (This is           │
│  DISORDERS (15% to 20%         thought to be undesirable in the│
│  reduction of total cholesterol, prevention and treatment of  │
│  10% to 15% reduction of LDL   atherosclerosis.)              │
│  cholesterol when used in      Diarrhea, indigestion (10%)    │
│  conjunction with a                                            │
│  low-cholesterol diet)                                         │
└─────────────────────────────────────────────────────────────┘
```

▷ **Principal Uses**

As a Single Drug Product: Used for the reduction of abnormally high blood levels of cholesterol (type IIa) that have not responded to adequate control of diet, weight, diabetes and hypothyroidism.

How This Drug Works: Not completely known. It is thought that this drug may inhibit the absorption of dietary cholesterol, may inhibit the early stages of cholesterol production in the liver and may increase the rate of LDL cholesterol destruction and elimination.

Available Dosage Forms and Strengths
Tablets — 250 mg, 500 mg

▷ **Usual Adult Dosage Range:**   250 mg to 500 mg twice daily. **Note: Actual dosage and administration schedule must be determined by the physician for each patient individually.**

▷ **Dosing Instructions:**   Take with the morning and evening meals. The tablet may be crushed for administration.

Usual Duration of Use: Continual use on a regular schedule for 3 to 6 months is usually necessary to determine this drug's effectiveness in lowering cholesterol blood levels. Long-term use (months to years) requires periodic evaluation of response and dosage adjustment. Consult your physician on a regular basis.

▷ **This Drug Should Not Be Taken If**
• you have had an allergic reaction to it previously.
• you have had a heart attack (myocardial infarction) recently.

▷ **Inform Your Physician Before Taking This Drug If**
• you are pregnant.
• you have a history of heart disease, heart rhythm disorder or abnormal electrocardiogram.
• you have impaired liver function or gallstones.

Possible Side-Effects (natural, expected and unavoidable drug actions)
None.

▷ **Possible Adverse Effects** (unusual, unexpected and infrequent reactions)
If any of the following develop, consult your physician promptly for guidance.
Mild Adverse Effects
Allergic Reactions: Rash, itching, swelling (angioedema) of face, mouth, hands or feet.
Headache, dizziness, numbness or tingling in extremities.
Indigestion, excessive gas, abdominal discomfort, nausea, vomiting, diarrhea.
Serious Adverse Effects
Idiosyncratic Reactions: Dizziness, fainting, chest pain, heart palpitations.
Altered electrocardiogram in some individuals.

▷ **Possible Effects on Sexual Function**
Altered timing and pattern of menstruation.
Impotence (rare).

Possible Effects on Laboratory Tests
Blood eosinophil count: increased (allergic reaction).
Blood total cholesterol, HDL and LDL cholesterol levels: decreased.
Blood triglyceride levels: decreased.
Blood uric acid level: increased (in women only).

CAUTION
1. Report promptly the development of chest pain, heart palpitations, dizziness or faintness.
2. Comply fully with all recommendations for periodic measurements of blood cholesterol and triglyceride levels. These are essential to monitoring your response to treatment and determining the need for changes in dosage or medication.

Precautions for Use
By Infants and Children: Safety and effectiveness for use by those under 12 years of age have not been established.
By Those over 60 Years of Age: It is advisable to have an electrocardiogram before starting this drug and at intervals of 6 months until it is determined that there is no drug-induced alteration of heart function.

▷ **Advisability of Use During Pregnancy**
Pregnancy Category: B (tentative). See Pregnancy Code inside back cover.
Animal studies: No drug-induced birth defects found in rodents.
Human studies: Information from adequate studies of pregnant women is not available.
Use this drug only if clearly needed. Because of the long persistence of this drug in body tissues, it is recommended that the drug be discon-

tinued and that birth control be used for 6 months before attempting to establish pregnancy.

The manufacturer does not recommend the use of this drug during pregnancy.

Advisability of Use if Breast-Feeding

Presence of this drug in breast milk: Unknown.

Avoid drug or refrain from nursing.

Habit-Forming Potential: None.

Effects of Overdosage: Abdominal distress, nausea, vomiting, diarrhea.

Possible Effects of Long-Term Use: Decrease in high density (HDL) cholesterol blood levels; increase in triglyceride blood levels.

Suggested Periodic Examinations While Taking This Drug (at physician's discretion)

Measurements of blood levels of total cholesterol, HDL and LDL cholesterol fractions and triglycerides.

Electrocardiograms (selectively).

▷ **While Taking This Drug, Observe the Following**

Foods: Follow the low-cholesterol diet prescribed by your physician.

Beverages: No restrictions.

▷ *Alcohol:* No interactions expected.

Tobacco Smoking: No interactions expected.

▷ *Other Drugs*

Probucol may *decrease* the effects of

• chenodiol (Chenix), and impair its effectiveness in the treatment of gallstones.

▷ *Driving, Hazardous Activities:* This drug may cause dizziness or faintness in sensitive individuals. Restrict activities as necessary.

Aviation Note: The use of this drug *is usually not a disqualification* for piloting. Consult a designated Aviation Medical Examiner.

Exposure to Sun: No restrictions.

Discontinuation: Do not discontinue this drug without your physician's knowledge and guidance. Abrupt withdrawal may be followed by prompt and excessive increase in blood cholesterol levels.

PROCAINAMIDE
(proh kayn A mide)

Introduced: 1950

Prescription: USA: Yes
Canada: Yes

Available as Generic: USA: Yes
Canada: No

Class: Antiarrhythmic

Controlled Drug: USA: No
Canada: No

Brand Names: Procamide SR, Procan SR, Pronestyl, Pronestyl-SR

BENEFITS versus RISKS

Possible Benefits	*Possible Risks*
EFFECTIVE TREATMENT OF SELECTED HEART RHYTHM DISORDERS	NARROW TREATMENT RANGE INDUCTION OF SYSTEMIC LUPUS ERYTHEMATOSUS SYNDROME in 20% of long-term users Provocation of abnormal heart rhythms Blood cell disorders: insufficient white blood cells and platelets

---

▷ **Principal Uses**

As a Single Drug Product: This drug is classified as a Type 1 antiarrhythmic agent, similar to disopyramide and quinidine in its actions. It is used primarily to abolish and prevent the recurrence of premature beats arising in the atria (upper chambers) and the ventricles (lower chambers) of the heart. It is also useful in the treatment and prevention of atrial fibrillation, atrial flutter and abnormally rapid heart rates (tachycardia) that originate in the atria or the ventricles.

How This Drug Works: By slowing the activity of the pacemaker and delaying the transmission of electrical impulses through the conduction system and muscle of the heart, this drug assists in restoring normal heart rate and rhythm.

Available Dosage Forms and Strengths

Capsules — 250 mg, 375 mg, 500 mg
Injections — 100 mg per ml, 500 mg per ml
Tablets — 250 mg, 375 mg, 500 mg
Tablets, prolonged-action — 250 mg, 500 mg, 750 mg, 1000 mg

▷ **Usual Adult Dosage Range:** Dose varies according to indication for use.
Premature atrial or ventricular contractions: 250 to 500 mg/3 hours.
Paroxysmal atrial tachycardia: initially, 1250 mg, followed in 1 hour by

750 mg; then 500 to 1000 mg/2 hours as needed and tolerated. Atrial fibrillation and flutter: the heart should be digitalized first; then initiate procainamide with 1250 mg, followed in 1 hour by 750 mg; follow with 500 to 1000 mg/2 hours as needed and tolerated. For maintenance: 500 to 1000 mg/4 to 6 hours. The total daily dosage should not exceed 6000 mg. **Note: Actual dosage and administration schedule must be determined by the physician for each patient individually.**

▷ **Dosing Instructions:**   Preferably taken on an empty stomach, 1 hour before or 2 hours after eating. However, it may be taken with or following food to reduce stomach irritation. The regular capsules may be opened and the regular tablets may be crushed for administration; however, the prolonged-action tablets should be swallowed whole without alteration.

Usual Duration of Use: Continual use on a regular schedule for 24 to 48 hours is usually necessary to determine this drug's effectiveness in correcting or preventing responsive rhythm disorders. Long-term use requires supervision and periodic evaluation by your physician. Consult your physician on a regular basis.

▷ **This Drug Should Not Be Taken If**
   • you have had an allergic reaction to it previously.
   • you have second-degree or third-degree heart block (determined by electrocardiogram).

▷ **Inform Your Physician Before Taking This Drug If**
   • you are allergic to procaine (Novocain) or to other local anesthetics of the "-caine" drug class, such as those commonly used for glaucoma testing and for dental procedures.
   • you have had any unfavorable reactions to other antiarrhythmic drugs in the past.
   • you have a history of heart disease of any kind, especially "heart block."
   • you have a history of low blood pressure.
   • you have a history of lupus erythematosus.
   • you have a history of abnormally low blood platelet counts from any cause.
   • you have impaired liver or kidney function.
   • you have myasthenia gravis.
   • you have an enlarged prostate gland.
   • you are taking any form of digitalis or any diuretic drug that can cause excessive loss of body potassium (ask physician).
   • you plan to have surgery under general anesthesia in the near future.

Possible Side-Effects (natural, expected and unavoidable drug actions)
Drop in blood pressure in susceptible individuals.

▷ **Possible Adverse Effects** (unusual, unexpected and infrequent reactions)
   If any of the following develop, consult your physician promptly for guidance.

Mild Adverse Effects

Allergic Reactions: Skin rash, hives, itching, drug fever (see Glossary). Weakness, light-headedness.

Loss of appetite, bitter taste, indigestion, nausea, vomiting, diarrhea.

Serious Adverse Effects

Allergic Reactions: Systemic lupus erythematosuslike syndrome: fever, skin eruptions, joint and muscle pains, pleurisy. (This is reported to occur in at least 20% of users.) Idiosyncratic Reactions: Mental depression, hallucinations, psychotic behavior, hemolytic anemia (see Glossary).

Severe drop in blood pressure, fainting.

Asthmalike breathing difficulties.

Induction of new heart rhythm disturbances.

Inability to empty urinary bladder, prostatism (see Glossary).

Blood cell disorders: abnormally low white blood cell count, causing fever, sore throat, infections; abnormally low blood platelet count, causing abnormal bleeding or bruising.

▷ **Possible Effects on Sexual Function:**   None reported.

▷ **Adverse Effects That May Mimic Natural Diseases or Disorders**

Rare liver reaction may suggest viral hepatitis.

Natural Diseases or Disorders That May Be Activated by This Drug

Systemic lupus erythematosus, myasthenia gravis.

Possible Effects on Laboratory Tests

Complete blood cell counts: decreased red cells, hemoglobin, white cells and platelets; increased eosinophils.

Blood lupus erythematosus (LE) cells: positive.

Blood antinuclear antibodies (ANA): positive (in 50–80% of those using drug after 3 to 6 months).

Liver function tests: increased liver enzymes (ALT/GPT, AST/GOT and alkaline phosphatase), increased bilirubin.

Urine screening tests for drug abuse: *initial* test result may be falsely **positive**; *confirmatory* test result will be **negative.** (Test results depend upon amount of drug taken and testing method used.)

CAUTION

1. Thorough evaluation of your heart function (including electrocardiograms) is necessary prior to using this drug.
2. Periodic evaluation of your heart function is necessary to determine your response to this drug. Some individuals may experience worsening of their heart rhythm disorder and/or deterioration of heart function. Close monitoring of heart rate, rhythm and overall performance is essential.
3. Dosage must be adjusted carefully for each individual. Do not change your dosage without the knowledge and supervision of your physician.

4. Do not take any other antiarrhythmic drug while taking this drug unless directed to do so by your physician.

Precautions for Use
By Infants and Children: Blood cell counts should be monitored for loss of white blood cells.

By Those over 60 Years of Age: Reduced kidney function may require reduction in dosage. Observe carefully for light-headedness, dizziness, unsteadiness and tendency to fall.

▷ **Advisability of Use During Pregnancy**
Pregnancy Category: C (tentative). See Pregnancy Code inside back cover.
Animal studies: No information available.
Human studies: Information from adequate studies of pregnant women is not available.
Use this drug only if clearly needed.

Advisability of Use if Breast-Feeding
Presence of this drug in breast milk: Unknown.
Avoid drug or refrain from nursing.

Habit-Forming Potential: None.

Effects of Overdosage: Loss of appetite, nausea, vomiting, weakness, faintness, irregular heart rhythm, stupor, circulatory collapse, heart arrest.

Possible Effects of Long-Term Use: Lupus erythematosuslike syndrome (see above).

Suggested Periodic Examinations While Taking This Drug (at physician's discretion)
Complete blood cell counts.
Blood tests for the development of lupus erythematosus (LE) cells and antinuclear antibodies.
Electrocardiograms to monitor the full effect of this drug on the mechanisms that influence heart rate and rhythm.

▷ **While Taking This Drug, Observe the Following**
Foods: No restrictions.
Beverages: Avoid excessive intake of coffee, tea and cola beverages. Avoid iced drinks. May be taken with milk.
▷ *Alcohol:* Use caution until the combined effects have been determined. Alcohol can increase the blood-pressure-lowering effects of this drug.
Tobacco Smoking: Nicotine can cause irritability of the heart and reduce the effectiveness of this drug. Follow physician's advice regarding smoking.
▷ *Other Drugs*
Procainamide may *increase* the effects of
• antihypertensive drugs, and cause excessive lowering of blood pressure.

The following drugs may *increase* the effects of procainamide
- amiodirone.
- cimetidine (Tagamet).

▷ *Driving, Hazardous Activities:* This drug may cause dizziness or weakness. Restrict activities as necessary.

Aviation Note: The use of this drug *may be a disqualification* for piloting. Consult a designated Aviation Medical Examiner.

Exposure to Sun: No restrictions.

Exposure to Heat: Use caution. Hot environments are conducive to lower blood pressure.

Occurrence of Unrelated Illness: Disorders that cause vomiting, diarrhea or dehydration can affect this drug's action adversely. Report such developments promptly.

Discontinuation: This drug should not be discontinued abruptly following long-term use. Ask your physician for guidance regarding gradual dose reduction.

PROCHLORPERAZINE
(proh klor PER a zeen)

Introduced: 1956

Class: Strong tranquilizer, antiemetic, phenothiazines

Prescription: USA: Yes
Canada: Yes

Controlled Drug: USA: No
Canada: No

Available as Generic: USA: Yes
Canada: No

Brand Names: ✦Combid [CD], Compazine, ✦Stemetil

BENEFITS versus RISKS

Possible Benefits	*Possible Risks*
EFFECTIVE CONTROL OF ACUTE MENTAL DISORDERS in the majority of patients: beneficial effects on thinking, mood and behavior	SERIOUS TOXIC EFFECTS ON BRAIN with long-term use
EFFECTIVE CONTROL OF NAUSEA AND VOMITING	Liver damage with jaundice (infrequent)
Relief of anxiety and nervous tension	Rare blood cell disorders: abnormally low white cell and platelet counts

---

▷ **Principal Uses**

As a Single Drug Product: This member of the phenothiazine class is used primarily to relieve severe nausea and vomiting. Although it has sedative and antipsychotic effects characteristic of this class, it is used less often as a major tranquilizer.

How This Drug Works: Not completely established. Present theory is that by inhibiting the action of dopamine, this drug acts to correct an imbalance of nerve impulse transmissions that is thought to be responsible for certain mental disorders. By blocking the action of dopamine in the chemoreceptor trigger zone of the brain, this drug prevents excessive stimulation of the vomiting center.

Available Dosage Forms and Strengths
Capsules, prolonged-action — 10 mg, 15 mg, 30 mg
Injection — 5 mg per ml
Suppositories — 2.5 mg, 5 mg, 25 mg
Syrup — 5 mg per 5-ml teaspoonful
Tablets — 5 mg, 10 mg, 25 mg

▷ **Usual Adult Dosage Range:**   Initially, 5 mg/6 to 8 hours. If needed and tolerated, dose may be increased by 5 mg at intervals of 3 to 4 days. Usual range is 35 to 60 mg/24 hours. The total daily dosage should not exceed 150 mg. **Note: Actual dosage and administration schedule must be determined by the physician for each patient individually.**

▷ **Dosing Instructions:**   May be taken with or following food to reduce stomach irritation. The tablets may be crushed for administration. Prolonged-action capsules should be swallowed whole without alteration.

Duration of Use: Continual use on a regular schedule for 12 to 24 hours is usually necessary to determine this drug's effectiveness in controlling nausea and vomiting. If used for severe anxiety-tension states or acute psychotic behavior, a trial of several weeks is usually necessary to determine effectiveness. If not significantly beneficial within 6 weeks, it should be discontinued. Consult your physician on a regular basis.

▷ **This Drug Should Not Be Taken If**
  • you have had an allergic reaction to it previously.
  • you have active liver disease.
  • you have cancer of the breast.
  • you have a current blood cell or bone marrow disorder.

▷ **Inform Your Physician Before Taking This Drug If**
  • you are allergic or abnormally sensitive to any phenothiazine drug (see Drug Class, Section Four).
  • you have impaired liver or kidney function.
  • you have any type of seizure disorder.
  • you have diabetes, glaucoma or heart disease.
  • you have a history of lupus erythematosus.
  • you are taking any drug with sedative effects.
  • you plan to have surgery under general or spinal anesthesia in the near future.

Possible Side-Effects (natural, expected and unavoidable drug actions)
Drowsiness (usually during the first 2 weeks), orthostatic hypotension (see Glossary), blurred vision, dry mouth, nasal congestion, constipation, impaired urination.
Pink or purple coloration of urine, of no significance.

▷ **Possible Adverse Effects** (unusual, unexpected and infrequent reactions)
If any of the following develop, consult your physician promptly for guidance.
Mild Adverse Effects
Allergic Reactions: Skin rash, hives, low-grade fever.
Lowering of body temperature, especially in the elderly. (See Hypothermia in Glossary.)
Increased appetite and weight gain.
Dizziness, weakness, agitation, insomnia, impaired day and night vision.
Chronic constipation, fecal impaction.
Serious Adverse Effects
Allergic Reactions: Hepatitis with jaundice (see Glossary), usually between second and fourth week; high fever; asthma; anaphylactic reaction (see Glossary).
Idiosyncratic Reactions: Toxic dermatitis. Neuroleptic malignant syndrome (see Glossary).
Depression, disorientation, seizures.
Disturbances of heart rhythm, rapid heart rate.
Bone marrow depression (see Glossary): fever, sore throat, abnormal bleeding or bruising.
Parkinson-like disorders (see Glossary); muscle spasms of face, jaw, neck, back, extremities; extreme restlessness; slowed movements, muscle rigidity, tremors; tardive dyskinesias (see Glossary).

▷ **Possible Effects on Sexual Function**
Altered timing and pattern of menstruation.
Female breast enlargement with milk production.
Male breast enlargement and tenderness.
Inhibited ejaculation; priapism (see Glossary).
Causes false positive pregnancy test result.

▷ **Adverse Effects That May Mimic Natural Diseases or Disorders**
Nervous system reactions may suggest Parkinson's disease.
Liver reactions may suggest viral hepatitis.
Reactions resembling systemic lupus erythematosus can occur.

Natural Diseases or Disorders That May Be Activated by This Drug
Latent epilepsy, glaucoma, diabetes mellitus, prostatism (see Glossary).

Possible Effects on Laboratory Tests
White blood cell count: decreased.
Liver function tests: increased liver enzymes (ALT/GPT, AST/GOT and alkaline phosphatase), increased bilirubin.

CAUTION
1. Many over-the-counter medications (see OTC Drugs in Glossary) for allergies, colds and coughs contain drugs that can interact unfavorably with this drug. Ask your physician or pharmacist for guidance before using any such medications.
2. Antacids that contain aluminum and/or magnesium can prevent the absorption of this drug and reduce its effectiveness.
3. Obtain prompt evaluation of any change or disturbance of vision.

Precautions for Use

By Infants and Children: Do not use this drug in infants under 2 years of age, or in children of any age with symptoms suggestive of Reye syndrome (see Glossary). Children with acute illnesses ("flulike" infections, measles, chicken pox, etc.) are very susceptible to adverse effects when this drug is given to control nausea and vomiting.

By Those over 60 Years of Age: Small doses are advisable until individual response has been determined. You may be more susceptible to the development of drowsiness, lethargy, constipation, lowering of body temperature (hypothermia) and orthostatic hypotension (see Glossary). This drug can enhance existing prostatism (see Glossary). You may also be more susceptible to the development of Parkinson-like reactions and/or tardive dyskinesia (see discussion of these terms in Glossary). These reactions must be recognized early since they may become unresponsive to treatment and irreversible.

▷ ## Advisability of Use During Pregnancy

Pregnancy Category: C (tentative). See Pregnancy Code inside back cover.
Animal studies: Cleft palate reported in mouse and rat studies.
Human studies: No increase in birth defects reported in 2023 exposures. Information from adequate studies of pregnant women is not available.
Limit use to small and infrequent doses. Avoid drug during the last month because of possible effects on the newborn infant.

Advisability of Use if Breast-Feeding

Presence of this drug in breast milk: Yes, in small amounts.
Monitor nursing infant closely and discontinue drug or nursing if adverse effects develop.

Habit-Forming Potential: None.

Effects of Overdosage: Marked drowsiness, weakness, tremor, agitation, unsteadiness, deep sleep, coma, convulsions.

Possible Effects of Long-Term Use: Tardive dyskinesias. Eye changes: opacities in cornea or lens, retinal pigmentation.

Suggested Periodic Examinations While Taking This Drug (at physician's discretion)
Complete blood cell counts, especially between the fourth and tenth weeks of treatment.

Liver function tests, electrocardiograms.

Complete eye examinations—eye structures and vision.

Careful inspection of the tongue for early evidence of fine, involuntary, wavelike movements that could indicate the beginning of tardive dyskinesia.

▷ **While Taking This Drug, Observe the Following**

Foods: No restrictions.

Nutritional Support: A riboflavin (vitamin B-2) supplement should be taken with long-term use.

Beverages: No restrictions. May be taken with milk.

▷ *Alcohol:* Avoid completely. Alcohol can increase the sedative action of phenothiazines and accentuate their depressant effects on brain function and blood pressure. Phenothiazines can increase the intoxicating effects of alcohol.

Tobacco Smoking: Possible reduction of drowsiness from drug.

Marijuana Smoking: Moderate increase in drowsiness; accentuation of orthostatic hypotension; increased risk of precipitating latent psychoses, confusing the interpretation of mental status and drug responses.

▷ *Other Drugs*

Prochlorperazine may *increase* the effects of

• all sedative drugs, especially meperidine (Demerol), and cause excessive sedation.

• all atropinelike drugs, and cause nervous system toxicity.

Prochlorperazine may *decrease* the effects of

• guanethidine (Ismelin, Esimil), and reduce its effectiveness in lowering blood pressure.

Prochlorperazine *taken concurrently* with

• propranolol (Inderal) may cause increased effects of both drugs; monitor drug effects closely and adjust dosages as necessary.

The following drugs may *decrease* the effects of prochlorperazine

• antacids containing aluminum and/or magnesium.

• benztropine (Cogentin).

• trihexyphenidyl (Artane).

▷ *Driving, Hazardous Activities:* This drug can impair mental alertness, judgment and physical coordination. Avoid hazardous activities.

Aviation Note: The use of this drug *is a disqualification* for piloting. Consult a designated Aviation Medical Examiner.

Exposure to Sun: Use caution until sensitivity has been determined. Some phenothiazines can cause photosensitivity (see Glossary).

Exposure to Heat: Use caution and avoid excessive heat as much as possible. This drug may impair the regulation of body temperature and increase the risk of heat stroke.

Exposure to Cold: Use caution and dress warmly. This drug can increase the risk of hypothermia in the elderly.

Discontinuation: After a period of long-term use, do not discontinue this drug suddenly. Gradual withdrawal over 2 to 3 weeks under physician supervision is recommended.

PROMETHAZINE
(proh METH a zeen)

Introduced: 1945

Class: Antiemetic, antihistamines, phenothiazines

Prescription: USA: Yes
Canada: No

Controlled Drug: USA: No
Canada: No

Available as Generic: USA: Yes
Canada: Yes

Brand Names: ✦Histanil, K-Phen, Pentazine, Phenergan, Phenergan-D [CD], Phenergan w/Codeine [CD], ✦PMS Promethazine, Prorex

---

BENEFITS versus RISKS

Possible Benefits	*Possible Risks*
EFFECTIVE SYMPTOMATIC RELIEF OF ALLERGIC RHINITIS AND DERMATOSIS	EXCESSIVE SEDATION in sensitive individuals
Moderately effective prevention and treatment of motion sickness, nausea and vomiting	Atropinelike effects
Effective as mild sedative and hypnotic	Rare blood cell disorders: abnormally low white cell and platelet counts

---

▷ **Principal Uses**

As a Single Drug Product: This versatile drug shares the characteristics of two major drug classes, the antihistamines and the phenothiazines. It is used to provide symptomatic relief in allergic disorders (hay fever, hives, etc.), to control nausea and vomiting and to produce mild sedation.

As a Combination Drug Product [CD]: This drug is often combined with analgesics such as aspirin or codeine to enhance their pain-relieving action by producing mild sedation. It is also used in cough mixtures for its drying (antihistaminic) effect.

How This Drug Works: Not completely established. This drug reduces the intensity of the allergic response by blocking the action of histamine after it has been released from sensitized tissue cells. It reduces the sensitivity of the nerve endings in the labyrinth (inner ear) and blocks the transmission of excessive nerve impulses to the vomiting center in the brain. The way this drug produces sedation and light sleep is not known.

Available Dosage Forms and Strengths

Injections — 25 mg per ml, 50 mg per ml
Suppositories — 12.5 mg, 25 mg, 50 mg

　　　　Syrups — 6.25 mg per 5-ml teaspoonful (alcohol 7%), 25 mg per
　　　　　5-ml teaspoonful (alcohol 1.5%)
　　　Tablets — 12.5 mg, 25 mg, 50 mg

▷ **Usual Adult Dosage Range:**　12.5 to 25 mg/4 to 6 hours as needed. The total
daily dosage should not exceed 150 mg. **Note: Actual dosage and administration schedule must be determined by the physician for each
patient individually.**

▷ **Dosing Instructions:**　Preferably taken with or following food to reduce
stomach irritation. The tablets may be crushed for administration.

Usual Duration of Use:　Continual use on a regular schedule for 3 to 5 days
is usually necessary to determine this drug's effectiveness in relieving
allergic symptoms or controlling vomiting. If not effective within 5
days, it should be discontinued.

▷ **This Drug Should Not Be Taken If**
　• you have had an allergic reaction to it previously.
　• you have a blood cell or bone marrow disorder.
　• you have narrow-angle glaucoma (not adequately treated).

▷ **Inform Your Physician Before Taking This Drug If**
　• you are allergic or overly sensitive to any phenothiazine drug (see Drug
　　Class, Section Four).
　• you are taking any drugs with sedative effects.
　• you have a seizure disorder or bronchial asthma.
　• you have impaired liver function.
　• you have a history of peptic ulcer disease.
　• you have an enlarged prostate gland or prostatism (see Glossary).

Possible Side-Effects (natural, expected and unavoidable drug actions)
　Drowsiness (25% of users), lethargy, impaired concentration, dry mouth,
　constipation, impaired urination, reduced tolerance for contact lenses.

▷ **Possible Adverse Effects** (unusual, unexpected and infrequent reactions)
　**If any of the following develop, consult your physician promptly for
　guidance.**
　Mild Adverse Effects
　Allergic Reactions: Skin rash, hives.
　Headache, dizziness, unsteadiness, confusion, nervousness, excitation,
　　irritability, tremor, insomnia, numbness and tingling, blurred vision,
　　double vision, ringing in ears.
　Loss of appetite, stomach irritation, nausea, vomiting, diarrhea.
　Rapid heart rate, palpitation, low blood pressure.
　Chest tightness, asthmatic wheezing, thickening of bronchial secretions.
　Serious Adverse Effects
　Allergic Reactions: Drug-induced hepatitis with jaundice (see Glossary).
　Idiosyncratic Reactions: Euphoria, hysteria.

Nervous system reactions: Muscle spasms of the face, neck, back and extremities: rolling of the eyes, twisting of the neck, arching of the back, spasms of the hands and feet.

Blood cell disorders: abnormally low white blood cell and blood platelet counts, causing fever, sore throat, infections, abnormal bleeding or bruising (all very rare).

▷ **Possible Effects on Sexual Function:** None reported.

▷ **Adverse Effects That May Mimic Natural Diseases or Disorders**
Drug-induced hepatitis may suggest viral hepatitis.

Natural Diseases or Disorders That May Be Activated by This Drug
Latent epilepsy, glaucoma, prostatism (see Glossary).

Possible Effects on Laboratory Tests
White blood cell count: decreased.
Liver function tests: increased liver enzymes (ALT/GPT, AST/GOT and alkaline phosphatase), increased bilirubin.
Urine pregnancy tests: false positive result with Gravindex; false negative result with Prepuerin and Pap-test.

CAUTION
1. This drug should not be used alone to treat symptoms of lower respiratory tract disease, including asthma.
2. Avoid this drug for at least 5 days before skin testing for possible allergens.

Precautions for Use
By Infants and Children: This drug should not be used in premature or full-term newborn infants. The young child is especially sensitive to the nervous system effects of antihistamines and phenothiazines. Children with acute illnesses ("flulike" infections, measles, chicken pox, etc.) are very susceptible to muscular spasms of the face, neck, back or extremities when this drug is used to control nausea and vomiting. Avoid this drug completely during such infections; there is evidence to suggest that it may contribute to the development of Reye syndrome (see Glossary).

By Those over 60 Years of Age: You may be more susceptible to the development of drowsiness, dizziness and lethargy and to impaired thinking, judgment and memory. The sedative effect of this drug can cause a hypoactive syndrome that may be misinterpreted as senility or emotional depression. This drug can increase the symptoms of prostatism (see Glossary).

▷ **Advisability of Use During Pregnancy**
Pregnancy Category: B (tentative). See Pregnancy Code inside back cover.
Animal studies: No birth defects reported in rats.

Human studies: No significant increase in birth defects reported in 746 exposures to this drug.

Avoid use of this drug during the last 3 months; it can reduce certain blood clotting factors in the fetus and cause bleeding in the newborn infant.

Advisability of Use if Breast-Feeding
Presence of this drug in breast milk: Yes.
Avoid drug or refrain from nursing.

Habit-Forming Potential: None.

Effects of Overdosage: Marked drowsiness, weakness, unsteadiness, agitation, delirium, deep sleep, coma, seizures.

Possible Effects of Long-Term Use: The development of tolerance and loss of effectiveness.

Suggested Periodic Examinations While Taking This Drug (at physician's discretion)
Complete blood cell counts.

▷ **While Taking This Drug, Observe the Following**
Foods: No restrictions.
Beverages: No restrictions. May be taken with milk.
▷ *Alcohol:* Use extreme caution until the combined effects have been determined. The combination of alcohol and antihistamines can cause rapid and marked sedation.
Tobacco Smoking: No interactions expected.
▷ *Other Drugs*
Promethazine may *increase* the effects of
• all sedative drugs, and cause excessive sedation.
• atropine and atropinelike drugs (see Drug Class, Section Four).
▷ *Driving, Hazardous Activities:* This drug may cause dizziness or drowsiness. Restrict activities as necessary.
Aviation Note: The use of this drug *is a disqualification* for piloting. Consult a designated Aviation Medical Examiner.
Exposure to Sun: Use caution until sensitivity has been determined. This drug may cause photosensitivity (see Glossary).

PROPOXYPHENE
(proh POX i feen)

Introduced: 1955

Class: Analgesic, narcotic

Prescription: USA: Yes
Canada: Yes

Controlled Drug: USA: C-IV*
Canada: <N>

Available as Generic: Yes

Brand Names: Darvocet-N 50/100 [CD], Darvon, Darvon-N, Darvon w/ASA [CD], Darvon Compound [CD], Darvon Compound-65 [CD], Darvon-N w/ASA [CD], ✦Darvon-N Compound [CD], Dolene, Dolene AP-65 [CD], Dolene Compound-65 [CD], E-Lor [CD], ✦Novopropoxyn, ✦Novopropoxyn Compound [CD], Propacet-100 [CD], ✦642, Wygesic [CD]

BENEFITS versus RISKS

Possible Benefits	*Possible Risks*
EFFECTIVE RELIEF OF MILD TO MODERATE PAIN	POTENTIAL FOR HABIT FORMATION (DEPENDENCE)
	Sedative effects
	Drug-induced hepatitis (very rare)

▷ **Principal Uses**

As a Single Drug Product: This drug is used exclusively as an analgesic to relieve mild to moderate pain.

As a Combination Drug Product [CD]: It is available in combinations with acetaminophen and with aspirin. These milder pain relievers are added to enhance the analgesic effect and to reduce fever when present. Some combinations also contain caffeine to counteract the sedative effects of the analgesics.

How This Drug Works: Acting primarily as a depressant of certain brain functions, this drug suppresses the perception of pain and calms the emotional response to pain.

Available Dosage Forms and Strengths

Capsules — 32 mg, 65 mg
Oral suspension — 50 mg per 5-ml teaspoonful
Tablets — 100 mg

▷ **Usual Adult Dosage Range:** For propoxyphene: 65 mg/4 hours as needed. The total daily dosage should not exceed 390 mg. For propoxyphene napsylate (Darvon-N): 100 mg/4 hours as needed. The total daily dose should not exceed 600 mg. **Note: Actual dosage and administration schedule must be determined by the physician for each patient individually.**

*See Schedules of Controlled Drugs inside back cover.

▷ **Dosing Instructions:**   May be taken with or following food to reduce stomach irritation or nausea. The tablet may be crushed and the capsule may be opened for administration.

Usual Duration of Use: As required to control pain. Continual use should not exceed 5 to 7 days without interruption and reassessment of need.

▷ **This Drug Should Not Be Taken If**
- you have had an allergic reaction to any dosage form of it previously.
- you are having an acute attack of asthma.

▷ **Inform Your Physician Before Taking This Drug If**
- you have had an unfavorable reaction to any narcotic drug in the past.
- you have a history of drug abuse or alcoholism.
- you have chronic lung disease with impaired breathing.
- you have impaired liver or kidney function.
- you are taking any other drugs that have a sedative effect.

Possible Side-Effects (natural, expected and unavoidable drug actions)
Drowsiness, light-headedness, constipation.

▷ **Possible Adverse Effects** (unusual, unexpected and infrequent reactions)
If any of the following develop, consult your physician promptly for guidance.
Mild Adverse Effects
Allergic Reactions: Skin rash, itching.
Headache, dizziness, weakness, confusion, blurred vision.
Nausea, vomiting, abdominal discomfort.
Serious Adverse Effects
Allergic Reactions: Hepatitis with jaundice (see Glossary).
Paradoxical excitement, agitation, insomnia.

▷ **Possible Effects on Sexual Function:**   None reported.

Possible Effects on Laboratory Tests
Liver function tests: increased liver enzymes (ALT/GPT, AST/GOT and alkaline phosphatase), increased bilirubin.
Urine sugar tests: no effect with TesTape; false low results with Clinistix and Diastix.
Urine screening tests for drug abuse: may be **positive**. (Test results depend upon amount of drug taken and testing method used.)

▷ **Precautions for Use**
By Infants and Children: Safety and effectiveness for use by those under 12 years of age have not been established.
By Those over 60 Years of Age: Use small doses initially and increase dosage as needed and tolerated. Limit use to short-term treatment only. There may be increased susceptibility to the development of drowsiness, dizziness, unsteadiness, falling and constipation (possibly leading to fecal impaction).

▷ **Advisability of Use During Pregnancy**
Pregnancy Category: C (tentative). See Pregnancy Code inside back cover.
Animal studies: No birth defects due to this drug were found.
Human studies: Information from studies of pregnant women indicates
no significant increase in birth defects in 2914 exposures to this drug.
Use this drug only if clearly needed and in small, infrequent doses.

Advisability of Use if Breast-Feeding
Presence of this drug in breast milk: Yes, in small amounts.
Monitor nursing infant closely and discontinue drug or nursing if adverse effects develop.

Habit-Forming Potential: Psychological and/or physical dependence can
develop with use of large doses for an extended period of time.

Effects of Overdosage: Drowsiness, restlessness, agitation, nausea, vomiting, dry mouth, vertigo, weakness, lethargy, stupor, coma, seizures.

Possible Effects of Long-Term Use: Psychological and physical dependence, chronic constipation.

Suggested Periodic Examinations While Taking This Drug (at physician's
discretion)
None.

▷ **While Taking This Drug, Observe the Following**
Foods: No restrictions.
Beverages: No restrictions. May be taken with milk.
▷ *Alcohol:* Use extreme caution until the combined effects have been determined. Propoxyphene can intensify the intoxicating effects of alcohol,
and alcohol can intensify the depressant effects of propoxyphene on
brain function.
Tobacco Smoking: Heavy smoking may reduce the effectiveness of this
drug.
Marijuana Smoking: Increase in drowsiness and pain relief; impairment of
mental and physical performance.
▷ *Other Drugs*
Propoxyphene may ***increase*** the effects of
• other drugs with sedative effects.
• oral anticoagulants (Coumadin, etc.), and increase the risk of bleeding.
• carbamazepine (Tegretol), and increase its toxicity.
• doxepin (Sinequan), and increase its toxicity.
▷ *Driving, Hazardous Activities:* This drug can impair mental alertness, judgment, reaction time and physical coordination. Avoid hazardous activities accordingly.
Aviation Note: The use of this drug ***is a disqualification*** for piloting.
Consult a designated Aviation Medical Examiner.
Exposure to Sun: No restrictions.

Discontinuation: It is advisable to limit this drug to short-term use. If it is necessary to use it for extended periods of time, discontinuation should be gradual to minimize possible effects of withdrawal.

PROPRANOLOL
(proh PRAN oh lohl)

Introduced: 1966

Class: Antianginal, antiarrhythmic, antihypertensive, migraine preventive, beta-adrenergic blocker

Prescription: USA: Yes
  Canada: Yes

Controlled Drug: USA: No
  Canada: No

Available as Generic: Yes

Brand Names: ✦Apo-Propranolol, ✦Detensol, Inderal, Inderal-LA, Inderide [CD], Inderide LA [CD], Ipran, ✦Novopranol, ✦PMS Propranolol

---

BENEFITS versus RISKS

Possible Benefits	*Possible Risks*
EFFECTIVE, WELL-TOLERATED AS: ANTIANGINAL DRUG in effort-induced angina; ANTIARRHYTHMIC DRUG in certain heart rhythm disorders; ANTIHYPERTENSIVE DRUG in mild to moderate hypertension EFFECTIVE PREVENTION OF MIGRAINE HEADACHES Effective adjunct in the prevention of recurrent heart attack (myocardial infarction) Effective adjunct in the management of pheochromocytoma	CONGESTIVE HEART FAILURE in advanced heart disease Worsening of angina in coronary heart disease (if drug is abruptly withdrawn) Masking of low blood sugar (hypoglycemia) in drug-treated diabetes Provocation of asthma Rare blood cell disorders: low white cell and platelet counts

---

▷ **Principal Uses**

As a Single Drug Product: This first beta blocker drug is used primarily to treat several serious cardiovascular disorders: classical effort-induced angina, certain types of heart rhythm disturbance and high blood pressure. It is also beneficial in preventing the recurrence of heart attacks (myocardial infarction). In addition, it is used to reduce the frequency and severity of migraine headaches. Other uses (not "officially approved" at this time) include the control of physical manifestations of anxiety and nervous tension (as in stage fright), the control of familial tremors and the control of symptoms associated with markedly overactive thyroid gland function (thyrotoxicosis).

As a Combination Drug Product [CD]: This drug is available in combination with hydrochlorothiazide for the treatment of hypertension. This combination product includes two "step 1" drugs with different mechanisms of action; it is intended to provide greater effectiveness and convenience for long-term use.

How This Drug Works: By blocking certain actions of the sympathetic nervous system, this drug
- reduces the rate and contraction force of the heart, thus lowering the ejection pressure of the blood leaving the heart and reducing the oxygen requirement for heart function.
- reduces the degree of contraction of blood vessel walls, resulting in their relaxation and expansion and consequent lowering of blood pressure.
- prolongs the conduction time of nerve impulses through the heart, of benefit in the management of certain heart rhythm disorders.

Available Dosage Forms and Strengths
Capsules, prolonged-action — 60 mg, 80 mg, 120 mg, 160 mg
Concentrate — 80 mg/ml
Injection — 1 mg per ml
Oral solution — 4 mg/ml, 8 mg/ml
Tablets — 10 mg, 20 mg, 40 mg, 60 mg, 80 mg, 90 mg

▷ **Usual Adult Dosage Range:** Varies with indication.
Antianginal: Initially, 10 to 20 mg 3 or 4 times/day; increase dose gradually every 3 to 7 days as needed and tolerated. The total daily dosage should not exceed 320 mg.
Antiarrhythmic: 10 to 30 mg 3 or 4 times/day as needed and tolerated.
Antihypertensive: Initially, 40 mg twice/day; increase dose gradually as needed and tolerated. The total daily dosage should not exceed 640 mg.
Migraine headache prevention: Initially, 20 mg 4 times/day; increase dose gradually as needed and tolerated. The total daily dosage should not exceed 240 mg.**Note: Actual dosage and administration schedule must be determined by the physician for each patient individually.**

▷ **Dosing Instructions:** Preferably taken 1 hour before eating to maximize absorption. The tablet may be crushed for administration; to prevent harmless possible numbing effect, mix with soft food and swallow promptly. The prolonged-action capsules should be swallowed whole without alteration. Do not discontinue this drug abruptly.

Usual Duration of Use: Continual use on a regular schedule for 10 to 14 days is usually necessary to determine this drug's effectiveness in preventing angina, controlling heart rhythm disorders and lowering blood pressure. Maximal effectiveness may require continual use for 6 to 8 weeks. The long-term use of this drug (months to years) will be determined by the course of your symptoms over time and your response to the overall treatment program (weight reduction, salt restriction, smoking cessation, etc.). Consult your physician on a regular basis.

▷ **This Drug Should Not Be Taken If**
  • you have had an allergic reaction to it previously.
  • you have Prinzmetal's variant angina (coronary artery spasm).
  • you have congestive heart failure.
  • you have an abnormally slow heart rate or a serious form of heart block.
  • you are taking, or have taken within the past 14 days, any monoamine oxidase (MAO) type A inhibitor drug (see Drug Class, Section Four).

▷ **Inform Your Physician Before Taking This Drug If**
  • you have had an adverse reaction to any beta blocker drug in the past (see Drug Class, Section Four).
  • you have a history of serious heart disease, with or without episodes of heart failure.
  • you have a history of hay fever (allergic rhinitis), asthma, chronic bronchitis or emphysema.
  • you have a history of overactive thyroid function (hyperthyroidism).
  • you have a history of low blood sugar (hypoglycemia).
  • you have impaired liver or kidney function.
  • you have diabetes or myasthenia gravis.
  • you are currently taking any form of digitalis, quinidine or reserpine, or any calcium blocker drug (see Drug Class, Section Four).
  • you plan to have surgery under general anesthesia in the near future.

Possible Side-Effects (natural, expected and unavoidable drug actions)
  Lethargy and fatigability, cold extremities, slow heart rate, light-headedness in upright position (see orthostatic hypotension in Glossary).

▷ **Possible Adverse Effects** (unusual, unexpected and infrequent reactions)
  If any of the following develop, consult your physician promptly for guidance.
  Mild Adverse Effects
  Allergic Reactions: Skin rash, temporary loss of hair, drug fever (see Glossary).
  Headache, dizziness, insomnia, vivid dreams.
  Indigestion, nausea, vomiting, diarrhea.
  Serious Adverse Effects
  Idiosyncratic Reactions: Acute behavioral disturbances: disorientation, confusion, hallucinations, amnesia.
  Mental depression, anxiety.
  Chest pain, shortness of breath, precipitation of congestive heart failure.
  Induction of bronchial asthma (in asthmatic individuals).
  Rare blood cell disorders: abnormally low white blood cell count, causing fever and sore throat; abnormally low blood platelet count, causing abnormal bleeding or bruising.

▷ **Possible Effects on Sexual Function**

Decreased libido; impaired erection (28%); impotence (15%).
This drug has been found to have the highest incidence of libido reduction and erectile impairment of all beta blocker drugs.
Male infertility (inhibited sperm motility); Peyronie's disease (see Glossary).

▷ **Adverse Effects That May Mimic Natural Diseases or Disorders**

Reduced blood flow to extremities may resemble Raynaud's phenomenon (see Glossary).

Natural Diseases or Disorders That May Be Activated by This Drug

Prinzmetal's variant angina, Raynaud's disease, intermittent claudication, myasthenia gravis (questionable).

Possible Effects on Laboratory Tests

White blood cell count: occasionally decreased.
Blood platelet count: increased or decreased.
Bleeding time: increased.
Blood total cholesterol level: no effect in some; increased in others.
Blood HDL cholesterol level: no effect in some; decreased in others.
Blood LDL cholesterol level: no effect in some; increased and decreased in others.
Blood VLDL cholesterol level: no effect in some; increased in others.
Blood triglyceride levels: no effect in some; increased in others.
Blood glucose level: no effect in some; increased and decreased in others.
Glucose tolerance test (GTT): decreased.
Blood thyroid hormone levels: T^3—no effect in some, decreased in others; T^4—increased; free T^4—increased.
Blood uric acid level: no effect in some; increased in others.
Liver function tests: increased liver enzymes (ALT/GPT, AST/GOT and alkaline phosphatase); effects probably not due to liver damage.

CAUTION

1. ***Do not discontinue this drug suddenly*** without the knowledge and guidance of your physician. Carry a notation on your person that you are taking this drug.
2. Consult your physician or pharmacist before using nasal decongestants usually present in over-the-counter cold preparations and nose drops. These can cause sudden increases in blood pressure when taken concurrently with beta blocker drugs.
3. Report the development of any tendency to emotional depression.

Precautions for Use

By Infants and Children: Safety and effectiveness for use by those under 12 years of age have not been established. However, if this drug is used, observe for the development of low blood sugar (hypoglycemia) during periods of reduced food intake.
By Those over 60 Years of Age: Proceed ***cautiously*** with all antihypertensive drugs. Unacceptably high blood pressure should be reduced without

creating the risks associated with excessively low blood pressure. Start treatment with small doses, and monitor the blood pressure response frequently. Sudden, rapid and excessive reduction of blood pressure can predispose to stroke or heart attack. Observe for dizziness, unsteadiness, tendency to fall, confusion, hallucinations, depression or urinary frequency.

▷ **Advisability of Use During Pregnancy**

Pregnancy Category: C (tentative). See Pregnancy Code inside back cover.
Animal studies: No significant increase in birth defects due to this drug. Some toxic effects on embryo reported.
Human studies: Information from adequate studies of pregnant women is not available.
Avoid use of drug during the first 3 months if possible. Use this drug only if clearly needed. Ask your physician for guidance.

Advisability of Use if Breast-Feeding

Presence of this drug in breast milk: Yes.
Monitor nursing infant closely and discontinue drug or nursing if adverse effects develop.

Habit-Forming Potential: None.

Effects of Overdosage: Weakness, slow pulse, low blood pressure, fainting, cold and sweaty skin, congestive heart failure, possible coma and convulsions.

Possible Effects of Long-Term Use: Reduced heart reserve and eventual heart failure in susceptible individuals with advanced heart disease.

Suggested Periodic Examinations While Taking This Drug (at physician's discretion)

Complete blood cell counts.
Measurements of blood pressure, evaluation of heart function.

▷ **While Taking This Drug, Observe the Following**

Foods: No restrictions. Avoid excessive salt intake.
Beverages: No restrictions. May be taken with milk.
▷ *Alcohol:* Use with caution until the combined effect has been determined. Alcohol may exaggerate this drug's ability to lower the blood pressure and may increase its mild sedative effect.
Tobacco Smoking: Nicotine may reduce this drug's effectiveness in treating angina, heart rhythm disorders and high blood pressure. Smoking increases the rate of elimination of this drug and decreases its blood levels, especially in younger individuals. In addition, high doses of this drug may potentiate the constriction of the bronchial tubes caused by regular smoking.
▷ *Other Drugs*

Propranolol may *increase* the effects of
• other antihypertensive drugs, and cause excessive lowering of blood pressure. Dosage adjustments may be necessary.

- lidocaine (Xylocaine, etc.).
- reserpine (Ser-Ap-Es, etc.), and cause sedation, depression, slowing of the heart rate and lowering of the blood pressure.
- verapamil (Calan, Isoptin), and cause excessive depression of heart function; monitor this combination closely.

Propranolol may *decrease* the effects of

- theophyllines (Aminophyllin, Theo-Dur, etc.), and reduce their antiasthmatic effectiveness.

Propranolol *taken concurrently* with

- clonidine (Catapres) requires close monitoring for rebound high blood pressure if clonidine is withdrawn while propranolol is still being taken.
- epinephrine (Adrenalin, etc.) may cause marked rise in blood pressure and slowing of the heart rate.
- insulin requires close monitoring to avoid undetected hypoglycemia (see Glossary).

The following drugs may *increase* the effects of propranolol

- chlorpromazine (Thorazine, etc.).
- cimetidine (Tagamet).
- methimazole (Tapazole).
- propylthiouracil (Propacil).

The following drugs may *decrease* the effects of propranolol

- barbiturates (phenobarbital, etc.).
- indomethacin (Indocin), and possibly other "aspirin substitutes," may impair propranolol's antihypertensive effect.
- rifampin (Rifadin, Rimactane).

▷ *Driving, Hazardous Activities:* Use caution until the full extent of drowsiness, lethargy and blood pressure change have been determined.

Aviation Note: The use of this drug *may be a disqualification* for piloting. Consult a designated Aviation Medical Examiner.

Exposure to Sun: No restrictions.

Exposure to Heat: Caution advised. Hot environments can lower blood pressure and exaggerate the effects of this drug.

Exposure to Cold: Caution advised. Cold environments can enhance the circulatory deficiency in the extremities that may occur with this drug. The elderly should take precautions to prevent hypothermia (see Glossary).

Heavy Exercise or Exertion: It is advisable to avoid exertion that produces light-headedness, excessive fatigue or muscle cramping. The use of this drug may intensify the hypertensive response to isometric exercise.

Occurrence of Unrelated Illness: The fever that accompanies systemic infections can lower blood pressure and require adjustment of dosage. Illnesses that cause nausea or vomiting may interrupt the regular dosage schedule. Ask your physician for guidance.

Discontinuation: It is advisable to avoid sudden discontinuation of this drug in all situations; this is especially true in the presence of coronary artery disease. If possible, gradual reduction of dose over a period of 2 to 3 weeks is recommended. Ask your physician for specific guidance.

PYRIDOSTIGMINE
(peer id oh STIG meen)

Introduced: 1962

Class: Antimyasthenic

Prescription: USA: Yes
Canada: No

Controlled Drug: USA: No
Canada: No

Available as Generic: USA: No
Canada: No

Brand Names: Mestinon, Mestinon Timespan, Regonol

BENEFITS versus RISKS

Possible Benefits	*Possible Risks*
MODERATELY EFFECTIVE TREATMENT OF OCULAR AND MILD FORMS OF MYASTHENIA GRAVIS (symptomatic relief of muscle weakness)	Cholinergic crisis (overdose): excessive salivation, nausea, vomiting, stomach cramps, diarrhea, shortness of breath (asthmalike wheezing), excessive weakness

---

▷ **Principal Uses**

As a Single Drug Product: Used primarily to treat the ocular and milder forms of myasthenia gravis by providing temporary relief of muscle weakness and fatigability. It is most useful in long-term treatment when there is little or no difficulty in swallowing.

How This Drug Works: This drug inhibits cholinesterase, the enzyme that destroys acetylcholine. This results in higher levels of acetylcholine, the nerve transmitter that facilitates the stimulation of muscular activity. The net effects are increased muscle strength and endurance.

Available Dosage Forms and Strengths

Syrup — 60 mg per 5-ml teaspoonful (5% alcohol)
Tablets — 60 mg
Tablets, prolonged-action — 180 mg

▷ **Usual Adult Dosage Range:** Initially: 60 to 120 mg/3 to 4 hours; adjust dosage as needed and tolerated. Maintenance: 60 to 1500 mg/24 hours; the average dose is 600 mg/24 hours. Prolonged-action tablets: 180 to 540 mg once or twice a day, at least 6 hours apart. **Note: Actual dosage and administration schedule must be determined by the physician for each patient individually.**

▷ **Dosing Instructions:** Take with food or milk to reduce the intensity of side-effects. Larger portions of the daily maintenance dosage should be timed according to the pattern of fatigue and weakness. The syrup will permit a finer adjustment of dosage. The regular tablet may be crushed for administration. The prolonged-action tablet should be taken whole (not altered).

Usual Duration of Use: Continual use on a regular schedule (with dosage adjustment) for 10 to 14 days is usually necessary to determine this drug's effectiveness in relieving the symptoms of myasthenia gravis. Long-term use (months to years) requires periodic evaluation of response and dosage adjustment. Consult your physician on a regular basis.

▷ **This Drug Should Not Be Taken If**
  • you are known to be allergic to bromide compounds.

▷ **Inform Your Physician Before Taking This Drug If**
  • you are subject to heart rhythm disorders or bronchial asthma.
  • you have recurrent urinary tract infections.
  • you have prostatism (see Glossary).
  • you plan to have surgery under general anesthesia in the near future.

Possible Side-Effects (natural, expected and unavoidable drug actions)
  Small pupils, watering of eyes, slow pulse, excessive salivation, nausea, vomiting, stomach cramps, diarrhea, urge to urinate, increased sweating.

▷ **Possible Adverse Effects** (unusual, unexpected and infrequent reactions)
  If any of the following develop, consult your physician promptly for guidance.
  Mild Adverse Effects
  Allergic Reaction: Skin rash.
  Nervousness, anxiety, unsteadiness, muscle cramps or twitching.
  Loss of scalp hair.
  Serious Adverse Effects
  Confusion, slurred speech, seizures, difficult breathing (asthmatic wheezing).
  Increased muscle weakness or paralysis.
  Excessive vomiting or diarrhea may induce abnormally low blood potassium levels (hypokalemia). This will accentuate muscle weakness.

▷ **Possible Effects on Sexual Function:** None reported.

▷ **Adverse Effects That May Mimic Natural Diseases or Disorders**
  Seizures may suggest the possibility of epilepsy.

Natural Diseases or Disorders That May Be Activated by This Drug
  Latent bronchial asthma.

Possible Effects on Laboratory Tests
  None reported.

CAUTION
  1. Certain drugs can block the action of this drug and reduce its effec-

tiveness in treating myasthenia gravis. (See *Other Drugs* below.) Consult your physician before starting any new drug, prescription or over-the-counter.

2. The dosage schedule of this drug must be carefully individualized for each patient. Variations in response may occur from time to time. Because generalized muscle weakness is a major symptom of both myasthenia crisis (underdosage) and cholinergic crisis (overdosage), it may be difficult to recognize the correct cause. As a rule, weakness that begins within 1 hour after taking this drug probably represents overdosage; weakness that begins 3 or more hours after taking this drug is probably due to underdosage. Observe these time relationships and inform your physician.

3. During long-term use of this drug, observe for the possible development of resistance to the drug's therapeutic action (loss of effectiveness). Consult your physician regarding the advisability of discontinuing this drug for a few days to see if responsiveness can be restored.

Precautions for Use

By Infants and Children: The syrup form of this drug permits greater precision of dosage adjustment and ease of administration in this age group.

By Those over 60 Years of Age: The natural decline of kidney function with aging may require smaller doses to prevent accumulation of this drug to toxic levels.

▷ Advisability of Use During Pregnancy

Pregnancy Category: C (tentative). See Pregnancy Code inside back cover.
Animal studies: No information available.
Human studies: Information from adequate studies of pregnant women is not available.

There are no reports of birth defects due to the use of this drug during pregnancy. However, there are reports of significant muscular weakness in newborn infants whose mothers had taken this drug during pregnancy. Ask your physician for guidance.

Advisability of Use if Breast-Feeding

Presence of this drug in breast milk: Probably not.
Monitor nursing infant closely and discontinue drug or nursing if adverse effects develop.

Habit-Forming Potential: None.

Effects of Overdosage: Generalized muscular weakness, blurred vision, very small pupils, slow heart rate, difficult breathing (wheezing), excessive salivation, nausea, vomiting, stomach cramps, diarrhea, muscle cramps or twitching. This syndrome constitutes the cholinergic crisis.

Possible Effects of Long-Term Use: Development of tolerance (see Glossary) with loss of therapeutic effectiveness.

Pyridostigmine **909**

Suggested Periodic Examinations While Taking This Drug (at physician's
   discretion)
   Assessment of drug effectiveness and dosage schedule for optimal therapeutic results.

▷ **While Taking This Drug, Observe the Following**
   Foods: No restrictions.
   Beverages: No restrictions. May be taken with milk.
▷ *Alcohol:* Use caution until the combined effects are determined. Weakness
      and unsteadiness may be accentuated.
   Tobacco Smoking: No interactions expected.
▷ *Other Drugs*
      The following drugs may *decrease* the effects of pyridostigmine
      • atropine (belladonna).
      • clindamycin (Cleocin).
      • guanadrel (Hylorel).
      • guanethidine (Esimil, Ismelin).
      • procainamide (Procan SR, Pronestyl).
      • quinidine (Cardioquin, Duraquin, etc.).
      • quinine (Quinamm).
▷ *Driving, Hazardous Activities:* This drug may cause blurred vision, confu-
      sion or generalized weakness. Restrict activities as necessary.
   Aviation Note: The use of this drug *is a disqualification* for piloting.
      Consult a designated Aviation Medical Examiner.
   Exposure to Sun: No restrictions.
   Exposure to Heat: Use caution. This may cause excessive sweating and
      increased weakness.
   Exposure to Environmental Chemicals: Avoid excessive exposure (inhala-
      tion, skin contamination) to the insecticides Baygon, Diazinon and
      Sevin. These can accentuate the potential toxicity of this drug.
   Discontinuation: Do not discontinue this drug abruptly without your physi-
      cian's knowledge and guidance.

QUINACRINE
(KWIN a kreen)

Other Name: Mepacrine

Introduced: 1967

Class: Antiprotozoal, lupus suppressant

Prescription: USA: Yes
Canada: No

Controlled Drug: USA: No
Canada: No

Available as Generic: USA: No
Canada: No

Brand Name: Atabrine,

BENEFITS versus RISKS

Possible Benefits	*Possible Risks*
HIGHLY EFFECTIVE TREATMENT FOR GIARDIASIS (95% cure rate) Effective treatment for mild to moderate discoid lupus erythematosus	Infrequent adverse behavioral effects: irritability, mood changes, hallucinations, psychotic thinking Yellow discoloration of skin Rare corneal and retinal changes, hepatitis, aplastic anemia with high-dose and/or long-term use

---

▷ **Principal Uses**

As a Single Drug Product: Used primarily to (1) treat giardiasis (eradicate Giardia lamblia that are infecting the small intestine; (2) control the activity of skin lesions in discoid lupus erythematosus.

How This Drug Works: Not completely established. As an antiprotozoal, it is thought that this drug inhibits the functions of DNA and RNA and thus prevents reproduction of infecting organisms. As a lupus suppressant, it is thought that this drug impairs the activities of nucleoproteins that are responsible for inflammatory autoimmune reactions.

Available Dosage Forms and Strengths

Tablets — 100 mg

▷ **Usual Adult Dosage Range:** For giardiasis: 100 mg 3 times a day for 5 to 7 days.

For discoid lupus: 50 mg to 100 mg daily for several months.**Note: Actual dosage and administration schedule must be determined by the physician for each patient individually.**

▷ **Dosing Instructions:** Take after meals with a full glass of water, tea or fruit juice. The tablet may be crushed for administration; the bitter taste can be disguised by mixing with jam, jelly, honey or chocolate syrup. Take the full course prescribed.

Usual Duration of Use:
Continual use on a regular schedule for 5 to 7 days is usually necessary to determine this drug's effectiveness in curing giardiasis. Continual use on a regular schedule for up to 6 months is usually required to determine this drug's effectiveness in controlling the skin lesions of lupus. Long-term use (months to years) requires periodic evaluation of response and dosage adjustment. Consult your physician on a regular basis.

Currently a "Drug of Choice"
for treating symptomatic giardiasis (Giardia lamblia infection).

▷ **This Drug Should Not Be Taken If**
  • you have had an allergic reaction to it previously.
  • you have active liver disease.
  • you have active bone marrow disease or a blood cell disorder.

▷ **Inform Your Physician Before Taking This Drug If**
  • you are pregnant, planning pregnancy, or breast-feeding.
  • you have a history of liver disease or impaired liver function.
  • you have a history of bone marrow depression or blood cell disorder, especially drug-induced.
  • you have a history of mental disorder (psychosis).
  • you have any type of eye disorder or impaired vision.
  • you have a history of porphyria or psoriasis.
  • you are currently taking primaquine.

Possible Side-Effects
(natural, expected and unavoidable drug actions)
Yellow discoloration of skin, eyes and urine (of no significance).
Blue-black discoloration of palate and nails with long-term use (of no significance).

▷ **Possible Adverse Effects**
(unusual, unexpected and infrequent reactions)
If any of the following develop, consult your physician promptly for guidance.
Mild Adverse Effects
Allergic Reactions: Skin rashes, itching, peeling.
Headache, dizziness.
Loss of appetite, nausea, vomiting, stomach pain or cramping, diarrhea.
Low-grade fever, loss of scalp hair, joint and muscle aches.
Serious Adverse Effects
Allergic Reactions: Chronic dermatitis, exfoliative dermatitis.
Idiosyncratic Reactions: Heart rhythm disturbances; hemolytic anemia in those with glucose-6-phosphate dehydrogenase deficient red blood cells.

Acute behavioral reactions: excitement, agitation, hallucinations, nightmares, psychosis ("Mepacrine madness").
Corneal swelling and deposits, impaired vision.
Bone marrow depression (see Glossary): fatigue, weakness, fever, sore throat, abnormal bruising or bleeding.

▷ **Possible Effects on Sexual Function:**   None reported.

Possible Delayed Adverse Effects: Aplastic anemia (see Glossary) and retinal damage are rare occurrences after discontinuation of this drug.

▷ **Adverse Effects That May Mimic Natural Diseases or Disorders**
Yellow discoloration of skin and eyes may suggest jaundice.
Acute behavioral reactions may suggest unrelated neuropsychiatric disorder.

Natural Diseases or Disorders That May Be Activated by This Drug
Porphyria, psoriasis.

Possible Effects on Laboratory Tests
Complete blood cell counts: decreased red cells, hemoglobin, white cells and platelets; increased eosinophils (allergic reaction).
Liver function tests: increased liver enzymes (ALT/GPT, AST/GOT and alkaline phosphatase), increased bilirubin.

CAUTION
1. Following a course of treatment for giardia infection, it is advisable to perform 3 separate stool examinations taken 3 to 5 days apart, beginning 3 to 4 weeks after completion of medication. If these examinations are negative (indicating a cure), any persistent symptoms may be due to a lactose intolerance induced by the infection. This may persist for several weeks.
2. During the long-term use of this drug for the treatment of lupus, report promptly any changes in vision that occur so appropriate evaluation can be made.

Precautions for Use
By Infants and Children
: This drug is not well tolerated by this age group. Dosage schedules and treatment monitoring should be supervised by a qualified pediatrician.
By Those over 60 Years of Age: Adverse behavioral reactions are more likely to occur in this age group. Observe closely for nervous irritability, mood changes, sleep disturbances, or other signs of toxic mental effects. Report these promptly.

▷ **Advisability of Use During Pregnancy**
Pregnancy Category: C (tentative). See Pregnancy Code inside back cover.
Animal studies: Rat studies reveal increased fetal deaths but no birth defects.
Human studies: Information from adequate studies of pregnant women

is not available. There has been one report of an infant born with hydrocephalus and an absent kidney possibly attributable to the use of this drug during pregnancy.

If possible, this drug should be avoided during the entire pregnancy.

Advisability of Use if Breast-Feeding
Presence of this drug in breast milk: Yes.
Avoid drug or refrain from nursing.

Habit-Forming Potential: None.

Effects of Overdosage: Seizures, low blood pressure, heart rhythm abnormalities, circulatory collapse.

Possible Effects of Long-Term Use: Yellow discoloration of skin, eyes and urine.
Blue-black discoloration of palate and nails.
Chronic dermatitis.
Retinal pigmentation and damage with impaired vision.
Drug-induced hepatitis.

Suggested Periodic Examinations While Taking This Drug
(at physician's discretion)
Complete blood cell counts, liver function tests.
Complete eye examinations *before* start of long-term drug use and every 3 to 6 months during use.

▷ **While Taking This Drug, Observe the Following**
Foods: No restrictions.
Beverages: No restrictions. May be taken with milk.
▷ *Alcohol:* Use with caution. This combination may cause a mild disulfiram-like reaction (see Glossary).
Tobacco Smoking: No interactions expected.
▷ *Other Drugs*
Quinacrine may *increase* the effects of
• primaquine and increase its toxic potential.
▷ *Driving, Hazardous Activities:* This drug may cause dizziness. Restrict activities as necessary.
Aviation Note: The use of this drug **may be a disqualification** for piloting. Consult a designated Aviation Medical Examiner.
Exposure to Sun: No restrictions.
Discontinuation: During the long-term use of this drug for lupus, if no significant benefit is apparent after 6 months, this drug should be discontinued.

QUINIDINE
(KWIN i deen)

Introduced: 1918

Class: Antiarrhythmic

Prescription: USA: Yes
Canada: No

Controlled Drug: USA: No
Canada: No

Available as Generic: Yes

Brand Names: ✦Apo-Quinidine, ✦Biquin Durules, Cardioquin, Cin-Quin, Duraquin, ✦Novoquinidine, Quinaglute Dura-Tabs, ✦Quinate, Quinidex Extentabs, ✦Quinobarb [CD]*, Quinora

---

BENEFITS versus RISKS

Possible Benefits	*Possible Risks*
EFFECTIVE TREATMENT OF SELECTED HEART RHYTHM DISORDERS	NARROW TREATMENT RANGE FREQUENT ADVERSE EFFECTS (30% of users) NUMEROUS ALLERGIC AND IDIOSYNCRATIC REACTIONS Dose-related toxicity Provocation of abnormal heart rhythms Abnormally low blood platelet count (rare)

▷ **Principal Uses**

As a Single Drug Product: Used primarily to control the following types of abnormal heart rhythm: atrial fibrillation and flutter, paroxysmal atrial tachycardia, paroxysmal ventricular tachycardia, premature atrial and ventricular contractions.

As a Combination Drug Product [CD]: This drug is available (in Canada) in combination with a barbiturate, a mild sedative that is added to allay the anxiety and nervous tension that often accompany heart rhythm disorders.

How This Drug Works: By slowing the activity of the pacemaker and delaying the transmission of electrical impulses through the conduction system and muscle of the heart, this drug assists in restoring normal heart rate and rhythm.

Available Dosage Forms and Strengths

Capsules — 200 mg, 300 mg
Injections — 80 mg, 200 mg per ml
Tablets — 100 mg, 200 mg, 275 mg, 300 mg
Tablets, prolonged-action — 300 mg, 324 mg, 330 mg

*Quinobarb contains phenylethylbarbiturate, a sedative of the barbiturate class.

▷ **Usual Adult Dosage Range:** Test dose: 200 mg, then observe for 2 hours for evidence of idiosyncrasy.
Dose varies with indication:
Premature atrial or ventricular contractions: 200 to 300 mg 3 or 4 times/day.
Paroxysmal atrial tachycardia: 400 to 600 mg/2 to 3 hours until paroxysm is terminated.
Atrial flutter: digitalize first; then individualize dosage schedule as appropriate.
Atrial fibrillation: digitalize first; then try 200 mg/2 to 3 hours for 5 to 8 doses; increase dose daily until normal rhythm is restored or toxic effects develop.
Maintenance schedule: 200 to 300 mg 3 or 4 times/day. The total daily dosage should not exceed 4000 mg.**Note: Actual dosage and administration schedule must be determined by the physician for each patient individually.**

▷ **Dosing Instructions:** Preferably taken on an empty stomach to achieve high blood levels rapidly. However, it may be taken with or following food to reduce stomach irritation. The regular tablets may be crushed and the capsules opened for administration. The prolonged-action forms should be swallowed whole without alteration.

Usual Duration of Use: Continual use on a regular schedule for 2 to 4 days is usually necessary to determine this drug's effectiveness in correcting or preventing responsive abnormal rhythms. Long-term use (months to years) requires supervision and periodic evaluation by your physician. Consult your physician on a regular basis.

▷ **This Drug Should Not Be Taken If**
- you have had an allergic or idiosyncratic reaction to any dosage form of it previously.
- you currently have an acute infection of any kind.

▷ **Inform Your Physician Before Taking This Drug If**
- you have coronary artery disease or myasthenia gravis.
- you have a history of hyperthyroidism.
- you have had a deficiency of blood platelets in the past from any cause.
- you are now taking, or have taken recently, any digitalis preparation (digitoxin, digoxin, etc.).
- you plan to have surgery under general anesthesia in the near future.

Possible Side-Effects (natural, expected and unavoidable drug actions)
Drop in blood pressure, may be marked in sensitive individuals.

▷ **Possible Adverse Effects** (unusual, unexpected and infrequent reactions)
If any of the following develop, consult your physician promptly for guidance.
Mild Adverse Effects
Allergic Reactions: Skin rash, hives, itching, drug fever (rare).

Dose-related toxicity (cinchonism): blurred vision, ringing in the ears, loss of hearing, dizziness.

Nausea, vomiting, diarrhea (20% to 30% of users).

Serious Adverse Effects

Allergic Reactions: Severe skin reactions, hemolytic anemia (see Glossary), joint and muscle pains, anaphylactic reaction (see Glossary), reduced blood platelet count, drug-induced hepatitis (see Glossary).

Idiosyncratic Reactions: Skin rash, rapid heart rate, acute delirium and combative behavior, difficult breathing.

Heart conduction abnormalities.

Optic neuritis, impaired vision.

Abnormally low white blood cell count: fever, sore throat, infections.

▷ **Possible Effects on Sexual Function:**   None reported.

▷ **Adverse Effects That May Mimic Natural Diseases or Disorders**
Drug-induced hepatitis may suggest viral hepatitis.

Natural Diseases or Disorders That May Be Activated by This Drug
Systemic lupus erythematosus, myasthenia gravis, psoriasis (in sensitive individuals).

Possible Effects on Laboratory Tests
Complete blood cell counts: decreased red cells, hemoglobin, white cells and platelets; increased eosinophils (allergic reaction); marked increase of white blood cells in association with "quinidine fever" (very rare).

Antinuclear antibodies (ANA): positive.

Prothrombin time: increased (when taken concurrently with warfarin).

Liver function tests: increased liver enzymes (ALT/GPT, AST/GOT and alkaline phosphatase), increased bilirubin.

CAUTION

1. The effects of this drug are very unpredictable because of the wide variation in response from person to person. Dosage adjustments must be based upon individual reaction. Notify your physician of any events that you suspect may be drug related.
2. It is advisable to carry a card of personal identification that includes a notation that you are taking this drug.

Precautions for Use
By Infants and Children: A test for drug idiosyncrasy should be made before starting treatment with this drug. If there is no beneficial response after 3 days of adequate dosage, this drug should be discontinued.

By Those over 60 Years of Age: Small doses are mandatory until your individual response has been determined. Observe for the development of light-headedness, dizziness, weakness or sense of impending faint. Use caution to prevent falls.

▷ **Advisability of Use During Pregnancy**
Pregnancy Category: C (tentative). See Pregnancy Code inside back cover.
Animal studies: No information available.
Human studies: Information from adequate studies of pregnant women
is not available. No birth defects have been reported following use of
this drug during pregnancy.
Use this drug only if clearly needed.

Advisability of Use if Breast-Feeding
Presence of this drug in breast milk: Yes.
Avoid drug or refrain from nursing.

Habit-Forming Potential: None.

Effects of Overdosage: Nausea, vomiting, ringing in the ears, headache,
jerky eye movements, double vision, altered color vision, confusion,
delirium, hot skin, seizures, coma.

Possible Effects of Long-Term Use: None reported.

Suggested Periodic Examinations While Taking This Drug (at physician's
discretion)
Complete blood cell counts, electrocardiograms.

▷ **While Taking This Drug, Observe the Following**
Foods: No restrictions.
Beverages: No restrictions. May be taken with milk.
▷   *Alcohol:* Use caution until the combined effects have been determined.
Alcohol may enhance the blood-pressure-lowering effects of this drug.
Tobacco Smoking: Nicotine can increase irritability of the heart and aggra-
vate rhythm disorders. Avoid all forms of tobacco.
▷   *Other Drugs*
Quinidine may *increase* the effects of
• anticoagulants (Coumadin, etc.), and increase the risk of bleeding.
• digitoxin and digoxin (Lanoxin), and cause digitalis toxicity.
The following drugs may *increase* the effects of quinidine
• amiodarone.
• cimetidine (Tagamet).
The following drugs may *decrease* the effects of quinidine
• barbiturates (phenobarbital, etc.).
• phenytoin (Dilantin).
• rifampin (Rifadin, Rimactane).
▷   *Driving, Hazardous Activities:* This drug may cause dizziness and alter vision. Restrict activities as necessary.
Aviation Note: The use of this drug *may be a disqualification* for piloting.
Consult a designated Aviation Medical Examiner.
Exposure to Sun: No restrictions.

RAMIPRIL
(ra MI pril)

Introduced: 1985

Prescription: USA: Yes

Available as Generic: No

Brand Name: Altace

Class: Antihypertensive, ACE inhibitor

Controlled Drug: USA: No

BENEFITS versus RISKS

Possible Benefits	*Possible Risks*
EFFECTIVE CONTROL OF MILD TO SEVERE HIGH BLOOD PRESSURE	Headache (5.4%), dizziness (2.2%), fatigue (2.0%) Low blood pressure (0.5%) Allergic swelling of face, tongue or vocal cords (angioedema) (0.3%)

▷ **Principal Uses**

As a Single Drug Product

Used primarily to treat all degrees of high blood pressure, alone or concurrently with thiazide-type diuretics. Mild to moderate high blood pressure usually responds to low doses; severe high blood pressure may require higher doses, with greater risk of serious adverse effects.

How This Drug Works: Not completely known. It is thought that by blocking certain enzyme systems that influence arterial function, this drug contributes to the relaxation of arterial walls throughout the body and thus lowers the resistance to blood flow that causes high blood pressure. This, in turn, reduces the workload of the heart and improves its performance.

Available Dosage Forms and Strengths

Capsules — 1.25 mg, 2.5 mg, 5 mg, 10 mg

▷ **Usual Adult Dosage Range:**   Initially 2.5 mg once daily for 2 to 4 weeks. Usual maintenance dose is 2.5 to 20 mg/day in a single dose or in 2 divided doses. If taking diuretics: Either discontinue the diuretic for 3 days before initiating this drug, or begin treatment with 1.25 mg of this drug.

Total daily dose should not exceed 5 mg if kidney function is significantly impaired. **Note: Actual dosage and administration schedule must be determined by the physician for each patient individually.**

▷ **Dosing Instructions:**   Take on an empty stomach or with food, at same time each day. The capsule may be opened for administration.

Usual Duration of Use: Continual use on a regular schedule for 2 to 4 weeks is usually necessary to determine this drug's effectiveness in controlling high blood pressure. The proper treatment of high blood pressure usually requires the long-term use of effective medications. Consult your physician on a regular basis.

▷ **This Drug Should Not Be Taken If**
  • you have had an allergic reaction to it previously.
  • you have a history of angioedema (a serious allergic reaction) from any cause.
  • you have active liver disease.
  • you have an abnormally high level of blood potassium.

▷ **Inform Your Physician Before Taking This Drug If**
  • you have had an unfavorable reaction to other angiotensin-converting enzyme (ACE) drugs previously: captopril (Capoten), enalapril (Vasotec), lisinopril (Prinivil, Zestril).
  • you are pregnant, planning pregnancy, or breast-feeding.
  • you have impaired liver or kidney function.
  • you have scleroderma or systemic lupus erythematosus.
  • you have any form of heart disease.
  • you have diabetes.
  • you are taking any of the following drugs: other antihypertensives, diuretics, nitrates or potassium supplements.
  • you plan to have surgery under general anesthesia in the near future.

Possible Side-Effects (natural, expected and unavoidable drug actions)
  Dizziness (2.2%), light-headedness (0.5%).

▷ **Possible Adverse Effects** (unusual, unexpected and infrequent reactions)
  If any of the following develop, consult your physician promptly for guidance.
  Mild Adverse Effects
  Allergic Reactions: Skin rash, itching.
  Headache (5.4%), fatigue (2%), drowsiness, nervousness, numbness and tingling, insomnia.
  Chest pain, palpitation, drug-induced cough (12%).
  Indigestion, stomach pain, nausea (1.1%), vomiting, diarrhea.
  Excessive sweating, joint and muscle aches.
  Serious Adverse Effects
  Allergic Reactions: Swelling (angioedema) of face, tongue and/or vocal cords: can be life threatening (0.3%).

▷ **Possible Effects on Sexual Function:**   Rare report of impotence (0.4%).

Possible Effects on Laboratory Tests
  Complete blood cell counts: decreased red cells and hemoglobin (0.4% using this drug alone; 1.5% using this drug and a diuretic); decreased white cells, increased eosinophils (both rare).
  Blood potassium level: increased (1%).

Liver function tests: increased liver enzymes (ALT/GPT, AST/GOT and alkaline phosphatase), increased bilirubin.

Kidney function tests: increased blood urea nitrogen (BUN) (0.5% using this drug alone; 3% using this drug and a diuretic); increased creatinine (1.2% using this drug alone; 1.5% using this drug and a diuretic).

CAUTION
1. Consult your physician regarding the advisability of discontinuing other antihypertensive drugs (especially diuretics) for 1 week before starting this drug.
2. **Report promptly** any indications of infection (fever, sore throat), and any indications of water retention (weight gain, puffiness, swollen feet or ankles).
3. Do not use a salt substitute without your physician's knowledge and approval. (Many salt substitutes contain potassium.)
4. It is advisable to obtain blood cell counts and urine analyses **before** starting this drug.
5. Notify your physician promptly if pregnancy occurs.

Precautions for Use
By Infants and Children: Safety and effectiveness for use by those in this age group have not been established.

By Those over 60 Years of Age: Small doses are advisable until tolerance has been determined. Sudden and excessive lowering of blood pressure can predispose to stroke or heart attack in those with impaired brain circulation or coronary artery heart disease.

▷ Advisability of Use During Pregnancy
Pregnancy Category: D (tentative). See Pregnancy Code inside back cover.

Animal studies: Fetal kidney defects found in rat studies; retarded growth found in mouse studies..

Human studies: Information from adequate studies of pregnant women is not available. However, drugs of this class taken during the last 6 months of pregnancy have been reported to cause serious fetal defects: skull and facial malformations, limb deformities, lung defects and kidney failure.

This drug should not be used during pregnancy.

Advisability of Use if Breast-Feeding
Presence of this drug in breast milk: Yes.

Avoid drug or refrain from nursing.

Habit-Forming Potential: None.

Effects of Overdosage: Excessive drop in blood pressure—light-headedness, dizziness, fainting.

Possible Effects of Long-Term Use: Gradual increase in blood potassium level.

Suggested Periodic Examinations While Taking This Drug (at physician's discretion)

Before starting drug: Complete blood cell counts; urine analysis with measurement of protein content; blood potassium level.

During use of drug: Blood cell counts; measurements of blood potassium.

▷ **While Taking This Drug, Observe the Following**

Foods: Consult physician regarding salt intake.

Nutritional Support: Do not take potassium supplements unless directed by your physician.

Beverages: No restrictions. May be taken with milk.

▷ *Alcohol:* Use caution until combined effect has been determined. Alcohol may enhance the blood-pressure-lowering effect of this drug.

Tobacco Smoking: No interactions expected.

▷ *Other Drugs*

Ramipril *taken concurrently* with

- lithium (Lithane, Lithotab, etc.) may cause increased blood lithium levels and symptoms of lithium toxicity. Monitor lithium levels closely.
- potassium preparations (K-Lyte, Slow-K, etc.) may cause increased blood levels of potassium with risk of serious heart rhythm disturbances.
- potassium-sparing diuretics: amiloride (Moduretic), spironolactone (Aldactazide), triamterene (Dyazide) may cause increased blood levels of potassium with risk of serious heart rhythm disturbances.

▷ *Driving, Hazardous Activities:* Usually no restrictions. Be aware of possible drops in blood pressure with resultant dizziness or faintness.

Aviation Note: The use of this drug *may be a disqualification* for piloting. Consult a designated Aviation Medical Examiner.

Exposure to Sun: Caution advised. A similar drug of this class can cause photosensitivity.

Exposure to Heat: Caution advised. Avoid excessive perspiring with resultant loss of body water and drop in blood pressure.

Occurrence of Unrelated Illness: Report promptly any disorder that causes nausea, vomiting or diarrhea. Fluid and chemical imbalances must be corrected as soon as possible.

RANITIDINE
(ra NI te deen)

Introduced: 1981

Class: Antiulcer, H-2 receptor blocker

Prescription: USA: Yes
Canada: Yes

Controlled Drug: USA: No
Canada: No

Available as Generic: No

Brand Name: Zantac

Warning: The brand names Zantac and Xanax are similar and can be mistaken for each other; this can lead to serious medication errors. These names represent very different drugs. Zantac (a large white tablet) is the generic drug ranitidine; it is used to treat peptic ulcer disease. Xanax (white, yellow, blue oval tablets) is the generic drug alprazolam; it is a mild tranquilizer. Verify that you are taking the correct drug.

BENEFITS versus RISKS

Possible Benefits	*Possible Risks*
EFFECTIVE TREATMENT OF PEPTIC ULCER DISEASE: relief of symptoms, acceleration of healing, prevention of recurrence	Drug-induced hepatitis (rare)
	Confusion (in severely ill elderly patients)
CONTROL OF HYPERSECRETORY STOMACH DISORDERS	Rare blood cell disorders
Beneficial in treatment of reflux esophagitis	

▷ **Principal Uses**

As a Single Drug Product: Used primarily in the treatment of peptic ulcer disease, both benign stomach (gastric) ulcer and duodenal ulcer. It is used specifically to hasten the healing of ulcer and to prevent recurrence. Also used to control the excessive production of stomach acid in the Zollinger-Ellison syndrome. Though its effectiveness has not been fully established, this drug is also widely used in the management of esophagitis (as with hiatal hernia) and upper gastrointestinal bleeding.

How This Drug Works: By blocking the action of histamine, this drug effectively inhibits the secretion of stomach acid and thus creates a more favorable environment for the healing of peptic ulcers.

Available Dosage Forms and Strengths
Injection — 0.5 mg per ml, 25 mg per ml

Syrup — 15 mg per ml (7.5% alcohol)
Tablets — 150 mg, 300 mg

▷ **Usual Adult Dosage Range:** For active peptic ulcer and hypersecretory states: 150 mg 2 times daily, 12 hours apart. For prevention of recurrent ulcer: 150 mg at bedtime. **Note: Actual dosage and administration schedule must be determined by the physician for each patient individually.**

▷ **Dosing Instructions:** To obtain the longest period of stomach acid reduction, this drug should be taken with or immediately following meals. The tablet may be crushed for administration.

Usual Duration of Use: Continual use on a regular schedule for 4 to 6 weeks is usually necessary to determine this drug's effectiveness in healing active peptic ulcer. Long-term use (1 to 8 years) for prevention of ulcer recurrence requires individual consideration by your physician.

▷ **This Drug Should Not Be Taken If**
  • you have had an allergic reaction to any dosage form of it previously.

▷ **Inform Your Physician Before Taking This Drug If**
  • you are allergic to cimetidine (Tagamet).
  • you have impaired liver or kidney function.
  • you are taking an oral anticoagulant.

Possible Side-Effects (natural, expected and unavoidable drug actions)
  None reported.

▷ **Possible Adverse Effects** (unusual, unexpected and infrequent reactions)
  If any of the following develop, consult your physician promptly for guidance.
  Mild Adverse Effects
  Allergic Reaction: Skin rash.
  Headache, malaise, dizziness.
  Nausea, constipation, diarrhea.
  Serious Adverse Effects
  Idiosyncratic Reaction: Confusion in the elderly and debilitated.
  Drug-induced hepatitis (see Glossary).
  Bone marrow depression (see Glossary)—weakness, fever, sore throat, abnormal bleeding or bruising.

▷ **Possible Effects on Sexual Function:** Decreased libido, impotence, male breast enlargement and tenderness (all rare).

▷ **Adverse Effects That May Mimic Natural Diseases or Disorders**
  Liver reactions may suggest viral hepatitis.

Possible Effects on Laboratory Tests
  Blood eosinophil count: increased (allergic reaction).
  White blood cell count: decreased.

Blood thyroid hormone levels: T^4 and free T^4 decreased.

Urine screening tests for drug abuse: *initial* test result may be falsely **positive**; *confirmatory* test result will be **negative**. (Test results depend upon amount of drug taken and testing method used.)

CAUTION

1. Do not discontinue this drug abruptly. (Ulcer activation and perforation have occurred following abrupt cessation of cimetidine, a closely related drug.)
2. After discontinuation of this drug, inform your physician promptly if you experience a return of symptoms indicative of ulcer reactivation.

Precautions for Use

By Infants and Children: Safety and effectiveness for use by those under 12 years of age have not been established.

By Those over 60 Years of Age: Observe for the development of nervous agitation or confusion. This drug may contribute to the formation of stomach phytobezoars (masses of undigested vegetable fibers). Individuals with poor chewing ability (missing teeth) and those who have had partial gastrectomy or vagotomy (stomach surgery) are most susceptible. Observe for loss of appetite, stomach fullness, nausea and vomiting.

▷ Advisability of Use During Pregnancy

Pregnancy Category: B (tentative). See Pregnancy Code inside back cover.

Animal studies: No birth defects reported.

Human studies: Information from adequate studies of pregnant women is not available.

Use this drug only if clearly needed. Ask physician for guidance.

Advisability of Use if Breast-Feeding

Presence of this drug in breast milk: Yes.

Avoid drug or refrain from nursing.

Habit-Forming Potential: None.

Effects of Overdosage: Confusion, delirium, slurred speech, flushing, sweating, drowsiness, muscle twitching, seizures, coma.

Possible Effects of Long-Term Use: None reported.

Suggested Periodic Examinations While Taking This Drug (at physician's discretion)

Complete blood cell counts, liver function tests.

▷ While Taking This Drug, Observe the Following

Foods: Protein-rich foods produce maximal stomach acid secretion. Follow the diet prescribed to derive optimal benefit from this drug.

Beverages: No restrictions. May be taken with milk.

▷ *Alcohol:* No interactions with drug. However, alcoholic beverages increase stomach acidity and can reduce the effectiveness of this drug.

▷ *Other Drugs*

Ranitidine may *increase* the effects of
- oral anticoagulants, and increase the risk of bleeding.

▷ *Driving, Hazardous Activities:* This drug may cause dizziness. Restrict activities as necessary.

Aviation Note: The use of this drug *may be a disqualification* for piloting. Consult a designated Aviation Medical Examiner.

Exposure to Sun: No restrictions.

Discontinuation: Do not discontinue this drug suddenly if taken for peptic ulcer disease. Consult physician for withdrawal instructions. This drug does not provide an extended protective effect. Be alert to the possibility of ulcer recurrence anytime after discontinuation. Studies show recurrence rates of 50%–90% within 1 year.

RIFAMPIN
(RIF am pin)

Other Name: Rifampicin

Introduced: 1967

Class: Antibiotic, rifamycins

Prescription: USA: Yes
Canada: Yes

Controlled Drug: USA: No
Canada: No

Available as Generic: No

Brand Names: Rifadin, Rifamate [CD], Rimactane, Rimactane/INH Dual Pack [CD], ✦Rofact

---

BENEFITS versus RISKS

Possible Benefits	*Possible Risks*
EFFECTIVE TREATMENT OF TUBERCULOSIS in combination with other drugs EFFECTIVE PREVENTION OF MENINGITIS by the elimination of meningococcus from the throat of carriers	DRUG-INDUCED HEPATITIS DRUG-INDUCED NEPHRITIS Flulike syndrome Rare blood cell disorder: abnormally low blood platelet count

---

▷ **Principal Uses**

As a Single Drug Product: This antibiotic drug is used primarily to treat active tuberculosis. It is usually given concurrently with other antitubercular drugs to enhance its effectiveness. It is also used to eliminate the meningitis germ (meningococcus) from the throats of healthy carriers so it cannot be spread to others. It is not effective in the treatment of active meningitis.

As a Combination Drug Product [CD]: This drug is available in combination with isoniazid, another antitubercular drug that delays the development of drug-resistant strains of the tuberculosis germ.

How This Drug Works: This drug prevents the growth and multiplication of susceptible tuberculosis organisms by blocking specific enzyme systems that are involved in the formation of essential proteins.

Available Dosage Forms and Strengths
Capsules — 150 mg, 300 mg

▷ **Usual Adult Dosage Range:** For tuberculosis: 600 mg once/day. For meningococcus carriers: 600 mg once/day for 4 days. The total daily dosage should not exceed 600 mg. **Note: Actual dosage and administration schedule must be determined by the physician for each patient individually.**

▷ **Dosing Instructions:** Preferably taken with 8 ounces of water on an empty stomach (1 hour before or 2 hours after eating). However, it may be taken with food if necessary to reduce stomach irritation. The capsule may be opened and the contents mixed with applesauce or jelly for administration.

Usual Duration of Use: Continual use on a regular schedule for several months is usually necessary to determine this drug's effectiveness in promoting recovery from tuberculosis. Long-term use (possibly 1 to 2 years) requires ongoing supervision and periodic evaluation by your physician. Consult your physician on a regular basis.

▷ **This Drug Should Not Be Taken If**
 • you have had an allergic reaction to it previously.
 • you have active liver disease.

▷ **Inform Your Physician Before Taking This Drug If**
 • you are pregnant.
 • you have a history of liver disease or impaired liver function.
 • you consume alcohol daily.
 • you are taking an oral contraceptive. (An alternate method of contraception is advised.)
 • you are taking an anticoagulant.

Possible Side-Effects (natural, expected and unavoidable drug actions)
Red, orange or brown discoloration of tears, sweat, saliva, sputum, urine or stool. Yellow discoloration of the skin (not jaundice). Note: In the absence of symptoms indicating illness, any discoloration is a harmless drug effect and does not indicate toxicity.
Possible fungal superinfections (see Glossary).

▷ **Possible Adverse Effects** (unusual, unexpected and infrequent reactions)
  If any of the following develop, consult your physician promptly for guidance.
  Mild Adverse Effects
    Allergic Reactions: Skin rash, hives, itching, drug fever (see Glossary).
    Headache, drowsiness, dizziness, blurred vision, impaired hearing, vague numbness and tingling.
    Loss of appetite, heartburn, nausea, vomiting, abdominal cramps, diarrhea.
  Serious Adverse Effects
    Flulike syndrome: fever, chills, headache, dizziness, musculoskeletal pain, difficult breathing.
    Drug-induced liver damage, with or without jaundice.
    Drug-induced kidney damage: impaired urine production, bloody or cloudy urine.
    Excessively low blood platelet count: abnormal bleeding or bruising.

▷ **Possible Effects on Sexual Function**
    Altered timing and pattern of menstruation.
    Decreased effectiveness of oral contraceptives taken concurrently.

▷ **Adverse Effects That May Mimic Natural Diseases or Disorders**
    Liver reactions may suggest viral hepatitis.
    Kidney reactions may suggest an infectious nephritis.

Possible Effects on Laboratory Tests
    Complete blood cell counts: decreased red cells, hemoglobin, white cells and platelets; increased eosinophils (allergic reaction).
    Prothrombin time: increased (when taken concurrently with warfarin).
    Liver function tests: increased liver enzymes (ALT/GPT, AST/GOT and alkaline phosphatase), increased bilirubin.

CAUTION
  1. This drug may permanently discolor soft contact lenses.
  2. This drug may reduce the effectiveness of oral contraceptives; unplanned pregnancy could occur; an alternate method of contraception is advised.
  3. When this drug is used alone in the treatment of tuberculosis, bacterial strains that are resistant to this drug can develop rapidly. This drug should only be used in conjunction with other antitubercular drugs.
  4. To ensure the best possible response to treatment, take the full course of medication prescribed; this may be for several months or years.

Precautions for Use
  By Infants and Children: Monitor closely for possible liver toxicity or deficiency of blood platelets.
  By Those over 60 Years of Age: Natural changes in body composition and

function make you more susceptible to the adverse effects of this drug. Report promptly any indications of possible drug toxicity.

▷ **Advisability of Use During Pregnancy**
Pregnancy Category: C (tentative). See Pregnancy Code inside back cover.
Animal studies: Cleft palate and spinal defects reported in rodent studies.
Human studies: Information from adequate studies of pregnant women is not available.
If possible, avoid use of drug during the first 3 months.

Advisability of Use if Breast-Feeding
Presence of this drug in breast milk: Yes.
Avoid drug or refrain from nursing.

Habit-Forming Potential: None.

Effects of Overdosage: Nausea, vomiting, drowsiness, unconsciousness, severe liver damage, jaundice.

Possible Effects of Long-Term Use: Superinfections, fungal overgrowth of mouth or tongue.

Suggested Periodic Examinations While Taking This Drug (at physician's discretion)
Complete blood cell counts, liver and kidney function tests.
Hearing acuity tests if hearing loss is suspected.

▷ **While Taking This Drug, Observe the Following**
Foods: No restrictions.
Beverages: No restrictions.
▷ *Alcohol:* It is best to avoid alcohol completely to reduce the risk of potential liver toxicity.
Tobacco Smoking: No interactions expected.
▷ *Other Drugs*
Rifampin may ***decrease*** the effects of
• anticoagulants (Coumadin, etc.), and reduce their effectiveness.
• beta blockers: metoprolol, propranolol.
• cortisonelike drugs (see Drug Class, Section Four).
• cyclosporine.
• digitoxin.
• methadone (Dolophine).
• mexiletine (Mexitil).
• oral contraceptives.
• phenytoin (Dilantin).
• progestins.
• quinidine.
• sulfonylureas: chlorpropamide, tolbutamide.
• theophyllines (Aminophyllin, Theo-Dur, etc.).
The following drugs may ***decrease*** the effects of rifampin
• aminosalicylic acid (PAS), and reduce its antitubercular effectiveness.

▷ *Driving, Hazardous Activities:* This drug may cause dizziness, drowsiness, impaired vision and impaired hearing. Restrict activities as necessary.

Aviation Note: The use of this drug **may be a disqualification** for piloting. Consult a designated Aviation Medical Examiner.

Exposure to Sun: No restrictions.

Discontinuation: It is advisable not to interrupt or discontinue this drug without consulting your physician. Intermittent administration can increase the possibility of developing allergic reactions.

SELEGILINE
(se LEDGE i leen)

Other Name: Deprenyl

Introduced: 1981

Class: Antiparkinsonism, mono-amine oxidase (MAO) type B inhibitor

Prescription: USA: Yes

Controlled Drug: USA: No

Available as Generic: USA: No

Brand Name: Eldepryl

BENEFITS versus RISKS
Possible Benefits   *Possible Risks*

Possible Benefits	*Possible Risks*
ADDITIVE RELIEF OF SYMPTOMS OF PARKINSON'S DISEASE when used concurrently with levodopa/carbidopa (Sinemet) PERMITS UP TO 30% REDUCTION IN SINEMET DOSAGE with resultant decrease in adverse effects	ABNORMAL INVOLUNTARY MOVEMENTS (12%) HALLUCINATIONS (5.4%) INITIAL FALL IN BLOOD PRESSURE/ORTHOSTATIC HYPOTENSION (1.8%)

▷ **Principal Uses**

As a Single Drug Product: Used solely as an adjunct to levodopa/carbidopa treatment of Parkinson's disease for those individuals who experience intolerable abnormal movements (dyskinesia) and/or increasing "on-off" episodes due to loss of effectiveness of levodopa. The addition of selegiline (1) permits reduction of the daily dose of levodopa (by 25% to 30%) with consequent lessening of dyskinesia and erratic drug response, and (2) provides additional relief of parkinsonian symptoms.

How This Drug Works: By (1) inhibiting monoamine oxidase type B, the enzyme that inactivates dopamine in the brain, and by (2) slowing the restorage of released dopamine at nerve terminals, this drug helps to correct the deficiency of dopamine that is responsible for the rigidity, tremor and sluggish movement characteristic of Parkinson's disease.

Available Dosage Forms and Strengths
Tablets — 5 mg

▷ **Usual Adult Dosage Range**

5 mg once or twice daily. The usual maintenance dose is 5 mg after breakfast and 5 mg after lunch. A total daily dose of 10 mg is adequate to achieve optimal benefit from this drug. Higher doses do not result in further improvement and are not advised.

During the gradual introduction of selegiline, the concurrent dose of levodopa/carbidopa (Sinemet) may be cautiously decreased in accord with your physician's instructions. Concurrent Sinemet dosage should be reduced by 10% to 20% when selegiline is started. **Note: Actual dosage and administration schedule must be determined by the physician for each patient individually.**

▷ **Dosing Instructions:** Take with food or milk to reduce stomach irritation. The tablet may be crushed for administration.

Usual Duration of Use: Continual use on a regular schedule for 4 to 6 weeks is usually necessary to determine this drug's effectiveness in controlling the symptoms of Parkinson's disease and permitting reduction of levodopa/carbidopa dosage. Long-term use (months to years) requires periodic evaluation of response and dosage adjustment. Consult your physician on a regular basis.

Possible Advantages of This Drug

It may provide a more effective and uniform control of parkinsonian symptoms and a significant reduction of some adverse effects associated with long-term levodopa therapy. Fifty to 60% of users show improvement.

It does not lose its effectiveness with long-term use.

It does not require avoidance of foods containing tyramine, as is necessary with monoamine oxidase (MAO) type A inhibitors.

It causes no life-threatening or irreversible adverse effects.

▷ **This Drug Should Not Be Taken If**
- you have had an allergic reaction to it previously.
- you have Huntington's disease, hereditary (essential) tremor or tardive dyskinesia (see Glossary).
- you are pregnant or breast-feeding.

▷ **Inform Your Physician Before Taking This Drug If**
- you have constitutionally low blood pressure.
- you have peptic ulcer disease.

- you have a history of heart rhythm disorder.
- you are taking any antihypertensive drugs or antipsychotic drugs (see Drug Classes, Section Four).

Possible Side-Effects (natural, expected and unavoidable drug actions)
Weakness (0.3%), orthostatic hypotension (see Glossary) (1.8%), dry mouth (2%), insomnia (1.5%).

▷ **Possible Adverse Effects** (unusual, unexpected and infrequent reactions)
If any of the following develop, consult your physician promptly for guidance.
Mild Adverse Effects
Headache (2%), dizziness (2.2%), agitation (2.5%).
Palpitations (0.2%), fainting (0.1%).
Altered taste (0.1%), nausea and vomiting (7%), stomach pain (4%).
Serious Adverse Effects
Dyskinesias: abnormal involuntary movements (12%).
Confusion and hallucinations (5.4%), depression (0.4%), psychosis (0.2%), vivid dreams (2%).
Aggravation of peptic ulcer (0.2%), gastrointestinal bleeding (0.2%).

▷ **Possible Effects on Sexual Function:**   None reported.

▷ **Adverse Effects That May Mimic Natural Diseases or Disorders**
Effects on mental function and behavior may resemble psychotic disorders.

▷ **Natural Diseases or Disorders That May Be Activated by This Drug**
Peptic ulcer disease.

Possible Effects on Laboratory Tests
None reported.

CAUTION
1. This drug can initiate dyskinesias and can intensify existing dyskinesias. Observe carefully for the development of tremors, twitching or abnormal, involuntary movements of any kind. Report these promptly.
2. This drug potentiates the effects of levodopa. When this drug is added to current levodopa treatment, adverse effects of levodopa may develop or be intensified. It is necessary to reduce the dose of levodopa by 10% to 20% when treatment with selegiline begins.
3. Inform your physician promptly if you become pregnant or plan pregnancy. The manufacturer does not recommend the use of this drug during pregnancy.

Precautions for Use
By Infants and Children: This drug is not utilized by this age group.
By Those over 60 Years of Age: This drug is well tolerated by the elderly. Observe closely for any tendency to light-headedness or faintness, especially on arising from a lying or sitting position.

▷ **Advisability of Use During Pregnancy**
Pregnancy Category: B (tentative). See Pregnancy Code inside back cover.
Animal studies: No birth defects due to this drug were found in rat studies.
Human studies: Information from adequate studies of pregnant women is not available. The manufacturer advises that this drug should not be taken during pregnancy.

Advisability of Use if Breast-Feeding
Presence of this drug in breast milk: Unknown.
Avoid drug or refrain from nursing.

Habit-Forming Potential: None.

Effects of Overdosage: Nausea, vomiting, palpitations, low blood pressure, agitation, severe involuntary movements, hallucinations.

Possible Effects of Long-Term Use: None reported.

Suggested Periodic Examinations While Taking This Drug (at physician's discretion)
Regular evaluation of drug response, heart function and blood pressure status.

▷ **While Taking This Drug, Observe the Following**
Foods: No restrictions.
Beverages: No restrictions. May be taken with milk.
▷ *Alcohol:* Use caution until the combined effects have been determined. Alcohol may exaggerate the blood-pressure-lowering and sedative effects of this drug.
Tobacco Smoking: No interactions expected.
▷ *Other Drugs*
Selegiline *taken concurrently* with
• antihypertensive drugs (and other drugs that can lower blood pressure) requires careful monitoring for excessive drops in pressure. Dosage adjustments may be necessary.
• meperidine (Demerol) may cause a life-threatening reaction of unknown cause; avoid this combination.
The following drugs may *decrease* the effects of selegiline and diminish its effectiveness
• chlorprothixene (Taractan).
• haloperidol (Haldol).
• metoclopramide (Reglan).
• phenothiazines (see Drug Class, Section Four).
• reserpine (Ser-Ap-Es, etc.), in high doses.
• thiothixene (Navane).
▷ *Driving, Hazardous Activities:* This drug may cause dizziness, drowsiness, impaired coordination or fainting. Restrict activities as necessary.
Aviation Note: The use of this drug *is a disqualification* for piloting. Consult a designated Aviation Medical Examiner.

Exposure to Sun: No restrictions.

Exposure to Heat: Use caution until the combined effects have been determined. Hot environments can cause lowering of blood pressure.

Discontinuation: Do not discontinue this drug abruptly. Sudden withdrawal can cause prompt increase in parkinsonian symptoms and deterioration of control. Consult your physician regarding a schedule for gradual withdrawal and concurrent adjustment of Sinemet or other appropriate drugs.

SPIRONOLACTONE
(speer on oh LAK tohn)

Introduced: 1959

Class: Diuretic

Prescription: USA: Yes
Canada: Yes

Controlled Drug: USA: No
Canada: No

Available as Generic: USA: Yes
Canada: No

Brand Names: Aldactone, Aldactazide [CD], Alatone, ✦Novospiroton, ✦Novospirozine [CD], ✦Sincomen

---

BENEFITS versus RISKS

Possible Benefits	*Possible Risks*
EFFECTIVE PREVENTION OF POTASSIUM LOSS when used adjunctively with other diuretics	ABNORMALLY HIGH BLOOD POTASSIUM LEVEL with excessive use
EFFECTIVE DIURETIC IN REFRACTORY CASES OF FLUID RETENTION when used adjunctively with other diuretics	Enlargement of male breast tissue Masculinization effects in women: excessive hair growth, deepening of the voice

---

▷ **Principal Uses**

As a Single Drug Product: This mild diuretic is used as part of the treatment program for the management of congestive heart failure and disorders of the liver and kidney that are accompanied by excessive fluid retention (edema). It is also used in conjunction with other measures to treat high blood pressure. It is used primarily in situations where it is advisable to prevent loss of potassium from the body.

As a Combination Drug Product [CD]: This drug is available in combination with hydrochlorothiazide, a different kind of diuretic that promotes the loss of potassium from the body. Spironolactone is used in this combination to counteract the potassium-wasting effect of the thiazide diuretic.

How This Drug Works: Not completely established. It is thought that by inhibiting the action of aldosterone (an adrenal gland hormone), this drug prevents the reabsorption of sodium and the excretion of potassium by the kidney. Thus the drug promotes the excretion of sodium (and water with it) and the retention of potassium.

Available Dosage Forms and Strengths
Tablets — 25 mg, 50 mg, 100 mg

▷ **Usual Adult Dosage Range:**   Initially, 25 to 100 mg/day for 5 days. The dose is then adjusted according to individual response. The usual maintenance dose is 50 to 200 mg/day, divided into 2 to 4 doses. The total daily dosage should not exceed 400 mg. **Note: Actual dosage and administration schedule must be determined by the physician for each patient individually.**

▷ **Dosing Instructions:**   May be taken with or following meals to promote absorption of the drug and to reduce stomach irritation. The tablet may be crushed for administration. Intermittent or alternate day use is recommended to minimize the possibility of sodium and potassium imbalance.

Usual Duration of Use: Continual use on a regular schedule for 5 to 10 days is usually necessary to determine this drug's effectiveness in clearing edema, and for 2 to 3 weeks to determine its effect on hypertension. Long-term use (months to years) requires supervision and periodic evaluation by your physician. Consult your physician on a regular basis.

▷ **This Drug Should Not Be Taken If**
   • you have had an allergic reaction to it previously.
   • you have severely impaired liver or kidney function.

▷ **Inform Your Physician Before Taking This Drug If**
   • you have a history of liver or kidney disease.
   • you have diabetes.
   • you are taking any of the following: an anticoagulant, antihypertensives, a digitalis preparation, another diuretic, lithium or a potassium preparation.
   • you plan to have surgery under general anesthesia in the near future.

Possible Side-Effects (natural, expected and unavoidable drug actions)
Abnormally high blood potassium levels (42%), abnormally low blood sodium levels (12%), dehydration (17%).

▷ **Possible Adverse Effects** (unusual, unexpected and infrequent reactions)
   If any of the following develop, consult your physician promptly for guidance.
   Mild Adverse Effects
   Allergic Reactions: Skin rash, hives, itching, drug fever (see Glossary).

Headache, dizziness, unsteadiness, weakness, drowsiness, lethargy, confusion.

Dry mouth, nausea, vomiting, diarrhea.

Serious Adverse Effects

Allergic Reaction: Abnormally low blood platelet count (rare).

Symptomatic potassium excess: confusion, numbness and tingling in lips and extremities, fatigue, weakness, shortness of breath, slow heart rate, low blood pressure.

Masculine pattern of hair growth and deepening of the voice in women.

Stomach ulceration with bleeding (rare).

▷ **Possible Effects on Sexual Function**

Decreased libido (close to 100%); impaired erection or impotence (30%).

Male breast enlargement and tenderness (close to 100% with high doses).

Female breast enlargement (100% with high doses); altered timing and pattern of menstruation; postmenopausal bleeding.

Decreased vaginal secretion.

Possible Effects on Laboratory Tests

White blood cell count: decreased (one report only).

Blood platelet count: decreased.

Prothrombin time: decreased.

Blood potassium level: increased.

Blood uric acid level: no effect in some; increased and decreased in others.

CAUTION

1. Do not take potassium supplements or increase your intake of potassium-rich foods while taking this drug.
2. Do not discontinue this drug abruptly unless abnormally high blood levels of potassium develop.
3. Ordinary doses of aspirin (600 mg) may reverse the diuretic effect of this drug. Observe response to this drug combination.
4. Avoid the excessive use of salt substitutes that contain potassium; these are a potential cause of potassium excess.

Precautions for Use

By Infants and Children: Limit the continual use of this drug in children to 1 month. Observe closely for indications of potassium accumulation.

By Those over 60 Years of Age: The natural decline in kidney function may predispose to potassium retention in the body. Limit continual use of this drug to periods of 2 to 3 weeks. Observe for indications of potassium excess: slow heart rate, irregular heart rhythms, low blood pressure, confusion, drowsiness. The excessive use of diuretics can cause harmful loss of body water (dehydration), increased viscosity of the blood and an increased tendency of the blood to clot, predisposing to stroke, heart attack or thrombophlebitis.

▷ **Advisability of Use During Pregnancy**
   Pregnancy Category: D (tentative). See Pregnancy Code inside back cover.
   Animal studies: This drug causes feminization of male rat fetuses.
   Human studies: Information from adequate studies of pregnant women
   is not available.
   This drug should not be used during pregnancy unless a very serious
   complication of pregnancy occurs for which this drug is significantly
   beneficial.

Advisability of Use if Breast-Feeding
   Presence of this drug in breast milk: A metabolic byproduct (canrenone)
   is present.
   Avoid drug or refrain from nursing.

Habit-Forming Potential: None.

Effects of Overdosage: Thirst, drowsiness, fatigue, weakness, nausea, vomiting, confusion, irregular heart rhythm, low blood pressure.

Possible Effects of Long-Term Use: Potassium accumulation to abnormally high blood levels. Male breast enlargement.

Suggested Periodic Examinations While Taking This Drug (at physician's
   discretion)
   Measurements of blood sodium, potassium and chloride levels.
   Kidney function tests.

▷ **While Taking This Drug, Observe the Following**
   Foods: No restrictions. Avoid excessive restriction of salt.
   Beverages: No restrictions. May be taken with milk.
▷ *Alcohol:* Use with caution until the combined effects have been determined.
      Alcohol may enhance the drowsiness and the blood-pressure-lowering
      effect of this drug.
   Tobacco Smoking: No interactions expected.
▷ *Other Drugs*
      Spironolactone may *increase* the effects of
      • digoxin (Lanoxin).
      Spironolactone may *decrease* the effects of
      • anticoagulants (Coumadin, etc.).
      Spironolactone *taken concurrently* with
      • captopril (Capoten) may cause excessively high blood potassium levels.
      • digitoxin (Crystodigin) may cause either increased or decreased digi-
        toxin effects (unpredictable).
      • lithium may cause accumulation of lithium to toxic levels.
      • potassium preparations may cause excessively high blood potassium
        levels.
      The following drugs may *decrease* the effects of spironolactone
      • aspirin may reduce its diuretic effectiveness.
▷ *Driving, Hazardous Activities:* This drug may cause dizziness and drowsi-
      ness. Restrict activities as necessary.

Aviation Note: The use of this drug *may be a disqualification* for piloting. Consult a designated Aviation Medical Examiner.

Exposure to Sun: No restrictions.

Discontinuation: With high dosage or prolonged use, it is advisable to withdraw this drug gradually. Ask your physician for guidance.

SUCRALFATE
(soo KRAL fayt)

Introduced: 1978

Prescription: USA: Yes
    Canada: Yes

Available as Generic: No

Brand Names: Carafate, ✚Sulcrate

Class: Antiulcer

Controlled Drug: USA: No
    Canada: No

BENEFITS versus RISKS

Possible Benefits	*Possible Risks*
EFFECTIVE TREATMENT IN PEPTIC ULCER DISEASE	Constipation
	Skin rash, hives, itching
No serious adverse effects	
No significant drug interactions	

▷ **Principal Uses**

As a Single Drug Product: Used exclusively in the management of peptic ulcer disease to promote healing of both stomach (gastric) and duodenal ulcer. It is effective when used alone, but may be used in conjunction with antacids when these are needed for pain relief. It is also used to prevent ulcer recurrence.

How This Drug Works: Not completely established. It is thought that this drug promotes ulcer healing by several mechanisms: (1) the formation of a protective coating over the ulcer site to prevent further erosion by stomach acid; (2) the inhibition of the digestive action of pepsin; (3) the protection of injured tissue at the ulcer margins; (4) the stimulation of active healing (tissue repair).

Available Dosage Forms and Strengths
    Tablets — 0.5 gram, 1 gram

▷ **Usual Adult Dosage Range:** 1 gram 4 times/day. **Note: Actual dosage and administration schedule must be determined by the physician for each patient individually.**

▷ **Dosing Instructions:**   Take with water on an empty stomach at least 1 hour before or 2 hours after each meal and at bedtime. Swallow the tablets whole; do not alter or chew. Take the full course prescribed.

Usual Duration of Use: Continual use on a regular schedule for 6 to 8 weeks is usually necessary to determine this drug's effectiveness in promoting the healing of peptic ulcers. Use beyond 8 weeks must be determined by your physician.

▷ **This Drug Should Not Be Taken If**
- you have had an allergic reaction to it previously.

▷ **Inform Your Physician Before Taking This Drug If**
- you have chronic constipation.
- you are taking any other drugs at this time.

Possible Side-Effects (natural, expected and unavoidable drug actions)
Constipation (2.2%).

▷ **Possible Adverse Effects** (unusual, unexpected and infrequent reactions)
If any of the following develop, consult your physician promptly for guidance.
Mild Adverse Effects
Allergic Reactions: Skin rash, hives, itching.
Dizziness, light-headedness, drowsiness.
Dry mouth, indigestion, nausea, cramping, diarrhea.
Serious Adverse Effects
None reported.

▷ **Possible Effects on Sexual Function:**   None reported.

Possible Effects on Laboratory Tests
None reported.

CAUTION
1. If antacids are needed to relieve ulcer pain, do not take them within half an hour before or 1 hour after the dose of sucralfate.
2. This drug may impair the absorption of other drugs if they are taken close together. It is advisable to avoid taking any other drugs within 2 hours of taking sucralfate. This applies especially to cimetidine (Tagamet), phenytoin (Dilantin) and tetracyclines.

▷ **Advisability of Use During Pregnancy**
Pregnancy Category: B (tentative). See Pregnancy Code inside back cover.
Animal studies: No birth defects due to this drug reported in mouse, rat and rabbit studies.
Human studies: Information from adequate studies of pregnant women is not available.
Because only very small amounts of this drug are absorbed, it is probably safe for use at any time during pregnancy. However, it should be used only if clearly needed. Ask your physician for guidance.

Advisability of Use if Breast-Feeding
　　Presence of this drug in breast milk: Unknown.
　　Monitor nursing infant closely and discontinue drug or nursing if adverse effects develop.

Habit-Forming Potential:　None.

Effects of Overdosage:　Nausea, stomach cramping, possible diarrhea.

Possible Effects of Long-Term Use:　Deficiencies of vitamins A, D, E and K due to impaired absorption from the intestine.

Suggested Periodic Examinations While Taking This Drug (at physician's discretion)
　　None required.

▷ **While Taking This Drug, Observe the Following**
　　Foods: No restrictions. Follow diet prescribed by your physician.
　　Beverages: No restrictions. This drug is preferably taken with water.
▷　*Alcohol:* No interactions with drug expected. However, alcohol is best avoided because of its irritant effect on the stomach.
　　Tobacco Smoking: No interactions expected. However, nicotine can delay ulcer healing and reduce the effectiveness of this drug. Avoid all forms of tobacco.
▷　*Other Drugs*
　　Sucralfate may *decrease* the effects of
　　　• cimetidine (Tagamet).
　　　• digoxin (Lanoxin).
　　　• phenytoin (Dilantin, etc.).
　　　• tetracycline (Achromycin, Tetracyn, etc.).
　　　• warfarin (Coumadin, etc.), and reduce its effectiveness as an anticoagulant.
▷　*Driving, Hazardous Activities:* This drug may cause dizziness or drowsiness. Restrict activities as necessary.
　　Aviation Note: The use of this drug *may be a disqualification* for piloting. Consult a designated Aviation Medical Examiner.
　　Exposure to Sun: No restrictions.

SULFAMETHOXAZOLE
(sul fa meth OX a zohl)

Introduced: 1961

Class: Anti-infective, sulfonamides

Prescription: USA: Yes
Canada: Yes

Controlled Drug: USA: No
Canada: No

Available as Generic: Yes

Brand Names: ✦Apo-Sulfamethoxazole, ✦Apo-Sulfatrim [CD], ✦Apo-Sulfatrim DS [CD], Azo Gantanol [CD], Bactrim [CD], Bactrim DS [CD], Bethaprim [CD], Comoxol [CD], Cotrim [CD], Gantanol, ✦Novotrimel [CD], ✦Novotrimel DS [CD], ✦Protrin [CD], ✦Protrin DF [CD], ✦Roubac [CD], Septra [CD], Septra DS [CD], ✦Uro Gantanol [CD], Uroplus DS [CD], Uroplus SS [CD]

BENEFITS versus RISKS

Possible Benefits	*Possible Risks*
EFFECTIVE ANTIMICROBIAL ACTION against susceptible bacteria and protozoa	Allergic reactions: mild to severe skin reactions, anaphylaxis, myocarditis
	Rare blood cell disorders: aplastic anemia, hemolytic anemia, abnormally low white cell and platelet counts
	Drug-induced liver damage
	Drug-induced kidney damage

▷ **Principal Uses**

As a Single Drug Product: This member of the sulfonamide class is used to treat a variety of bacterial and protozoal infections. It is most commonly used to treat certain infections of the urinary tract.

As a Combination Drug Product [CD]: This drug is available in combination with phenazopyridine, an analgesic drug that relieves the discomfort associated with acute infections of the urinary bladder and urethra. This combination provides early symptomatic relief while the underlying infection is being eradicated. This drug is also available in combination with another antibacterial drug—trimethoprim. This combination is quite effective in the treatment of certain types of middle ear infection, bronchitis, pneumonia and certain infections of the intestinal tract and the urinary tract.

How This Drug Works: This drug prevents the growth and multiplication of susceptible bacteria by interfering with their formation of folic acid, an essential nutrient.

Available Dosage Forms and Strengths
Oral suspension — 500 mg per 5-ml teaspoonful
Tablets — 500 mg, 1 gram

▷ **Usual Adult Dosage Range:**   Initially, 2 grams; then 1 gram every 8 to 12 hours, depending upon the severity of the infection. The total daily dosage should not exceed 3 grams. **Note: Actual dosage and administration schedule must be determined by the physician for each patient individually.**

▷ **Dosing Instructions:**   Preferably taken on an empty stomach, 1 hour before or 2 hours after eating. However, it may be taken with or following food to reduce stomach irritation. The tablet may be crushed for administration.

Usual Duration of Use: Continual use on a regular schedule for 4 to 7 days is usually necessary to determine this drug's effectiveness in controlling responsive infections. Treatment should be continued until the patient is free of symptoms for 48 hours. Limit treatment to no more than 14 days if possible.

Currently a "Drug of Choice"
(when combined with trimethoprim) for preventing pneumonia (due to pneumocystis carinii) in patients with AIDS.

▷ **This Drug Should Not Be Taken If**
  • you are allergic to *any* sulfonamide drug (see Drug Class, Section Four).
  • you are in the last month of pregnancy.
  • you are breast-feeding.

▷ **Inform Your Physician Before Taking This Drug If**
  • you are allergic to any sulfonamide derivative: acetazolamide, thiazide diuretics, sulfonylurea antidiabetic drugs (see Drug Classes, Section Four).
  • you are allergic by nature: history of hay fever, asthma, hives, eczema.
  • you have impaired liver or kidney function.
  • you have a personal or family history of porphyria.
  • you have had a drug-induced blood cell or bone marrow disorder in the past.
  • you are currently taking any oral anticoagulant, antidiabetic drug or phenytoin.
  • you plan to have surgery under pentothal anesthesia while taking this drug.

Possible Side-Effects (natural, expected and unavoidable drug actions)
Brownish coloration of the urine, of no significance.
Superinfections, bacterial or fungal (see Glossary).

▷ **Possible Adverse Effects** (unusual, unexpected and infrequent reactions)
If any of the following develop, consult your physician promptly for guidance.

Mild Adverse Effects

Allergic Reactions: Skin rashes, hives, itching, localized swellings, reddened eyes.

Headache, dizziness, unsteadiness, ringing in the ears.

Loss of appetite, irritation of the mouth and tongue, nausea, vomiting, abdominal pain, diarrhea.

Serious Adverse Effects

Allergic Reactions: Drug fever (see Glossary), swollen glands, painful joints, anaphylaxis (see Glossary). Allergic reaction in the heart muscle (myocarditis), allergic pneumonitis, allergic hepatitis. Severe skin reactions.

Idiosyncratic Reaction: Hemolytic anemia (see Glossary).

Bone marrow depression (see Glossary): fatigue, weakness, fever, sore throat, abnormal bleeding or bruising.

Pancreatitis; kidney damage: bloody or cloudy urine, reduced urine volume.

Psychotic reactions, hallucinations, seizures, hearing loss, peripheral neuropathy (see Glossary).

▷ **Possible Effects on Sexual Function:**   None reported.

▷ **Adverse Effects That May Mimic Natural Diseases or Disorders**

Liver reactions may suggest viral hepatitis.

Lung reactions may suggest an infectious pneumonia.

Natural Diseases or Disorders That May Be Activated by This Drug

Goiter, acute intermittent porphyria, polyarteritis nodosa, systemic lupus erythematosus (questionable).

Possible Effects on Laboratory Tests

Complete blood cell counts: decreased red cells, hemoglobin, white cells and platelets; increased eosinophils (allergic reaction).

Prothrombin time: increased (when taken concurrently with warfarin).

Liver function tests: increased liver enzymes (ALT/GPT, AST/GOT and alkaline phosphatase), increased bilirubin.

CAUTION

1. A large intake of water (up to 2 quarts daily) is necessary to ensure an adequate volume of urine.
2. Shake liquid dosage forms thoroughly before measuring each dose.

Precautions for Use

By Infants and Children: This drug should not be used in infants under 2 months of age.

By Those over 60 Years of Age: Small doses taken at longer intervals often achieve adequate blood and tissue drug levels. Observe for the development of reduced urine volume, fever, sore throat, abnormal bleeding or bruising or skin irritation with itching, particularly in the anal or genital regions.

▷ **Advisability of Use During Pregnancy**
Pregnancy Category: C (tentative). See Pregnancy Code inside back cover.
Animal studies: Cleft palate and skeletal birth defects reported in mice and rats.
Human studies: No increase in birth defects reported in 4584 exposures to various sulfonamides during pregnancy.
Avoid use of drug during the last month of pregnancy because of possible adverse effects on the newborn infant.

Advisability of Use if Breast-Feeding
Presence of this drug in breast milk: Yes.
Avoid drug or refrain from nursing.

Habit-Forming Potential: None.

Effects of Overdosage: Headache, dizziness, nausea, vomiting, abdominal cramping, toxic fever, coma, jaundice, kidney failure.

Possible Effects of Long-Term Use: Superinfections, bacterial or fungal. Development of goiter, with or without hypothyroidism. Excessive loss of vitamin C via urine.

Suggested Periodic Examinations While Taking This Drug (at physician's discretion)
Complete blood cell counts, weekly for the first 8 weeks.
Urine analysis weekly.
Liver and kidney function tests.

▷ **While Taking This Drug, Observe the Following**
Foods: No restrictions.
Beverages: No restrictions. May be taken with milk.
▷ *Alcohol:* Use caution until the combined effect has been determined. Sulfonamide drugs can increase the intoxicating effects of alcohol.
Tobacco Smoking: No interactions expected.
▷ *Other Drugs*
Sulfamethoxazole may *increase* the effects of
  • anticoagulants (Coumadin, etc.), and increase the risk of bleeding.
  • sulfonylureas (see Drug Class, Section Four), and increase the risk of hypoglycemia.
Sulfamethoxazole may *decrease* the effects of
  • cyclosporine, and reduce its immunosuppressive effect.
  • penicillins.
▷ *Driving, Hazardous Activities:* This drug may cause dizziness. Restrict activities as necessary.
Aviation Note: The use of this drug *may be a disqualification* for piloting. Consult a designated Aviation Medical Examiner.
Exposure to Sun: Use caution until sensitivity has been determined. Some sulfonamide drugs can cause photosensitivity (see Glossary).

SULFASALAZINE
(sul fa SAL a zeen)

Introduced: 1949

Class: Bowel anti-inflammatory, sulfonamides

Prescription: USA: Yes
Canada: Yes

Controlled Drug: USA: No
Canada: No

Available as Generic: USA: Yes
Canada: No

Brand Names: Azaline, Azulfidine, Azulfidine EN-tabs, ✦PMS Sulfasalazine, ✦PMS Sulfasalazine E.C., ✦Salazopyrin, ✦SAS-Enema, ✦SAS Enteric-500, SAS-500

BENEFITS versus RISKS

Possible Benefits	*Possible Risks*
EFFECTIVE SUPPRESSION OF INFLAMMATORY BOWEL DISEASE SYMPTOMATIC RELIEF IN TREATMENT OF REGIONAL ENTERITIS AND ULCERATIVE COLITIS	Allergic reactions: mild to severe skin reactions Rare blood cell disorders: aplastic anemia, hemolytic anemia, abnormally low white cell and platelet counts Drug-induced liver damage Drug-induced kidney damage

---

▷ **Principal Uses**

As a Single Drug Product: This member of the sulfonamide class is used exclusively to treat inflammatory disease of the lower intestinal tract: regional enteritis (Crohn's disease) and ulcerative colitis. It is usually taken by mouth, but may also be used in retention enemas.

How This Drug Works: Not completely established. Possible methods of this drug's action include
- an anti-inflammatory action that suppresses the formation of prostaglandins (and related compounds), tissue substances that induce inflammation, tissue destruction and diarrhea.
- an anti-infective action that may prevent the growth and multiplication of certain infective agents in the intestine and colon. (This method of action is questionable.)

Available Dosage Forms and Strengths
Oral suspension — 250 mg per 5-ml teaspoonful
Tablets — 500 mg
Tablets, enteric-coated — 500 mg

▷ **Usual Adult Dosage Range:**   Initially, 1 to 2 grams every 6 to 8 hours until symptoms are adequately controlled. For maintenance, 500 mg/6 hours. The total daily dosage should not exceed 12 grams. **Note: Actual dosage and administration schedule must be determined by the physician for each patient individually.**

▷ **Dosing Instructions:**   Preferably taken with 8 ounces of water on an empty stomach, 1 hour before or 2 hours after eating. However, it may be taken with or following food to reduce stomach irritation. Intervals between doses (day and night) should be no longer than 8 hours. The regular tablet may be crushed for administration; the enteric-coated tablet should be swallowed whole without alteration.

Usual Duration of Use: Continual use on a regular schedule for 1 to 3 weeks is usually necessary to determine this drug's effectiveness in controlling the symptoms of regional enteritis or ulcerative colitis. Long-term use (months to years) requires supervision and periodic evaluation by your physician. Consult your physician on a regular basis.

▷ **This Drug Should Not Be Taken If**
  • you are allergic to *any* sulfonamide drug (see Drug Class, Section Four), or to aspirin (or other salicylates).
  • you are in the last month of pregnancy.
  • you are breast-feeding.

▷ **Inform Your Physician Before Taking This Drug If**
  • you are allergic to any sulfonamide derivative: acetazolamide, thiazide diuretics, sulfonylurea antidiabetic drugs (see Drug Classes, Section Four).
  • you are allergic by nature: history of hay fever, asthma, hives, eczema.
  • you have impaired liver or kidney function.
  • you have a personal or family history of porphyria.
  • you have had a drug-induced blood cell or bone marrow disorder in the past.
  • you are currently taking any oral anticoagulant, antidiabetic drug or phenytoin.
  • you plan to have surgery under pentothal anesthesia while taking this drug.

Possible Side-Effects (natural, expected and unavoidable drug actions)
  Brownish coloration of the urine, of no significance.
  Superinfections, bacterial or fungal (see Glossary).

▷ **Possible Adverse Effects** (unusual, unexpected and infrequent reactions)
  If any of the following develop, consult your physician promptly for guidance.
  Mild Adverse Effects
  Allergic Reactions: Skin rashes, hives, itching.
  Headache, dizziness.

Loss of appetite, irritation of the mouth and tongue, nausea, vomiting, abdominal pain, diarrhea.

Serious Adverse Effects

Allergic Reactions: Drug fever (see Glossary), swollen glands, painful joints, anaphylaxis (see Glossary). Allergic pneumonitis, allergic hepatitis. Severe skin reactions.

Idiosyncratic Reaction: Hemolytic anemia (see Glossary).

Bone marrow depression (see Glossary): fatigue, weakness, fever, sore throat, abnormal bleeding or bruising.

Pancreatitis; kidney damage: bloody or cloudy urine, reduced urine volume.

Peripheral neuropathy (see Glossary).

▷ **Possible Effects on Sexual Function:**   Decreased production of sperm, reversible infertility.

▷ **Adverse Effects That May Mimic Natural Diseases or Disorders**

Liver reactions may suggest viral hepatitis.

Lung reactions may suggest an infectious pneumonia.

Natural Diseases or Disorders That May Be Activated by This Drug

Goiter, acute intermittent porphyria.

Possible Effects on Laboratory Tests

Complete blood cell counts: decreased red cells, hemoglobin, white cells and platelets; increased eosinophils (allergic reaction).

Liver function tests: increased liver enzymes (ALT/GPT, AST/GOT and alkaline phosphatase), increased bilirubin.

Sperm count: decreased; abnormal sperm common; effects reversible on discontinuation of drug.

CAUTION

1. A large intake of water (up to 2 quarts daily) is necessary to ensure an adequate volume of urine.
2. Shake liquid dosage forms thoroughly before measuring each dose.

Precautions for Use

By Infants and Children: Safety and effectiveness for use by those under 2 years of age have not been established.

By Those over 60 Years of Age: Observe for the development of reduced urine volume, fever, sore throat, abnormal bleeding or bruising or skin irritation with itching, particularly in the anal or genital regions.

▷ **Advisability of Use During Pregnancy**

Pregnancy Category: C (tentative). See Pregnancy Code inside back cover.

Animal studies: Cleft palate and skeletal birth defects due to sulfonamides reported in mice and rats.

Human studies: No increase in birth defects reported in 4584 exposures to various sulfonamides during pregnancy.

Avoid use of drug during the last month of pregnancy because of possible adverse effects on the newborn infant.

Advisability of Use if Breast-Feeding
Presence of this drug in breast milk: Yes.
Avoid drug or refrain from nursing.

Habit-Forming Potential: None.

Effects of Overdosage: Headache, dizziness, nausea, vomiting, abdominal cramping, toxic fever, coma, jaundice, kidney failure.

Possible Effects of Long-Term Use: Development of goiter, with or without hypothyroidism. An orange-yellow discoloration of the skin has been reported. This is not jaundice.

Suggested Periodic Examinations While Taking This Drug (at physician's discretion)
Complete blood cell counts, weekly for the first 8 weeks.
Urine analysis weekly.
Liver and kidney function tests.

▷ **While Taking This Drug, Observe the Following**
Foods: No restrictions. Follow prescribed diet.
Beverages: No restrictions. May be taken with milk.
▷ *Alcohol:* Use caution until the combined effect has been determined. Sulfonamide drugs can increase the intoxicating effects of alcohol.
Tobacco Smoking: No interactions expected.
▷ *Other Drugs*
Sulfasalazine may *increase* the effects of
• anticoagulants (Coumadin, etc.), and increase the risk of bleeding.
• sulfonylureas (see Drug Class, Section Four), and increase the risk of hypoglycemia.
Sulfasalazine may *decrease* the effects of
• digoxin (Lanoxin).
▷ *Driving, Hazardous Activities:* This drug may cause dizziness. Restrict activities as necessary.
Aviation Note: The use of this drug *may be a disqualification* for piloting. Consult a designated Aviation Medical Examiner.
Exposure to Sun: Use caution until sensitivity has been determined. Some sulfonamide drugs can cause photosensitivity (see Glossary).

SULFISOXAZOLE
(sul fi SOX a zohl)

Introduced: 1949

Prescription: USA: Yes
Canada: Yes

Available as Generic: Yes

Class: Anti-infective, sulfonamides

Controlled Drug: USA: No
Canada: No

Brand Names: ✦Apo-Sulfisoxazole, Azo Gantrisin [CD], Eryzole [CD], Gantrisin, Lipo Gantrisin, ✦Novosoxazole, Pediazole [CD]

BENEFITS versus RISKS

Possible Benefits	*Possible Risks*
EFFECTIVE ANTIMICROBIAL ACTION against susceptible bacteria and protozoa	Allergic reactions: mild to severe skin reactions, anaphylaxis Rare blood cell disorders: aplastic anemia, hemolytic anemia, abnormally low white cell and platelet counts Drug-induced liver damage Drug-induced kidney damage

---

▷ **Principal Uses**

As a Single Drug Product: This member of the sulfonamide class is used to treat a variety of bacterial and protozoal infections. It is most commonly used to treat certain infections of the urinary tract.

As a Combination Drug Product [CD]: This drug is available in combination with phenazopyridine, an analgesic drug that relieves the discomfort associated with acute infections of the urinary bladder and urethra. This combination provides early symptomatic relief while the underlying infection is being eradicated.

How This Drug Works: This drug prevents the growth and multiplication of susceptible bacteria by interfering with their formation of folic acid, an essential nutrient.

Available Dosage Forms and Strengths
Emulsion, prolonged-action — 1 gram per 5-ml teaspoonful
Eye drops — 4%
Eye ointment — 4%
Injection — 400 mg per ml
Pediatric suspension — 500 mg per 5-ml teaspoonful
Syrup — 500 mg per 5-ml teaspoonful
Tablets — 500 mg

▷ **Usual Adult Dosage Range:** Initially, 2 to 4 grams; then 750 to 1500 mg (1.5 grams) every 4 hours, or 1 to 2 grams every 6 hours, depending upon the severity of the infection. The total daily dosage should not exceed

12 grams. **Note: Actual dosage and administration schedule must be determined by the physician for each patient individually.**

▷ **Dosing Instructions:** Preferably taken with 8 ounces of water on an empty stomach, 1 hour before or 2 hours after eating. However, it may be taken with or following food to reduce stomach irritation. The tablet may be crushed for administration.

Usual Duration of Use: Continual use on a regular schedule for 7 to 10 days is usually necessary to determine this drug's effectiveness in controlling responsive infections. Treatment should be continued until the patient is free of symptoms for 48 hours. Limit treatment to no more than 14 days if possible.

▷ **This Drug Should Not Be Taken If**
• you are allergic to *any* sulfonamide drug (see Drug Class, Section Four).
• you are in the last month of pregnancy.
• you are breast-feeding.

▷ **Inform Your Physician Before Taking This Drug If**
• you are allergic to any sulfonamide derivative: acetazolamide, thiazide diuretics, sulfonylurea antidiabetic drugs (see Drug Classes, Section Four).
• you are allergic by nature: history of hay fever, asthma, hives, eczema.
• you have impaired liver or kidney function.
• you have a personal or family history of porphyria.
• you have had a drug-induced blood cell or bone marrow disorder in the past.
• you are currently taking any oral anticoagulant, antidiabetic drug or phenytoin.
• you plan to have surgery under pentothal anesthesia while taking this drug.

Possible Side-Effects (natural, expected and unavoidable drug actions)
Brownish coloration of the urine, of no significance.
Superinfections, bacterial or fungal (see Glossary).

▷ **Possible Adverse Effects** (unusual, unexpected and infrequent reactions)
If any of the following develop, consult your physician promptly for guidance.
Mild Adverse Effects
Allergic Reactions: Skin rashes, hives, itching, localized swellings, reddened eyes.
Headache, dizziness, unsteadiness, ringing in the ears.
Loss of appetite, irritation of the mouth and tongue, nausea, vomiting, abdominal pain, diarrhea.
Serious Adverse Effects
Allergic Reactions: Drug fever (see Glossary), swollen glands, painful joints, anaphylaxis (see Glossary). Allergic hepatitis. Severe skin reactions.

Idiosyncratic Reaction: Hemolytic anemia (see Glossary).

Bone marrow depression (see Glossary): fatigue, weakness, fever, sore throat, abnormal bleeding or bruising.

Kidney damage: bloody or cloudy urine, reduced urine volume.

Peripheral neuropathy (see Glossary).

▷ **Possible Effects on Sexual Function:** None reported.

▷ **Adverse Effects That May Mimic Natural Diseases or Disorders**
Liver reactions may suggest viral hepatitis.

Natural Diseases or Disorders That May Be Activated by This Drug
Goiter, acute intermittent porphyria.

Possible Effects on Laboratory Tests
Complete blood cell counts: decreased red cells, hemoglobin, white cells and platelets; increased eosinophils (allergic reaction).

Blood lupus erythematosus (LE) cells: positive.

Blood amylase and lipase levels: increased (pancreatitis).

Liver function tests: increased liver enzymes (ALT/GPT, AST/GOT and alkaline phosphatase), increased bilirubin.

CAUTION
1. A large intake of water (up to 2 quarts daily) is necessary to ensure an adequate volume of urine.
2. Shake liquid dosage forms thoroughly before measuring each dose.

Precautions for Use
By Infants and Children: This drug should not be used in infants under 2 months of age.

By Those over 60 Years of Age: Small doses taken at longer intervals often achieve adequate blood and tissue drug levels. Observe for the development of reduced urine volume, fever, sore throat, abnormal bleeding or bruising or skin irritation with itching, particularly in the anal or genital regions.

▷ **Advisability of Use During Pregnancy**
Pregnancy Category: C (tentative). See Pregnancy Code inside back cover.

Animal studies: Cleft palate and skeletal birth defects due to sulfonamides reported in mice and rats.

Human studies: No increase in birth defects reported in 4287 exposures to this drug during pregnancy.

Avoid use of drug during the last month of pregnancy because of possible adverse effects on the newborn infant.

Advisability of Use if Breast-Feeding
Presence of this drug in breast milk: Yes.

Avoid drug or refrain from nursing.

Habit-Forming Potential: None.

Effects of Overdosage: Headache, dizziness, nausea, vomiting, abdominal cramping, toxic fever, coma, jaundice, kidney failure.

Possible Effects of Long-Term Use: Superinfections, bacterial or fungal. Development of goiter, with or without hypothyroidism. Excessive loss of vitamin C via urine.

Suggested Periodic Examinations While Taking This Drug (at physician's discretion)
Complete blood cell counts, weekly for the first 8 weeks.
Urine analysis weekly.
Liver and kidney function tests.

▷ **While Taking This Drug, Observe the Following**
Foods: No restrictions.
Beverages: No restrictions. May be taken with milk.
▷ *Alcohol:* Use caution until the combined effect has been determined. Sulfonamide drugs can increase the intoxicating effects of alcohol.
Tobacco Smoking: No interactions expected.
▷ *Other Drugs*
Sulfisoxazole may ***increase*** the effects of
• anticoagulants (Coumadin, etc.), and increase the risk of bleeding.
• sulfonylureas (see Drug Class, Section Four), and increase the risk of hypoglycemia.
Sulfisoxazole may ***decrease*** the effects of
• penicillins.
▷ *Driving, Hazardous Activities:* This drug may cause dizziness. Restrict activities as necessary.
Aviation Note: The use of this drug ***may be a disqualification*** for piloting. Consult a designated Aviation Medical Examiner.
Exposure to Sun: Use caution until sensitivity has been determined. Some sulfonamide drugs can cause photosensitivity (see Glossary).

SULINDAC
(sul IN dak)

Introduced: 1976

Class: Mild analgesic, anti-inflammatory

Prescription: USA: Yes
Canada: Yes

Controlled Drug: USA: No
Canada: No

Available as Generic: Yes

Brand Name: Clinoril

```
┌─────────────────────────────────────────────────────────────┐
│                  BENEFITS versus RISKS                        │
│                                                               │
│    Possible Benefits              Possible Risks              │
│  EFFECTIVE RELIEF OF MILD    Gastrointestinal pain, ulceration,│
│    TO MODERATE PAIN AND        bleeding (rare)                │
│    INFLAMMATION              Rare liver damage                │
│                             Rare kidney damage               │
│                             Rare bone marrow depression      │
│                               (aplastic anemia)              │
│                                                               │
└─────────────────────────────────────────────────────────────┘
```

▷ **Principal Uses**

As a Single Drug Product: Used primarily to relieve mild to moderately severe pain associated with (1) rheumatoid arthritis and osteoarthritis; (2) acute and chronic gout; and (3) bursitis, tendinitis and related disorders.

How This Drug Works: Not completely established. It is thought that this drug reduces the tissue concentrations of prostaglandins (and related compounds), substances involved in the production of inflammation and pain.

Available Dosage Forms and Strengths

Tablets — 150 mg, 200 mg

▷ **Usual Adult Dosage Range:**   150 to 200 mg twice/day, 12 hours apart. The total daily dosage should not exceed 400 mg. **Note: Actual dosage and administration schedule must be determined by the physician for each patient individually.**

▷ **Dosing Instructions:**   Preferably taken on an empty stomach, 1 hour before or 2 hours after eating. However, it may be taken with or after food if necessary to reduce stomach irritation. Take with a full glass of water and remain upright (do not lie down) for 30 minutes. The tablet may be crushed for administration.

Usual Duration of Use: Continual use on a regular schedule for 2 to 3 weeks is usually necessary to determine this drug's effectiveness in relieving the discomfort of arthritis. Acute gout usually responds within 7 days. Shoulder bursitis or tendinitis usually responds within 7 to 14 days. Long-term use (months to years) requires supervision and periodic evaluation by your physician. Consult your physician on a regular basis.

▷ **This Drug Should Not Be Taken If**
- you have had an allergic reaction to it previously.
- you are subject to asthma or nasal polyps caused by aspirin.
- you have active peptic ulcer disease or any form of gastrointestinal bleeding.

- you have a bleeding disorder or a blood cell disorder.
- you have severe impairment of liver or kidney function.

▷ **Inform Your Physician Before Taking This Drug If**
- you are allergic to aspirin or to other aspirin substitutes.
- you have a history of peptic ulcer disease or any type of bleeding disorder.
- you have impaired liver or kidney function.
- you have high blood pressure or a history of heart failure.
- you are taking any of the following: acetaminophen, aspirin or other aspirin substitutes, anticoagulants, oral antidiabetic drugs.

Possible Side-Effects (natural, expected and unavoidable drug actions)
Fluid retention (edema).
Drowsiness in sensitive individuals.

▷ **Possible Adverse Effects** (unusual, unexpected and infrequent reactions)
If any of the following develop, consult your physician promptly for guidance.
Mild Adverse Effects
Allergic Reactions: Skin rash, hives, itching.
Headache, dizziness, mild numbness and tingling, blurred vision, ringing in the ears.
Mouth sores, indigestion, nausea, vomiting, constipation, diarrhea.
Serious Adverse Effects
Allergic Reactions: Anaphylactic reaction (see Glossary), severe skin reactions.
Idiosyncratic Reactions: Drug-induced pneumonitis with fever.
Active peptic ulcer, with or without bleeding.
Liver damage with jaundice (see Glossary).
Kidney damage with reduced urine formation (very rare).
Rare bone marrow depression (see Glossary): fatigue, weakness, fever, sore throat, abnormal bleeding or bruising.

▷ **Possible Effects on Sexual Function**
Vaginal bleeding (less than 1%).
Male breast enlargement (causal relationship not established).

Possible Delayed Adverse Effects: Mild anemia due to "silent" blood loss from the stomach (less than that caused by aspirin).

▷ **Adverse Effects That May Mimic Natural Diseases or Disorders**
Liver reaction may suggest viral hepatitis.

Natural Diseases or Disorders That May Be Activated by This Drug
Peptic ulcer disease, ulcerative colitis.

Possible Effects on Laboratory Tests
Complete blood cell counts: decreased red cells, hemoglobin, white cells and platelets.

Liver function tests: increased liver enzymes (ALT/GPT, AST/GOT and alkaline phosphatase), increased bilirubin.

CAUTION
1. Dosage should always be limited to the smallest amount that produces reasonable improvement.
2. This drug may mask early indications of infection. Inform your physician if you think you are developing an infection of any kind.

Precautions for Use
By Infants and Children: Safety and effectiveness for use by those under 12 years of age have not been established.

By Those over 60 Years of Age: Small doses are advisable until tolerance is determined. Observe for any indications of liver or kidney toxicity, fluid retention, dizziness, confusion, impaired memory, stomach bleeding or constipation.

▷ **Advisability of Use During Pregnancy**
Pregnancy Category: C (tentative). See Pregnancy Code inside back cover.
Animal studies: A low incidence of birth defects has been reported but not confirmed.

Human studies: Information from adequate studies of pregnant women is not available.

The manufacturer does not recommend the use of this drug during pregnancy.

Advisability of Use if Breast-Feeding
Presence of this drug in breast milk: Unknown.
Avoid drug or refrain from nursing.

Habit-Forming Potential: None.

Effects of Overdosage: Stomach irritation, nausea, vomiting, diarrhea.

Possible Effects of Long-Term Use: Fluid retention.

Suggested Periodic Examinations While Taking This Drug (at physician's discretion)
Complete blood cell counts, liver and kidney function tests, complete eye examinations if vision is altered in any way.

▷ **While Taking This Drug, Observe the Following**
Foods: No restrictions.
Beverages: No restrictions. May be taken with milk.
▷   *Alcohol:* Use with caution. The irritant action of alcohol on the stomach lining, added to the irritant action of this drug in sensitive individuals, can increase the risk of stomach ulceration and/or bleeding.
Tobacco Smoking: No interactions expected.
▷   *Other Drugs*
Sulindac may *increase* the effects of
• acetaminophen (Tylenol, etc.), and increase the risk of kidney damage; avoid prolonged use of this combination.

- anticoagulants (Coumadin, etc.), and increase the risk of bleeding; monitor prothrombin time, adjust dose accordingly.

Sulindac *taken concurrently* with the following drugs may increase the risk of bleeding; avoid these combinations:
- aspirin.
- dipyridamole (Persantine).
- indomethacin (Indocin).
- sulfinpyrazone (Anturane).
- valproic acid (Depakene).

▷ *Driving, Hazardous Activities:* This drug may cause drowsiness or dizziness. Restrict activities as necessary.

Aviation Note: The use of this drug *may be a disqualification* for piloting. Consult a designated Aviation Medical Examiner.

Exposure to Sun: No restrictions.

TAMOXIFEN
(ta MOX i fen)

Introduced: 1973

Class: Antiestrogen, anticancer

Prescription: USA: Yes
Canada: Yes

Controlled Drug: USA: No
Canada: No

Available as Generic: No

Brand Names: Nolvadex, ✦Nolvadex-D, ✦Tamofen

BENEFITS versus RISKS

Possible Benefits	*Possible Risks*
EFFECTIVE ADJUNCTIVE TREATMENT IN ADVANCED BREAST CANCER in 30% to 40% of cases	Severe increase in tumor or bone pain, transient Thromophlebitis, pulmonary embolism Abnormally high blood calcium levels Eye changes: corneal opacities, retinal injury

---

▷ **Principal Uses**

As a Single Drug Product: Used primarily as an alternative to estrogens and androgens (male sex hormones) to treat advanced breast cancer in postmenopausal women. It is also used to stimulate ovulation in premenopausal women with infertility.

How This Drug Works: Not completely established. It is thought that by blocking the uptake of estradiol (estrogen), this drug removes or reduces a stimulus to breast cancer cells.

Available Dosage Forms and Strengths
Tablets — 10 mg, 20 mg (in Canada)

▷ **Usual Adult Dosage Range:**   10 to 20 mg twice/day, morning and evening. **Note: Actual dosage and administration schedule must be determined by the physician for each patient individually.**

▷ **Dosing Instructions:**   May be taken either on an empty stomach or with food. The tablet may be crushed for administration.

Usual Duration of Use: Continual use on a regular schedule for 4 to 10 weeks is usually necessary to determine this drug's effectiveness in controlling the growth and spread of advanced breast cancer. In the presence of bone involvement, treatment for several months may be required to evaluate effectiveness. Long-term use (months to years) requires supervision and periodic evaluation by your physician. Consult your physician on a regular basis.

▷ **This Drug Should Not Be Taken If**
- you have had a serious allergic or adverse reaction to it previously.
- you have active phlebitis.
- you have a significant deficiency of white blood cells or blood platelets.

▷ **Inform Your Physician Before Taking This Drug If**
- you have a history of thrombophlebitis or pulmonary embolism.
- you have a history of abnormally high blood calcium levels.
- you have a history of any type of blood cell or bone marrow disorder.
- you have cataracts or other visual impairment.
- you have impaired liver function.
- you plan to have surgery in the near future.

Possible Side-Effects (natural, expected and unavoidable drug actions)
Hot flashes, fluid retention, weight gain.

▷ **Possible Adverse Effects** (unusual, unexpected and infrequent reactions)
If any of the following develop, consult your physician promptly for guidance.
Mild Adverse Effects
Allergic Reaction: Skin rash.
Headache, dizziness, drowsiness, depression, fatigue, confusion.
Nausea, vomiting, itching in genital area, loss of hair.
Serious Adverse Effects
Initial "flare" of severe pain in tumor or involved bone.
Development of thrombophlebitis, risk of pulmonary embolism.
Eye changes: corneal opacities, retinal injury.
Development of abnormally high blood calcium levels.
Transient decreases in white blood cells and blood platelets.

▷ **Possible Effects on Sexual Function**
Premenopausal: altered timing and pattern of menstruation.
Postmenopausal: vaginal bleeding.

This drug may be effective in treating the following conditions:
- male infertility due to abnormally low sperm counts.
- male breast enlargement and tenderness.
- chronic female breast pain (mastalgia).

Possible Effects on Laboratory Tests
Complete blood cell counts: decreased red cells, hemoglobin, white cells and platelets.
Blood calcium level: increased.
Blood thyroid hormone levels: T^3, T^4 and free T^4 increased.
Liver function tests: increased liver enzyme (AST/GOT), increased bilirubin (one case report).
Sperm count: increased.

CAUTION
1. If this drug is used prior to your menopause, it may induce ovulation and predispose to pregnancy. Since this drug should not be used during pregnancy, some method of contraception (other than oral contraceptives) is advised.
2. Do not take any form of estrogen while taking this drug; estrogens can inhibit tamoxifen's effectiveness.

▷ **Advisability of Use During Pregnancy**
Pregnancy Category: X (tentative). See Pregnancy Code inside back cover.
Animal studies: No birth defects due to this drug reported.
Human studies: Information from adequate studies of pregnant women is not available.
This drug can have estrogenic effects. It should not be used during pregnancy.

Advisability of Use if Breast-Feeding
Presence of this drug in breast milk: Unknown.
Avoid drug or refrain from nursing.

Habit-Forming Potential: None.

Effects of Overdosage: No information available.

Possible Effects of Long-Term Use: Development of abnormally high blood calcium levels.

Suggested Periodic Examinations While Taking This Drug (at physician's discretion)
Complete blood cell counts, measurements of blood calcium levels.
Complete eye examinations if impaired vision occurs.

▷ **While Taking This Drug, Observe the Following**
Foods: No restrictions.
Beverages: No restrictions. May be taken with milk.
▷ *Alcohol:* No interactions expected.
Tobacco Smoking: No interactions expected.

▷   *Other Drugs*
The following drugs may ***decrease*** the effects of tamoxifen
- estrogens.
- oral contraceptives (those that contain estrogens).

▷   *Driving, Hazardous Activities:* This drug may cause dizziness or drowsiness. Restrict activities as necessary.
Aviation Note: The use of this drug ***may be a disqualification*** for piloting. Consult a designated Aviation Medical Examiner.
Exposure to Sun: No restrictions.

TEMAZEPAM
(tem AZ e pam)

Introduced: 1978   **Class:** Hypnotic, benzodiazepines

Prescription: USA: Yes   **Controlled Drug:** USA: C-IV*
　　Canada: Yes   　　Canada: No

Available as Generic: USA: Yes
　　Canada: No

Brand Names: Razepam, Restoril, Temaz

BENEFITS versus RISKS

Possible Benefits	*Possible Risks*
EFFECTIVE HYPNOTIC after 4 weeks of continual use	Habit-forming potential with long-term use
Wide margin of safety with therapeutic doses	Minor impairment of mental functions ("hangover" effect)

▷ **Principal Uses**
As a Single Drug Product: This member of the benzodiazepine class of "minor tranquilizers" is used exclusively as a bedtime sedative to induce sleep.

How This Drug Works: It is thought that this drug produces a calming effect by enhancing the action of the nerve transmitter gamma-aminobutyric acid (GABA), which in turn blocks the arousal of higher brain centers and helps to induce sleep.

Available Dosage Forms and Strengths
Capsules — 15 mg, 30 mg

▷ **Usual Adult Dosage Range:** 15 to 30 mg at bedtime. Total daily dosage should not exceed 90 mg. **Note: Actual dosage and administration**

*See Schedules of Controlled Drugs inside back cover.

schedule must be determined by the physician for each patient individually.

▷ **Dosing Instructions:** Preferably taken on an empty stomach to hasten absorption and induce sleep rapidly. The capsule may be opened for administration. Do not discontinue this drug abruptly if taken for more than 4 weeks.

Usual Duration of Use: Periods of 3 to 5 nights intermittently, repeated as needed with appropriate dosage adjustment. Avoid uninterrupted and prolonged use. The duration of use should not exceed 2 weeks without reappraisal of continued need.

▷ **This Drug Should Not Be Taken If**
- you have had an allergic reaction to it previously.
- you have acute narrow-angle glaucoma, inadequately treated.

▷ **Inform Your Physician Before Taking This Drug If**
- you are allergic to any benzodiazepine drug (see Drug Class, Section Four).
- you have a history of alcoholism or drug abuse.
- you are pregnant or planning pregnancy.
- you have impaired liver or kidney function.
- you have a history of serious depression or mental disorder.
- you are taking other drugs with sedative effects.
- you have any of the following: asthma, emphysema, epilepsy, myasthenia gravis.

Possible Side-Effects (natural, expected and unavoidable drug actions)
"Hangover" effects on arising: drowsiness, lethargy and unsteadiness.

▷ **Possible Adverse Effects** (unusual, unexpected and infrequent reactions)
If any of the following develop, consult your physician promptly for guidance.
Mild Adverse Effects
Allergic Reactions: Skin rash, hives.
Dizziness, fainting, slurred speech, nausea, indigestion.
Serious Adverse Effects
Idiosyncratic Reactions: Nervousness, talkativeness, irritability, apprehension, euphoria, excitement, hallucinations.

▷ **Possible Effects on Sexual Function:** None reported.

Possible Effects on Laboratory Tests
Urine screening tests for drug abuse: may be **positive**. (Test results depend upon amount of drug taken and testing method used.)

CAUTION
1. This drug should not be discontinued abruptly if it has been taken continually for more than 4 weeks.
2. The concurrent use of some over-the-counter drug products that con-

tain antihistamines (allergy and cold preparations, sleep aids) can cause excessive sedation in sensitive individuals.

3. Regular nightly use of any hypnotic drug should be avoided.
4. If you experience a "hangover" effect, avoid hazardous activities (driving, etc.) and the use of alcohol.

Precautions for Use
By Infants and Children: Safety and effectiveness for use by those under 18 years of age have not been established.

By Those over 60 Years of Age: It is advisable to use smaller doses (15 mg) at first to determine your response. Observe for the possible development of lethargy, indifference, fatigue, weakness, unsteadiness, disturbing dreams, nightmares and paradoxical reactions of excitement, agitation, anger, hostility and rage.

▷ Advisability of Use During Pregnancy
Pregnancy Category: X (tentative). See Pregnancy Code inside back cover.
Animal studies: Rib defects reported in rats; skull and rib defects reported in rabbits.
Human studies: Information from adequate studies of pregnant women is not available.
Avoid use during entire pregnancy.

Advisability of Use if Breast-Feeding
Presence of this drug in breast milk: Probably yes.
Avoid drug or refrain from nursing.

Habit-Forming Potential: This drug can produce psychological and/or physical dependence (see Glossary) if used in large doses for an extended period of time. Avoid continual use.

Effects of Overdosage: Marked drowsiness, weakness, feeling of drunkenness, staggering gait, tremor, stupor progressing to deep sleep or coma.

Possible Effects of Long-Term Use: Psychological and/or physical dependence.

Periodic Examinations While Taking This Drug (at physician's discretion) Complete blood cell counts during long-term use.

▷ While Taking This Drug, Observe the Following
Foods: No restrictions.
Beverages: Avoid excessive intake of caffeine-containing beverages (coffee, tea, cola) within 4 hours of taking this drug. May be taken with milk.
▷ *Alcohol:* Use with extreme caution until the combined effect has been determined. Alcohol may increase the absorption of this drug and add to its depressant effects on the brain. It is advisable to avoid alcohol completely throughout the day and night if it is necessary to drive or to engage in any hazardous activity.
Tobacco Smoking: Heavy smoking may reduce the hypnotic action of this drug.

Marijuana Smoking: Increased sedation and significant impairment of intellectual and physical performance.
▷ *Other Drugs*
Temazepam may *increase* the effects of
• digoxin (Lanoxin), and cause digoxin toxicity.
• phenytoin (Dilantin), and cause phenytoin toxicity.
Temazepam may *decrease* the effects of
• levodopa (Sinemet, etc.), and reduce its effectiveness in treating Parkinson's disease.
The following drugs may *increase* the effects of temazepam
• cimetidine (Tagamet).
• disulfiram (Antabuse).
• isoniazid (INH, Rifamate, etc.).
• oral contraceptives.
• valproic acid (Depakene).
The following drugs may *decrease* the effects of temazepam
• rifampin (Rimactane, etc.).
• theophylline (Aminophylline, Theo-Dur, etc.).
▷ *Driving, Hazardous Activities:* This drug can impair mental alertness, judgment, physical coordination and reaction time. Avoid hazardous activities accordingly.
Aviation Note: The use of this drug *is a disqualification* for piloting. Consult a designated Aviation Medical Examiner.
Exposure to Sun: No restrictions.
Exposure to Heat: Use caution until the effect of excessive perspiration is determined. Because of reduced urine volume, this drug may accumulate in the body and produce effects of overdosage.
Discontinuation: Avoid sudden discontinuation if this drug has been taken for over 4 weeks without interruption. Dosage should be tapered gradually to prevent a withdrawal syndrome that could include depression, confusion, hallucinations, tremor, seizures, muscle cramping, sweating and vomiting.

TERAZOSIN
(ter AY zoh sin)

Introduced: 1987   **Class:** Antihypertensive

Prescription: USA: Yes   **Controlled Drug:** USA: No

Available as Generic: No

Brand Name: Hytrin

```
┌─────────────────────────────────────────────────────────┐
│                   BENEFITS versus RISKS                    │
│                                                            │
│      Possible Benefits              Possible Risks         │
│  EFFECTIVE TREATMENT OF       "First dose" drop in blood   │
│    MILD TO MODERATE             pressure with fainting (1%)│
│    HYPERTENSION when used     Fluid retention (5.5%)       │
│    alone or in combination    Rapid heart rate (1.9%)      │
│    with other antihyperten-                                │
│    sive drugs                                              │
└─────────────────────────────────────────────────────────┘
```

▷ **Principal Uses**

As a Single Drug Product: Used primarily as a "step 1" antihypertensive drug to initiate treatment of mild to moderate hypertension. Also used in conjunction with other drugs to treat moderate to severe hypertension.

How This Drug Works: It is thought that by blocking certain actions of the sympathetic nervous system, this drug causes direct relaxation and expansion of blood vessel walls, thus lowering the pressure of the blood within the vessels.

Available Dosage Forms and Strengths

Tablets — 1 mg, 2 mg, 5 mg

▷ **Usual Adult Dosage Range:** Initiate treatment with a "test dose" of 1 mg to determine the patient's response within the first 2 hours. If tolerated satisfactorily, increase dose cautiously (as needed and tolerated) up to 5 mg/24 hours taken as a single dose at bedtime. Total daily dosage should not exceed 20 mg. **Note: Actual dosage and administration schedule must be determined by the physician for each patient individually.**

▷ **Dosing Instructions:** Preferably taken at bedtime to avoid orthostatic hypotension (see Glossary). May be taken without regard to food. The tablet may be crushed for administration.

Usual Duration of Use: Continual use on a regular schedule for 6 to 8 weeks is usually necessary to determine this drug's effectiveness in controlling hypertension. Long-term use (months to years) requires supervision and periodic evaluation by your physician. Consult your physician on a regular basis.

Possible Advantages of This Drug

May be used to initiate treatment.
Usually effective with once-a-day dosage.
Rarely causes depression or impotence.
Does not alter blood cholesterol, potassium or sugar.

▷ **This Drug Should Not Be Taken If**

• you have had an allergic reaction to it previously.
• you are experiencing mental depression.

- you have angina (active coronary artery disease) and you are not taking a beta-blocking drug. (Consult your physician.)

▷ **Inform Your Physician Before Taking This Drug If**
- you have experienced orthostatic hypotension (see Glossary) when using other antihypertensive drugs.
- you have a history of mental depression.
- you have impaired circulation to the brain, or a history of stroke.
- you have coronary artery disease.
- you have active liver disease or impaired liver function.
- you have impaired kidney function.
- you plan to have surgery under general anesthesia in the near future.

Possible Side-Effects (natural, expected and unavoidable drug actions)
Orthostatic hypotension (1.3%), drowsiness (5.4%), salt and water retention (5.5%), dry mouth, nasal congestion (5.9%), constipation.

▷ **Possible Adverse Effects** (unusual, unexpected and infrequent reactions)
If any of the following develop, consult your physician promptly for guidance.
Mild Adverse Effects
Allergic Reaction: Skin rash.
Headache (16.2%), dizziness (19.3%), fatigue (6.9%), weakness (11.3%), nervousness (2.3%), sweating, numbness and tingling (2.9%), blurred vision (1.6%).
Palpitation (4.3%), rapid heart rate (1.9%), shortness of breath (3.1%).
Nausea (4.4%), vomiting, diarrhea, abdominal pain.
Serious Adverse Effects
Mental depression (0.3%).

▷ **Possible Effects on Sexual Function:**   Impotence (1.2%).

Natural Diseases or Disorders That May Be Activated by This Drug
Latent coronary artery insufficiency.

Possible Effects on Laboratory Tests
Blood total cholesterol, LDL and VLDL cholesterol levels: decreased.
Blood HDL cholesterol level: no effect.
Blood triglyceride levels: no effect.

CAUTION
1. Observe for the possible "first dose" response of precipitous drop in blood pressue, with or without fainting; this usually occurs within 30 to 90 minutes. Limit initial doses to 1 mg taken at bedtime for the first 3 days; remain supine after taking these trial doses.
2. Impaired kidney function may increase your sensitivity to this drug and require smaller than usual doses.
3. Consult your physician if you plan to use over-the-counter remedies

for allergic rhinitis or head colds; these preparations contain drugs that may interact with terazosin.

Precautions for Use

By Infants and Children: Safety and effectiveness for use by those under 12 years of age have not been established.

By Those over 60 Years of Age: Begin treatment with no more than 1 mg/ day for the first 3 days. Subsequent increases in dose must be very gradual and carefully supervised by your physician. The occurrence of orthostatic hypotension can cause unexpected falls and injury; sit or lie down promptly if you feel light-headed or dizzy. Report any indications of dizziness or chest pain promptly.

▷ **Advisability of Use During Pregnancy**

Pregnancy Category: C (tentative). See Pregnancy Code inside back cover.
Animal studies: No birth defects found in rat or rabbit studies.
Human studies: Information from adequate studies of pregnant women is not available.
Use this drug only if clearly needed. Ask your physician for guidance.

Advisability of Use if Breast-Feeding

Presence of this drug in breast milk: Unknown.
Monitor nursing infant closely and discontinue drug or nursing if adverse effects develop.

Habit-Forming Potential: None.

Effects of Overdosage: Orthostatic hypotension, headache, generalized flushing, rapid heart rate, extreme weakness, irregular heart rhythm, circulatory collapse.

Possible Effects of Long-Term Use: None reported.

Suggested Periodic Examinations While Taking This Drug (at physician's discretion)
Measurements of blood pressure in lying, sitting and standing positions.
Measurements of body weight to detect fluid retention.

▷ **While Taking This Drug, Observe the Following**

Foods: No restrictions. Avoid excessive salt intake.
Beverages: No restrictions. May be taken with milk.
▷ *Alcohol:* Use with extreme caution until the combined effects have been determined. Alcohol can exaggerate the blood-pressure-lowering actions of this drug and cause excessive reduction.
Tobacco Smoking: Nicotine can contribute significantly to this drug's ability to intensify coronary insufficiency in susceptible individuals. All forms of tobacco should be avoided.
▷ *Other Drugs*
The following drugs may *increase* the effects of terazosin
• beta-adrenergic-blocking drugs (see Drug Class, Section Four); the se-

verity and duration of the "first dose" hypotensive response may be increased.

The following drugs may *decrease* the effects of terazosin

• estrogens.

• indomethacin (Indocin).

▷ *Driving, Hazardous Activities:* This drug may cause dizziness or drowsiness. Restrict activities as necessary.

Aviation Note: The use of this drug *is a disqualification* for piloting. Consult a designated Aviation Medical Examiner.

Exposure to Sun: No restrictions.

Exposure to Cold: Use caution until combined effect has been determined. Cold environments may increase this drug's ability to cause coronary insufficiency (angina) and hypothermia (see Glossary) in susceptible individuals.

Heavy Exercise or Exertion: Excessive exertion can augment this drug's ability to induce angina. See Angina in Section Two.

Discontinuation: If you are taking this drug as part of your treatment program for congestive heart failure, do not discontinue it abruptly. Ask your physician for guidance.

TERBUTALINE
(ter BYU ta leen)

Introduced: 1974

Class: Antiasthmatic, bronchodilator

Prescription: USA: Yes
Canada: Yes

Controlled Drug: USA: No
Canada: No

Available as Generic: No

Brand Names: Brethaire, Brethine, Bricanyl, ✦Bricanyl Spacer

BENEFITS versus RISKS	
Possible Benefits	*Possible Risks*
VERY EFFECTIVE RELIEF OF BRONCHOSPASM	Increased blood pressure Fine hand tremor Irregular heart rhythm (with excessive use)

▷ **Principal Uses**

As a Single Drug Product: To relieve acute bronchial asthma and to reduce the frequency and severity of chronic, recurrent asthmatic attacks; also used to relieve reversible bronchospasm associated with chronic bronchitis and emphysema.

How This Drug Works: By stimulating certain sympathetic nerve terminals, this drug acts to dilate those bronchial tubes that are in sustained constriction, thereby increasing the size of the airway and improving the ability to breathe.

Available Dosage Forms and Strengths
Aerosol — 0.2 mg/actuation, 0.25 mg/actuation (Canada)
Injection — 1 mg per ml
Tablets — 2.5 mg, 5 mg

▷ **Usual Adult Dosage Range:** Aerosol: 0.4 mg taken in 2 separate inhalations 1 minute apart; repeat every 4 to 6 hours as needed. Tablets: 2.5 to 5 mg taken 3 times/day, 6 hours apart. The total daily dosage should not exceed 15 mg. **Note: Actual dosage and administration schedule must be determined by the physician for each patient individually.**

▷ **Dosing Instructions:** May be taken on empty stomach or with food or milk. Tablets may be crushed for administration. For aerosol, follow the written instructions carefully. Do not overuse.

Usual Duration of Use: According to individual requirements. Do not use beyond the time necessary to terminate episodes of asthma.

Possible Advantages of This Drug
Rapid onset of action.
Long duration of action.
Highly effective relief of asthma.

▷ **This Drug Should Not Be Taken If**
 • you have had an allergic reaction to any dosage form of it previously.
 • you currently have an irregular heart rhythm.
 • you are taking, or have taken within the past 2 weeks, any monoamine oxidase (MAO) type A inhibitor drug (see Drug Class, Section Four).

▷ **Inform Your Physician Before Taking This Drug If**
 • you are overly sensitive to other drugs that stimulate the sympathetic nervous system.
 • you are currently using epinephrine (Adrenalin, Primatene Mist, etc.) to relieve asthmatic breathing.
 • you have a seizure disorder.
 • you have any type of heart or circulatory disorder, especially high blood pressure or coronary heart disease.
 • you have diabetes or an overactive thyroid gland (hyperthyroidism).
 • you are taking any form of digitalis or any stimulant drug.

Possible Side-Effects (natural, expected and unavoidable drug actions)
Aerosol: dryness or irritation of mouth or throat, altered taste. Tablet: nervousness, tremor, palpitation.

▷ **Possible Adverse Effects** (unusual, unexpected and infrequent reactions)
   If any of the following develop, consult your physician promptly for guidance.
   Mild Adverse Effects
   Headache, dizziness, drowsiness, restlessness, insomnia.
   Rapid, pounding heartbeat; increased sweating; muscle cramps in arms and legs.
   Nausea, heartburn, vomiting.
   Serious Adverse Effects
   Rapid or irregular heart rhythm, intensification of angina, increased blood pressure.

▷ **Possible Effects on Sexual Function:**   None reported.

Natural Diseases or Disorders That May Be Activated By This Drug
   Latent coronary artery disease, diabetes or high blood pressure.

Possible Effects on Laboratory Tests
   Blood total cholesterol and LDL cholesterol levels: no effect.
   Blood HDL cholesterol level: increased.
   Blood triglyceride levels: no effect.
   Blood thyroid hormone levels: T^3 increased; T^4 decreased; free T^4 no effect.

CAUTION
1. Concurrent use of this drug by aerosol inhalation with beclomethasone aerosol (Beclovent, Vanceril) may increase the risk of toxicity due to fluorocarbon propellants. It is advisable to use this aerosol 20 to 30 minutes *before* beclomethasone aerosol. This will reduce the risk of toxicity and will enhance the penetration of beclomethasone.
2. *Avoid excessive use of aerosol inhalation.* The excessive or prolonged use of this drug by inhalation can reduce its effectiveness and cause serious heart rhythm disturbances, including cardiac arrest.
3. Do not use this drug concurrently with epinephrine. These two drugs may be used alternately if an interval of 4 hours is allowed between doses.
4. If you do not respond to your usually effective dose, ask your physician for guidance. Do not increase the size or frequency of the dose without your physician's approval.

Precautions for Use
   By Infants and Children: Safety and effectiveness for use by those under 12 years of age have not been established.
   By Those over 60 Years of Age: Avoid excessive and continual use. If acute asthma is not relieved promptly, other drugs will have to be tried. Observe for the development of nervousness, palpitations, irregular heart rhythm and muscle tremors. Use with extreme caution if you have hardening of the arteries, heart disease or high blood pressure.

▷ **Advisability of Use During Pregnancy**
   Pregnancy Category: B (tentative). See Pregnancy Code inside back cover.
      Animal studies: No significant birth defects reported in mouse and rat studies.
      Human studies: Information from adequate studies of pregnant women is not available.
      Use only if clearly needed. Ask your physician for guidance.

Advisability of Use if Breast-Feeding
   Presence of this drug in breast milk: Yes.
   Monitor nursing infant closely and discontinue drug or nursing if adverse effects develop.

Habit-Forming Potential: None.

Effects of Overdosage: Nervousness, palpitation, rapid heart rate, sweating, headache, tremor, vomiting, chest pain.

Possible Effects of Long-Term Use: Loss of effectiveness. See *CAUTION* category above.

Suggested Periodic Examinations While Taking This Drug (at physician's discretion)
   Blood pressure measurements, evaluation of heart status.

▷ **While Taking This Drug, Observe the Following**
   Foods: No restrictions.
   Beverages: Avoid excessive use of caffeine-containing beverages: coffee, tea, cola, chocolate.
▷ *Alcohol:* No interactions expected.
   Tobacco Smoking: No interactions expected.
▷ *Other Drugs*
      Terbutaline *taken concurrently* with
      • monoamine oxidase (MAO) type A inhibitor drugs may cause excessive increase in blood pressure and undesirable heart stimulation (see Drug Class, Section Four).
      The following drugs may *decrease* the effects of terbutaline
      • beta blocker drugs may impair its effectiveness (see Drug Class, Section Four).
▷ *Driving, Hazardous Activities:* Usually no restrictions. Use caution if excessive nervousness or dizziness occurs.
   Aviation Note: The use of this drug *is a disqualification* for piloting. Consult a designated Aviation Medical Examiner.
   Exposure to Sun: No restrictions.
   Heavy Exercise or Exertion: Use caution. Excessive exercise can induce asthma in sensitive individuals.

TERFENADINE
(ter FEN a deen)

Introduced: 1977

Prescription: USA: Yes
Canada: No

Available as Generic: No

Brand Names: Seldane, Seldane-D

Class: Antihistamines

Controlled Drug: USA: No
Canada: No

BENEFITS versus RISKS

Possible Benefits	*Possible Risks*
EFFECTIVE RELIEF OF ALLERGIC RHINITIS AND ALLERGIC SKIN DISORDERS	Infrequent headache Mild fatigue Minor digestive disturbances Slight atropinelike effects

---

▷ **Principal Uses**

As a Single Drug Product: Used primarily to provide symptomatic relief in allergic and related disorders: seasonal and perennial allergic rhinitis (hay fever), allergic conjunctivitis and vasomotor rhinitis; also in hives and localized swellings (angioedema) of allergic origin.

How This Drug Works: Antihistamines reduce the intensity of the allergic response by blocking the action of histamine after it has been released from sensitized tissue cells in the eyes, nose and skin.

Available Dosage Forms and Strengths
Suspension — 30 mg per 5-ml teaspoonful (Canada)
Tablets — 60 mg

▷ **Usual Adult Dosage Range:**   60 mg every 8 to 12 hours as needed. The total daily dosage should not exceed 360 mg. **Note: Actual dosage and administration schedule must be determined by the physician for each patient individually.**

▷ **Dosing Instructions:**   May be taken with food or milk to prevent stomach irritation. The tablet may be crushed for administration.

Usual Duration of Use: Continual use on a regular schedule for 2 to 3 days is usually necessary to determine this drug's effectiveness in relieving the symptoms of allergic rhinitis and dermatosis. It may be necessary to take this drug throughout the entire pollen season, depending upon individual sensitivity. However, antihistamines should not be taken continually (without interruption) for long-term use. Limit their use to periods that require symptomatic relief. Consult your physician on a regular basis.

Possible Advantages of This Drug
>   Fast onset of action, relief within one hour.
>   No loss of effectiveness with continual use.
>   No drowsiness or impaired mental function that is so characteristic of
>   other antihistamines.

▷ **This Drug Should Not Be Taken If**
>   • you have had an allergic reaction to any dosage form of it previously.
>   • you are currently undergoing allergy skin tests.

▷ **Inform Your Physician Before Taking This Drug If**
>   • you have had any allergic reactions or unfavorable responses to the
>   previous use of antihistamines.

Possible Side-Effects (natural, expected and unavoidable drug actions)
>   Dry nose, mouth or throat.

▷ **Possible Adverse Effects** (unusual, unexpected and infrequent reactions)
>   **If any of the following develop, consult your physician promptly for
>   guidance.**
>   *Mild Adverse Effects*
>   Allergic Reactions: Skin rash, itching.
>   Headache, nervousness, fatigue.
>   Increased appetite, indigestion, nausea, vomiting.
>   *Serious Adverse Effects*
>   None reported.

▷ **Possible Effects on Sexual Function**
>   Altered timing and pattern of menstruation.
>   Female breast enlargement with milk production.

Possible Effects on Laboratory Tests
>   None reported.

CAUTION
>   1. Discontinue this drug 4 days before diagnostic skin testing proce-
>   dures in order to prevent false negative test results.
>   2. Do not use this drug if you have active bronchial asthma, bronchitis
>   or pneumonia. It may thicken bronchial mucus and make it more
>   difficult to remove (by absorption or coughing).

Precautions for Use
>   *By Infants and Children:* Safety and effectiveness for use by those under 12
>   years of age have not been established.
>   *By Those over 60 Years of Age:* You may be more susceptible to the develop-
>   ment of headache and fatigue. Use smaller doses at longer intervals if
>   necessary.

▷ **Advisability of Use During Pregnancy**
>   *Pregnancy Category:* C (tentative). See Pregnancy Code inside back cover.
>   Animal studies: No birth defects due to this drug reported.

Human studies: Information from adequate studies of pregnant women is not available.

Use this drug only if clearly needed. Ask your physician for guidance.

Advisability of Use if Breast-Feeding
Presence of this drug in breast milk: Unknown.

Avoid drug or refrain from nursing.

Habit-Forming Potential: None.

Effects of Overdosage: No information available. No serious or threatening effects expected.

Possible Effects of Long-Term Use: None reported.

Suggested Periodic Examinations While Taking This Drug (at physician's discretion)
None required.

▷ ### While Taking This Drug, Observe the Following
Foods: No restrictions.

Beverages: No restrictions. May be taken with milk.

▷ *Alcohol:* No interactions expected.

Tobacco Smoking: No interactions expected.

▷ *Other Drugs:* No significant interactions reported to date.

Hazardous Activities: No restrictions.

Aviation Note: The use of this drug *is probably not a disqualification* for piloting. Consult a designated Aviation Medical Examiner.

Exposure to Sun: No restrictions.

TETRACYCLINE
(te trah SI kleen)

Introduced: 1953

Class: Antibiotic, tetracyclines

Prescription: USA: Yes
Canada: Yes

Controlled Drug: USA: No
Canada: No

Available as Generic: Yes

Brand Names: Achromycin, Achromycin V, ✦Apo-Tetra, Cyclopar, ✦Medi-cycline, Mysteclin-F [CD], ✦Neo-Tetrine, Nor-Tet, ✦Novotetra, Panmycin, Retet, Robitet, Sumycin, Tetra-C, Tetracyn, Tetralan, Tetram, Tropicycline

```
                    BENEFITS versus RISKS

      Possible Benefits                    Possible Risks
  EFFECTIVE TREATMENT OF           ALLERGIC REACTIONS, mild to
  INFECTIONS due to susceptible      severe: ANAPHYLAXIS,
  bacteria and protozoa              DRUG-INDUCED HEPATITIS
                                     (rare)
                                   Drug-induced colitis
                                   Superinfections (bacterial or
                                     fungal)
                                   Rare blood cell disorders:
                                     hemolytic anemia, abnormally
                                     low white cell and platelet
                                     counts
```

▷ **Principal Uses**

As a Single Drug Product: This member of the tetracycline drug class is used primarily to (1) treat a broad range of infections caused by susceptible bacteria and protozoa (short-term use); and (2) treat severe, resistant pustular acne (long-term use).

As a Combination Drug Product [CD]: This drug is available in combination with amphotericin B, an antifungal antibiotic that is provided to reduce the risk of developing an overgrowth of yeast organisms (superinfection) of the gastrointestinal tract.

How This Drug Works: This drug prevents the growth and multiplication of susceptible bacteria by interfering with their formation of essential proteins.

Available Dosage Forms and Strengths
                    Capsules — 100 mg, 250 mg, 500 mg
                    Ointment — 3%
       Ointment, ophthalmic — 10 mg per gram
            Solution, topical — 2.2 mg per ml
     Suspension, ophthalmic — 10 mg per ml
            Suspension, oral — 125 mg per 5-ml teaspoonful
                    Tablets — 250 mg, 500 mg

▷ **Usual Adult Dosage Range:**   250 to 500 mg/6 hours, or 500 to 1000 mg/12 hours. The total daily dosage should not exceed 4000 mg (4 grams). **Note: Actual dosage and administration schedule must be determined by the physician for each patient individually.**

▷ **Dosing Instructions:**   Preferably taken on an empty stomach, 1 hour before or 2 hours after eating. However, to reduce stomach irritation it may be taken with crackers that contain insignificant amounts of iron, calcium, magnesium or zinc. Avoid all dairy products for 2 hours before and after taking this drug. Take at the same time each day, with a full glass of water. Take the full course prescribed. The tablet may be crushed and the capsule may be opened for administration.

Usual Duration of Use: The time required to control the acute infection and be free of fever and symptoms for 48 hours. This varies with the nature of the infection. Long-term use (months to years, as for treatment of acne) requires supervision and periodic evaluation. Consult your physician on a regular basis.

Currently a "Drug of Choice"
for the initial treatment of early Lyme disease. (Note: Children under 8 years of age and pregnant/breast-feeding women should use penicillin instead of tetracycline.)

▷ **This Drug Should Not Be Taken If**
   • you are allergic to any tetracycline drug (see Drug Class, Section Four).
   • you are pregnant or breast-feeding.

▷ **Inform Your Physician Before Taking This Drug If**
   • it is prescribed for a child under 8 years of age.
   • you have a history of liver or kidney disease.
   • you have systemic lupus erythematosus.
   • you are taking any penicillin drug.
   • you are taking any anticoagulant drug.
   • you plan to have surgery under general anesthesia in the near future.

Possible Side-Effects (natural, expected and unavoidable drug actions)
Superinfections (see Glossary), often due to yeast organisms. These can occur in the mouth, intestinal tract, rectum and/or vagina, resulting in rectal and vaginal itching.

▷ **Possible Adverse Effects** (unusual, unexpected and infrequent reactions)
If any of the following develop, consult your physician promptly for guidance.
Mild Adverse Effects
Allergic Reactions: Skin rash, hives, itching of hands and feet, swelling of face or extremities.
Loss of appetite, stomach irritation, nausea, vomiting, diarrhea.
Irritation of mouth or tongue, "black tongue," sore throat, abdominal cramping or pain.
Serious Adverse Effects
Allergic Reactions: Anaphylactic reaction (see Glossary), asthma, fever, swollen joints and lymph glands.
Drug-induced hepatitis with jaundice.
Permanent discoloration and/or malformation of teeth when taken under 8 years of age, including unborn child and infant.
Impaired vision, increased intracranial pressure.
Drug-induced colitis.
Rare blood cell disorders: hemolytic anemia (see Glossary); abnormally low white blood cell count, causing fever, sore throat and infections; abnormally low blood platelet count, causing abnormal bleeding or bruising.

▷ **Possible Effects on Sexual Function:**   Decreased effectiveness of oral contraceptives taken concurrently (several case reports of pregnancy).

▷ **Adverse Effects That May Mimic Natural Diseases or Disorders**
Drug-induced hepatitis may suggest viral hepatitis.

Natural Diseases or Disorders That May Be Activated by This Drug
Systemic lupus erythematosus.

Possible Effects on Laboratory Tests
Complete blood cell counts: decreased red cells, hemoglobin, white cells and platelets; increased eosinophils (allergic reaction).
Blood lupus erythematosus (LE) cells: positive.
Blood amylase level: increased (toxic effect in pregnant women).
Liver function tests: increased liver enzymes (ALT/GPT, AST/GOT and alkaline phosphatase), increased bilirubin.
Kidney function tests: increased blood creatinine and urea nitrogen (BUN) levels (kidney damage).
Urine sugar tests: false positive results with Benedict's solution and Clinitest.

CAUTION
1. Antacids, dairy products and preparations containing aluminum, bismuth, calcium, iron, magnesium or zinc can prevent adequate absorption of this drug and reduce its effectiveness significantly.
2. Troublesome and persistent diarrhea can develop in sensitive individuals. If diarrhea persists for more than 24 hours, discontinue this drug and consult your physician.
3. If surgery under general anesthesia is required while taking this drug, the choice of anesthetic agent must be considered carefully to prevent serious kidney damage.

Precautions for Use
By Infants and Children: If possible, tetracyclines should not be given to children under 8 years of age because of the risk of permanent discoloration and deformity of the teeth. Rarely, young infants may develop increased intracranial pressure within the first 4 days of receiving this drug. Tetracyclines may inhibit normal bone growth and development.
By Those over 60 Years of Age: Dosage must be carefully individualized and based upon determinations of kidney function. Natural skin changes may predispose to severe and prolonged itching reactions in the genital and anal regions.

▷ **Advisability of Use During Pregnancy**
Pregnancy Category: D (tentative). See Pregnancy Code inside back cover.
Animal studies: Tetracycline causes limb defects in rats, rabbits and chickens.
Human studies: Information from studies of pregnant women indicates that this drug can cause impaired development and discoloration of teeth and other developmental defects.
It is advisable to avoid this drug completely during entire pregnancy.

Advisability of Use if Breast-Feeding
Presence of this drug in breast milk: Yes.
Avoid drug or refrain from nursing.

Habit-Forming Potential: None.

Effects of Overdosage: Stomach burning, nausea, vomiting, diarrhea.

Possible Effects of Long-Term Use: Superinfections; rarely, impairment of bone marrow, liver or kidney function.

Suggested Periodic Examinations While Taking This Drug (at physician's discretion)
Complete blood cell counts, liver and kidney function tests.
During extended use, sputum and stool examinations may detect early superinfection due to yeast organisms.

▷ **While Taking This Drug, Observe the Following**
Foods: Avoid cheeses, yogurt, ice cream, iron-fortified cereals and supplements and meats for 2 hours before and after taking this drug. Calcium and iron can combine with this drug and reduce its absorption significantly.
Beverages: Avoid all forms of milk for 2 hours before and after taking this drug.
▷ *Alcohol:* No interactions expected. However, it is best avoided if you have active liver disease.
Tobacco Smoking: No interactions expected.
▷ *Other Drugs*
Tetracyclines may *increase* the effects of
• oral anticoagulants, and make it necessary to reduce their dosage.
• digoxin (Lanoxin), and cause digitalis toxicity.
• lithium (Eskalith, Lithane, etc.), and increase the risk of lithium toxicity.
Tetracyclines may *decrease* the effects of
• oral contraceptives, and impair their effectiveness in preventing pregnancy.
• penicillins, and impair their effectiveness in treating infections.
Tetracyclines *taken concurrently* with
• methoxyflurane anesthesia may impair kidney function.
The following drugs may *decrease* the effects of tetracyclines
• antacids (aluminum and magnesium preparations, sodium bicarbonate, etc.) may reduce drug absorption.
• iron and mineral preparations may reduce drug absorption.
▷ *Driving, Hazardous Activities:* Usually no restrictions. However, this drug may cause nausea or diarrhea. Restrict activities as necessary.
Aviation Note: The use of this drug *may be a disqualification* for piloting. Consult a designated Aviation Medical Examiner.
Exposure to Sun: Use caution until sensitivity has been determined. Some tetracyclines can cause photosensitivity (see Glossary).

THEOPHYLLINE
(thee OFF i lin)

Other Names: Aminophylline, oxtriphylline

Introduced: 1929

Class: Antiasthmatic, broncho-dilator, xanthines

Prescription: USA: Yes
Canada: No

Controlled Drug: USA: No
Canada: No

Available as Generic: Yes

Brand Names: Accurbron, Amesec [CD], Brondecon [CD], Bronkaid Tablets [CD], Bronkodyl, Bronkolixir [CD], Bronkotabs [CD], Choledyl, Constant-T, Elixicon, Elixophyllin, LaBID, Lodrane, Marax [CD], Marax DF [CD], Mudrane GG Elixir & Tablets [CD], Mudrane Tablets [CD], ♣PMS Theophylline, ♣Pulmophylline, Quadrinal [CD], Quibron [CD], Quibron Plus [CD], Quibron-T Dividose, ♣Quibron-T/SR, Respbid, Slo-bid, Slo-bid Gyrocaps, Slo-Phyllin, Slo-Phyllin GG [CD], Slo-Phyllin Gyrocaps, Somophyllin-CRT, Somophyllin-DF, Somophyllin-T, ♣Somophyllin-12, Sustaire, ♣Tedral Preparations [CD], Theobid Duracaps, Theochron, Theo-Dur, Theolair, Theophyl-SR, Theo-24, Theovent, Theox

---

BENEFITS versus RISKS

Possible Benefits	*Possible Risks*
EFFECTIVE RELIEF OF ACUTE BRONCHIAL ASTHMA	NARROW TREATMENT RANGE
MODERATELY EFFECTIVE CONTROL OF CHRONIC, RECURRENT BRONCHIAL ASTHMA	FREQUENT STOMACH DISTRESS
Moderately effective symptomatic relief in chronic bronchitis and emphysema	Gastrointestinal bleeding
	Central nervous system toxicity, seizures
	Heart rhythm disturbances

▷ **Principal Uses**

As a Single Drug Product: Used primarily to relieve the shortness of breath and wheezing characteristic of acute bronchial asthma, and to prevent the recurrence of asthmatic episodes. It is also useful in relieving the asthmaticlike symptoms that are associated with some types of chronic bronchitis and emphysema.

As a Combination Drug Product [CD]: This drug is available in combination with several other drugs that are beneficial in the overall management of bronchial asthma and related conditions. Ephedrine is added to enhance the bronchodilator effects; guaifenesin is added to provide an expectorant effect that thins the mucus secretions in the bronchial tubes; mild sedatives such as phenobarbital are added to allay the anxiety that often accompanies acute attacks of asthma.

How This Drug Works: By inhibiting the enzyme phosphodiesterase, this drug produces an increase in the tissue chemical cyclic AMP. This causes relaxation of the muscles in the bronchial tubes and blood vessels of the lung, resulting in relief of bronchospasm, expanded lung capacity and improved lung circulation.

Available Dosage Forms and Strengths

Capsules — 100 mg, 200 mg, 250 mg
Capsules, prolonged-action — 50 mg, 60 mg, 75 mg, 100 mg, 125 mg, 130 mg, 200 mg, 250 mg, 260 mg, 300 mg
Elixir — 80 mg, 150 mg per 15-ml tablespoonful
Oral solution — 80 mg, 160 mg per 15-ml tablespoonful
Oral suspension — 300 mg per 15-ml tablespoonful
Syrup — 80 mg, 150 mg per 15-ml tablespoonful
Tablets — 100 mg, 125 mg, 200 mg, 250 mg, 300 mg
Tablets, prolonged-action — 100 mg, 200 mg, 250 mg, 300 mg, 400 mg, 450 mg, 500 mg

▷ **Usual Adult Dosage Range:** Because of its potential toxicity, this drug is given according to body weight. For acute asthma: Initially, 6 mg/kg as the first dose; then 3 mg/kg every 6 hours for 12 hours; then 3 mg/kg every 8 hours as needed. For maintenance: 16 mg/kg/24 hours, or 400 mg/24 hours, whichever is less, taken in 3 or 4 divided doses at intervals of 6 to 8 hours. The total daily dosage should not exceed 900 mg. **Note: Actual dosage and administration schedule must be determined by the physician for each patient individually.**

▷ **Dosing Instructions:** May be taken with or following food to reduce stomach irritation. The regular capsules may be opened and the regular tablets may be crushed for administration. The prolonged action dosage forms should be swallowed whole and not altered.

Usual Duration of Use: Continual use on a regular schedule for 48 to 72 hours is usually necessary to determine this drug's effectiveness in controlling the breathing impairment associated with bronchial asthma and chronic lung disease. Long-term use (months to years) requires supervision and periodic evaluation by your physician. Consult your physician on a regular basis.

▷ **This Drug Should Not Be Taken If**
  • you have had an allergic reaction to it previously.
  • you have active peptic ulcer disease.
  • you have an uncontrolled seizure disorder.

▷ **Inform Your Physician Before Taking This Drug If**
  • you have had an unfavorable reaction to any xanthine drug previously (see Drug Class, Section Four).
  • you have a seizure disorder of any kind.

- you have a history of peptic ulcer disease.
- you have impaired liver or kidney function.
- you have hypertension, heart disease or any type of heart rhythm disorder.

Possible Side-Effects (natural, expected and unavoidable drug actions)
Nervousness, insomnia, rapid heart rate, increased urine volume.

▷ **Possible Adverse Effects** (unusual, unexpected and infrequent reactions)
If any of the following develop, consult your physician promptly for guidance.
Mild Adverse Effects
Allergic Reactions: Skin rash, hives.
Headache, dizziness, irritability, tremor, fatigue, weakness.
Loss of appetite, nausea, vomiting, abdominal pain, diarrhea, excessive thirst.
Flushing of face.
Serious Adverse Effects
Idiosyncratic Reactions: Marked anxiety, confusion, behavioral disturbances.
Central nervous system toxicity: muscle twitching, seizures.
Heart rhythm abnormalities, rapid breathing, low blood pressure.
Gastrointestinal bleeding.

▷ **Possible Effects on Sexual Function:**   None reported.

Natural Diseases or Disorders That May Be Activated by This Drug
Latent peptic ulcer disease.

Possible Effects on Laboratory Tests
Blood uric acid level: increased.
Fecal occult blood test: positive (large doses may cause stomach bleeding).

CAUTION
1. This drug should not be taken concurrently with other antiasthmatic drugs unless you are directed to do so by your physician. Serious overdosage could result.
2. It has been reported that influenza vaccine may delay the elimination of this drug and cause accumulation to toxic levels.

Precautions for Use
By Infants and Children: Observe for indications of toxicity: irritability, agitation, tremors, lethargy, fever, vomiting, rapid heart rate and breathing, seizures.
By Those over 60 Years of Age: Start treatment with small doses until your tolerance has been determined. You may be more susceptible to the development of stomach irritation, nausea, vomiting or diarrhea. When used concurrently with coffee (caffeine) or with nasal decongestants, this drug may cause excessive stimulation and a hyperactivity syndrome.

▷ **Advisability of Use During Pregnancy**
    Pregnancy Category: C (tentative). See Pregnancy Code inside back cover.
      Animal studies: Significant birth defects due to this drug reported in
      mice.
      Human studies: Information from adequate studies of pregnant women
      is not available. No increase in birth defects reported in 394 exposures
      to this drug.
      Avoid this drug during the first 3 months. Use it otherwise only if clearly
      needed. Ask your physician for guidance.

Advisability of Use if Breast-Feeding
    Presence of this drug in breast milk: Yes.
    Avoid drug or refrain from nursing.

Habit-Forming Potential: None.

Effects of Overdosage: Nausea, vomiting, restlessness, irritability, confusion, delirium, seizures, high fever, weak pulse, coma.

Possible Effects of Long-Term Use: Gastrointestinal irritation.

Suggested Periodic Examinations While Taking This Drug (at physician's
    discretion)
    Measurement of blood theophylline levels, especially with high dosage or
    long-term use. (See Therapeutic Drug Monitoring in Section One.)

▷ **While Taking This Drug, Observe the Following**
    Foods: No restrictions.
    Beverages: Avoid excessive use of caffeine-containing beverages: coffee, tea,
    cola; this combination could cause nervousness and insomnia.
▷   *Alcohol:* No interactions expected. May have additive effect on stomach
    irritation.
    Tobacco Smoking: May hasten the elimination of this drug and reduce its
    effectiveness. Higher doses may be necessary to maintain a therapeutic
    blood level.
▷   *Other Drugs*
    Theophylline may *decrease* the effects of
    • lithium (Lithane, Lithobid, etc.), and reduce its effectiveness.
    Theophylline *taken concurrently* with
    • halothane (anesthesia) may cause heart rhythm abnormalities.
    • phenytoin (Dilantin) may cause decreased effects of both drugs.
    The following drugs may *increase* the effects of theophylline
    • allopurinol (Lopurin, Zyloprim).
    • cimetidine (Tagamet).
    • ciprofloxacin (Cipro).
    • erythromycin (E-Mycin, Erythrocin, etc.).
    • oral contraceptives.
    • troleandomycin (TAO).
    The following drugs may *decrease* the effects of theophylline
    • barbiturates (phenobarbital, etc.).

- beta blocker drugs (see Drug Class, Section Four).
- rifampin (Rifadin, Rimactane, etc.).

▷ *Driving, Hazardous Activities:* This drug may cause dizziness. Restrict activities as necessary.

Aviation Note: The use of this drug *may be a disqualification* for piloting. Consult a designated Aviation Medical Examiner.

Exposure to Sun: No restrictions.

Occurrence of Unrelated Illness: Acute viral respiratory infections can delay the elimination of this drug significantly. Observe closely for indications of toxicity and the need to reduce dosage or lengthen the dosage interval.

Discontinuation: Avoid prolonged and unnecessary use of this drug. When you have achieved an asthma-free state, withdraw this drug gradually over several days.

THIORIDAZINE
(thi oh RID a zeen)

Introduced: 1959

Class: Strong tranquilizer, phenothiazines

Prescription: USA: Yes
Canada: Yes

Controlled Drug: USA: No
Canada: No

Available as Generic: USA: Yes
Canada: Yes

Brand Names: ♦Apo-Thioridazine, Mellaril, Mellaril-S, Millazine, ♦Novoridazine, ♦PMS Thioridazine

---

BENEFITS versus RISKS

Possible Benefits	*Possible Risks*
EFFECTIVE CONTROL OF ACUTE MENTAL DISORDERS in the majority of patients: beneficial effects on thinking, mood and behavior	SERIOUS TOXIC EFFECTS ON BRAIN with long-term use
Relief of anxiety, agitation and tension	Liver damage with jaundice (infrequent)
Possibly effective in the management of the hyperactivity syndrome in children	Rare blood cell disorders: abnormally low white blood cell count

---

▷ **Principal Uses**

As a Single Drug Product: This antipsychotic drug is used primarily in the management of the following conditions: moderate to marked depression with significant anxiety and nervous tension; agitation, anxiety, depression and exaggerated fears in the elderly; severe behavioral problems in children characterized by hyperexcitability, combativeness, short attention span and rapid swings in mood.

How This Drug Works: Not completely established. Present theory is that by inhibiting the action of dopamine in certain brain centers, this drug acts to correct an imbalance of nerve impulse transmissions that is thought to be responsible for certain mental disorders.

Available Dosage Forms and Strengths
Concentrate — 30 mg, 100 mg per ml
Oral suspension — 25 mg, 100 mg per 5-ml teaspoonful
Tablets — 10 mg, 15 mg, 25 mg, 50 mg, 100 mg, 150 mg, 200 mg

▷ **Usual Adult Dosage Range:**   Initially, 25 to 100 mg 3 times/day. Dose may be increased by 25 to 50 mg at 3 to 4 day intervals as needed and tolerated. Usual dosage range is 200 to 800 mg daily, divided into 2 to 4 doses. The total daily dosage should not exceed 800 mg. **Note: Actual dosage and administration schedule must be determined by the physician for each patient individually.**

▷ **Dosing Instructions:**   May be taken with or following meals to reduce stomach irritation. The tablets may be crushed for administration.

Usual Duration of Use: Continual use on a regular schedule for 3 to 4 weeks is usually necessary to determine this drug's effectiveness in controlling psychotic disorders. If not significantly beneficial within 6 weeks, it should be discontinued. Long-term use (months to years) requires periodic evaluation of response, appropriate dosage adjustment and consideration of continued need. Consult your physician on a regular basis.

▷ **This Drug Should Not Be Taken If**
   • you are allergic to any of the drugs bearing the brand names listed above.
   • you have active liver disease.
   • you have cancer of the breast.
   • you have a current blood cell or bone marrow disorder.

▷ **Inform Your Physician Before Taking This Drug If**
   • you are allergic or abnormally sensitive to any phenothiazine drug (see Drug Class, Section Four).
   • you have impaired liver or kidney function.
   • you have any type of seizure disorder.
   • you have diabetes, glaucoma or heart disease.
   • you have a history of lupus erythematosus.

- you are taking any drug with sedative effects.
- you plan to have surgery under general or spinal anesthesia in the near future.

Possible Side-Effects (natural, expected and unavoidable drug actions)
Drowsiness (usually during the first 2 weeks), orthostatic hypotension (see Glossary), blurred vision, dry mouth, nasal congestion, constipation, impaired urination.
Pink or purple coloration of urine, of no significance.

▷ **Possible Adverse Effects** (unusual, unexpected and infrequent reactions)
If any of the following develop, consult your physician promptly for guidance.
Mild Adverse Effects
Allergic Reactions: Skin rash, hives, low-grade fever.
Lowering of body temperature, especially in the elderly. (See Hypothermia in Glossary.)
Increased appetite and weight gain.
Weakness, agitation, insomnia, impaired day and night vision.
Chronic constipation, fecal impaction.
Serious Adverse Effects
Allergic Reactions: Hepatitis with jaundice (see Glossary), severe skin reactions.
Idiosyncratic Reactions: Neuroleptic malignant syndrome (see Glossary).
Depression, disorientation, seizures, loss of peripheral vision.
Rapid heart rate, heart rhythm disorders.
Blood cell disorders: reduced white blood cell count (more common in the elderly).
Nervous system reactions: Parkinson-like disorders (see Glossary), severe restlessness, muscle spasms involving the face and neck, tardive dyskinesia (see Glossary).

▷ **Possible Effects on Sexual Function**
Decreased male and female libido; inhibited ejaculation (49% to 60%); impotence (54%); impaired female orgasm; priapism (see Glossary).
Male breast enlargement and tenderness.
Female breast enlargement with milk production.
Altered timing and pattern of menstruation.
False positive pregnancy test results.

▷ **Adverse Effects That May Mimic Natural Diseases or Disorders**
Nervous system reactions may suggest true Parkinson's disease.
Liver reactions may suggest viral hepatitis.
Reactions resembling systemic lupus erythematosus can occur.

Natural Diseases or Disorders That May Be Activated by This Drug
Latent epilepsy, glaucoma, diabetes mellitus, prostatism (see Glossary).

Possible Effects on Laboratory Tests

Complete blood cell counts: decreased red cells, hemoglobin, white cells and platelets.

Liver function tests: increased liver enzymes (ALT/GPT, AST/GOT and alkaline phosphatase), increased bilirubin.

Urine pregnancy tests: falsely positive result with Prognosticon.

CAUTION

1. Many over-the-counter medications (see OTC Drugs in Glossary) for allergies, colds and coughs contain drugs that can interact unfavorably with this drug. Ask your physician or pharmacist for guidance before using any such medications.
2. Antacids that contain aluminum and/or magnesium can prevent the absorption of this drug and reduce its effectiveness.
3. Obtain prompt evaluation of any change or disturbance of vision.

Precautions for Use

By Infants and Children: Use of this drug is not recommended in children under 2 years of age. Do not use this drug in the presence of symptoms suggestive of Reye syndrome (see Glossary). Children with acute infectious diseases ("flulike" infections, chicken pox, measles, etc.) are more prone to develop muscular spasms of the face, back and extremities when this drug is given for any reason.

By Those over 60 Years of Age: Small doses are advisable until individual response has been determined. You may be more susceptible to the development of drowsiness, lethargy, constipation, lowering of body temperature (hypothermia) and orthostatic hypotension (see Glossary). This drug can enhance existing prostatism (see Glossary). You may also be more susceptible to the development of Parkinson-like reactions and/or tardive dyskinesia (see discussion of these terms in Glossary). These reactions must be recognized early since they may become unresponsive to treatment and irreversible.

▷ **Advisability of Use During Pregnancy**

Pregnancy Category: C (tentative). See Pregnancy Code inside back cover.

Animal studies: The results of rodent studies are conflicting.

Human studies: No increase in birth defects reported in 23 exposures. Information from adequate studies of pregnant women is not available.

Avoid drug during the first 3 months. Use it otherwise only if clearly needed. Ask your physician for guidance.

Advisability of Use if Breast-Feeding

Presence of this drug in breast milk: Yes, in minute amounts.

Monitor nursing infant closely and discontinue drug or nursing if adverse effects develop.

Habit-Forming Potential: None.

Effects of Overdosage: Marked drowsiness, weakness, tremor, agitation, unsteadiness, deep sleep, coma, convulsions.

Possible Effects of Long-Term Use: Opacities in the cornea or lens of the eye, pigmentation of the retina. Tardive dyskinesia (see Glossary).

Suggested Periodic Examinations While Taking This Drug (at physician's discretion)
Complete blood cell counts, especially between the fourth and tenth weeks of treatment.
Liver function tests, electrocardiograms.
Complete eye examinations—eye structures and vision.
Careful inspection of the tongue for early evidence of fine, involuntary, wavelike movements that could indicate the beginning of tardive dyskinesia.

▷ **While Taking This Drug, Observe the Following**
Foods: No restrictions.
Nutritional Support: A riboflavin (vitamin B-2) supplement should be taken with long-term use.
Beverages: No restrictions. May be taken with milk.
▷ *Alcohol:* Avoid completely. Alcohol can increase the sedative action of phenothiazines and accentuate their depressant effects on brain function and blood pressure. Phenothiazines can increase the intoxicating effects of alcohol.
Tobacco Smoking: Possible reduction of drowsiness from drug.
Marijuana Smoking: Moderate increase in drowsiness; accentuation of orthostatic hypotension; increased risk of precipitating latent psychoses, confusing the interpretation of mental status and drug responses.
▷ *Other Drugs*
Thioridazine may *increase* the effects of
• all sedative drugs, especially meperidine (Demerol), and cause excessive sedation.
• all atropinelike drugs, and cause nervous system toxicity.
Thioridazine may *decrease* the effects of
• guanethidine (Ismelin, Esimil), and reduce its effectiveness in lowering blood pressure.
Thioridazine *taken concurrently* with
• lithium (Lithobid, Lithotabs) may impair the effectiveness of lithium and cause nervous system toxicity.
The following drugs may *decrease* the effects of thioridazine
• antacids containing aluminum and/or magnesium.
• barbiturates (see Drug Class, Section Four).
• benztropine (Cogentin).
• disulfiram (Antabuse).
• trihexyphenidyl (Artane).
▷ *Driving, Hazardous Activities:* This drug can impair mental alertness, judgment and physical coordination. Avoid hazardous activities.

Aviation Note: The use of this drug *is a disqualification* for piloting. Consult a designated Aviation Medical Examiner.

Exposure to Sun: Use caution until sensitivity has been determined. Some phenothiazines can cause photosensitivity (see Glossary).

Exposure to Heat: Use caution and avoid excessive heat as much as possible. This drug may impair the regulation of body temperature and increase the risk of heat stroke.

Exposure to Cold: Use caution and dress warmly. This drug can increase the risk of hypothermia in the elderly.

Discontinuation: After a period of long-term use, do not discontinue this drug suddenly. Gradual withdrawal over 2 to 3 weeks under physician supervision is recommended. Do not discontinue this drug without your physician's knowledge and approval.

THIOTHIXENE
(thi oh THIX een)

Introduced: 1967

Class: Strong tranquilizer, thioxanthenes

Prescription: USA: Yes
Canada: Yes

Controlled Drug: USA: No
Canada: No

Available as Generic: USA: Yes
Canada: No

Brand Name: Navane

BENEFITS versus RISKS

Possible Benefits	*Possible Risks*
EFFECTIVE CONTROL OF ACUTE MENTAL DISORDERS in the majority of patients: beneficial effects on thinking, mood and behavior	SERIOUS TOXIC EFFECTS ON BRAIN with long-term use
Liver damage with jaundice (rare)
Rare blood cell disorders: abnormally low white blood cell count

---

▷ **Principal Uses**

As a Single Drug Product: This antipsychotic drug is used to ameliorate the psychotic thinking and behavior associated with acute psychoses of unknown nature, episodes of mania and paranoia, and acute schizophrenia.

How This Drug Works: Not completely established. Present theory is that, by inhibiting the action of dopamine, this drug acts to correct an imbalance of nerve impulse transmissions that is thought to be responsible for certain mental disorders.

Available Dosage Forms and Strengths
Capsules — 1 mg, 2 mg, 5 mg, 10 mg, 20 mg
Concentrate — 5 mg per ml
Injections — 2 mg, 5 mg per ml

▷ **Usual Adult Dosage Range:**   Initially, 2 to 5 mg 2 or 3 times daily. Dose may be increased by 2 mg at 3 to 4 day intervals as needed and tolerated. Usual dosage range is 20 to 30 mg daily. The total daily dosage should not exceed 60 mg. **Note: Actual dosage and administration schedule must be determined by the physician for each patient individually.**

▷ **Dosing Instructions:**   May be taken with or following meals to reduce stomach irritation. The capsules may be opened for administration. The liquid concentrate must be diluted just before administration by adding it to 8 ounces of water, milk, fruit juice or carbonated beverage.

Usual Duration of Use: Continual use on a regular schedule for several weeks is usually necessary to determine this drug's effectiveness in controlling psychotic disorders. If not significantly beneficial within 6 weeks, it should be discontinued. Long-term use (months to years) requires periodic evaluation of response, appropriate dosage adjustment and consideration of continued need. Consult your physician on a regular basis.

▷ **This Drug Should Not Be Taken If**
• you have had an allergic reaction to it previously.
• you have active liver disease.
• you have cancer of the breast.
• you have a current blood cell or bone marrow disorder.

▷ **Inform Your Physician Before Taking This Drug If**
• you are allergic or abnormally sensitive to other thioxanthene drugs or any phenothiazine drug (see Drug Classes, Section Four).
• you have impaired liver or kidney function.
• you have any type of seizure disorder.
• you have diabetes, glaucoma or heart disease.
• you have a history of lupus erythematosus.
• you are taking any drug with sedative effects.
• you drink alcohol daily.
• you plan to have surgery under general or spinal anesthesia in the near future.

Possible Side-Effects (natural, expected and unavoidable drug actions)
Mild drowsiness (usually during the first 2 weeks), orthostatic hypotension (see Glossary), blurred vision, dry mouth, nasal congestion, constipation, impaired urination.

▷ **Possible Adverse Effects** (unusual, unexpected and infrequent reactions)
If any of the following develop, consult your physician promptly for guidance.

Mild Adverse Effects

Allergic Reactions: Skin rash, hives, itching.

Lowering of body temperature, especially in the elderly. (See Hypothermia in Glossary.)

Fluid retention, weight gain.

Dizziness, weakness, agitation, insomnia, impaired vision.

Nausea, vomiting.

Serious Adverse Effects

Allergic Reactions: Rare hepatitis with jaundice (see Glossary), anaphylactic reaction (see Glossary).

Idiosyncratic Reactions: Paradoxical worsening of psychotic symptoms. Development of the neuroleptic malignant syndrome (see Glossary). Depression, disorientation, seizures, deposits in cornea and lens.

Rapid heart rate, heart rhythm disorders.

Blood cell disorders: reduced white blood cell count.

Nervous system reactions: Parkinson-like disorders (see Glossary), severe restlessness, muscle spasms involving the face and neck, tardive dyskinesia (see Glossary).

▷ **Possible Effects on Sexual Function**

Altered timing and pattern of menstruation.

Impotence (rare).

Male breast enlargement and tenderness.

Female breast enlargement with milk production.

▷ **Adverse Effects That May Mimic Natural Diseases or Disorders**

Nervous system reactions may suggest true Parkinson's disease or Reye syndrome (see Glossary).

Liver reactions may suggest viral hepatitis.

Natural Diseases or Disorders That May Be Activated by This Drug

Latent epilepsy, glaucoma, prostatism (see Glossary).

Possible Effects on Laboratory Tests

Complete blood cell counts: decreased red cells, hemoglobin, white cells and platelets; increased eosinophils.

Blood glucose level: increased and decreased (fluctuations).

Liver function tests: increased liver enzymes (ALT/GPT, AST/GOT and alkaline phosphatase), increased bilirubin.

Urine pregnancy tests: falsely positive result with some tests.

CAUTION

1. Many over-the-counter medications (see OTC Drugs in Glossary) for allergies, colds and coughs contain drugs that can interact unfavorably with this drug. Ask your physician or pharmacist for guidance before using any such medications.

2. Antacids that contain aluminum and/or magnesium may prevent the absorption of this drug and reduce its effectiveness.
3. Obtain prompt evaluation of any change or disturbance of vision.

Precautions for Use
By Infants and Children: Use of this drug is not recommended in children under 12 years of age. Do not use this drug in the presence of symptoms suggestive of Reye syndrome (see Glossary). Children with acute infectious diseases ("flulike" infections, chicken pox, measles, etc.) are more prone to develop muscular spasms of the face, back and extremities when this drug is given.

By Those over 60 Years of Age: Small doses are advisable until individual response has been determined. You may be more susceptible to the development of drowsiness, lethargy, constipation, lowering of body temperature (hypothermia) and orthostatic hypotension (see Glossary). This drug can enhance existing prostatism (see Glossary). You may also be more susceptible to the development of Parkinson-like reactions and/or tardive dyskinesia (see discussion of these terms in Glossary). These reactions must be recognized early since they may become unresponsive to treatment and irreversible.

▷ ## Advisability of Use During Pregnancy
Pregnancy Category: B (tentative). See Pregnancy Code inside back cover.
Animal studies: No birth defects reported in rats, rabbits or monkeys.
Human studies: Information from adequate studies of pregnant women is not available.
Avoid drug during the first 3 months if possible. Avoid during the last month because of possible effects on the newborn infant.

Advisability of Use if Breast-Feeding
Presence of this drug in breast milk: Unknown.
Avoid drug or refrain from nursing.

Habit-Forming Potential: None.

Effects of Overdosage: Marked drowsiness, weakness, tremor, agitation, unsteadiness, deep sleep, coma, convulsions.

Possible Effects of Long-Term Use: Opacities in the cornea or lens of the eye, pigmentation of the retina. Tardive dyskinesia (see Glossary).

Suggested Periodic Examinations While Taking This Drug (at physician's discretion)
Complete blood cell counts, especially between the fourth and tenth weeks of treatment.
Liver function tests, electrocardiograms.
Complete eye examinations—eye structures and vision.
Careful inspection of the tongue for early evidence of fine, involuntary, wavelike movements that could indicate the beginning of tardive dyskinesia.

▷ **While Taking This Drug, Observe the Following**

Foods: No restrictions.

Beverages: No restrictions. May be taken with milk.

▷   *Alcohol:* Avoid completely. Alcohol can increase the sedative action of thio-thixene and accentuate its depressant effects on brain function and blood pressure. Thiothixene can increase the intoxicating effects of alcohol.

Tobacco Smoking: No interactions expected.

Marijuana Smoking: Moderate increase in drowsiness; accentuation of or-thostatic hypotension; increased risk of precipitating latent psychoses, confusing the interpretation of mental status and drug responses.

▷   *Other Drugs*

Thiothixene may *increase* the effects of
- all sedative drugs, especially barbiturates and narcotic analgesics, and cause excessive sedation.
- all atropinelike drugs, and cause nervous system toxicity.

Thiothixene may *decrease* the effects of
- guanethidine (Ismelin, Esimil), and reduce its effectiveness in lowering blood pressure.

The following drugs may *decrease* the effects of thiothixene
- antacids containing aluminum and/or magnesium.
- barbiturates (see Drug Class, Section Four).
- benztropine (Cogentin).
- trihexyphenidyl (Artane).

▷   *Driving, Hazardous Activities:* This drug can impair mental alertness, judg-ment and physical coordination. Avoid hazardous activities.

Aviation Note: The use of this drug *is a disqualification* for piloting. Consult a designated Aviation Medical Examiner.

Exposure to Sun: Use caution until sensitivity has been determined. This drug can cause photosensitivity (see Glossary).

Exposure to Heat: Use caution and avoid excessive heat as much as possible. This drug may impair the regulation of body temperature and increase the risk of heat stroke.

Exposure to Cold: Use caution and dress warmly. This drug can increase the risk of hypothermia in the elderly.

Discontinuation: After a period of long-term use, do not discontinue this drug suddenly. Gradual withdrawal over 2 to 3 weeks under physician supervision is recommended. Do not discontinue this drug without your physician's knowledge and approval. The relapse rate of schizo-phrenia after discontinuation is 50% to 60%.

THYROID
(THI royd)

Introduced: 1896

Prescription: USA: Yes
Canada: Yes

Available as Generic: Yes

Class: Thyroid hormones

Controlled Drug: USA: No
Canada: No

Brand Names: Armour Thyroid, Proloid, S-P-T, Thyrar, Thyroid Strong, Thyroid USP Enseals

---

BENEFITS versus RISKS

Possible Benefits	*Possible Risks*
EFFECTIVE REPLACEMENT THERAPY IN STATES OF THYROID HORMONE DEFICIENCY (HYPOTHYROIDISM) EFFECTIVE TREATMENT OF SIMPLE GOITER AND CHRONIC THYROIDITIS EFFECTIVE TREATMENT OF THYROID GLAND CANCER	Intensification of angina in presence of coronary artery disease

---

▷ **Principal Uses**

As a Single Drug Product: This natural form of thyroid hormones (derived from animal thyroid glands) is used primarily to correct a deficiency of these hormones (hypothyroidism). In the absence of true thyroid deficiency, the use of this drug to treat nonspecific fatigue, obesity, infertility or slow growth is inappropriate and possibly harmful.

How This Drug Works: Not completely established. By altering the processes of cellular chemistry that store energy in an inactive (reserve) form, this drug makes more energy available for biochemical activity and increases the rate of cellular metabolism of all tissues throughout the body.

Available Dosage Forms and Strengths

Capsules — 65 mg, 130 mg, 195 mg, 325 mg
Tablets — 16 mg, 32 mg, 65 mg, 98 mg, 100 mg, 130 mg, 195 mg, 200 mg, 260 mg, 325 mg
Tablets, enteric-coated — 32 mg, 65 mg, 130 mg
Tablets, sugar-coated — 32 mg, 65 mg, 130 mg, 195 mg

▷ **Usual Adult Dosage Range:** Initially, 60 mg/day; increase dose by 60 mg at intervals of 1 month as needed and tolerated. The usual maintenance dose is 60 to 180 mg/day. **Note: Actual dosage and administration schedule must be determined by the physician for each patient individually.**

▷ **Dosing Instructions:**   Preferably taken in the morning on an empty stomach to ensure maximal absorption and uniform results. The capsules may be opened and the uncoated tablets may be crushed for administration. The enteric-coated tablets should not be altered.

▷ **While Taking This Drug, Observe the Following**
Foods: No restrictions.
Beverages: No restrictions.
▷ *Alcohol:* No interactions expected.
Tobacco Smoking: No interactions expected.
▷ *Other Drugs*
Thyroid may *increase* the effects of
• warfarin (Coumadin), and increase the risk of bleeding; reduction in the dosage of anticoagulant is usually necessary.
Thyroid may *decrease* the effects of
• digoxin (Lanoxin), when correcting hypothyroidism; a larger dose of digoxin may be needed.
Thyroid *taken concurrently* with
• all antidiabetic drugs (insulin and sulfonylureas) may require an increase in the dosage of the antidiabetic agent to obtain proper control of blood sugar levels. After correct doses of both drugs have been determined, a reduction in the dose of thyroid may require a simultaneous reduction in the dose of the antidiabetic drug to prevent hypoglycemia.
• tricyclic antidepressants (see Drug Class, Section Four) may cause an increase in the activity of both drugs; monitor for indications of overdosage of each drug.
The following drugs may *decrease* the effects of thyroid
• cholestyramine (Cuemid, Questran) may reduce its absorption; intake of the two drugs should be separated by 5 hours.
▷ *Driving, Hazardous Activities:* No restrictions.
Aviation Note: The use of this drug is probably not a disqualification for piloting. Consult a designated Aviation Medical Examiner.
Exposure to Sun: No restrictions.
Exposure to Heat: This drug may decrease individual tolerance to warm environments, increasing discomfort due to heat. Consult your physician if you develop symptoms of overdosage during the warm months of the year.
Heavy Exercise or Exertion: Use caution if you have angina (coronary artery disease). This drug may increase the frequency or severity of angina during physical activity.
Discontinuation: This drug must be taken continually on a regular schedule to correct thyroid deficiency. Do not discontinue it without consulting your physician.

Note: The information categories provided in this Profile are appropriate for thyroid preparations derived from natural sources. For specific information that is normally found in those categories that have been omitted from this Profile, the reader is referred to the Drug Profile of Thyroxine which follows. Thyroxine is a chemically pure form of the principal thyroid hormone; its actions and effects are representative of both natural and synthetic thyroid preparations.

THYROXINE
(thi ROX een)

Other Names: Levothyroxine, L-thyroxine, T-4

Introduced: 1953

Class: Thyroid hormones

Prescription: USA: Yes
Canada: Yes

Controlled Drug: USA: No
Canada: No

Available as Generic: USA: Yes
Canada: No

Brand Names: ✦Eltroxin, Euthroid [CD], Levothroid, Levoxine, Synthroid, Thyrolar [CD]

BENEFITS versus RISKS	
Possible Benefits	*Possible Risks*
EFFECTIVE REPLACEMENT THERAPY IN STATES OF THYROID HORMONE DEFICIENCY (HYPOTHYROIDISM) EFFECTIVE TREATMENT OF SIMPLE GOITER AND CHRONIC THYROIDITIS EFFECTIVE TREATMENT OF THYROID GLAND CANCER	Intensification of angina in presence of coronary artery disease Drug-induced hyperthyroidism (with excessive dosage)

▷ **Principal Uses**

As a Single Drug Product: This synthetic thyroid hormone is used primarily to correct thyroid deficiency (hypothyroidism). In addition, it is used to suppress thyroid function in the treatment of simple goiter and the management of Hashimoto's thyroiditis. It is also of value as adjunctive therapy in the management of thyroid gland cancer.

As a Combination Drug Product [CD]: This thyroid hormone is available in combination with the other principal thyroid hormone, liothyronine, in a preparation that resembles the natural hormone material produced by the thyroid gland.

How This Drug Works: Not completely established. By altering the processes of cellular chemistry that store energy in an inactive (reserve) form, this drug makes more energy available for biochemical activity and increases the rate of cellular metabolism of all tissues throughout the body.

Available Dosage Forms and Strengths
   Injections — 100 mcg per ml, 200 mcg per vial
   Tablets — 0.0125 mg, 0.025 mg, 0.05 mg, 0.075 mg, 0.1 mg, 0.112 mg, 0.125 mg, 0.15 mg, 0.175 mg, 0.2 mg, 0.3 mg

▷ **Usual Adult Dosage Range:** Initially, 0.05 to 0.10 mg/day. The dose may be increased at intervals of 2 to 3 weeks as needed and tolerated. The usual maintenance dose is 0.025 to 0.3 mg/day. The total daily dosage should not exceed 0.4 mg. **Note: Actual dosage and administration schedule must be determined by the physician for each patient individually.**

▷ **Dosing Instructions:** Preferably taken in the morning on an empty stomach to ensure maximal absorption and uniform results. The tablets may be crushed for administration.

Usual Duration of Use: Continual use on a regular schedule for 4 to 6 weeks is usually necessary to determine this drug's effectiveness in correcting the symptoms of thyroid deficiency. Long-term use (months to years, possibly for life) requires supervision and periodic evaluation by your physician. Consult your physician on a regular basis.

▷ **This Drug Should Not Be Taken If**
   • you have had an allergic reaction to it previously.
   • you are recovering from a recent heart attack; ask your physician for guidance.
   • you are using it to lose weight and your thyroid function is normal (no deficiency).

▷ **Inform Your Physician Before Taking This Drug If**
   • you have high blood pressure, any form of heart disease or diabetes.
   • you have a history of Addison's disease or adrenal gland deficiency.
   • you are taking any antiasthmatic medications.
   • you are taking an anticoagulant.

Possible Side-Effects (natural, expected and unavoidable drug actions)
   None if dosage is adjusted correctly.

▷ **Possible Adverse Effects** (unusual, unexpected and infrequent reactions)
   If any of the following develop, consult your physician promptly for guidance.
   Mild Adverse Effects
   Allergic Reactions: Skin rash, hives.
   Headache in sensitive individuals, even with proper dosage adjustment.

Serious Adverse Effects

Increased frequency or intensity of angina in the presence of coronary artery disease.

Note: Other adverse effects are manifestations of excessive dosage. See Effects of Overdosage category.

▷ **Possible Effects on Sexual Function**

Altered menstrual pattern during dosage adjustments.

Possibly beneficial in treating impaired sexual function that is associated with true hypothyroidism.

Natural Diseases or Disorders That May Be Activated by This Drug

Latent coronary artery insufficiency (angina), diabetes.

Possible Effects on Laboratory Tests

Prothrombin time: increased (when taken concurrently with warfarin).
Blood total cholesterol, HDL and LDL cholesterol levels: decreased.
Blood triglyceride levels: no effect.
Blood glucose level: increased.
Blood thyroid hormone levels: increased T^3, T^4 and free T^4.
Blood thyroid stimulating hormone (TSH) level: decreased.

CAUTION

1. The need for and response to thyroid hormone treatment varies greatly from person to person. Careful supervision of individual response is necessary to determine correct dosage. Do not change your dosage schedule without consulting your physician.
2. In the absence of verified thyroid deficiency, this drug should not be used to treat nonspecific fatigue, obesity, infertility or slow growth. Such use is inappropriate and could be harmful.

Precautions for Use

By Infants and Children: To facilitate normal growth and development, the thyroid-deficient child often requires higher dosage than the adult. A transient loss of hair may occur during the early months of treatment.

By Those over 60 Years of Age: This drug must be used cautiously by this age group. Usually the requirements for thyroid hormone replacement are about 25% lower than in younger adults. Observe closely for any indications that suggest possible overdosage.

▷ **Advisability of Use During Pregnancy**

Pregnancy Category: A (tentative). See Pregnancy Code inside back cover.

Animal studies: Cataract formation reported in rat studies. Other defects reported in rabbit and guinea pig studies.

Human studies: Thyroid hormones do not reach the fetus (cross the placenta) in significant amounts. Clinical experience has shown that appropriate use of thyroid hormones causes no adverse effects on the fetus.

Use this drug only if clearly needed and with carefully adjusted dosage.

Advisability of Use if Breast-Feeding
Presence of this drug in breast milk: Yes, in minimal amounts.
Breast-feeding is considered safe with correctly adjusted dosage.

Habit-Forming Potential: None.

Effects of Overdosage: Headache, sense of increased body heat, nervousness, increased sweating, hand tremors, insomnia, rapid and irregular heart action, diarrhea, muscle cramping, weight loss.

Possible Effects of Long-Term Use: Bone loss (osteoporosis) in the lumbar vertebrae (spine).

Suggested Periodic Examinations While Taking This Drug (at physician's discretion)
Measurement of thyroid hormone levels in blood.

▷ **While Taking This Drug, Observe the Following**
Foods: No restrictions.
Beverages: No restrictions.
▷ *Alcohol:* No interactions expected.
Tobacco Smoking: No interactions expected.
▷ *Other Drugs*
Thyroxine may *increase* the effects of
• warfarin (Coumadin), and increase the risk of bleeding; reduction in the dosage of anticoagulant is usually necessary.
Thyroxine may *decrease* the effects of
• digoxin (Lanoxin), when correcting hypothyroidism; a larger dose of digoxin may be needed.
Thyroxine *taken concurrently* with
• all antidiabetic drugs (insulin and sulfonylureas) may require an increase in the dosage of the antidiabetic agent to obtain proper control of blood sugar levels. After correct doses of both drugs have been determined, a reduction in the dose of thyroid may require a simultaneous reduction in the dose of the antidiabetic drug to prevent hypoglycemia.
• tricyclic antidepressants (see Drug Class, Section Four) may cause an increase in the activity of both drugs; monitor for indications of overdosage of each drug.
The following drugs may *decrease* the effects of thyroxine
• cholestyramine (Cuemid, Questran) may reduce its absorption; intake of the two drugs should be separated by 5 hours.
▷ *Driving, Hazardous Activities:* No restrictions.
Aviation Note: The use of this drug is probably not a disqualification for piloting. Consult a designated Aviation Medical Examiner.
Exposure to Sun: No restrictions.
Exposure to Heat: This drug may decrease individual tolerance to warm environments, increasing discomfort due to heat. Consult your physician if you develop symptoms of overdosage during the warm months of the year.

Heavy Exercise or Exertion: Use caution if you have angina (coronary artery disease). This drug may increase the frequency or severity of angina during physical activity.

Discontinuation: This drug must be taken continually on a regular schedule to correct thyroid deficiency. Do not discontinue it without consulting your physician.

TIMOLOL
(TI moh lohl)

Introduced: 1972

Class: Antianginal, antiglaucoma, antihypertensive, migraine preventive, beta-adrenergic blocker

Prescription: USA: Yes
Canada: Yes

Controlled Drug: USA: No
Canada: No

Available as Generic: USA: Yes
Canada: No

Brand Names: Blocadren, Timolide [CD], Timoptic

BENEFITS versus RISKS

Possible Benefits	*Possible Risks*
EFFECTIVE, WELL-TOLERATED AS: ANTIANGINAL DRUG in effort-induced angina; ANTIGLAUCOMA DRUG in open-angle glaucoma; ANTIHYPERTENSIVE DRUG in mild to moderate hypertension EFFECTIVE PREVENTION OF MIGRAINE HEADACHES Effective adjunct in the prevention of recurrent heart attack (myocardial infarction)	CONGESTIVE HEART FAILURE in advanced heart disease Worsening of angina in coronary heart disease (if drug is abruptly withdrawn) Masking of low blood sugar (hypoglycemia) in drug-treated diabetes Provocation of asthma

---

▷ **Principal Uses**

As a Single Drug Product: This member of the beta blocker drug class is used primarily to treat (1) classical effort-induced angina, certain types of heart rhythm disturbance and high blood pressure; (2) increased internal eye pressure and chronic open-angle glaucoma. It is also beneficial in preventing the recurrence of heart attacks (myocardial infarction). In addition, it is used to reduce the frequency and severity of migraine headaches.

As a Combination Drug Product [CD]: This drug is available in combination with hydrochlorothiazide for the treatment of hypertension. This combination product includes two "step 1" drugs with different mechanisms of action; it is intended to provide greater effectiveness and convenience for long-term use.

How This Drug Works: By blocking certain actions of the sympathetic nervous system, this drug

- reduces the rate and contraction force of the heart, thus lowering the ejection pressure of the blood leaving the heart and reducing the oxygen requirement for heart function.
- reduces the degree of contraction of blood vessel walls, resulting in their relaxation and expansion and consequent lowering of blood pressure.
- prolongs the conduction time of nerve impulses through the heart, of benefit in the management of certain heart rhythm disorders.
- slows the formation of fluid (aqueous humor) in the anterior chamber of the eye and improves its drainage from the eye, thus lowering the internal eye pressure.

Available Dosage Forms and Strengths
Eye solutions — 0.25%, 0.5%
    Tablets — 5 mg, 10 mg, 20 mg

▷ **Usual Adult Dosage Range:** Varies with indication.
Antianginal and antihypertensive: Initially, 10 mg 2 times/day; increase dose gradually every 7 days as needed and tolerated. Usual maintenance dose is 10 to 20 mg twice/day. The total daily dosage should not exceed 60 mg.
Migraine headache prevention: Initially, 10 mg 2 times/day; increase dose as needed to 10 mg in the morning and 20 mg at night.
Recurrent heart attack prevention: 10 mg twice/day.
Antiglaucoma: 1 drop in affected eye every 12 to 24 hours.**Note: Actual dosage and administration schedule must be determined by the physician for each patient individually.**

▷ **Dosing Instructions:** Preferably taken 1 hour before eating to maximize absorption. The tablet may be crushed for administration. Do not discontinue this drug abruptly.

Usual Duration of Use: Continual use on a regular schedule for 10 to 14 days is usually necessary to determine this drug's effectiveness in preventing angina, controlling heart rhythm disorders and lowering blood pressure. Maximal effectiveness may require continual use for 6 to 8 weeks. The long-term use of this drug (months to years) will be determined by the course of your symptoms over time and your response to the overall treatment program (weight reduction, salt restriction, smoking cessation, etc.). Consult your physician on a regular basis.

Currently a "Drug of Choice"
for initiating treatment of hypertension with a single drug.

▷ **This Drug Should Not Be Taken If**
- you have had an allergic reaction to it previously.
- you have Prinzmetal's variant angina (coronary artery spasm).
- you have congestive heart failure.
- you have an abnormally slow heart rate or a serious form of heart block.
- you are taking, or have taken within the past 14 days, any monoamine oxidase (MAO) type A inhibitor drug (see Drug Class, Section Four).

▷ **Inform Your Physician Before Taking This Drug If**
- you have had an adverse reaction to any beta blocker drug in the past (see Drug Class, Section Four).
- you have a history of serious heart disease, with or without episodes of heart failure.
- you have a history of hay fever (allergic rhinitis), asthma, chronic bronchitis or emphysema.
- you have a history of overactive thyroid function (hyperthyroidism).
- you have a history of low blood sugar (hypoglycemia).
- you have impaired liver or kidney function.
- you have diabetes or myasthenia gravis.
- you are currently taking any form of digitalis, quinidine or reserpine, or any calcium blocker drug (see Drug Class, Section Four).
- you plan to have surgery under general anesthesia in the near future.

Possible Side-Effects (natural, expected and unavoidable drug actions)
Lethargy and fatigability, cold extremities, slow heart rate, light-headedness in upright position (see Orthostatic Hypotension in Glossary).

▷ **Possible Adverse Effects** (unusual, unexpected and infrequent reactions)
If any of the following develop, consult your physician promptly for guidance.
Mild Adverse Effects
Allergic Reactions: Skin rash, itching.
Loss of hair involving the scalp, eyebrows and/or eyelashes. This effect can occur with use of the oral tablets or the eye drops (used to treat glaucoma). Regrowth occurs with discontinuation of this drug.
Headache, dizziness, visual disturbances, vivid dreams.
Indigestion, nausea, vomiting, diarrhea.
Numbness and tingling in extremities.
Serious Adverse Effects
Allergic Reactions: Laryngospasm, severe dermatitis.
Idiosyncratic Reactions: Acute behavioral disturbances: depression, hallucinations.
Chest pain, shortness of breath, precipitation of congestive heart failure.
Induction of bronchial asthma (in asthmatic individuals).
Masking of warning signs of impending low blood sugar (hypoglycemia) in drug-treated diabetes.

▷ **Possible Effects on Sexual Function**
Decreased libido, impaired erection, impotence.
Note: All of these effects can occur with the use of timolol eye drops at recommended dosage.

▷ **Adverse Effects That May Mimic Natural Diseases or Disorders**
Reduced blood flow to extremities may resemble Raynaud's phenomenon (see Glossary).

Natural Diseases or Disorders That May Be Activated by This Drug
Prinzmetal's variant angina, Raynaud's disease, intermittent claudication, myasthenia gravis (questionable).

Possible Effects on Laboratory Tests
None reported.

CAUTION
1. *Do not discontinue this drug suddenly* without the knowledge and guidance of your physician. Carry a notation on your person that you are taking this drug.
2. Consult your physician or pharmacist before using nasal decongestants usually present in over-the-counter cold preparations and nose drops. These can cause sudden increases in blood pressure when taken concurrently with beta blocker drugs.
3. Report the development of any tendency to emotional depression (rare with this drug).

Precautions for Use
By Infants and Children: Safety and effectiveness for use by those under 12 years of age have not been established. However, if this drug is used, observe for the development of low blood sugar (hypoglycemia) during periods of reduced food intake.
By Those over 60 Years of Age: Proceed *cautiously* with all antihypertensive drugs. Unacceptably high blood pressure should be reduced without creating the risks associated with excessively low blood pressure. Start treatment with small doses, and monitor the blood pressure response frequently. Sudden, rapid and excessive reduction of blood pressure can predispose to stroke or heart attack. Observe for dizziness, unsteadiness, tendency to fall, confusion, hallucinations, depression or urinary frequency.

▷ **Advisability of Use During Pregnancy**
Pregnancy Category: C (tentative). See Pregnancy Code inside back cover.
Animal studies: No significant increase in birth defects due to this drug.
Human studies: Information from adequate studies of pregnant women is not available.
Avoid use of drug during the first 3 months if possible. Use this drug only if clearly needed. Ask your physician for guidance.

Advisability of Use if Breast-Feeding
Presence of this drug in breast milk: Probably yes.

Monitor nursing infant closely and discontinue drug or nursing if adverse effects develop.

Habit-Forming Potential: None.

Effects of Overdosage: Weakness, slow pulse, low blood pressure, fainting, cold and sweaty skin, congestive heart failure, possible coma and convulsions.

Possible Effects of Long-Term Use: Reduced heart reserve and eventual heart failure in susceptible individuals with advanced heart disease.

Suggested Periodic Examinations While Taking This Drug (at physician's discretion)
Complete blood cell counts (because of adverse effects of other drugs of this class).
Measurements of blood pressure, evaluation of heart function.

▷ **While Taking This Drug, Observe the Following**
Foods: No restrictions. Avoid excessive salt intake.
Beverages: No restrictions. May be taken with milk.
▷ *Alcohol:* Use with caution until the combined effect has been determined. Alcohol may exaggerate this drug's ability to lower the blood pressure and may increase its mild sedative effect.
Tobacco Smoking: Nicotine may reduce this drug's effectiveness in treating angina, heart rhythm disorders and high blood pressure. In addition, high doses of this drug may potentiate the constriction of the bronchial tubes caused by regular smoking.
▷ *Other Drugs*
Timolol may *increase* the effects of
• other antihypertensive drugs, and cause excessive lowering of blood pressure. Dosage adjustments may be necessary.
• lidocaine (Xylocaine, etc.).
• reserpine (Ser-Ap-Es, etc.), and cause sedation, depression, slowing of the heart rate and lowering of the blood pressure.
• verapamil (Calan, Isoptin), and cause excessive depression of heart function; monitor this combination closely.
Timolol may *decrease* the effects of
• theophyllines (Aminophyllin, Theo-Dur, etc.), and reduce their antiasthmatic effectiveness.
Timolol *taken concurrently* with
• clonidine (Catapres) requires close monitoring for rebound high blood pressure if clonidine is withdrawn while timolol is still being taken.
• epinephrine (Adrenalin, etc.) may cause marked rise in blood pressure and slowing of the heart rate.
• insulin requires close monitoring to avoid undetected hypoglycemia (see Glossary).
The following drugs may *increase* the effects of timolol
• chlorpromazine (Thorazine, etc.)

- cimetidine (Tagamet).
- methimazole (Tapazole).
- propylthiouracil (Propacil).

The following drugs may *decrease* the effects of timolol

- barbiturates (phenobarbital, etc.).
- indomethacin (Indocin), and possibly other "aspirin substitutes," may impair timolol's antihypertensive effect.
- rifampin (Rifadin, Rimactane).

▷ *Driving, Hazardous Activities:* Use caution until the full extent of dizziness, lethargy and blood pressure change have been determined.

Aviation Note: The use of this drug *may be a disqualification* for piloting. Consult a designated Aviation Medical Examiner.

Exposure to Sun: No restrictions.

Exposure to Heat: Caution advised. Hot environments can lower blood pressure and exaggerate the effects of this drug.

Exposure to Cold: Caution advised. Cold environments can enhance the circulatory deficiency in the extremities that may occur with this drug. The elderly should take precautions to prevent hypothermia (see Glossary).

Heavy Exercise or Exertion: It is advisable to avoid exertion that produces light-headedness, excessive fatigue or muscle cramping. The use of this drug may intensify the hypertensive response to isometric exercise.

Occurrence of Unrelated Illness: The fever that accompanies systemic infections can lower blood pressure and require adjustment of dosage. Illnesses that cause nausea or vomiting may interrupt the regular dosage schedule. Ask your physician for guidance.

Discontinuation: It is advisable to avoid sudden discontinuation of this drug in all situations; this is especially true in the presence of coronary artery disease. If possible, gradual reduction of dose over a period of 2 to 3 weeks is recommended. Ask your physician for specific guidance.

TOCAINIDE
(toh KAY nide)

Introduced: 1976

Class: Antiarrhythmic

Prescription: USA: Yes
Canada: Yes

Controlled Drug: USA: No
Canada: No

Available as Generic: USA: No
Canada: No

Brand Name: Tonocard

BENEFITS versus RISKS

Possible Benefits	*Possible Risks*
EFFECTIVE TREATMENT OF SELECTED HEART RHYTHM DISORDERS (ventricular)	DRUG-INDUCED HEART RHYTHM DISORDERS (10.9%)
	CONGESTIVE HEART FAILURE (4%)
	Rare blood cell disorders: aplastic anemia, abnormally low white blood cell and platelet counts
	Drug-induced lung damage

▷ **Principal Uses**

As a Single Drug Product: This drug is classified as a Type 1 antiarrhythmic agent, similar to procainamide and quinidine in its actions. It is used primarily to correct and prevent the recurrence of (1) abnormally rapid heart rates (tachycardia) that arise in the ventricles (lower heart chambers); and (2) premature beats arising in the ventricles.

How This Drug Works: By slowing the transmission of electrical impulses throughout the conduction system of the heart, this drug assists in restoring normal heart rate and rhythm.

Available Dosage Forms and Strengths

Tablets — 400 mg, 600 mg

▷ **Usual Adult Dosage Range:** Do not take a loading dose. Initiate treatment with 400 mg/8 hours. If needed and tolerated, the dose may be increased gradually to 600 mg/8 hours. The total daily dosage should not exceed 2400 mg. **Note: Actual dosage and administration schedule must be determined by the physician for each patient individually.**

▷ **Dosing Instructions:** May be taken without regard to meals, but may be taken with or following food if desired to reduce stomach irritation. Take at same time each day to obtain uniform results. The tablet may be crushed for administration.

Usual Duration of Use: Continual use on a regular schedule for 1 to 2 weeks is usually necessary to determine this drug's effectiveness in correcting or preventing responsive rhythm disorders. Long-term use requires supervision and periodic evaluation by your physician. Consult your physician on a regular basis.

▷ **This Drug Should Not Be Taken If**
- you have had an allergic reaction to it previously.
- you are allergic to local anesthetics of the Novocain type.
- you have second-degree or third-degree heart block (with no pacemaker).

▷ **Inform Your Physician Before Taking This Drug If**
- you have had any unfavorable reactions to other antiarrhythmic drugs in the past.
- you have a history of heart disease of any kind, especially heart block.
- you have impaired liver or kidney function.
- you are taking any form of digitalis, a potassium supplement or any diuretic drug that can cause excessive loss of body potassium (ask physician).

Possible Side-Effects (natural, expected and unavoidable drug actions)
Flushing, increased sweating, light-headedness.
The onset of tremors indicates that the dose is reaching the maximum that can be tolerated.

▷ **Possible Adverse Effects** (unusual, unexpected and infrequent reactions)
If any of the following develop, consult your physician promptly for guidance.
Mild Adverse Effects
Allergic Reactions: Skin rash (8%), hives, itching.
Headache (4%), dizziness (15%), visual disturbance (1.5%), fatigue (0.8%), tremor (8%), numbness (9%).
Loss of appetite, indigestion, nausea (14%), vomiting (4%), diarrhea (4%).
Serious Adverse Effects
Idiosyncratic Reactions: Confusion, disorientation, hallucinations (2.7%).
Drug-induced heart rhythm disorders (10%), congestive heart failure (4%), shortness of breath, palpitations, chest pain.
Drug-induced lung damage: pneumonitis and fibrosis, causing cough and breathing difficulty. (Usually occurs after 3 to 18 weeks of drug use.)
Bone marrow depression (see Glossary): fatigue, weakness, fever, sore throat, abnormal bleeding or bruising. (Usually occurs after 2 to 12 weeks of drug use.)

▷ **Possible Effects on Sexual Function:**   None reported.

▷ **Adverse Effects That May Mimic Natural Diseases or Disorders**
Lung reactions may suggest an infectious bronchitis or pneumonia.

Possible Effects on Laboratory Tests
Complete blood cell counts: decreased red cells, hemoglobin, white cells and platelets (rare—less than 0.2% of users).
Blood lupus erythematosus (LE) cells: positive (rare).
Blood antinuclear antibodies (ANA): positive (rare).
Liver function tests: increased liver enzymes (ALT/GPT and AST/GOT).

CAUTION
1. Thorough evaluation of your heart function (including electrocardiograms) is necessary prior to using this drug.
2. Periodic evaluation of your heart function is necessary to determine

your response to this drug. Some individuals may experience worsening of their heart rhythm disorder and/or deterioration of heart function. Close monitoring of heart rate, rhythm and overall performance is essential.

3. Dosage must be adjusted carefully for each individual. Do not change your dosage without the knowledge and supervision of your physician.

4. Do not take any other antiarrhythmic drug while taking this drug unless directed to do so by your physician.

Precautions for Use

By Infants and Children: Safety and effectiveness for use by those under 12 years of age have not been established. Initial use of this drug requires hospitalization and supervision by a qualified cardiologist.

By Those over 60 Years of Age: Reduced kidney function may require reduction in dosage. Observe carefully for light-headedness, dizziness, unsteadiness and tendency to fall.

▷ Advisability of Use During Pregnancy

Pregnancy Category: C (tentative). See Pregnancy Code inside back cover.

Animal studies: No birth defects reported in rat or rabbit studies; however, an increase in fetal resorptions, stillbirths and abortions was reported.

Human studies: Information from adequate studies of pregnant women is not available.

Avoid this drug during first 3 months. Use this drug only if clearly needed. Ask your physician for guidance.

Advisability of Use if Breast-Feeding

Presence of this drug in breast milk: Unknown.

Avoid drug or refrain from nursing.

Habit-Forming Potential: None.

Effects of Overdosage: Impaired urination, constipation, marked drop in blood pressure, abnormal heart rhythms, slow heart rate, congestive heart failure, seizures.

Possible Effects of Long-Term Use: None reported.

Suggested Periodic Examinations While Taking This Drug (at physician's discretion)

Electrocardiograms, complete blood cell counts, measurements of potassium blood levels.

▷ While Taking This Drug, Observe the Following

Foods: No restrictions. Ask physician regarding need for salt restriction and advisability of eating potassium-rich foods.

Beverages: No restrictions. May be taken with milk.

▷ *Alcohol:* Use caution until the combined effects have been determined. Alcohol can increase the blood-pressure-lowering effects of this drug.

Tobacco Smoking: Nicotine can cause irritability of the heart and reduce the effectiveness of this drug. Follow physician's advice regarding smoking.

▷ *Other Drugs*

Tocainide may *increase* the effects of
- antihypertensive drugs, and cause excessive lowering of blood pressure.
- beta blocker drugs (see Drug Class, Section Four).

The following drugs may *decrease* the effects of tocainide
- diuretics that promote potassium loss.

▷ *Driving, Hazardous Activities:* This drug may cause dizziness or blurred vision. Restrict activities as necessary.

Aviation Note: The use of this drug *may be a disqualification* for piloting. Consult a designated Aviation Medical Examiner.

Exposure to Sun: No restrictions.

Occurrence of Unrelated Illness: Disorders that cause vomiting, diarrhea or dehydration can affect this drug's action adversely. Report such developments promptly.

Discontinuation: This drug should not be discontinued abruptly following long-term use. Ask your physician for guidance regarding gradual dose reduction.

TOLAZAMIDE
(tohl AZ a mide)

Introduced: 1966

Class: Antidiabetic, sulfonylureas

Prescription: USA: Yes

Controlled Drug: USA: No

Available as Generic: Yes

Brand Names: Ronase, Tolamide, Tolinase

BENEFITS versus RISKS

Possible Benefits	*Possible Risks*
Assistance in regulating blood sugar in noninsulin-dependent diabetes (adjunctive to appropriate diet and weight control)	HYPOGLYCEMIA, severe and prolonged Drug-induced liver damage Rare bone marrow depression (see Glossary) Hemolytic anemia (see Glossary)

▷ **Principal Uses**

As a Single Drug Product: To assist in the control of mild to moderately severe type II diabetes mellitus (adult, maturity-onset) that does not require insulin, but that cannot be adequately controlled by diet alone.

How This Drug Works: It is thought that this drug (1) stimulates the release of insulin (by a pancreas that is capable of responding to stimulation), and (2) enhances the utilization of insulin by appropriate tissues.

Available Dosage Forms and Strengths
Tablets — 100 mg, 250 mg, 500 mg

▷ **Usual Adult Dosage Range:**   Initially, 100 to 250 mg daily with breakfast. At 7 day intervals, the dose may be increased by increments of 100 to 250 mg daily as needed and tolerated. The total daily dosage should not exceed 1000 mg (1 gram). A "loading" or priming dose is not necessary and should not be given. **Note: Actual dosage and administration schedule must be determined by the physician for each patient individually.**

▷ **Dosing Instructions:**   If the daily maintenance dose is found to be more than 500 mg, the total dose should be divided into 2 equal doses: the first taken with the morning meal, the second with the evening meal. The tablet may be crushed for administration.

Usual Duration of Use: Continual use on a regular schedule for several weeks is usually necessary to determine this drug's effectiveness in controlling diabetes. Failure to respond to maximal doses within 1 month constitutes a primary failure. Up to 10% of those who respond initially may develop secondary failure of the drug later. The duration of effective use can only be determined by periodic measurement of the blood sugar. Consult your physician on a regular basis.

▷ **This Drug Should Not Be Taken If**
• you have had an allergic reaction to it previously.
• you have severe impairment of liver or kidney function.
• you are pregnant.

▷ **Inform Your Physician Before Taking This Drug If**
• you are allergic to other sulfonylurea drugs or to "sulfa" drugs. (See Drug Classes, Section Four).
• your diabetes has been unstable or "brittle" in the past.
• you do not know how to recognize or treat hypoglycemia (see Glossary).
• you have a history of congestive heart failure, peptic ulcer disease, cirrhosis of the liver, hypothyroidism or porphyria.

Possible Side-Effects (natural, expected and unavoidable drug actions)
If drug dosage is excessive or food intake is delayed or inadequate, abnormally low blood sugar (hypoglycemia) will occur as a predictable drug effect.

▷ **Possible Adverse Effects** (unusual, unexpected and infrequent reactions)
If any of the following develop, consult your physician promptly for guidance.
Mild Adverse Effects
Allergic Reactions: Skin rash, hives, itching, drug fever.
Headache, ringing in the ears.
Indigestion, heartburn, nausea, vomiting, diarrhea.
Serious Adverse Effects
Allergic Reactions: Hepatitis with jaundice (see Glossary).
Idiosyncratic Reactions: Hemolytic anemia (see Glossary); disulfiram-like reaction with concurrent use of alcohol (see Glossary), infrequent with this drug.
Bone marrow depression (see Glossary): fatigue, weakness, fever, sore throat, abnormal bleeding or bruising.

▷ **Possible Effects on Sexual Function**
None reported.

▷ **Adverse Effects That May Mimic Natural Diseases or Disorders**
Liver reactions may suggest viral hepatitis.

Possible Effects on Laboratory Tests
Complete blood cell counts: decreased red cells, hemoglobin, white cells and platelets.
Blood glucose level: decreased.
Liver function tests: increased liver enzymes (ALT/GPT, AST/GOT and alkaline phosphatase), increased bilirubin.

CAUTION
1. This drug must be regarded as only one part of the total program for the management of your diabetes. It is not a substitute for a properly prescribed diet and regular exercise.
2. Over a period of time (usually several months), this drug may lose its effectiveness in controlling blood sugar levels. Periodic follow-up examinations are necessary to monitor all aspects of response to drug treatment.

Precautions for Use
By Infants and Children: This drug is not effective in type I (juvenile, growth-onset) insulin-dependent diabetes.
By Those over 60 Years of Age: This drug should be used with caution in this age group. Start treatment with 100 mg/day; increase dosage cautiously and monitor closely to prevent hypoglycemic reactions. Repeated episodes of hypoglycemia in the elderly can cause brain damage.

▷ **Advisability of Use During Pregnancy**
Pregnancy Category: C (tentative). See Pregnancy Code inside back cover.
Animal studies: No birth defects due to this drug reported in rats.

Human studies: Information from adequate studies of pregnant women is not available.

Because uncontrolled blood sugar levels during pregnancy are associated with a higher incidence of birth defects, many experts recommend that insulin (instead of an oral agent) be used as necessary to control diabetes during the entire pregnancy.

Use during pregnancy is not recommended by the manufacturer.

Advisability of Use if Breast-Feeding

Presence of this drug in breast milk: Probably yes.

Avoid drug or refrain from nursing.

Habit-Forming Potential: None.

Effects of Overdosage: Symptoms of mild to severe hypoglycemia: headache, light-headedness, faintness, nervousness, confusion, tremor, sweating, heart palpitation, weakness, hunger, nausea, vomiting, stupor progressing to coma.

Possible Effects of Long-Term Use: Reduced function of the thyroid gland (hypothyroidism). Reports of increased frequency and severity of heart and blood vessel diseases associated with long-term use of this class of drugs are highly controversial and inconclusive. A direct cause-and-effect relationship (see Glossary) is tenuous. Ask your physician for guidance.

Suggested Periodic Examinations While Taking This Drug (at physician's discretion)

Complete blood cell counts, liver function tests, thyroid function tests, periodic evaluation of heart and circulatory system.

▷ **While Taking This Drug, Observe the Following**

Foods: Follow the diabetic diet prescribed by your physician.

Beverages: As directed in the diabetic diet. May be taken with milk.

▷ *Alcohol:* Use with extreme caution until the combined effect has been determined. Alcohol can exaggerate this drug's hypoglycemic effect. This drug infrequently causes a marked intolerance of alcohol resulting in a disulfiramlike reaction (see Glossary): facial flushing, sweating, palpitation.

Tobacco Smoking: No interactions expected.

▷ *Other Drugs*

The following drugs may *increase* the effects of tolazamide

- aspirin, and other salicylates.
- cimetidine (Tagamet).
- clofibrate (Atromid S).
- fenfluramine (Pondimin).
- monoamine oxidase (MAO) type A inhibitor drugs (see Drug Class, Section Four).
- phenylbutazone (Butazolidin).
- ranitidine (Zantac).

The following drugs may *decrease* the effects of tolazamide

- beta blocker drugs (see Drug Class, Section Four).
- bumetanide (Bumex).
- diazoxide (Proglycem).
- ethacrynic acid (Edecrin).
- furosemide (Lasix).
- phenytoin (Dilantin).
- thiazide diuretics (see Drug Class, Section Four).

▷ *Driving, Hazardous Activities:* Regulate your dosage schedule, eating schedule and physical activities very carefully to prevent hypoglycemia. Be able to recognize the early symptoms of hypoglycemia so you can avoid hazardous activities and take corrective measures.

Aviation Note: Diabetes *is a disqualification* for piloting. Consult a designated Aviation Medical Examiner.

Exposure to Sun: Use caution until sensitivity has been determined. Some drugs of this class can cause photosensitivity (see Glossary).

Occurrence of Unrelated Illness: Acute infections, illnesses causing vomiting or diarrhea, serious injuries and surgical procedures can interfere with diabetic control and may require the use of insulin. If any of these conditions occur, consult your physician promptly.

Discontinuation: Because of the possibility of secondary failure, it is advisable to evaluate the continued benefit of this drug every 6 months.

TOLBUTAMIDE
(tohl BYU ta mide)

Introduced: 1956   **Class:** Antidiabetic, sulfonylureas

Prescription: USA: Yes   **Controlled Drug:** USA: No
    Canada: Yes   Canada: No

Available as Generic: Yes

Brand Names: ✦Apo-Tolbutamide, ✦Mobenol, ✦Novobutamide, Oramide, Orinase

Warning: The brand names Orinase, Ornade and Ornex are similar and can be mistaken for each other; this can lead to serious medication errors. These names represent very different drugs. Orinase (a white tablet) is the generic drug tolbutamide; it is used to treat diabetes. Ornade (a red capsule containing colored beads) is a combination of chlorpheniramine and phenylpropanolamine; it is used to treat nasal and sinus congestion. Ornex (a blue caplet) is a combination of acetaminophen and phenylpropanolamine; it is used to treat headcolds and sinus pain. Verify that you are taking the correct drug.

```
┌─────────────────────────────────────────────────────────────────────┐
│                      BENEFITS versus RISKS                            │
│                                                                       │
│        Possible Benefits                    Possible Risks            │
│    Assistance in regulating blood      HYPOGLYCEMIA, severe and       │
│      sugar in noninsulin-dependent       prolonged                    │
│      diabetes (adjunctive to           Drug-induced liver damage      │
│      appropriate diet and weight       Rare bone marrow depression    │
│      control)                            (See Glossary)               │
│                                        Hemolytic anemia (See Glossary)│
└─────────────────────────────────────────────────────────────────────┘
```

▷ **Principal Uses**

As a Single Drug Product: To assist in the control of mild to moderately severe type II diabetes mellitus (adult, maturity-onset) that does not require insulin, but that cannot be adequately controlled by diet alone.

How This Drug Works: It is thought that this drug (1) stimulates the release of insulin (by a pancreas that is capable of responding to stimulation), and (2) enhances the utilization of insulin by appropriate tissues.

Available Dosage Forms and Strengths

Tablets — 250 mg, 500 mg

▷ **Usual Adult Dosage Range:**   Initially, 500 mg twice a day. The dose may be increased or decreased every 48 to 72 hours until the minimal amount required for satisfactory control is determined. The usual range is 500 to 2000 mg/24 hours. The total daily dosage should not exceed 3000 mg (3 grams). A "loading" or priming dose is not necessary and should not be given. **Note: Actual dosage and administration schedule must be determined by the physician for each patient individually.**

▷ **Dosing Instructions:**   May be taken with food (morning and evening meals) to reduce stomach irritation. The tablet may be crushed for administration.

Usual Duration of Use: Continual use on a regular schedule for several weeks is usually necessary to determine this drug's effectiveness in controlling diabetes. Failure to respond to maximal doses within 1 month constitutes a primary failure. Up to 15% of those who respond initially may develop secondary failure of the drug within the first year. The duration of effective use can only be determined by periodic measurement of the blood sugar. Consult your physician on a regular basis.

▷ **This Drug Should Not Be Taken If**
- you have had an allergic reaction to it previously.
- you have severe impairment of liver or kidney function.
- you are pregnant.

▷ **Inform Your Physician Before Taking This Drug If**
- you are allergic to other sulfonylurea drugs or to "sulfa" drugs. (See Drug Classes, Section Four).

- your diabetes has been unstable or "brittle" in the past.
- you do not know how to recognize or treat hypoglycemia (see Glossary).
- you have a history of congestive heart failure, peptic ulcer disease, cirrhosis of the liver, hypothyroidism or porphyria.

Possible Side-Effects (natural, expected and unavoidable drug actions)
If drug dosage is excessive or food intake is delayed or inadequate, abnormally low blood sugar (hypoglycemia) will occur as a predictable drug effect.

▷ **Possible Adverse Effects** (unusual, unexpected and infrequent reactions)
If any of the following develop, consult your physician promptly for guidance.
Mild Adverse Effects
Allergic Reactions: Skin rash, hives, itching, drug fever.
Headache, ringing in the ears, weakness.
Indigestion, heartburn, nausea, vomiting.
Serious Adverse Effects
Allergic Reactions: Hepatitis with jaundice (see Glossary).
Idiosyncratic Reactions: Hemolytic anemia (see Glossary); disulfiram-like reaction with concurrent use of alcohol (see Glossary), infrequent with this drug.
Bone marrow depression (see Glossary): fatigue, weakness, fever, sore throat, abnormal bleeding or bruising.

▷ **Possible Effects on Sexual Function**
None reported.

▷ **Adverse Effects That May Mimic Natural Diseases or Disorders**
Liver reactions may suggest viral hepatitis.

Natural Diseases or Disorders That May Be Activated by This Drug
Acute intermittent porphyria (see Glossary).

Possible Effects on Laboratory Tests
Complete blood cell counts: decreased red cells, hemoglobin, white cells and platelets.
Blood glucose level: decreased.
Liver function tests: increased liver enzymes (ALT/GPT, AST/GOT and alkaline phosphatase), increased bilirubin.

CAUTION
1. This drug must be regarded as only one part of the total program for the management of your diabetes. It is not a substitute for a properly prescribed diet and regular exercise.
2. Over a period of time (usually several months), this drug may lose its effectiveness in controlling blood sugar levels. Periodic follow-up examinations are necessary to monitor all aspects of response to drug treatment.

Precautions for Use
By Infants and Children: This drug is not effective in type I (juvenile, growth-onset) insulin-dependent diabetes.
By Those over 60 Years of Age: This drug should be used with caution in this age group. Start treatment with 500 mg/day; increase dosage cautiously and monitor closely to prevent hypoglycemic reactions. Repeated episodes of hypoglycemia in the elderly can cause brain damage.

▷ **Advisability of Use During Pregnancy**
Pregnancy Category: C (tentative). See Pregnancy Code inside back cover.
Animal studies: Ocular and bone birth defects reported in rat studies.
Human studies: Information from adequate studies of pregnant women is not available.
Because uncontrolled blood sugar levels during pregnancy are associated with a higher incidence of birth defects, many experts recommend that insulin (instead of an oral agent) be used as necessary to control diabetes during the entire pregnancy.
Use during pregnancy is not recommended by the manufacturer.

Advisability of Use if Breast-Feeding
Presence of this drug in breast milk: Yes.
Avoid drug or refrain from nursing.

Habit-Forming Potential: None.

Effects of Overdosage: Symptoms of mild to severe hypoglycemia: headache, light-headedness, faintness, nervousness, confusion, tremor, sweating, heart palpitation, weakness, hunger, nausea, vomiting, stupor progressing to coma.

Possible Effects of Long-Term Use: Reduced function of the thyroid gland (hypothyroidism). Reports of increased frequency and severity of heart and blood vessel diseases associated with long-term use of this class of drugs are highly controversial and inconclusive. A direct cause-and-effect relationship (see Glossary) is tenuous. Ask your physician for guidance.

Suggested Periodic Examinations While Taking This Drug (at physician's discretion)
Complete blood cell counts, liver function tests, thyroid function tests, periodic evaluation of heart and circulatory system.

▷ **While Taking This Drug, Observe the Following**
Foods: Follow the diabetic diet prescribed by your physician.
Beverages: As directed in the diabetic diet. May be taken with milk.
▷ *Alcohol:* Use with extreme caution until the combined effect has been determined. Alcohol can exaggerate this drug's hypoglycemic effect. This drug infrequently causes a marked intolerance of alcohol resulting in

a disulfiramlike reaction (see Glossary): facial flushing, sweating, palpitation.

Tobacco Smoking: No interactions expected.

▷ *Other Drugs*

The following drugs may *increase* the effects of tolbutamide
- aspirin, and other salicylates.
- chloramphenicol (Chloromycetin).
- cimetidine (Tagamet).
- clofibrate (Atromid S).
- fenfluramine (Pondimin).
- monoamine oxidase (MAO) type A inhibitor drugs (see Drug Class, Section Four).
- phenylbutazone (Butazolidin).
- ranitidine (Zantac).
- sulfonamide drugs (see Drug Class, Section Four).

The following drugs may *decrease* the effects of tolbutamide
- beta blocker drugs (see Drug Class, Section Four).
- bumetanide (Bumex).
- diazoxide (Proglycem).
- ethacrynic acid (Edecrin).
- furosemide (Lasix).
- phenytoin (Dilantin).
- rifampin (Rifadin, Rimactane).
- thiazide diuretics (see Drug Class, Section Four).

▷ *Driving, Hazardous Activities:* Regulate your dosage schedule, eating schedule and physical activities very carefully to prevent hypoglycemia. Be able to recognize the early symptoms of hypoglycemia so you can avoid hazardous activities and take corrective measures.

Aviation Note: Diabetes *is a disqualification* for piloting. Consult a designated Aviation Medical Examiner.

Exposure to Sun: Use caution until sensitivity has been determined. Some drugs of this class can cause photosensitivity (see Glossary).

Occurrence of Unrelated Illness: Acute infections, illnesses causing vomiting or diarrhea, serious injuries and surgical procedures can interfere with diabetic control and may require the use of insulin. If any of these conditions occur, consult your physician promptly.

Discontinuation: Because of the possibility of secondary failure, it is advisable to evaluate the continued benefit of this drug every 6 months.

TOLMETIN
(TOHL met in)

Introduced: 1976

Class: Mild analgesic, anti-inflammatory

Prescription: USA: Yes
Canada: Yes

Controlled Drug: USA: No
Canada: No

Available as Generic: No

Brand Names: Tolectin, Tolectin DS, Tolectin 600

BENEFITS versus RISKS

Possible Benefits	*Possible Risks*
EFFECTIVE RELIEF OF MILD TO MODERATE PAIN AND INFLAMMATION	Increased blood pressure (3–9%) Gastrointestinal pain, ulceration, bleeding (rare) Rare liver damage Rare kidney damage Rare blood cell disorders: hemolytic anemia, abnormally low white blood cell and platelet counts

---

▷ **Principal Uses**

As a Single Drug Product: Used primarily to relieve mild to moderately severe pain and inflammation associated with (1) acute and chronic rheumatoid arthritis; (2) osteoarthritis; and (3) juvenile rheumatoid arthritis.

How This Drug Works: Not completely established. It is thought that this drug reduces the tissue concentrations of prostaglandins (and related compounds), substances involved in the production of inflammation and pain.

Available Dosage Forms and Strengths
Capsules — 400 mg
Tablets — 200 mg, 600 mg

▷ **Usual Adult Dosage Range:** Initially, 400 mg 3 times/day. For maintenance: adjust dosage from 600 mg to 1600 mg daily as needed, taken in 3 or 4 divided doses. The total daily dosage should not exceed 2000 mg (2.0 grams) for rheumatoid arthritis, or 1600 mg (1.6 grams) for osteoarthritis. **Note: Actual dosage and administration schedule must be determined by the physician for each patient individually.**

▷ **Dosing Instructions:** Preferably taken on an empty stomach, 1 hour before or 2 hours after eating. However, it may be taken with or after food if necessary to reduce stomach irritation. Take with a full glass of water and remain upright (do not lie down) for 30 minutes. Schedule dosing to include one in the morning and one at bedtime. The capsule may be opened and the tablet may be crushed for administration.

Usual Duration of Use: Continual use on a regular schedule for 1 to 2 weeks is usually necessary to determine this drug's effectiveness in relieving the discomfort of arthritis. Long-term use (months to years) requires supervision and periodic evaluation by your physician. Consult your physician on a regular basis.

▷ **This Drug Should Not Be Taken If**
  • you have had an allergic reaction to it previously.
  • you are subject to asthma or nasal polyps caused by aspirin.
  • you have active peptic ulcer disease or any form of gastrointestinal bleeding.
  • you have a bleeding disorder or a blood cell disorder.
  • you have severe impairment of liver or kidney function.

▷ **Inform Your Physician Before Taking This Drug If**
  • you are allergic to aspirin or to other aspirin substitutes.
  • you have a history of peptic ulcer disease or any type of bleeding disorder.
  • you have impaired liver or kidney function.
  • you have high blood pressure or a history of heart failure.
  • you are taking any of the following: acetaminophen, aspirin or other aspirin substitutes, anticoagulants, oral antidiabetic drugs.

Possible Side-Effects (natural, expected and unavoidable drug actions)
  Fluid retention (edema).
  Drowsiness in sensitive individuals.

▷ **Possible Adverse Effects** (unusual, unexpected and infrequent reactions)
  If any of the following develop, consult your physician promptly for guidance.
  Mild Adverse Effects
  Allergic Reactions: Skin rash, hives, itching.
  Headache, dizziness, blurred vision, ringing in the ears.
  Mouth sores, indigestion, nausea, vomiting, constipation, diarrhea.
  Serious Adverse Effects
  Allergic Reactions: Anaphylactic reaction (see Glossary), severe skin reactions.
  Active peptic ulcer, with or without bleeding.
  Liver damage with jaundice (see Glossary).
  Kidney damage with painful urination, bloody urine, reduced urine formation.
  Abnormally low white blood cell count: fever, sore throat.
  Abnormally low blood platelet count: abnormal bleeding or bruising.

▷ **Possible Effects on Sexual Function**
None reported.

Possible Delayed Adverse Effects: Mild anemia due to "silent" blood loss from the stomach (less than that caused by aspirin).

▷ **Adverse Effects That May Mimic Natural Diseases or Disorders**
Liver reaction may suggest viral hepatitis.

Natural Diseases or Disorders That May Be Activated by This Drug
Peptic ulcer disease, ulcerative colitis.

Possible Effects on Laboratory Tests
Complete blood cell counts: decreased red cells, hemoglobin, white cells and platelets.
Bleeding time: increased.
Blood potassium level: increased.
Blood urea nitrogen (BUN) level: increased.
Liver function tests: increased liver enzymes (ALT/GPT, AST/GOT and alkaline phosphatase), increased bilirubin.

CAUTION
1. Dosage should always be limited to the smallest amount that produces reasonable improvement.
2. This drug may mask early indications of infection. Inform your physician if you think you are developing an infection of any kind.

Precautions for Use
By Infants and Children: Safety and effectiveness for use by those under 2 years of age have not been established.
By Those over 60 Years of Age: Small doses are advisable until tolerance is determined. Observe for any indications of liver or kidney toxicity, fluid retention, dizziness, confusion, impaired memory, stomach bleeding or constipation.

▷ **Advisability of Use During Pregnancy**
Pregnancy Category: B (tentative). See Pregnancy Code inside back cover.
Animal studies: No birth defects due to this drug reported.
Human studies: Information from adequate studies of pregnant women is not available.
The manufacturer does not recommend the use of this drug during pregnancy.

Advisability of Use if Breast-Feeding
Presence of this drug in breast milk: Unknown.
Avoid drug or refrain from nursing.

Habit-Forming Potential: None.

Effects of Overdosage: Stomach irritation, nausea, vomiting, diarrhea.

Possible Effects of Long-Term Use: Fluid retention.

Suggested Periodic Examinations While Taking This Drug (at physician's discretion)
   Complete blood cell counts, liver and kidney function tests, complete eye examinations if vision is altered in any way.

▷ **While Taking This Drug, Observe the Following**
   Foods: No restrictions.
   Beverages: No restrictions. May be taken with milk.
▷   *Alcohol:* Use with caution. The irritant action of alcohol on the stomach lining, added to the irritant action of this drug in sensitive individuals, can increase the risk of stomach ulceration and/or bleeding.
   Tobacco Smoking: No interactions expected.
▷   *Other Drugs*
      Tolmetin may ***increase*** the effects of
      • acetaminophen (Tylenol, etc.), and increase the risk of kidney damage; avoid prolonged use of this combination.
      • anticoagulants (Coumadin, etc.), and increase the risk of bleeding; monitor prothrombin time, adjust dose accordingly.
      Tolmetin ***taken concurrently*** with the following drugs may increase the risk of bleeding; avoid these combinations:
      • aspirin.
      • dipyridamole (Persantine).
      • indomethacin (Indocin).
      • sulfinpyrazone (Anturane).
      • valproic acid (Depakene).
▷   *Driving, Hazardous Activities:* This drug may cause drowsiness or dizziness. Restrict activities as necessary.
   Aviation Note: The use of this drug ***may be a disqualification*** for piloting. Consult a designated Aviation Medical Examiner.
   Exposure to Sun: No restrictions.

TRAZODONE
(TRAZ oh dohn)

Introduced: 1967

Class: Antidepressants

Prescription: USA: Yes
   Canada: Yes

Controlled Drug: USA: No
   Canada: No

Available as Generic: USA: Yes
   Canada: No

Brand Name: Desyrel, Trialodine

```
┌─────────────────────────────────────────────────────────────┐
│                    BENEFITS versus RISKS                      │
│                                                               │
│      Possible Benefits              Possible Risks            │
│   EFFECTIVE TREATMENT IN        Adverse behavioral effects:   │
│     ALL TYPES OF DEPRESSIVE        confusion, disorientation, │
│     ILLNESS, with or without       delusions, hallucinations (all │
│     anxiety                        infrequent)                │
│                                 Potential for inducing heart  │
│                                    rhythm disorders (in individuals │
│                                    with heart disease)        │
└─────────────────────────────────────────────────────────────┘
```

▷ **Principal Uses**

As a Single Drug Product: Used to provide symptomatic relief in all types of depression, with or without anxiety or agitation. The primary intent is to initiate restoration of normal mood with a minimum of adverse drug effects.

How This Drug Works: Not completely established. It is thought that this drug increases the availability of the nerve impulse transmitter serotonin within certain brain centers and thereby relieves the symptoms of emotional depression.

Available Dosage Forms and Strengths

Tablets — 50 mg, 100 mg, 150 mg, 300 mg

▷ **Usual Adult Dosage Range:** Initially, 50 mg 3 times/day. The dose may be increased by 50 mg daily at intervals of 3 or 4 days as needed and tolerated. The total daily dosage should not exceed 400 mg. **Note: Actual dosage and administration schedule must be determined by the physician for each patient individually.**

▷ **Dosing Instructions:** Best taken with food to improve absorption. The tablet may be crushed for administration. If excessive drowsiness or dizziness occurs, it is advisable to take a larger portion of the total daily dose at bedtime and to divide the remaining amount into 2 or 3 smaller doses to be taken during the day.

Usual Duration of Use: Continual use on a regular schedule for 2 to 4 weeks is usually necessary to determine this drug's effectiveness in relieving the symptoms of depression. Long-term use (weeks to months) requires supervision and periodic evaluation by your physician. Consult your physician on a regular basis.

▷ **This Drug Should Not Be Taken If**
- you have had an allergic reaction to it previously.
- you are recovering from a recent heart attack (myocardial infarction).
- you are taking, or have taken within the past 14 days, any monoamine oxidase (MAO) type A inhibitor drug (see Drug Class, Section Four).

▷ **Inform Your Physician Before Taking This Drug If**
- you have a history of any of the following: alcoholism, epilepsy, heart disease (especially heart rhythm disorders).
- you have impaired liver or kidney function.
- you are taking any antihypertensive drugs.
- you plan to have surgery under general anesthesia in the near future.

Possible Side-Effects (natural, expected and unavoidable drug actions)
Drowsiness, light-headedness, blurred vision, dry mouth, constipation.

▷ **Possible Adverse Effects** (unusual, unexpected and infrequent reactions)
If any of the following develop, consult your physician promptly for guidance.
Mild Adverse Effects
Allergic Reaction: Skin rash.
Headache, dizziness, fatigue, impaired concentration, nervousness, tremors.
Rapid heart rate, palpitations.
Peculiar taste, stomach discomfort, nausea, vomiting, diarrhea.
Muscular aches and pains.
Serious Adverse Effects
Behavioral effects: Confusion, anger, hostility, disorientation, impaired memory, delusions, hallucinations, nightmares.
Irregular heart rhythms, low blood pressure, fainting.

▷ **Possible Effects on Sexual Function**
Decreased male libido; increased female libido.
Inhibited ejaculation, impotence, priapism (see Glossary).
Altered timing and pattern of menstruation.

Possible Effects on Laboratory Tests
None reported.

CAUTION
1. If you experience a significant degree of mouth dryness while using this drug, consult your dentist regarding the risk of gum erosion or tooth decay. Ask for his guidance in ways to keep the mouth comfortably moist.
2. It is advisable to withhold this drug if electroconvulsive therapy (ECT) is to be used.

Precautions for Use
By Infants and Children: Safety and effectiveness for use by those under 18 years of age have not been established.
By Those over 60 Years of Age: During the first two weeks of treatment, observe for the development of restlessness, agitation, excitement, forgetfulness, confusion or disorientation. Be aware of possible unsteadiness and incoordination that may predispose to falling. This drug may enhance prostatism (see Glossary).

▷ **Advisability of Use During Pregnancy**
Pregnancy Category: C (tentative). See Pregnancy Code inside back cover.
Animal studies: Fetal deaths and birth defects reported.
Human studies: Information from adequate studies of pregnant women
is not available.
Avoid this drug completely during the first 3 months. Use otherwise only
if clearly needed. Ask your physician for guidance.

Advisability of Use if Breast-Feeding
Presence of this drug in breast milk: Yes.
Avoid drug or refrain from nursing.

Habit-Forming Potential: None.

Effects of Overdosage: Marked drowsiness, weakness, confusion, tremors,
low blood pressure, rapid heart rate, stupor, coma, possible seizures.

Possible Effects of Long-Term Use: None reported.

Suggested Periodic Examinations While Taking This Drug (at physician's
discretion)
Complete blood cell counts. (This drug may cause slight reductions in
white blood cell counts. This should be monitored closely if infection,
sore throat or fever develops.)
Serial blood pressure readings and electrocardiograms.

▷ **While Taking This Drug, Observe the Following**
Foods: No restrictions.
Beverages: No restrictions. May be taken with milk.
▷ *Alcohol:* Avoid completely. This drug can increase markedly the intoxicating effects of alcohol and accentuate its depressant action on brain
functions.
Tobacco Smoking: No interactions expected.
▷ *Other Drugs*
Trazodone may *increase* the effects of
• antihypertensive drugs, and cause excessive lowering of blood pres-
sure; dosage adjustments may be necessary.
• drugs with sedative effects, and cause excessive sedation.
• phenytoin (Dilantin), by raising its blood level; observe for phenytoin
toxicity.
▷ *Driving, Hazardous Activities:* This drug may cause dizziness or drowsiness.
Restrict activities as necessary.
Aviation Note: The use of this drug *is a disqualification* for piloting.
Consult a designated Aviation Medical Examiner.
Exposure to Sun: No restrictions.
Discontinuation: It is advisable to discontinue this drug gradually. Ask your
physician for guidance in dosage reduction over an appropriate period
of time.

TRIAMTERENE
(tri AM ter een)

Introduced: 1964

Prescription: USA: Yes
  Canada: Yes

Class: Diuretic

Controlled Drug: USA: No
  Canada: No

Available as Generic: No

Brand Names: ✦Apo-Triazide [CD], Dyazide [CD], Dyrenium, Maxzide [CD], Maxzide-25 [CD], ✦Novotriamzide [CD]

BENEFITS versus RISKS

Possible Benefits	*Possible Risks*
EFFECTIVE PREVENTION OF POTASSIUM LOSS when used adjunctively with other diuretics	ABNORMALLY HIGH BLOOD POTASSIUM LEVEL with excessive use
EFFECTIVE DIURETIC IN REFRACTORY CASES OF FLUID RETENTION when used adjunctively with other diuretics	Rare blood cell disorders: megaloblastic anemia, abnormally low white blood cell and platelet counts

---

▷ **Principal Uses**

As a Single Drug Product: This mild diuretic is used as part of the treatment program for the management of congestive heart failure and disorders of the liver and kidney that are accompanied by excessive fluid retention (edema). It is also used in conjunction with other measures to treat high blood pressure. It is used primarily in situations where it is advisable to prevent loss of potassium from the body.

As a Combination Drug Product [CD]: This drug is available in combination with hydrochlorothiazide, a different kind of diuretic that promotes the loss of potassium from the body. Triamterene is used in this combination to counteract the potassium-wasting effect of the thiazide diuretic.

How This Drug Works: Not completely established. It is thought that by inhibiting the enzyme system that initiates the sodium-potassium exchange process, this drug prevents the reabsorption of sodium and the excretion of potassium by the kidney. Thus the drug promotes the excretion of sodium (and water with it) and the retention of potassium.

Available Dosage Forms and Strengths
  Capsules — 50 mg, 100 mg

▷ **Usual Adult Dosage Range:** Initially, 100 mg twice daily. The dose is then adjusted according to individual response. The usual maintenance dose is 100 to 200 mg/day, divided into 2 doses. The total daily dosage should not exceed 300 mg. **Note: Actual dosage and administration** schedule must be determined by the physician for each patient individually.

▷ **Dosing Instructions:** May be taken with or following meals to promote absorption of the drug and to reduce stomach irritation. The capsule may be opened for administration. Intermittent or alternate-day use is recommended to minimize the possibility of sodium and potassium imbalance.

Usual Duration of Use: Continual use on a regular schedule for 3 to 5 days is usually necessary to determine this drug's effectiveness in clearing edema, and for 2 to 3 weeks to determine its effect on hypertension. Long-term use (months to years) requires supervision and periodic evaluation by your physician. Consult your physician on a regular basis.

▷ **This Drug Should Not Be Taken If**
  • you have had an allergic reaction to it previously.
  • you have severely impaired liver or kidney function.

▷ **Inform Your Physician Before Taking This Drug If**
  • you have a history of liver or kidney disease.
  • you have diabetes or gout.
  • you are taking any of the following: antihypertensives, a digitalis preparation, another diuretic, lithium or a potassium preparation.
  • you plan to have surgery under general anesthesia in the near future.

Possible Side-Effects (natural, expected and unavoidable drug actions)
  With excessive use: abnormally high blood potassium levels, abnormally low blood sodium levels, dehydration.
  Blue coloration of the urine (of no significance).

▷ **Possible Adverse Effects** (unusual, unexpected and infrequent reactions)
  If any of the following develop, consult your physician promptly for guidance.
  Mild Adverse Effects
  Allergic Reactions: Skin rash, itching.
  Headache, dizziness, unsteadiness, weakness, drowsiness, lethargy.
  Dry mouth, nausea, vomiting, diarrhea.
  Serious Adverse Effects
  Allergic Reaction: Anaphylactic reaction (see Glossary).
  Symptomatic potassium excess: confusion, numbness and tingling in lips and extremities, fatigue, weakness, shortness of breath, slow heart rate, low blood pressure.
  Rare blood cell disorders: megaloblastic anemia, causing weakness and fatigue; abnormally low white blood cell count, causing infection, fever or sore throat; abnormally low blood platelet count, causing abnormal bleeding or bruising.

▷ **Possible Effects on Sexual Function:** None reported.

Possible Effects on Laboratory Tests
Complete blood cell counts: decreased red cells, hemoglobin, white cells and platelets; increased eosinophils (allergic reaction).
Blood glucose level: increased in diabetics.
Blood lithium level: increased.
Blood potassium level: increased.
Blood uric acid level: increased in 17% of users.
Kidney function tests: increased blood creatinine and urea nitrogen (BUN) levels (kidney damage).

CAUTION
1. Do not take potassium supplements or increase your intake of potassium-rich foods while taking this drug.
2. Do not discontinue this drug abruptly unless abnormally high blood levels of potassium develop.
3. Avoid the liberal use of salt substitutes that contain potassium; these are a potential cause of potassium excess.

Precautions for Use
By Infants and Children: This drug is not recommended for use in children.
By Those over 60 Years of Age: The natural decline in kidney function may predispose to potassium retention in the body. Limit continual use of this drug to periods of 2 to 3 weeks. Observe for indications of potassium excess: slow heart rate, irregular heart rhythms, low blood pressure, confusion, drowsiness. The excessive use of diuretics can cause harmful loss of body water (dehydration), increased viscosity of the blood and an increased tendency of the blood to clot, predisposing to stroke, heart attack or thrombophlebitis.

▷ **Advisability of Use During Pregnancy**
Pregnancy Category: B (tentative). See Pregnancy Code inside back cover.
Animal studies: No birth defects due to this drug reported.
Human studies: Information from adequate studies of pregnant women is not available.
This drug should not be used during pregnancy unless a very serious complication of pregnancy occurs for which this drug is significantly beneficial.

Advisability of Use if Breast-Feeding
Presence of this drug in breast milk: Yes.
Avoid drug or refrain from nursing.

Habit-Forming Potential: None.

Effects of Overdosage: Thirst, drowsiness, fatigue, weakness, nausea, vomiting, confusion, irregular heart rhythm, low blood pressure.

Possible Effects of Long-Term Use: Potassium accumulation to abnormally high blood levels.

Suggested Periodic Examinations While Taking This Drug (at physician's discretion)

Complete blood cell counts.

Measurements of blood sodium, potassium and chloride levels.

Kidney function tests.

▷ **While Taking This Drug, Observe the Following**

Foods: No restrictions. Avoid excessive restriction of salt.

Beverages: No restrictions. May be taken with milk.

▷ *Alcohol:* Use with caution until the combined effects have been determined. Alcohol may enhance the drowsiness and the blood-pressure-lowering effect of this drug.

Tobacco Smoking: No interactions expected.

▷ *Other Drugs*

Triamterene may *increase* the effects of

• amantadine (Symmetrel).

• digoxin (Lanoxin).

Triamterene *taken concurrently* with

• captopril (Capoten) may cause excessively high blood potassium levels.

• indomethacin (Indocin) may increase the risk of kidney damage.

• lithium may cause accumulation of lithium to toxic levels.

• potassium preparations may cause excessively high blood potassium levels.

▷ *Driving, Hazardous Activities:* This drug may cause dizziness and drowsiness. Restrict activities as necessary.

Aviation Note: The use of this drug *may be a disqualification* for piloting. Consult a designated Aviation Medical Examiner.

Exposure to Sun: Use caution until your sensitivity has been determined. This drug may cause photosensitivity (see Glossary).

Discontinuation: With high dosage or prolonged use, it is advisable to withdraw this drug gradually. Sudden discontinuation may cause rebound potassium excretion and resultant potassium deficiency. Ask your physician for guidance.

TRIAZOLAM
(tri AY zoh lam)

Introduced: 1974

Class: Hypnotic, benzodiazepines

Prescription: USA: Yes
Canada: Yes

Controlled Drug: USA: C-IV*
Canada: No

Available as Generic: USA: No
Canada: No

Brand Name: Halcion

*See Schedules of Controlled Drugs inside back cover.

```
┌─────────────────────────────────────────────────────────────┐
│                    BENEFITS versus RISKS                      │
│                                                               │
│      Possible Benefits              Possible Risks            │
│  Possibly effective hypnotic with   SIGNIFICANT "NEXT-DAY"    │
│    short duration of action           MEMORY IMPAIRMENT and   │
│                                       AMNESIA                 │
│                                     Adverse behavioral effects:│
│                                       confusion, hallucinations,│
│                                       bizarre behavior.       │
│                                     Habit-forming potential with│
│                                       long-term use.          │
└─────────────────────────────────────────────────────────────┘
```

▷ **Note:** Recent studies have established that this drug is often ineffective in improving sleep when used at the recommended dose of 0.25 mg; however, this dose commonly causes serious impairment of memory and periods of amnesia during the day following its use. A consensus is emerging that this drug does not have an adequate benefit-to-risk ratio.

▷ **Principal Uses**

As a Single Drug Product: This member of the benzodiazepine class of "minor tranquilizers" is used exclusively as a bedtime sedative to induce sleep. It may be useful in the short-term management of insomnia characterized by difficulty in falling asleep, frequent awakenings during the night and early morning awakening.

How This Drug Works: It is thought that this drug produces a calming effect by enhancing the action of the nerve transmitter gamma-aminobutyric acid (GABA), which in turn blocks the arousal of higher brain centers and helps to induce sleep.

Available Dosage Forms and Strengths

Tablets — 0.125 mg, 0.25 mg

▷ **Usual Adult Dosage Range:** 0.125 to 0.25 mg at bedtime. The total daily dosage should not exceed 0.5 mg. **Note: Actual dosage and administration schedule must be determined by the physician for each patient individually.**

▷ **Dosing Instructions:** Preferably taken on an empty stomach to hasten absorption and induce sleep rapidly. The tablet may be crushed for administration. Do not discontinue this drug abruptly if taken for more than 4 weeks.

Usual Duration of Use: Periods of 3 to 5 nights intermittently, repeated as needed with appropriate dosage adjustment. Avoid uninterrupted and prolonged use. The duration of use should not exceed 2 weeks without reappraisal of continued need.

▷ **This Drug Should Not Be Taken If**
- you have had an allergic reaction to it previously.
- you are currently experiencing a significant mental disorder.

▷ **Inform Your Physician Before Taking This Drug If**
- you are allergic to any benzodiazepine drug (see Drug Class, Section Four).
- you have a history of alcoholism or drug abuse.
- you are pregnant or planning pregnancy.
- you have impaired liver or kidney function.
- you have a history of serious depression or mental disorder.
- you are taking other drugs with sedative effects.
- you have any of the following: asthma, emphysema, epilepsy, myasthenia gravis.

Possible Side-Effects (natural, expected and unavoidable drug actions)
"Hangover" effects on arising: drowsiness (14%), lethargy and unsteadiness (4.6%).

▷ **Possible Adverse Effects** (unusual, unexpected and infrequent reactions)
If any of the following develop, consult your physician promptly for guidance.
Mild Adverse Effects
Allergic Reactions: Skin rash, itching.
Headache, dizziness, fatigue, blurred vision.
Nausea, indigestion, constipation, diarrhea.
Serious Adverse Effects
Idiosyncratic Reactions: Nervousness, talkativeness, irritability, apprehension, euphoria, excitement, confusion, hallucinations, bizarre behavior.
Mental depression.
Significant "next-day" memory impairment and amnesia. This is more frequent and more pronounced following the use of this drug than following the use of other drugs of this class.

▷ **Possible Effects on Sexual Function:**   None reported.

Possible Effects on Laboratory Tests
Urine screening tests for drug abuse: may be **positive**. (Test results depend upon amount of drug taken and testing method used.)

CAUTION
1. This drug should not be discontinued abruptly if it has been taken continually for more than 4 weeks.
2. The concurrent use of some over-the-counter drug products that contain antihistamines (allergy and cold preparations, sleep aids) can cause excessive sedation in sensitive individuals.
3. Regular nightly use of any hypnotic drug should be avoided.
4. If you experience a "hangover" effect, avoid hazardous activities (driving, etc.) and the use of alcohol.
5. This drug should not be used by those with a history of schizophrenia.

Precautions for Use

By Infants and Children: Safety and effectiveness for use by those under 18 years of age have not been established.

By Those over 60 Years of Age: It is advisable to use smaller doses (0.125 mg) at first to determine your response. Observe for the possible development of lethargy, indifference, fatigue, weakness, unsteadiness, disturbing dreams, nightmares and paradoxical reactions of excitement, agitation, anger, hostility and rage.

▷ **Advisability of Use During Pregnancy**

Pregnancy Category: X (tentative). See Pregnancy Code inside back cover.

Animal studies: Benzodiazepines cause significant birth defects in test animals.

Human studies: Information from adequate studies of pregnant women is not available.

Avoid use during entire pregnancy.

Advisability of Use if Breast-Feeding

Presence of this drug in breast milk: Probably yes.

Avoid drug or refrain from nursing.

Habit-Forming Potential: This drug can produce psychological and/or physical dependence (see Glossary) if used in large doses for an extended period of time. Avoid continual use.

Effects of Overdosage: Marked drowsiness, weakness, feeling of drunkenness, staggering gait, tremor, stupor progressing to deep sleep or coma.

Possible Effects of Long-Term Use: Psychological and/or physical dependence.

Periodic Examinations While Taking This Drug (at physician's discretion)

Complete blood cell counts during long-term use.

▷ **While Taking This Drug, Observe the Following**

Foods: No restrictions.

Beverages: Avoid excessive intake of caffeine-containing beverages (coffee, tea, cola) within 4 hours of taking this drug. May be taken with milk.

▷ *Alcohol:* Use with extreme caution until the combined effect has been determined. Alcohol may increase the absorption of this drug and add to its depressant effects on the brain. It is advisable to avoid alcohol completely throughout the day and night if it is necessary to drive or to engage in any hazardous activity.

Tobacco Smoking: Heavy smoking may reduce the hypnotic action of this drug.

Marijuana Smoking: Increased sedation and significant impairment of intellectual and physical performance.

▷ *Other Drugs*

Triazolam may *increase* the effects of

- digoxin (Lanoxin), and cause digoxin toxicity.
- phenytoin (Dilantin), and cause phenytoin toxicity.

Triazolam may *decrease* the effects of
- levodopa (Sinemet, etc.), and reduce its effectiveness in treating Parkinson's disease.

The following drugs may *increase* the effects of triazolam
- cimetidine (Tagamet).
- disulfiram (Antabuse).
- isoniazid (INH, Rifamate, etc.).
- oral contraceptives.
- valproic acid (Depakene).

The following drugs may *decrease* the effects of triazolam
- rifampin (Rimactane, etc.).
- theophylline (Aminophylline, Theo-Dur, etc.).

▷ *Driving, Hazardous Activities:* This drug can impair mental alertness, judgment, physical coordination and reaction time. Avoid hazardous activities accordingly.

Aviation Note: The use of this drug *is a disqualification* for piloting. Consult a designated Aviation Medical Examiner.

Exposure to Sun: No restrictions.

Exposure to Heat: Use caution until the effect of excessive perspiration is determined. Because of reduced urine volume, this drug may accumulate in the body and produce effects of overdosage.

Discontinuation: Avoid sudden discontinuation if this drug has been taken for over 4 weeks without interruption. Dosage should be tapered gradually to prevent a withdrawal syndrome that could include depression, confusion, hallucinations, tremor, seizures, muscle cramping, sweating and vomiting.

TRIFLUOPERAZINE
(tri floo oh PER a zeen)

Introduced: 1958

Class: Strong tranquilizer, phenothiazines

Prescription: USA: Yes
Canada: Yes

Controlled Drug: USA: No
Canada: No

Available as Generic: USA: Yes
Canada: No

Brand Names: ✦Apo-Trifluoperazine, ✦Novoflurazine, ✦Solazine, Stelazine, Suprazine, ✦Terfluzine

```
┌─────────────────────────────────────────────────────────────┐
│                   BENEFITS versus RISKS                       │
│                                                               │
│   Possible Benefits              Possible Risks               │
│ EFFECTIVE CONTROL OF          SERIOUS TOXIC EFFECTS ON        │
│   ACUTE MENTAL DISORDERS        BRAIN with long-term use      │
│   in the majority of patients: Liver damage with jaundice     │
│   beneficial effects on thinking, (infrequent)                │
│   mood and behavior           Rare blood cell disorders:      │
│                                 abnormally low red and white  │
│                                 blood cell and platelet counts│
└─────────────────────────────────────────────────────────────┘
```

▷ **Principal Uses**

As a Single Drug Product: This antipsychotic drug is used primarily to treat psychotic thinking and behavior associated with acute psychoses of unknown nature, mania, paranoid states and acute schizophrenia. It is most effective in those who are withdrawn and apathetic and in those with agitation, delusions and hallucinations.

How This Drug Works: Not completely established. Present theory is that by inhibiting the action of dopamine, this drug acts to correct an imbalance of nerve impulse transmissions that is thought to be responsible for certain mental disorders.

Available Dosage Forms and Strengths

    Concentrate — 10 mg per ml

    Injection — 2 mg per ml

    Tablets — 1 mg, 2 mg, 5 mg, 10 mg

▷ **Usual Adult Dosage Range:** Initially, 1 or 2 mg twice daily. The dose may be increased by 1 or 2 mg at 3 to 4 day intervals as needed and tolerated. Usual dosage range is 10 to 30 mg daily. The total daily dosage should not exceed 40 mg. **Note: Actual dosage and administration schedule must be determined by the physician for each patient individually.**

▷ **Dosing Instructions:** May be taken with or following meals to reduce stomach irritation. The tablets may be crushed for administration.

Usual Duration of Use: Continual use on a regular schedule for several weeks is usually necessary to determine this drug's effectiveness in controlling psychotic disorders. If not significantly beneficial within 6 weeks, it should be discontinued. Long-term use (months to years) requires periodic evaluation of response, appropriate dosage adjustment and consideration of continued need. Consult your physician on a regular basis.

▷ **This Drug Should Not Be Taken If**

- you are allergic to any of the drugs bearing the brand names listed above.
- you have active liver disease.

- you have cancer of the breast.
- you have a current blood cell or bone marrow disorder.

▷ **Inform Your Physician Before Taking This Drug If**
- you are allergic or abnormally sensitive to any phenothiazine drug (see Drug Class, Section Four).
- you have impaired liver or kidney function.
- you have any type of seizure disorder.
- you have diabetes, glaucoma or heart disease.
- you have a history of lupus erythematosus.
- you are taking any drug with sedative effects.
- you plan to have surgery under general or spinal anesthesia in the near future.

Possible Side-Effects (natural, expected and unavoidable drug actions)
Drowsiness (usually during the first 2 weeks), orthostatic hypotension (see Glossary), blurred vision, dry mouth, nasal congestion, constipation, impaired urination.
Pink or purple coloration of urine, of no significance.

▷ **Possible Adverse Effects** (unusual, unexpected and infrequent reactions)
If any of the following develop, consult your physician promptly for guidance.
Mild Adverse Effects
Allergic Reactions: Skin rash, hives, low-grade fever.
Lowering of body temperature, especially in the elderly. (See Hypothermia in Glossary.)
Increased appetite and weight gain.
Dizziness, weakness, agitation, insomnia, impaired day and night vision.
Chronic constipation, fecal impaction.
Serious Adverse Effects
Allergic Reactions: Hepatitis with jaundice (see Glossary), severe skin reactions, anaphylactic reaction (see Glossary).
Idiosyncratic Reactions: Neuroleptic malignant syndrome (see Glossary).
Depression, disorientation, seizures, loss of peripheral vision.
Rapid heart rate, heart rhythm disorders.
Blood cell disorders: significant reduction in all cellular elements of the blood (reduced counts of red cells, white cells and blood platelets). (See Bone Marrow Depression in the Glossary.)
Nervous system reactions: Parkinsonlike disorders (see Glossary), severe restlessness, muscle spasms involving the face and neck, tardive dyskinesia (see Glossary) (10% to 20%).

▷ **Possible Effects on Sexual Function**
Altered timing and pattern of menstruation.
Male breast enlargement and tenderness.
Female breast enlargement with milk production.

Spontaneous male orgasm, paradoxical (1 case reported).
Inhibited ejaculation, painful ejaculation, priapism (see Glossary).
Delayed female orgasm.

▷ **Adverse Effects That May Mimic Natural Diseases or Disorders**
Nervous system reactions may suggest true Parkinson's disease.
Liver reactions may suggest viral hepatitis.
Reactions resembling systemic lupus erythematosus may occur.

Natural Diseases or Disorders That May Be Activated by This Drug
Latent epilepsy, glaucoma, diabetes mellitus, prostatism (see Glossary).

Possible Effects on Laboratory Tests
Complete blood cell counts: decreased red cells, hemoglobin, white cells
and platelets.
Liver function tests: increased liver enzymes (ALT/GPT, AST/GOT and
alkaline phosphatase), increased bilirubin.
Urine pregnancy tests: falsely positive result with some.

CAUTION
1. Many over-the-counter medications (see OTC Drugs in Glossary) for
allergies, colds and coughs contain drugs that can interact unfavorably with this drug. Ask your physician or pharmacist for guidance
before using any such medications.
2. Antacids that contain aluminum and/or magnesium may prevent
the absorption of this drug and reduce its effectiveness.
3. Obtain prompt evaluation of any change or disturbance of vision.

Precautions for Use
By Infants and Children: Use of this drug is not recommended in children
under 6 years of age. Do not use this drug in the presence of symptoms
suggestive of Reye syndrome (see Glossary). Children with acute infectious diseases ("flulike" infections, chicken pox, measles, etc.) are more
prone to develop muscular spasms of the face, back and extremities
when this drug is given.
By Those over 60 Years of Age: Small doses are advisable until individual
response has been determined. You may be more susceptible to the
development of drowsiness, lethargy, constipation, lowering of body
temperature (hypothermia) and orthostatic hypotension (see Glossary). This drug may enhance existing prostatism (see Glossary). You
may also be more susceptible to the development of Parkinson-like
reactions and/or tardive dyskinesia (see discussion of these terms in
Glossary). These reactions must be recognized early since they may
become unresponsive to treatment and irreversible.

▷ **Advisability of Use During Pregnancy**
Pregnancy Category: C (tentative). See Pregnancy Code inside back cover.
Animal studies: Significant birth defects reported in mouse and rat stud-
ies.
Human studies: No increase in birth defects reported in 700 exposures.

Information from adequate studies of pregnant women is not available.

Avoid drug during the first 3 months; avoid during the last month because of possible adverse effects on the newborn infant.

Advisability of Use if Breast-Feeding
Presence of this drug in breast milk: Yes, in minute amounts.
Monitor nursing infant closely and discontinue drug or nursing if adverse effects develop.

Habit-Forming Potential: None.

Effects of Overdosage: Marked drowsiness, weakness, tremor, agitation, unsteadiness, deep sleep, coma, convulsions.

Possible Effects of Long-Term Use: Tardive dyskinesia (see Glossary).

Suggested Periodic Examinations While Taking This Drug (at physician's discretion)
Complete blood cell counts, especially between the fourth and tenth weeks of treatment.
Liver function tests, electrocardiograms.
Complete eye examinations eye structures and vision.
Careful inspection of the tongue for early evidence of fine, involuntary, wavelike movements that could indicate the beginning of tardive dyskinesia.

▷ **While Taking This Drug, Observe the Following**
Foods: No restrictions.
Nutritional Support: A riboflavin (vitamin B-2) supplement should be taken with long-term use.
Beverages: No restrictions. May be taken with milk.
▷ *Alcohol:* Avoid completely. Alcohol can increase the sedative action of phenothiazines and accentuate their depressant effects on brain function and blood pressure. Phenothiazines can increase the intoxicating effects of alcohol.
Tobacco Smoking: Possible reduction of drowsiness from drug.
Marijuana Smoking: Moderate increase in drowsiness; accentuation of orthostatic hypotension; increased risk of precipitating latent psychoses, confusing the interpretation of mental status and drug responses.
▷ *Other Drugs*
Trifluoperazine may *increase* the effects of
• all sedative drugs, especially narcotic analgesics, and cause excessive sedation.
• all atropinelike drugs, and cause nervous system toxicity.
Trifluoperazine may *decrease* the effects of
• guanethidine (Ismelin, Esimil), and reduce its effectiveness in lowering blood pressure.
Trifluoperazine *taken concurrently* with
• lithium (Lithobid, Lithotabs) may impair the effectiveness of lithium and cause nervous system toxicity.

The following drugs may *decrease* the effects of trifluoperazine
- antacids containing aluminum and/or magnesium.
- barbiturates (see Drug Class, Section Four).
- benztropine (Cogentin).
- disulfiram (Antabuse).
- trihexyphenidyl (Artane).

▷ *Driving, Hazardous Activities:* This drug can impair mental alertness, judgment and physical coordination. Avoid hazardous activities.

Aviation Note: The use of this drug *is a disqualification* for piloting. Consult a designated Aviation Medical Examiner.

Exposure to Sun: Use caution until sensitivity has been determined. Some phenothiazines can cause photosensitivity (see Glossary).

Exposure to Heat: Use caution and avoid excessive heat as much as possible. This drug may impair the regulation of body temperature and increase the risk of heat stroke.

Exposure to Cold: Use caution and dress warmly. This drug can increase the risk of hypothermia in the elderly.

Discontinuation: After a period of long-term use, do not discontinue this drug suddenly. Gradual withdrawal over 2 to 3 weeks under physician supervision is recommended. Do not discontinue this drug without your physician's knowledge and approval. The relapse rate of schizophrenia after discontinuation is 50% to 60%.

TRIMETHOPRIM
(tri METH oh prim)

Introduced: 1966

Class: Anti-infective

Prescription: USA: Yes
Canada: Yes

Controlled Drug: USA: No
Canada: No

Available as Generic: USA: Yes
Canada: No

Brand Names: ✦Apo-Sulfatrim [CD], ✦Apo-Sulfatrim DS [CD], Bactrim [CD], Bactrim DS [CD], Bethaprim [CD], Comoxol [CD], ✦Coptin [CD], Cotrim [CD], ✦Novotrimel [CD], ✦Novotrimel DS [CD], Proloprim, ✦Protrin [CD], ✦Protrin DF [CD], ✦Roubac [CD], Septra [CD], Septra DS [CD], Trimpex, Uroplus DS [CD], Uroplus SS [CD]

BENEFITS versus RISKS	
Possible Benefits	*Possible Risks*
EFFECTIVE TREATMENT OF INFECTIONS due to susceptible microorganisms	Rare blood cell disorders: megaloblastic anemia, methemoglobinemia, abnormally low white blood cell and platelet counts

▷ **Principal Uses**

As a Single Drug Product: Used primarily to treat the initial episode of certain infections of the urinary tract that are not complicated by the presence of kidney stones or obstructions to the normal flow of urine. It is sometimes used to prevent the recurrence of such infections.

As a Combination Drug Product
[CD]:

This drug is available in combination with sulfamethoxazole; the generic name co-trimoxazole is used in some countries to identify this combination. It is very effective in the treatment of certain urinary tract infections, middle ear infections, chronic bronchitis, acute enteritis and certain types of pneumonia.

How This Drug Works: This drug prevents the growth and multiplication of susceptible infecting organisms by inactivating the enzyme systems that are necessary for the formation of essential nuclear elements and cell proteins.

Available Dosage Forms and Strengths

Tablets — 100 mg, 200 mg
Tablets — 80 mg combined with 400 mg of sulfamethoxazole
Tablets — 160 mg combined with 800 mg of sulfamethoxazole
Oral suspension — 40 mg combined with 200 mg of sulfamethoxazole per 5-ml teaspoonful

▷ **Usual Adult Dosage Range:**   100 mg every 12 hours for 10 days. For certain pneumonias, the same dose is given every 6 hours. The total daily dosage should not exceed 640 mg. **Note: Actual dosage and administration schedule must be determined by the physician for each patient individually.**

▷ **Dosing Instructions:**   May be taken without regard to meals. However, it may also be taken with or following food if necessary to reduce stomach irritation. The tablet may be crushed for administration.

Usual Duration of Use: Continual use on a regular schedule for 7 to 14 days is usually necessary to determine this drug's effectiveness in controlling responsive infections. The actual duration of use will depend upon the nature of the infection.

Currently a "Drug of Choice"
(when combined with sulfamethoxazole) for preventing pneumonia (due to pneumocystis carinii) in patients with AIDS.

▷ **This Drug Should Not Be Taken If**
• you have had an allergic reaction to it previously.
• you have an anemia due to folic acid deficiency.

▷ **Inform Your Physician Before Taking This Drug If**
• you have a history of folic acid deficiency.

- you have impaired liver or kidney function.
- you are pregnant or breast-feeding.

Possible Side-Effects (natural, expected and unavoidable drug actions)
None with short-term use.

▷ **Possible Adverse Effects** (unusual, unexpected and infrequent reactions)
If any of the following develop, consult your physician promptly for guidance.
Mild Adverse Effects
Allergic Reactions: Skin rash (2.9%), itching, drug fever.
Headache, abnormal taste, sore mouth or tongue, loss of appetite, nausea, vomiting, abdominal cramping, diarrhea.
Serious Adverse Effects
Allergic Reactions: Severe dermatitis with peeling of skin.
Blood cell disorders: megaloblastic anemia, methemoglobinemia, abnormally low white blood cell and platelet counts. (All are rare.)

▷ **Possible Effects on Sexual Function:** None reported.

Possible Effects on Laboratory Tests
Complete blood cell counts: decreased red cells, hemoglobin, white cells and platelets.
Prothrombin time: increased (when taken concurrently with warfarin).

CAUTION
1. Certain strains of bacteria that cause urinary tract infections can develop resistance to this drug. If you do not show significant improvement within 10 days, consult your physician.
2. Comply with your physician's request for periodic blood counts during long-term therapy.

Precautions for Use
By Infants and Children: Safety and effectiveness for use by those under 2 months of age have not been established.
By Those over 60 Years of Age: The natural decline in liver and kidney function may require smaller doses. If you develop itching reactions in the genital or anal areas, report this promptly.

▷ **Advisability of Use During Pregnancy**
Pregnancy Category: C (tentative). See Pregnancy Code inside back cover.
Animal studies: Birth defects due to this drug reported in rat and rabbit studies.
Human studies: Information from adequate studies of pregnant women is not available.
Avoid use of drug during the first 3 months and during the last 2 weeks of pregnancy. Use this drug otherwise only if clearly needed. Ask your physician for guidance.

Advisability of Use if Breast-Feeding
Presence of this drug in breast milk: Yes.
Avoid drug or refrain from nursing.

Habit-Forming Potential: None.

Effects of Overdosage: Headache, dizziness, confusion, depression, nausea, vomiting, bone marrow depression, possible liver toxicity with jaundice.

Possible Effects of Long-Term Use: Impaired production of red and white blood cells and blood platelets.

Suggested Periodic Examinations While Taking This Drug (at physician's discretion)
Complete blood cell counts.

▷ **While Taking This Drug, Observe the Following**
Foods: No restrictions.
Beverages: No restrictions. May be taken with milk.
▷ *Alcohol:* No interactions expected.
Tobacco Smoking: No interactions expected.
▷ *Other Drugs*
Trimethoprim may *increase* the effects of
• phenytoin (Dilantin), and cause phenytoin toxicity.
The following drugs may *decrease* the effects of trimethoprim
• rifampin (Rifadin, Rimactane).
▷ *Driving, Hazardous Activities:* No restrictions.
Aviation Note: The use of this drug is probably not a disqualification for piloting. Consult a designated Aviation Medical Examiner.
Exposure to Sun: No restrictions.

VALPROIC ACID
(val PROH ik)

Introduced: 1967   **Class:** Anticonvulsant

Prescription: USA: Yes   **Controlled Drug:** USA: No
Canada: Yes   Canada: No

Available as Generic: USA: Yes
Canada: No

Brand Names: Depa, Depakene, Depakote, Deproic

BENEFITS versus RISKS

Possible Benefits	*Possible Risks*
EFFECTIVE CONTROL OF MULTIPLE SEIZURE TYPES: ABSENCE SEIZURES, TONIC-CLONIC SEIZURES, MYOCLONIC SEIZURES, PSYCHOMOTOR SEIZURES when used adjunctively with other antiseizure drugs	LIVER TOXICITY, infrequent but may be severe Rare reduction of blood platelets and impaired platelet function with risk of bleeding

---

▷ **Principal Uses**

As a Single Drug Product: Used effectively in the management of the following types of epilepsy: simple and complex absence seizures (petit mal); tonic-clonic seizures (grand mal); myoclonic seizures; complex partial seizures (psychomotor, temporal lobe epilepsy). It is sometimes used adjunctively with other anticonvulsants as needed.

How This Drug Works: Not completely established. It is thought that by increasing the availability of the nerve impulse transmitter gamma-aminobutyric acid (GABA), this drug suppresses the spread of abnormal electrical discharges that cause seizures.

Available Dosage Forms and Strengths

Capsules — 250 mg
Capsules, sprinkle — 125 mg
Syrup — 250 mg per 5-ml teaspoonful
Tablets, enteric-coated — 125 mg, 250 mg, 500 mg

▷ **Usual Adult Dosage Range:**   Initially, 15 mg/kg/24 hours. The dose is increased cautiously by 5 to 10 mg/kg/24 hours every 7 days as needed and tolerated. *The usual daily dose is from 1000 mg to 1600 mg in divided doses.* The total daily dosage should not exceed 60 mg/kg. **Note: Actual dosage and administration schedule must be determined by the physician for each patient individually.**

▷ **Dosing Instructions:**   Preferably taken 1 hour before meals. However, it may be taken with or following food if necessary to prevent stomach irritation. The regular capsule should not be opened and the tablet should not be crushed for administration. The sprinkle-capsule may be opened and the contents sprinkled on soft food for administration. Do not administer the syrup in carbonated beverages. It may be diluted in water or milk.

Usual Duration of Use: Continual use on a regular schedule for 2 weeks is usually necessary to determine this drug's effectiveness in reducing the frequency and severity of seizures. Long-term use (months to years) requires supervision and periodic evaluation by your physician. Consult your physician on a regular basis.

▷ **This Drug Should Not Be Taken If**
- you have had an allergic reaction to it previously.
- you have active liver disease.
- you have an active bleeding disorder.

▷ **Inform Your Physician Before Taking This Drug If**
- you have a history of liver disease or impaired liver function.
- you have a history of any type of bleeding disorder.
- you are pregnant or planning pregnancy.
- you have myasthenia gravis.
- you are taking any of the following drugs: anticoagulants; other anticonvulsants; antidepressants, either the tricyclic type or monoamine oxidase (MAO) type A inhibitors (see Drug Classes, Section Four).
- you plan to have surgery or dental extraction in the near future.

Possible Side-Effects (natural, expected and unavoidable drug actions)
Drowsiness and lethargy (5%).

▷ **Possible Adverse Effects** (unusual, unexpected and infrequent reactions)
If any of the following develop, consult your physician promptly for guidance.
Mild Adverse Effects
Allergic Reaction: Skin rash (rare).
Headache, dizziness, confusion, unsteadiness, slurred speech.
Nausea, indigestion, stomach cramps, diarrhea.
Temporary loss of scalp hair.
Serious Adverse Effects
Idiosyncratic Reactions: Bizarre behavior, hallucinations.
Drug-induced hepatitis with jaundice (see Glossary).
Drug-induced pancreatitis.
Possible Reye syndrome (see Glossary).
Reduced formation of blood platelets and impaired function of platelets, with increased risk of abnormal bleeding.

▷ **Possible Effects on Sexual Function**
Altered timing and pattern of menstruation.
Female breast enlargement with milk production.
Decreased libido.
Decreased effectiveness of oral contraceptives taken concurrently (6%).

▷ **Adverse Effects That May Mimic Natural Diseases or Disorders**
Liver reactions may suggest viral hepatitis.

Possible Effects on Laboratory Tests
Complete blood cell counts: decreased white cells and platelets. Bleeding time: increased.
Prothrombin time: increased.

Blood amylase level: increased (possible pancreatitis).

Liver function tests: increased liver enzymes (ALT/GPT, AST/GOT and alkaline phosphatase), increased bilirubin.

CAUTION

1. The capsules and tablets should be swallowed whole without alteration to avoid irritation of the mouth and throat.
2. This drug can impair normal blood clotting mechanisms. In the event of injury, dental extraction, or need for surgery, inform your physician or dentist that you are taking this drug.
3. Because this drug can impair the normal function of blood platelets, it is advisable to avoid aspirin (which has the same effect).
4. Over-the-counter drug products that contain antihistamines (allergy and cold remedies, sleep aids) can enhance the sedative effects of this drug.

Precautions for Use

By Infants and Children: The concurrent use of aspirin with this drug can cause abnormal bleeding or bruising. Children with mental retardation, organic brain disease or severe seizure disorders may be at increased risk for severe liver toxicity while taking this drug. Observe closely for the development of fever that could indicate the onset of a drug-induced Reye syndrome (see Glossary). Avoid concurrent use of clonazepam (Clonopin); the combined use could result in continuous petit mal episodes.

By Those over 60 Years of Age: Start treatment with small doses and increase dosage cautiously. Observe closely for excessive sedation, confusion or unsteadiness that could predispose to falling and injury.

▷ **Advisability of Use During Pregnancy**

Pregnancy Category: D (tentative). See Pregnancy Code inside back cover.

Animal studies: Palate and skeletal birth defects reported in mouse, rat and rabbit studies.

Human studies: Information from adequate studies of pregnant women is not available. There have been several reports of birth defects attributed to the use of this drug during early pregnancy.

Consult your physician regarding the advantages and disadvantages of using this drug. If it is used, it is advisable to keep the dose as low as possible.

Advisability of Use if Breast-Feeding

Presence of this drug in breast milk: Yes, in small amounts.

Monitor nursing infant closely and discontinue drug or nursing if adverse effects develop.

Habit-Forming Potential: None.

Effects of Overdosage: Increased drowsiness, weakness, unsteadiness, confusion, stupor progressing to coma.

Possible Effects of Long-Term Use: None reported.

Suggested Periodic Examinations While Taking This Drug (at physician's discretion)

Complete blood cell counts and baseline liver function tests should be done before treatment is started. During treatment, blood counts should be repeated every month and liver function tests repeated every 2 months.

▷ **While Taking This Drug, Observe the Following**

Foods: No restrictions.

Beverages: Do not administer the syrup in carbonated beverages; this could liberate the valproic acid and irritate the mouth and throat. This drug may be taken with milk.

▷   *Alcohol:* Use extreme caution until the combined effects have been determined. Alcohol can increase the sedative effect of this drug. Also, this drug can increase the depressant effects of alcohol on brain function.

Tobacco Smoking: No interactions expected.

▷   *Other Drugs*

Valproic acid may *increase* the effects of

- anticoagulants (Coumadin, etc.), and increase the risk of bleeding.
- antidepressants, both monoamine oxidase (MAO) type A inhibitors and tricyclics, and cause toxicity.
- phenobarbital, and cause barbiturate intoxication.
- phenytoin (Dilantin), and cause phenytoin toxicity.

Valproic acid *taken concurrently* with

- antiplatelet drugs: aspirin, dipyridamole (Persantine), sulfinpyrazone (Anturane) may enhance the inhibition of platelet function and increase the risk of bleeding.

▷   *Driving, Hazardous Activities:* This drug may cause drowsiness, dizziness or confusion. Restrict activities as necessary.

Aviation Note: The use of this drug *is a disqualification* for piloting. Consult a designated Aviation Medical Examiner.

Exposure to Sun: No restrictions.

Discontinuation: **Do not discontinue this drug suddenly.** Abrupt withdrawal can cause repetitive seizures that are difficult to control.

VERAPAMIL
(ver AP a mil)

Introduced: 1967

Class: Antianginal, antiarrhythmic, antihypertensive, calcium channel blocker

Prescription: USA: Yes
Canada: Yes

Controlled Drug: USA: No
Canada: No

Available as Generic: USA: Yes
Canada: No

Brand Names: Calan, Calan SR, Isoptin, Isoptin SR, Verelan

BENEFITS versus RISKS

Possible Benefits	*Possible Risks*
EFFECTIVE PREVENTION OF BOTH MAJOR TYPES OF ANGINA	Congestive heart failure
	Low blood pressure (2.9%)
	Heart rhythm disturbance
EFFECTIVE CONTROL OF HEART RATE IN CHRONIC ATRIAL FIBRILLATION AND FLUTTER	Fluid retention (1.7%)
	Liver damage without jaundice (very rare)
EFFECTIVE PREVENTION OF PAROXYSMAL ATRIAL TACHYCARDIA (PAT)	
EFFECTIVE TREATMENT OF HYPERTENSION	

▷ **Principal Uses**

As a Single Drug Product: Used primarily to treat (1) angina pectoris due to coronary artery spasm (Prinzmetal's variant angina) that occurs spontaneously and is not associated with exertion; (2) classical angina-of-effort (due to atherosclerotic disease of the coronary arteries) in individuals who have not responded to or cannot tolerate the nitrates and beta blocker drugs customarily used to treat this disorder; (3) abnormally rapid heart rate due to chronic atrial fibrillation or flutter; (4) recurrent paroxysmal atrial tachycardia; and (5) primary hypertension.

How This Drug Works: Not completely established. It is thought that by blocking the normal passage of calcium through certain cell walls (which is necessary for the function of nerve and muscle tissue), this drug slows the spread of electrical activity through the conduction system of the heart and inhibits the contraction of coronary arteries and peripheral arterioles. As a result of these combined effects, this drug

- prevents spontaneous spasm of the coronary arteries (Prinzmetal's type of angina).
- reduces the rate and contraction force of the heart during exertion, thus lowering the oxygen requirement of the heart muscle; this reduces the occurrence of effort-induced angina (classical angina pectoris).
- reduces the degree of contraction of peripheral arterial walls, resulting in their relaxation and consequent lowering of blood pressure. This further reduces the work load of the heart during exertion and contributes to the prevention of angina.
- slows the rate of electrical impulses through the conduction system of the heart and thereby prevents excessively rapid heart action (tachycardia).

Available Dosage Forms and Strengths
Capsules, prolonged-action — 120 mg, 240 mg
Injection — 5 mg per 2 ml
Tablets — 40 mg, 80 mg, 120 mg
Tablets, prolonged-action — 180 mg, 240 mg

▷ **Usual Adult Dosage Range:**   Initially, 80 mg 3 or 4 times daily. The dose may be increased gradually at 1 to 7 day intervals as needed and tolerated. The usual maintenance dose is from 240 mg to 480 mg daily in 3 or 4 divided doses. The prolonged-action dosage forms permit once-a-day dosing. The total daily dosage should not exceed 480 mg. Once-a-day treatment may be initiated with 1 prolonged-action capsule of 120 mg or 1 tablet of 180 mg.**Note: Actual dosage and administration schedule must be determined by the physician for each patient individually.**

▷ **Dosing Instructions:**   Preferably taken with meals and with food at bedtime. The regular tablet may be crushed for administration. The prolonged-action dosage forms (capsules and tablets) should be swallowed whole and not altered. Verelan capsules may be taken without regard to food intake.

Usual Duration of Use: Continual use on a regular schedule for 2 to 4 weeks is usually necessary to determine this drug's effectiveness in reducing the frequency and severity of angina. Reduction of elevated blood pressure may be apparent within the first 1 to 2 weeks. For long-term use (months to years), determine the smallest effective dose; this requires supervision and periodic evaluation by your physician. Consult your physician on a regular basis.

Possible Advantages of This Drug
No adverse effects on blood levels of glucose, potassium or uric acid.
Does not increase blood cholesterol or triglyceride levels.
Does not impair capacity for exercise.

Currently a "Drug of Choice"
for (1) initiating treatment of hypertension with a single drug; (2)treating hypertension in Afro-Americans.

▷ **This Drug Should Not Be Taken If**
  • you have had an allergic reaction to it previously.
  • you have active liver disease.
  • you have a "sick sinus" syndrome (and do not have an artificial pace-maker).
  • you have been told that you have a second-degree or third-degree heart block.
  • you have low blood pressure systolic pressure below 90.

▷ **Inform Your Physician Before Taking This Drug If**
  • you have had an unfavorable response to any calcium blocker drug in the past.
  • you are currently taking any other drugs, especially digitalis or a beta blocker drug (see Drug Class, Section Four).
  • you have had a recent stroke or heart attack.
  • you have a history of congestive heart failure or heart rhythm dis-orders.
  • you have impaired liver or kidney function.
  • you have a history of drug-induced liver damage.

Possible Side-Effects (natural, expected and unavoidable drug actions)
Low blood pressure (2.9%), fluid retention (1.7%).

▷ **Possible Adverse Effects** (unusual, unexpected and infrequent reactions)
   If any of the following develop, consult your physician promptly for guidance.
Mild Adverse Effects
Allergic Reactions: Skin rash, hives, itching, aching joints.
Headache (1.8%), dizziness (3.6%), fatigue (1.1%).
Nausea (1.6%), indigestion, constipation (6.3%).
Serious Adverse Effects
Serious disturbances of heart rate and/or rhythm, congestive heart fail-ure (0.9%).
Drug-induced liver damage without jaundice (very rare).

▷ **Possible Effects on Sexual Function**
Altered timing and pattern of menstruation.
Male breast enlargement and tenderness.
Impotence (20%).

Possible Effects on Laboratory Tests
Blood total cholesterol and HDL cholesterol levels: no effect in some; decreased in others.
Blood LDL cholesterol level: no effect.
Blood triglyceride levels: no effect.
Glucose tolerance test (GTT): decreased.
Liver function tests: increased liver enzymes (ALT/GPT and AST/GOT), increased bilirubin (one case report).

CAUTION
  1. Be sure to inform all physicians and dentists you consult that you are

taking this drug. Note the use of this drug on your card of personal identification.
2. You may use nitroglycerin and other nitrate drugs as needed to relieve acute episodes of angina pain. However, if you detect that your angina attacks are becoming more frequent or intense, notify your physician promptly.
3. If this drug is used concurrently with a beta blocker drug, you may develop excessively low blood pressure.
4. This drug may cause swelling of the feet and ankles. This may not be indicative of either heart or kidney dysfunction.

Precautions for Use
By Infants and Children: Safety and effectiveness for use by those under 12 years of age have not been established.
By Those over 60 Years of Age: You may be more susceptible to the development of weakness, dizziness, fainting and falling. Take necessary precautions to prevent injury. Report promptly any changes in your pattern of thirst and urination.

▷ **Advisability of Use During Pregnancy**
Pregnancy Category: C (tentative). See Pregnancy Code inside back cover.
Animal studies: Toxic effects on the embryo and retarded growth of the fetus (but no birth defects) reported in rat studies.
Human studies: Information from adequate studies of pregnant women is not available.
Avoid this drug during the first 3 months. Use during the last 6 months only if clearly needed. Ask your physician for guidance.

Advisability of Use if Breast-Feeding
Presence of this drug in breast milk: Possibly yes.
Avoid drug or refrain from nursing.

Habit-Forming Potential: None.

Effects of Overdosage: Flushed and warm skin, sweating, light-headedness, irritability, rapid heart rate, low blood pressure, loss of consciousness.

Possible Effects of Long-Term Use: None reported.

Suggested Periodic Examinations While Taking This Drug (at physician's discretion)
Evaluations of heart function, including electrocardiograms; liver and kidney function tests, with long-term use.

▷ **While Taking This Drug, Observe the Following**
Foods: No restrictions. Avoid excessive salt intake.
Beverages: No restrictions. May be taken with milk.
▷ *Alcohol:* Use with caution until combined effects have been determined. Alcohol may exaggerate the drop in blood pressure experienced by some individuals.

Tobacco Smoking: Nicotine can reduce the effectiveness of this drug. Avoid all forms of tobacco.

Marijuana Smoking: Possible reduced effectiveness of this drug; mild to moderate increase in angina; possible changes in electrocardiogram, confusing interpretation.

▷ *Other Drugs*

Verapamil may *increase* the effects of
- carbamazepine (Tegretol), and cause carbamazepine toxicity.
- digitoxin and digoxin, and cause digitalis toxicity.

Verapamil *taken concurrently* with
- beta blocker drugs (see Drug Class, Section Four) may affect heart rate and rhythm adversely. Careful monitoring by your physician is necessary if these drugs are taken concurrently.

The following drugs may *increase* the effects of verapamil
- cimetidine (Tagamet).

▷ *Driving, Hazardous Activities:* Usually no restrictions. This drug may cause dizziness. Restrict activities as necessary.

Aviation Note: Coronary artery disease *is a disqualification* for piloting. Consult a designated Aviation Medical Examiner.

Exposure to Sun: Use caution until sensitivity has been determined. This drug may cause photosensitivity (see Glossary).

Exposure to Heat: Caution advised. Hot environments can exaggerate the blood-pressure-lowering effects of this drug. Observe for light-headedness or weakness.

Heavy Exercise or Exertion: This drug may improve your ability to be more active without resulting angina pain. Use caution and avoid excessive exercise that could impair heart function in the absence of warning pain.

Discontinuation: Do not discontinue this drug abruptly. Consult your physician regarding gradual withdrawal to prevent the development of rebound angina.

WARFARIN
(WAR far in)

Introduced: 1941

Prescription: USA: Yes
Canada: Yes

Available as Generic: USA: Yes
Canada: No

Class: Anticoagulant, coumarins

Controlled Drug: USA: No
Canada: No

Brand Names: ✦Athrombin-K, Carfin, Coumadin, Panwarfin, Sofarin, ✦Warfilone

> **BENEFITS versus RISKS**
>
> | *Possible Benefits* | *Possible Risks* |
> |---|---|
> | EFFECTIVE PREVENTION OF BOTH ARTERIAL AND VENOUS THROMBOSIS EFFECTIVE PREVENTION OF EMBOLIZATION IN THROMBOEMBOLIC DISORDERS | NARROW TREATMENT RANGE Dose-related bleeding (5% to 7%) Skin and soft tissue hemorrhage with tissue death (rare) |

▷ **Principal Uses**

As a Single Drug Product: Used exclusively for its anticoagulant effect in treating the following conditions: (1) acute thrombosis (clot) or thrombophlebitis of the deep veins; (2) acute pulmonary embolism, resulting from blood clots that originate anywhere in the body; (3) atrial fibrillation, to prevent clotting of blood inside the heart that could result in embolization of small clots to any part of the body; (4) acute myocardial infarction (heart attack), to prevent clotting and embolization; (5) transient ischemic attack (TIA), a temporary reduction of blood flow to a part of the brain; used here to reduce the risk of repeated attacks or possible stroke. Other possible uses include the long-term prevention of recurrent heart attack, and prevention of embolization from the heart in those individuals with artificial heart valves.

How This Drug Works: The coumarin anticoagulants interfere with the production of four essential blood clotting factors by blocking the action of vitamin K. This leads to a deficiency of these clotting factors in circulating blood and inhibits blood clotting mechanisms.

Available Dosage Forms and Strengths

Injection — 50 mg/vial

Tablets — 1 mg, 2 mg, 2.5 mg, 5 mg, 7.5 mg, 10 mg

▷ **Usual Adult Dosage Range:**   Initially, 10 to 15 mg daily for 2 to 3 days. A large loading dose is inappropriate and may be hazardous. For maintenance, 2 to 10 mg/day. The dosage is adjusted according to the prothrombin time. **Note: Actual dosage and administration schedule must be determined by the physician for each patient individually.**

▷ **Dosing Instructions:**   Preferably taken when the stomach is empty, and at the same time each day to ensure uniform results. The tablet may be crushed for administration.

Usual Duration of Use: Continual use on a regular schedule for 3 to 5 days is usually necessary to determine this drug's effectiveness in providing significant anticoagulation. An additional 10 to 14 days is required to determine the optimal maintenance dose for each individual. Long-term use (months to years) requires supervision and periodic evaluation by your physician. Consult your physician on a regular basis.

▷ **This Drug Should Not Be Taken If**
  • you have had an allergic reaction to it previously.
  • you have an active peptic ulcer or active ulcerative colitis.
  • you have had a recent stroke.

▷ **Inform Your Physician Before Taking This Drug If**
  • you are now taking *any other drugs,* either prescription drugs or over-the-counter drug products.
  • you are pregnant or planning pregnancy.
  • you have a history of a bleeding disorder.
  • you have high blood pressure.
  • you have abnormally heavy or prolonged menstrual bleeding.
  • you have diabetes.
  • you are using an indwelling catheter.
  • you have impaired liver or kidney function.
  • you plan to have surgery or dental extraction in the near future.

Possible Side-Effects (natural, expected and unavoidable drug actions)
  Minor episodes of bleeding may occur even though dosage and prothrombin times are well within the recommended range.

▷ **Possible Adverse Effects** (unusual, unexpected and infrequent reactions)
  If any of the following develop, consult your physician promptly for guidance.
  Mild Adverse Effects
  Allergic Reactions: Skin rash, hives.
  Loss of scalp hair.
  Loss of appetite, nausea, vomiting, cramping, diarrhea.
  Serious Adverse Effects
  Allergic Reaction: Drug fever (see Glossary).
  Idiosyncratic Reactions: Bleeding into skin and soft tissues causing gangrene of breast, toes and localized areas anywhere (rare).
  Abnormal bleeding from nose, gastrointestinal tract, urinary tract or uterus.

▷ **Possible Effects on Sexual Function:**   None reported.

▷ **Adverse Effects That May Mimic Natural Diseases or Disorders**
  Drug-induced fever may suggest infection.

Natural Diseases or Disorders That May Be Activated by This Drug
  Bleeding from "silent" peptic ulcer, intestinal or bladder polyp or tumor.

Possible Effects on Laboratory Tests
  Complete blood cell counts: decreased red cells, hemoglobin and white cells.
  Bleeding time: increased.

Prothrombin time: increased.
Blood uric acid level: increased (in men). ·
Liver function tests: increased liver enzymes (ALT/GPT, AST/GOT and alkaline phosphatase).

CAUTION
1. Always carry with you a card of personal identification that includes a statement that *you are taking an anticoagulant drug.*
2. While taking this drug, always consult your physician *before* starting any new drug, changing the dosage schedule of any drug or discontinuing any drug.

Precautions for Use
By Those over 60 Years of Age: Small doses are mandatory until your individual sensitivity has been determined. Observe regularly for indications of excessive drug effects: prolonged bleeding from shaving cuts, bleeding gums, bloody urine, rectal bleeding, excessive bruising.

▷ **Advisability of Use During Pregnancy**
Pregnancy Category: X. See Pregnancy Code inside back cover.
Animal studies: Fetal hemorrhage and death due to this drug reported in mice.
Human studies: Information from studies of pregnant women indicates fetal defects and fetal hemorrhage due to this drug.
The manufacturers state that this drug is contraindicated during entire pregnancy.

Advisability of Use if Breast-Feeding
Presence of this drug in breast milk: Yes.
Avoid drug or refrain from nursing.

Habit-Forming Potential: None.

Effects of Overdosage: Episodes of bleeding from minor surface bleeding (nose, gums, small lacerations) to major internal bleeding: vomiting blood, bloody urine or stool.

Possible Effects of Long-Term Use: None reported.

Suggested Periodic Examinations While Taking This Drug (at physician's discretion)
Regular determinations of prothrombin time are essential to safe dosage and proper control.
Urine analyses for blood.

▷ **While Taking This Drug, Observe the Following**
Foods: A larger intake than usual of foods rich in vitamin K may reduce the effectiveness of this drug and make larger doses necessary. Foods rich in vitamin K include: asparagus, bacon, beef liver, cabbage, cauliflower, fish, green leafy vegetables.
Beverages: No restrictions. May be taken with milk.

▷ *Alcohol:* Limit alcohol to one drink daily. Note: Heavy users of alcohol with liver damage may be very sensitive to anticoagulants and require smaller than usual doses.

Tobacco Smoking: Heavy smokers may require relatively larger doses of this drug.

▷ *Other Drugs*

Warfarin may *increase* the effects of
- phenytoin (Dilantin).

The following drugs may *increase* the effects of warfarin
- amiodarone.
- androgens.
- cephalosporins.
- chloral hydrate.
- cimetidine.
- clofibrate.
- dextrothyroxine.
- disulfiram.
- glucagon.
- metronidazole.
- phenylbutazone.
- quinidine.
- salicylates.
- sulfinpyrazone.
- sulfonamides.
- thyroid hormones.

The following drugs may *decrease* the effects of warfarin
- barbiturates.
- carbamazepine.
- cholestyramine.
- ethchlorvynol.
- glutethimide.
- griseofulvin.
- rifampin.
- vitamin K.

▷ *Driving, Hazardous Activities:* No restrictions.

Aviation Note: The use of this drug *is a disqualification* for piloting. Consult a designated Aviation Medical Examiner.

Exposure to Sun: No restrictions.

Discontinuation: Do not discontinue this drug abruptly unless abnormal bleeding occurs. Ask your physician for guidance regarding gradual reduction in dosage over a period of 3 to 4 weeks.

ZIDOVUDINE
(zi DOH vyoo deen)

Other Names: AZT, azidothymidine, Compound S

Introduced: 1987   **Class:** Antiviral

Prescription: USA: Yes   **Controlled Drug:** USA: No
    Canada: Yes   Canada: No

Available as Generic: USA: No
    Canada: No

Brand Name: Retrovir

BENEFITS versus RISKS

Possible Benefits	*Possible Risks*
SIGNIFICANTLY DELAYED PROGRESSION OF DISEASE IN AIDS INFECTED INDIVIDUALS WITHOUT SYMPTOMS PROLONGATION OF LIFE AND REDUCED INCIDENCE OF INFECTIONS IN TREATING ACTIVE AIDS AND AIDS-RELATED COMPLEX	SERIOUS BONE MARROW DEPRESSION (see Glossary) Brain toxicity Lip, mouth and tongue sores

---

▷ **Principal Uses**

As a Single Drug Product: Used primarily to treat selected patients who have acquired immunodeficiency syndrome (AIDS) or acquired immunodeficiency syndrome-related complex (ARC) caused by human immunodeficiency virus (HIV); it is used specifically to treat those with interstitial plasma cell pneumonia or a marked deficiency of helper T-lymphocytes. This drug is not a cure for AIDS, and it does not reduce the risk of transmission of AIDS infection to others through sexual contact or contamination of blood.

How This Drug Works: By interfering with essential enzyme systems, this drug is thought to prevent the growth and reproduction of HIV particles within tissue cells, thus limiting the severity and extent of HIV infection.

Available Dosage Forms and Strengths
    Capsules — 100 mg
    Injection — 10 mg per ml
       Syrup — 50 mg per 5-ml teaspoonful

▷ **Usual Adult Dosage Range:** For asymptomatic HIV infection: 100 mg/4 hours while awake (500 mg/day).

For symptomatic HIV infection: Initially 200 mg/4 hours throughout the day and night (no omission for activities or sleep) for 1 month. Smaller and larger doses may be used according to individual patient characteristics. After 1 month, the dose may be reduced to 100 mg/4 hours. **Note: Actual dosage and administration schedule must be determined by the physician for each patient individually.**

▷ **Dosing Instructions:** Preferably taken on an empty stomach, but may be taken with or following food. Take exactly as prescribed. The capsule may be opened and the contents mixed with food just prior to administration.

Usual Duration of Use: Continual use on a regular schedule for 10 to 12 weeks is usually necessary to determine this drug's effectiveness in improving the course of symptomatic AIDS infection. Long-term use requires periodic evaluation of response and dosage adjustment. Consult your physician on a regular basis.

▷ **This Drug Should Not Be Taken If**
  • you have had a serious allergic reaction to it previously.
  • you have a serious degree of uncorrected bone marrow depression.

▷ **Inform Your Physician Before Taking This Drug If**
  • you have a history of either folic acid or vitamin B-12 deficiency.
  • you have impaired liver or kidney function.

Possible Side-Effects (natural, expected and unavoidable drug actions)
None reported.

▷ **Possible Adverse Effects** (unusual, unexpected and infrequent reactions)
If any of the following develop, consult your physician promptly for guidance.
Mild Adverse Effects
Allergic Reactions: Skin rash, hives, itching.
Headache (50%), weakness (20%), drowsiness, dizziness, nervousness, insomnia.
Nausea (50%), stomach pain (20%), diarrhea (12%), loss of appetite and vomiting (5% to 11%), altered taste, lip sores, swollen mouth or tongue.
Muscle aches (8%), fever, sweating.
Serious Adverse Effects
Confusion, loss of speech, twitching, tremors, seizures (representing brain toxicity).
Bone marrow depression (see Glossary): fatigue, weakness, fever, sore throat, abnormal bleeding or bruising. Anemia occurs most commonly after 4 to 6 weeks of treatment; abnormally low white blood cell counts occur after 6 to 8 weeks of treatment.

▷ **Possible Effects on Sexual Function**
None reported.

Possible Delayed Adverse Effects: Significant anemia and deficient white blood cell counts may develop after this drug has been discontinued.

▷ **Adverse Effects That May Mimic Natural Diseases or Disorders**
Seizures may suggest the possibility of epilepsy.

Possible Effects on Laboratory Tests
Complete blood cell counts: decreased red cells, hemoglobin, white cells and platelets.

CAUTION
1. This drug is not a cure for AIDS or AIDS-related complex. Nor does it protect completely against other infections or complications. Follow your physician's instructions and take all medications exactly as prescribed.
2. This drug does not reduce the risk of transmitting AIDS to others through sexual contact or contamination of the blood. The use of an effective condom is mandatory. Needles for drug administration should not be shared.

Precautions for Use
By Infants and Children: Effectiveness for use by those under 12 years of age has not been established. However, the FDA has authorized use of zidovudine syrup in HIV-infected children from 3 months to 12 years of age. For further information call 1–800-829-PEDS.
By Those over 60 Years of Age: Impaired kidney function will require dosage reduction.

▷ **Advisability of Use During Pregnancy**
Pregnancy Category: C (tentative). See Pregnancy Code inside back cover.
Animal studies: Rat studies reveal no birth defects.
Human studies: Information from adequate studies of pregnant women is not available.
Consult your physician for specific guidance.

Advisability of Use if Breast-Feeding
Presence of this drug in breast milk: Unknown.
Avoid drug or refrain from nursing.

Habit-Forming Potential: None.

Effects of Overdosage: Nausea, vomiting, diarrhea, bone marrow depression.

Possible Effects of Long-Term Use: Serious anemia and loss of white blood cells.

Suggested Periodic Examinations While Taking This Drug (at physician's discretion)

Complete blood cell counts before starting treatment and weekly thereafter until tolerance is established. Continual monitoring for bone marrow depression is necessary during entire course of treatment.

▷ **While Taking This Drug, Observe the Following**

Foods: No restrictions.

Beverages: No restrictions. May be taken with milk.

▷   *Alcohol:* No interactions expected.

Tobacco Smoking: No interactions expected.

▷   *Other Drugs*

The following drugs may *increase* the effects of zidovudine and enhance its toxicity

- acetaminophen.
- acyclovir.
- aspirin.
- benzodiazepines (see Drug Class, Section Four).
- cimetidine.
- indomethacin.
- morphine.
- probenecid.
- sulfonamides (see Drug Class, Section Four).

▷   *Driving, Hazardous Activities:* This drug may cause dizziness or fainting. Restrict activities as necessary.

Aviation Note: The use of this drug *is a disqualification* for piloting. Consult a designated Aviation Medical Examiner.

Exposure to Sun: No restrictions.

Discontinuation: Do not discontinue this drug without your physician's knowledge and guidance.

DRUG CLASSES

Drug Classes

Throughout the Drug Profiles in Section Three reference is made to various drug classes. The reader may be advised to consult Section Four to become familiar with the drugs which belong to a particular class of drugs that share important characteristics in their chemical composition or in their actions within the body. Often it is important to know that *any* drug (or *all* drugs) within a given class can be expected to behave in a particular way. Such information may be useful in preventing interactions that could reduce the effectiveness of the drugs in use or result in unanticipated and sometimes hazardous adverse effects.

The presentation of each Drug Class is divided into two listings. The upper list contains the more widely recognized brand names of the drugs within the class; the lower list contains the generic names of the class members. In some instances the number of brand names in use is so large that a complete listing is not possible. In such cases, to be certain that you are consulting the correct drug class, determine the generic name of the drug that concerns you and consult the lower list to see if it is included there. The generic name listing is sufficiently complete to serve the scope of this book.

The following page lists the names of all the Drug Classes included in this section.

LIST OF DRUG CLASSES

Amphetaminelike Drugs
Analgesics, Mild
Analgesics, Strong (Narcotic Drugs)
Antiacne Drugs
Antiallergic Drugs
Antianginal Drugs
Antiarthritic/Anti-inflammatory
    Drugs (Aspirin Substitutes)
Antiasthmatic Drugs
    (Bronchodilators)
Antibiotics
Anticoagulants
Antidepressants
Antidiabetics, Oral (Sulfonylureas)
Antidiarrheal Drugs
Antiepileptic Drugs
    (Anticonvulsants)
Antiglaucoma Drugs
Antigout Drugs
Antihistamines
Antihypertensives
Anti-infective Drugs
    (Nonantibiotic-Antimicrobials)
Anti-itching Drugs (Antipruritics)
Anti-Motion Sickness/Antinausea
    Drugs (Antiemetics)
Antiparkinsonism Drugs
Antispasmodics, Synthetic
Appetite Suppressants (Anorexiants)
Atropinelike Drugs
Barbiturates
Benzodiazepines
Beta-Adrenergic-Blocking Drugs
    (Beta Blockers)
Calcium Channel-Blocking Drugs
    (Calcium Blockers)

Cephalosporins
Cholesterol-Reducing Drugs
Cortisonelike Drugs (Adrenocortical
    Steroids)
Cough Suppressants (Antitussives)
Decongestants
Digitalis Preparations
Diuretics
Female Sex Hormones
Fever-Reducing Drugs
    (Antipyretics)
Heart Rhythm Regulators
    (Antiarrhythmic Drugs)
Histamine (H-2)-Blocking Drugs
    (H-2 Blockers)
Male Sex Hormones (Androgens)
Monoamine Oxidase (MAO)
    Inhibitor Drugs
Muscle Relaxants
Nitrates
Penicillins
Phenothiazines
Salicylates
Sedatives/Sleep Inducers,
    Nonbarbiturate (Hypnotics)
Sulfonamides ("Sulfa" Drugs)
Sulfonylureas
Tetracyclines
Thiazide Diuretics
Tranquilizers, Mild (Antianxiety
    Drugs)
Tranquilizers, Strong (Antipsychotic
    Drugs)
Vasodilators
Xanthines

AMPHETAMINELIKE DRUGS

BRAND NAMES

Amodex	Didrex	Ritalin
Benzedrine	Fastin	Tenuate
Biphetamine	Ionamin	Tepanil
Desoxyn	Obalan	Tora
Dexatrim	Plegine	Wilpowr
Dexedrine	Preludin	

GENERIC NAMES

amphetamine	methylphenidate
benzphetamine	phendimetrazine
dextroamphetamine	phenmetrazine
diethylpropion	phentermine
levamphetamine	phenylpropanolamine
methamphetamine	

ANALGESICS, MILD

BRAND NAMES

Anaprox	Hycodan	Talwin
A.S.A. Preparations	Indocin	Taper
Darvocet	Motrin	Tempra
Darvon	Nebs	Tylenol
Datril	Percodan	Valadol

GENERIC NAMES

acetaminophen	naproxen
aspirin	oxycodone
codeine	paregoric
hydrocodone	pentazocine
ibuprofen	propoxyphene
indomethacin	

ANALGESICS, STRONG
(Narcotic Drugs)

BRAND NAMES

Demerol
Dilaudid
Dolophine
Leritine

GENERIC NAMES

anileridine
hydromorphone
meperidine
methadone
morphine

ANTIACNE DRUGS

BRAND NAMES

Accutane
Achromycin V
Eryderm
Lucidol
Retin-A

GENERIC NAMES

benzoyl peroxide
erythromycin
isotretinoin
tetracycline
tretinoin

ANTIALLERGIC DRUGS

See: Antihistamines
       Cortisonelike Drugs

ANTIANGINAL DRUGS

BRAND NAMES

Calan
Cardene
Cardizem
Cartrol
Corgard
Inderal
Isoptin
Isordil

Nitrostat
Peritrate
Procardia
Tenormin

GENERIC NAMES

beta blockers (see Class)
diltiazem
nicardipine

nifedipine
nitrates (see Class)
verapamil

ANTIARTHRITIC/ANTI-INFLAMMATORY DRUGS

(Aspirin Substitutes)

BRAND NAMES

Ansaid
Clinoral
Dolobid
Feldene
Indocin
Meclomen
Motrin

Nalfon
Naprosyn
Orudis
Suprol
Tolectin
Voltaren

GENERIC NAMES

diclofenac
diflunisal
fenoprofen
flurbiprofen
ibuprofen
indomethacin
ketoprofen

meclofenamate
naproxen
piroxicam
sulindac
suprofen
tolmetin

ANTIASTHMATIC DRUGS

(Bronchodilators)

BRAND NAMES

Aarane
Adrenalin
Alupent
Aminodur
Brethine
Bricanyl
Bronkodyl
Bronkometer
Bronkosol
Bronkotabs
Choledyl

Elixophyllin
Intal
Isuprel
Lufyllin
Maxair
Medihaler-Epi
Medihaler-Iso
Metaprel
Neothylline
Norisodrine

Proternol
Proventil
Slo-Phyllin
Somophylline
Sus-Phrine
Theolair
Tornalate
Vaponefrin
Ventolin

GENERIC NAMES

albuterol
aminophylline
bitolterol
cromolyn
dyphylline
ephedrine
epinephrine

isoetharine
isoproterenol
metaproterenol
oxtriphylline
pirbuterol
terbutaline
theophylline

ANTIBIOTICS

BRAND NAMES

See respective Classes listed under Generic Names.

GENERIC NAMES

cephalosporins
chloramphenicol
clindamycin
erythromycins

lincomycin
penicillins
rifampin
tetacyclines

ANTICOAGULANTS

Coumarin Class

BRAND NAMES

Coumadin
Dicumarol
Liquamar
Panwarfin
Sintrom
Tromexan

GENERIC NAMES

acenocoumarol
dicumarol
phenprocoumon
warfarin

Indandione Class

BRAND NAMES

Danilone
Dipaxin
Eridione
Hedulin
Miradon

GENERIC NAMES

anisindione
diphenadione
phenindione

ANTIDEPRESSANTS
Bicyclic Antidepressants

BRAND NAMES

Prozac

GENERIC NAMES

fluoxetine

Tricyclic Antidepressants

BRAND NAMES

Adapin	Pamelor
Asendin	Pertofrane
Aventyl	Presamine
Elavil	Sinequan
Endep	Surmontil
Janimine	Tofranil
Norpramin	Vivactil

GENERIC NAMES

amitriptyline	imipramine
amoxapine	nortriptyline
desipramine	protriptyline
doxepin	trimipramine

Tetracyclic Antidepressants

BRAND NAMES

Ludiomil

GENERIC NAMES

maprotiline

Other Antidepressants

BRAND NAMES

Desyrel

GENERIC NAMES

trazodone

ANTIDIABETICS, ORAL

Sulfonylurea Class

BRAND NAMES

Chloronase   Glucotrol
DiaBeta   Micronase
Diabinese   Mobenol
Dimelor   Orinase
Dymelor   Stabinol
Euglucon   Tolinase

GENERIC NAMES

acetohexamide
chlorpropamide
glipizide
glyburide
tolazamide
tolbutamide

ANTIDIARRHEAL DRUGS

BRAND NAMES

Donnagel
Imodium
Kaopectate
Lomotil
Parepectolin

GENERIC NAMES

atropine
diphenoxylate
kaolin
loperimide
paregoric
pectin

ANTIEPILEPTIC DRUGS

(Anticonvulsants)

BRAND NAMES

Depakene	Mysoline
Diamox	Tegretol
Dilantin	Valium
Klonopin	Zarontin
Luminal	

GENERIC NAMES

acetazolamide	phenobarbital
carbamazepine	phenytoin
clonazepam	primidone
diazepam	valproic acid
ethosuximide	

ANTIGLAUCOMA DRUGS

BRAND NAMES

Betoptic
Diamox
Glaucon
Isopto-carpine
Timoptic

GENERIC NAMES

acetazolamide
betaxolol
epinephrine
pilocarpine
timolol

ANTIGOUT DRUGS

<u>BRAND NAMES</u>

Anaprox
Anturane
Benemid
Clinoril
Naprosyn
Zyloprim

<u>GENERIC NAMES</u>

allopurinol
colchicine
naproxen
probenecid
sulfinpyrazone
sulindac

ANTIHISTAMINES

<u>BRAND NAMES</u>

Actidil
Atarax
Benadryl
Bonine
Chlor-Trimeton
Clistin
Decapryn
Dimetane
Dramamine

Hismanal
Hispril
Histadyl
Histalon
Inhiston
Marezine
Neo-Antergan
Norflex

Optimine
Periactin
Phenergan
Pyribenzamine
Seldane
Tavist
Trimeton
Vistaril

<u>GENERIC NAMES</u>

astemizole
azatadine
brompheniramine
carbinoxamine
chlorpheniramine
clemastine
cyclizine
cyproheptadine

dimenhydrinate
diphenhydramine
diphenylpyraline
doxylamine
hydroxyzine
meclizine
methapyrilene

orphenadrine
pheniramine
promethazine
pyrilamine
terfenidine
tripelennamine
triprolidine

ANTIHYPERTENSIVES

BRAND NAMES

Aldomet	Esidrix	Minipress
Altace	Eutonyl	Naqua
Anhydron	Exna	Naturetin
Apresoline	HydroDiuril	Normodyne
Blocadren	Hygroton	Prinivil
Capoten	Hytrin	Renese
Cardene	Inderal	Saluron
Cardura	Inversine	Sectral
Cartrol	Ismelin	Serpasil
Catapres	Kerlone	Tenex
Corgard	Lasix	Tenormin
Diuril	Levatol	Trandate
DynaCirc	Loniten	Vasotec
Enduron	Lopressor	Visken
Esbaloid	Lozol	Zestril

GENERIC NAMES

bendroflumethiazide	cyclothiazide	methyclothiazide
benzthiazide	doxazosin	methyldopa
beta blockers (see Class)	enalapril	minoxidil
	furosemide	nicardipine
bethanidine	guanethidine	pargyline
calcium channel blockers (see Class)	guanfacine	penbutolol
	hydralazine	polythiazide
	hydrochlorothiazide	prazosin
captopril	hydroflumethiazide	reserpine
chlorothiazide	indapamide	ramipril
chlorthalidone	lisinopril	terazosin
clonidine	mecamylamine	trichlormethiazide

ANTI-INFECTIVE DRUGS

(Nonantibiotic-Antimicrobials)

BRAND NAMES

Bactrim	Gantrisin
Cipro	Macrodantin
Flagyl	NegGram
Floxin	Noroxin
Furadantin	Septra

GENERIC NAMES

ciprofloxacin
metronidazole
nalidixic acid
nitrofurantoin
norfloxacin
ofloxacin
sulfonamides (see Class)
trimethoprim

ANTI-ITCHING DRUGS

(Antipruritics)

BRAND NAMES

Atarax
Cortaid
Dermolate
Periactin
Temaril
Vistaril

GENERIC NAMES

cortisonelike drugs (see Class)
cyproheptadine
hydroxyzine
trimeprazine

ANTI-MOTION SICKNESS/ANTINAUSEA DRUGS

(Antiemetics)

BRAND NAMES

Antivert	Compazine	Phenergan
Atarax	Dexedrine	Thorazine
Benadryl	Dramamine	Tigan
Bonine	Marezine	Vistaril

GENERIC NAMES

chlorpromazine	meclizine
cyclizine	prochlorperazine
dextroamphetamine	promethazine
dimenhydrinate	scopolamine
diphenhydramine	trimethobenzamide
hydroxyzine	

ANTIPARKINSONISM DRUGS

BRAND NAMES

Akineton	Kemadrin	Parsidol
Artane	Larodopa	Permax
Bendopa	Levodopa	Phenoxene
Biodopa	Norflex	Pipanol
Cogentin	Pagitane	Sinemet
Disipal	Parda	Symmetrel
Dopar	Parlodel	Tremin
Eldepryl		

GENERIC NAMES

amantadine	levodopa
benztropine	orphenadrine
biperiden	pergolide
bromocriptine	procyclidine
chlorphenoxamine	selegiline
cycrimine	trihexyphenidyl
ethopropazine	

ANTISPASMODICS, SYNTHETIC

Antrenyl	Nacton	Quarzan
Banthine	Pamine	Robinul
Bentyl	Pathilon	Tral
Cantil	Prantal	Trocinate
Darbid	Pro-Banthine	

clidinium	isopropamide	poldine
dicyclomine	mepenzolate	propantheline
diphemanil	methantheline	thiphenamil
glycopyrrolate	methscopolamine	tridihexethyl
hexocyclium	oxyphenonium	

APPETITE SUPPRESSANTS

(Anorexiants)

Dexedrine	Preludin
Dietac	Pre-Sate
Fastin	Sanorex
Ionamin	Tenuate
Plegine	Tepanil
Pondimin	

chlorphentermine	phendimetrazine
dextroamphetamine	phenmetrazine
diethylpropion	phentermine
fenfluramine	phenylpropanolamine
mazindol	

ATROPINELIKE DRUGS

The drugs included in the following groups may exhibit atropinelike (anticholinergic) action. This can be important in the management of certain diseases and in potential interactions with other drugs used concurrently.

All drugs containing:

atropine	Antidepressants, tricyclic
belladonna	Antihistamines (some)
hyoscyamine	Antiparkinsonism Drugs
scopolamine	(some)
	Antispasmodics, Synthetic
	Muscle Relaxants (some)

BARBITURATES

BRAND NAMES

Alurate	Mebaral
Amytal	Nembutal
Butisol	Sandoptal
Lotusate	Seconal
Luminal	Sombulex

GENERIC NAMES

amobarbital	mephobarbital
aprobarbital	pentobarbital
butabarbital	phenobarbital
butalbital	secobarbital
hexobarbital	talbutal

BENZODIAZEPINES

Ativan	Paxipam
Centrax	Restoril
Dalmane	Serax
Halcion	Tranxene
Klonopin	Valium
Libritabs	Verstran
Librium	Xanax

GENERIC NAMES

alprazolam	halazepam
chlordiazepoxide	lorazepam
clonazepam	oxazepam
clorazepate	prazepam
diazepam	temazepam
flurazepam	triazolam

BETA-ADRENERGIC-BLOCKING DRUGS
(Beta Blockers)

BRAND NAMES

Blocadren	Lopressor
Cartrol	Normodyne
Corgard	Sectral
Inderal	Tenormin
Kerlone	Trandate
Levatol	Visken

GENERIC NAMES

acebutolol	nadolol
atenolol	penbutolol
betaxolol	pindolol
carteolol	propranolol
labetalol	timolol
metoprolol	

CALCIUM CHANNEL-BLOCKING DRUGS
(Calcium Blockers)

BRAND NAMES

Calan
Cardene
Cardizem
DynaCirc
Isoptin
Procardia

GENERIC NAMES

diltiazem
isradipine
nicardipine
nifedipine
verapamil

CEPHALOSPORINS

BRAND NAMES

Anspor
Ceclor
Ceftin
Ceporex
Duricef

Keflex
Novolexin
Suprax
Ultracef
Velosef

GENERIC NAMES

cefaclor
cefadroxil
cefixime
cefuroxime
cephalexin
cephradine

CHOLESTEROL-REDUCING DRUGS

BRAND NAMES

Atromid S   Lopid
Choloxin   Lorelco
Colestid   Mevacor
Cytellin   Nicobid
                   Questran

GENERIC NAMES

cholestyramine   gemfibrozil
clofibrate   lovastatin
colestipol   niacin
dextrothyroxine   probucol
                        sitosterols

CORTISONELIKE DRUGS

(Adrenocortical Steroids)

BRAND NAMES

Aristocort   Dexamethadrone   Meticorten
Colisone   Dexasone   Novadex
Cortef   Gammacorten   Novapred
Cortril   Hexadrol   Paracort
Decadron   Hydeltra   Prednis
Delta-Cortef   Hydrocortone   Servisone
Deltasone   Inflamase   Sterane
Deltra   Kenacort   Valisone
Deronil   Maxidex   Vanceril
Dexameth   Medrol   Wescopred

GENERIC NAMES

beclomethasone   methylprednisolone
betamethasone   prednisolone
cortisone   prednisone
dexamethasone   triamcinolone
hydrocortisone

COUGH SUPPRESSANTS

(Antitussives)

BRAND NAMES

Benylin   Phenergan
Benylin DM   Tessalon
Dilaudid   Tussionex
Hycodan

GENERIC NAMES

benzonatate   hydrocodone
codeine   hydromorphone
dextromethorphan   promethazine
diphenhydramine

DECONGESTANTS

BRAND NAMES

Afrin   Privine
Gluco-Fedrin   Propadrine
Neo-Synephrine   Sudafed
Novafed   Tyzine
Otrivin

GENERIC NAMES

ephedrine   pseudoephedrine
naphazoline   tetrahydrozoline
oxymetazoline   xylometazoline
phenylephrine
phenylpropanolamine

DIGITALIS PREPARATIONS

BRAND NAMES

Crystodigin	Lanoxicaps
Digifortis	Lanoxin
Digiglusin	Purodigin
Gitaligin	

GENERIC NAMES

digitalis	digoxin
digitoxin	gitalin

DIURETICS

BRAND NAMES

Aldactone	Hygroton
Bumex	Lasix
Diamox	Lozol
Diulo	Midamor
Diuril	Zaroxolyn
Dyrenium	(See Thiazide Brand Names)
Edecrin	

GENERIC NAMES

acetazolamide	indapamide
amiloride	metolazone
bumetanide	spironolactone
chlorthalidone	thiazides (see Class)
ethacrynic acid	triamterene
furosemide	

FEMALE SEX HORMONES

BRAND NAMES

Estrogens
Delestrogen
DES
Estinyl
Estrace
Estrovis
Evex
Feminone
Ogen
Premarin
TACE

Progestogens
Amen
Curretab
Megace
Micronor
Morlutin
Ovrette
Provera

GENERIC NAMES

Estrogens
chlorotrianisene
diethylstilbestrol
estradiol
estrogens, conjugated
estrogens, esterified
estropipate
ethinyl estradiol
quinestrol

Progestogens
medroxyprogesterone
megestrol
norethindrone
norgestrel

FEVER-REDUCING DRUGS

(Antipyretics)

BRAND NAMES

Anaprox
Clinoril
Indocin
Motrin
Nalfon

Naprosyn
Ponstel
Rufen
Tolectin
Tylenol

GENERIC NAMES

acetaminophen
aspirin
fenoprofen

ibuprofen
indomethacin
mefenamic acid

naproxen
sulindac
tolmetin

HEART RHYTHM REGULATORS

(Antiarrhythmic Drugs)

BRAND NAMES

Calan	Pronestyl
Crystodigin	Purodigin
Inderal	Quinaglute
Isoptin	Quinidex
Lanoxin	Quinora
Mexitil	Tambocor
Norpace	Tonocard
Procan SR	

GENERIC NAMES

digitoxin	procainamide
digoxin	propranolol
disopyramide	quinidine
flecainide	tocainide
mexiletine	verapamil

HISTAMINE (H-2)-BLOCKING DRUGS

(H-2 Blockers)

BRAND NAMES

Axid
Pepcid
Tagamet
Zantac

GENERIC NAMES

cimetidine
famotidine
nizatidine
ranitidne

MALE SEX HORMONES

(Androgens)

BRAND NAMES

Android	Oratestin
Android F	Ora-Testryl
Depo-Testosterone	Oreton
Halotestin	Oreton Methyl
Metandren	Testred

GENERIC NAMES

fluoxymesterone
methyltestosterone
testosterone

MONOAMINE OXIDASE (MAO) INHIBITOR DRUGS

MAO Type A Inhibitors

(Food restrictions apply)

BRAND NAMES

Actomol	Marsilid
Catron	Nardil
Drazine	Niamid
Eutonyl	Parnate
Furoxone	Tersavid
Marplan	

GENERIC NAMES

furazolidone	phenelzine
iproniazid	pheniprazine
isocarboxazid	phenoxypropazine
mebanazine	piohydrazine
nialamide	tranylcypromine
pargyline	

MAO Type B Inhibitors
(Food restrictions do not apply)

Eldepryl

selegiline

MUSCLE RELAXANTS

Equanil   Rela
Flexeril   Robaxin
Lioresal   Skelaxin
Norflex   Soma
Paraflex   Valium
Parafon Forte

baclofen   meprobamate
carisoprodol   metaxalone
chlorzoxazone   methocarbamol
cyclobenzaprine   orphenadrine
diazepam

NITRATES

Cardilate   Nitro-Bid   Peritrate
Isordil   Nitroglyn   SK-Petn
Laserdil   Nitrospan   Sorbide
Neo-Corovas   Nitrostat   Sorbitrate

erythrityl tetranitrate
isosorbide dinitrate
nitroglycerin
pentaerythritol tetranitrate

PENICILLINS

BRAND NAMES

Alpen	Omnipen	Principen
Amcill	Orbenin	Prostaphlin
Amoxil	Pathocil	Spectrobid
Bactocil	Penbritin	Tegopen
Dynapen	Pentids	Unipen
Geocillin	Pen-Vee K	V-Cillin K
Geopen	Polycillin	Veracillin
Larotid	Polymox	

GENERIC NAMES

amoxicillin	dicloxacillin
ampicillin	nafcillin
bacampicillin	oxacillin
carbenicillin	penicillin G
cloxacillin	penicillin V

PHENOTHIAZINES

BRAND NAMES

Chlor-PZ	Proketazine	Tacaryl
Compazine	Prolixin	Temaril
Largon	Promatar	Thorazine
Levoprome	Quide	Tindal
Mellaril	Repoise	Torecan
Parsidol	Serentil	Trilafon
Permitil	Sparine	Vesprin
Phenergan	Stelazine	

GENERIC NAMES

acetophenazine	methdilazine	propiomazine
butaperazine	methotrimeprazine	thiethylperazine
carphenazine	perphenazine	thioridazine
chlorpromazine	piperacetazine	trifluoperazine
ethopropazine	procholorperazine	triflupromazine
fluphenazine	promazine	trimeprazine
mesoridazine	promethazine	

SALICYLATES

BRAND NAMES

Arthropan   Empirin
Bufferin   Magan
Causalin   Neocylate
Ecotrin   Uracel

GENERIC NAMES

aspirin
choline salicylate
magnesium salicylate
potassium salicylate
sodium salicylate

SEDATIVES/SLEEP INDUCERS, NONBARBITURATE

(Hypnotics)

BRAND NAMES

Carbrital   Halcion   Restoril
Dalmane   Noctec   Somnafac
Doriden   Noludar   Sopor
Dorimide   Parest   Valmid
Felsules   Placidyl

GENERIC NAMES

carbromal   glutethimide
chloral hydrate   methyprylon
ethchlorvynol   temazepam
ethinamate   triazolam
flurazepam

SULFONAMIDES
("Sulfa" Drugs)

<u>BRAND NAMES</u>

Azulfidine   Gantanol   Sonilyn
Coco-Diazine   Gantrisin   Suladyne
Cosulfa   Kynex   Thiosulfil
Dagenan   Madribon   Triple Sulfas
Diamox   Midicel   Urobiotic
Elkosin   Neotrizine

<u>GENERIC NAMES</u>

acetazolamide   sulfamethazine   sulfapyridine
sulfachlorpyridazine sulfamethizole   sulfasalazine
sulfadiazine   sulfamethoxazole   sulfisomidine
sulfadimethoxine   sulfamethoxy-   sulfisoxazole
sulfamerazine   pyridazine   trisulfapyrimidines

SULFONYLUREAS
<u>BRAND NAMES</u>

Chloronase   Micronase
DiaBeta   Mobenol
Diabinese   Novobutamide
Dimelor   Orinase
Dymelor   Tolbutone
Euglucon   Tolinase
Glucotrol

<u>GENERIC NAMES</u>

acetohexamide
chlorpropamide
glipizide
glyburide
tolazamide
tolbutamide

TETRACYCLINES

BRAND NAMES

Achromycin	Rondomycin	Tetracyn
Aureomycin	Steclin	Vectrin
Declomycin	Sumycin	Velacycline
Minocin	Terramycin	Vibramycin
Panmycin	Tetrachel	

GENERIC NAMES

chlortetracycline	minocycline
demeclocycline	oxytetracycline
doxycycline	rolitetracycline
methacycline	tetracycline

THIAZIDE DIURETICS

BRAND NAMES

Anhydron	Hydrazide	Naqua
Chemhydrazide	Hydrid	Naturetin
Diucardin	Hydrite	Neocodema
Diuchlor	Hydro-Aquil	Novohydrazide
Diuril	Hydrodiuretex	Oretic
Duretic	HydroDiuril	Renese
Edemol	Hydrosaluret	Saluron
Enduron	Hydrozide	Thiuretic
Esidrix	Metahydrin	Urozide
Exna		

GENERIC NAMES

bendroflumethiazide	hydroflumethiazide
benzthiazide	methyclothiazide
chlorothiazide	polythiazide
cyclothiazide	trichlormethiazide
hydrochlorothiazide	

TRANQUILIZERS, MILD

(Antianxiety Drugs)

BRAND NAMES

Atarax	Miltown	Tybatran
Buspar	Paxipam	Ultran
Deprol	Serax	Valium
Equanil	Trancopal	Vistaril
Fenarol	Tranxene	Xanax
Librium		

GENERIC NAMES

alprazolam	halazepam
benactyzine	hydroxyzine
buspirone	meprobamate
chlordiazepoxide	oxazepam
chlormezanone	phenaglycodol
clorazepate	tybamate
diazepam	

TRANQUILIZERS, STRONG

(Antipsychotic Drugs)

BRAND NAMES

Carbolith	Lithonate	Sandril
Clozaril	Lithotabs	Serpasil
Eskalith	Loxitane	Taractan
Haldol	Moban	(See Phenothiazines, Brand
Lithane	Navane	Names)

GENERIC NAMES

chlorprothixene	molindone
clozapine	phenothiazines (see Class)
haloperidol	reserpine
lithium	thiothixene
loxapine	

VASODILATORS

BRAND NAMES

Arlidin   Pavabid
Cerespan   Vasodilan
Cyclospasmol   Vasospan
Ethatab

GENERIC NAMES

cyclandelate
ethaverine
isoxsuprine
nylidrin
papaverine

XANTHINES

BRAND NAMES

Aminodur   Quibron-T
Bronkodyl   Slo-Phyllin
Choledyl   Theo-Dur
Droxine   Theolixir
Elixophylline   Theovent

GENERIC NAMES

aminophylline
dyphylline
oxtriphylline
theophylline

A GLOSSARY
OF
DRUG-RELATED TERMS

Glossary

Addiction The traditional term used to identify the irresistible craving for and compulsive use of habit-forming drugs. The more recent preference for the term *dependence* has served to clarify the distinction between habituation and addiction. Drugs capable of producing addiction do so by interacting with the biochemistry of the brain in such a way that they assume a working role. This physical incorporation of the drug into the fundamental processes of brain tissue function is responsible for the agony of the "withdrawal syndrome"—the intense mental and physical pain experienced by the addict when intake of the drug is stopped abruptly. Thus addiction is a *physical dependence.* (See DEPENDENCE for a further account of physical and psychological dependence.)

Adverse Effect or Reaction An abnormal, unexpected, infrequent and usually unpredictable injurious response to a drug. Used in this restrictive sense, the term *adverse reaction* does *not* include effects of a drug which are normally a part of its pharmacological action, even though such effects may be undesirable and unintended. (See SIDE-EFFECT.) Adverse reactions are of three basic types: those due to drug *allergy,* those caused by individual *idiosyncrasy* and those representing *toxic* effects of drugs on tissue structure and function (see ALLERGY, IDIOSYNCRASY and TOXICITY).

Allergy (Drug) An abnormal mechanism of drug response that occurs in individuals who produce injurious antibodies* that react with foreign

---

*Antibodies are special tissue proteins that combine with substances foreign to the body. Protective antibodies destroy bacteria and neutralize toxins. Injurious antibodies, reacting with foreign substances, cause the release of histamine, the principal chemical responsible for allergic reactions.

substances—in this instance, a drug. The person who is allergic by nature and has a history of hay fever, asthma, hives or eczema is more likely to develop drug allergies. Allergic reactions to drugs take many forms: skin eruptions of various kinds, fever, swollen glands, painful joints, jaundice, interference with breathing, acute collapse of circulation, etc. Drug allergies can develop gradually over a long period of time, or they can appear with dramatic suddenness and require life-saving intervention.

Analgesic A drug that is used primarily to relieve pain. Analgesics are of three basic types: (1) Simple, nonnarcotic analgesics that relieve pain by suppressing the local production of prostaglandins and related substances; examples are acetaminophen, aspirin and the large group of nonsteroidal anti-inflammatory drugs known as aspirin substitutes (Motrin, Advil, Naprosyn, etc.). (2) Narcotic analgesics or opioids ("like opium" derivatives) that relieve pain by suppressing its perception in the brain; examples are morphine, codeine and hydrocodone (natural derivatives of opium), and meperidine or pentazocine (synthetic drug products). (3) Local anesthetics that prevent or relieve pain by rendering sensory nerve endings insensitive to painful stimulation; an example is the urinary tract analgesic phenazopyridine (Pyridium).

Anaphylactic (Anaphylactoid) Reaction A group of symptoms which represent (or resemble) a sometimes overwhelming and dangerous allergic reaction due to extreme hypersensitivity to a drug. Anaphylactic reactions, whether mild, moderate or severe, often involve several body systems. Mild symptoms consist of itching, hives, nasal congestion, nausea, abdominal cramping and/or diarrhea. Sometimes these precede more severe symptoms such as choking, shortness of breath and sudden loss of consciousness (usually referred to as anaphylactic shock).

Characteristic features of anaphylactic reaction must be kept in mind. It can result from a very small dose of drug; it develops suddenly, usually within a few minutes after taking the drug; it can be rapidly progressive and can lead to fatal collapse in a short time if not reversed by appropriate treatment. A developing anaphylactic reaction is a true medical emergency. Any adverse effect that appears within 20 minutes after taking a drug should be considered the early manifestation of a possible anaphylactic reaction. Obtain medical attention immediately! (See ALLERGY, DRUG and HYPERSENSITIVITY.)

Antihypertensive A drug used to lower excessively high blood pressure. The term *hypertension* denotes blood pressure above the normal range. It does not refer to excessive nervous or emotional tension. The term *antihypertensive* is sometimes used erroneously as if it had the same meaning as *antianxiety* (or tranquilizing) drug action.

Today there are more than 100 drug products in use for treating hypertension. Those most frequently prescribed for long-term use fall into three major groups:

drugs that increase urine production (the diuretics)
drugs that relax blood vessel walls
drugs that reduce the activity of the sympathetic nervous system

Regardless of their mode of action, all these drugs share an ability to lower the blood pressure. It is important to remember that many other drugs can interact with antihypertensive drugs: some add to their effect and cause excessive reduction in blood pressure; others interfere with their action and reduce their effectiveness. Anyone who is taking medications for hypertension should consult with his or her physician whenever drugs are prescribed for the treatment of other conditions as well.

Antipyretic A drug that is used to treat fever because of its ability to lower body temperature that is elevated above the normal. Antipyretics relieve fever through their effects on the temperature regulating center in the hypothalamus of the brain. Their actions cause dilation of the blood vessels (capillary beds) in the skin, bringing overheated blood to the surface for cooling; in addition, the sweat glands are stimulated to provide copious perspiration that cools the body further through evaporation. An antipyretic drug may also be analgesic (acetaminophen), or analgesic and anti-inflammatory (aspirin).

Aplastic Anemia A form of bone marrow failure in which the production of all 3 types of blood cells is seriously impaired (also known as pancytopenia). Aplastic anemia can occur spontaneously from unknown causes, but about one-half of reported cases are induced by certain drugs or chemicals. The symptoms reflect the consequences of inadequate supplies of all 3 blood cell types: deficiency of red blood cells (anemia) results in fatigue, weakness and pallor; deficiency of white blood cells (leukopenia) predisposes to infections; deficiency of blood platelets (thrombocytopenia) leads to spontaneous bruising and hemorrhage. Treatment is difficult and the outcome unpredictable. Even with the best of care, approximately 50% of cases end fatally.

These drugs and chemicals are known to be capable of inducing aplastic anemia:

acetazolamide	meprobamate
anticancer drugs	methimazole
aspirin	oxyphenbutazone
benzene (solvent)	penicillin
carbamazepine	phenacetin
carbon tetrachloride (solvent)	phenylbutazone
chlordane (insecticide)	phenytoin
chlordiazepoxide	primidone
chloromycetin	promazine
chlorothiazide	quinacrine
chlorpheniramine	sulfonamides
chlorpromazine	tetracyclines
chlorpropamide	thiouracil
colchicine	tolbutamide
DDT (insecticide)	triflupromazine
indomethacin	trimethadione
lithium	tripelennamine
mephenytoin	

Although aplastic anemia is a rare consequence of drug treatment (3 in 100,000 users of quinacrine, for example), anyone taking a drug capable of inducing it should have complete blood cell counts periodically if the drug is to be used over an extended period of time.

Bioavailability The measurable characteristics of a drug product (usually a tablet or a capsule) that represent how rapidly the active drug ingredient is absorbed into the bloodstream and to what extent it is absorbed. Two types of measurements—(1) blood levels of the drug at certain time intervals after administration, and (2) the duration of the drug's presence in the blood—indicate how much of the drug is available for biological activity and for how long.

Another method of determining a drug product's bioavailability is to measure (1) the cumulative amount of the drug (or any breakdown product after transformation) that is excreted in the urine, and (2) the rate of drug accumulation in the urine.

The two major factors that govern a drug product's bioavailability are the chemical and physical characteristics (the formulation) of the dosage form given, and the functional state of the digestive system of the individual who takes it. A drug product that disintegrates rapidly in a normally functioning stomach and small intestine produces blood levels of the absorbed drug quite promptly. Such a drug product can be demonstrated to possess good bioavailability.

Specially designed laboratory tests are now available to evaluate a drug product's potential bioavailability when taken by the "average" individual.

Bioequivalence It is generally accepted that the ability of a drug product to produce its intended therapeutic effect is directly related to its bioavailability. When a particular drug is marketed by several manufacturers, often in a variety of dosage forms, it is critically important that the drug product selected for use be one that possesses the bioavailability necessary to be effective therapeutically. Substantial variations occur among manufacturers in the formulation of their drug products. Although the principal drug ingredient of products from different firms may be identical chemically, it cannot be assumed that these products possess equal bioavailability and are therefore equal therapeutically.

The bioavailability of any drug product is governed to a large extent by the physical characteristics of its formulation; these in turn determine how rapidly and how completely the drug product disintegrates and releases its active drug component(s) for absorption into the bloodstream. Drug products that contain the same principal drug ingredient but are combined with different inert additives, are coated with different substances or are enclosed in capsules of different composition may or may not possess the same bioavailability. Those that do are said to be bioequivalent, and can be relied upon to be equally effective in achieving therapeutic results.

If you consider having your prescription filled with the generic equivalent of a brand name drug product, ask your physician *and* pharmacist for guidance. This decision requires professional judgment in each case. In many treatment situations, reasonable differences in the bioavailability patterns among drug products are acceptable. In some situations, however, because of the serious nature of the illness, or because it is mandatory that blood levels of the drug be maintained within a narrowly defined range, it is essential to use the drug product that has been demonstrated to possess reliable bioavailability.

Blood Platelets The smallest of the three types of blood cells produced by the bone marrow. Platelets are normally present in very large numbers. Their primary function is to assist the process of normal blood clotting so as to prevent excessive bruising and bleeding in the event of injury. When present in proper numbers and functioning normally, platelets preserve the retaining power of the walls of the smaller blood vessels. By initiating appropriate clotting processes in the blood, platelets seal small points of leakage in the vessel walls, thereby preventing spontaneous bruising or bleeding (that which is unprovoked by trauma).

Certain drugs and chemicals may reduce the number of available blood platelets to abnormally low levels. Some of these drugs act by suppressing platelet formation; other drugs hasten their destruction. When the number of functioning platelets falls below a critical level, blood begins to leak through the thin walls of smaller vessels. The outward evidence of this leakage is the spontaneous appearance of scattered bruises in the skin of the thighs and legs. This is referred to as purpura. Bleeding may occur anywhere in the body, internally as well as superficially into the tissues immediately beneath the skin.

Bone Marrow Depression A serious reduction in the ability of the bone marrow to carry on its normal production of blood cells. This can occur as an adverse reaction to the toxic effect of certain drugs and chemicals on bone marrow components. When functioning normally, the bone marrow produces the majority of the body's blood cells. These consist of three types: the red blood cells (erythrocytes), the white blood cells (leukocytes) and the blood platelets (thrombocytes). Each type of cell performs one or more specific functions, all of which are indispensable to the maintenance of life and health.

Drugs that are capable of depressing bone marrow activity can impair the production of all types of blood cells simultaneously or of only one type selectively. Periodic examinations of the blood can reveal significant changes in the structure and number of the blood cells that indicate a possible drug effect on bone marrow activity.

Impairment of the production of red blood cells leads to anemia, a condition of abnormally low red cells and hemoglobin. This causes weakness, loss of energy and stamina, intolerance of cold environments and shortness of breath on physical exertion. A reduction in the formation of white blood cells can impair the body's immunity and lower its resistance to infection. These changes may result in the development of fever, sore throat or pneumonia. When the formation of blood platelets is suppressed to abnormally low levels, the blood loses its ability to quickly seal small points of leakage in blood vessel walls. This may lead to episodes of unusual and abnormal spontaneous bruising or to prolonged bleeding in the event of injury.

Any of these symptoms can occur in the presence of bone marrow depression. They should alert both patient and physician to the need for prompt studies of blood and bone marrow.

Brand Name The registered trade name given to a drug product by its manufacturer. Many drugs are marketed by more than one manufacturer or distributor. Each company adopts a distinctive trade name to distinguish its brand of the generic drug from that of its competitors. Thus a brand name designates a proprietary drug—one that is protected by patent or copyright. Generally brand names are shorter, easier to pronounce and more readily remembered than their generic counterparts.

Cause-and-Effect Relationship A possible causative association between a drug and an observed biologic event—most commonly a side-effect or an adverse effect. Knowledge of a drug's full spectrum of effects (wanted and unwanted) is highly desirable when weighing its benefits and risks in any treatment situation. However, it is often impossible to establish with certainty that a particular drug is the primary agent responsible for a suspected adverse effect. In the evaluation of every cause-and-effect relationship, therefore, meticulous consideration must be given to such factors as the time sequence of drug administration and possible reaction, the use of multiple drugs, possible interactions among these drugs, the effects of the disease under treatment, the physiological and psychological characteristics of the patient and the possible influence of unrecognized disorders and malfunctions.

The majority of adverse drug reactions occur sporadically, unpredictably and infrequently in the general population. A *definite* cause-and-effect relationship between drug and reaction is established when (1) the adverse effect immediately follows administration of the drug; or (2) the adverse effect disappears after the drug is discontinued (dechallenge) and promptly reappears when the drug is used again (rechallenge); or (3) the adverse effects are clearly the expected and predictable toxic consequences of drug overdosage.

In contrast to the obvious "causative" (definite) relationship, there exists a large gray area of "probable," "possible" and "coincidental" associations that are clouded by varying degrees of uncertainty. These classifications usually apply to alleged drug reactions that require a relatively long time to develop, are of low incidence and for which there are no clear-cut objective means of demonstrating a causal mechanism that links drug and reaction. Clarification of cause-and-effect relationships in these uncertain groups requires carefully designed observation over a long period of time, followed by sophisticated statistical analysis. Occasionally the public is alerted to a newly found "relationship" based upon suggestive but incomplete data. Though early warning is clearly in the public interest, such announcements should make clear whether the presumed relationship is based upon definitive criteria or is simply inferred because the use of a drug and an observed event were found to occur together within an appropriate time frame.

The most competent techniques for evaluating cause-and-effect relationships of adverse drug reactions have been devised by the Division of Tissue Reactions to Drugs, a research unit of the Armed Forces Institute of Pathology. Based upon a highly critical examination of all available evidence, the Division's study of 2800 drug-related deaths yielded the following levels of certainty regarding cause-and-effect relationship:

No association	5.0%
Coincidental	14.5%
Possible	33.0%
Probable	30.0%
Causative	17.5%

It is significant that expert evaluation of 2800 drug-related cases concluded that only 47.5% could be substantiated as definitely or probably causative.

Contraindication A condition or disease that precludes the use of a particular drug. Some cointraindications are *absolute,* meaning that the use of the drug would expose the patient to extreme hazard and therefore cannot be justified. Other contraindications are *relative,* meaning that the condition or disease does not entirely bar the use of the drug but requires that, before the decision to use the drug is made, special consideration be given to factors which could aggravate existing disease, interfere with current treatment or produce new injury.

Dependence The preferred term used to identify the drug-dependent states of *psychological dependence* (or *habituation*), and *physical dependence* (or *addiction*). In addition, a third kind of drug-dependence can be included under this term. This might be called *functional dependence*—the need to use a drug continuously in order to sustain a particular body function, the impairment of which causes annoying symptoms of varying degree and significance.

    Psychological dependence is a form of neurotic behavior. Its principal characteristic is an obsession to satisfy a particular desire, be it one of self-gratification or one of escape from some real or imagined distress. Psychological dependence is a very human trait that is seen often in many socially acceptable patterns and practices such as entertainment, gambling, sports and collecting. A common form of this dependence in today's culture is the increasing reliance upon drugs to help in coping with the everyday problems of living: pills for frustration, disappointment, nervous stomach, tension headache and insomnia. The 20 million smokers of marijuana have found it to be a drug that eases their stress, one whose effectiveness fosters habit (psychological dependence) but not addiction.

    Physical dependence, which is true addiction, includes two elements: habituation and tolerance. Addicting drugs provide relief from anguish and pain swiftly and effectively; they also induce a physiological tolerance that requires increasing dosage or repeated use if they are to remain effective. These two features foster the continued need for the drug and lead to its becoming a functioning component in the biochemistry of the brain. As this occurs, the drug assumes an "essential" role in ongoing chemical processes. (Thus some authorities prefer the term *chemical dependence.*) Sudden removal of the drug from the system causes a major upheaval in body chemistry and provokes a withdrawal syndrome—the intense mental and physical pain experienced by the addict when intake of the drug is stopped abruptly—that is the hallmark of addiction.

Functional dependence differs significantly from both psychological and physical dependence. It occurs when a drug effectively relieves an annoying or distressing condition and the particular body function involved becomes increasingly dependent upon the action of the drug to provide a sense of well-being. Drugs which are capable of inducing functional dependence are used primarily for the relief of symptoms. They do not act on the brain to produce alteration of mood or consciousness as do those drugs with potential for either psychological or physical dependence. The most familiar example of functional dependence is the "laxative habit." Some types of constipation are made worse by the wrong choice of laxative, and natural function gradually fades as the colon becomes more and more dependent upon the action of certain laxative drugs.

Disulfiramlike (Antabuselike) Reaction The symptoms that result from the interaction of alcohol and any drug that is capable of provoking the pattern of response typical of the "Antabuse effect." The interacting drug interrupts the normal decomposition of alcohol by the liver and thereby permits the accumulation of a toxic by-product that enters the bloodstream. When sufficient levels of both alcohol and drug are present in the blood the reaction occurs. It consists of intense flushing and warming of the face, a severe throbbing headache, shortness of breath, chest pains, nausea, repeated vomiting, sweating and weakness. If the amount of alcohol ingested has been large enough, the reaction may progress to blurred vision, vertigo, confusion, marked drop in blood pressure and loss of consciousness. Severe reactions may lead to convulsions and death. The reaction can last from 30 minutes to several hours, depending upon the amount of alcohol in the body. As the symptoms subside, the individual is exhausted and usually sleeps for several hours.

Diuretic A drug that alters kidney function to increase the volume of urine. Diuretics use several different mechanisms to increase urine volume, and these, in turn, have different effects on body chemistry. Diuretics are used primarily to (1) remove excess water from the body (as in congestive heart failure and some types of liver and kidney disease), and (2) treat hypertension by promoting the excretion of sodium from the body.

Dosage Forms and Strengths This information category in the individual Drug Profiles (Section Three) uses several abbreviations to designate measurements of weight and volume. These are

mcg — microgram — 1,000,000th of a gram (weight)
mg — milligram — 1000th of a gram (weight)
ml — milliliter — 1000th of a liter (volume)
gm — gram   — 1000 milligrams (weight)

There are approximately 65 mg in 1 grain.
There are approximately 5 ml in 1 teaspoonful.
There are approximately 15 ml in 1 tablespoonful.

There are approximately 30 ml in 1 ounce.

1 milliliter of water weighs 1 gram.

There are approximately 454 grams in 1 pound.

Drug, Drug Product Terms often used interchangeably to designate a medicine (in any of its dosage forms) used in medical practice. Strictly speaking, the term *drug* refers to the single chemical entity that provokes a specific response when placed within a biological system—the "active" ingredient. A *drug product* is the manufactured dosage form—tablet, capsule, elixir, etc.—that contains the active drug intermixed with inactive ingredients to provide for convenient administration.

Drug products which contain only one active ingredient are referred to as single entity drugs. Drug products with two or more active ingredients are called combination drugs (designed < CD > in the lists of brand names in the Drug Profiles, Section Three).

Drug Class A group of drugs that are similar in chemistry, method of action and use in treatment. Because of their common characteristics, many drugs within a class will produce the same side-effects and have similar potential for provoking related adverse reactions and interactions. However, significant variations among members within a drug class can occur. This sometimes allows the physician an important degree of selectivity in choosing a drug if certain beneficial actions are desired or particular side-effects are to be minimized.

Examples: Antihistamines, phentothiazines, tetracyclines (see Section Four).

Drug Fever The elevation of body temperature that occurs as an unwanted manifestation of drug action. Drugs can induce fever by several mechanisms; these include allergic reactions, drug-induced tissue damage, acceleration of tissue metabolism, constriction of blood vessels in the skin with resulting decrease in loss of body heat and direct action on the temperature-regulating center in the brain.

The most common form of drug fever is that associated with allergic reactions. It may be the only allergic manifestation apparent, or it may be part of a complex of allergic symptoms that can include skin rash, hives, joint swelling and pain, enlarged lymph glands, hemolytic anemia or hepatitis. The fever usually appears about 7 to 10 days after starting the drug and may vary from low-grade to alarmingly high levels. It may be sustained or intermittent, but it usually persists for as long as the drug is taken. In previously sensitized individuals drug fever may occur within 1 or 2 hours after taking the first dose of medication.

While many drugs are capable of producing fever, the following are more commonly responsible:

allopurinol	iodides
antihistamines	isoniazid
atropinelike drugs	methyldopa
barbiturates	nadalol
coumarin anticoagulants	novobiocin
hydralazine	para-aminosalicylic acid

penicillin
pentazocine
phenytoin
procainamide

propylthiouracil
quinidine
rifampin
sulfonamides

Extension Effect An unwanted but predictable drug response that is a logical consequence of mild to moderate overdosage. An extension effect is an exaggeration of the drug's normal pharmacological action; it can be thought of as a mild form of dose-related toxicity (see OVERDOSAGE and TOXICITY).

Example: The continued "hangover" of drowsiness and mental sluggishness that persists after arising in the morning is a common extension effect of a long-acting sleep-inducing drug (hypnotic) taken the night before.

Example: The persistent intestinal cramping and diarrhea that result from too generous a dose of laxative are extension effects of the drug's anticipated action.

Generic Name The official, common or public name used to designate an active drug entity, whether in pure form or in dosage form. Generic names are coined by committees of officially appointed drug experts and are approved by governmental agencies for national and international use. Thus they are nonproprietary. Many drug products are marketed under the generic name of the principal active ingredient and bear no brand name of the manufacturer.

While the total number of prescriptions written in the United States in 1986 increased by 0.6%, prescriptions specifying the *generic name* of the drug increased by 8.6%. Generically written prescriptions now account for 13.5% of all new prescriptions written in the United States. The drugs most commonly prescribed by generic name are listed below, ranked in descending order of the number of new prescriptions issued.

amoxicillin
penicillin VK
ampicillin
tetracycline
prednisone

erythromycin
hydrochlorothiazide
acetaminophen/codeine
doxycycline
phenobarbital

Habituation A form of drug dependence based upon strong psychological gratification rather than the physical (chemical) dependence of addiction. The habitual use of drugs that alter mood or relieve minor discomforts results from a compulsive need to feel pleasure and satisfaction or to escape the manifestations of emotional distress. The abrupt cessation of habituating drugs does not produce the withdrawal syndrome seen in addiction. Thus habituation is a *psychological dependence.* (See DEPENDENCE for a further account of psychological and physical dependence.)

Hemolytic Anemia A form of anemia (deficient red blood cells and hemoglobin) resulting from the premature destruction (hemolysis) of circulating red blood cells. Several mechanisms can be responsible for the development of hemolytic anemia; among these is the action of certain drugs and chemicals. Some individuals are susceptible to hemolytic anemia because of a genetic deficiency in the makeup of their red blood cells. If such people are given certain antimalarial drugs, sulfa drugs or numerous other drugs, some of their red cells will disintegrate on contact with the drug. (About 10% of American blacks have this genetic trait.)

Another type of drug-induced hemolytic anemia is a form of drug allergy. Many drugs in wide use (including quinidine, methyldopa, levodopa and chlorpromazine) are known to cause hemolytic destruction of red cells as a hypersensitivity (allergic) reaction.

Hemolytic anemia can occur abruptly (with evident symptoms) or silently. The acute form lasts about 7 days and is characterized by fever, pallor, weakness, dark-colored urine and varying degrees of jaundice (yellow coloration of eyes and skin). When drug-induced hemolytic anemia is mild, involving the destruction of only a small number of red blood cells, there may be no symptoms to indicate its presence. Such episodes are detected only by means of laboratory studies (see IDIOSYNCRASY and ALLERGY, DRUG).

Hepatitislike Reaction Changes in the liver, induced by certain drugs, which closely resemble those produced by viral hepatitis. The symptoms of drug-induced hepatitis and virus-induced hepatitis are often so similar that the correct cause cannot be established without precise laboratory studies.

Hepatitis due to drugs may be a form of drug allergy (as in reaction to many of the phenothiazines), or it may represent a toxic adverse effect (as in reaction to some of the monoamine oxidase inhibitor drugs). Liver reactions of significance usually result in jaundice and represent serious adverse effects (see JAUNDICE).

Hypersensitivity A term subject to varying usages for many years. One common use has been to identify the trait of overresponsiveness to drug action, that is, an intolerance to even small doses. Used in this sense, the term indicates that the nature of the response is appropriate but the degree of response is exaggerated.

The term is more widely used today to identify a state of allergy. To have a *hypersensitivity* to a drug is to be *allergic* to it (see ALLERGY, DRUG).

Some individuals develop cross-hypersensitivity. This means that once a person has developed an allergy to a certain drug, that person will experience an allergic reaction to other drugs which are closely related in chemical composition.

Example: The patient was known to be *hypersensitive* by nature, having a history of seasonal hay fever and asthma since childhood. His *allergy* to tetracycline developed after his third course of treatment. This drug *hypersensitivity* manifested itself as a diffuse, measleslike rash.

Hypnotic A drug that is used primarily to induce sleep. There are several classes of drugs that have hypnotic effects: antihistamines, barbiturates, benzodiazepines and several unrelated compounds. Within the past 15 years the benzodiazepines, because of their relative safety and lower potential for inducing dependence, have largely replaced the barbiturates

as the most commonly used hypnotics. The body usually develops a tolerance to the hypnotic effect after several weeks of continual use. To maintain their effectiveness, hypnotics should be used intermittently for short
periods of time.

Hypoglycemia A condition in which the amount of glucose (a sugar) in the
blood is below the normal range. Since normal brain function is dependent upon an adequate supply of glucose, reducing the level of glucose
in the blood below a critical point will cause serious impairment of brain
activity. The resulting symptoms are characteristic of the hypoglycemic
state. Early indications are headache, a sensation resembling mild drunkenness and an inability to think clearly. These may be accompanied by
hunger. As the level of blood glucose continues to fall, nervousness and
confusion develop. Varying degrees of weakness, numbness, trembling,
sweating and rapid heart action follow. If sugar is not provided at this
point and the blood glucose level drops further, impaired speech, incoordination and unconsciousness, with or without convulsions, will follow.

Hypoglycemia in any stage requires prompt recognition and treatment. Because of the potential for injury to the brain, the mechanisms
and management of hypoglycemia should be understood by all who use
drugs capable of producing it.

Hypothermia A state of the body characterized by an unexpected decline of
internal body temperature to levels significantly below the norm of 98.6
degrees F or 37 degrees C. By definition, hypothermia means a body
temperature of less than 95 degrees F or 35 degrees C. The elderly and
debilitated are more prone to develop hypothermia if clothed inadequately and exposed to cool environments. Most episodes are initiated by
room temperatures below 65 degrees F or 18.3 degrees C. The condition
often develops suddenly, can mimic a stroke and has a mortality rate of
50%. Some drugs, such as phenothiazines, barbiturates and benzodiazepines, are conducive to the development of hypothermia in susceptible
individuals.

Idiosyncrasy An abnormal mechanism of drug response that occurs in individuals who have a peculiar defect in their body chemistry (often hereditary) which produces an effect totally unrelated to the drug's normal
pharmacological action. Idiosyncrasy is not a form of allergy. The actual
chemical defects responsible for certain idiosyncratic drug reactions are
well understood; others are not.

Example: Approximately 100 million people in the world (including
10% of American blacks) have a specific enzyme deficiency in their red
blood cells that causes these cells to disintegrate when exposed to drugs
such as sulfonamides (Gantrisin, Kynex), nitrofurantoin (Furadantin,
Macrodantin), probenecid (Benemid), quinine and quinidine. As a result
of this reaction, these drugs (and others) can cause a significant anemia
in susceptible individuals.

Example: Approximately 5% of the population of the United States
is susceptible to the development of glaucoma on prolonged use of
cortisone-related drugs (see Cortisone Drug Class in Section Four).

Immunosuppressive A drug that significantly impairs (suppresses) the functions of the body's immune system. In some instances, immunosuppression is an intended drug effect as in the use of cyclosporine to prevent the immune system from rejecting a transplanted heart or kidney. In other instances, it is an unwanted side-effect as in the long-term use of cortisonelike drugs (to control chronic asthma) that suppresses the immune system sufficiently to permit reactivation of a dormant tuberculosis. Immunosuppressant drugs are being used to treat several chronic disorders that are thought to be autoimmune diseases, notably advanced rheumatoid arthritis, ulcerative colitis and systemic lupus erythematosus.

Interaction An unwanted change in the body's response to a drug that results when a second drug that is capable of altering the action of the first is administered at the same time. Some drug interactions can enhance the effect of either drug, producing an overresponse similar to overdosage. Other interactions may reduce drug effectiveness and cause inadequate response. A third type of interaction can produce a seemingly unrelated toxic response with no associated increase or decrease in the pharmacological actions of the interacting drugs.

Theoretically, many drugs can interact with one another, but in reality drug interactions are comparatively infrequent. Many interactions can be anticipated, and the physician can make appropriate adjustments in dosage to prevent or minimize unintended fluctuations in drug response.

Jaundice A yellow coloration of the skin (and the white portion of the eyes) that occurs when excessive bile pigments accumulate in the blood as a result of impaired liver function. Jaundice can be produced by several mechanisms. It may occur as a manifestation of a wide variety of diseases, or it may represent an adverse reaction to a particular drug. At times it is difficult to distinguish between disease-induced jaundice and drug-induced jaundice.

Jaundice due to a drug is always a serious adverse effect. Anyone taking a drug that is capable of causing jaundice should watch closely for any significant change in the color of urine or feces. Dark discoloration of the urine and paleness (lack of color) of the stool may be early indications of a developing jaundice. Should either of these symptoms occur, it is advisable to discontinue the drug and notify the prescribing physician promptly. Diagnostic tests are available to clarify the nature of the jaundice.

Lupus Erythematosus (LE) A serious disease of unknown cause that occurs in two forms, one limited to the skin (discoid LE) and the other involving several body systems (systemic LE). Both forms occur predominantly in young women. About 5% of cases of the discoid form convert to the systemic form. Basically, systemic LE is a disorder of the body's immune system which may result in chronic, progressive inflammation and destruction of the connective tissue framework of the skin, blood vessels, joints, brain, heart muscle, lungs and kidneys. Altered proteins in the blood lead to the formation of antibodies which react with certain organ tissues to produce the inflammation and destruction characteristic of the disease. A reduction in the number of white blood cells and blood platelets often occurs. The course of systemic LE is usually quite protracted and unpredictable. While no cure is known, satisfactory management may be achieved in some cases by the judicious use of cortisonelike drugs.

Several drugs in wide use are capable of initiating a form of systemic LE quite similar to that which occurs spontaneously. (More than 100 cases due to the use of procainamide have been reported.) Suggestive symptoms may appear as early as 2 weeks or as late as 8 years after starting the responsible drug. The initial symptoms usually consist of low-grade fever, skin rashes of various kinds, aching muscles and multiple joint pains. Chest pains (pleurisy) are fairly common. Enlargement of the lymph glands occurs less frequently. Symptoms usually subside following discontinuation of the responsible drug, but laboratory evidence of the reaction may persist for many months.

Drugs known to induce systemic LE include:

chlorpromazine

clofibrate

hydralazine

isoniazid

oral contraceptives

penicillamine

phenolphthalein

phenothiazines (some)

phenylbutazone

phenytoin

practolol

procainamide

thiouracil

Neuroleptic Malignant Syndrome (NMS) A rare, serious, sometimes fatal idiosyncratic reaction to the use of neuroleptic (antipsychotic) drugs. The principal features of the reaction are hyperthermia (temperatures of 102 to 104 degress F), marked muscle rigidity and coma. Other symptoms include rapid heart rate and breathing, profuse sweating, tremors and seizures. Two thirds of reported cases occurred in men, one third in women. The mortality rate is 15% to 20%.

The following drugs have a potential for inducing this reaction:

amitriptyline + perphenazine (Triavil)

amoxapine (Asendin)

chlorpromazine (Thorazine)

chlorprothixene (Taractan)

clomipramine (Anafranil)

fluphenazine (Permitil, Prolixin)

haloperidol (Haldol)

imipramine (Tofranil, etc.)

levodopa + carbidopa (Sinemet)

loxapine (Loxitane)

metoclopramide (Reglan, Octamide)

molindone (Moban)

perphenazine (Etrafon, Trilafon)

pimozide (Orap)

prochlorperazine (Compazine)

thioridazine (Mellaril)

thiothixene (Navane)

trifluoperazine (Stelazine)

trimeprazine (Temaril)

Orthostatic Hypotension A type of low blood pressure that is related to body position or posture (also called postural hypotension). The individual who is subject to orthostatic hypotension may have a normal blood pressure while lying down, but on sitting upright or standing he will experience sudden sensations of lightheadedness, dizziness and a feeling of impending faint that compel him to return quickly to a lying position. These symptoms are manifestations of inadequate blood flow (oxygen supply) to the brain due to an abnormal delay in the rise in blood pressure that always occurs as the body adjusts the circulation to the erect position.

Many drugs (especially the stronger antihypertensives) may cause orthostatic hypotension. Individuals who experience this drug effect should report it to their physician so that appropriate dosage adjustment can be made to minimize it. Failure to correct or to compensate for these sudden drops in blood pressure can lead to severe falls and injury.

The tendency to orthostatic hypotension can be reduced by avoiding sudden standing, prolonged standing, vigorous exercise and exposure to hot environments. Alcoholic beverages should be used cautiously until their combined effect with the drug in use has been determined.

Overdosage The meaning of this term should not be limited to the concept of doses that clearly exceed the normal dosage range recommended by the manufacturer. The optimal dose of many drugs (that amount which gives the greatest benefit with least distress) varies greatly from person to person. What may be an average dose for the majority of individuals will be an overdose for some and an underdose for others. Numerous factors, such as age, body size, nutritional status and liver and kidney function, have significant influence on dosage requirements. Drugs with narrow safety margins often produce indications of overdosage if something delays the regular elimination of the customary daily dose. In this instance, overdosage results from accumulation of prescribed daily doses. Massive overdosage—as occurs with accidental ingestion of drugs by children or with suicidal intention by adults—is referred to as poisoning.

Over-the-Counter (OTC) Drugs Drug products that can be purchased without prescription. Many are available in food stores, variety stores and newsstands as well as in conventional drug stores. Because of the unrestricted availability of these drugs, many people do not look upon OTC medicines as drugs. But drugs they are! And like the more potent drug products that are sold only on prescription, they are chemicals that are capable of a wide variety of actions on biological systems. Within the last 30 years, many OTC drugs have assumed greater importance because of their ability to interact unfavorably with some widely used prescription drugs. Serious problems in drug management can arise when (1) the patient fails to inform the physician of the OTC drug(s) he is taking ("because they really aren't drugs") and (2) the physician fails to specify that his question about what medicines are being taken currently *includes all OTC drugs.* During any course of treatment, whether medical or surgical, the patient should consult with the physician regarding any OTC drug that he wishes to take.

The major classes of OTC drugs for internal use include:

allergy medicines (antihistamines)
antacids
antiworm medicines
aspirin and aspirin combinations
aspirin substitutes
asthma aids
cold medicines (decongestants)
cough medicines
diarrhea remedies
digestion aids
diuretics
iron preparations

laxatives
menstrual aids
motion sickness remedies
pain relievers
reducing aids
salt substitutes
sedatives and tranquilizers
sleeping pills
stimulants (caffeine)
sugar substitutes (saccharin)
tonics
vitamins

Paradoxical Reaction An unexpected drug response that is not consistent with the known pharmacology of the drug and may in fact be the opposite of the intended and anticipated response. Such reactions are due to individual sensitivity or variability and can occur in any age group. They are seen more commonly, however, in children and the elderly.

Example: An 80-year-old man was admitted to a nursing home following the death of his wife. He had difficulty adjusting to his new environment and was restless, agitated and irritable. He was given a trial of the tranquilizer diazepam (Valium) to relax him, starting with small doses. On the second day of medication he became confused and erratic in behavior. The dose of diazepam was increased. On the third day he began to wander aimlessly, talked incessantly in a loud voice and displayed anger and hostility when attempts were made to help him. Suspecting the possibility of a paradoxical reaction, the diazepam was discontinued. All behavioral disturbances gradually subsided within 3 days.

Parkinson-like Disorders (Parkinsonism) A group of symptoms that resembles those caused by Parkinson's disease, a chronic disorder of the nervous system also known as shaking palsy. The characteristic features of parkinsonism include a fixed, emotionless facial expression (masklike in appearance), a prominent trembling of the hands, arms or legs and stiffness of the extremities that limits movement and produces a rigid posture and gait.

Parkinsonism is a fairly common adverse effect that occurs in about 15% of all patients who take large doses of strong tranquilizers (notably the phenothiazines) or use them over an extended period of time. If recognized early, the Parkinson-like features will lessen or disappear with reduced dosage or change in medication. In some instances, however, Parkinson-like changes may become permanent, requiring appropriate medication for their control.

Peripheral Neuritis (Peripheral Neuropathy) A group of symptoms that results from injury to nerve tissue in the extremities. A variety of drugs and chemicals are capable of inducing changes in nerve structure or function. The characteristic pattern consists of a sensation of numbness and tingling that usually begins in the fingers and toes and is accompanied by an altered sensation to touch and vague discomfort ranging from aching sensations to burning pain. Severe forms of peripheral neuritis may include loss of muscular strength and coordination.

A relatively common form of peripheral neuritis is that seen with the long-term use of isoniazid in the treatment of tuberculosis. If vitamin B-6 (pyridoxine) is not given concurrently with isoniazid, peripheral neuritis may occur in sensitive individuals. Vitamin B-6 can be both preventive and curative in this form of drug-induced peripheral neuritis.

Since peripheral neuritis can also occur as a late complication following many viral infections, care must be taken to avoid assigning a cause-and-effect relationship to a drug which is not responsible for the nerve injury (see CAUSE-AND-EFFECT RELATIONSHIP).

Peyronie's Disease A permanent deformity of the penis caused by the formation of dense fibrous (scarlike) tissue within the system of penile vessels that become engorged with blood during the process of erection. During sexual arousal, this inelastic fibrous tissue causes a painful downward bowing of the penis that hampers or precludes satisfactory intercourse. This condition has been associated with the use of phenytoin (Dilantin, etc.) and with most members of the beta blocker class of drugs (see Drug Class, Section Four).

Pharmacology The medical science that relates to the development and use of medicinal drugs, their composition and action in animals and man. Used in its broadest sense, pharmacology embraces the related sciences of medicinal chemistry, experimental therapeutics and toxicology.

Example: The widely used sulfonylurea drugs (Diabinese, Dymelor, Orinase, Tolinase) are effective in the treatment of some forms of diabetes because of the accidental discovery that some of their parent "sulfa" drugs produced hypoglycemia (low blood sugar) during their early therapeutic trials as anti-infectives. Subsequent investigation of the mechanisms of action (*pharmacology*) of these drugs revealed that they are capable of stimulating the pancreas to release more insulin.

Pharmacological studies on another group of "sulfa" related drugs—the thiazide diuretics—revealed that they could induce the kidney to excrete more water and salt in the urine. This drug action is of great value in treating high blood pressure and heart failure.

Photosensitivity A drug-induced change in the skin that results in the development of a rash or exaggerated sunburn on exposure to the sun or ultraviolet lamps. The reaction is confined to uncovered areas of skin, providing a clue to the nature of its cause. (See Table 3 in Section Six.)

Porphyria The porphyrias are a group of hereditary disorders characterized by excessive production of prophyrins, essential respiratory pigments of the body. (One porphyrin is a component of hemoglobin, the pigment of red blood cells.) Two forms of porphyria—acute intermittent porphyria and cutaneous porphyria—can be activated by the use of certain drugs. Acute intermittent porphyria involves damage to the nervous system; an acute attack can include fever, rapid heart rate, vomiting, pain in the abdomen and legs, hallucinations, seizures, paralysis and coma. Twenty-three drugs (or drug classes) can induce an acute attack; among these are the barbiturates, "sulfa" drugs, chlordiazepoxide (Librium), chlorpropamide (Diabinese), methyldopa (Aldomet) and phenytoin (Dilantin). Cutaneous porphyria involves damage to the skin and liver. An episode can include reddening and blistering of the skin, followed by crust formation, scarring and excessive hair growth; repeated liver damage can lead to cirrhosis. This form of porphyria can be precipitated by chloroquine, estrogen, oral contraceptives and excessive iron.

Priapism The prolonged, painful erection of the penis usually unassociated with sexual arousal or stimulation. It is caused by obstruction to the outflow (drainage) of blood through the veins at the root of the penis. Erection may persist for 30 minutes to a few hours and then subside spontaneously; or it may persist for up to 30 hours and require surgical drainage of blood from the penis for relief. More than half of the episodes of priapism induced by drugs result in permanent impotence. Sickle cell anemia (or trait) may predispose to priapism; individuals with this disorder should avoid all drugs that may induce priapism.

Drugs reported to induce priapism include the following:

anabolic steroids (male hormonelike drugs: Anadrol, Anavar, Android, Halotestin, Metandren, Oreton, Testred, Winstrol)
chlorpromazine (Thorazine)
cocaine
guanethidine (Ismelin)
haloperidol (Haldol)
heparin
levodopa (Sinemet)
molindone (Moban)
prazosin (Minipress)
prochlorperazine (Compazine)
trazodone (Desyrel)
trifluoperazine (Stelazine)
warfarin (Coumadin)

Prostatism This term refers to the difficulties associated with an enlarged prostate gland. As the prostate enlarges (a natural development in aging men), it constricts the urethra (outflow passage) where it joins the urinary bladder and impedes urination. This causes a reduction in the size and force of the urinary stream, hesitancy in starting the flow of urine, interruption of urination and incomplete emptying of the bladder. Atropine and drugs with atropinelike effects can impair the bladder's ability to compensate for the obstructing prostate gland, thus intensifying all of the above symptoms.

Raynaud's Phenomenon This term refers to intermittent episodes of reduced blood flow into the fingers or toes, with resulting paleness, discomfort, numbness and tingling. It is due to an exaggerated constriction of the small arteries that supply blood to the digits. Characteristically an attack is precipitated either by emotional stress or exposure to cold. It can occur as part of a systemic disorder (lupus erythematosus, scleroderma), or it can occur without apparent cause (Raynaud's disease). Some widely used drugs, notably beta-adrenergic blockers and products that contain ergotamine, are conducive to the development of Raynaud-like symptoms in predisposed individuals.

Reye (Reye's) Syndrome An acute, often fatal, childhood illness characterized by swelling of the brain and toxic degeneration of the liver. It usually develops during recovery from a flulike infection, measles or chickenpox. Symptoms include fever, headache, delirium, loss of consciousness and seizures. It is one of the 10 major causes of death in children aged 1 to 10 years. Evidence to date suggests that the syndrome may be due to the combined effects of viral infection and chemical toxins (possibly drugs) in a genetically predisposed child. Drugs that have been used just prior to the onset of symptoms include acetaminophen, aspirin, antibiotics and antiemetics (drugs to control nausea and vomiting). Although it has not been definitely established that drugs actually cause Reye syndrome, it is thought that they may contribute to its development or adversely affect its course. Current recommendations are to avoid the use of acetaminophen, aspirin and antiemetic drugs in children with flulike infections, chickenpox or measles.

Secondary Effect A by-product or complication of drug use which does not occur as part of the drug's primary pharmacological activity. Secondary effects are unwanted consequences and may therefore be classified as adverse effects.

Example: The reactivation of dormant tuberculosis can be a *secondary effect* of long-term cortisone administration for arthritis. Cortisone and related drugs (see Drug Class, Section Four) suppress natural immunity and lower resistance to infection.

Example: The cramping of leg muscles can be a *secondary effect* of diuretic (urine-producing) drug treatment for high blood pressure. Excessive loss of potassium through increased urination renders the muscle vulnerable to painful spasm during exercise.

Side-Effect A normal, expected and predictable response to a drug that accompanies the principal (intended) response sought in treatment. Side-effects are part of a drug's pharmacological activity and thus are unavoidable. Most side-effects are undesirable. The majority cause minor annoyance and inconvenience; some may cause serious problems in managing certain diseases; a few can be hazardous.

Example: The drug propantheline (Pro-Banthine) is used to treat peptic ulcer because one of the consequences of its pharmacological action is the reduction of acid formation in the stomach (an intended effect). Other consequences can include blurring of near vision, dryness of the mouth and constipation. These are *side-effects.*

Superinfection (Suprainfection) The development of a second infection that is superimposed upon an initial infection currently under treatment. The superinfection is caused by organisms that are not susceptible to the killing action of the drug(s) used to treat the original (primary) infection. Superinfections usually occur during or immediately following treatment with a broad spectrum antibiotic—one that is capable of altering the customary balance of bacterial populations in various parts of the body. The disturbance of this balance permits the overgrowth of organisms that normally exist in numbers too small to cause disease. The superinfection may also require treatment, using those drugs that are effective against the offending organism.

> *Example:* Recurrent infections of the kidney and bladder often require repeated courses of treatment with a variety of anti-infective drugs. When these are taken by mouth they can suppress the normally dominant types of bacteria present in the colon and rectum, encouraging the overgrowth of yeast organisms which are capable of causing *colitis*. When this occurs, colitis is a *superinfection*.

Tardive Dyskinesia A late-developing, drug-induced disorder of the nervous system characterized by involuntary bizarre movements of the eyelids, jaws, lips, tongue, neck and fingers. It occurs after long-term treatment with the more potent drugs used in the management of serious mental illness. While it may occur in any age group, it is more common in the middle-aged and the elderly. Older, chronically ill women are particularly susceptible to this adverse drug effect. Once developed, the pattern of uncontrollable chewing, lip puckering and repetitive tongue protruding (fly-catching movement) appears to be irreversible. No consistently satisfactory treatment or cure is available. To date, there is no way of identifying beforehand the individual who may develop this distressing reaction to drug treatment, and there is no known prevention. Fortunately, the persistent dyskinesia (abnormal movement) is not accompanied by further impairment of mental function or deterioration of intelligence. It is ironic, however, that the patient who shows significant improvement in his mental illness but is unfortunate enough to develop tardive dyskinesia may have to remain hospitalized because of a reaction to a drug that was given to make it possible for him to leave the hospital.

Tolerance An adaptation by the body that lessens responsiveness to a drug on continuous administration. Body tissues become accustomed to the drug's presence and react to it less vigorously. Tolerance can be beneficial or harmful in treatment.

> *Examples:* Beneficial tolerance occurs when the hay fever sufferer finds that the side-effect of drowsiness gradually disappears after 4 or 5 days of continuous use of antihistamines.

> Harmful tolerance occurs when the patient with "shingles" (herpes zoster) finds that the usual dose of codeine is no longer sufficient to relieve pain and that the need for increasing dosage creates a risk of physical dependence or addiction.

Toxicity The capacity of a drug to dangerously impair body functions or to damage body tissues. Most drug toxicity is related to total dosage: the larger the overdose, the greater the toxic effects. Some drugs, however, can produce toxic reactions when used in normal doses. Such adverse effects are not due to allergy or idiosyncrasy; in many instances their mechanisms are not fully understood. Toxic effects due to overdosage are generally a harmful extension of the drug's normal pharmacological actions and—to some extent—are predictable and preventable. Toxic reactions which occur with normal dosage are unrelated to the drug's known pharmacology and for the most part are unpredictable and unexplainable.

Tyramine A chemical present in many common foods and beverages that causes no difficulties to body functioning under normal circumstances. The main pharmacological action of tyramine is to raise the blood pressure. Normally, enzymes present in many body tissues neutralize this action of tyramine in the quantities in which it is consumed in the average diet. The principal enzyme responsible for neutralizing the blood-pressure-elevating action of tyramine (and chemicals related to it) is monoamine oxidase (MAO) type A. Monoamine oxidase type A serves an important regulatory function that helps to balance several of the chemical processes in the body that control certain activities of the nervous system. Stabilization of the blood pressure is one of these activities. If the action of monoamine oxidase type A is blocked, chemical substances like tyramine function unopposed, and relatively small amounts can cause alarming and dangerous elevations of blood pressure.

Several drugs in use today are capable of blocking the action of monoamine oxidase type A. These drugs are commonly referred to as monoamine oxidase (MAO) type A inhibitors (see Drug Class, Section Four). If an individual is taking one of these drugs and his diet includes foods or beverages that contain a significant amount of tyramine, he may experience a sudden increase in blood pressure. Before this interaction of food and drug was understood, several deaths due to brain hemorrhage occurred in persons taking MAO type A inhibitor drugs as a result of an extreme elevation of blood pressure following a meal of tyramine-rich foods.

It should be noted also that MAO inhibitor drugs can interact with many other drugs and cause serious adverse effects. Consult your physician before taking *any* drug concurrently with one that can inhibit the action of monoamine oxidase, type A or B.

Any protein-containing food that has undergone partial decomposition may present a hazard because of its increased tyramine content. The following foods and beverages have been reported to contain varying amounts of tyramine. Unless their tyramine content is known to be insignificant, they should be avoided altogether while taking a MAO type A inhibitor drug. Consult your physician about the advisability of using any of the foods or beverages on these lists if you are taking such drugs.

FOODS

BEVERAGES

Aged cheeses of all kinds*

AvocadoBanana skins

Bean curd

Bologna

"Bovril" extract

Broad bean pods

Chicken liver (unless fresh and
  used at once)

Chocolate

Figs, canned

Fish, canned

Fish, dried and salted

Herring, pickled

Liver, if not very fresh

"Marmite" extract

Meat extracts

Meat tenderizers

Pepperoni

Raisins

Raspberries

Salami

Shrimp paste

Sour cream

Soy sauce

Yeast extracts

Beer (unpasteurized)

Chianti wine

Sherry wine

Vermouth

NOTE: *Any* high-protein food that is aged or has undergone breakdown by putrefaction probably contains tyramine and could produce a hypertensive crisis in anyone taking MAO type A inhibiting drugs.

*Cottage cheese, cream cheese and processed cheese are safe to eat.

TABLES OF DRUG
INFORMATION

TABLE 1

Your Drugs and Behavior

In addition to producing side-effects that can alter mood and disturb emotional stability, some drugs are capable of inducing unexpected and unpredictable patterns of abnormal thinking and behavior. Such responses are relatively infrequent, but the nature and degree of mental disturbance can, at times, be quite alarming and potentially dangerous for both patient and family. It is now well recognized that such paradoxical responses are often of an idiosyncratic nature, and that the individual with a history of a serious mental or emotional disorder is more likely to experience bizarre reactions involving disturbed behavior.

It is often difficult to judge whether a particular aberration of thought or behavior is primarily a feature of the disorder under treatment or an effect of one (or more) drugs the patient may be taking at the time. If in doubt, it is advisable to discontinue any drug with potential for such side-effects and observe for changes during a drug-free period.

Drugs reported to impair *concentration* and/or *memory*

antihistamines*
antiparkinsonism drugs*
barbiturates*
benzodiazepines*
isoniazid

monoamine oxidase inhibitor
 drugs*
phenytoin
primidone
scopolamine

Drugs reported to cause *confusion, delirium* or *disorientation*

acetazolamide
aminophylline
antidepressants*
antihistamines*
atropinelike drugs*
barbiturates*
benzodiazepines*
bromides
carbamazepine
chloroquine
cimetidine
cortisonelike drugs*
cycloserine
digitalis

digitoxin
digoxin
disulfiram
ethchlorvynol
ethinamate
fenfluramine
glutethimide
isoniazid
levodopa
meprobamate
para-aminosalicylic acid
phenelzine
phenothiazines*
phenytoin

*See Drug Class, Section Four.

Drugs reported to cause *confusion, delirium* or *disorientation* (cont.)

piperazine
primidone
propranolol

reserpine
scopolamine

Drugs reported to cause *paranoid thinking*

bromides
cortisonelike drugs*
diphenhydramine

disulfiram
isoniazid
levodopa

Drugs reported to cause *schizophreniclike behavior*

amphetamines*
ephedrine
fenfluramine

phenmetrazine
phenylpropanolamine

Drugs reported to cause *maniclike behavior*

antidepressants*
cortisonelike drugs*
levodopa

monoamine oxidase inhibitor
    drugs*

Less apparent—but no less important—are the mood-altering *side-effects* of some drugs which are prescribed primarily for altogether unrelated conditions, with no intention of modifying emotional status. In keeping with the wide variation of individual response to the primary and intended effects of drugs, it is to be expected that the emotional and behavioral secondary effects will also be quite unpredictable and will vary enormously from person to person. However, the following experiences have been observed with sufficient frequency to establish recognizable patterns.

Drugs reported to cause *nervousness* (anxiety and irritability)

amantadine
amphetaminelike drugs* (appetite
    suppressants)
antihistamines*
caffeine
chlorphenesin

cortisonelike drugs*
ephedrine
epinephrine
isoproterenol
levodopa
liothyronine (in excessive dosage)

*See Drug Class, Section Four.

Drugs reported to cause *nervousness* (cont.)

methylphenidate
methysergide
monoamine oxidase inhibitor
  drugs*
nylidrin

oral contraceptives
theophylline
thyroid (in excessive dosage)
thyroxine (in excessive dosage)

Drugs reported to cause *emotional depression*

amantadine
amphetamine* (on withdrawal)
benzodiazepines*
carbamazepine
chloramphenicol
cortisonelike drugs*
cycloserine
digitalis
digitoxin
digoxin
diphenoxylate
estrogens
ethionamide
fenfluramine (on withdrawal)
fluphenazine
guanethidine

haloperidol
indomethacin
isoniazid
levodopa
methsuximide
methyldopa
methysergide
metoprolol
oral contraceptives
phenylbutazone
procainamide
progesterones
propranolol
reserpine
sulfonamides*
vitamin D (in excessive dosage)

Drugs reported to cause *euphoria*

amantadine
aminophylline
amphetamines
antihistamines* (some)
antispasmodics, synthetic*
aspirin
barbiturates*
benzphetamine
chloral hydrate
clorazepate
codeine
cortisonelike drugs*
diethylpropion
diphenoxylate
ethosuximide

flurazepam
haloperidol
levodopa
meprobamate
methysergide
monoamine oxidase inhibitor
  drugs*
morphine
pargyline
pentazocine
phenmetrazine
propoxyphene
scopalamine
tybamate

*See Drug Class, Section Four.

Drugs reported to cause *excitement*

acetazolamide
amantadine
amphetaminelike drugs*
antidepressants*
antihistamines*
atropinelike drugs*
barbiturates* (paradoxical response)
benzodiazepines* (paradoxical response)
cortisonelike drugs
cycloserine
diethylpropion
digitalis
ephedrine
epinephrine
ethinamate (paradoxical response)
ethionamide
glutethimide (paradoxical response)
isoniazid
isoproterenol
levodopa
meperidine and MAO inhibitor drugs*
methyldopa and MAO inhibitor drugs*
methyprylon (paradoxical response)
nalidixic acid
orphenadrine
quinine
scopolamine

*See Drug Class, Section Four.

TABLE 2

Your Drugs and Vision

Approximately 3.5% of all adverse drug effects involve impairment of vision or damage to structures of the eye. Some effects, such as blurring of vision or double vision, may occur shortly after starting a drug. These quickly disappear with adjustment of dosage. More subtle and serious effects, such as the development of cataracts or damage to the retina or optic nerve, may not occur until a drug has been in continuous use for an extended period of time. Some of these changes are irreversible. If you are taking a drug that can affect the eye in any way, you are urged to report promptly any eye discomfort or change in vision so that appropriate evaluation can be made and corrective action taken as soon as possible.

Drugs reported to cause *blurring of vision*

acetazolamide
antiarthritic/anti-inflammatory
   drugs
antidepressants*
antihistamines*
atropinelike drugs*
chlorthalidone
ciprofloxacin
cortisonelike drugs*

diethylstilbestrol
etretinate
fenfluramine
norfloxacin
oral contraceptives
phenytoin
sulfonamides*
tetracyclines*
thiazide diuretics*

Drugs reported to cause *double vision*

antidepressants*
antidiabetic drugs*
antihistamines*
aspirin
barbiturates*
benzodiazepines*
bromides
carbamazepine
carisoprodol
chloroquine
chlorprothixene
ciprofloxacin
clomiphene
colchicine

colistin
cortisonelike drugs*
digitalis
digitoxin
digoxin
ethionamide
ethosuximide
etretinate
guanethidine
hydroxychloroquine
indomethacin
isoniazid
levodopa
mephenesin

*See Drug Class, Section Four.

Drugs reported to cause *double vision* (cont.)

methocarbamol
methsuximide
morphine
nalidixic acid
nitrofurantoin
norfloxacin
oral contraceptives
orphenadrine
oxyphenbutazone
pentazocine

phenothiazines*
phensuximide
phenylbutazone
phenytoin
primidone
propranolol
quinidine
sedatives/sleep inducers*
thiothixene
tranquilizers*

Drugs reported to cause *farsightedness*

ergot
penicillamine

sulfonamides* (possibly)
tolbutamide (possibly)

Drugs reported to cause *nearsightedness*

acetazolamide
aspirin
carbachol
chlorthalidone
codeine
cortisonelike drugs*
ethosuximide
methsuximide
morphine

oral contraceptives
penicillamine
phenothiazines*
phensuximide
spironolactone
sulfonamides*
tetracyclines*
thiazide diuretics*

Drugs reported to *alter color vision*

acetaminophen
amodiaquine
amyl nitrite
aspirin
atropine
barbiturates*
belladonna
chloramphenicol
chloroquine
chlorpromazine
chlortetracycline

ciprofloxacin
cortisonelike drugs*
digitalis
digitoxin
digoxin
disulfiram
epinephrine
ergotamine
erythromycin
ethchlorvynol
ethionamide

*See Drug Class, Section Four.

Drugs reported to *alter color vision* (cont.)

fluphenazine
furosemide
hydroxychloroquine
indomethacin
isocarboxazid
isoniazid
mephenamic acid
mesoridazine
methysergide
nalidixic acid
norfloxacin
oral contraceptives
oxyphenbutazone
paramethadione
pargyline
penicillamine
pentylenetetrazol
perphenazine
phenacetin

phenylbutazone
primidone
prochlorperazine
promazine
promethazine
quinacrine
quinidine
quinine
reserpine
sodium salicylate
streptomycin
sulfonamides*
thioridazine
tranylcypromine
trifluoperazine
triflupromazine
trimeprazine
trimethadione

Drugs reported to cause *sensitivity to light* (photophobia)

antidiabetic drugs*
atropinelike drugs*
bromides
chloraquine
ciprofloxacin
clomiphene
digitoxin
doxepin
ethambutol
ethionamide
ethosuximide
etretinate
hydroxychloroquine

mephenytoin
methsuximide
monoamine oxidase inhibitor
    drugs*
nalidixic acid
norfloxacin
oral contraceptives
paramethadione
phenothiazines*
quinidine
quinine
tetracyclines*
trimethadione

Drugs reported to cause *halos around lights*

amyl nitrite
chloroquine
cortisonelike drugs*
digitalis

digitoxin
digoxin
hydrochloroquine
nitroglycerin

*See Drug Class, Section Four.

Drugs reported to cause *halos around lights* (cont.)

norfloxacin
oral contraceptives
paramethadione

phenothiazines*
quinacrine
trimethadione

Drugs reported to cause *visual hallucinations*

amantadine
amphetaminelike drugs*
amyl nitrite
antihistamines*
aspirin
atropinelike drugs*
barbiturates*
benzodiazepines*
bromides
carbamazepine
cephalexin
cephaloglycin
chloroquine
cycloserine
digitalis
digoxin
disulfiram
ephedrine
furosemide
griseofulvin

haloperidol
hydroxychloroquine
indomethacin
isosorbide
levodopa
nialamide
oxyphenbutazone
pargyline
pentazocine
phenothiazines*
phenylbutazone
phenytoin
primidone
propranolol
quinine
sedatives/sleep inducers*
sulfonamides*
tetracyclines*
tricyclic antidepressants*
tripelennamine

Drugs reported to impair the use of *contact lenses*

brompheniramine
carbinoxamine
chlorpheniramine
cyclizine
cyproheptadine
dexbrompheniramine
dexchlorpheniramine

dimethindene
diphenhydramine
diphenpyraline
furosemide
oral contraceptives
terfenadine
tripelennamine

Drugs reported to cause *cataracts* or *lens deposits*

allopurinol
busulfan
chlorpromazine

chlorprothixene
cortisonelike drugs*
fluphenazine

*See Drug Class, Section Four.

Drugs reported to cause *cataracts* or *lens deposits* (cont.)

mesoridazine
methotrimeprazine
perphenazine
phenmetrazine
pilocarpine
prochlorperazine
promazine

promethazine
thioridazine
thiothixene
trifluoperazine
triflupromazine
trimeprazine

*See Drug Class, Section Four.

TABLE 3

Your Drugs and the Sun: Photosensitivity

Some drugs are capable of sensitizing the skin of some individuals to the action of ultraviolet light. This can cause uncovered areas of the skin to react with a rash or exaggerated burn on exposure to sun or ultraviolet lamps. If you are taking any of the following drugs, ask your physician for guidance and use caution with regard to sun exposure.

acetohexamide	lincomycin
amitriptyline	maprotiline
amoxapine	mesoridazine
barbiturates	methacycline
bendroflumethiazide	methotrexate
carbamazepine	nalidixic acid
chlordiazepoxide	nortriptyline
chloroquine	oral contraceptives
chlorothiazide	oxyphenbutazone
chlorpromazine	oxytetracycline
chlorpropamide	perphenazine
chlortetracycline	phenobarbital
chlorthalidone	phenylbutazone
clindamycin	phenytoin
cyproheptadine	prochlorperazine
demeclocycline	promazine
desipramine	promethazine
diethylstilbestrol	protriptyline
diltiazem	pyrazinamide
diphenhydramine	sulfonamides
doxepin	tetracycline
doxycycline	thioridazine
estrogen	tolazamide
fluphenazine	tolbutamide
glyburide	tranylcypromine
gold preparations	triamterene
griseofulvin	trifluoperazine
hydrochlorothiazide	trimeprazine
hydroflumethiazide	trimipramine
imipramine	triprolidine
isotretinoin	

TABLE 4
Your Drugs and Sexuality

It is now well established that certain drugs have the potential for affecting sexual functions in a variety of unintended ways. Many commonly prescribed drugs can cause both obvious and subtle effects on one or more aspects of sexual expression. Patients are usually unaware that changes in sexual performance or response may be related to medications they are taking. If they should suspect it, they are often reluctant to discuss the possible association with their physician. In some situations, the sexual dysfunction may be a natural consequence of the disorder under treatment or of a concurrent and undetected disorder, possibilities often overlooked by both practitioner and patient. It is well known that disorders such as diabetes, kidney failure, hypertension, depression and alcoholism may reduce libido and cause failure of erection. In addition, many of the drugs commonly used to treat these conditions may have the ability to augment a subclinical sexual dysfunction through unavoidable pharmacological activity. Such situations require the closest cooperation between therapist and patient in order to correctly assess the possible cause-and-effect relationships and to modify the treatment program appropriately.

Possible Drug Effects on Male Sexuality

1. Increased libido
   androgens (replacement therapy in deficiency states)
   baclofen (Lioresal)
   chlordiazepoxide (Librium) (antianxiety effect)
   diazepam (Valium) (antianxiety effect)
   haloperidol (Haldol)
   levodopa (Larodopa, Sinemet) (may be an indirect effect due to improved sense of well-being)

2. Decreased libido
   antihistamines
   barbiturates
   chlordiazepoxide (Librium) (sedative effect)
   chlorpromazine (Thorazine) 10% to 20% of users
   cimetidine (Tagamet)
   clofibrate (Atromid-S)
   clonidine (Catapres) 10% to 20% of users
   danazol (Danocrine)
   diazepam (Valium) (sedative effect)
   disulfiram (Antabuse)
   estrogens (therapy for prostatic cancer)
   fenfluramine (Pondimin)
   heroin

licorice
medroxyprogesterone (Provera)
methyldopa (Aldomet) 10% to 15% of users
perhexilene (Pexid)
prazosin (Minipress) 15% of users
propranolol (Inderal) rarely
reserpine (Serpasil, Ser-Ap-Es)
spironolactone (Aldactone)
tricyclic antidepressants (TAD's)

3. Impaired erection (impotence)
anticholinergics
antihistamines
baclofen (Lioresal)
barbiturates (when abused)
beta blockers (see Drug Class, Section Four)
chlordiazepoxide (Librium) (in high dosage)
chlorpromazine (Thorazine)
cimetidine (Tagamet)
clofibrate (Atromid-S)
clonidine (Catapres) 10% to 20% of users
cocaine
diazepam (Valium) (in high dosage)
digitalis and its glycosides
disopyramide (Norpace)
disulfiram (Antabuse) (uncertain)
estrogens (therapy for prostatic cancer)
ethacrynic acid (Edecrin) 5% of users
ethionamide (Trecator-SC)
fenfluramine (Pondimin)
furosemide (Lasix) 5% of users
guanethidine (Ismelin)
haloperidol (Haldol) 10% to 20% of users
heroin
hydroxyprogesterone (therapy for prostatic cancer)
licorice
lithium (Lithonate)
marijuana
mesoridazine (Serentil)
methantheline (Banthine)
methyldopa (Aldomet) 10% to 15% of users
monoamine oxidase (MAO) type A inhibitors, 10% to 15% of users
perhexilene (Pexid)
prazosin (Minipres) infrequently
reserpine (Serpasil, Ser-Ap-Es)
spironolactone (Aldactone)
thiazide diuretics, 5% of users

thioridazine (Mellaril)
tricyclic antidepressants (TAD's)

4. Impaired ejaculation
anticholinergics
barbiturates (when abused)
chlorpromazine (Thorazine)
clonidine (Catapres)
estrogens (therapy for prostatic cancer)
guanethidine (Ismelin)
heroin
mesoridazine (Serentil)
methyldopa (Aldomet)
monoamine oxidase (MAO) type A inhibitors
phenoxybenzamine (Dibenzyline)
phentolamine (Regitine)
reserpine (Serpasil, Ser-Ap-Es)
thiazide diuretics
thioridazine (Mellaril)
tricyclic antidepressants (TAD's)

5. Decreased testosterone
adrenocorticotropic hormone (ACTH)
barbiturates
digoxin (Lanoxin)
haloperidol (Haldol)
  increased testosterone with low dosage
  decreased testosterone with high dosage
lithium (Lithonate)
marijuana
medroxyprogesterone (Provera)
monoamine oxidase (MAO) type A inhibitors
spironolactone (Aldactone)

6. Impaired spermatogenesis (reduced fertility)
adrenocorticosteroids (prednisone, etc.)
androgens (moderate to high dosage, extended use)
antimalarials
aspirin (abusive, chronic use)
chlorambucil (Leukeran)
cimetidine (Tagamet)
colchicine
co-trimoxazole (Bactrim, Septra)
cyclophosphamide (Cytoxan)
estrogens (therapy for prostatic cancer)
marijuana
medroxyprogesterone (Provera)
methotrexate

monoamine oxidase (MAO) type A inhibitors
niridazole (Ambilhar)
nitrofurantoin (Furadantin)
spironolactone (Aldactone)
sulfasalazine (Azulfidine)
testosterone (moderate to high dosage, extended use)
vitamin C (in doses of 1 gram or more)

7. Testicular disorders
    Swelling
        tricyclic antidepressants (TAD's)
    Inflammation
        oxyphenbutazone (Tandearil)
    Atrophy
        androgens (moderate to high dosage, extended use)
        chlorpromazine (Thorazine)
        cyclophosphamide (Cytoxan) (in prepubescent boys)
        spironolactone (Aldactone)

8. Penile disorders
    Priapism (see Glossary)
        anabolic steroids (male hormonelike drugs)
        chlorpromazine (Thorazine)
        cocaine
        guanethidine (Ismelin)
        haloperidol (Haldol)
        heparin
        levodopa (Sinemet)
        molindone (Moban)
        prazosin (Minipress)
        prochlorperazine (Compazine)
        trazodone (Desyrel)
        trifluoperazine (Stelazine)
        warfarin (Coumadin)
    Peyronie's disease (see Glossary)
        beta blocker drugs (see Drug Class, Section Four)
        phenytoin (Dilantin, etc.)

9. Gynecomastia (excessive development of the male breast)
    androgens (partial conversion to estrogen)
    BCNU
    busulfan (Myleran)
    chlormadinone
    chlorpromazine (Thorazine)
    chlortetracycline (Aureomycin)
    cimetidine (Tagamet)
    clonidine (Catapres) (infrequently)
    diethylstilbestrol (DES)
    digitalis and its glycosides

estrogens (therapy for prostatic cancer)
ethionamide (Trecator-SC)
griseofulvin (Fulvicin, etc.)
haloperidol (Haldol)
heroin
human chorionic gonadotropin
isoniazid (INH, Nydrazid)
marijuana
mestranol
methyldopa (Aldomet)
phenelzine (Nardil)
reserpine (Serpasil, Ser-Ap-Es)
spironolactone (Aldactone)
thioridazine (Mellaril)
tricyclic antidepressants (TAD's)
vincristine (Oncovin)

10. Feminization (loss of libido, impotence, gynecomastia, testicular atrophy)
    conjugated estrogens (Premarin, etc.)

11. Precocious puberty
    anabolic steroids
    androgens
    isoniazid (INH)

Possible Drug Effects on Female Sexuality

1. Increased libido
    androgens
    chlordiazepoxide (Librium) (antianxiety effect)
    diazepam (Valium) (antianxiety effect)
    mazindol (Sanorex)
    oral contraceptives (freedom from fear of pregnancy)

2. Decreased libido
    See list of drug effects on male sexuality. Some of these *may* have
    potential for reducing libido in the female. The literature is sparse on
    this subject.

3. Impaired arousal and orgasm
    anticholinergics
    clonidine (Catapres)
    methyldopa (Aldomet)
    monoamine oxidase inhibitors (MAOI's)
    tricyclic antidepressants (TAD's)

4. Breast enlargement
    penicillamine
    tricyclic antidepressants (TAD's)

5. Galactorrhea (spontaneous flow of milk)
   amphetamine
   chlorpromazine (Thorazine)
   cimetidine (Tagamet)
   haloperidol (Haldol)
   heroin
   methyldopa (Aldomet)
   metoclopramide (Reglan)
   oral contraceptives
   phenothiazines
   reserpine (Serpasil, Ser-Ap-Es)
   sulpiride (Equilid)
   tricyclic antidepressants (TAD's)

6. Ovarian failure (reduced fertility)
   anesthetic gases (operating room staff)
   cyclophosphamide (Cytoxan)
   cytostatic drugs
   danazol (Danacrine)
   medroxyprogesterone (Provera)

7. Altered menstruation (menstrual disorders)
   adrenocorticosteroids (prednisone, etc.)
   androgens
   barbiturates (when abused)
   chlorambucil (Leukeran)
   chlorpromazine (Thorazine)
   cyclophosphamide (Cytoxan)
   danazol (Danocrine)
   estrogens
   ethionamide (Trecator-SC)
   haloperidol (Haldol)
   heroin
   isoniazid (INH, Nydrazid)
   marijuana
   medroxprogesterone (Provera)
   oral contraceptives
   phenothiazines
   progestins
   radioisotopes
   rifampin (Rifadin, Rifamate, Rimactane)
   spironolactone (Aldactone)
   testosterone
   thioridazine (Mellaril)
   vitamin A (in excessive dosage)

8. Virilization (acne, hirsutism, lowering of voice, enlargement of clitoris)
   anabolic drugs
   androgens

haloperidol (Haldol)
oral contraceptives (lowering of voice)

9. Precocious puberty
estrogens (in hair lotions)
isoniazid (INH, Nydrazid)

TABLE 5

Your Drugs and Alcohol

Beverages containing alcohol may interact unfavorably with a wide variety of drugs. The most important (and most familiar) interaction occurs when the depressant action on the brain of sedatives, sleep-inducing drugs, tranquilizers and narcotic drugs is intensified by alcohol. Alcohol may also reduce the effectiveness of some drugs, and it can interact with certain other drugs to produce toxic effects. Some drugs may increase the intoxicating effects of alcohol, producing further impairment of mental alertness, judgment, physical coordination and reaction time.

While drug interactions with alcohol are generally predictable, the intensity and significance of these interactions can vary greatly from one individual to another and from one occasion to another. This is because many factors influence what happens when drugs and alcohol interact. These factors include individual variations in sensitivity to drugs (including alcohol), the chemistry and quantity of the drug, the type and amount of alcohol consumed and the sequence in which drug and alcohol are taken. If you need to use any of the drugs listed in the following tables, you should ask your physician for guidance concerning the use of alcohol.

Drugs with which it is advisable to avoid alcohol completely

Drug name or class	Possible interaction with alcohol
amphetamines	excessive rise in blood pressure with alcoholic beverages containing tyramine**
antidepressants*	excessive sedation, increased intoxication
barbiturates*	excessive sedation
bromides	confusion, delirium, increased intoxication
calcium carbamide	disulfiramlike reaction**
carbamazepine	excessive sedation
chlorprothixene	excessive sedation
chlorzoxazone	excessive sedation
disulfiram	disulfiram reaction**
ergotamine	reduced effectiveness of ergotamine
fenfluramine	excessive stimulation of nervous system with some beers and wines
furazolidone	disulfiramlike reaction**
haloperidol	excessive sedation

*See Drug Class, Section Four.
**See Glossary.

Drug name or class	Possible interaction with alcohol
MAO inhibitor drugs*	excessive rise in blood pressure with alcoholic beverages containing tyramine**
meperidine	excessive sedation
meprobamate	excessive sedation
methotrexate	increased liver toxicity and excessive sedation
metronidazole	disulfiramlike reaction**
narcotic drugs	excessive sedation
oxyphenbutazone	increased stomach irritation and/or bleeding
pentazocine	excessive sedation
pethidine	excessive sedation
phenothiazines*	excessive sedation
phenylbutazone	increased stomach irritation and/or bleeding
procarbazine	disulfiramlike reaction**
propoxyphene	excessive sedation
reserpine	excessive sedation, orthostatic hypotension**
sleep-inducing drugs (hypnotics)	excessive sedation
carbromal	
chloral hydrate	
ethchlorvynol	
ethinamate	
glutethimide	
flurazepam	
methaqualone	
methyprylon	
temazepam	
triazolam	
thiothixene	excessive sedation
tricyclic antidepressants*	excessive sedation, increased intoxication
trimethobenzamide	excessive sedation

Drugs with which alcohol should be used only in small amounts (use cautiously until combined effects have been determined)

Drug name or class	Possible interaction with alcohol
acetaminophen (Tylenol, etc.)	increased liver toxicity
amantadine	excessive lowering of blood pressure

*See Drug Class, Section Four.
**See Glossary.

Drug name or class	Possible interaction with alcohol
antiarthritic/anti-inflammatory drugs	increased stomach irritation and/or bleeding
anticoagulants (coumarins)*	increased anticoagulant effect
antidiabetic drugs (sulfonylureas)*	increased antidiabetic effect, excessive hypoglycemia**
antihistamines*	excessive sedation
antihypertensives*	excessive orthostatic hypotension**
aspirin (large doses or continuous use)	increased stomach irritation and/or bleeding
benzodiazepines*	excessive sedation
carisoprodol	increased alcoholic intoxication
diethylpropion	excessive nervous system stimulation with alcoholic beverages containing tyramine**
dihydroergotoxine	excessive lowering of blood pressure
diphenoxylate	excessive sedation
dipyridamole	excessive lowering of blood pressure
diuretics*	excessive orthostatic hypotension**
ethionamide	confusion, delirium, psychotic behavior
fenoprofen	increased stomach irritation and/or bleeding
griseofulvin	flushing and rapid heart action
ibuprofen	increased stomach irritation and/or bleeding
indomethacin	increased stomach irritation and/or bleeding
insulin	excessive hypoglycemia**
iron	excessive absorption of iron
isoniazid	decreased effectiveness of isoniazid, increased incidence of hepatitis
lithium	increased confusion and delirium (avoid all alcohol if any indication of lithium overdosage)
methocarbamol	excessive sedation
methotrimeprazine	excessive sedation
methylphenidate	excessive nervous system stimulation with alcoholic beverages containing tyramine**
metoprolol	excessive orthostatic hypotension**
nalidixic acid	increased alcoholic intoxication

*See Drug Class, Section Four.
**See Glossary.

Drug name or class	**Possible interaction with alcohol**
naproxen	increased stomach irritation and/or bleeding
nicotinic acid	possible orthostatic hypotension**
nitrates* (vasodilators)	possible orthostatic hypotension**
nylidrin	increased stomach irritation
orphenadrine	excessive sedation
phenelzine	increased alcoholic intoxication
phenoxybenzamine	possible orthostatic hypotension**
phentermine	excessive nervous system stimulation with alcoholic beverages containing tyramine**
phenytoin	decreased effect of phenytoin
pilocarpine	prolongation of alcohol effect
prazosin	excessive lowering of blood pressure
primidone	excessive sedation
propranolol	excessive orthostatic hypotension**
sulfonamides*	increased alcoholic intoxication
sulindac	increased stomach irritation and/or bleeding
tolmetin	increased stomach irritation and/or bleeding
tranquilizers (mild)	excessive sedation
chlordiazepoxide	
clorazepate	
diazepam	
hydroxyzine	
meprobamate	
oxazepam	
phenaglycodol	
tybamate	
tranylcypromine	increased alcoholic intoxication

Drugs capable of producing a disulfiramlike reaction** when used concurrently with alcohol

antidiabetic drugs (sulfonylureas)*
calcium carbamide
chloral hydrate
chloramphenicol
disulfiram
furazolidone
metronidazole

nifuroxine
nitrofurantoin
procarbazine
quinacrine
sulfonamides*
tinidazole
tolazoline

*See Drug Class, Section Four.
**See Glossary.

TABLE 6

High-Potassium Foods

Diuretic drugs that cause loss of potassium from the body are often used to treat conditions that also require a reduced intake of sodium. The high-potassium foods listed below have been selected for their compatibility with a sodium restricted diet (500 to 1000 mg of sodium daily).

Beverages

orange juice
prune juice
skim milk

tea
tomato juice
whole milk

Breads and Cereals

brown rice
cornbread
griddle cakes
muffins

oatmeal
shredded wheat
waffles

Fruits

apricot
avocado
banana
fig
honeydew melon

mango
orange
papaya
prune

Meats

beef
chicken
codfish
flounder
haddock
halibut

liver
pork
rockfish
salmon
turkey
veal

Vegetables

baked beans
lima beans
mushrooms
navy beans
parsnips

radishes
squash
sweet potato
tomato
white potato

Sources

The following sources were consulted in the compilation and revision of this book:

Adverse Drug Reaction Bulletin. Edited by D. M. Davies. Meditext, Weybridge, Surrey, United Kingdom, 1991.

AMA Department of Drugs, *AMA Drug Evaluations,* 6th ed. Chicago: American Medical Association, 1986.

Andreoli, T. E., Carpenter, C. C. J., Plum, F., Smith, L. H., eds., *Cecil Essentials of Medicine.* Philadelphia: W. B. Saunders Co., 1986.

Arndt, K. A., *Manual of Dermatologic Therapeutics,* 4th ed. Boston: Little, Brown and Co., 1989.

Atkinson, A. J., Ambre, J. J., *Kalman and Clark's Drug Assay, The Strategy of Therapeutic Drug Monitoring,* 2nd ed. New York: Masson Publishing USA, 1985.

Avery, G. S., ed., *Drug Treatment,* 2nd ed. Sydney, Australia: ADIS Press, 1980.

Berkow, R., ed., *The Merck Manual,* 15th ed. Rahway, New Jersey: Merck Sharp & Dohme Research Laboratories, 1987.

Bevan, J. A., ed., *Essentials of Pharmacology.* Hagerstown, Maryland: Harper & Row, 1976.

Billups, N. F., ed., *American Drug Index 1991.* Philadelphia: J. B. Lippincott Co., 199'.

Branch, W. T., *Office Practice of Medicine,* 2nd ed. Philadelphia: W. B. Saunders Co., 1987.

Briggs, G. G., Bodendorfer, T. W., Freeman, R. K., Yaffee, S. J., *Drugs in Pregnancy and Lactation.* Baltimore: Williams & Wilkins, 1983.

Brooke, M. H., *A Clinician's View of Neuromuscular Diseases,* 2nd ed. Baltimore: Williams & Wilkins, 1986.

Canadian Pharmaceutical Association, *Compendium of Pharmaceuticals and Specialties,* 24th ed. Ottawa: Canadian Pharmaceutical Association, 1990.

Cape, Ronald, *Aging: Its Complex Management.* Hagerstown, Maryland: Harper & Row, 1978.

Clin-Alert. Medford, New Jersey: Clin-Alert, Inc., 1989–1991.

Davies, D. M., ed., *Textbook of Adverse Drug Reactions*, 2nd ed. New York: Oxford University Press, 1981.

Diamond, S., Dalessio, D. J., eds., *The Practicing Physician's Approach to Headache*, 4th ed. Baltimore: Williams & Wilkins, 1986.

Drug Interaction Facts. Edited by D. S. Tatro. St. Louis: Facts and Comparisons Division, J. B. Lippincott Co., 1991.

Drug Interactions Newsletter. Edited by P. D. Hansten, J. R. Horn. Spokane, Washington: Applied Therapeutics, Inc., 1991.

Drug Newsletter. Edited by B. R. Olin. St. Louis: Facts and Comparisons Division, J. B. Lippincott Co., 1991.

Drug Therapy, Physicians Prescribing Update. Lawrenceville, NJ: Excerpta Medica, 1991.

Dukes, M. N. G., ed., Meyler's Side Effects of Drugs, 11th ed. Amsterdam: Excerpta Medica, 1988.

Encyclopedia of Associations, 23rd ed., Vol. 1, Part 2. Detroit: Gale Research, Inc., 1991.

Facts and Comparisons. Edited by B. R. Olin. St. Louis: Facts and Comparisons Division, J. B. Lippincott Co., 1991.

F.D.A. Drug Bulletin. Rockville, Maryland: Department of Health and Human Services, Food and Drug Administration.

Fraunfelder, F. T., *Drug-Induced Ocular Side Effects and Drug Interactions*. Philadelphia: Lea & Febiger, 1976.

Goodman, L. S., Gilman, A., eds., *The Pharmacological Basis of Therapeutics*, 8th ed. New York: Macmillan, 1990.

Greenberger, N. J., Arvanitakis, C., Hurwitz, A., *Drug Treatment of Gastrointestinal Disorders*. New York: Churchill Livingstone, 1978.

Hansten, P. D., *Drug Interactions*, 6th ed. Philadelphia: Lea & Febiger, 1991.

Heinonen, O. P., Slone, D., Shapiro, S., *Birth Defects and Drugs in Pregnancy*. Littleton, Massachusetts: PSG Publishing Co., 1977.

Hollister, L. E., *Clinical Pharmacology of Psychotherapeutic Drugs*, 2nd ed. New York: Churchill Livingstone, 1983.

Huff, B. B., ed., *The Physicians' Desk Reference*, 45th ed. Oradell, New Jersey: Medical Economics Company, 1991.

International Drug Therapy Newsletter. Edited by F. J. Ayd. Baltimore: Ayd Medical Communications, 1991.

Jefferson, J. W., Greist, J. H., *Primer of Lithium Therapy*. Baltimore: Williams & Wilkens, 1977.

Journal of the American Medical Association. Edited by G. D. Lundberg. Chicago: American Medical Association, 1991.

Klippel, J. H., ed., Systemic Lupus Erythematosus. *Rheumatic Disease Clinics of North America*, Vol. 14, No. 1, April, 1988. Philadelphia: W. B. Saunders Co.

Koller, W. C., ed., *Handbook of Parkinson's Disease*. New York: Marcel Dekker, 1987.

Kolodny, R. C., Masters, W. H., Johnson, V. E., *Textbook of Sexual Medicine*. Boston: Little, Brown and Co., 1979.

Lawrence, R. A., *Breast-Feeding*. St. Louis: Mosby, 1980.

Lieberman, M. L., *The Sexual Pharmacy*. New York: New American Library, 1988.

Long, J. W., *Clinical Management of Prescription Drugs*. Philadelphia: Harper & Row, 1984.

McEvoy, G. K., ed., *American Hospital Formulary Service, Drug Information 90*. Bethesda, Maryland: American Society of Hospital Pharmacists, 1990.

Maddin, S., ed., *Current Dermatologic Therapy*. Philadelphia: W. B. Saunders Co., 1982.

The Medical Letter on Drugs and Therapeutics. Edited by H. Aaron. New Rochelle, New York: The Medical Letter, Inc., 1991.

Melmon, K. L., Morrelli, H. F., *Clinical Pharmacology,* 2nd ed. New York: Macmillan, 1978.

Messerli, F. H., ed., *Current Clinical Practice.* Philadelphia: W. B. Saunders Co., 1987.

Mohler, S. R., *Medication and Flying: A Pilot's Guide.* Boston: Boston Publishing Co., 1982.

The New England Journal of Medicine. Edited by A. S. Relman. Boston: The Massachusetts Medical Society, 1991.

Patient Drug Facts. Edited by B. R. Olin. St. Louis: Facts and Comparisons Division, J. B. Lippincott Co., 1991.

Postgraduate Medicine, The Journal of Applied Medicine for the Primary Care Physician. Minneapolis: McGraw-Hill, Inc., 1991.

Raj, P. P., *Practical Management of Pain.* Chicago: Year Book Medical Publishers, Inc., 1986.

Rakel, R. E., ed., *Conn's Current Therapy 1991.* Philadelphia: W. B. Saunders Co., 1991.

Rational Drug Therapy, Pharmacology for Physicians. Bethesda, Maryland: American Society for Pharmacology and Experimental Therapeutics, 1990.

Reynolds, J. E. F., ed. *Martindale, The Extra Pharmacopoeia,* 29th ed. London: The Pharmaceutical Press, 1989.

Rodman, M. J., Smith, D. W., *Clinical Pharmacology in Nursing.* Philadelphia: J. B. Lippincott Co., 1984.

Rogers, C. S., McCue, J. D., eds., *Managing Chronic Disease.* Oradell, New Jersey: Medical Economics Books, 1987.

Sauer, G. C., *Manual of Skin Diseases,* 5th ed. Philadelphia: J. B. Lippincott Co., 1985.

Schardein, J. L., *Drugs As Teratogens.* Cleveland: CRC Press, 1976.

Shepard, T. H., *Catalog of Teratogenic Agents,* 6th ed. Baltimore: Johns Hopkins University Press, 1989.

Smith, L. H., Thier, S. O., *Pathophysiology, The Biological Principles of Disease,* 2nd ed. Philadelphia: W. B. Saunders Co., 1985.

Speight, T. M., ed., *Avery's Drug Treatment,* 3rd ed. Auckland: ADIS Press, 1987.

Swash, M., Schwartz, M. S., *Neuromuscular Diseases,* 2nd ed. Berlin: Springer-Verlag, 1988.

Tuchmann-Duplessis, H., *Drug Effects on the Fetus.* Sydney, Australia: ADIS Press, 1975.

USAN 1989 and the USP Dictionary of Drug Names. Edited by M. C. Griffiths. Rockville, Maryland: United States Pharmacopeial Convention, Inc., 1988.

USP Dispensing Information 1991, 11th ed., Vol. 1, *Drug Information for the Health Care Provider.* Rockville, Maryland: United States Pharmacopeial Convention, 1991.

Utian, W. H., *Menopause in Modern Perspective.* New York: Appleton-Century-Crofts, 1980.

Wartak, J., *Drug Dosage and Administration.* Baltimore: University Park Press, 1983.

Worley, R. J., ed., *Clinical Obstetrics and Gynecology,* Vol. 24, No. 1: *Menopause.* Hagerstown, Maryland: Harper & Row, 1981.

Young, D. S., *Effects of Drugs on Clinical Laboratory Tests.* Washington: AACC Press, 1990.

Index

This index contains all the brand and generic drug names included in Section Three and the names and alternative names of the disorders and conditions for which drug management is described in Section Two.

Brand names of drugs appear in italic type and are capitalized.

Each brand name is followed by the generic name of its Drug Profile in Section Three.

The symbol [CD] indicates that the brand name represents a combination drug that contains the generic drug components listed below it. To be fully familiar with any combination drug [CD], it is necessary to read the Drug Profile of each of the components listed. The brand name of a combination drug *may* or *may not* appear in the brand name list of each Drug Profile that is cited in the index as a component of a particular combination drug. The index listing of component drugs for any combination drug product represents the manufacturer's formulation of that brand at the time this information was compiled for publication.

The symbol ✦ before the brand name of a combination drug indicates that the brand name is used in both the United States and Canada, but that the ingredients in the combination product in each country differ. The Canadaian drug is marked with the symbol ✦ to distinguish it from the American drug which has the same name.

A generic name with no page designation indicates an active component of a combination drug for which there is no Profile in Section Three. It is included to alert you to its presence, should you wish to consult your physician regarding its significance.

Accurbron, theophylline, 976
Accutane, isotretinoin, 605
acebutolol, 163
Acetazolam, acetazolamide, 167
acetazolamide, 167
acetylsalicylic acid. *See* aspirin, 210
Achromycin, tetracycline, 971
Achromycin V, tetracycline, 971
acne, 30
acne vulgaris. *See* acne, 30
Actifed w/Codeine [CD]
   CONTAINS
   codeine, 378
   pseudoephedrine*
   triprolidine*
acyclovir, 171
Adalat, nifedipine, 748
Adapin, doxepin, 465
Adrenalin, epinephrine, 476
adrenaline. *See* epinephrine, 476
Advil, ibuprofen, 571
affective disorder: depressive phase of
      manic-depressive disorder. *See*
      depression, 60
AIDS, 171, 352, 945, 1039, 1050
Ak-Chlor, chloramphenicol, 302
Ak-Cide [CD]
   CONTAINS
   prednisolone, 865
   sulfacetamide*
Ak-Dex, dexamethasone, 414
Ak-Tate, prednisolone, 865
Ak-Zol, acetazolamide, 167
Alatone, spironolactone, 933
Alazine, hydralazine, 550
albuterol, 174

Aldactazide [CD]
   CONTAINS
   hydrochlorothiazide, 554
   spironolactone, 933
Aldactone, spironolactone, 933
Aldoclor [CD]
   CONTAINS
   chlorothiazide, 316
   methyldopa, 677
Aldomet, methyldopa, 677
Aldoril D30/D50 [CD]
   CONTAINS
   hydrochlorothiazide, 554
   methyldopa, 677
Aldoril-15/25 [CD]
   CONTAINS
   hydrochlorothiazide, 554
   methyldopa, 677
*Alka-Seltzer Effervescent Pain Reliever &
      Antacid* [CD]
   CONTAINS
   aspirin, 210
   citric acid*
   sodium bicarbonate*
Alka-Seltzer Plus [CD]
   CONTAINS
   aspirin, 210
   chlorpheniramine*
   phenylpropanolamine*
Allerdryl, diphenhydramine, 443
Alloprin, allopurinol, 177
allopurinol, 83, 177
Almocarpine, pilocarpine, 840
alpha-methyldopa. *See* methyldopa, 677
alprazolam, 180
Altace, ramipril, 918

*The symbol [CD] indicates that the brand name given is a combination drug consisting of generic
drug components listed below it. If there is no page numbering following the name of the generic
drug component, there is no Drug Profile for that ingredient in this book.

*The symbol [CD] indicates that the brand name given is a combination drug consisting of generic
drug components listed below it. If there is no page numbering following the name of the generic
drug component, there is no Drug Profile for that ingredient in this book.

hydrocodone, 559
phenylephrine*
Biohisdine DHC [CD]
CONTAINS
diphenylpyraline*
hydrocodone, 559
phenylephrine*
Biquin Durules, quinidine, 914
bitolterol, 249
Blocadren, timolol, 996
Bonamine, meclizine, 647
Bonine, meclizine, 647
Brethaire, terbutaline, 965
Brethine, terbutaline, 965
Brevicon, oral contraceptives,
    780
Bricanyl, terbutaline, 965
Bricanyl Spacer, terbutaline, 965
bromocriptine, 134, 252
bronchial asthma. *See* asthma, 41
Brondecon [CD]
CONTAINS
guaifenesin*
theophylline, 976
Bronkaid Mist, epinephrine, 476
Bronkaid Mistometer, epinephrine,
    476
Bronkaid Tablets [CD]
CONTAINS
ephedrine*
guaifenesin*
theophylline, 976
Bronkodyl, theophylline, 976
Bronkolixir [CD]
CONTAINS
ephedrine*
guaifenesin*
phenobarbital, 825
theophylline, 976
Bronkotabs [CD]
CONTAINS
ephedrine*
guaifenesin*
phenobarbital, 825
theophylline, 976
Bufferin [CD]
CONTAINS
aspirin, 210
magnesium carbonate*
Bufferin Arthritis Strength [CD]
CONTAINS
aspirin, 210
magnesium carbonate*

Bufferin Extra Strength [CD]
CONTAINS
aspirin, 210
magnesium carbonate*
Bufferin w/Codeine [CD]
CONTAINS
aspirin, 210
codeine, 378
magnesium carbonate*
bumetanide, 256
Bumex, bumetanide, 256
Buspar, buspirone, 260
buspirone, 260
Butazolidin, phenylbutazone, 830
Butibel [CD]
CONTAINS
atropine, 224
butabarbital*
Butone [CD]
CONTAINS
malgadrate*
phenylbutazone, 830
Byclomine, dicyclomine, 428

Cafergot [CD]
CONTAINS
caffeine*
ergotamine, 481
Cafergot PB [CD]
CONTAINS
atropine, 224
caffeine*
ergotamine, 481
pentobarbital*
Caladryl [CD]
CONTAINS
calamine*
diphenhydramine, 443
Calan, verapamil, 1041
Calan SR, verapamil, 1041
calcium, 128
Cama Arthritis Pain Reliever [CD]
CONTAINS
aluminum hydroxide*
aspirin, 210
Capoten, captopril, 263
Capozide [CD]
CONTAINS
captopril, 263
hydrochlorothiazide, 554
captopril, 263
Carafate, sucralfate, 937
carbamazepine, 77, 267

*The symbol [CD] indicates that the brand name given is a combination drug consisting of generic drug components listed below it. If there is no page numbering following the name of the generic drug component, there is no Drug Profile for that ingredient in this book.

*The symbol [CD] indicates that the brand name given is a combination drug consisting of generic drug components listed below it. If there is no page numbering following the name of the generic drug component, there is no Drug Profile for that ingredient in this book.

*The symbol [CD] indicates that the brand name given is a combination drug consisting of generic drug components listed below it. If there is no page numbering following the name of the generic drug component, there is no Drug Profile for that ingredient in this book.

*The symbol [CD] indicates that the brand name given is a combination drug consisting of generic drug components listed below it. If there is no page numbering following the name of the generic drug component, there is no Drug Profile for that ingredient in this book.

*The symbol [CD] indicates that the brand name given is a combination drug consisting of generic drug components listed below it. If there is no page numbering following the name of the generic drug component, there is no Drug Profile for that ingredient in this book.

*The symbol [CD] indicates that the brand name given is a combination drug consisting of generic drug components listed below it. If there is no page numbering following the name of the generic drug component, there is no Drug Profile for that ingredient in this book.

*The symbol [CD] indicates that the brand name given is a combination drug consisting of generic drug components listed below it. If there is no page numbering following the name of the generic drug component, there is no Drug Profile for that ingredient in this book.

*The symbol [CD] indicates that the brand name given is a combination drug consisting of generic drug components listed below it. If there is no page numbering following the name of the generic drug component, there is no Drug Profile for that ingredient in this book.

*The symbol [CD] indicates that the brand name given is a combination drug consisting of generic drug components listed below it. If there is no page numbering following the name of the generic drug component, there is no Drug Profile for that ingredient in this book.

*The symbol [CD] indicates that the brand name given is a combination drug consisting of generic drug components listed below it. If there is no page numbering following the name of the generic drug component, there is no Drug Profile for that ingredient in this book.

About the Author

JAMES W. LONG, M.D., was born in Allentown, Pennsylvania. He received his premedical education from the University of Maryland and his medical degree from the George Washington University School of Medicine in Washington, D.C. For twenty years he was in the private practice of internal medicine in the Washington metropolitan area, and for over thirty-five years he was a member of the faculty of the George Washington University School of Medicine. He has served with the Food and Drug Administration, the National Library of Medicine, and the Bureau of Health Manpower of the National Institutes of Health. Prior to his retirement, Dr. Long was director of Health Services for the National Science Foundation in Washington. He lives in Oxford, Maryland.

Dr. Long's involvement in drug information activities includes service on the H.E.W. Task Force on Prescription Drugs, on the F.D.A. Task Force on Adverse Drug Reactions, as a delegate-at-large to the U.S. Pharmacopeial Convention, as editorial consultant for *Hospital Formulary,* as a director of the Drug Information Association, and as a member of the Toxicology Information Program Committee of the National Research Council/National Academy of Sciences. He was consultant to the Food and Drug Administration, serving as advisor to their staff on the development of patient package inserts. He is also the author of numerous articles in professional journals. *The Essential Guide to Prescription Drugs* is an outgrowth of his conviction that the general public needs and is entitled to practical drug information which is the equivalent of the professional "package insert." He believes the patient can be reasonably certain of using medications with the least risk and the greatest benefit only when the patient has all the relevant information about the drugs he or she is taking.

Schedules of Controlled Drugs*

Schedule I: Non-medicinal substances with high abuse potential and dependence liability. Used for research purposes only. Examples: heroin, marijuana, LSD. Not legally available for medicinal use by prescription.

Schedule II: Medicinal drugs in current use that have the highest abuse potential and dependence liability. Examples: opium derivatives (morphine, codeine, etc.), meperidine (Demerol), amphetamines (Dexedrine), short-acting barbiturates (Amytal, Nembutal, Seconal). A written prescription is required. Telephoned prescribing is prohibited. No refills are allowed.

Schedule III: Medicinal drugs with abuse potential and dependence liability less than Schedule II drugs but greater than Schedule IV or V drugs. Examples: codeine, hydrocodone and paregoric in combination with one or more non-narcotic drugs, some hypnotics (Doriden, Noludar), some appetite suppressants (Didrex, Tenuate, Sanorex). A telephoned prescription is permitted, to be converted to written form by the dispensing pharmacist. Prescriptions must be renewed every 6 months. Refills are limited to 5.

Schedule IV: Medicinal drugs with less abuse potential and dependence liability than Schedule III drugs. Examples: pentazocine (Talwin), propoxyphene (Darvon), all benzodiazepines (Librium, Valium, etc.), certain hypnotics (Placidyl, Noctec, Valmid, etc.). Prescription requirements are the same as for Schedule III.

Schedule V: Medicinal drugs with the lowest abuse potential and dependence liability. Examples: diphenoxylate (Lomotil), loperamide (Imodium). Drugs requiring a prescription are handled the same as any non-scheduled prescription drug. Some non-prescription drugs can be sold only with approval of the pharmacist; the buyer is required to sign a log of purchase at the time the drug is dispensed. Examples: codeine and hydrocodone in combination with other active, non-narcotic drugs, sold in preparations that contain limited quantities for control of cough and diarrhea.

*Under jurisdiction of the Controlled Substances Act of 1970.

Advisability of Drug Use During Pregnancy

Definitions of FDA Pregnancy Categories*

Category A: Adequate and well-controlled studies in pregnant women are **negative** for fetal abnormalities. Risk to the fetus is remote.

Category B: Animal reproduction studies are **negative** for fetal abnormalities. Information from adequate and well-controlled studies in pregnant women is not available.

OR

Animal reproduction studies are **positive** for fetal abnormalities. Adequate and well-controlled studies in pregnant women are **negative** for fetal abnormalities. Risk to the fetus is relatively unlikely.

Category C: Animal reproduction studies are **positive** for fetal abnormalities. Information from adequate and well-controlled studies in pregnant women is not available.

OR

Information from animal reproduction studies **and** from adequate and well-controlled studies in pregnant women is not available. Possible benefits of the drug are thought to justify potential risks to the fetus.

Category D: Studies in pregnant women and/or pre-marketing (investigational) or post-marketing experience demonstrate **positive** evidence of human fetal risk. The drug is needed in serious disease or in life-threatening situations where safer drugs are ineffective or cannot be used.

Category X: Animal reproduction studies and/or human pregnancy studies are **positive** for fetal abnormalities.

OR

Studies in pregnant women and/or pre-marketing (investigational) or post-marketing experience demonstrate **positive** evidence of human fetal risk.

AND

Potential risks to the fetus outweigh possible benefits of the drug. Use is **contraindicated.**

*Adapted from the Federal Register statement in Vol. 44, No. 124, Tuesday, June 26, 1979.